Surgery of the Liver, Bile Ducts and Pancreas in Children

Second edition

Surgery of the Liver, Bile Ducts and Pancreas in Children

Second edition

Edited by

Edward R Howard MS FRCS (Eng & Edin)
Emeritus Professor, Department of Paediatric Surgery,
King's College Hospital, London, UK

Mark D Stringer BSc MS FRCS FRCP FRCPCH
Consultant Paediatric Surgeon, St James's University
Hospital, Leeds, UK

Paul M Colombani MD
Chief of Pediatric Surgery, Johns Hopkins University
School of Medicine, Baltimore, MD, USA

A member of the Hodder Headline Group
LONDON   NEW YORK   NEW DELHI

First published in Great Britain in 1991 by
Butterworth-Heinemann Ltd as *Surgery of the Liver Disease in Children*

This edition published in 2002 by
Arnold, a member of the Hodder Headline Group,
338 Euston Road, London NW1 3BH

http://www.arnoldpublishers.com

Distributed in the United States of America by
Oxford University Press Inc.,
198 Madison Avenue, New York, NY 10016
Oxford is a registered trademark of Oxford University Press

British Library Cataloguing in Publication Data
A catalogue record for this book is available from the British Library

Library of Congress Cataloging-in-Publication Data
A catalog record for this book is available from the Library of Congress

ISBN 0 340 76129 6 (hb)

1 2 3 4 5 6 7 8 9 10

Publisher: Nick Dunton
Development Editor: Michael Lax
Production Editor: Rada Radojicic
Production Controller: Martin Kerans
Cover Design: Mouse Mat Design

Typeset in 10/12 Minion by Phoenix Photosetting, Chatham, Kent
Printed and bound in Italy by Giunti Industrie Grafiche

What do you think about this book? Or any other Arnold title?
Please send your comments to feedback.arnold@hodder.co.uk

This book is dedicated to all of our young patients and their families

When we find Nature herself practising 'experimental pathology,' it is well worth our while to investigate, as fully as we can, the conditions under which she works and the results of her experiments.

(John Thomson, 1892, preface to *Congenital Obliteration of the Bile Ducts*, Edinburgh)

The liver, because of its unforgiving and extraordinarily difficult surgical anatomy and complex physiology, will remain the Mount Everest of organs for surgeons.

(James Foster, 1991, History of liver surgery, *Archives of Surgery* **126**, 381)

Contents

Contributors

SN Cenk Büyükünal MD
Professor of Pediatric Surgery, Department of Pediatric Surgery, Cerrahpasa Medical Faculty, University of Istanbul, Turkey

Adela T Casas-Melley MD
Alfred I duPont Hospital for Children, Wilmington, DE, USA

Patricia Collins BSc PhD RGN
Senior Lecturer in Anatomy, Anglo-European College of Chiropractic, Bournemouth, UK

Paul M Colombani MD
Chief of Pediatric Surgery, Johns Hopkins University School of Medicine, Baltimore, MD, USA

Mark Davenport ChM FRCS (Paeds) FRCPS (Glas) FRCS (Eng)
Consultant Paediatric Hepatobiliary Surgeon, Department of Paediatric Surgery, King's College Hospital, London, UK

Stephen P Dunn MD
Chief, Division of Solid Organ Transplantation, Alfred I duPont Hospital for Children, Wilmington, DE, USA

Frederic Gauthier MD
Chef de Service, Service de Chirurgie Infantile, Centre Hospitalier Universitaire Bicêtre, Paris, France

David Green MB BS FRCA MBA
Consultant Anaesthetist, King's College Hospital, London, UK

Sarah Helps BSc DClinPsy CPsychol
Chartered Clinical Psychologist, Mary Sheridan Centre for Child Health, London, UK

Edward R Howard MS FRCS (Eng & Edin)
Emeritus Professor, Department of Paediatric Surgery, King's College Hospital, London, UK

VT Joseph FRCSEd FRACS MMed (Surgery) FAMS
Chairman, Division of Paediatric Surgery, KK Women's and Children's Hospital, Singapore

John Karani BSc FRCR
Consultant Radiologist, Department of Radiology, King's College Hospital, London, UK

Max R Langham Jr MD
Professor and Chief, Division of Pediatric Surgery, University of Florida College of Medicine, Director, Pediatric Liver Transplant Program, Gainesville, FL, USA

Patricia McClean MD FRCP FRCPCH
Consultant Paediatric Hepatologist, Children's Liver Centre, St James's University Hospital, Leeds, UK

Ryoji Ohi MD
Professor and Chief, Department of Pediatric Surgery, Tohoku University School of Medicine, Aobaku, Sendai, Japan

Charles N Paidas MD
Associate Professor of Surgery, Division of Pediatric Surgery, Johns Hopkins University School of Medicine, Baltimore, MD, USA

Walter Pegoli Jr MD
Chief, Section of Pediatric Surgery, University of Rochester Medical Center, Rochester, NY, USA

Myrddin Rees MS FRCS
Consultant Hepatobiliary Surgeon, North Hampshire Hospital, Basingstoke, UK

Mohamed Rela FRCS
Consultant Transplant Surgeon, Department of Transplantation, Liver Unit, King's College Hospital, London, UK

Frederick J Rescorla MD
Professor of Surgery, Section of Pediatric Surgery, Indiana University School of Medicine, JW Riley Hospital for Children, Indianapolis, IN, USA

Kathleen B Schwarz MD
Medical Director, Pediatric Liver Center, Johns Hopkins University School of Medicine, Baltimore, MD, USA

Mark D Stringer BSc MS FRCS FRCP FRCPCH
Consultant Paediatric Surgeon, St James's University Hospital, Leeds, UK

Riccardo A Superina MD CM FRCS(C)
Director of Transplant Surgery, Children's Memorial Hospital, Professor of Surgery, Northwestern University, Chicago, IL, USA

Andrew Taylor MD
Professor and Chair, Department of Radiology, University of Wisconsin School of Medicine, Madison, WI, USA

Steven L Werlin MD
Professor of Pediatrics, The Children's Hospital of Wisconsin, Medical College of Wisconsin, Milwaukee, WI, USA

Preface

It is now 10 years since the publication of the first edition of this book, devoted to the surgery of liver disease in children. The preface to that edition pointed out that the subspecialty of pediatric hepatobiliary surgery had been established for only two decades. During that relatively short time there had been major advances in the understanding and management of all of the major hepatobiliary diseases, including biliary atresia, portal hypertension and liver tumors. The significant role of non-operative management in pediatric liver trauma was evolving, and liver transplantation in children was gathering momentum, although experience was very limited.

Many innovations in the management of hepatobiliary conditions have occurred during the last 10 years. Refinements in magnetic resonance imaging, and the feasibility of endoscopic cholangiography in even the smallest infants, have enhanced the accuracy of investigation. A wider understanding of the anatomy of the liver has encouraged the development of safe segmental resection, which is useful both in the treatment of liver tumors and in the preparation of small liver grafts for transplantation into infants and young children. Liver transplantation and portoenterostomy have emerged as complementary procedures in biliary atresia, and chemotherapy regimens, developed through large multicenter trials in Europe and North America, have continued to improve the outlook of children with malignant liver tumors.

Other important developments within pediatric hepatobiliary surgery during this period have included the refinement of prognostic criteria, the publication of long-term results of surgery and an understanding of the long-term complications of treatment. The impact of nutritional factors and psychosocial aspects has been more widely appreciated, and there is now a greater emphasis on quality of life.

The editors have attempted to include discussion of all of these topics in this second edition. By inviting contributions from surgeons and physicians in North America, the UK, Japan, France, Singapore and Turkey we have tried to maintain a broad international perspective. We are greatly indebted to these authors. In addition, the book has been enlarged to include a comprehensive section on pancreatic disorders and trauma, conditions that are closely related to the hepatobiliary system. With so many congenital abnormalities, we considered that the book would be enriched by an overview of the embryology of the liver, biliary tract and pancreas. For a few topics we have accepted some repetition of material, largely where this highlights divergent opinion or where it is part of an overall conceptual approach.

As in the first edition, this book is not intended to be a manual of operative surgery, although key points of surgical technique are discussed. The text has been constructed first to review the diagnosis, management and outcome of specific conditions, and second to provide comprehensive and up-to-date summaries and references. We hope that the analyses of long-term results and complications will be helpful when counseling parents on the implications of hepatopancreatobiliary disorders, and that the book will be of value to physicians, surgeons and other members of today's multidisciplinary teams. Finally, we hope that the text will prove useful to those colleagues who treat adults with hepatobiliary disease, especially since they will be caring for an increasing number of our patients in the future.

Edward R Howard
Mark D Stringer
Paul M Colombani
July 2001

Acknowledgments

We are deeply indebted to our colleagues in surgery, medicine, anesthesiology and basic science who provided such expert contributions to this edition. They have helped to produce what we hope is a comprehensive and international account of all of the main areas of pediatric hepatobiliary and pancreatic surgery.

Michael Lax provided unflagging and kindly editorial assistance and expertise, as well as successfully co-ordinating contributions from authors, illustrators and editors. We also wish to thank our publisher, Edward Arnold, and Nicholas Dunton, Executive Director, who was persuaded by our arguments for a second edition of *Surgery of the Liver Disease in Children*. The book has been enhanced by a complete revision of the illustrations, and special gratitude is due to Charon Tec Pvt. Ltd, Chennai, India for this work. We are also grateful to Rada Radojicic and Carrie Walker for their unstinting efforts during the production phase of the book.

Finally, we thank our families. Without their support and encouragement our endeavors would not have been possible.

PART 1

Anatomy, physiology and investigation

Surgical anatomy of the liver and bile ducts

MYRDDIN REES

As recently as 1991, James Foster wrote 'The liver confounds the surgeon's dependence on anatomy.' This confusion is partly based on the deceptive surface anatomy, which bears little resemblance to the complex internal distribution of the tributaries of the hepatic arteries, portal veins and bile ducts on the one hand and the efferent hepatic veins on the other. However, the evolution of surgical techniques together with continued improvements in radiological imaging over the past 50 years now present the hepatobiliary surgeon with an unrivalled opportunity to tackle the most complex procedures, based on a firm grasp of detailed hepatic anatomy pertaining to each case.

HISTORICAL REVIEW (TABLE 1.1)

The earliest anatomical records of the liver emanate from Mesopotamia around 3000 to 2000 BC. The Babylonians and Assyrians regarded the liver as the seat of the soul (Jastrow, 1914) – hence the words 'liver' in English and 'leber' in German are derived from the verb 'to live'. The art of hepatoscopy evolved as a means of divination whereby the livers of sacrificed animals were studied for unusual signs that would predict a favorable or disastrous outcome in, for example, forthcoming battles. The key for such predictions was provided by a clay model of a sheep's liver with interpretive inscriptions on the different anatomical parts. An example dating from the seventh century BC can be seen in the British Museum (Milnes Walker, 1966).

The earliest medically relevant description of hepatic anatomy came from Herophilus (334–280 BC) as cited by Galen (Galen, 1956 translation by Singer). His contem-

porary Erasistratus (310–250 BC) in Alexandria coined the term 'parenchyma' (meaning 'to pour in beside'), and was the first to propose the nature of an intrahepatic capillary bed (Chen and Chen, 1984). This work was further developed by Galen (130–200 AD), who suggested that the liver lobes spread out like the fingers of a hand, but this was never fully explained (McClusky *et al.*, 1997).

In 1654, Francis Glisson from Cambridge University, England, published his landmark paper *Anatomia Hepatis* (Glisson, 1654). Although Johannes Walaeus had written in 1640 that the branches of the celiac artery, portal vein and bile ducts all lie together in a common sheath, it is to Glisson that we owe the first thorough description, and he applied the name 'capsule' to that structure. Glisson's publication contained no fewer than 45 chapters on the liver, based on careful dissection and removal of the parenchyma with small sticks to expose the anatomical detail. He described clearly divisions of the portal vein as we understand it today. To quote:

> the portal vein enters the liver and after it has penetrated it for about the length of a thumb, it is carried part on the right and part on the left, and then it is fashioned as it were into a fold – and from there it is divided into five wide branches; of these four are diffused far and wide through the substance of the liver, but the fifth leads straight towards the protuberance (namely the caudate).

He also perfused the liver with warm water colored by milk, and by observations of the subsequent outflow he predicted the presence of tiny vascular channels connecting the portal and hepatic venous systems (Milnes Walker, 1966). The colossal paper by Glisson that forms the basis of segmental anatomy was largely forgotten for

Table 1.1 *Landmark events in the history of liver surgery and use of anatomical principles*

1882	Langenbuch	First successful cholecystectomy
1886	Lius	First elective resection, but 67-year-old woman died from uncontrolled hemorrhage
1887	Langenbuch	First successful liver resection, despite return to theatre to control bleeding
1889	Ponfick	First observation in animal experiments of survival and subsequent regeneration of up to 75% liver removal
1892	Keen	Described first successful formal liver resection in the USA, and coined use of thumbnail to aid dissection
1903	Anschutz	First formal description of finger fracture dissection
1908	Hogarth Pringle	Described pinch inflow occlusion which 'helped' in four cases of hepatic trauma and subsequently in animal experiments
1909	Von Haberer	Ligated left hepatic artery before dissecting left lobe
1910	Wendell	Tied off right hepatic artery and right hepatic duct before resecting a large adenoma
1939	Meyer-May and Tung	Ligated specific vessels within liver parenchyma as they were encountered – so-called 'controlled resection'
1940	Cattell	First successful removal of colorectal metastases
1944	Donovan and Santulli	Specifically tied off left hepatic artery, left hepatic duct and left portal vein before resecting sarcoma in 7-year-old boy
1948	Raven	Reported formal resection along falciform ligament for colorectal metastases
1952	Lortat-Jacob and Robert	Performed a formal right hepatectomy with preliminary division of vessels
1952	Quttlebaum	Performed a right hepatectomy after formal ligation of hilum
1953	Ogilvy	Described use of blunt end of hemostat for fracturing the liver
1955	Honjo and Araki	Reported anatomical right lobectomy for metastatic carcinoma procedure performed in 1949
1956	Hepp-Couinaud	Approach to left hepatic duct
1957	Goldsmith and Woodburne	Described anatomical basis for modern liver resection
1966	Heaney	Total vascular occlusion with cross-clamping of abdominal aorta at level of diaphragm and inferior vena cava below liver
1968	Starzl	First successful orthotopic liver transplant
1975	Starzl	Described safe technique for massive liver resection (so-called trisegmentectomy or extended right hepatectomy)
1975	Starzl	Reported reduced-size liver transplant
1978	Huguet	Demonstrated safety of normothermic hepatic vascular exclusion for up to 60 minutes
1982	Bismuth	Landmark paper on 'segmental' approach to liver resection
1984	Hodgson	Description of use of ultrasonic 'scalpel' in liver transection
1984	Bismuth and Houssin	More extensive reports of reduced-size transplantation
1988	Pichlmayr	First split-liver transplantation
1989	Raia, Nery and Mies	First living (but unsuccessful) donor transplant
1990	Strong	First successful living donor transplant
1990	Pichlmayr	First 'on-the-bench' liver surgery

300 years. The fact that it was written in Latin and was never translated partly explains why it never achieved the acclaim it deserved. Hugo Rex re-explored the segmentation of the liver (Rex, 1988), although his findings were mostly based on mammalian livers.

The clearest early description of the division of the liver into nearly equal right and left halves based on a 'line passing from the fundus of the gallbladder to the exit of the hepatic veins' was that by James Cantlie (Cantlie, 1897). A surgeon and anatomist, he based his conclusions on clinical and experimental evidence sup-

ported by arterial injection techniques. His concept of the liver consisting of two nearly equal halves was confirmed by two fellows at the Mayo Clinic, McIndoe and Counsellor, who in 1927 used corrosion injection techniques in 12 cadaveric livers and examination of 30 other specimens. In the early 1950s, Hjortsjö (1951) and separately Elias and Petty (1952) made a further attempt to divide the liver into segments, but the credit for a detailed and complete account of the liver anatomy as currently understood and used by liver surgeons is due to Healey and Schroy (1953) and Couinaud (1954)

(Figures 1.1a and b). Healey and Schroy in their first paper based their subdivisions of the liver on the division of the hepatic duct. A subsequent publication in the same year by Healey *et al.* (1953) described the prevailing and identical pattern of arterial division. A third article by John Healey (1954) reviewed the anatomy of the biliary, arterial (Figure 1.2) and portal vein divisions as well as the hepatic veins. He highlighted the need for this knowledge to form the basis of radical hepatic surgery, a principle which was developed further by Goldsmith and Woodburne (1957). In contrast, Couinaud in Paris based his segments of the liver on the divisions of the portal vein and its interdigitations with the three hepatic veins. The Couinaud 'segments' were popularized in a paper by Bismuth *et al.* (1982) that depicted the surgical removal of these segments – 'segment-orientated resection'.

There were two fundamental differences between the accounts of Healey and Schroy (1953) and Couinaud (1954). First, the subdivisions of the left liver differed substantially in the second-order areas – the so-called sectors of Couinaud. Couinaud regarded the left half of the liver as being divided into two parts, namely medial and lateral sectors, along a plane passing through the left hepatic vein. He justified this view by regarding the portal vein branch to segment 2 as being a terminal branch. Botero and Strasberg (1998) have given a compelling account of why the division of the left side of the liver through the umbilical fissure as proposed by Healey is anatomically logical, and it certainly fits with what one encounters as a liver surgeon.

The second difference concerned the terminology used – identical areas of the liver were given different names (see Figure 1.3). The subsequent use of the equivalent liver resection terminology has served to confuse the hepatobiliary world for the last 50 years – what Strasberg has described as hepatic babel (Strasberg, 1997). The Americans and Japanese used the terminology of Healey and Schroy, while the Europeans largely followed that of Couinaud. At the annual meeting of the International Hepato Pancreatico Biliary Association (IHPBA) in Brisbane in 2000, a working party of the scientific committee proposed a new terminology for both liver anatomy and resections. As a compromise, the nomenclature of Couinaud segments 1–8 is retained, although the description of left-side anatomy by Healey and Schroy is adopted, with 'sections' replacing 'sectors'. Note also that the use of Roman numerals to depict segments is abandoned in order to enable all countries to follow the same numerical system. This proposal was accepted and is now

(b)

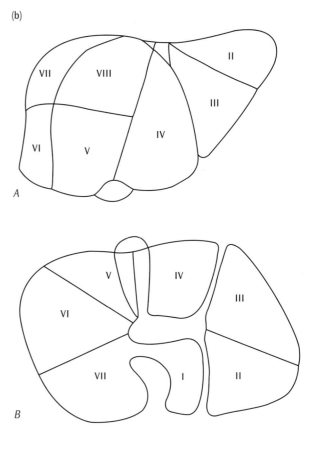

Figure 1.1b *Segmentation of the liver according to Couinaud. (Reproduced from Bismuth et al., 1982.) A, superior view – segment VIII is visible only on this view; B, inferior view – segment I is visible only on this view.*

(a)

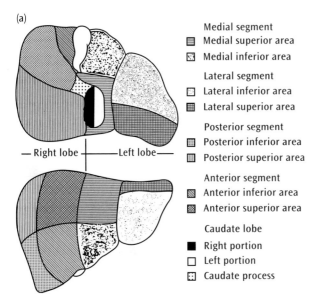

Medial segment
▤ Medial superior area
◪ Medial inferior area

Lateral segment
☐ Lateral inferior area
▦ Lateral superior area

Posterior segment
▩ Posterior inferior area
▥ Posterior superior area

Anterior segment
▨ Anterior inferior area
▧ Anterior superior area

Caudate lobe
■ Right portion
☐ Left portion
⊡ Caudate process

— Right lobe —— Left lobe —

Figure 1.1a *Divisions of the liver. Note that the visceral surface is shown in upper drawing and parietal surface in lower drawing. (Reproduced from Healey and Schroy, 1953.)*

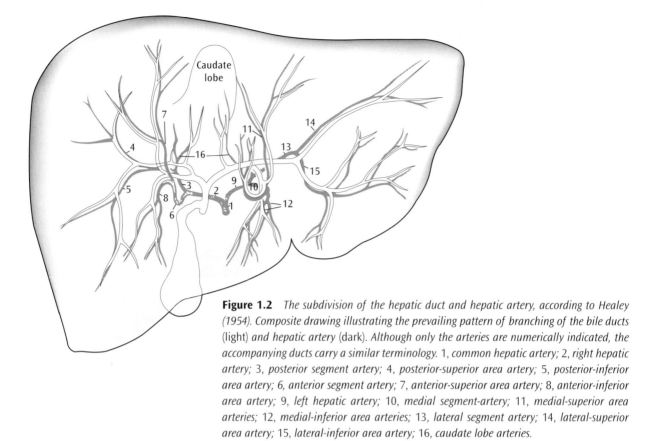

Figure 1.2 *The subdivision of the hepatic duct and hepatic artery, according to Healey (1954). Composite drawing illustrating the prevailing pattern of branching of the bile ducts (light) and hepatic artery (dark). Although only the arteries are numerically indicated, the accompanying ducts carry a similar terminology. 1, common hepatic artery; 2, right hepatic artery; 3, posterior segment artery; 4, posterior-superior area artery; 5, posterior-inferior area artery; 6, anterior segment artery; 7, anterior-superior area artery; 8, anterior-inferior area artery; 9, left hepatic artery; 10, medial segment-artery; 11, medial-superior area arteries; 12, medial-inferior area arteries; 13, lateral segment artery; 14, lateral-superior area artery; 15, lateral-inferior area artery; 16, caudate lobe arteries.*

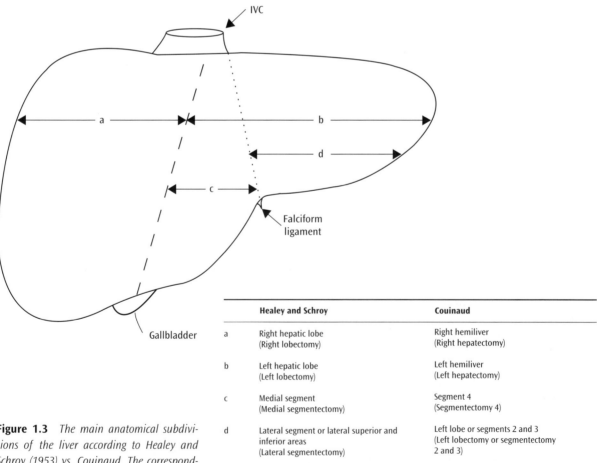

Figure 1.3 *The main anatomical subdivisions of the liver according to Healey and Schroy (1953) vs. Couinaud. The corresponding resection terminology is shown in parentheses.*

	Healey and Schroy	Couinaud
a	Right hepatic lobe (Right lobectomy)	Right hemiliver (Right hepatectomy)
b	Left hepatic lobe (Left lobectomy)	Left hemiliver (Left hepatectomy)
c	Medial segment (Medial segmentectomy)	Segment 4 (Segmentectomy 4)
d	Lateral segment or lateral superior and inferior areas (Lateral segmentectomy)	Left lobe or segments 2 and 3 (Left lobectomy or segmentectomy 2 and 3)
a and c	Anterior, posterior and medial segments (Right trisegmentectomy)	Right lobe (Right lobectomy)

recommended for worldwide use. The detailed account depicted below follows these guidelines.

INTRAHEPATIC SURGICAL ANATOMY

The first glimpse of the liver by a surgeon either at laparoscopy or at laparotomy is dominated by its peritoneal attachments. Superiorly, the falciform ligament is continued as the umbilical ligament (ligamentum teres) to the anterior abdominal wall. On either side, two folds of peritoneum fuse as the so-called left and right triangular ligaments. The surgical relevance of these three ligaments is simply the need to divide them in order to mobilize the liver. Only in this way can adequate exposure be obtained during resection. Similarly, for trauma to the right hemiliver, the peritoneal attachments on that side require division in order to control hemorrhage by packs placed behind and in front of the liver – the appropriately named 'sandwich technique' of packing. The next important peritoneal layer is the reflection of the lesser omentum around the portal structures entering the hilum of the liver – the so-called hepatoduodenal ligament. Division of this peritoneal layer allows the first view of relevant anatomy in the approach to the hilum. The common bile duct lies anteriorly and to the right, and the common hepatic artery lies anteriorly and to the left. The portal vein lies posteriorly with an immediately obvious small branch to the right caudate area.

The prevailing pattern of intrahepatic division of these three portal structures is now described using IHPBA-adopted terminology. Two roughly equal halves of the liver (the right side actually constitutes 55–60%) are defined by the right and left branches – the so-called first-order divisions of Healey and Schroy. All three structures divide within the hilum but outside the liver. Right-sided structures have a very short extrahepatic course (1–3 cm), with the left-sided branches being much longer. A common feature on both sides is that as the three portal structures enter the liver substance they are surrounded by the fibrous sheath of Walaeus, an extension from the Glissonian capsule. Resection techniques that rely on intrahepatic dissection (Tung, 1957; Launois and Jamieson, 1992) therefore result in the appropriate branches of hepatic duct, portal vein and hepatic artery being divided en masse within their sheath. Conversely, extrahepatic or hilar dissection requires each portal structure to be suture-ligated individually. This extension of vascular biliary fibrous sheaths continues to surround the second- and third-order branches of the portal vein, hepatic duct, hepatic artery, terminating in separate functional units or segments.

The right branches are usually short and run an almost vertical course (Figure 1.4a). The left portal vein and left hepatic duct lie in a more horizontal position at the hilum before entering the umbilical recess, where they become more vertical. The change in direction reflects the embryological derivation of the left portal vein (see Chapter 7). The horizontal course and more superior position of the left hepatic duct are exploited in bile duct reconstruction, etc. By 'lowering the hilar plate' (Hepp and Couinaud, 1956) the duct is easily exposed, especially when dilated. The left hepatic artery usually comes off early and lies on the medial or left aspect of the umbilical recess. This is very useful in radical extended right hepatectomies where the arterial blood supply to segments 2 and 3 is safely preserved.

The surgical demarcation of right and left hemilivers may be defined on the liver surface by a line connecting the gallbladder fundus to the insertion of the middle hepatic vein into the inferior vena cava (IVC) (Cantlie's line). This may be marked by cautery and confirmed by intraoperative ultrasound. The middle hepatic vein lies in the intended plane separating the right and left hemilivers. The direction of this 'midplane of the liver' follows the gallbladder fossa and is usually 20–30° from the vertical. Thus packs placed behind the right liver convert the midplane to a near vertical direction, which is easier to follow surgically when performing, say, a right hemihepatectomy.

The second-order divisions divide the liver into four areas, which are now called sections (Strasberg, 1999) – a medial and lateral section on the left and an anterior and posterior section on the right (Figure 1.4b).[1]

On the right side, the so-called second-order divisions dictate a right anterior and right posterior sectional (sectoral) duct with its attendant artery and portal vein. The two sections so defined lie anteriorly and posteriorly as seen in the patient at laparotomy and prior to mobilization. Separating the two is the right intersectional (intersectoral) plane, which lies in a true horizontal direction and is identified by the right hepatic vein on intraoperative ultrasound. The inferior limit of this plane lies midway between the gallbladder fundus and the most lateral peritoneal attachment of the liver, and runs to the insertion point of the right hepatic vein with the vena cava.

On the left side, the hepatic ducts and arteries predominantly divide into lateral and medial (sectional) branches. The functional division into medial and lateral sections is easily defined by the falciform ligament. The left portal vein takes a more vertical course in the umbilical recess (often covered by a variable bridge of liver tissue) and gives off third-order branches directly.

The third-order branches divide the liver into the 'segments' that have become universally known as Couinaud segments (Figure 1.4c) ('areas' of Healey and Schroy, 'subsegments' of Goldsmith and Woodburne). On the

---

[1] These correspond to Couinaud sectors on the right but not on the left. In practice, most surgeons either misinterpreted or ignored Couinaud's work and regarded the left sectors as described – which corresponds to surgically relevant divisions.

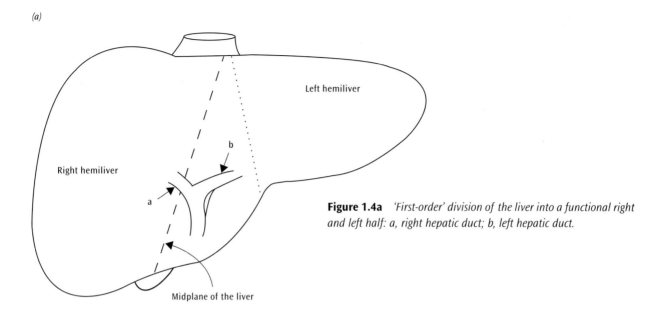

(a)

Left hemiliver

Right hemiliver

b

a

Midplane of the liver

Figure 1.4a *'First-order' division of the liver into a functional right and left half: a, right hepatic duct; b, left hepatic duct.*

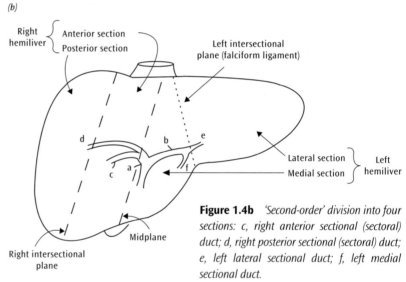

(b)

Right hemiliver { Anterior section / Posterior section

Left intersectional plane (falciform ligament)

d

b

e

c a

f

Lateral section } Left hemiliver / Medial section

Midplane

Right intersectional plane

Figure 1.4b *'Second-order' division into four sections: c, right anterior sectional (sectoral) duct; d, right posterior sectional (sectoral) duct; e, left lateral sectional duct; f, left medial sectional duct.*

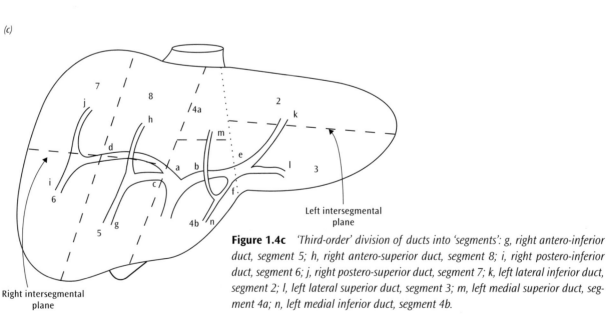

(c)

7

8

j

h

/4a

2

k

d

m

a b

e

i

c

l

3

6

f

g

4b n

5

Left intersegmental plane

Right intersegmental plane

Figure 1.4c *'Third-order' division of ducts into 'segments': g, right antero-inferior duct, segment 5; h, right antero-superior duct, segment 8; i, right postero-inferior duct, segment 6; j, right postero-superior duct, segment 7; k, left lateral inferior duct, segment 2; l, left lateral superior duct, segment 3; m, left medial superior duct, segment 4a; n, left medial inferior duct, segment 4b.*

right side the anterior and posterior divisions each give off superior and inferior branches. The anterior inferior branch is the segmental supply to segment 5, the anterior superior branch is the segmental supply to segment 8, the postero-inferior branch is to segment 6, and the postero-superior branch is to segment 7. The intersegmental plane between 5, 6 and 7, 8 is the most difficult to define surgically. It lies roughly halfway along the convex surface of the liver, and may be more easily defined by intraoperative ultrasound. Some surgeons advocate methylene blue injection of the relevant segmental vessels, although the author finds this messy and unnecessary.

On the left side, the segmental branching follows a similar pattern for ducts and arteries. The superior branch of the lateral sectional ducts supplies segment 3, and the inferior branch of the lateral sectional ducts supplies segment 2. The portal vein branch to segment 2 comes off the main portal vein at the base of the umbilical recess, with the branch to segment 3 arising more vertically within the recess. On the medial side, Scheele proposed a similar division into a superior branch supplying segment 4a and an inferior branch to segment 4b (Scheele, 1989). This schema of anatomy was clearly described by Healey and Schroy, and is probably the most commonly used subdivision in segment-oriented hepatic surgery. The ability to preserve half of segment 4 (as 4a or 4b) allows preservation of approximately 10% of functioning liver tissue, which may have important surgical applications when performing extended right

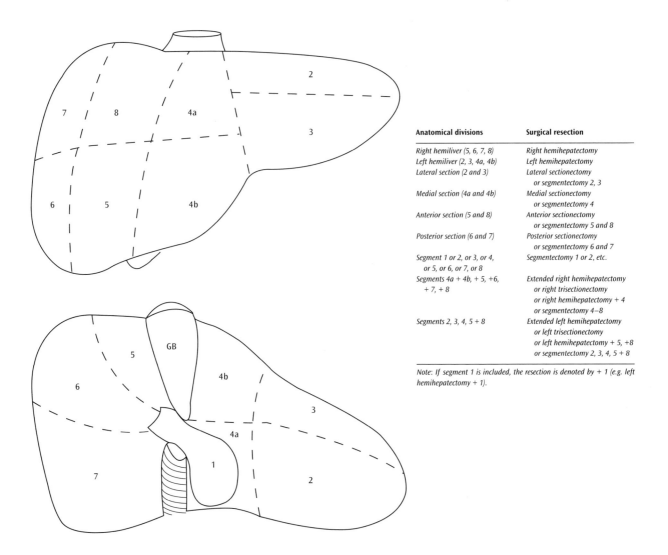

Anatomical divisions	Surgical resection
Right hemiliver (5, 6, 7, 8)	Right hemihepatectomy
Left hemiliver (2, 3, 4a, 4b)	Left hemihepatectomy
Lateral section (2 and 3)	Lateral sectionectomy or segmentectomy 2, 3
Medial section (4a and 4b)	Medial sectionectomy or segmentectomy 4
Anterior section (5 and 8)	Anterior sectionectomy or segmentectomy 5 and 8
Posterior section (6 and 7)	Posterior sectionectomy or segmentectomy 6 and 7
Segment 1 or 2, or 3, or 4, or 5, or 6, or 7, or 8	Segmentectomy 1 or 2, etc.
Segments 4a + 4b, + 5, +6, + 7, + 8	Extended right hemihepatectomy or right trisectionectomy or right hemihepatectomy + 4 or segmentectomy 4–8
Segments 2, 3, 4, 5 + 8	Extended left hemihepatectomy or left trisectionectomy or left hemihepatectomy + 5, +8 or segmentectomy 2, 3, 4, 5 + 8

Note: If segment 1 is included, the resection is denoted by + 1 (e.g. left hemihepatectomy + 1).

Figure 1.5 *Anatomical division of the liver, and the nomenclature of corresponding surgical resections. The numbers correspond to the numbered segments of the liver.*

hepatectomies (i.e. resection 4–8). It is also utilized in radical resection of gallbladder cancer (i.e. resection of segments 4b, 5 and 6).

The least understood aspect of hepatic anatomy is the caudate lobe (i.e. segment 1). Advances in surgical technique, particularly for hilar cholangiocarcinoma, mandate that this area of the liver be clearly appreciated. The caudate lies behind the hilum and in front of the inferior vena cava. It is bounded superiorly by the entrance of the middle hepatic vein (Heloury et al., 1988). There is usually an obvious extension to the right – the so-called 'right caudate process'. The body of the caudate is not normally visible, but a variably sized left caudate 'lobe' is easily visible immediately behind the peritoneum of the lesser sac and lying in front of the vena cava.

The arterial and portal supply and biliary drainage of the caudate have been extensively investigated and described by Healey and Schroy (1953) and by Couinaud (1954). Mizumoto et al. (1986) also studied the caudate lobe in 106 cadavers. Heloury et al. (1988) further contributed to our understanding of the caudate as viewed by intraoperative ultrasound. Most authors are agreed that there are generally two or three ducts, arteries and portal vein branches to the caudate. In Healey and Schroy's study, the entire caudate lobe drained into both right and left hepatic ducts in 78% of cases. Note also that the ductal drainage of the right caudate process is predominantly to the right posterior sectional duct (80% of cases in Mizumoto's study). The portal vein branches – two to three in number – are usually the most prominent and easily found surgically. The branch at the origin of the right portal vein to the right caudate process is constant and easily damaged. It is best divided early during hilar dissection for right hepatectomy. The caudate branch from the left portal vein is also easily identifiable during hilar dissection. In most instances of left hemihepatectomy (not including segment 1) the left caudate branch is preserved. In contrast, when segment 1 is to be included in a left resection, the portal and arterial branches are best divided early.

In summary, from a surgical perspective the bulk of the liver is divided into eight segments (2, 3, 4a, 4b, 5, 6, 7 and 8) and a caudate area (1) is further subdivided into three parts (right and left process and body) (Figure 1.5).

The ability to remove these areas separately – the so-called segment-oriented approach – has revolutionized hepatic surgery (Bismuth et al., 1982). Although line diagrams of the different segments are of necessity an oversimplification, an important and largely ignored paper by Gupta et al. (1977) demonstrated that the accepted distribution of size between the segments only occurred in 48% of cases. Using corrosion casts of 85 cadaveric livers, those researchers identified eight other variations in size of the different segments. Some of these variations may be obvious – for example, small segment 2 and 3. Less obvious is the variability in the extent of segments 4a and 4b, and even more so the subdivision within the right hemiliver. In particular, small segments 6 and 7 may be crucial when extended left hepatectomy is undertaken. The more complex hepatic resections therefore require a thorough assessment of the relative size of the individual segments. This may be further complicated by atrophy or hypertrophy with attendant rotation of the anatomy.

Hepatic veins

The hepatic veins are the structures that are most easily damaged during hepatic transection. In addition, knowledge of their position and draining areas has assumed greater importance as hepatic surgeons have become more adventurous in their resectional techniques. The veins are best identified by intraoperative ultrasound or by reference to late phase-contrast-enhanced CT scans. There is usually a large right hepatic vein draining segments 6 and 7 predominantly, and also part of segments 5 and 8 (Healey, 1954). The right hepatic vein lies in the intersectional plane of the right hemiliver. It receives many tributaries, although not in its short, extrahepatic course. Exposure of this vein is simplified by the preliminary division of the many (6–10) short draining veins that run posteriorly (in pairs, left and right) between the liver and the inferior vena cava. In addition, the hepatocaval ligament must be divided formally. This ligament (said to be avascular, although it invariably conceals a vein) is a 1–3 cm fibrous extension of Glisson's capsule between the right side of the vena cava and the posterior aspect of the liver. It may contain an extension of the caudate lobe (Heloury et al., 1988), and occasional vestigial, tiny bile ducts are encountered. There is a larger postero-inferior vein draining segment 6 directly into the vena cava in up to 25% of cases ('accessory right hepatic vein'). The size of this vein is inversely related to the size of the right hepatic vein. When present, it allows sacrifice of the right and middle hepatic veins in central resections, and is the basis for 'parenchymal-sparing' resections in patients with cirrhosis (Makuuchi et al., 1987).

As described above, the midplane of the liver is occupied by the middle hepatic vein, which in 90% of cases joins the left hepatic vein before insertion into the vena cava (Figure 1.6). The middle hepatic vein drains segments 4 and 5 and part of segment 8. The latter branch may cause troublesome bleeding during parenchymal transection for a right hemihepatectomy. The left hepatic vein drains segments 2 and 3 and may occasionally consist of two separate veins. An important vein that assumes prominence in extended right hepatectomy is the umbilical vein (Scheele, 1989). This vein joins the junctional groove between the middle and left hepatic vein. It will drain segment 4b or 4a if the middle hepatic vein is of necessity removed during transection, and it is easily identified by intraoperative ultrasound. There are

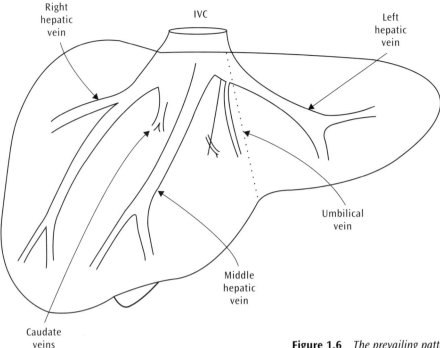

Figure 1.6   *The prevailing pattern of hepatic veins.*

clear communications between the main veins. Occasionally, parts of the liver may become temporarily congested at the conclusion of an extended hepatectomy, but this usually settles over a period of 10–15 minutes.

In addition to the usual intrahepatic anatomy described above, there are a number of important variations. A detailed account of these is beyond the scope of this chapter, but may be found in Couinaud's excellent book, which serves as the ultimate reference text (Couinaud, 1981, 1989).

Most of the surgically relevant anatomical variations involve the bile ducts, which are unforgiving if damaged or unsecured – a persisting bile leak or non-drainage of an area is to be regarded as technical failure. Left duct drainage is particularly complex, and assumes importance in living donor and reduced-size liver transplantation. The segment 3 duct follows an oblique course towards the porta hepatis, where it joins the (usually larger) segment 2 duct to form the lateral sectional duct. The union of these two lateral segmental ducts occurs in line with the falciform ligament in 50% of cases. It may also be placed to the right (42% of cases) or the left (8% of cases) of this left intersectional plane.

Ductal drainage of segments 4a and 4b (usually two to each area) was the most complex arrangement encountered by Healey and Schroy (1953). In the majority of cases (60%), all four ducts join to form a single medial sectional duct. In 24% of cases the superior duct has a separate drainage with a single trunk for the other three ducts. In 10% of cases the ducts to segment 4a and 4b drain separately, and finally in 6% two ducts drain sepa-

rately and two drain by a common stem. There are also variations with regard to the site of drainage of the segment 4a and 4b ducts.

EXTRAHEPATIC ANATOMY AND ANOMALIES

The biliary tree

The usual confluence of right and left hepatic ducts to form a common hepatic duct occurs in 72% of cases (Healey and Schroy, 1953) (Figure 1.7). Biliary surgeons also identify a so-called triple confluence (12% of cases in Couinaud's findings) of the left hepatic duct with the right and left sectional (sectoral) ducts. An important variation is the union of a right sectional (sectoral) duct with the left hepatic duct (according to Couinaud, 4% of cases involving the right posterior sectional duct, and 1% involving the anterior sectional duct.) This duct is prone to accidental damage during left hemihepatectomy, or

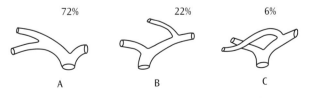

Figure 1.7   *The prevailing pattern of bile duct confluence. (Reproduced from Healey and Schroy, 1953.)*

resection for gallbladder cancer or hilar cholangiocarcinoma. A detailed pre- or perioperative cholangiogram is advocated in such resections (Professor Russell Strong, Brisbane, personal communication).

The common hepatic duct is joined at a variable level by the cystic duct to form the common bile duct. Occasionally the cystic duct will join the right hepatic duct. Usually the cystic duct joins the right side of the common hepatic duct at an acute angle (68% of cases according to Moosman and Coller, 1951). In 4% of cases the cystic duct joins the common duct on its anterior surface, and in 7% posteriorly. In nearly 20% of cases the cystic duct runs parallel to the common hepatic duct, united with it by fibrous connective tissue, for a variable distance ranging from 10 mm to over 25 mm (Moosman and Coller, 1951). In 2% of cases the cystic duct takes a spiral course (anterior or posterior) to join the left side of the common duct. The latter two instances make exploration of the common bile duct particularly difficult, and can lead to problems if unrecognized at liver transplantation (Koneru et al., 1989). The cystic duct length and diameter vary greatly (from 4 mm to 65 mm in length, and from 3 mm to 9 mm in diameter; Moosman and Coller, 1951).

Together with the common hepatic duct, the cystic duct forms the base (medial) and inferior margin of the so-called Calot's triangle, respectively. The superior border in Calot's original description (Rocko et al., 1981) was formed by the cystic artery. However, it has become generally accepted that a better working definition of Calot's triangle is a superior border occupied by the inferior surface of the right hemiliver. Dissection of this area – a crucial part of cholecystectomy – endangers a number of structures, in particular the right hepatic artery, aberrant right hepatic artery and accessory or replaced sectional ducts that join the common hepatic or, rarely, the cystic duct. The cystic duct leads to the neck of the gallbladder, usually lying in the cystic fossa that denotes the midplane of the liver. The biliary reservoir ranges from 18 mL to 150 mL in volume, and is adherent to dense connective tissue overlying Glisson's capsule. Occasionally there may be a mesentery or, more awkwardly, a gallbladder deeply embedded in liver substance. Rarely, the gallbladder may lie on the left side of the liver. Other recognized but rare anomalies (Gross, 1936) include a bilobed gallbladder, duplication of the gallbladder and cystic duct, diverticula and hepatic ducts that drain directly into the gallbladder.

The common bile duct (mean diameter 6 mm, although it has a tendency to be greater in the elderly) passes downwards in front of the portal vein and then diverges behind the first part of the duodenum and the head of the pancreas. The duct then inclines to the right to open into the duodenum approximately 10 cm from the pylorus. The common bile duct frequently joins the main pancreatic duct within the wall of the duodenum to form a short common channel which is 2–7 mm long (ampulla of Vater). Other variations include a separate opening for the two ducts (a variable distance apart), or a long common channel formed by union of the ducts before they enter the duodenal wall (Figure 1.8). This long common channel has been implicated in the etiology of choledochal cysts (see Chapter 10) and biliary pancreatitis. The distal part of the duct is surrounded by choledochal muscle – the so-called papilla – which is easily seen and felt on the medial wall of the second part of the duodenum.

Hepatic arteries

The hepatic artery supplies 25–30% of the total afferent flow, although it supplies about 50% of the available oxygen. It is long established that hepatic artery occlusion, ligation and embolization can usually be well tolerated in the intact liver, but if they occur in the transplanted liver, hepatic or biliary necrosis inevitably follows.

The common hepatic artery arises from the celiac axis in approximately 80% of cases. As it passes upwards to

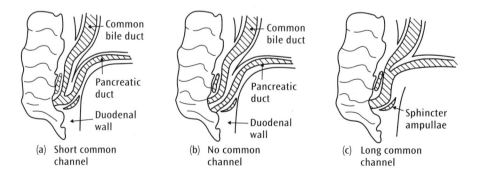

Figure 1.8 *Diagram showing the different types of union of the common bile duct and the main pancreatic duct. (a) Most frequently both ducts share a short common channel within the wall of the duodenum. (b) Each duct may have a separate opening, occasionally as much as 2 cm apart. (c) Both ducts may unite to form a long common channel before entering the duodenum.*

the hilum of the liver, it gives off the right gastric and gastroduodenal arteries to form the common hepatic artery 'proper'. Division into the right and left hepatic arteries occurs at a variable level, but either way, at the hilum the right and left hepatic arteries usually lie posterior to the ducts.

Aberrant right and left hepatic arteries may be *accessory* to (in addition to) or *replacement* to the usual vessels. The latter is usual, and division will therefore devascularize the part of the liver to which they are distributed. On the left side the commonest variant is an accessory left hepatic artery, found in 18% of cases, arising from the left gastric artery. Its course along the lesser omentum is easily seen, and in extended right hepatectomy it is a comforting sight.

An aberrant right hepatic artery occurs in about 20% of cases (four out of five as replacement and one out of five as accessory; Moosman and Coller, 1951), and typically reaches the liver by passing dorsal to the portal vein and then lying on the right side of the common hepatic duct. In the majority of cases (76%) the superior mesenteric is the source of an aberrant right hepatic artery. The cystic artery (86% single, 14% double) is usually a branch of the right hepatic artery, and typically passes behind the bile ducts and cephalad to the cystic duct. Variations of this course are not uncommon.

The blood supply to the supraduodenal part of the common bile duct is precarious. Elegant studies by Northover and Terblanche (1979) have demonstrated an axial distribution with an average of eight small arteries, the most important of which run on the lateral and medial borders of the duct as the so-called '3 and 9 o'clock arteries'. Around 60% of the blood vessels run upwards from the retroduodenal and retroportal arteries, while 38% of the arteries run downwards from the right hepatic and cystic arteries. Only 2% are non-axial, arising directly from the main trunk of the hepatic artery.

In liver transplantation, the donor bile duct is more liable to become ischemic than the recipient duct, and this may be related to the length of the transplanted donor duct.

Portal vein

The valveless portal vein drains blood from the splanchnic area and is formed behind the neck of the pancreas by confluence of the splenic and superior mesenteric veins. It lies posteriorly in the hepatoduodenal ligament and is remarkably constant. The most common variation is a trifurcation, when the main trunk divides simultaneously into the right posterior sectional, right anterior sectional and left portal branches. Important but rare anomalies include abnormal position anterior to the head of the pancreas and duodenum, or entrance of the portal vein directly into the inferior vena cava. In the latter situation the hepatic artery is greatly enlarged as it is the sole source of blood supply to the liver. Extremely rare congenital strictures or malformations of the portal vein at the hilum may cause portal hypertension (see Chapter 20).

In summary, the dawn of the millennium has coincided with the coming of age of hepatic surgery. The evolution of surgical technique has matched our detailed appreciation of the finer points of hepatic anatomy. Moreover, the efforts of the scientific committee of the IHPBA should now allow hepatobiliary surgeons worldwide to communicate with each other.

Key references

Healey JE, Schroy PC. Anatomy of the biliary ducts within the human liver. Analysis of the prevailing pattern of branchings and the major variations of the biliary ducts. *Archives of Surgery* 1953; **66**: 599–615.

A landmark paper which provides a clear description of the detailed intrahepatic anatomy.

Couinaud C. *Surgical anatomy of the liver revisited*. Paris: privately published, 1989.

An essential booklet that should be on every hepatic surgeon's bookshelf as a reference for the rare anatomical anomalies that appear.

Bismuth H, Houssin D, Castaing D. Major and minor segmentectomies – 'reglées – in liver surgery. *World Journal of Surgery* 1982; **6**: 10–24.

This paper popularized the segment-oriented approach to liver surgery.

Scheele J. Segment-orientated resection of the liver: rationale and technique. In: Lygidakis NJ, Tytgat GNJ, Argner K (eds) *Hepatobiliary and pancreatic malignancies*. New York: Thieme Medical, 1989: 219–47.

The most elegant demonstration of what can be achieved in liver resection, in particular highlighting the subdivision of segment 4 into 4a and 4b and its relevance to surgeons.

Strasberg SM. Terminology of liver anatomy and liver resections: coming to grips with the hepatic babel. *Journal of the American College of Surgeons* 1997; **184**: 413–34.

A clear narrative on the previous confusion regarding the terminology of liver anatomy and liver surgery.

REFERENCES

Bismuth H, Houssin D, Castaing D. Major and minor segmentectomies – 'reglées' – in liver surgery. *World Journal of Surgery* 1982; **6**: 10–24.

Botero AC, Strasberg SM. Division of the left hemiliver in man: segments, sectors or sections. *Liver Transplantation and Surgery* 1998; **4**: 226–31.

Cantlie J. On a new arrangement of the right and left lobes of the liver. *Proceedings of the Anatomical Society of Great Britain and Ireland* 1897; **32**: i–ix.

Chen TS, Chen PS. *Understanding the liver: a history*. Westport, CT: Greenwood Press, 1984.

Couinaud C. Lobes et segments hépatiques nôtes sur architecture anatomique et chirurgicale du foie. *Presse Medicale* 1954; **62**: 709–12.

Couinaud C. Controlled hepatectomies and exposure of intrahepatic bile ducts. In: *Anatomical and technical study*. Paris: privately published, 1981.

Couinaud C. *Surgical anatomy of the liver revisited*. Paris: privately published, 1989.

Elias H, Petty D. Gross anatomy of the blood vessels and ducts within the human liver. *American Journal of Anatomy* 1952; **90**: 59–111.

Foster JH. History of liver surgery. *Archives of Surgery* 1991; **126**: 381–7.

Galen C (translated by C Singer). *On anatomical procedures*. London: Oxford University Press, 1956.

Glisson F. *Anatomia hepatis*. London: O. Pullein, 1654.

Goldsmith NA, Woodburne RT. Surgical anatomy pertaining to liver surgery. *Surgery, Gynecology and Obstetrics* 1957; **195**: 310–18.

Gross RE. Congenital anomalies of the gallbladder. A review of a hundred and forty-eight cases with a report of a double gallbladder. *Archives of Surgery* 1936; **32**: 131–62.

Gupta SC, Gupta CD, Arosa AK. Subsegmentation of the human liver. *Journal of Anatomy* 1977; **124**: 413–23.

Healey JE. Clinical anatomical aspects of radical hepatic surgery. *Journal of the International College of Surgeons* 1954; **22**: 542–9.

Healey JE, Schroy PC. Anatomy of the biliary ducts within the human liver. Analysis of the prevailing pattern of branchings and the major variations of the biliary ducts. *Archives of Surgery* 1953; **66**: 599–616.

Healey JE, Schroy P, Sorensen R. The intrahepatic distribution of the hepatic artery in man. *Journal of the International College of Surgeons* 1953; **20**: 133–48.

Heloury Y, Leborgne J, Rogez JM, Robert R, Barbin R, Hureau J. The caudate lobe of the liver. *Surgical and Radiological Anatomy* 1988; **10**: 83–91.

Hepp J, Couinaud C. L'abord et l'utilisation du canal hépatique gauche dans les réparations de la voie biliaire principale. *Presse Medicale* 1956; **64**: 947–8.

Hjortsjö CH. The topography of the intrahepatic duct system. *Acta Anatomica (Basel)* 1951; **11**: 599–615.

Jastrow M Jr. Medicine of the Babylonians and Syrians. *Proceedings of the Royal Society of Medicine* 1914; **7**: 109–76.

Koneru B, Zajko AB, Linda S *et al*. Obstructing mucocoele of the cystic duct after transplantation of the liver. *Surgery, Gynecology and Obstetrics* 1989; **168**: 394–6.

Launois B, Jamieson GG. The importance of Glisson's capsule and its sheaths in the intrahepatic approach to resection of the liver. *Surgery, Gynecology and Obstetrics* 1992; **174**: 7–10.

McClusky DA, Skandalakis LJ, Colborn GL, Skandalakis JE. Hepatic surgery and hepatic surgical anatomy: historical partners in progress. *World Journal of Surgery* 1997; **21**: 330–42.

McIndoe AH, Counsellor VS. The bilaterality of the liver. *Archives of Surgery* 1927; **15**: 589–612.

Makuuchi M, Hasegawa H, Yamazaki S, Takayasu K, Morigama N. The use of operative ultrasound as an aid to liver resection in patients with hepatocellular carcinoma. *World Journal of Surgery* 1987; **11**: 615–21.

Milnes Walker R. Francis Glisson and his capsule. *Annals of the Royal College of Surgeons of England* 1966; **38**: 71–91.

Mizumoto R, Kawarada Y, Suzuki H. Surgical treatment of hilar cholangiocarcinoma of the bile duct. *Surgery, Gynecology and Obstetrics* 1986; **162**: 153–8.

Moosman DA, Coller FA. Prevention of traumatic injury to the bile ducts. *American Journal of Surgery* 1951; **82**: 132–43.

Northover JMA, Terblanche J. A new look at the arterial blood supply of the bile duct in man and its surgical implications. *British Journal of Surgery* 1979; **66**: 379–84.

Rex H. Beiträge zur Morphologie der Säugerleber. *Gegenbauers Morphologisches Jahrbuch* 1988; **14**: 517–616.

Rocko JM, Swan KG, Gioia JM. Calot's triangle revisited. *Surgery, Gynecology and Obstetrics* 1981; **153**: 410–14.

Scheele J. Segment-orientated resection of the liver: rationale and technique. In: Lygidakis NJ, Tytgat GNJ, Argner K (eds) *Hepatobiliary and pancreatic malignancies: diagnosis, medical and surgical management*. New York: Thieme Medical, 1989: 219–47.

Strasberg SM. Terminology of liver anatomy and liver resections: coming to grips with the hepatic babel. *Journal of the American College of Surgeons* 1997; **184**: 413–34.

Strasberg SM. Terminology of hepatic anatomy and resections. *HPB* 1999; **1**: 191–201.

Tung TT. *Les resections majeures and mineures du foie*. Paris: Masson, 1957.

Physiological responses to surgery

CHARLES N PAIDAS

The liver has two major functions, namely synthesis and clearance. On the one hand, it is involved in the generation of substrate for energy, the synthesis and secretion of plasma proteins, and the production of bile. On the other, it is responsible for waste management or detoxification, bile turnover and reticuloendothelial clearance. The liver is a repository for vitamins (A, D and B_{12}) and iron. It is also involved in the modulation of the response to stress. Furthermore, it performs all of these functions through a dual circulation and metabolic control that is regulated by both the nervous system and hormones.

EMBRYOLOGICAL CORRELATIONS

Formation of a dual circulation and development of a system of bile ducts are two processes that are unique to liver embryogenesis. The liver is formed from foregut endodermal cells known as the hepatic diverticulum and the septum transversum, a mesenchymal cell and capillary network, during the third week of development (Larsen, 1993). It is this endoderm–mesenchymal interaction that probably induces a coordinated sequence of hepatic differentiation into a liver bud. Even at this embryonic stage, the liver resembles a series of cords with each cell capable of synthesizing protein earlier than recognition of hepatic morphology (Cascio and Zaret, 1991). Proliferation of the cellular cord structures through a circuit of veins (vitelline veins) that drain the digestive tract gives rise to the hepatic sinusoid. The vitelline veins fuse to form the portal vein and empty into the sinus venosus, and the sinus venosus becomes the

inferior vena cava (see Chapter 20). During *in-utero* life, a second series of venous channels called the umbilical veins supply nutrients and oxygenated blood flow to the embryo from the placenta (Figure 2.1). The right umbilical vein obliterates early in week six of development, and the left umbilical vein drains along with the left portal vein into the ductus venosus. The fetal liver receives blood from the umbilical vein, as well as from the hepatic artery and portal vein. Extrapolating human flow from that in lambs suggests that nearly 75% of total fetal blood flow comes from the umbilical vein, and the remainder is from portal (vitelline) blood (15–20%) and the hepatic artery (5–10%) (Edelstone *et al.*, 1978; Rudolph, 1983).

The pattern of distribution of both fetal hepatic blood flow and oxygen delivery is heterogeneous. In general, blood oxygen saturation is higher within the left lobe of the fetal liver, and this is consistent with the presence of higher levels of hematopoiesis within the left lobe (Emery, 1963). After birth, the *in-utero* ductus venosus circuit fibroses, forming the ligamentum teres and falciform ligament, and flow is disconnected via the umbilical vein. Closure of the ductus may take over 10 days after birth. Total liver blood flow decreases after birth in response to the reduction in umbilical vein flow. The major postnatal component of overall liver blood flow is portal blood. Relative to intrauterine flow, there is an increased contribution by the hepatic artery. Following birth, and only after establishment of the dual circulation to the liver, gene expression for albumin, gluconeogenic enzymes and cytochrome P-450 is present by 3 weeks, whereas alpha-fetoprotein (active during fetal life) expression declines (Tilghman and Belayew, 1983).

A common misconception arises with regard to inser-

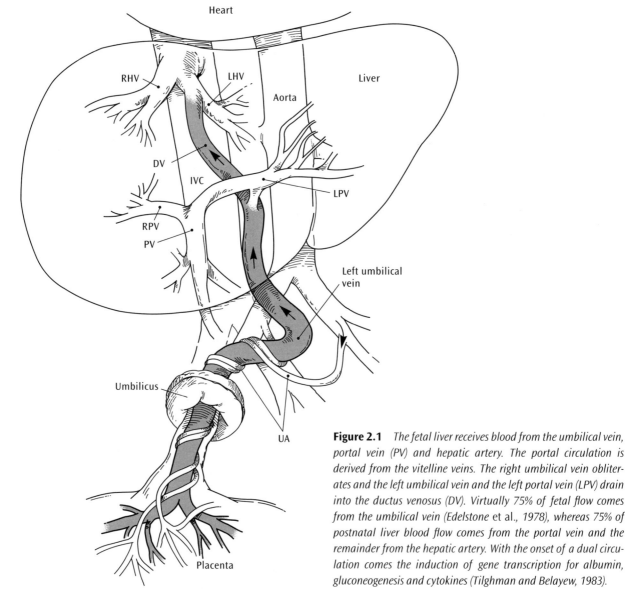

Figure 2.1 *The fetal liver receives blood from the umbilical vein, portal vein (PV) and hepatic artery. The portal circulation is derived from the vitelline veins. The right umbilical vein obliterates and the left umbilical vein and the left portal vein (LPV) drain into the ductus venosus (DV). Virtually 75% of fetal flow comes from the umbilical vein (Edelstone et al., 1978), whereas 75% of postnatal liver blood flow comes from the portal vein and the remainder from the hepatic artery. With the onset of a dual circulation comes the induction of gene transcription for albumin, gluconeogenesis and cytokines (Tilghman and Belayew, 1983).*

tion of an umbilical vein catheter. The umbilical vein catheter courses through the left lobe of the liver into the ductus venosus and then the inferior vena cava (IVC). Since the umbilical vein joins with the left portal vein to become the ductus venosus, technically the umbilical vein does not traverse the portal circulation but the catheter can indirectly obstruct portal flow. Thus portal vein thrombosis seen in the setting of an umbilical vein catheter is the result of the joining of portal and umbilical vein flow into the ductus venosus.

The second unique aspect of liver developmental physiology is the formation of bile ducts, canaliculi and bile itself without directly mixing with the circulation. Hepatocytes surrounding the portal vein begin to transform into ductular structures early in the sixth week of gestation (Moore, 1982). A ductal plate eventually forms from this first row and also from additional rows of hepa-

tocytes surrounding the portal vein. This process continues along branches of the portal vein until tubules and finally bile ducts are formed (Ruebner, 1990). Ductular epithelial cells are eventually distinguishable from hepatocytes by their cytokeratin content (Stosiek *et al.*, 1990). Eventually the ductular plates that are not connected to tubules are resorbed. By 40 weeks' gestation, a network of ductular plate tubules surrounds portal veins which connect to bile canaliculi and extrahepatic bile ducts (Van Eyken *et al.*, 1988). It is generally accepted that the ductal plate is the culprit in a number of intra- and extrahepatic newborn bile duct pathologies, including Caroli's disease, congenital hepatic fibrosis, biliary atresia and Alagille's syndrome (Desmet, 1991). Hepatocyte bile acid synthesis and ductular secretion of bile progressively increase in the postnatal period and through the first year of life (Heubi *et al.*, 1982).

Microcirculation

Microscopic anatomy is an important prelude to understanding the physiological response of the liver during normal metabolic events and episodes of stress. Classic microcirculatory anatomy has been described by Rappaport. He defines the acinus as the smallest functional unit of the liver (Rappaport *et al.* 1954; Rappaport, 1958) (Figure 2.2). The intrahepatic bile ductule, portal venule and hepatic arteriole parallel each other to form a triad at the periphery of each hepatic acinus. Sheets of sinusoids are exposed to blood from the portal venule within the triad, and ultimately blood leaves the acinus through the central (portal) or terminal hepatic venule. Union of the terminal hepatic venule and the portal venule occurs in the sinusoid. Shortly after birth and probably in response to the change in composition of blood flow, zonal distribution of metabolic processes begins within the liver acinus. Three zones define the space between the portal triad and the central or terminal hepatic venule. Unidirectional flow from the terminal portal venule to zone 1 exposes hepatocytes in this area to the highest portal pressure and oxygen tension, whereas zone 3 (pericentral sinusoids) is exposed to the lowest oxygen concentration. Hepatocytes surrounding zone 1 have the advantage with regard to nutrients and oxygen, and thus are most resistant to hypoxia and usually the first to regenerate (Gebhardt, 1992). Enzyme systems for all metabolic pathways are distributed within these zones. However, utilization is not uniform, but rather is a function of oxygen requirements, substrate gradients, blood flow and hormonal influences. This is termed functional or metabolic heterogeneity of the acinus (Gumucio, 1989; see Table 2.1).

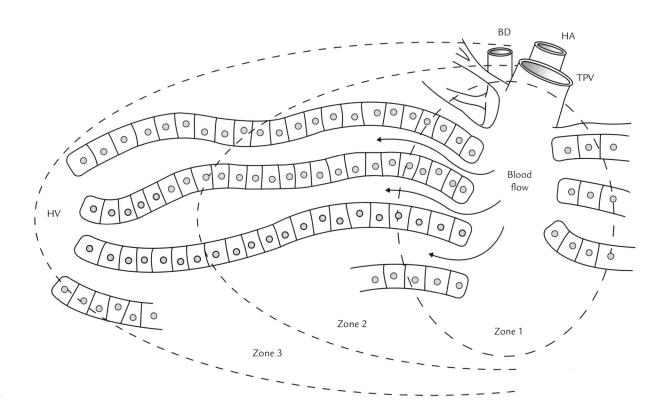

Figure 2.2 *Microcirculation. The classic functional unit of the liver is the acinus. Described by Rappaport, the acinus is bordered by the triad of terminal portal venule (TPV), bile ductule (BD) and hepatic arteriole (HA). Flow is unidirectional within the acinus from the triad to the hepatic venule (or central vein; HV) and ultimately hepatic veins. Three zones of metabolic function characterize the acinus. Zone 1 hepatocytes are exposed to the highest portal pressure and oxygen tension, and zone 3 to lowest oxygen tension (Gumucio, 1989).*

Table 2.1 *Functional zonation in the liver*

Periportal zone	Pericentral zone
Gluconeogenesis	Glycolysis
Glycogenesis	Lipogenesis
β-Oxidation of fatty acids	Ketogenesis
Cholesterol synthesis	Glutamine metabolism
Bile acid synthesis	Biotransformation
Ureagenesis	
Biotransformation	

Additional essential roles played by the liver include hepatic biotransformation, and heme, porphyrin and metal metabolism. These processes are heterogeneously distributed throughout the liver, and this accounts for selective zonal disruption during a toxic episode.

In general, the hepatic sinusoid is 7–15 μm in diameter and capable of increasing in size to 150–180 μm during stress (Paidas *et al.*, 1995). Pressure within the sinusoid is 2–3 mmHg. Hepatocytes vary between 10 and 30 μm in diameter. Their microvillar surface lines the perisinusoidal space. A portion of the plasma membrane is also dedicated to the bile canaliculus, which is separated from the perisinusoidal space by desmosomes and tight junctions.

Blood flow

The liver has a dual blood supply, with 75–80% of its blood flow coming from the portal vein and the remaining flow being contributed by the hepatic artery. A balance exists between these two systems such that total hepatic blood flow (100–130 mL/kg/minute) remains relatively constant, with the liver contributing 10–15% of total blood volume and accounting for 20–25% of total oxygen consumption. Moreover, in contrast to virtually every other organ in the body, metabolic demands not intra-organ oxygen requirements regulate hepatic blood flow (Granger *et al.*, 1975). Hepatic arterial resistance, portal venule resistance and total portal vein blood flow all contribute to overall liver blood flow. Even a transplanted liver has an analogous contribution to blood flow and similar autoregulation (Stieber *et al.*, 1991; Stevens *et al.*, 1992).

The volume of portal blood delivered to the liver is a function of the splanchnic (stomach, intestine, pancreas, spleen) circulation, hormones and bile salt pool. Although 75% of total liver blood flow is derived from the portal circulation, oxygen tension and portal pressure (7–10 mmHg) are both low. In an effort to accommodate the volume of blood that is delivered via the portal vein in the presence of such a low perfusion pressure, resistance within this circulation (i.e. resistance across the IVC and hepatic sinusoids) is very low.

In contrast to the portal oxygen tension and pressure, hepatic artery oxygen is equivalent to peripheral arterial oxygen partial pressure and systemic arterial blood pressure. Union of both of these circulations within the portal venule and the sinusoids and unidirectional flow sets up the oxygen gradient (50 μmol/L) from zones 1 to 3 within the hepatic lobule (Figure 2.2). Moreover, this gradient gives rise to centrilobular hypoxia such that during low-flow states (i.e. hypovolemic or hemorrhagic shock), the centrilobular area is affected first by ischemia (Gumucio, 1989). Oxidative enzymes within this centrilobular zone are also affected, and in addition to the low blood flow and oxygen tension, give rise to the hallmark of low-flow ischemia–centrilobular necrosis (Arcieli *et al.*, 1981; see Figure 2.2). This is extremely important for the newborn, in whom changes in oxygen tension can have dramatic effects on brain white matter and the cortex of the kidney. A classic example of centrilobular necrosis is the liver dysfunction produced by congestive heart failure. High right-sided venous pressure causes upstream elevation in hepatic venous pressure and sinusoidal edema. This leads to decreased hepatic arterial blood flow and oxygen delivery, as well as decreased arterial oxygen saturation, progressing to hypoxia and subsequent centrilobular necrosis (Paidas *et al.* 1995).

Ischemic hepatitis rather than overt centrilobular necrosis is a common accompaniment of congestive heart failure, hypovolemic and hemorrhagic shock, prolonged seizures, asphyxia and bypass (Paidas *et al.*, 1995). Transaminase activity increases by 48 hours after the insult, and alkaline phosphatase activity is usually normal. In response to elevated right-sided heart pressure, hepatomegaly, jaundice and coagulopathy can be seen (Garland *et al.*, 1988). Elevated creatine phosphokinase levels are indicative of global cardiac ischemia, and more often than not elevated serum creatinine levels highlight the associated renal hypoperfusion. Liver biopsy confirms the centrilobular necrosis and is temporally related to a decrease in transaminase levels towards normal values, simultaneous plateauing of bilirubin, and stabilization of coagulopathy (Mace *et al.*, 1985).

Although there is a well-described increase in hepatic arterial flow in response to reductions in portal flow, the opposite does not occur. This is because the changes in hepatic arterial flow have little effect on portal flow. Rather, any portocaval shunt or ligation of the mesenteric artery is followed by increased hepatic arterial blood flow, not increased portal vein blood flow (Legare and Lautt, 1987). Similarly, autoregulation controls hepatic arterial flow, not portal flow. In the newborn, hepatic arterial blood flow, as in the brain and kidney cortex, is preserved during systemic hypotension or reduced portal flow. It is only when hypotension becomes severe that both total liver blood flow and oxygen delivery are compromised. During this state of severe systemic hypotension, hepatic arterial blood flow is increased as a compensatory response despite any reduction in portal blood flow. This is called the hepatic artery buffer response (Lautt, 1983). Metabolic needs do not appear to affect this response, but rather it is portal flow that alters hepatic arterial resistance. Portal flow regulates hepatic artery flow via adenosine, which is released from hepatocytes and is a potent vasodilator. Adenosine accumulates near the hepatic arteriole resistance vessels, resulting in hepatic arteriolar vasodilatation and increased hepatic arteriolar flow (Lautt and Greenway, 1987). It is currently not known whether any other vasodilators, such as inducible nitric oxide synthase (iNOS), participate in the hepatic buffer response. Extrinsic humoral regulators such as gastrin, glucagon secretion and bile salts and α-adrenergic-receptor stimulation can control hepatic arterial blood flow (Richardson and Withrington, 1981).

Pathophysiological flow secondary to several types of obstruction involving the liver (intrahepatic vs. extrahepatic) have important clinical correlations both in the newborn and in the older child (Bernstein and Brown, 1962). Primary hepatocyte failure is a classic example of the consequences of altered acinar flow. Also known as hepatocellular failure, this process is characterized by jaundice, steatorrhea, encephalopathy and endocrine disorders. Laboratory alterations include a low serum albumin, low fibrinogen, prolonged coagulation times, anemia, and elevated bilirubin levels (Gottlieb et al., 1986). Frequent infections (derived from bacteria in the gastrointestinal tract) are the result of an inadequate reticuloendothelial system. Obstruction within the parenchyma is typically a post-sinusoidal blockade by fibrosis (Kirn et al., 1983). This means that the portal pressure rises from the normal range of 5–10 mmHg to levels above 18 mmHg. Portal systemic shunts develop as a result of the increased pressure, and this gives rise to the characteristic varices. The sequelae of portal hypertension include the development of ascites, hypersplenism and eventual hyperdynamic cardiac output state. The ascites results from the very low colloidal pressure and sodium retention. The sudden appearance of ascites, abdominal pain and hepatomegaly is associated with Budd–Chiari syndrome (Ludwig et al., 1990). This syndrome is caused by hepatic vein obstruction (Campbell and Punch, 1998). Veno-occlusive disease is classically described as narrowing of terminal hepatic venules in the absence of abnormal hepatic veins or inferior vena cava. The commonest presentation is that following bone-marrow transplantation (McDonald et al., 1984).

Innervation

The innervation of the liver consists of sympathetic fibers from T7-T10, vagus and phrenic nerves (Lautt, 1980). Sympathetic α-adrenergic stimulation causes both hepatic artery and portal vein constriction, whereas parasympathetic stimulation seems to have no effect on overall liver blood flow. Each of these nerves makes a contribution to hepatic artery, portal vein and bile duct within the liver. Denervation of liver following a transplantation harvest has no effect on intrinsic hepatic autoregulation (Ryckman et al., 1994).

Bile duct physiology

Bile ducts are derived from hepatocytes, and their canaliculi drain from intrahepatic ducts, lobar ducts and ultimately to the common hepatic duct. A separate capillary network surrounds the biliary system, which also terminates in the sinusoid. This capillary network is important for both secretion and absorption of bile (Yamamoto et al., 1985). Bile serves to eliminate bilirubin and cholesterol, and it also facilitates the absorption of both lipids and fat-soluble vitamins from the terminal ileum. Secretion of bile is energy and oxygen dependent, yet except under conditions of profound reduction of blood flow (i.e. shock) it is independent of liver blood flow (Nolan, 1981). Secretion occurs both from the canaliculus and directly from the ducts. In general, nearly 80% of bile is produced directly from the hepatocyte and the remainder is secreted from the ducts. The composition of bile is shown in Box 2.1. Bile has a water content of 80–85%. Sodium is the most important cation, and the electrolyte composition resembles that of lactated Ringer's solution at all ages. Therefore the replacement fluid of choice for bile is lactated Ringer's solution. Vagal stimulation increases bile output, whereas sympathetic stimulation decreases flow of both blood and bile. The most important regulatory component of bile flow is its linear relationship to bile acid synthesis by the hepatocyte. This production is in turn regulated by the return of bile salts to the liver through the enterohepatic circulation.

Box 2.1   *Characteristics of bile*

Bile flow 0.41–0.43 mL/minute in 70-kg man
Osmolality = 300 mOsm

Inorganic ions (meq/L)

Na$^+$	(140–165)	HCO$_3^-$	(15–55)
K$^+$	(3.8–5.8)	Ca^{2+}	(1.4–5.0)
Cl$^-$	(93–123)	Mg^{2+}	(1.5–3.0)

Organic solutes

Bile acids	Proteins
Cholesterol	IgA
Phospholipids	Bilirubin

Secretin – under chloride-channel regulation – is the major hormone responsible for very proximal (cholangiocyte) bile epithelial cell secretion, but others include epidermal growth factor and somatostatin (Nathanson and Boyer, 1991). Cholecystokinin, gastrin and glucagon increase bile flow at a site that is usually distal to the hepatocyte. The salts of the bile acids secreted into the intestine are reabsorbed into the enterohepatic circulation. Liver extracts the acids, transports them through the canalicular membrane and resecretes them back into bile. The canalicular membrane is the rate-limiting step for transport of bile acids (Meier, 1989). In addition, the membrane contains transporters for other components of bile and amino acids (Graf, 1983). The liver is quite efficient at this process, as evidenced by the very low serum levels of bile acids ($< 5\ \mu\text{mol/L}$).

Bile acids are synthesized from cholesterol in the liver, and they include cholic and chenodeoxycholic acids. Additional bile acids are synthesized from the intestine by bacterial dehydroxylation, including deoxycholic and lithocholic acids. All of these acids are conjugated to either of the amino acids taurine and glycine, facilitating ionization of the bile acids to deoxycholate and lithocholate and thus preventing their intestinal absorption. The conjugation of the bile acid facilitates solubilization of lipids by forming micelles and thereby enhancing their absorption. In children with ileal resection, short gut syndrome or motility disorders of the small intestine, bile acid absorption is reduced, resulting in significant diarrhea, steatorrhea and vitamin B_{12} deficiency. The resultant decrease in the bile acid pool is a hallmark of stone formation. Interestingly, babies whose mothers are treated with antenatal steroids to promote lung maturation show an increase in bile acids (Watkins et al., 1975).

Bilirubin, primarily derived from the breakdown of red blood cells, is bound to albumin in serum (not to be confused with conjugation). In the liver, bilirubin is released from albumin, detoxified first by a carrier-mediated transport system and then bound to X and Y transport systems. Within the hepatocyte, bilirubin is conjugated with glucuronic acid by glucuronyl tranferase and secreted into bile. Unconjugated hyperbilirubinemia includes neonatal disorders associated with sepsis (Zimmerman et al., 1979) and prematurity such as Crigler-Najjar syndrome and Gilbert's syndrome. Dubin-Johnson syndrome, rotor syndrome and prolonged parenteral nutrition are examples of conjugated hyperbilirubinemia. The latter can be caused by prolonged fasting, malnutrition, ischemia and reperfusion, as well as by positive pressure mechanical ventilation.

In the intestine, bilirubin is reduced by bacterial glucuronidase to urobilinogen, which is excreted in the stool. Urobilin is the oxidation product of bilirubin that gives stool its brown color. Urobilinogen is also absorbed in the intestinal tract, re-excreted into bile, and some is absorbed by the kidney and secreted in the urine. During states of stasis or biliary obstruction, urobilinogen cannot form and thus does not appear in the urine.

HEPATIC ULTRASTRUCTURE (FIGURE 2.3)

The liver represents 2–5% of total body weight and is composed of five different types of cells, namely

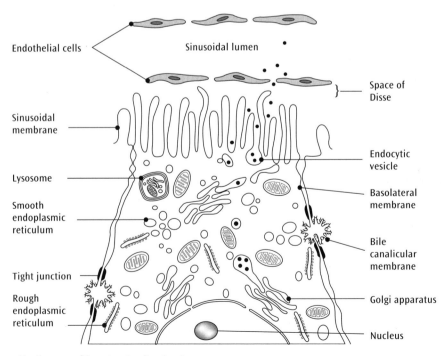

Figure 2.3 *Schematic diagram of hepatocyte ultrastructure.*

hepatocytes, Kupffer cells, stellate (Ito) cells, endothelial cells and biliary ductule epithelium (Box 2.2). Sinusoidal cells, Kupffer cells and biliary ductule epithelial cells each represent 10–15% of the total number of liver cells, leaving approximately 60% of the cellular mass as hepatocytes. The sinusoid is lined by endothelial cells and Kupffer cells.

Kupffer cells clear the bloodstream of old or damaged red blood cells, fibrin degradation products, cellular debris and endotoxins. Moreover, leukotrienes (Keppler et al., 1988), oxygen free radicals, interleukins and tumor necrosis factor can be produced and regulated by Kupffer cells (Paidas et al., 1995). Bacteria can be ingested by these cells via phagocytosis. They line the sinusoid and contain multiple enzymes that facilitate neutralization of foreign matter.

Endothelial cells are in direct contact with sinusoidal blood flow, but are also fenestrated and as such prevent the passage of particles above a certain size from passing into the space of Disse (Wisse et al., 1985; see below). Although difficult to distinguish from Kupffer cells, the fenestrations of endothelial cells make them identifiable and facilitate the protrusion of hepatocytes and microvilli, thus maximizing their surface area within the sinusoid. The handling of lipoproteins, vitamin A and endotoxins as well as cell-to-cell communication are all endothelial cell functions.

The stellate (Ito) cells are behind the sinusoids and have long finger-like projections that surround the hepatocytes. These cells store vitamin A, participate in connective tissue (collagen) synthesis and also secrete several growth factors in response to their interaction with both Kupffer and endothelial cells (Gressner, 1995; Michalopoulos and DeFrances, 1997). Because these cells have long projections surrounding the hepatocytes, it is speculated that they may have a regulatory role. However, to date this hypothesis has not been proven (Knook et al., 1982).

The space of Disse lies between the endothelial cell and the hepatocyte. It is that area between the endothelial cells and hepatocytes where the stellate cells, neurons, fibroblasts and abundant lymphatics are located. This space receives all of the large protein molecules that pass through the large pores of the endothelial cells. There are also lymphatic vessels that follow the terminal branching of the portal venule and communicate with the space of Disse. Lymphatic anatomy parallels portal and hepatic vein anatomy, forming in the perisinusoidal space of Disse and then draining into the cisterna chyli and ultimately into the thoracic duct. Direct lymphatic channels pass from the liver through the diaphragm and then to the thoracic duct. Cirrhosis, portal vein thrombosis, veno-occlusive disease, alterations in glycogen metabolism that act to plug the liver, and uncontrolled lipogenesis can all change the lymphatic pressure, resulting in ascites.

Each hepatocyte plasma membrane consists of a lipid bilayer in which a hydrophilic segment is oriented towards the sinusoid and a hydrophobic fatty acid tail is situated interiorly. Glycoproteins are interspersed within the membrane and they serve as tight junctions, receptors or carrier proteins. One important function of the plasma membrane is a process called endocytosis (Figure 2.3). This energy-requiring event involves the uptake of water or solute into the hepatocyte (pinocytosis), ingestion of larger molecules (parasites) by a process of phagocytosis, and receptor-mediated uptake of extracellular molecules. Because of the many functions of the hepatocyte, there is a definite polarity to the liver cells that corresponds to plasma membrane-dependent function. For example, the sinusoidal region of the membrane has a vast surface area studded with microvilli to enhance bidirectional active transport of water, proteins and carbon-containing (organic) and non-carbon-containing (inorganic) solutes. The basolateral area of the hepatocyte contains structural proteins that allow for attachment and cell–cell communication. Tight junctions are characteristic of this region. Finally, the canalicular region for processing of bile is situated away from

---

Box 2.2 *The cells of the liver and their functions*

Hepatocytes
  Ureagenesis
  Gluconeogenesis
  Protein synthesis
  Lipid metabolism
  Detoxification
  Bile formation
  Metabolism of prostaglandins and leukotrienes

Kupffer cells
  Modulation of protein synthesis of acute phase proteins
    and lipoproteins
  Phagocytosis of particles (viruses, bacteria, enzymes)
  Endotoxin clearance
  Cytokin secretion
  Antigen processing
  Catabolism of lipids and glycoproteins

Endothelial cells
  In direct contact with the sinusoidal circulation
  Macromolecule clearance
  Storage of vitamin A
  Metabolism of lipoproteins

Stellate cells
  Fat storage
  Vitamin A storage
  Collagen synthesis in normal and fibrotic liver

Biliary ductule epithelium
  Secretion of bile
  Absorption of water, bile

the region of blood flow and highlighted by microfilaments responsible for the formation of bile. Each region of the plasma membrane is characterized by certain membrane proteins. For example, alkaline phosphatase is located in the canalicular region, glucagon-stimulated adenylate cyclase is located in the sinusoidal domain and 5'-nucleotidase is located throughout the plasma membrane (Inoue *et al.*, 1983; Matsuura *et al.*, 1984; Meier *et al.*, 1984).

One important aspect of hepatocytes that matures following birth involves the reactions of cell-surface receptors by what was referred to earlier as receptor-mediated endocytosis. This process involves a ligand (e.g. insulin, insulin-like growth factor, growth hormone, lipoprotein or epidermal growth factor) and a hepatocyte receptor (corresponding to the ligand), typically on the sinusoidal aspect of the cell. A variety of intracellular second messengers (i.e. cyclic adenosine monophosphate or kinases) then activate additional pathways targeting destinations that function as trophic responses, facilitate the metabolism of fat and regulate gut immune function. Dissociation of the ligand–receptor complex involves endosomes, which facilitate recycling of the receptor.

Lysosomes are organelles that contain enzymes capable of incorporating and degrading intracellular protein. An example of this in the biliary system is the asialoglycoprotein that is secreted into bile. The microsomal fraction of the liver consists of the rough and smooth endoplasmic reticulum and the Golgi complex. The nucleus is the largest of the hepatocyte organelles. Mitochondria within the nucleus contain the enzymes for electron transport and synthesis of ATP in their inner membrane. As expected, liver mitochondria have substantial oxygen requirements and heavily populate zone 1 (Figure 2.2 and Table 2.1), due to its high oxygen tension.

The genes that encode all proteins are contained in every cell of the body. However, gene transcription dictates which proteins are synthesized by what cells. Thus hepatic protein synthesis is 'liver-specific.' Protein synthesis takes place in the ribosomes, which are located within the cytoplasm. The rough endoplasmic reticulum is responsible for synthesis and the smooth endoplasmic reticulum is responsible for intracellular transport. At any age, albumin is the most abundant protein synthesized by the liver. It has a half-life of approximately 22 days (Tavill *et al.*, 1968). Albumin binds to bilirubin, thyroid hormone, cortisol, testosterone, metals and a multitude of drugs, facilitating their transport through the circulation. Other transport proteins that are synthesized by the liver include transferrin, fibrinogen, prothrombin, haptoglobin, ferritin and ceruloplasmin. The microsomes are important for synthesis and transport of protein outside the cell (e.g. albumin, fibrinogen, cholesterol, bile salts), glucuronidation of drugs and steroids, esterification of fats and breakdown of glycogen.

METABOLISM

The liver plays a pivotal role in the metabolism and storage of ingested protein, lipid and carbohydrates for use both by the liver and by extrahepatic tissues. In addition, the liver receives metabolites from other tissues, mainly for the purpose of generating energy. These extrahepatically derived substrates include glycerol and fatty acids from fat, lactate and pyruvate from skeletal muscle, and red blood cells and alanine and other α-keto acids, also from skeletal muscle. Consistent with the liver's role in the traffic of metabolites and provision of energy, hepatocytes make two vital oxidative substrates for transport to extrahepatic tissues. These substrates are glucose formed via glycogenolysis and gluconeogenesis, and acetoacetate formed by the oxidation of adipose tissue-derived fatty acids. These pathways are oxygen dependent. In contrast, the liver (as well as any individual cell) is capable of generating energy in the form of ATP under anaerobic or hypoxic conditions through the Embden–Meyerhof pathway of glycolysis (Pilkis, 1991).

INTERMEDIARY METABOLISM (BOX 2.3)

Carbohydrates

The liver performs transcriptionally regulated specific carbohydrate functions consisting of the storage and breakdown of glycogen, gluconeogenesis (with a small contribution from the kidney), and conversion of other sugars (galactose and fructose) to glucose.

One of the central roles of the liver is that of maintaining blood glucose levels. *In utero*, alternative fuels in

---

Box 2.3 *Intermediary metabolism of the liver*

Carbohydrate
  Glycogenesis
  Gluconeogenesis*
  Conversion of galactose and fructose to glucose

Fat
  β-Oxidation of fatty acids*
  Cholesterol synthesis
  Lipoprotein and phospholipid synthesis
  Ketone body formation (acetoacetate and
    β-hydroxybutyrate)
  Conversion of carbohydrate and protein into fat

Protein
  Deamination of amino acids
  Ureagenesis
  Synthesis of acute phase proteins

* Not unique to the liver.

the form of amino acids and lactate are utilized and enzymes that phosphorylate glucose, such as glucokinase, are not transcribed. The glucose that is utilized in the fetus is phosphorylated by hexokinase to glucose-6-phosphate (Faulkner and Jones, 1976). The last step in hepatic glucose formation is catalyzed by the enzyme glucose-6-phosphatase, which is absent from fetal liver. Thus fetal liver directs gluconeogenic precursors into the hexose monophosphate or pentose shunt pathways for synthesis of nucleotides (purines) and nucleic acids, as well as glycogen formation (Jones, 1981). Postnatally, glucokinase mRNA levels increase, resulting in further production of glucose-6-phosphate and subsequent glycolytic flux to increase the production of glucose by the liver for energy (Walker, 1963). Enhanced gluconeogenesis and increased glucose production are observed in neonates whose birth weights are less than 1200 g (Keshen et al., 1997). Glucose is the sole energy source for red blood cells, because they lack mitochondria. In addition, it is the preferred energy source for the renal medulla, tissue macrophages and cerebral cortex (Lehninger et al., 1993).

With regard to carbohydrate metabolism, the liver's role is highlighted by two major pathways, namely glycogen metabolism and the formation of glucose via gluconeogenesis. During stress (e.g. systemic inflammatory response syndrome, injury), liver glycogen is depleted rapidly, so that glucose levels have to be maintained by gluconeogenesis (Parillo et al., 1990).

The major stimulus for glycogen formation is the plasma glucose concentration. High glucose levels induce glycogen synthetase and therefore glycogen synthesis, while simultaneously inhibiting any breakdown of glycogen (Figure 2.4). Insulin induced by the high plasma glucose levels also favors this reaction, as do corticosteroids. Furthermore, high glucose levels cause glucagon levels to decline and a simultaneous increase in glucokinase activity. Since this enzyme is specific to the liver, glucokinase activity plays a key role in phosphorylating glucose and glucogenic amino acids. Hepatic glycogen stores at birth are large enough to maintain blood glucose levels for 10–12 hours as glycogen is broken down (glycogenolysis). Infants with intrauterine growth retardation have a much lower capacity for glycogen storage, and consequently cannot avoid problems of hypoglycemia during the postnatal period (Lubchenco and Bard, 1971). Glucagon is a major stimulus to glycogenolysis through its second messenger, namely cyclic AMP. In addition, vasopressin, angiotensin, oxytocin and α-adrenergic stimulation activate glycogenolysis through a different second messenger system (Exton, 1987). Glycogenolysis utilizes a debranching enzyme and phosphorylase to make glucose. It is thought that glycogenolysis occurs in the newborn until gluconeogenic enzymes are transcribed. This process usually occurs during the first 10–12 hours postnatally (Gain et al., 1981). Although the same system is found in muscle, hormonal control and the enzyme glucokinase distinguish the specific role of the liver.

Glucose-6-phosphate (Figure 2.4) is a key intermediate for entry into the hexose monophosphate shunt, glycogen synthesis, gluconeogenesis and glycolysis. Its fate is dependent on substrate requirements. Postnatally, there is a reciprocal relationship in the liver with regard to glycolysis (which is dependent on glucokinase) and gluconeogenesis (which is dependent on phosphoenolpyruvate carboxykinase, PEPCK) which is dependent on the substrate delivered to the liver. A low carbohydrate state stimulates glucagon and PEPCK, thus favoring glucose production. However, a high carbohydrate state favors the stimulation of insulin and induction of glucokinase, resulting in glucose utilization (Perdereau et al., 1990).

The vast majority of gluconeogenic capability occurs in the liver, with a small contribution by the kidney because of ammonia metabolism and acid–base balance. However, only these two organs make glucose (Figure 2.5 below). The most important precursors are pyruvate, lactate and glucogenic amino acids (all but leucine). Even-chain fatty acids and ketone bodies are not themselves gluconeogenic precursors, but rather they supply energy for gluconeogenic precursors and thus activate hepatic gluconeogenesis. Propionyl-CoA, which is formed from the final oxidation and cleavage of odd-chain fatty acids, is a gluconeogenic substrate. The pathway of gluconeogenesis consumes 6 moles of ATP for each mole of glucose synthesized. Gluconeogenesis involves multiple steps in both the mitochondria and cytoplasm, beginning with conversion of pyruvate to oxaloacetate, followed by conversion to phosphoenolpyruvate via PEPCK.

Three reactions distinguish gluconeogenesis from its counterpart reverse reaction for breaking down glucose, which is known as glycolysis. The rate-limiting reaction involves conversion of pyruvate to phosphoenolpyruvate by PEPCK. The postnatal appearance of PEPCK is the result of both a rise in glucagon and a fall in insulin (Lyonnet et al., 1988). This enzyme is transcriptionally regulated and highly dependent on nutritional state (Liu et al., 1991). The environment and physiological status of the patient also influences PEPCK. PEPCK is suppressed in systemic inflammatory response syndrome, sepsis and severe injury and illness (Deutschman et al., 1993). A family of polypeptide proteins called heat shock or stress proteins is expressed in response to such stresses (DeMaio, 1999). Expression of PEPCK is preserved after endotoxin administration in the presence of heat shock proteins. This effect appears to be mediated by a rapid recovery of the enzyme at the level of transcription (Paidas et al., submitted). Ketogenesis is affected by rates of gluconeogenesis because of the supply of oxaloacetate. When gluconeogenesis is accelerated, the mitochondrial oxaloacetate supply is decreased. Thus acetyl-CoA is inhibited from entering the citric acid cycle.

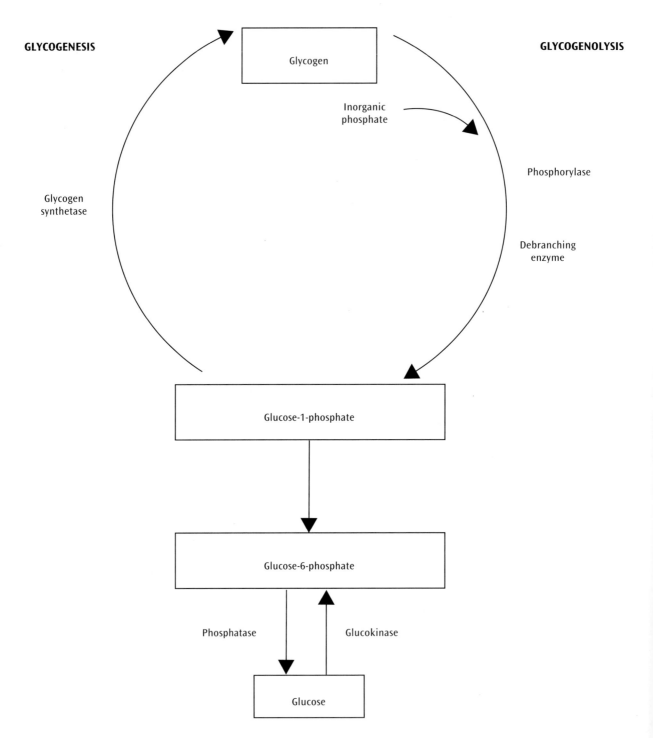

GLYCOGENESIS

GLYCOGENOLYSIS

Glycogen

Inorganic
phosphate

Phosphorylase

Glycogen
synthetase

Debranching
enzyme

Glucose-1-phosphate

Glucose-6-phosphate

Phosphatase

Glucokinase

Glucose

Figure 2.4 *Summary of hepatic glycogenesis and glycogenolysis. Glycogen synthetase, the rate-limiting enzyme for glycogenesis, is stimulated by glucose and insulin and inhibited by cyclic AMP and low glucose levels. Phosphorylase is stimulated by glucagon, epinephrine and cyclic AMP. Glucokinase is liver specific. Glucose-6-phosphate is an intermediate for the hexose shunt, glycolysis, gluconeogenesis and glycogenesis.*

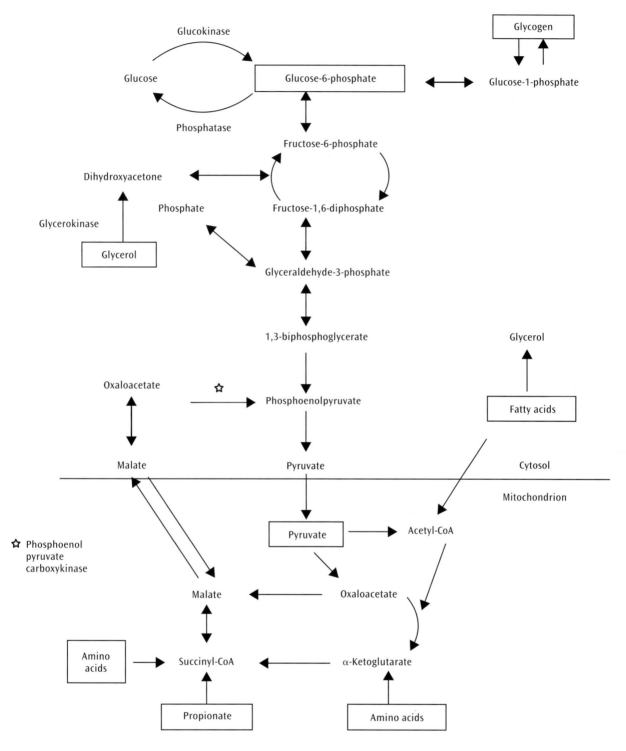

Figure 2.5 *Summary of gluconeogenesis. Gluconeogenic precursors include pyruvate, amino acids, propionate, glycogen, acetyl-CoA from fatty acids and glycerol. Gluconeogenesis is stimulated by glucagon, epinephrine and corticosteroids. Insulin suppresses gluconeogenesis.*

Glucagon, epinephrine and corticosteroids stimulate the regulatory enzymes and insulin suppresses gluconeogenesis (Kraus-Friedmann, 1984).

Two additional unique features of the liver involve the metabolism of galactose and fructose. Galactose is made from lactose (which is composed of glucose and galactose), and is used for the biosynthesis of glycoproteins and lipids. The fate of galactose includes formation of glycogen or glucose-6-phosphate for ultimate oxidation (Leloir, 1951; Gitzelmann and Hansen, 1980). Fructose is metabolized slightly by adipose tissue, but breakdown in the liver requires a specific enzyme, namely ketohexokinase. The fate of fructose is either conversion to pyruvate and acetyl-CoA for fatty acid synthesis, or glycogen formation, depending on the hormonal milieu and nutritional status (Van Schaftingen et al., 1980).

Fats

Hepatocytes have the capacity for β-oxidation of fatty acids, ketone body formation, conversion of both sugars and protein into fat, lipoprotein synthesis and cholesterol biosynthesis. Triacylglycerol, which represents nearly half of the total fatty acids in the blood, is broken down into fatty acids and glycerol. Oxidation of fatty acids can occur in liver, heart, muscle, lung, testis, brain and adipose tissue. Glycerol utilization requires glycerokinase, an enzyme that is only found in liver, kidney, intestine, adipose and breast tissue (Wakil et al., 1983). The liver generates most of its energy for intrahepatic processes from the oxidation of fatty acids.

Glucose and maternal ketones are precursors for fatty acid synthesis in utero which are stored as triacylglycerol (Seccombe et al., 1977). Storage of fat is short-lived because after birth the triacylglycerol is utilized, yielding both ATP and ketone bodies. Fats are broken down into glycerol and fatty acids. The glycerol can be used to synthesize glucose in the pathway of gluconeogenesis (Figure 2.5). However, each fatty acid is irreversibly broken down to acetyl-CoA to be used in the Kreb's cycle or for formation of ketone bodies (acetoacetate, acetone and β-hydroxybutyrate) (Figure 2.6). Ketones are a second major fuel source manufactured by the liver. Prolonged fasting in older children and stressed newborns has the capacity to generate ketones (in mitochondria and peroxisomes) from the breakdown of fatty acids derived from lipopolysis (Ozawa et al., 1983). The commonest ketone body is acetoacetate, which is used as a secondary fuel for brain tissue, muscle and renal cortex. In response to exogenous substrate, the liver has the capacity to store substrate both locally (in the form of glycogen) and at distant sites (as fatty acids, glycerol and lipoproteins). Alternatively, the acetoacetate can be transported to other tissues and reconverted into acetyl-CoA and oxidized in other tissues, or it can be broken down into acetone and CO_2 or reduced using NADH to form β-hydroxybutyrate. Collectively, it is the liver that is the sole source of these three ketone bodies which are then used by extrahepatic tissues (brain, muscle and renal cortex). Since acetoacetate and β-hydroxybutyrate are in equilibrium with the NAD/NADH ratio within the liver, where they are both formed, they have been used to measure redox potential and thus indicators of hepatic ischemia (Yamamoto et al., 1979; Paidas et al., 1995). During hypoxia there is a shortage of electron transport acceptors at the very end of the chain, and therefore NADH builds up and NAD is depleted, thus lowering the redox state of the hepatocyte.

Cholesterol synthesized in the liver is used for bile salt and lipoprotein synthesis. Cholesterol can also be synthesized by the adrenal cortex, aorta, skin, intestine and testis, but it is predominantly the liver that controls the turnover and transport of cholesterol. Acetyl-CoA is the source of all carbon atoms for cholesterol synthesis. Insulin and thyroid hormone both stimulate synthesis of cholesterol, whereas corticosteroids and glucagon inhibit cholesterol synthesis (Dempsey, 1974). Very-low-density lipoproteins manufactured by the liver transport cholesterol from the liver and diet for extrahepatic tissue utilization. Cholesterol is eliminated by conversion to bile acids (enterohepatic circulation) and/or by excretion as sterols in the feces. Phospholipids, which are also uniquely specific to the liver, are transported by lipoproteins into the circulation.

Protein metabolism

Transamination, oxidative deamination, formation of urea and synthesis of proteins and amino acids are all features of protein metabolism which for the most part are unique to the liver. A small amount (relative to the role of the liver) of transamination and deamination occurs in the kidney. In a similar manner to the zonation of glycolysis and gluconeogenesis, there exists a metabolic zonation of enzymes for amino acid and nucleic acid metabolism. One important example is glutamine synthetase. Located in the pericentral region of the acinus, this enzyme catalyzes the reaction of glutamate with ammonia to form glutamine (Figure 2.7). In extrahepatic tissues, this is the pathway by which ammonia is eliminated.

In the liver, catabolism of protein first involves removal of the amino group by transamination to an α-keto acid to form glutamate, alanine or aspartate (Figure 2.7). These amino acids can transfer their amino groups as ammonia into the urea cycle within the liver. The ammonia enters the urea cycle, and glutamic acid, under the action of a synthetase and in the presence of blood ammonia, forms glutamine. Thus this interconversion enables free ammonia to be scavenged for use in the urea cycle.

Urea is made from 1 mole of ammonia, 1 mole of carbon dioxide and 1 mole of the amino group of aspartate (Figure 2.8). Five enzymes are included in the cycle, with the first two steps performed only within the liver. These

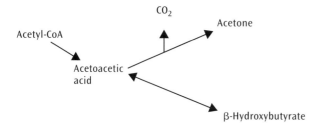

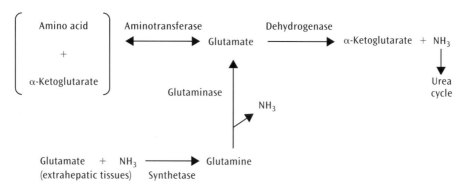

Figure 2.6 *Ketone body formation. The oxidation of fatty acids results in the production of acetyl-CoA. If oxaloacetate is available, then acetyl-CoA enters the citric acid cycle. If the oxaloacetate supply is low (e.g. due to starvation, diabetes or sepsis), two molecules of acetyl-CoA condense to form acetoacetate. Acetoacetate can reversibly form β-hydroxybutyrate or be decarboxylated to form acetone. Both acetoacetic acid and β-hydroxybutyrate account for the ketoacidosis associated with diabetes and severe starvation.*

Figure 2.7 *Transamination and disposal of ammonia. Amino groups derived from amino acids are transferred to glutamate within the hepatocyte cytosol. Glutamate is then transferred into the mitochondria, where it undergoes deamination to form α-ketoglutarate (available for the citric acid cycle) and ammonia (available for the urea cycle). Extrahepatic ammonia combines with glutamate to form glutamine, which readily enters hepatocyte mitochondria, where the amino group is removed for entry into the urea cycle.*

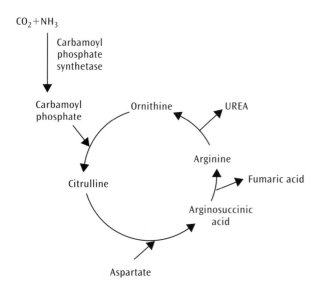

Figure 2.8 *Summary of urea synthesis. Ammonia (NH₃) is derived from amino acids, nucleic acids, extrahepatic conversion of glutamine to glutamate, and intestinal bacterial degradation of urea. Periportal hepatic enzymes for urea synthesis are the largest producers of urea. The molecules of ammonia that contribute to urea are derived from blood ammonia and aspartate. Regulation of the urea cycle is a function of the amount of ammonia produced. The rate-limiting enzyme is carbamoyl phosphate synthetase.*

first two enzymes are carbamyl phosphate and ornithine transcarbamylase, respectively. Regulation of the urea cycle is coordinated through the amount of ammonia delivered to the liver. This is a function of dietary protein intake, starvation (increased protein degradation), sepsis and severe injury. The rate-limiting enzyme is the carbamylphosphate synthetase.

Glutamate can also transfer its amino group to pyruvate, forming alanine and regenerating α-ketoglutarate. The α-ketoglutarate is preserved for subsequent transamination, and the alanine is taken up by the liver, where the amino group of alanine is transferred back to α-ketoglutarate again, forming glutamate and pyruvate. Ultimately, the ammonia from glutamate is transferred into the urea cycle and pyruvate can enter the gluconeogenic pathway. Pyruvate, a glucogenic precursor, is converted to glucose, leaves the liver, and enters muscle as a substrate for glycolysis, thus completing the glucose–alanine cycle (Snell, 1980; Figure 2.9).

Although all tissues can use glutamine formation as the principal pathway for removal of ammonia, the liver uses the urea cycle for ammonia removal. Urea is released into the bloodstream and excreted by the kidney. Other sources of ammonia include deamination of amino acids and nucleic acids, and bacterial degradation of urea in the intestinal tract.

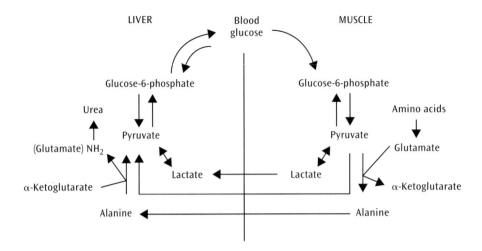

Figure 2.9 *Interconversion of lactate, pyruvate, alanine and glucose: the glucose–alanine and lactic acid (Cori) cycle. Muscle-derived lactate can be converted to pyruvate and transaminated to alanine using an amino group from glutamate. Muscle-derived lactate or alanine can enter the liver and be converted to glucose via glucose-6-phosphate. The ammonia produced from deamination of alanine in the liver enters the urea cycle. These two cycles combine to cycle glucose from liver to muscle and alanine from muscle to liver. The net effect is also a transfer of nitrogen to the liver and energy from liver to muscle.*

ENERGY AND METABOLIC REGULATION

The liver generates energy in the form of ATP for transport, synthesis and biotransformation. It also responds to hormonal and substrate influences to meet the needs of many tissues, such as generating acetoacetate and glucose by gluconeogenesis and glycogenolysis. Interestingly, most if not all of the energy and substrate intermediates are not utilized by the liver, but rather are destined for use by extrahepatic tissues. Thus although other tissues may utilize pathways in common with the liver (Box 2.3 above), the latter appears to be the conductor during normal life and at times of stress.

The generation of high-energy phosphates in the form of ATP and the priority that each cell must give to this event are vital to cellular metabolism and should not be taken for granted in the newborn, growing child or adolescent. Even in the octagenarian, ATP consumption exceeds ATP stores (Hirai *et al.*, 1984). Thus for intermediary metabolism, ion transport, cell-surface endocytosis and cell–cell communication, energy provision in the form of these high-energy phosphates is paramount. Generation of ATP is an oxygen-dependent (aerobic) process that occurs in the mitochondria through a series of steps that all culminate in the process of oxidative phosphorylation. Regardless of the substrate (i.e. glycogen, glycerol or fatty acid) or the condition that yields an excess of substrate (i.e. lactic acid during ischemia or hypoperfusion), the steps are the same and they include entry into the citric acid cycle, followed by generation of reducing equivalents of pyridine nucleotides (NADH and NADPH) and finally electron transport and oxidative phosphorylation.

Substrate flux though any metabolic pathway is affected by the concentration of the substrate and by both hormone and allosteric regulation, all of which occur within seconds to minutes. Enzyme levels, by virtue of the need for transcriptional and translational events, take hours to affect substrate flux. Substrate level regulation occurs by the substrate/product ratio or mass action. Allosteric regulation is dependent on another signal related to the given pathway. Metabolic regulation can be regarded as having both an acute and a more chronic capacity for adaptation or change. The simplest examples of unstressed regulation are the events that occur secondary to nutritional intake. Regardless of any stress that is imposed on a child, storage and mobilization of energy are dependent on the fed and fasted state.

THE FED STATE (BOX 2.4; CLEMENS AND PAIDAS, 1997)

After a meal, the tendency to store free glucose, amino acids and lipids (as glycerol and triacylglycerol) is high. The hormonal milieu in the fed state (insulin > glucagon) also favors storage. In effect there is little need for both liberation of glucose and *de-novo* synthesis of glucose (gluconeogenesis). Moreover, in skeletal muscle the fed state (high insulin) favors both uptake of glucose and its flux through glycolysis. Acetyl-CoA derived from glucose breakdown to pyruvate in the mitochondria increases in the fed state, as does oxaloacetate, and both of these compounds cause cytoplasmic citrate levels to rise, leading to fatty acid synthesis. Fatty acid synthesis causes malonyl-CoA levels to increase, and this step in regulation is important because malonyl-CoA effectively shuts off fatty acid degradation. Ingested glucose fuels the pentose shunt pathway which generates the cofactor NADPH from NADP necessary for fatty acid synthesis. Hepatic fatty acid synthesis is simultaneously accompanied by adipose tissue stimulation of fat synthesis and inhibition of fatty acid breakdown. Amino acids are stored in the fed state, and those that are catabolized serve as substrates which facilitate fatty acid synthesis.

THE FASTED STATE (BOX 2.4; CLEMENS AND PAIDAS, 1997)

Glucose and other dietary substrates are reduced in the fasted state. The liver responds by no longer storing but releasing substrate for the maintenance of blood glucose levels, and it shifts the energy fuels to fatty acids and ketone bodies. Gluconeogenesis is also increased within the liver because of reduced substrate availability and a shift in the insulin/glucagon ratio, which now favors high glucagon, during fasting. Catecholamines are also stimulated in response to the stress of starvation. The net hormonal effect results in increased rates of glycolysis, gluconeogenesis and lipolysis. In premature infants and older children who are deprived of nutritional substrate during times of stress, liver glycogen is rapidly depleted and gluconeogenesis is the sole source for glucose-dependent cells, namely brain, renal medulla and red blood cells. Ketosis (acetoacetate and acetyl-CoA) occurs during prolonged fasting and chronic stress (sepsis). Oxaloacetate is now depleted and no longer present as a precursor for gluconeogenesis, and together with acetyl-

CoA can no longer combine to enter the citric acid cycle. Acetyl-CoA, which is abundant because of the breakdown of fatty acids during starvation, is shunted into the formation of both acetoacetate and acetate, causing ketosis.

THE LIVER IN THE RESPONSE TO STRESS

Inflammation, sepsis and severe trauma all lead to an increased requirement for energy, a significant oxidative stress and a unique liver-specific response at both the metabolic and microcirculatory level.

At the level of intermediary metabolism, the hepatic response to stress (i.e. endotoxin) is associated with increased rates of glycolytic flux and subsequent lactic acidosis (Lang, et al., 1983, 1984). This response is also associated with increased glucose utilization by Kupffer cells and extrahepatic cells, including neutrophils and vascular endothelial cells (Meszaros et al., 1991). These events occur in the absence of any hemodynamic instability associated with hypotension (Long et al., 1976). Moreover, the increase in glucose consumption is associated with lactic acidosis and a narrowed arteriovenous oxygen content. Thus the hepatocytes' ability to use oxygen is compromised during stress. Microvascular studies have elucidated heterogeneous zonal perfusion resulting in mismatch of oxygen delivery, and blood flow resulting in the narrowed arteriovenous oxygen gradients and lactic acid release from hepatocytes exposed to endotoxin or ischemia (Bauer et al., 1994; Clemens et al., 1994a, b). Nitric oxide (the inducible not constitutive form) is upregulated during stress, and its product of the reaction with superoxide, peroxynitrite, impairs electron transport and the citric acid cycle enzyme aconitase (which converts citrate to isocitrate) (Hausladen and Fridovich, 1994). The deleterious effect of this substance is a profound reduction in reactions that can generate reducing equivalents (NADH) and thus form ATP. In effect, what is created is a scenario similar to hypoxia and prolonged starvation in which ketone body formation prevails, as well as a persistent dependence on anaerobic glycolysis (lactic acid cycle) and recycling by gluconeogenesis through the glucose–alanine cycle (Figure 2.9). In fact, in an effort to provide for continued glucose production in a state of glycogen depletion, substrate availability and hormonal milieu both favor accelerated gluconeogensis during stress (Gump et al., 1974, 1975; Long et al., 1976). Despite the accelerated rate of gluconeogensis during endotoxemia, mild injury or illness, the liver's capacity for glucose production remains simultaneously impaired. Hormone-stimulated gluconeogenesis is also attenuated during endotoxemia, regardless of the substrate used (Paidas and Clemens, 1994). Even in the newborn, if hypotension is associated with the response, a state of intractable hypoglycemia may ensue

---

Box 2.4 *Comparison of metabolic events during the fed and fasted state*

Fed state
 Overall goal is storage of exogenous substrate
 Insulin/glucagon ratio is high
 Gluconeogenesis is suppressed
 Skeletal muscle uptake of glucose
 Fatty acid synthesis is increased
 Adipose tissue lipogenesis is increased

Fasted state
 Endogenous substrate becomes energy fuel
 Endogenous ketogenesis
 Insulin/glucagon ratio is low
 Gluconeogenesis is increased
 Glycolysis is increased
 Lipolysis is increased
 Glycogenolysis is increased

(Clemens *et al.*, 1984). In the case of the bile ducts, the vascular permeability associated with the release of the proinflammatory cytokines results in cholestasis (Utili *et al.*, 1976). Jaundice and conjugated hyperbilirubinemia together with elevated transaminases occur in response to the endotoxin (Franson *et al.*, 1985; Brooks *et al.*, 1991).

As a result of protein breakdown (in muscle) following such stresses, there is profound ureagenesis and negative nitrogen balance. The proinflammatory cytokines, interleukins 1 and 8, and tumor necrosis factor-alpha (TNF-α) all help to sustain this proteolytic response in both children and adults (Sullivan *et al.*, 1992; Lin *et al.*, 2000). The resulting free amino acids are used in gluconeogenesis (Figure 2.9). Fat utilization is impaired because of the degree of hypoxia. Moreover, adipocyte lipase and lipoprotein lipase are poorly activated and thus mobilization of fat, fatty acids and glycerol is impaired (Nelson and Spitzer, 1985; Price *et al.*, 1986). This impairment of fat metabolism in the face of poor glucose utilization leads to increased dependence on proteolysis, glycogenolysis, gluconeogenesis and ureagenesis (Long, *et al.*, 1976).

The liver has the capacity both to initiate and to neutralize the response to stress. The hepatic response to stress (i.e. endotoxin) is initiated by the release of cytokines (i.e. tumor necrosis factor and interleukins 1 and 8) by Kupffer and endothelial cells (Billiau and Vandekerckhove, 1991). Kupffer cells are the main source of non-circulating phagocytic cells in the body. In addition to the cytokines, a series of counter-regulatory hormones (cortisol, glucagon and catecholamines) are stimulated, which suppress both growth hormone and insulin (Fong *et al.*, 1990).

In response to stress, the liver increases the synthesis of a family of proteins known as acute phase reactants (Schreiber *et al.*, 1982, 1983; Table 2.2). Clinically, plasma levels of the acute phase protein C-reactive protein (CRP) have been correlated with the magnitude of acute stress in the neonate (Chwals *et al.*, 1992). Resolution of the acute stress is accompanied by a decrease in plasma CRP levels (Chwals *et al.*, 1993). It appears that in the recovery phase of sepsis, on evaluation of the acute phase C-reactive

protein, preterm infants show a more rapid return to normal levels compared with term infants (Tueting *et al.*, 1999).

Simultaneously with the synthesis of acute phase proteins there is a decrease in the expression of other hepatic proteins, such as albumin. For this reason, these down-regulated genes during stress have been termed negative acute phase proteins. The balance between up- and down-regulation of gene expression during stress has been termed the 'adaptive response to stress', which is the result of the limited cellular capacity for gene expression (Wang *et al.*, 1995). The function of the acute phase proteins is to neutralize the response to stress. For example, phagocytic cells secrete proteolytic proteins during infection, which are directed to destroying the pathogen. However, these lytic agents can also damage the host cells. Smooth muscle contraction in response to the cytokines results in decreased perfusion and chemotaxis for white blood cells to release proteases. Acute phase proteins such as trypsin inhibitor can neutralize these proteases (Table 2.2). In addition, other acute phase proteins can act as scavengers of free radicals and cytokines. The acute phase protein fibrinogen is necessary for the coagulation process. In contrast to the zonation observed in many of the hepatic pathways for intermediary metabolism, acute phase protein synthesis is distributed throughout all zones of the acinus (Schreiber *et al.*, 1970). Interestingly, both term and preterm infants can mount a similar counter-regulatory and acute phase response (Anand *et al.*, 1985, 1990).

Biotransformation (BOX 2.5)

Biotransformation involves the liver's ability to metabolize intracellular proteins such as heme and steroids. Cytochrome P-450 (located in the microsomes) catalyzes oxidation, deamination, dealkylation and hydroxylation. This enzyme is important for the metabolism of both drugs and toxins. This sets up a second phase of conjugation by some of the other biotransformation enzymes. The cytochrome P-450 proteins have the potential to generate toxic metabolites. This detoxification system is significant in children, in whom drugs such as acetaminophen, isoniazid and phenothiazines can generate

Table 2.2 *Pattern of acute phase proteins after stress*

Increased levels	Decreased levels
Alpha-1-antitrypsin	Albumin
Fibrinogen	Prealbumin
C-reactive protein	Retinol-binding protein
Haptaglobin	
Ceruloplasmin	
α_1-Acid glycoprotein	
α_2-Macroglobulin	
Transferrin	

Box 2.5 *Components of biotransformation*

Cytochrome P-450
Uridine diphosphate (UDP)-glucuronyl transferase
Glutathione-S-transferase
Sulphotransferase

free radicals that may injure the hepatic ultrastructure. Conjugation of UDP-glucuronic acid by its transferase (a process known as glucuronidation) facilitates the metabolism of acetaminophen, bilirubin, testosterone and aspirin. Glutathione-S-transferase conjugates acetaminophen, bile acids, heme and bilirubin from plasma to liver. The sulphotransferases catalyze the transfer of sulphate groups from proteins such as thyroxine, bile acids and acetaminophen.

The liver participates not only in the detoxification of exogenous compounds but also in that of endogenous molecules. Ammonia is detoxified by the enzymes of the urea cycle (Figure 2.8 above). Heme, which forms the center of both hemoglobin and myoglobin molecules, is formed from glycine and succinate. Porphyrinogens are intermediates of heme metabolism which, when oxidized, form porphyrins that are excreted in excess in children with inherited enzyme defects (porphyria). In addition, acquired states of porphyria can occur following estrogen replacement, alcohol intoxication or heavy metal exposure (e.g. lead poisoning).

The liver and bone marrow constitute the two largest repositories of iron in the body at all ages (Sherlock and Dooley, 1993). Iron is conjugated in blood by transferrin and, after internalization, it dissociates with transferrin, binds to apoferritin and is then called ferritin. Ferritin is the protein-bound non-toxic form of iron. Free iron can cause injury by the formation of free radicals. This is kept in check through the excretion of stored iron by gastrointestinal epithelial cells. Hemochromatosis is the condition in which absorption and storage of iron are uncoupled. In the liver this can cause cirrhosis and hepatocellular cancer (Walker *et al.*, 1975).

Regeneration

Partial hepatectomy is the historical model that has facilitated the study of the coordinated response of the liver to regenerate (Michalopoulos and DeFrances, 1997). We now know that the response is dependent on the magnitude of the liver removed (Starzl *et al.*, 1993), but even a 10% hepatectomy can induce a regenerative response. The regenerative response in the liver is defined as DNA synthesis (proliferation) of all cell types (Figure 2.10). Hepatocytes begin to proliferate first, followed by biliary cells, Kupffer cells and stellate cells, and ending with the sinusoidal endothelial cells. The kinetics of the response appear to begin with DNA synthesis 24 hours after partial hepatectomy. Proliferation begins in the periportal area, and by 36–48 hours it is pericentral (Rabes *et al.*, 1976). By 7 days, the regenerated liver appears as sinusoidal plates that are not one cell layer thick as is characteristic of normal liver, but two layers thick. In a rat liver model of regeneration, a single hepatocyte has the capacity to regenerate 50 rat livers (Overturf *et al.*, 1997). Equally important is the fact that each regenerated hepatocyte has the capacity to perform all of its functions. A number of mitogens, either alone or in combination, stimulate the regenerative process. These include hepatocyte growth factor, TNF-α, IL-6, epidermal growth factor, transforming growth factor-β (Beer-Stolz and Michalopoulos, 1997), norepinephrine and insulin (Michalopoulos and DeFrances, 1997). Termination of DNA synthesis usually ends by 3 days, and alterations in histology follow. Transforming growth factor-β1 appears to be one of the terminating mitogens for the response (Petersen *et al.*, 1994).

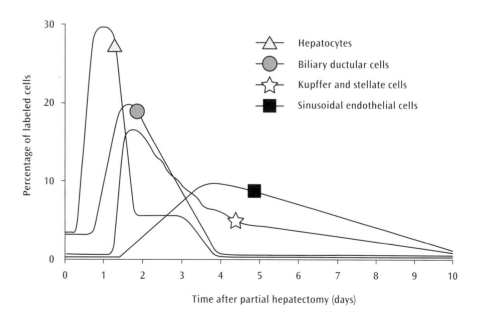

Figure 2.10 *Appearance of hepatic cell types during regeneration.*

Key references

Jungermann K, Katz N. Functional hepatocellular heterogeneity. *Hepatology* 1982; **2**: 385–95.

Metabolic compartmentation is defined within the context of the function of each of the three acinar zones. The liver achieves its tasks of solute regulation and bile turnover by virtue of its heterogeneity.

Lin E, Calvano SE, Lowry SF. Surgical research review: inflammatory cytokines and cell response in surgery. *Surgery* 2000; **127**: 117–26.

A recent literature review, this paper highlights the cytokine response to injury, its sources and interactions. It brings together the role of all cytokines in the systemic inflammatory response.

Rappaport AM, Borowy ZJ, Lougheed WM, Lotto WN. Subdivision of hexagonal liver lobules into a structural and functional unit: role in hepatic physiology and pathology. *Anatomical Record* 1954; **119**: 11–34.

This classic paper is the original description of the acinus as the functional unit of the liver. The acinus and therefore all hepatocytes are perfused by a terminal portal venule and hepatic arteriole. Moreover, the acinus was divided into three zones, all with unidirectional flow culminating within the hepatic venule.

Schreiber G, Howlett G. Synthesis and secretion of acute-phase proteins. In: Glaumann H, Peters T Jr, Redman C (eds) *Plasma protein secretion by the liver*. London: Academic Press, 1983: 423–49.

This article is a detailed discussion of the acute phase proteins whose plasma concentrations are increased or decreased in response to stress.

REFERENCES

Anand KJ, Brown MJ, Bloom SR *et al.* Studies on the hormonal regulation of fuel metabolism in the human newborn infant undergoing anesthesia and surgery. *Hormone Research* 1985; **22**: 115–28.

Anand KJ, Hansen DD, Hickey PR. Hormonal metabolic stress responses in neonates undergoing cardiac surgery. *Anesthesiology* 1990; **73**: 661–70.

Arcieli JM, Moore GW, Hutchins GM. Hepatic morphology in cardiac dysfunction: a clinicopathologic study of 1000 subjects at autopsy. *American Journal of Pathology* 1981; **104**: 159–66.

Bauer M, Zhang JX, Bauer I *et al.* Endothelin-1-induced alterations of hepatic microcirculation: sinusoidal and extrasinusoidal sites of action. *American Journal of Physiology* 1994; **267**: G143.

Beer-Stolz D, Michalopoulos GK. Synergistic enhancement of EGF, but not HGF, stimulated hepatocyte motility by TGF-beta 1 *in vitro. Journal of Cell Physiology* 1997; **170**: 57–68.

Bernstein J, Brown AK. Sepsis and jaundice in early infancy. *Pediatrics* 1962; **29**: 873–82.

Billiau A, Vandekerckhove F. Cytokines and their interaction with other inflammatory mediators in the pathogenesis of sepsis and septic shock. *European Journal of Clinical Investigation* 1991; **21**: 559–73.

Brooks GS, Zimbler AG, Bodenheimer HC, Burchard KW. Patterns of liver test abnormalities in patients with surgical sepsis. *American Surgeon* 1991; **57**: 656–61.

Campbell DA, Punch JD, Budd–Chiari syndrome. In: Cameron J (ed.) *Current surgical therapy*, 6th edn. St Louis, MO: Mosby, 1998: 398–401.

Cascio S, Zaret KS. Hepatocyte differentiation initiates during endodermal–mesenchymal interactions prior to liver formation. *Development* 1991; **113**: 217–25.

Chwals WJ, Fernandez ME, Charles BJ *et al.* Serum visceral protein levels reflect protein-calorie repletion in neonates recovering from major surgery. *Journal of Pediatric Surgery* 1992; **27**: 317–20.

Chwals WJ, Fernandez ME, Jamie AC, Charles BJ. Relationship of metabolic indexes to postoperative mortality in surgical infants. *Journal of Pediatric Surgery* 1993; **28**: 819–22.

Clemens MG, Paidas CN. Metabolism. In: Oldham KT, Colombani PM, Foglia RP (eds) *Surgery of infants and children: scientific principles and practice*. Philadelphia, PA: Lippincott-Raven Publishers, 1997: 117–26.

Clemens MG, Chaudry IH, Daigneau N *et al.* Insulin resistance and depressed gluconeogenic capability during early hyperglycemic sepsis. *Journal of Trauma* 1984; **24**: 701–8.

Clemens MG, Bauer M, Gingalewski C *et al.* Hepatic intercellular communication in shock and inflammation. *Shock* 1994a; **2**: 1–9.

Clemens MG, Bauer M, Gingalewski C *et al.* Heterogeneity of hepatocellular response: role of intercellular communication. In: Faist E, Schildberg F, Baue A (eds) *Host defense dysfunction in trauma, shock and sepsis*, 2nd edn. Berlin: Springer Verlag, 1994b: 1–9.

DeMaio A. Heat shock proteins: facts, thoughts and dreams. *Shock* 1999; **11**: 1–12.

Dempsey ME. Regulation of steroid biosynthesis. *Annual Review of Biochemistry* 1974; **43**: 967–90.

Desmet VJ. Embryology of the liver and intrahepatic biliary tract, and an overview of malformations of the bile duct. In: McIntyre N, Benhamou J-P, Bircher J *et al.* (eds) *The Oxford textbook of clinical hepatology. Vol. 1.* Oxford: Oxford University Press, 1991; 497–519.

Deutschman SC, De Maio A, Buchman TG, Clemens MG. Sepsis-induced alterations in levels of mRNA coding for phosphoenolpyruvate carboxykinase: the role of insulin and glucagon. *Circulatory Shock* 1993; **40**: 295–302.

Edelstone DI, Rudolph AM, Heymann MA. Liver and ductus

venosus blood flows in fetal lambs *in utero*. *Circulation Research* 1978; **42**: 426–33.

Emery JL. Functional asymmetry of the liver. *Annals of the New York Academy of Sciences* 1963; **111**: 37–44.

Exton JH. Mechanisms of hormonal regulation of hepatic glucose metabolism. *Diabetes/Metabolism Reviews* 1987; **3**: 163–83.

Faulkner A, Jones CT. Hexokinase isoenzymes in tissues of the adult and developing guinea pig. *Archives of Biochemistry and Biophysics* 1976; **175**: 477–86.

Fong Y, Moldawer LL, Shires GT *et al*. The biologic characteristics of cytokines and their implication in surgical injury. *Surgery, Gynecology and Obstetrics* 1990; **170**: 363–78.

Franson TR, Hierholzer WJ Jr, LaBreque DR. Frequency and characteristics of hyperbilirubinemia associated with bacteremia. *Reviews of Infectious Diseases* 1985; **7**: 1–9.

Gain KR, Malthus R, Watts C. Glucose homeostatis during the prenatal period in normal rats and rats with a glycogen storage disorder. *Journal of Clinical Investigation* 1981; **67**: 1569–73.

Garland JS, Werlin SL, Rice TB. Ischemic hepatitis in children: diagnosis and clinical course. *Critical Care Medicine* 1988; **16**: 1209–12.

Gebhardt R. Metabolic zonation of the liver: regulation and implications for liver function. *Pharmacology and Therapeutics* 1992; **53**: 275–354.

Gitzelmann R, Hansen RG. Galactose metabolism, hereditary defects and their clinical significance. In: Burman D, Holton JB, Pennock CA (eds) *Inherited disorders of carbohydrate metabolism*. Baltimore, MD: University Park Press, 1980: 61–87.

Gottlieb JE, Menashe PI, Cruz E. Gastrointestinal complications in critically ill patients: the intensivists' overview. *American Journal of Gastroenterology* 1986; **81**: 227–38.

Graf J. Canalicular bile-salt independent bile formation: concepts and clues from electrolyte transport in rat liver. *American Journal of Physiology* 1983; **244**: G233–46.

Granger HJ, Goodman AH, Cook BH. Metabolic models of microcirculatory regulation. *Federal Proceedings* 1975; **34**: 2025–30.

Gressner AM. Cytokines and cellular crosstalk involved in the activation of fat-storing cells. *Journal of Hepatology* 1995; **22 (Supplement 2)**: 28–36.

Gump FE, Long C, Killian P *et al*. Studies of glucose intolerance in septic injured patients. *Journal of Trauma* 1974; **14**: 378.

Gump FE, Long CL, Geiger JW *et al*. The significance of altered gluconeogenesis in surgical catabolism. *Journal of Trauma* 1975; **15**: 704.

Gumucio JJ. Hepatocyte heterogeneity: the coming of age from the description of a biological curiosity to a partial understanding of its physiological meaning and regulation. *Hepatology* 1989; **9**: 154–60.

Hausladen A, Fridovich I. Superoxide and peroxynitrite

inactivate aconitases but nitric oxide does not. *Journal of Biological Chemistry* 1994; **269**: 29405–8.

Heubi JE, Balistreri WF, Suchy FJ. Bile salt metabolism in the first year of life. *Journal of Laboratory and Clinical Medicine* 1982; **100**: 127–36.

Hirai F, Aoyama H, Ohtoshi M *et al*. Significance of mitochondrial enhancement in hepatic energy metabolism in relation to alterations in hemodynamics in septic pigs with severe peritonitis. *European Surgical Research* 1984; **16**: 148–55.

Inoue M, Kinne R, Tran T, Biempica L, Arias IM. Rat liver canalicular membrane vesicles. Isolation and topological characterization. *Journal of Biological Chemistry* 1983; **258**: 5183–8.

Jones CT. Comparative aspects of hepatic glucose metabolism during foetal development. *Biochemical Society Transactions* 1981; **9**: 375–6.

Keppler D, Huber M, Baumert T. Leukotrienes as mediators in diseases of the liver. *Seminars in Liver Disease* 1988; **8**: 3547–63.

Keshen T, Miller R, Jahoor F, Jaksic T, Reeds PJ. Glucose production and gluconeogenesis are negatively related to body weight in mechanically ventilated, very-low-birth-weight neonates. *Pediatric Research* 1997; **41**: 132–8.

Kirn A, Gut JP, Bingen A, Steffan AM. Murine hepatitis induced by frog virus 3: a model for studying the effect of sinusoidal cell damage on the liver. *Hepatology* 1983; **3**: 105–11.

Knook DL, Seffelaar AM, de Leeuw AM. Fat-storing cells of the rat liver. Their isolation and purification. *Experimental Cell Research* 1982; **139**: 468–71.

Kraus-Friedmann N. Hormonal regulation of hepatic gluconeogenesis. *Physiological Reviews* 1984; **64**: 170–259.

Lang CH, Bagby GJ, Bornside GH *et al*. Sustained hypermetabolic sepsis in rats: characterization of the model. *Journal of Surgical Research* 1983; **35**: 201–10.

Lang CH, Bagby GJ, Spitzer JJ. Carbohydrate dynamics in the hypermetabolic septic rat. *Metabolism* 1984; **33**: 959–63.

Larsen WJ. Development of the gastrointestinal tract. In: Schmitt WR (ed.) *Human embryology*. New York: Churchill Livingstone, 1993: 205–34.

Lautt WW. Hepatic nerves – a review of their functions and effects. *Canadian Journal of Physiology and Pharmacology* 1980; **58**: 105–23.

Lautt WW. Relationship between hepatic blood flow and overall metabolism: the hepatic arterial buffer response. *Federation Proceedings* 1983; **42**: 1662–6.

Lautt WW, Greenway CV. Conceptual review of the hepatic vascular bed. *Hepatology* 1987; **7**: 952–63.

Legare DJ, Lautt WW. Hepatic venous resistance site in the dog: localization and validation of intrahepatic pressure measurements. *Canadian Journal of Physiology and Phamacology* 1987; **65**: 352–9.

Lehninger AL, Nelson DL, Cox MM. Glycolysis and the

catabolism of hexoses. In: *Principles of biochemistry*, 2nd edn. New York: Worth Publishers, 1993; 400–45.

Leloir LF. The enzymatic transformation of uridine diphosphate glucose into a galactose derivative. *Archives of Biochemistry and Biophysics* 1951; **33**: 186–95.

Lin E, Calvano SE, Lowry SF. Inflammatory cytokines and cell response in surgery. *Surgery* 2000; **127**: 117–26.

Liu J, Park EA, Gurney AL, Roesler WJ, Hanson RW. Cyclic AMP induction of phosphoenolpyruvate carboxykinase (GTP) gene transcription is mediated by multiple promoter elements. *Journal of Biological Chemistry* 1991; **266**: 19095–102.

Long CL, Kinney JM, Geiger JW. Nonsuppressability of gluconeogenesis by glucose in septic patients. *Metabolism* 1976; **25**: 193–201.

Lubchenco LO, Bard H. Incidence of hypoglycemia in newborn infants classified by birth weight and gestational age. *Pediatrics* 1971; **47**: 831–8.

Ludwig J, Hashimoto E, McGill DB et al. Classification of hepatic venous outflow obstruction: ambiguous terminology of the Budd–Chiari syndrome. *Mayo Clinic Proceedings* 1990; **65**: 51–5.

Lyonnet S, Coupe C, Girard J et al. In-vivo regulation of glycolytic and gluconeogenic enzyme gene expression in newborn rat liver. *Journal of Clinical Investigation* 1988; **81**: 1682–9.

McDonald GB, Sharma P, Matthews DE et al. Veno-occlusive disease of the liver after bone marrow transplantation: diagnosis, incidence and predisposing factors. *Hepatology* 1984; **4**: 116–22.

Mace S, Borkat G, Liebman J. Hepatic dysfunction and cardiovascular abnormalities: occurrence in infants, children and young adults. *American Journal of Disease in Childhood* 1985; **139**: 60–5.

Matsuura E, Eto S, Kata K, Tashiro Y. Ferritin immunoelectron microscopic localization of 5′-nucleotidase on rat liver cell surface. *Journal of Cell Biology* 1984; **99**: 166–73.

Meier PJ. The bile secretory pole of hepatocytes. *Journal of Hepatology* 1989; **9**: 124–9.

Meier PJ, Sztul ES, Reuben A, Boyer JL. Structural and functional polarity of canalicular and basolateral plasma membrane vesicles isolated in high yield from rat liver. *Journal of Cell Biology* 1984; **98**: 991–1000.

Meszaros K, Bojta J, Bautista AP et al. Glucose utilization by Kupffer cells, endothelial cells and granulocytes in endotoxemic rat liver. *American Journal of Physiology* 1991; **260**: G7–12.

Michalopoulos GK, DeFrances MC. Liver regeneration. *Science* 1997; **276**: 60–66.

Moore KL. The digestive system. In: *The developing human*, 3rd edn. Philadelphia, PA: WB Saunders, 1982: 231–3.

Nathanson MH, Boyer JL. Mechanisms and regulation of bile secretion. *Hepatology* 1991; **14**: 551.

Nelson KM, Spitzer JA. Alteration of adipocyte calcium homeostasis by *Escherichia coli* endotoxin. *American Journal of Physiology* 1985; **248**: R331.

Nolan JP. Endotoxin, reticuloendothelial function and liver injury. *Hepatology* 1981; **1**: 458–65.

Overturf K, Al-Dhalimy M, Ou CN et al. Serial transplantation reveals the stem-cell-like regenerative potential of adult mouse hepatocytes. *American Journal of Pathology* 1997; **151**: 1273–80.

Ozawa K, Kamlyama Y, Kimura K et al. Contribution of the arterial blood ketone body ratio to elevated plasma amino acids in hepatic encephalopathy of surgical patients. *American Journal of Surgery* 1983; **146**: 299.

Paidas CN, Clemens MG. Hormone effects on hepatic substrate preference in sepsis. *Shock* 1994; **1**: 94–100.

Paidas CN, Mattei P, Clemens MG, Schleien C. Splanchnic function in heart disease. In: Nichols DG, Cameron DE, Greeley WJ, Lappe DG, Ungerleider RM, Wetzel RC (eds) *Critical care heart disease in infants and children*. St Louis, MO: Mosby, 1995: 143–55.

Paidas CN, Mooney ML, Theodorakis NG et al. Accelerated recovery after endotoxic challenge in heat shock pretreated mice. *American Journal of Physiology* (in press).

Parillo JE, Parker MM, Natanson C et al. Septic shock in humans: advances in the understanding of pathogenesis, cardiovascular dysfunction and therapy. *Annals of Internal Medicine* 1990; **113**: 227–42.

Perdereau D, Narkewicz M, Coupe C et al. Hormonal control of specific gene expression in the rat liver during the suckling–weaning transition. *Advances in Enzyme Regulation* 1990; **30**: 91–108.

Petersen B, Yee CJ, Bowen W, Zarnegar R, Michalopoulos GK. Distinct morphological and mito-inhibitory effects induced by TGF-beta-1, HGF and EGF on mouse, rat and human hepatocytes. *Cell Biology and Toxicology* 1994; **10**: 219–30.

Pilkis SJ. Hepatic gluconeogenesis/glycolysis: regulation and structure/function relationships of substrate cycle enzymes. *Annual Review of Nutrition* 1991; **11**: 465–515.

Price SR, Olivecrona T, Pekala PH. Regulation of lipoprotein lipase synthesis by recombinant tumor necrosis factor: the primary regulatory role of the hormone 3T3-L1 adipocytes. *Archives of Biochemistry and Biophysics* 1986; **251**: 738.

Rabes HM, Wirsching R, Tuczek HV, Iseler G. Analysis of cell cycle compartments of hepatocytes after partial hepatecomy. *Cell Tissue Kinetics* 1976; **9**: 517–32.

Rappaport AM. The structural and functional unit in the human liver (liver acinus). *Anatomical Record* 1958; **130**: 673–86.

Rappaport AM, Borowy ZJ, Laugheed WM, Lotto WN. Subdivision of hexagonal liver lobules into a structural and functional unit: role in hepatic physiology and pathology. *Anatomical Record* 1954; **119**: 11–34.

Richardson PDI, Withrington PG. Liver blood flow. II. Effects of drugs and hormones on liver blood flow. *Gastroenterology* 1981; **81**: 356–79.

Rudolph AM. Hepatic and ductus venosus blood flows during fetal life. *Hepatology* 1983; **3**: 254–8.

Ruebner BH *et al.* Development and transformation of the ductal plate in the developing human liver. *Pediatric Pathology and Laboratory Medicine* 1990; **10**: 55–68.

Ryckman FC, Ziegler MM, Pedersen SH, Dittrich V, Balistreri WF. Liver transplantation in children. In: Suchy FJ, Sokol RJ, Balistreri WF (eds) *Liver disease in children*. St Louis, MO: Mosby, 1994: 930–50.

Schreiber G, Lesch R, Weinssen U, Zahringer J. The distribution of albumin synthesis throughout the liver lobule. *Journal of Cell Biology* 1970; **47**: 285–9.

Schreiber G, Howlett G, Nagashima M *et al.* The acute phase response of plasma protein synthesis during experimental inflammation. *Journal of Biological Chemistry* 1982; **257**: 10271–7.

Seccombe DW, Harding PG, Possmayer F. Fetal utilization of maternally derived ketone bodies for lipogenesis in the rat. *Biochimica et Biophysica Acta* 1977; **488**: 402–16.

Sherlock S, Dooley J. *Diseases of the liver and biliary system*, 9th edn. Oxford: Blackwell Scientific Publications, 1993.

Snell K. Muscle alanine synthesis and hepatic gluconeogenesis. *Biochemical Society Transactions* 1980; **8**: 205.

Starzl TE, Fung J, Tsakis A *et al.* Baboon-to-human liver transplantation. *Lancet* 1993; **341**: 65–71.

Stevens LH, Emond JC, Piper JB *et al.* Hepatic artery thrombosis in infants. *Transplantation* 1992; **53**: 396–9.

Stieber AC, Zetti G, Todo S *et al.* The spectrum of portal vein thrombosis in liver transplantation. *Annals of Surgery* 1991; **213**: 199–206.

Stosiek P, Kasper M, Karsten U. Expression of cytokeratin 19 during human liver organogenesis. *Liver* 1990; **10**: 59–63.

Sullivan JS, Kilpatrick L, Costarino AT, Lee SC, Harris MC. Correlation of plasma cytokine elevations with mortality rate in children with sepsis. *Journal of Pediatrics* 1992; **120**: 510–15.

Tavill AS, Craigie A, Rosenoer WM. The measurement of the synthetic rate of albumin in man. *Clinical Science* 1968; **34**: 1–28.

Tilghman SM, Belayew A. Transcriptional control of the murine albumin-alphafetoprotein locus during development. *Proceedings of the National Academy of Sciences of the USA* 1983; **79**: 5254–7.

Tueting JL, Byerley LO, Chwals WJ. Anabolic recovery relative to degree of prematurity after acute injury in neonates. *Journal of Pediatric Surgery* 1999; **34**: 13–17.

Utili R, Abernathy CO, Zimmerman HJ. Cholestatic effects of *Escherichia coli* endotoxin on the isolated perfused rat liver. *Gastroenterology* 1976; **70**: 248–53.

Van Eyken P, Sciot R, Callea F *et al.* The development of the intrahepatic bile ducts in man: a keratin immunohistochemical study. *Hepatology* 1988; **8**: 1586–95.

Van Schaftingen E, Hue L, Hers HG. Control of the fructose-6-phosphate/fructose-1,6-bisphosphate cycle in isolated hepatocytes by glucose and glucagon. *Biochemical Journal* 1980; **192**: 887.

Wakil SJ, Stoops JK, Joshi VC. Fatty acid synthesis and its regulation. *Annual Review of Biochemistry* 1983; **52**: 537–79.

Walker DG. On the presence of two soluble glucose phosphorylating enzymes in adult liver and the development of one of these after birth. *Biochimica et Biophysica Acta* 1963; **77**: 209–26.

Walker GO, Jacobs A, Worwood M *et al.* Iron absorption in normal subjects and patients with idiopathic haemochromatosis: relationship with serum ferritin concentration. *Gut* 1975; **16**: 188–92.

Walters GO, Jacobs A, Worwood M, Trevett D, Thomson W. Iron absorption in normal subjects and patients with idiopathic haemachromatosis: relationship with serum ferritin concentration. *Gut* 1975; **16**: 188–92.

Wang K, Deutschman CS, Clemens MG, De Maio A. Reciprocal expression of acute phase genes and phosphoenolpyruvate carboxykinase (PEPCK) during acute inflammation. *Shock* 1995; **3**: 204–9.

Watkins JB, Szczepanik P, Gould JB *et al.* Bile salt metabolism in the human premature infant. Preliminary observations of pool size and synthesis rate following prenatal administration of dexamethasone and phenobarbital. *Gastroenterology* 1975; **69**: 706–13.

Wisse E, De Zanger RB, Charels K *et al.* The liver sieve: considerations concerning the structure and function of endothelial fenestrae, the sinusoidal wall and the space of Disse. *Hepatology* 1985; **5**: 683–92.

Yamamoto M, Tanaka J, Ozawa K *et al.* Significance of acetoacetate/β-hydroxybutyrate ratio in arterial blood as an indicator of the severity of hemorrhagic shock. *Journal of Surgical Research* 1979; **28**: 124.

Yamamoto K, Fisher MM, Phillips MJ. Hilar biliary plexus in human liver. A comparative study of the intrahepatic bile ducts in man and animals. *Laboratory Investigation* 1985; **52**: 103–6.

Zimmerman HJ, Fang M, Utili R *et al.* Jaundice due to bacterial infection. *Gastroenterology* 1979; **77**: 362–74.

3

Investigation of the liver and biliary system

JOHN KARANI

LABORATORY STUDIES

Bilirubin

The majority of newborn infants develop a serum unconjugated bilirubin concentration greater than 34 μmol/L, but this physiological jaundice resolves spontaneously within 10–14 days. Although some surgical conditions, such as meconium retention or high intestinal obstruction, can occasionally cause an unconjugated hyperbilirubinemia, the vast majority of pathological causes are medical, and it is beyond the scope of this book to discuss in detail the medical investigations that may be required. The reader is directed to the comprehensive review by Roberts (1999).

The surgeon's role is to identify those patients in whom there is a significant obstructive component to the jaundice, and who would benefit from operative relief. Speed of investigation is imperative in infancy. Conjugated hyperbilirubinemia is always pathological, but it is important to remember that the child with cholestasis may present with symptoms and signs other than jaundice. Possible presentations include intraventricular hemorrhage due to bleeding, sepsis with ascites or spontaneous rupture of the bile duct.

DIFFERENTIAL DIAGNOSES OF JAUNDICE

Examples of medical causes include the following:

- intrauterine acquired infection;
- metabolic disorders;
- chromosomal abnormalities;
- familial disorders;
- inspissated bile syndrome;
- parenteral alimentation.

Examples of surgical causes include the following:

- biliary atresia;
- spontaneous perforation of the bile duct;
- choledochal cyst;
- rare causes (e.g. gallstones, extrinsic bile duct compression, reduplication of the bile duct).

Enzymes

Alanine aminotransferase (ALT) is found almost exclusively in the liver, whereas aspartate aminotransferase (AST) also occurs in the muscle, heart and kidneys. Rises in these enzymes indicate liver cell damage, but they are non-specific and correlate poorly with the extent of the disease. Gamma-glutamyl transpeptidase (GGT) is located in the hepatocyte and biliary epithelium and is also a non-specific indicator of liver disease. Levels are normally raised up to three times higher than those found in adults. Serum alkaline phosphatase is also normally raised during growth, but further elevation may reflect obstruction or inflammation of the biliary epithelium.

Alpha-fetoprotein

Alpha-fetoprotein is a major plasma protein in early fetal development, and reaches its highest level after 13 weeks' gestation. Thereafter the level falls rapidly until 6 weeks of age, and then more gradually until normal levels are reached by 2 years of age. Although markedly raised levels are characteristic of hepatoblastoma or hepatoma, moderate elevations can occur with other liver diseases.

IMAGING STUDIES

Imaging studies are now a key component in the investigation of pediatric hepatobiliary disease. Our understanding of the pathogenesis and natural history of these disorders has been paralleled by the development and introduction of these radiological techniques into clinical practice. Today, advances in ultrasound, computed tomography, magnetic resonance imaging and invasive vascular and biliary techniques have allowed a clear demonstration of vascular and biliary anatomy and an accuracy in the detection of small liver tumors that would not have been possible a decade ago. The challenge for hepatobiliary surgeons, hepatologists and radiologists is to learn the appropriate use of this technology, which continues to evolve through the manipulation of physical rather than biological principles. An understanding of the limitations of individual techniques is as important to the radiologist as recognizing their diagnostic potential. Experience has shown that no imaging technique stands alone, and although imaging-based protocols are of value, they have to be tailored to the individual child. Although didactic algorithms of investigation can be used as a guide, there will always be variance in observation, equipment and radiological experience that may adversely affect or advance the diagnostic pathway.

The role of imaging is first to detect abnormalities referable to the clinical presentation, second to predict the pathology, and finally to stage the disorder as a prelude to the treatment of the disease. This may be primarily surgical or medical, but there is increasing recognition of the role of interventional radiological techniques in the treatment of many liver disorders in infancy and childhood.

This chapter will describe the techniques available and their applicability to both common and rare disorders of the liver and pancreas.

TECHNIQUES

Plain radiographs

Conventional radiographs have been largely superseded by other techniques, but they should not be omitted and their merits should not be overlooked. Calcification within the liver is always pathological, and occurs in association with both primary and secondary hepatic tumors. Approximately 5% of primary liver tumors show calcification or ossification, and this feature has

been attributed to all of the main primary tumors. It is a characteristic feature of hepatoblastoma, and well recognized as a sign of response to chemotherapy. Calcification is also a recognized feature of other primary tumors, including hemangioendothelioma, cavernous hemangioma and hepatocellular carcinoma. In addition, it may be present in hepatic metastases from neuroblastoma, osteosarcoma, leiomyosarcoma, rhabdomyosarcoma, lymphoma and embryonal testicular tumors. Hepatic calcification may also be present in hydatid disease and the granulomatous disorders of the liver, which include tuberculosis, histoplasmosis and brucellosis.

Further pathological observations that may be made on a plain abdominal radiograph include the presence of gas in the portal venous system or biliary tree.

The chest radiograph is of particular importance in tumor staging when metastases to the lung parenchyma or mediastinum may be visible. A 'normal' chest radiograph does not exclude intrathoracic metastatic disease, but if it is abnormal, with evidence of metastatic disease, then computed tomography, which is the most sensitive technique for detection of pulmonary nodules, can be excluded from the investigative sequence.

The chest radiograph is equally important for assessing the pulmonary manifestations of liver disease, which include hepatopulmonary syndrome from portal hypertension, and interstitial or airways disease that may be present as part of a multisystem disorder (cystic fibrosis is one such example).

Pulmonary infection in acute or chronic liver failure and following liver transplantation carries a significant morbidity. The chest radiograph remains the principal investigation for early recognition of infection, assessing the extent, characterizing its likely etiology and monitoring the response to antimicrobial therapy.

Plain radiographs also play an integral role in assessing the skeletal manifestations of the individual liver disorders. These may form part of a multisystem developmental disorder, as illustrated by Alagille's syndrome, which includes defects of vertebral segmentation and abnormalities of the third and fourth digits in association with biliary hypoplasia, cardiac abnormalities and abnormal facies. Alternatively, they may be acquired as a sequela of the metabolic disturbance of liver dysfunction. The skeletal changes of rickets resulting from severe liver cholestasis provide the best example in this group.

Radionuclide imaging

Radionuclide studies for the assessment of biliary excretion play an important role in the investigation of jaundice and in the follow-up of children who have undergone previous biliary surgery. These scans provide a dynamic representation of bile flow, and can confirm the normal excretion of isotope through a normal biliary tree from canalicular level to a normally functioning gallbladder and extrahepatic biliary tree. Technetium-99m-labeled iminodiacetic acid (IDA) derivatives form the basis of these compounds. The di-isopropyl compound, DISIDA, is the preferred derivative because of its maximum concentration in the liver, low renal excretion and unconjugated excretion into the biliary system. An enhanced concentration in the liver can be achieved if phenobarbitone (5 mg/kg) is given for 3 days prior to the test. After an intravenous injection of DISIDA, imaging is carried out at 5-minute intervals in the first hour and then at hourly intervals for 10 hours. If excretion to the bowel is delayed, imaging is repeated at 24 hours. Scanning after 24 hours is impractical because of the short half-life of technetium-99m-labeled compounds. In a normal study there will be visualization of the bile ducts 10–20 minutes after the injection and of the small bowel within 30–40 minutes. The current main indications for excretion scintigraphy are confirmation of bile duct patency in neonatal jaundice, demonstration of postoperative bile leaks, and the assessment of the differential functional status of the native liver and graft following auxiliary liver transplantation.

Ultrasound

Ultrasound is the pre-eminent first-line technique for the investigation of hepatobiliary disorders in infancy and childhood. It does not involve ionizing radiation, and it is accepted that in standard use it has no harmful biological effects. Although it is dependent on equipment and interpretative expertise, most departments now have high-quality equipment with regular update programs to encompass the continuing developments in ultrasound technology.

High-frequency sound waves are emitted from a transducer, transmitted through the body, and reflected or transmitted at different tissue interfaces. The same transducer detects the reflections, and an image of the insonated structures is displayed. The resolution allows lesions of less than 5 mm to be detected. The character of the lesion is important, particularly in determining whether it is cystic or solid and whether it is associated with increased vascularity on interrogation with spectral, color-flow or contrast-enhanced Doppler techniques. The importance of ultrasound in the preoperative and intraoperative assessment of liver tumors also lies in its ability to map the relationship of a tumor to the portal and hepatic venous anatomy, thereby defining its segmental anatomy according to the classical eight functional segments defined by Couinaud (see Chapter 1).

A major role for ultrasound has emerged in the investigation of jaundice in neonates, infants and children. The key question is to confirm or refute the presence of bile duct dilatation. This may be segmental, as in the developmental choledochal anomalies, or it may involve the intra- and extrahepatic biliary tree, as in the inspissated bile plug syndrome, where the level of obstruction and the reflective intraductal plug or gallstones may be seen.

In neonates with conjugated hyperbilirubinemia, it is important to define those with an acquired or developmental abnormality that requires surgical intervention. In extrahepatic biliary atresia, full mapping of the biliary system may not be possible and a 'normal' ultrasound does not exclude the diagnosis. However, there may be supportive signs. These include the presence of a hypoplastic gallbladder, intrahepatic bile lakes or other developmental anomalies, including situs inversus, polysplenia, malrotation or a preduodenal portal vein as part of the biliary atresia splenic malformation syndrome (see Chapter 8). Equally important is the assessment of the liver parenchyma to determine whether this is normal or whether there is evidence of established cirrhosis with nodular regeneration. It may also be possible to detect a deposition disorder, such as glycogen storage disease, where the ultrasound appearances of highly reflective parenchyma may be pathognomonic.

In the investigation of portal hypertension, particularly in children presenting with their first variceal hemorrhage, the importance of ultrasound lies in distinguishing those with cirrhosis and those with 'normal' livers but with presinusoidal venous occlusion and cavernous transformation of the portal vein. The etiology may be determined by accurate mapping of the intra- and extrahepatic portal vein with Doppler studies, which may also allow the investigator to determine whether portosystemic shunting is a potential therapeutic option. Splenomegaly, ascites, peritoneal thickening and varices may be present in both of the disease categories.

In addition to defining the anatomy of the portal venous system, the use of Doppler studies is important for confirming blood flow in the portal vein and its velocity characteristics. This is of particular importance in the pre- and postoperative assessment of patients undergoing liver transplantation. Graft surveillance for the early recognition of vascular and biliary complications is an important component of optimization of graft function (see Chapter 30). Doppler studies are also useful for confirming shunt patency and reversal of the signs of portal hypertension after portosystemic shunt surgery.

Computed tomography (FIGURE 3.1)

A computed tomography (CT) examination of the liver is incomplete without contrast enhancement, which increases the sensitivity of lesion detection. Identification of a focal liver lesion is dependent on its differing tissue characteristics and vascularity compared with the surrounding liver. The vascular supply to the liver is complex, with two-thirds of inflow from the portal vein and the remainder from the hepatic artery.

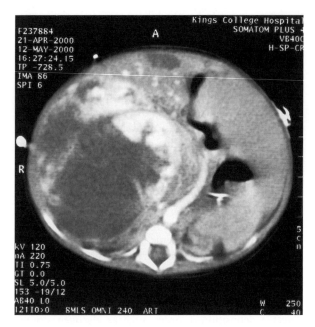

Figure 3.1 *Arterial phase computed tomography (CT) demonstrating a peripherally arterialized tumor in the right lobe of the liver in an infant. There is evidence of centripetal enhancement and a hyperplastic feeding artery, which are characteristic features of a hemangioendothelioma.*

This unique dual circulation is balanced by reciprocity of flow, which is reflected in the distribution of intravascular contrast agents within liver tissue and vasculature. The iodinated non-ionic contrast agents in CT, gadolinium salts in magnetic resonance imaging and microbubble contrast agents in ultrasound scans all exhibit the same time–distribution characteristics in the liver.

Tumors of the liver can be categorized by their vascular properties. In broad terms they are associated with enhanced arterialization, interruption of portal venous flow, arterioportal shunting and arteriohepatic venous shunting. Their characteristics in the arterial phase at 25 seconds following injection, in the portal phase at 60 seconds and in the delayed (or equilibrium) phase are diagnostic features which can be used to predict their pathology.

CT is the method most commonly used for intra- and extrahepatic staging of primary malignant tumors of the liver as well as monitoring the response to chemotherapy (see Chapter 18). Local and retroperitoneal lymph node involvement is readily diagnosed, as is extra-abdominal spread to the central nervous system and thorax. CT also allows visualization of the hepatic and portal veins when planning surgical resection or when assessing liver trauma on an organ injury scale (see Chapter 26).

Magnetic resonance imaging

Magnetic resonance imaging (MRI) uses non-ionizing radiation (radiofrequency) within a strong magnetic field. The absorbed energy is released from the cell nuclei in a specific manner that is proportional to proton density, allowing differentiation of soft tissues. This results in a change in the magnetic field that is translated into a 'signal' of varying intensity which is plotted to produce a representation of a slice through the body. These signals can be presented in any plane, and may therefore be imaged in the axial, coronal or sagittal plane without mathematical reconstruction of the dataset. There are no known harmful biological effects, and repeat imaging is therefore acceptable. As with CT, fast techniques lead to a reduction in misregistration artifacts, resulting in enhanced resolution of the liver. The terminology of MRI is often complex, but a simple principle is to regard T1-weighted images as defining the anatomy and contrast-enhanced vascular characteristics of a lesion, and T2-weighted images as defining its inherent water content.

Hemangiomas, with their slow-flowing blood, and simple cysts therefore give a uniform high signal on the T2-weighted acquisition. On this sequence solid tumors are isointense or of non-uniform, marginally higher signal than the surrounding liver.

Extended MRI techniques include vascular imaging techniques of magnetic resonance arteriography/venography (MRA and MRV) (see Figure 3.2) and magnetic resonance cholangiopancreatography (MRCP), which allow non-invasive imaging of the hepatic vasculature, biliary and pancreatic ducts. These techniques rely on the enhancement and 'water' properties of the

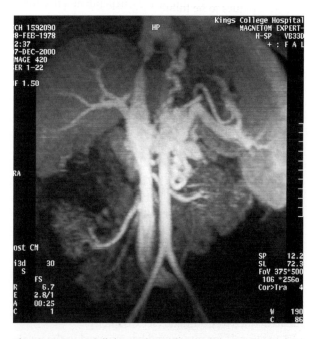

Figure 3.2 *Gadolinium-enhanced magnetic resonance (MR) angiography and venography defining the arterial, portal venous and caval anatomy in a transplant recipient. A tight suprahepatic venous stenosis has been defined which was successfully treated by balloon dilatation.*

structures. High-signal ('bright bile') techniques are utilized in MRCP and commonly use T2-weighted, breath-hold sequences with repeated or single acquisition. Image manipulation allows rotation of the summated image and display of the cholangiogram to best advantage (see Figure 3.3). The diagnostic sensitivity of the techniques varies according to pathology, and in particular whether the disease results in dilatation of the biliary system. For example, disorders such as choledochal cysts or choledocholithiasis that result in bile duct dilatation will be more reliably demonstrated than the subtle duct changes of sclerosing cholangitis. The latter may only be present at third- and fourth-order intrahepatic duct level. Chemical shift techniques allow differentiation of focal fat from other causes of focal pathology.

Tissue-specific agents have been developed in MRI. Super-paramagnetic agents (SPIOs, ferroxumides) contain iron particles that are phagocytosed in the liver by Kuppfer cells. Following intravenous administration, normal liver parenchyma will return low-signal intensity with accumulation of these iron particles and non-liver cell tumors as an area without uptake and higher signal intensity. Manganese (mangafodipir trisodium, MnDpDp) is an agent that is metabolized by hepatocytes. It can be used to widen the signal window between the normal liver and a metastasis, or as a method for defining lesions such as hepatomas or adenomas, where increased uptake may be seen on delayed scans at 24 hours. Careful technique, patient cooperation and experienced interpretation are necessary for the potential of these techniques to be fulfilled in everyday practice.

Arteriography

Although non-invasive mapping of the hepatic vascular anatomy (arterial, portal and hepatic venous) can be achieved with MRI, multislice CT and ultrasound, there remains a requirement for invasive vascular techniques both for diagnosis and as a prelude to intervention. The morbidity of angiography, which should not be overstated, has been significantly reduced by the use of non-ionic low-osmolality contrast media which carry a lower risk of hypersensitivity, tissue toxicity and renal failure. This has been coupled with improved registration and resolution using digital techniques. Arterial dissection and thrombosis are still potential complications, but are reduced by the use of high-flow, small-caliber catheters and heparinization during the procedure. Any invasive procedure should be preceded by a clinical risk/benefit analysis, but with careful technique and an experienced operator they carry a low morbidity.

In children with primary liver tumors, arteriography provides detailed information about their circulation (see Chapter 18). Characteristically, malignant tumors exhibit a neovascular circulation with new vessel formation, arterial or portal venous encasement and arteriovenous shunting (see Figure 3.4). Arteriography also defines the level and volume of intrahepatic shunting of the primary vascular disorders of the liver, such as infantile epithelioid hemangioendothelioma and developmental arterioportal shunts (see Chapter 15). Furthermore, anatomical variants that may influence the surgical approach to liver transplantation or surgical resection are delineated. The commonest of these

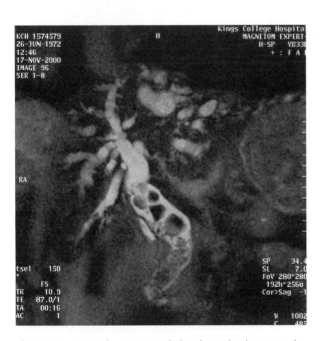

Figure 3.3 *Magnetic resonance cholangiography demonstrating calculi within a dilated common duct.*

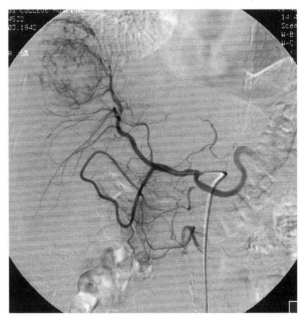

Figure 3.4 *Hepatic arteriography demonstrating the neovascular arterial characteristics of a hepatocellular carcinoma in the right lobe of the liver.*

include the replaced right hepatic artery as the first division of the superior mesenteric artery and the left hepatic artery arising from the left gastric artery.

Arterial catheterization is also a prelude to embolization as a therapy for liver tumors, a method of abating hemorrhage following blunt or penetrating hepatic trauma, and a technique for the closure of developmental intrahepatic vascular shunts. Useful occlusive agents include tissue glues, thrombin, polyvinyl alcohol and metallic coils, the choice of agent being dependent on the size and level of shunt and whether it involves an end or anastomotic artery.

Portal venography

The portal venous system can be mapped by direct or indirect portography. The latter depends on imaging the venous return following splenic or superior mesenteric artery injection using digital subtraction techniques. Shunt therapy in cirrhosis or presinusoidal venous occlusion is directed by the extent of involvement of the portal venous system. The key issue is whether there is a segment of portal, superior mesenteric or splenic vein which will allow portosystemic shunting, either surgical or via transjugular intrahepatic portosystemic shunt placement (TIPS) that will completely decompress both the portomesenteric and splenoportal venous system.

Various patterns have been described, including the following:

- occlusion of the main portal vein and first-order intrahepatic divisions;
- occlusion of the main portal vein and all intrahepatic divisions;
- total occlusion of the portal venous system.

Characteristically, venous collaterals termed cavernous transformation replace the occluded portal vein (Figure 3.5) (see Chapter 20).

The two main techniques of direct portography are splenic and transhepatic venography. Splenic venography is performed by injecting contrast through a 23-gauge Chiba needle that is inserted into the splenic tissue via an intercostal route, and sequential digital image registration. The procedure demands careful technique and interpretation. A collateral circulation will be demonstrated in the presence of extrahepatic portal vein occlusion, but the superior mesenteric vein will not be shown unless there is retrograde flow. The portogram will reflect the pattern of variceal flow, and the portal vein may not opacify if there is severe portal hypertension with hepatofugal flow into retroperitoneal splenoportal shunts and short gastric varices.

An alternative method depends on the percutaneous transhepatic cannulation of the intrahepatic portal venous system. This maneuver is also a prelude to portal vein dilatation or stenting in cases of segmental portal

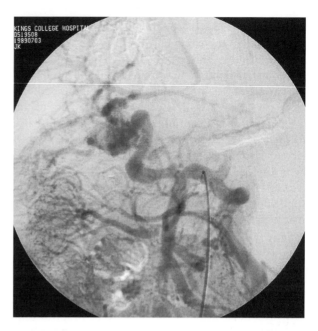

Figure 3.5 *Indirect portography demonstrating cavernous transformation of the portal vein with bridging portal venous collaterals reconstituting intrahepatic portal venous radicals.*

occlusion or stenosis that may occur as complications of liver transplantation.

PORTAL PRESSURE MEASUREMENTS

In addition to defining the anatomy of the portal venous system, a key part of the investigation of portal hypertension is the measurement of portal pressure. A direct pressure measurement may be taken during splenic or transhepatic portal venography. A pressure of 7–14 mmHg represents mild, a pressure of 15–30 mmHg represents moderate and a pressure higher than 30 mmHg represents severe portal hypertension. Alternatively, a quantification of the 'bleeding risk' can be deduced from the hepatic venous pressure gradient (HVPG), which represents the difference between the free and wedged hepatic venous pressure. This is measured using the technique of transvenous catheterization of the hepatic veins, and if it is greater than 12 mmHg, the patient is placed in a 'high-risk bleeding' category.

Cavography and hepatic venography

This technique is often coupled with pressure measurements as the method of diagnosing the cause and level in hepatic venous outflow obstruction which may complicate prothrombotic disorders, chemotherapy or liver transplantation. The diagnosis of Budd–Chiari syndrome is made by demonstrating the replacement of the main hepatic veins with a 'spider's web' of hepatic venous collaterals (see Figure 3.6). If a hemodynamically significant

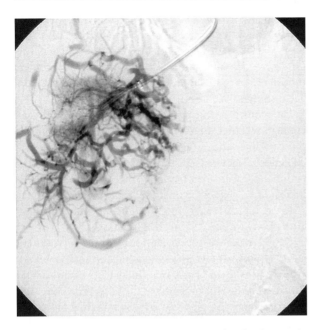

Figure 3.6 *Hepatic venography demonstrating the characteristic 'spider's web' of venous collaterals replacing the main hepatic veins in Budd–Chiari syndrome.*

stenosis is demonstrated either at a hepatic vein orifice or within the suprahepatic inferior vena cava, then balloon dilatation or stent placement is often curative.

Direct cholangiography

Direct visualization of the bile ducts is achieved by either percutaneous (PTC) or endoscopic retrograde (ERC) cholangiography. The choice of technique is dependent on the pathology and on local expertise. The techniques are complementary, not competitive.

Percutaneous cholangiography is indicated if there has been previous surgery with disconnection of the bile duct and the formation of a biliary–enteric anastomosis with, for example, a retrocolic Roux loop. This type of biliary drainage will be present after the correction of many congenital biliary abnormalities, including biliary atresia and choledochal cysts, and in most techniques of liver transplantation used for pediatric recipients. PTC can define the pattern of bile flow and the site of any biliary fistula. With the use of saline irrigation, it also allows the clearance of the bile duct of inspissated bile. As in adults, it is important to exclude coagulopathy and to administer antibiotic prophylaxis in order to avoid the potential complication of septic shock. General anesthesia is almost always required in children. Direct puncture of the intrahepatic bile ducts is usually achieved, but occasionally delayed bile duct filling occurs indirectly by diffusion of contrast from a sinusoidal injection. Opacification can also be achieved by direct puncture of the gallbladder, but there may be incomplete demonstration of the intrahepatic bile ducts if there is rapid flow

through the papilla, or if the obstruction is proximal to the cystic duct. Technically, it is important to map the biliary system fully, recognizing the normal anatomical variants and the developmental patterns at the pancreaticobiliary junction that are a key diagnostic feature of choledochal anomalies (see Chapter 10). Failure to opacify the bile ducts and the visualization of hyperplastic lymphatics are supportive diagnostic features of biliary atresia.

If obstructive bile duct pathology is confirmed, then it may be possible to intubate the bile ducts to facilitate balloon dilatation, stent insertion or clearance of calculi (Figure 3.7). With the development of the neonatal endoscope, ERCP is now possible in all age groups and across the whole range of biliary disorders. It is of particular value in the investigation of persistent conjugated neonatal jaundice, when the diagnosis of biliary atresia can be excluded if the biliary tree is visualized. This obviates the need for exploratory laparotomy and operative cholangiography in difficult cases in which biopsy and non-invasive imaging have failed to establish a diagnosis. ERCP in this age group can also be used for diagnosis of conditions such as biliary hypoplasia, sclerosing cholangitis or Caroli malformation. As in adults, the technique can be extended to allow therapeutic intervention, including sphincterotomy, extraction of calculi, balloon dilatation of strictures and stent insertion. Complications include pancreatitis, hemorrhage and sepsis.

Biopsy techniques

Needle biopsy and expert histopathological interpretation are fundamental for the correct diagnosis of pediatric disorders. Biopsy can be performed with sedation

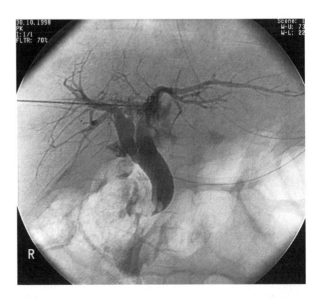

Figure 3.7 *Percutaneous cholangiogram demonstrating an inspissated bile plug obstructing the distal bile duct of an infant who presented with obstructive jaundice.*

and local anesthesia or under general anesthetic. Imaging with CT or ultrasound allows the targeting of focal lesions in the liver and safer guidance in diffuse liver disease if there is ascites or a coagulopathy. Image guidance is also indicated if the axis of the liver is abnormal following liver resection or segmental liver transplantation, when an anterior rather than a lateral intercostal route may be more appropriate. Either the Menghini or Trucut needle can be used. If there is a severe coagulopathy and a histological diagnosis is mandatory, then a transjugular biopsy is performed after transvenous catheterization of the hepatic veins. All of these approaches allow plugging of the biopsy track with occlusive agents, but this addition to the procedure is not indicated routinely.

The overall mortality of liver biopsy is less than 0.01%, but as with any invasive procedure a careful risk/benefit analysis should be undertaken and the importance of the consenting process should not be underestimated. Vascular complications include hemorrhage that may be intrahepatic, subcapsular or intraperitoneal, hemobilia and arteriovenous fistula. Further complications include biliary peritonitis, cholangitis and septic shock. The risk of inadvertent injury to adjacent organs as a complication is reduced by the use of image guidance. Continuing hemorrhage demands immediate operative or radiological intervention.

Drainage techniques

CT or ultrasound guidance allows accurate placement of drainage catheters or aspiration of collections. The choice of technique depends on the route of access and the modality that best demonstrates the pathology and its relationship to any adjacent organs. Fine-needle introduction techniques that allow graded placement of large drains are safe, carry a low morbidity and obviate the need for further surgical intervention. Specific indications include bile leaks, intrahepatic abscesses and collections following interstitial or hemorrhagic pancreatitis.

PRINCIPLES OF INVESTIGATION

This section summarizes how these techniques are applied in a clinical context and describes the characteristic features of some disorders.

Jaundice in infancy

Neonatal jaundice that persists beyond 14–21 days requires radiological investigation. Although the vast majority of these babies will have physiological jaundice, it is important to distinguish those in whom there is a conjugated hyperbilirubinemia and a structural biliary abnormality from those with parenchymal 'medical' causes where the imaging may be normal at presentation. The latter group will include the neonatal hepatitis syndrome, intrauterine infection, endocrine disorders, inborn errors of metabolism, cystic fibrosis and the storage disorders.

Ultrasound is the primary investigation and it will confirm whether there is duct dilatation. If the latter is present, then the differential diagnosis will include a choledochal cyst or inspissated bile plug syndrome. If the jaundice persists, then percutaneous cholangiography is indicated to define the anatomy as a prelude to reconstructive biliary surgery and to allow the potential clearance of any inspissated bile by saline irrigation.

If there is no bile duct dilatation and there is persistent jaundice with acholic stools, then the diagnosis of biliary atresia has to be confirmed or refuted. Early diagnosis and surgery improve the outcome of the Kasai procedure, and therefore there should be no delay in initiating radiological investigation (see Chapter 8). Radiological features that indicate a diagnosis of biliary atresia are as follows:

1 an ultrasound examination confirming the absence of dilated ducts, presence of an atretic gallbladder, bile lakes or other congenital abnormalities (e.g. polysplenia, malrotation, situs inversus);
2 failure of biliary excretion into the gut by 24 hours on an HIDA scan.

Neither of these tests is individually pathognomonic, but in combination with characteristic histological features on biopsy they will confirm the diagnosis in the vast majority of infants. Endoscopic cholangiography is reserved for those in whom the diagnosis remains in doubt following non-invasive imaging and biopsy.

Jaundice in older children

Liver disease in children older than 6 months may be acute or chronic. The aims of radiology are to distinguish between these and to define the etiology in individuals with chronic liver disease. The diagnosis of chronic liver disease is commonly made by clinical presentation and signs, but all of the non-invasive imaging techniques have the capability to confirm the clinical impression by demonstrating architectural changes within the hepatic parenchyma and signs of portal hypertension. However, it should be noted that ascites might be a manifestation of acute liver failure of any cause, hepatitis and acute pre- or posthepatic venous obstruction.

The diagnosis of an acquired or developmental biliary disorder is based on the presence of segmental duct dilatation demonstrated on ultrasound scan. PTC or ERCP, preceded by MRCP, is then indicated to determine whether there are characteristic ductal changes of a cholangiopathy such as sclerosing cholangitis with ductal irregularity, stricturing, or focal dilatation affecting the intra- or extrahepatic biliary tree. Alternatively, there may be evidence of choledocholithiasis with common duct calculi, or the characteristic features of a choledochal cyst with an anomalous pancreaticobiliary junction.

The diagnosis of drug-induced liver disease, the metabolic disorders, chronic hepatitis and other causes of either acute or chronic liver failure is made by serological means, and the role of radiology is to provide corroborative data by assessing the potential complications, and to exclude any correctable pathology. Equally, the value of a 'normal' examination should not be underestimated.

Radiological surveillance in chronic liver disease

Radiological surveillance is necessary to determine any signs of hepatic decompensation or the development of portal hypertension, and for the early detection of a hepatocellular carcinoma. Regular ultrasound examination should detect these complications and allow the appropriate selection of recipients and timing of liver transplantation. Sepsis, variceal hemorrhage and hepatic ischemia are factors that may adversely affect the outcome of transplantation, so their prompt recognition and treatment is of the utmost importance.

Any focal nodule that develops in the presence of cirrhosis demands investigation. Although the histopathological spectrum of a nodule will include nodular regeneration and adenomatous hyperplasia, it is the development of a hepatocellular carcinoma that will adversely affect survival if left untreated. Hepatocellular carcinomas of diameter less than 4 cm arising in the presence of cirrhosis are cured by liver transplantation. Hepatocellular carcinomas are characterized by pathological arterialization that can be reliably detected by dual-phase CT with arterial and portal phase studies, arterial gadolinium-enhanced T1-weighted MRI sequences, enhanced uptake at 24 hours following MnDpDP T1-weighted MRI sequences, and arteriography where the features of a nodular hepatocellular are characteristic. These techniques are often complementary, and all of them may be necessary to avoid a false-positive diagnosis, particularly if the child has well-compensated cirrhosis and the 'tumor' would be the only indication for early transplantation.

Prior to transplantation it is necessary to confirm the anatomy and patency of the portal venous system, initially by Doppler ultrasound scan and then proceeding to MRV or indirect portography if there is possible occlusion.

Liver masses

Primary liver tumors account for only 3% of all tumors in children, but they account for 15% of abdominal neoplasms. Two-thirds of these tumors are malignant.

The aims of radiology are first to define the tumor, second to predict the histological type, and third to stage the tumor accurately.

Although all of the tumors exhibit variable characteristics, there are key radiological signs which, if recognized, will lead to an accurate diagnosis. No imaging technique is pre-eminent, and the most important factor is the interpretative summation of the findings by an experienced pediatric hepatobiliary radiologist.

The specific characteristics of the individual tumors are summarized below.

MALIGNANT LESIONS

Hepatoblastoma (Figure 3.8)

USS Homogenous, encapsulated tumor that may be associated with portal venous or caval invasion.

CT Predominantly hypodense in the unenhanced and portal phase studies, with scattered segments of pathological arterialization in the arterial phase. Calcification/ossification is present in up to 40% of cases. Lymph node or pulmonary metastases are detected in 40% of cases at presentation.

MRI Low signal on T1-weighted sequences, heterogeneous signal on T2-weighted sequences and variable enhancement.

CT and MRI depict segmental and vascular anatomy. Arteriography is reserved for those cases with vascular invasion where operability for resection or transplantation remains in question.

Hepatocellular carcinoma

USS Hypoechoic nodule or diffuse area of heterogeneous parenchyma with venous invasion.

CT/MRI Arterialized tumor that becomes hypodense in the portal phase. Nodular or diffuse pattern with evidence of venous invasion.

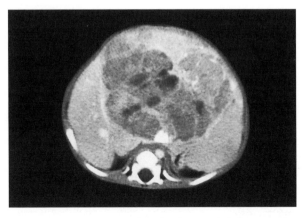

Figure 3.8 *CT demonstrating the characteristic features of a centrally placed hepatoblastoma. Note the characteristic appearances of mixed attenuation with areas of ossification.*

ANGIO Neovascular blush with irregular vessels and pathological venous shunting.

All techniques may show evidence of cirrhosis and portal hypertension. This is a 'field change' process, and therefore multifocal nodular disease is common.

Embryonal angiosarcoma

USS Echogenic myxoid matrix with increased vascularity.

CT/MRI Hypodense on CT, hypointense on T1-weighted sequences, hyperintense on T2-weighted sequences as the tumor has a cystic myxoid matrix with a pseudocapsule. Pathological arterialization in enhanced studies with venous invasion.

ANGIO Arterialized hypervascular tumor with venous invasion.

Rhabdomyosarcoma

USS Large central mass with periportal infiltration and biliary obstruction.

CT Hypodense central mass with local invasion of hepatic vasculature and adjacent viscera.

MRI Central mass that is hypointense on T1-weighted sequences, hyperintense on T2-weighted sequences with biliary and venous invasion.

BENIGN LESIONS

Infantile hemangioendothelioma

USS Single or multiple hypoechoic masses.

CT/MRI Hypervascular tumor on CT that is hyperintense on T2-weighted MRI sequences. All techniques demonstrate hypertrophy of the hepatic artery, dilatation of the hepatic veins and hypoplasia of the infrahepatic aorta. Punctate calcification is a variable feature. The tumor may be characterized by a low-volume shunt, and a pattern of centripetal enhancement with 'filling in' on the delayed phase may be seen.

ANGIO Confirms the level and volume of the shunt, the pattern of arterial supply and the potential for arterial embolization.

Mesenchymal hamartoma (Figure 3.9)

USS Multiloculate mass with cystic matrix.

CT/MRI Complex solid and cystic matrix with cystic component of high signal on T2-weighted sequences. No vascular invasion or significant vascular enhancement.

Hepatic adenoma

USS Focal hyperechoic mass with areas of hemorrhage and necrosis.

CT Hypodense, enhancing nodule in the arterial phase with central hemorrhage.

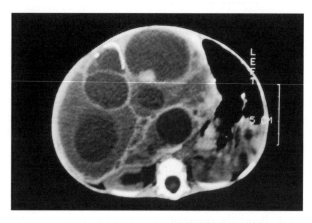

Figure 3.9 *CT demonstrating the characteristic features of a mesenchymal hamartoma, with a multiseptate mass replacing the right lobe of the liver.*

MRI Focal enhancing tumor of increased signal on T1-weighted and T2-weighted sequences, and increased uptake on delayed scans with MnDpDp enhancement.

ANGIO Hypervascular tumor. Abnormal parenchyma with deposition of fat due to glycogen storage disorders or anabolic steroid therapy may be evident as a predisposing condition. The imaging findings of a hemoperitoneum may be evident if the tumor has ruptured.

Focal nodular hyperplasia

USS Variable echogenicity, but commonly isoechoic with normal liver. Hypervascular on Doppler sonography.

CT/MRI Often contains a central scar, and is characterized by intense arterial enhancement equilibrating with normal liver in the portal phase.

ANGIO Arterialized tumor with centrifugal arterial supply creating a 'spoke-wheel' pattern with organized venous drainage.

The role of biopsy is to diagnose the lesions with indeterminate radiological characteristics and to confirm the histological diagnosis before commencing chemotherapy in tumors such as hepatoblastoma. Accurate staging and application of these techniques should ensure that children are not subjected to unnecessary laparotomy because of understaging of disease, and that those children who will benefit from curative surgery are appropriately selected.

Transplantation

The role of radiology in the pretransplant assessment is generally not one of diagnosis, but rather recognition of the sequels of longstanding liver disease or the associated anomalies that may alter the surgical approach or indeed contraindicate transplantation. The importance of defining the anatomy and patency of the portal venous system and early detection of hepatocellular carcinomas has already been stated.

Postoperatively, both diagnostic and interventional radiology are key to optimization of graft function. Although the incidence of the more common vascular and biliary complications has been reduced by improved surgical technique and experience, the development of innovative surgical techniques of segmental, split-liver, auxiliary and live-related transplantation has brought with it a new dimension of potential complications.

Early recognition and treatment of the vascular complications is key to graft survival, with Doppler ultrasound being the pre-eminent technique for confirming vascular integrity of the anastomoses. Corroborative non-invasive evidence can be obtained with CT and MRI when the parenchyma can be assessed for focal necrosis, but in the acute situation arteriography is indicated. Not only will this confirm the diagnosis, but the procedure can be extended to thrombolysis, angioplasty or stenting of an arterial or portal vein stenosis, depending on the findings.

Biliary complications include anastomotic strictures, diffuse cholangiopathy or bile leaks, all of which may be seen with ischemic liver injury (see Chapter 30). Cholestasis, cholangitis or non-specific biochemical indicators are often the presenting features. Ultrasound may be misleading, as dilatation of the ducts within the graft is a variable feature. More commonly a high-pressure/low-volume system develops proximal to the stricture. Consequently, direct cholangiography – either endoscopic for end-to-end biliary reconstruction or percutaneous for Roux-loop anastomoses – is performed, proceeding to balloon dilatation or stenting if a stricture is confirmed. This approach obviates the need for further biliary reconstruction in the majority of pediatric recipients.

Trauma

In liver trauma, CT is the single most important factor permitting safe non-operative management following blunt abdominal trauma. It allows a non-invasive method for classification of injury on an organ injury scale. Although splenic laceration is twice as common as liver laceration, it carries a significantly higher morbidity, with coexistent splenic and liver injury in up to 45% of patients. Diaphragmatic, splenic and CNS injuries are present in up to 15% of children with liver trauma and, if present, increase the mortality from 0.4% to up to 15%. 'Missed' radiological injuries resulting from suboptimal technique or misinterpretation have a measurable adverse impact on outcome, so imaging assessment needs to be complete. It should define the lobar and segmental extent of the liver injury, determine whether there is continued hemorrhage (Figures 3.10a and b) and recognize any other sites of organ injury.

Hepatic arteriography is used to define a site of continued hemorrhage, particularly if this follows surgical intervention. Any site of arterial hemorrhage can then be effectively embolized with occlusive agents, minimizing the territory of ischemia in the liver.

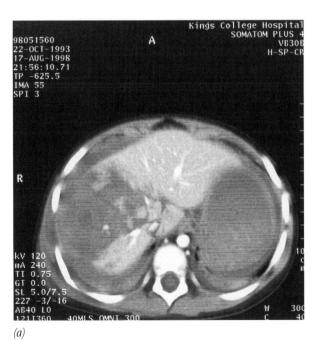

(a)

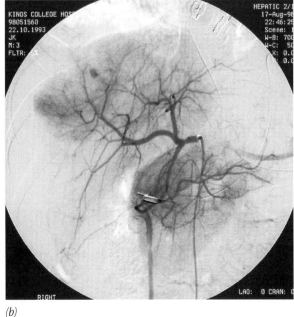

(b)

Figure 3.10 *A radiological assessment of liver trauma. (a) This CT scan defines the planes of a laceration across the right lobe, with a hemoperitoneum. (b) Subsequent arteriography confirms the site of hemorrhage with a traumatic pseudoaneurysm of the right hepatic artery. The aneurysm was treated successfully by selective embolization.*

Pancreatitis

One of the main aims of imaging in pancreatitis is to assess the severity of the chronic inflammatory change by demonstration of pancreatic calcification and duct dilatation or the sequelae of acute pancreatitis. These would include pancreatic necrosis, peripancreatic collections, cystic change or the vascular complications of pseudoaneurysm formation, and segmental portal hypertension from splenic vein occlusion. The value of CT in demonstrating these pathological changes is well documented.

Second, imaging should be directed towards confirming or refuting the presence of calculus disease or a developmental anomaly of the pancreaticobiliary ductal apparatus as predisposing causes. The latter group would include pancreas divisum and choledochal anomalies with long common channels. MRCP proceeding to direct cholangiography are the techniques used to define these potentially correctable causes.

REFERENCES

Roberts EA. The jaundiced baby. In: Kelly DA (ed.) *Diseases of the liver and biliary system in children*. Oxford: Blackwell Science, 1999: 11–45.

PART 2

Perioperative management

4

Anesthesia and perioperative care

DAVID GREEN

This chapter considers anesthesia and aspects of perioperative care in children undergoing surgery for liver disease.

PATHOPHYSIOLOGY AND PHARMACOLOGY

The liver, liver dysfunction and anesthesia

The liver has five main groups of functions:

- synthetic – producing clotting factors, acute phase proteins and albumin;
- metabolic – glucose control and control of acid-base balance;
- metabolizing – most drugs, and substances such as ammonia;
- excretion – bilirubin and drugs excreted in the bile;
- infection control – a major role in the reticuloendothelial monocyte macrophage system.

The consequences of liver failure can be seen in varying degrees in all of these five groups. They do not necessarily progress together. In general, the most obvious sign is jaundice, but increasing dysfunction such as bleeding and metabolic changes will be seen as liver failure progresses. When assessing and anesthetizing a patient with 'liver disease', due regard should be given to the degree to which these functions are disturbed. Physiological responses of the liver to surgery are discussed in Chapter 2. This chapter will concentrate on responses that are specifically related to anesthesia and the immediate perioperative period.

DRUG METABOLISM AND THE LIVER

The liver is the most important site for drug metabolism, and its role is mainly to convert active, highly lipophilic drugs to an inactive, water-soluble form that allows efficient renal and biliary elimination. This takes place in two main phases. Phase 1 utilizes the cytochrome P-450 mixed function oxidase system, causing oxidation, reduction and hydrolysis, and phase 2 involves conjugation with a variety of substances (e.g. sulphate and glucuronide). In this context, it should be noted that hepatic acinar blood flows from the periportal region to the centrilobular hepatic vein. Blood in zone 1 of the acinus (nearest to the portal venular and hepatic arteriolar tributaries) contains high levels of oxygen and nutrients, which decrease as blood flow moves away from this region through the sinusoids to zone 3 nearest the centrilobular hepatic vein (see Figure 2.2). The enzyme systems that subserve phase 2 reactions are predominantly located in zone 1, and are thus less affected by reductions in blood flow and hepatic damage than the enzymes which subserve phase 1 reactions, which are located near zone 3.

Other enzymes are both present in the liver (e.g. esterases) and produced by it (e.g. pseudocholinesterase), and may therefore be affected by parenchymal liver disease.

It should be remembered that, in advanced liver disease, increased *pharmacodynamic* sensitivity to the action of drugs such as sedatives and opioids may be seen in addition to the effects of liver disease on their *pharmacokinetics*.

Two factors must therefore be considered when examining the effect of hepatic metabolism in pediatric anesthesia, namely age and the effect of liver disease itself.

Age factors that affect pharmacokinetics

Together with deficient phase 2 glucuronidation, an alteration in drug-handling ability may be present in the neonatal and infant liver. This defect is unpredictable, but certainly drugs such as chloramphenicol must be avoided. In general, hepatic clearance is reduced and half-life of elimination ($T_{\frac{1}{2}\,elim.}$) is increased. Therefore smaller doses must be given at longer intervals. Unpredictable pharmacokinetics *and* pharmacodynamics mean that anesthetic drugs must be used with great circumspection in infants, particularly those with liver disease. In general, both phase 1 and phase 2 reactions are at or above adult levels by about 3 months of age (see below).

Pharmacokinetic alterations in liver disease

The presence of hepatic dysfunction could be expected to have profound effects on the actions and use of many drugs. Although one must differentiate between hepatocellular damage (as in neonatal hepatitis and cirrhosis) and obstructive jaundice (as in biliary atresia, inspissated bile syndrome and biliary atresia), both frequently co-exist in the pediatric patient. For example, the patient presenting for the Kasai procedure or portoenterostomy may have severe obstructive jaundice together with established cirrhosis.

Volume of distribution of a drug (V_d)

The volume of distribution of a drug (V_d) simply represents the dilutional effect of an abstract volume, unrelated to any anatomical body compartment, on a drug when administered. V_d is calculated by dividing the dose of the drug administered by the theoretical concentration of the drug, on a semilogarithmic concentration/time plot, extrapolated back to time zero.

$$V_d = dose/concentration, \text{ or}$$
$$\text{Loading dose} = V_d \times desired\ concentration.$$

The V_d of lipid-soluble drugs is usually unaffected by liver disease. However, the V_d of water-soluble drugs is often increased due to sodium and water retention consequent upon activation of the renin–angiotensin–aldosterone axis and increased levels of antidiuretic hormone (ADH).

Clearance (Cl)

Most drugs used in anesthesia and intensive care are metabolized by first-order kinetics (i.e. the amount metabolized is proportional to the drug's concentration). Metabolism thus equals a *constant* multiplied by concentration. This constant is *clearance*, and it has the units of flow (volume per unit time). Thus:

$$\text{Amount metabolized (maintenance dose)} =$$
$$clearance \times concentration.$$

Total body clearance includes both hepatic and renal contributions. Although we are only concerned with the effects of liver disease in this chapter, many patients in hepatic failure will have coexisting renal problems. For water-soluble drugs, the kidney is the main site of drug elimination. Thus:

$$\text{Total body clearance (Cl)} = \text{hepatic clearance (HCl)} +$$
$$\text{renal clearance (RCl).}$$

The following equations show the relationship between HCl, hepatic blood flow (HBF) and extraction ratio (ER). ER is a measure of the extent of the liver's capacity to metabolize a drug. A high ER equates with a drug which undergoes extensive hepatic metabolism due to high enzyme activity, and vice versa. ER is expressed as the ratio of the amount of drug being delivered to the liver, Ci (if the drug is given orally this would be the amount absorbed into the portal venous system) minus the amount leaving the liver, Co (i.e. after 'first-pass' metabolism) divided by Ci:

$$ER = (Ci - Co)/Ci.$$

HCl is simply the product of HBF and ER:

$$HCl = HBF \times ER.$$

Thus if HBF is 1500 mL/minute and the extraction ratio is 50%, then Cl is equal to 750 mL/minute.

$T_{\frac{1}{2}}$ elimination ($T_{\frac{1}{2}\,elim.}$)

This is the time taken for the concentration in the plasma to fall by one half. $T_{\frac{1}{2}\,elim.}$ is dependent on both V_d and Cl of the drug. Thus:

$$T_{\frac{1}{2}\,elim.} = (V_d/Cl) \times 0.693.$$

An increase in $T_{\frac{1}{2}\,elim.}$, and thus in the duration of drug action, can therefore be due to either an increase in V_d or a reduction in Cl, or a combination of both.

Drugs handled by the liver are often divided into 'flow limited' and 'capacity or enzyme limited'.

Flow-limited drugs

These include most opioids, propofol, local anesthetics, and beta-blockers such as propranolol and labetalol where the ER, and thus the HCl and total Cl of the drug, is high and therefore very dependent on HBF. These drugs usually undergo significant 'first-pass metabolism' if given orally, and consequently have a low bioavailability by this route. A fall in HBF (due to hypovolemia or cirrhosis) and ER (e.g. due to severe hepatic failure or cirrhosis) results in decreased Cl and thus a prolonged $T_{\frac{1}{2}\,elim.}$ and duration of action. This is exacerbated in portal hypertension (PHT) by portosystemic shunting, which may involve up to 60% of drug in the portal venous blood bypassing the liver, decreasing HCl still further. Drug-induced changes in enzyme activity (either inhibition or induction) have little effect (see next section).

Capacity- or enzyme-limited drugs

These include drugs such as diazepam, lorazepam, theophylline and thiopentone which have much lower

ERs and therefore HCls than flow-limited drugs. Their metabolism depends much more on the intrinsic metabolic activity, which may be affected by parenchymal disease *and* by enzyme induction and inhibition. Clearly, since both HBF and enzyme activity are reduced in cirrhotic liver disease, HCl of both groups of drugs is reduced. The decrease in HCl of the flow-limited drug lignocaine correlates more closely with the severity of liver disease than the capacity- or enzyme-limited drug theophylline (Colli *et al.*, 1988). In fact, the extent of lignocaine metabolism has been suggested as a 'dynamic' measure of donor hepatic function pre-operatively in determining graft survival (Oellerich *et al.*, 1989).

Some drugs, such as alfentanil, midazolam, pethidine and metoprolol, seem to be both flow and enzyme limited, and are therefore affected by changes in HBF and enzyme activity.

Protein binding

The plasma concentration of the acute phase protein, α1-acid glycoprotein, which binds basic drugs, may be elevated in acute liver failure, and increased protein binding of drugs such as lignocaine and propranolol should be anticipated. On the other hand, although the levels of albumin, which binds acidic drugs, may be low in advanced liver disease, protein binding correlates poorly with albumin levels and with the degree of liver dysfunction. Changes in plasma protein concentration will have a more pronounced effect on the distribution and pharmacological action of a highly protein-bound drug with a small V_d and a narrow therapeutic index. This does not apply to most of the drugs that are used in anesthesia (Carton *et al.*, 1994).

Choice of anesthetic drugs

Hepatic dysfunction in the child presenting for anesthesia is rarely of sufficient severity to affect one's choice of anesthetic, and most of the commonly used agents may be utilized. In general, greater reliance should be placed on short-acting analgesics, such as remifentanil, which are unaffected by liver disease (Navapurkar *et al.*, 1998) and inhalational agents such as isoflurane and desflurane for maintenance, as they undergo very little metabolism in the body. The latter are used in preference to 'fixed' drugs given by the intravenous route, which can accumulate in liver disease for the reasons mentioned in the previous section.

INHALATIONAL AGENTS

The ideal agent

In children with hepatic disease who are undergoing major abdominal surgery, the choice of agent is complex. The features of an ideal inhalational agent include the following:

- absence of hepatotoxicity;
- absence of metabolism, in order to minimize the effects of reduced hepatic function;
- absence of deleterious effects on splanchnic blood flow (SBF), in order to minimize reduction of HBF, especially during periods of hemorrhage and possible hypotension;
- maintenance of hepatic oxygen delivery and balance of hepatic arterial and portal venous flow;
- minimal effects on cardiovascular dynamics.

Hepatic function is already compromised, and may be further affected by a reduction in SBF during prolonged abdominal surgery, with the possibility of major hemodynamic disturbance due to hepatic mobilization and fluid and blood loss during the procedure. In addition, it must be remembered that repeated anesthetics are likely to be necessary in the ensuing years (e.g. for injection of esophageal varices due to portal hypertension).

Halothane hepatitis

This is a well-recognized phenomenon (Bottiger *et al.*, 1976). However, its incidence in children is known to be much lower than that in adults. Although hepatitis is believed to be more common with halothane vs. isoflurane, due to increased metabolism of the former (up to 40% vs. 0.2%), decreased halothane metabolism in children does not explain this reduced incidence, as it is similar to that in adults (Wark *et al.*, 1990). A review from the Hospital for Sick Children, Great Ormond Street, London, revealed an incidence of about 1 per 82 000 halothane anesthetics (Wark, 1983). There seems to be little evidence to support the avoidance of halothane simply on the grounds of hepatitis risk in this group of patients. Despite the spectre of hepatitis and the claimed advantages of sevoflurane, halothane will remain the agent of choice in most pediatric patients for many anesthetists (Walton, 1986; Sarner *et al.*, 1995; Welborn *et al.*, 1996; Bacher *et al.*, 1997). Isoflurane is metabolized to a very small extent by comparison with halothane and sevoflurane, and is therefore preferable according to this criterion. Desflurane is metabolized even less, showing a tenfold reduction compared with isoflurane (Ghantous *et al.*, 1991; Koblin, 1992), so is theoretically even more appropriate for these cases.

Effects of inhalational anesthetics on hepatic and splanchnic blood flow

Until the advent of sevoflurane and desflurane, isoflurane had usually been considered the agent of choice in cases where preservation of HBF and SBF was required. HBF and the hepatic artery buffer response are maintained better in the presence of isoflurane than with halothane and enflurane. Recent single and multi-agent studies have compared the effects of the newer inhalational anesthetics with isoflurane on HBF and SBF in animals, human volunteers and patients with and without underlying hepatic disease or hemorrhage. These studies are briefly reviewed here.

Animal studies

A comparative study of isoflurane vs. ketamine, enflurane and halothane in the cirrhotic rat model concluded that isoflurane was the most efficient agent in maintaining splanchnic circulation in hypovolemia (Debaene *et al.*, 1990). Another study investigated the effects of desflurane on systemic and splanchnic hemodynamics, oxygen (O_2) delivery and O_2 uptake, tissue oxygenation (as monitored by surface PO_2 electrodes) and hepatic oxygen-dependent intermediary metabolism (hepatic lactate uptake, intestinal lactate production and ketone-body ratio) in the pig. Total HBF decreased in a dose-dependent manner. Although oxygen deliveries of whole body, liver and small intestine were markedly reduced at both concentrations, respective oxygen uptake values did not change significantly. No evidence for severe tissue hypoxia could be found. Although desflurane had no adverse effects on hepatic and small intestinal metabolic function, these data indicate that hepatic and small intestinal oxygen reserve capacity is impaired by desflurane (Armbruster *et al.*, 1997).

Human volunteer studies and studies performed prior to surgery

Isoflurane has a more favorable effect on hepatic circulation than halothane (Kanaya *et al.*, 1995). A study using sevoflurane applied sensitive markers of renal and hepatic function to determine the safety of prolonged (8-hour), high-concentration (3% end-tidal) sevoflurane anesthesia in human volunteers. It was concluded that prolonged sevoflurane anesthesia administered to volunteers in a fresh gas flow of 2 L/minute did not result in clinically significant changes in biochemical markers of renal or hepatic dysfunction (Ebert *et al.*, 1998a, b). The potential toxicity of prolonged desflurane anesthesia in 13 young men was studied, and it was concluded that desflurane did not have greater toxicity than currently used inhaled anesthetics and, because of its lesser metabolism, might have less or no toxicity (Weiskopf *et al.*, 1992).

Patients undergoing major surgery without underlying hepatic disease

SBF is reduced to a greater extent by halothane than by isoflurane and desflurane, and this reduction is exacerbated by hemorrhage (Jacob *et al.*, 1991). In another study during prolonged anesthesia for head and neck surgery, HBF was more favorably maintained by isoflurane (Murray *et al.*, 1992). One study compared the effects of desflurane and equipotent doses of isoflurane and halothane on total HBF (tHBF). A significant decrease in tHBF was found in all patients regardless of the inhalation agent used, and its relationship to cardiac output also decreased significantly. No difference was found between the groups with regard to tHBF and hemodynamics. It was concluded that all of the inhalation agents included in the study significantly decreased tHBF during anesthesia (Schindler *et al.*, 1996).

Desflurane has similar hemodynamic effects to isoflurane. The effects of desflurane anesthesia vs. isoflurane have been compared on small bowel and hepatic microcirculatory flow during major surgery using laser Doppler flowmetry in a prospective, randomized, single-blind, crossover study. Desflurane anesthesia at 1 MAC (minimum alveolar concentration) was associated with significantly greater gut blood flow than 1 MAC of isoflurane. These differences could not be explained by systemic hemodynamic differences. The similarity in tHBF between groups implies an intact hepatic artery buffer response with desflurane and isoflurane (O'Riordan *et al.*, 1997).

Patients with underlying hepatic disease

A total of 40 patients with hepatic disease were studied and received either desflurane or isoflurane. It was concluded that laboratory values did not change significantly from pre- to postoperative state within 24 hours of anesthesia, and no differences in these changes were found between desflurane and isoflurane (Zaleski *et al.*, 1993).

Comment For the reasons stated above, although there seems to be little reason to avoid the use of halothane for induction of anesthesia, there is some evidence in favor of sevoflurane. For maintenance, on the grounds of minimal metabolism and equivalent effects on HBF, SBF and cardiac performance to isoflurane, desflurane in air and oxygen would seem to be a reasonable choice. As yet there is no definitive comparative study which has suggested superiority of either isoflurane, desflurane or sevoflurane for maintenance of anesthesia in children with liver disease.

NEUROMUSCULAR BLOCKERS

There is no reason to avoid the use of suxamethonium in these patients in circumstances where it has distinct advantages (e.g. rapid sequence induction and intubation). The intermediate-acting agents, such as vecuronium and atracurium, are suitable in cases where a longer duration of neuromuscular blockade is required. However, although the action of vecuronium is not prolonged in patients with alcoholic liver disease (Arden *et al.*, 1988), it is in patients with obstructive jaundice (Orko *et al.*, 1988), and therefore atracurium and cisatracurium (one of the stereoisomers of atracurium, but with less histamine release) are the agents of choice in procedures where biliary obstruction is prominent (Simpson and Green, 1986; De Wolf *et al.*, 1996).

OPIOIDS

Effect of age

Opioid analgesia in pediatrics is a vexed question, particularly in the neonate (Lloyd-Thomas, 1990). Evidence suggests that infants handle fentanyl as well as adults, with no greater incidence of respiratory depression postoperatively (Hertzka *et al.*, 1989). Indeed, clearance may be greater in this age group than in adults (Singleton *et al.*, 1987). A higher rate of clearance of sufentanil in children suggests that they would also require relatively larger maintenance doses than adults (Guay *et al.*, 1992).

A review of the English-language literature evaluated current knowledge of the metabolism and pharmacokinetics of morphine in children (Kart *et al.*, 1997). Unfortunately, such studies have not included children with liver disease. The majority of preterm neonates are capable of glucuronidating morphine, but birth weight, gestational and postnatal age influence the glucuronidation capability. Lynn *et al.* (1998) studied the clearance of morphine in postoperative infants and children who had undergone major non-cardiac surgery. From these and previous studies it was concluded that the volume of distribution of morphine was approximately 2.5 L/kg and was unrelated to age. A loading dose of 0.05 mg/kg is therefore appropriate in order to achieve an effective concentration in the range 10–20 ng/mL (0.01–0.02 mg/L). However, clearance (and therefore $T_{\frac{1}{2}\,elim.}$) ranges from about 3 mL/minute/kg in preterm babies up to 50 mL/minute/kg in children aged 6 months to 1 year. This would result in a $T_{\frac{1}{2}\,elim.}$ ranging from 0.6 to 10 hours. Maintenance infusion rates could thus vary from 6 to 60 µg/kg/hour. Time to equilibration following changes in infusion rate in preterm babies could be as long as 40 to 50 hours, or for a 6-month-old infant as little as 2 to 3 hours (three to four times the half-life). Great caution is obviously needed when managing such variability in metabolism and elimination of morphine.

Effect of liver disease

The metabolism of most opioids is flow-limited (see above). A decreased clearance, prolongation of the $T_{\frac{1}{2}\,elim.}$ and increased duration of action have been demonstrated for morphine in adults with cirrhosis (Crotty *et al.*, 1989), although not for sufentanil (Chauvin *et al.*, 1989). The latter may be accounted for by the existence of extrahepatic sites for sufentanil metabolism but not for alfentanil (Raucoules-Aime *et al.*, 1997). In mild to moderate liver disease, a reduction in oral dosage is necessitated by an increase in oral bioavailability, which may be increased by up to threefold, due not only to decreased extraction by the liver but also to portosystemic shunting. This applies particularly to pethidine and pentazocine. Drugs given by the sublingual route (e.g. buprenorphine) or parenterally require little adjustment of the dosage in mild to moderate disease. However, in moderate to severe liver disease, HBF and thus clearance fall still further, leading to a marked prolongation of $T_{\frac{1}{2}\,elim.}$. An increase in the dosage interval together with careful titration is then required.

Postoperative analgesia

Based on the information on morphine presented in the previous section, a simple formula is to put the weight in kilograms of morphine diluted in a 50-mL syringe of water and run the infusion rate at 0.25 mL/hour (for the preterm infant) rising to 2 mL/hour (for a healthy 6-month-old). This gives a range of 5–40 µg/kg/hour. In severe liver disease with encephalopathy due to increased pharmacodynamic sensitivity, these drugs must be avoided or at the very least they must be precisely titrated intravenously.

SEDATIVES

Drugs that undergo phase 1 and 2 metabolism (e.g. diazepam and midazolam) are more affected by liver disease than those which undergo primarily phase 2 metabolism, such as lorazepam (see above). Cytochrome P-450 inhibitors such as cimetidine can profoundly decrease the metabolism of midazolam. Midazolam has a $T_{\frac{1}{2}\,elim.}$ of approximately 1.5 to 3 hours, but this may be prolonged in patients with renal or hepatic dysfunction (Nordt and Clark, 1997). The cytochrome P-450 enzyme system occurs in both the liver and the kidney, and it has been proposed that some extrahepatic metabolism of midazolam may occur (Park *et al.*, 1989; Wandel *et al.*, 1994). The pharmacokinetics of midazolam in anesthetized, well-compensated, adult cirrhotic patients vs. controls have been studied (Trouvin *et al.*, 1988). Although V_d remained unaltered, the Cl of about 600 mL/minute was reduced by 25% and the $T_{\frac{1}{2}\,elim.}$ increased by 25% in these patients. This was relatively modest by comparison with diazepam, which has been shown to display an increase of 50% in $T_{\frac{1}{2}\,elim.}$. Thus in mild to moderate disease, midazolam and diazepam require a reduction in dosage, while lorazepam does not. Extreme caution is required in individuals with severe disease.

INDUCTION AGENTS

Propofol is a suitable agent for induction, as its overall pharmacokinetics, even when given by infusion to maintain general anesthesia in adults, are not affected in patients with moderate cirrhosis (Servin *et al.*, 1990). In a study of propofol infusion in pediatric patients without liver disease, recovery was slow because of the high infusion rates required to maintain satisfactory anesthesia and the large difference between the blood concentration required for anesthesia and that at which waking occurred (Short *et al.*, 1994). Propofol and sevoflurane induction have not been compared in the pediatric population with liver disease. Both agents would be suitable.

CARDIOPULMONARY FUNCTION

The presence of portal hypertension frequently leads to increased portosystemic flow and a propensity to gastrointestinal hemorrhage, which can result in severe hypovolemia and hypotension. Mild arterial hypoxemia in a child with liver disease can result from common, non-specific abnormalities such as atelectasis, pleural effusion and ascites.

Pulmonary function is also disturbed in disease associated with cirrhosis, such as cystic fibrosis. These patients require careful preoperative workup and assessment (see below). More severe hypoxemia is usually due to the hepatopulmonary syndrome (HPS), which is a triad of liver dysfunction, intrapulmonary vascular dilatation and severe hypoxia, usually refractory to oxygen therapy. This results in V/Q mismatch due to alteration of the perfusion (Q) component. The two mechanisms of V/Q mismatch are classified as precapillary vascular dilatation (type I) and intrapulmonary arteriovenous shunting (type II). The former is by far the commonest cause of HPS, and restoring normal liver blood flow and function by transplantation can improve oxygenation in the long term in this group (McCloskey et al., 1991). The causation of HPS is unclear, but it is thought to be due to an imbalance between vasodilator and vasoconstrictor elements in the lung, possibly associated with nitric oxide metabolism (Liu and Lee, 1999). The implications for anesthesia and transplantation in these patients have been reviewed elsewhere (Van Obbergh et al., 1998).

The hyperdynamic cardiovascular syndrome, with high cardiac output and low peripheral and pulmonary vascular resistance, which is frequently seen in adults, has not been so extensively documented in children.

RENAL FUNCTION

Profound alterations in the levels of renin, angiotensin, aldosterone and ADH result in alterations in fluid homeostasis. This is manifested as water and sodium retention due to impaired water and sodium excretion. The patients are often hyponatremic, with urinary sodium concentrations of less than 20 mmol/L. Some patients who present for transplantation in severe hepatic failure may be suffering from the hepatorenal syndrome and may require preoperative peritoneal dialysis. Successful transplantation usually reverses the changes.

ANESTHETIC TECHNIQUES FOR PEDIATRIC LIVER SURGERY

In the following sections, anesthetic techniques are described for procedures that are commonly required in pediatric liver surgery. An analysis of elective cases anesthetized by the author during the 10-year period from January 1989 to January 1999 is shown in Table 4.1. It can be seen that endoscopic sclerotherapy (injection of varices) is a commonly required procedure which is always performed under general anesthesia in the child (as opposed to the adult, in whom sedation is usually employed).

The demographic data for the patients are shown in Table 4.2.

Table 4.1 *Spectrum of elective pediatric liver surgery anesthetized by the author during the period from January 1989 to January 1999*

Category	Operation performed	Number
Intermediate	Esophagogastroduodenoscopy (OGD)	154
Intermediate	OGD and injection of varices	216
Intermediate	OGD and esophageal dilatation	9
Intermediate	OGD (total)	379
Major/plus	Hepaticoportoenterostomy (Kasai)	60
Major/plus	Choledochal cystectomy	17
Major/plus	Hepatic resection	6
Major/plus	Esophageal transection	1
Major/plus	Cholecystectomy (laparoscopic)	17 (10)
	Total Number Performed	480

Table 4.2 *Demographic data for the patients, and duration of surgery*

Demographic data	Mean	Minimum	Maximum	Total
Age (years)	6.1	0.1	16	—
ASA class	3	1	4	—
Weight (kg)	21	2	82	—
Duration (hours)	1.1	0.15	8	523

ASA, American Society of Anesthesiology.

Anesthesia for surgical correction of persistent jaundice in the infant

This has been the subject of a recent review, to which the reader is referred (Green et al., 2000).

DIFFERENTIAL DIAGNOSIS OF JAUNDICE IN THE NEWBORN

The differential diagnosis of persistent 'pathological' jaundice in the infant includes neonatal hepatitis, intrahepatic biliary hypoplasia, choledochal cyst and inspissated bile syndrome, as well as extrahepatic biliary atresia.

ASSOCIATED ABNORMALITIES

These are found in up to 20% of cases of extrahepatic biliary atresia, but they rarely concern the anesthetist. The *biliary atresia–splenic malformation syndrome* (also known as the *polysplenia syndrome*) is the most common, consisting of intestinal malrotation, preduodenal portal vein, polysplenia, situs inversus, absent inferior vena cava, cardiac defects and anomalous hepatic artery supply.

PREOPERATIVE PREPARATION

Vitamin K, 1.0 mg, is administered for at least 4 days intramuscularly (Yanofsky et al., 1984). Oral neomycin

(50 mg/kg) is given for 24 hours at 4-hourly intervals. Hemoglobin and clotting factors are checked, but it is rare for there to be significant coagulopathy except where the procedure is a re-exploration for a previous failed operation. One unit of blood (less than 5 days old if possible) is cross-matched. Clear fluids are administered for 24 hours and the patient is starved for 4 hours before scheduled arrival in the operating-room. An intravenous infusion is commenced either in the ward or more usually at induction of anesthesia.

ANESTHESIA

The patient is placed on a thermostatically controlled warming blanket and monitoring is attached (ECG, non-invasive blood pressure and pulse oximetry) prior to induction. Induction may be intravenous or inhalational (with halothane or sevoflurane). A reliable intravenous infusion is then started. This may prove difficult due to previous venepuncture attempts in the preoperative 'diagnostic' period. Blood loss can occasionally exceed 50% of estimated blood volume. (In re-explorations, at least two intravenous infusions are used together with central venous and intra-arterial pressure monitoring.) Nerve stimulator electrodes are placed over the median nerve at the elbow and a control 'train of four' is obtained prior to administration of the neuromuscular blocker.

Atracurium is the neuromuscular blocker of choice (Simpson and Green, 1986) and is administered at a dose of 0.6 mg/kg. This reliably produces complete neuromuscular blockade within 2 minutes, and lasts for about 45 minutes in these patients. Following tracheal intubation and insertion of a nasogastric tube (size 8 or 10 FG), maintenance of anesthesia is with isoflurane or desflurane, in air and oxygen with an FIO_2 of about 0.4. There is no evidence to date of any prolongation of the effect of atracurium with isoflurane vs. halothane (Green, 1991). The use of nitrous oxide is avoided, and this has resulted in a marked decrease in troublesome gut distension at the end of the procedure. The lungs are mechanically ventilated with humidified gases with end-tidal carbon dioxide maintained at about 3.5–4.5% (5–6 kPa). A rectal temperature probe is inserted. Intravenous antibiotics such as gentamicin (2.5 mg/kg) and cefoxitin (30 mg/kg) are administered as soon as possible after insertion of the intravenous cannula.

In the absence of nitrous oxide, morphine (0.1 mg/kg) is administered just prior to commencement of surgery, or remifentanil is given by infusion. During surgery, neuromuscular blockade is maintained with atracurium increments of 0.5–1 mg on visual reappearance of the first twitch of the 'train of four'. Maintenance crystalloid solutions must contain dextrose in order to avoid hypoglycemia. This can be administered as Plasmalyte or Hartmann's in 5% dextrose by a syringe driver at a rate of about 8 mL/kg/hour. In contrast to the case of adults

with obstructive jaundice, the use of diuretics or volume loading is not required for prevention of renal failure, as it is virtually unknown in this age group. Warmed blood is replaced as soon as it exceeds 10% of the estimated blood volume (EBV). Ascites is not usually a prominent feature in these cases, but if it is, 4.5% albumin in 0.9% sodium chloride or a suitable colloid such as Gelofusin may be administered to replace losses. Urine output is not formally assessed.

During the operation, the liver is mobilized by separating it from its ligamentous attachment to the undersurface of the diaphragm. This allows the undersurface to be rotated forwards, thereby giving the surgeon an excellent view of the porta hepatis. This mobilization may cause modest hypotension in about 50% of patients, due to kinking of the inferior vena cava behind the liver and obstruction to venous return. Additional intravenous fluids or blood and lightening of anesthesia may be necessary to maintain arterial blood pressure.

At the end of the procedure, neuromuscular function is assessed and neostigmine and atropine are administered as required. In a large percentage of patients, neostigmine is not needed (Simpson and Green, 1986). The trachea is extubated when the patient is breathing adequately and opening their eyes.

POSTOPERATIVE MANAGEMENT

The patient is returned, spontaneously ventilating with additional humidified oxygen, to the pediatric high-dependency unit. No patients have required postoperative mechanical ventilation. Monitoring of ECG, non-invasive blood pressure, temperature and pulse oximetry is continued, and intravenous fluids and blood given as required. Non-blood abdominal drainage loss is replaced with colloid, usually 4.5% albumin in 0.9% sodium chloride, and nasogastric drainage is continued until bowel activity is restored. Intravenous antibiotics are given for 5 days, watching for the appearance of increasing bilirubin and pyrexia as being indicative of ascending cholangitis, which must be vigorously treated as it often leads to significant morbidity. Long-term antibiotic prophylaxis with the use of oral antibiotics is frequently unsuccessful. However, oral neomycin may be useful in some cases (Mones et al., 1994).

ANALGESIA

Assessment of pain in this age group is fraught, and calculation of the 'right dose' and assessment of its effect is exceedingly difficult. Nevertheless, most workers advocate a regimen as indicated in the above section on opioids, backed up with a simple, five-point behavioral assessment pain scale. Despite cirrhosis and severe derangement of hepatic function tests due to cholestasis, hepatic synthetic and metabolic functions are relatively unimpaired and, as stated above, doses of opioid analgesics need little modification in this group of patients. Morphine is now the agent of choice at King's College Hospital, and is given in the regimen indicated above. However, since these patients are breathing spontaneously, *great care must be taken to avoid respiratory depression*. The sedation score is especially important, because excessive somnolence may precede severe respiratory depression (Lloyd-Thomas, 1995). Epidural analgesia with opioids has been used, but again severe respiratory depression requiring naloxone has been reported to occur 6 hours post injection, so these infants must also be closely monitored (Vila *et al.*, 1997).

Anesthesia for excision of choledochal cysts in the infant and child

Choledochal cysts represent a spectrum of congenital cystic anomalies involving the pancreaticobiliary system. Operation is by excision of the cyst and Roux-en-Y reconstruction of biliary drainage. Depending on age at presentation, anesthesia may be exactly as described for biliary atresia or a straightforward abdominal procedure at a later stage.

Anesthesia for hepatic resection

Around 80% of hepatic resections are performed for tumors, the majority of which are malignant. Hepatoblastoma is the most frequent type in children under 2 years of age, and hepatocellular carcinoma peaks at 10 years. It is important to note that the residual liver, following complete resection, is usually normal (unlike the situation in adults, where the remaining liver is often cirrhotic). Some hepatic neuroendocrine tumors have a marked propensity for intraluminal venous extension. These tumors present several anesthetic and surgical challenges, and may be resected with the use of cardiopulmonary bypass (Przybylo *et al.*, 1994).

In the Cleveland clinic series of 128 patients who underwent hepatic resection (1960–84), seven cases were pediatric (aged from 22 months to 19 years). Five of these seven cases had hepatocellular carcinoma. Despite massive involvement of the liver, subsequent chemotherapy may allow lobectomy to be performed at a later date with a good prognosis (Sesto *et al.*, 1987). The major indication in the adult is for isolated secondaries of colorectal carcinoma, while in the child metastatic tumors account for only 10% of cases (Didolkar *et al.*, 1989; Sesto *et al.*, 1987).

DIAGNOSIS AND PREOPERATIVE MANAGEMENT

Major hepatic resection in the presence of cirrhosis carries a high mortality from hepatic failure. A recent study of partial hepatectomy in adults with Child-Turcotte class B ($n = 46$) and C ($n = 17$) cirrhosis revealed major complications in 17 patients (27%), six (9.5%) of whom died within 1 month after surgery. The overall in-hospital death rate was 14.3%. Favorable factors for survival were Child class B, no transcatheter arterial embolization before surgery, young age, and low alanine aminotransferase levels before surgery. The study concluded that hepatic resection can provide a favorable result, especially in young patients with hepatocellular carcinoma complicating Child class B cirrhosis with low hepatitis activity, but that transcatheter arterial embolization before surgery should be avoided in such patients (Nagasue *et al.*, 1999).

It is obviously crucial to define whether the tumor is resectable, so CT scan and MRI, ultrasound and arteriography are performed, often under general anesthesia. The most important preoperative checks are hemoglobin, clotting profile, bleeding time, prothrombin time and partial thromboplastin time. It is necessary to crossmatch two to three times the EBV and to have fresh frozen plasma (FFP) and platelets available. Premedication is according to personal preference.

OPERATION

Refinement of our understanding of the surgical anatomy of the liver has allowed for more accurate dissection, a greater percentage of resectable tumors and reduced blood loss, which in earlier days accounted for a 25% mortality rate. Use of the Cavitron ultrasonic dissector (CUSA) has dramatically reduced peroperative blood loss, duration of operations, postoperative morbidity and mortality, ICU stay and overall hospital stay (Storck *et al.*, 1991; Thomson *et al.*, 1987). However, it may still be necessary to clamp the portal vein and hepatic artery (Pringle maneuver) to minimize excessive blood loss during critical parts of the dissection, and this can have profound effects on cardiovascular homeostasis and postoperative liver function. A new technique of hepatic resection without vascular occlusion using CUSA could decrease the morbidity in patients who have less hepatic functional reserve. It could also decrease intraoperative blood loss. This new technique avoids hepatic ischemic stress, and consequently extends the safety limits of major hepatectomy (Yamamoto *et al.*, 1999). Mobilization of the enlarged liver can also greatly restrict venous drainage, leading to reduced cardiac output and hypotension (thus the need for invasive arterial monitoring).

ANESTHESIA

Age at presentation for hepatic resection is from the neonatal period onwards. In the neonate and small infant, induction and maintenance proceed as for the Kasai procedure as described above. A conventional intravenous induction is appropriate for the older child. Monitoring is as for the Kasai procedure, including in addition a triple-lumen cannula (of appropriate size) for CVP measurement and administration of drugs and fluids, peripheral intravenous and invasive arterial blood pressure monitoring. Inotropes should be readily available. For smaller infants (< 10 kg body weight) it will be necessary to dilute ephedrine, epinephrine, calcium chloride and atropine.

Isoflurane or desflurane and air/oxygen have been found to be suitable together with analgesia (morphine, buprenorphine or remifentanil) and muscle relaxation with atracurium (by infusion and monitored with a peripheral nerve stimulator). Blood is replaced as it is lost. FFP will be necessary in the perioperative period in most cases. The following tests are performed at least every hour, and corrections are made as appropriate:

- Na^+ and K^+;
- hemoglobin and hematocrit (maintained at 30–35%);
- platelets (maintained at >50 000/mm³);
- clotting function, including prothrombin time (PT) and activated partial thromboplastin time (APTT);
- arterial blood gases;
- ionized calcium;
- blood glucose.

POSTOPERATIVE COURSE

Admission to intensive care will be required for all cases. The decision to continue intermittent positive-pressure ventilation (IPPV) will depend on individual circumstances. For the infant who has undergone massive hepatic resection it is mandatory, providing stability and enabling adequate opioid analgesia to be administered without danger of respiratory depression. It also facilitates surgical re-exploration, should this be required for bleeding in the immediate postoperative period. Major problems, apart from continued blood loss, include the following:

- normalization of clotting factors using FFP and platelets as necessitated by frequent measurement of clotting profiles;
- maintenance of ionized calcium;
- maintenance of normoglycemia – the reduced glycogen storage and gluconeogenic ability of the liver increase the possibility of hypoglycemia; 10% dextrose solutions are administered and glucose levels are checked on an hourly basis.

Anesthesia for surgical treatment of portal hypertension

Portal hypertension (PHT) is defined as blood pressure in the portal venous system exceeding 10 mmHg (normal value is < 7 mmHg). Although mainly used in adults to lower portal venous pressure, propranolol is well tolerated with minimal side-effects in pediatric patients with portal hypertension. Adherence and adequacy of dosage (> 1 mg/kg per day, more than twice daily dose

frequency) are important determinants of efficacy (Shashidhar *et al.*, 1999). Causes may be subdivided into three categories (Howard, 1991) as follows:

- prehepatic (extrahepatic) (e.g. portal venous thrombosis);
- intrahepatic (e.g. due to cirrhosis and congenital hepatic fibrosis);
- extrahepatic (e.g. Budd–Chiari syndrome – hepatic vein occlusion).

It is extremely important to make an accurate diagnosis of the cause. For example, Wilson's disease may be medically treated with regression of both the PHT and the underlying cirrhosis if commenced at an early stage.

CLINICAL IMPLICATIONS

Inability of blood to drain freely from the gut and spleen through the liver and into the systemic circulation leads to the following clinical features that are found in PHT:

1 *splenomegaly* due to poor venous drainage, one of the characteristic presenting features in children, and usually associated with thrombocytopenia;
2 *portosystemic shunting* through collaterals, particularly those in the lower esophagus and duodenum, which results in the following:
   - gastrointestinal hemorrhage, which can be sudden and catastrophic, requiring urgent expert medical and surgical treatment;
   - encephalopathy due to venous drainage from the gut bypassing the liver detoxifying processes (see above);
   - hypoxia if shunting occurs from the portal venous system into the pulmonary vein (see below);
   - failure to thrive and malnutrition due to gut wall edema consequent upon raised portal venous pressure;
   - ascites, exacerbated in particular by low serum albumin concentrations (<20–25 g/dL) in intrahepatic causes of PHT.

Treatment of gastrointestinal hemorrhage from esophageal varices

This is a medical emergency that requires urgent transfer of the patient to hospital. Reliable intravenous access with a wide-bore peripheral cannula is established, and blood is taken for group and cross-match and baseline hematological and biochemical investigations. Fluids are administered as appropriate based on clinical signs and results of investigations. The bleed may result in significant deterioration of hepatic function even in prehepatic causes of PHT, due to a further reduction in hepatic blood flow and the increased breakdown of blood products in the gut. Hemorrhage usually remits spontaneously for a time, but further measures may be necessary for control. These include reduction of splanchnic blood flow by propranolol and pitressin administration and balloon tamponade with a Sengstaken–Blakemore tube. In a study in adults, somatostatin infusion was found to be as effective as a Sengstaken–Blakemore tube in controlling acute variceal bleeding until an elective session of endoscopic sclerotherapy could be performed. However, larger studies are still needed to confirm this work (Jaramillo *et al.*, 1991).

If the bleeding resolves, further investigations can take place to assess the cause of the hemorrhage. However, to prevent recurrent bleeding, surgical treatment by endoscopic sclerotherapy is preferred.

ESOPHAGO-GASTRO-DUODENOSCOPY (OGD), DILATATION AND INJECTION OF VARICES (SCLEROTHERAPY)

The introduction of the flexible fiberoptic gastroscope, together with the ability to pass an injection needle through the biopsy channel, has enabled sclerosant solution (e.g. ethanolamine oleate) to be injected around and into the varices under direct vision. Endoscopic variceal sclerotherapy (EVS) has been regarded as the mainstay of therapy for bleeding esophageal varices in children (Stringer and Howard, 1991). However, recent data have shown that endoscopic variceal banding is just as efficacious and has fewer complications than EVS (Price *et al.*, 1996; Sasaki *et al.*, 1998). Both techniques result in a major reduction in variceal size and incidence of bleeding, and have thus revolutionized the diagnosis and treatment of esophageal varices in children. Esophageal transection and portosystemic shunting procedures, with their associated high morbidity and mortality, are rarely required to control bleeding.

INDICATIONS

An analysis of 50 children presenting for OGD over a 14-month period revealed that the main indication was for follow-up of patients who had undergone portoenterostomy in the first few months of life. Other causes, including portal vein thrombosis, congenital hepatic thrombosis and cystic fibrosis, are listed in Table 4.3. Most operations are performed for assessment and checking of variceal development or regression. However, repeated sclerotherapy can lead to stricture formation at the cardia, which may require esophageal dilatation. Following a bout of active bleeding, endoscopic sclerotherapy is performed at repeated intervals until control has been achieved.

A total of 76 procedures were performed, with some children undergoing as many as seven procedures in the 14-month period. On 27 of the 76 occasions injection of varices was required, in six cases dilatation was needed, and in 43 cases only an OGD was performed.

Table 4.3 *Indications for OGD in 50 consecutive children*

Indications	Numbers
Post-portoenterostomy	21
Portal venous thrombosis	10
Congenital hepatic thrombosis	4
Cystic fibrosis	3
Cryptogenic cirrhosis	1
Choledochal cyst	1
Miscellaneous (including dilatation)	10
Total	50

PREOPERATIVE ASSESSMENT AND MANAGEMENT

The underlying liver disease is usually well compensated with good nutritional status, absence of ascites and normal levels of albumin and bilirubin (Child's class A). However, recurrent episodes of variceal bleeding together with hypersplenism may result in low hemoglobin and platelets to a degree that requires preoperative transfusion. It is rare to perform this procedure on an actively bleeding child, as control is usually achievable by medical means in the short term, as described above. The child with cirrhosis and PHT resulting from cystic fibrosis will need respiratory assessment preoperatively, and physiotherapy and antibiotics in the perioperative period. This includes tracheal saline instillation and suction immediately following endotracheal tube insertion at induction and immediately prior to its removal at the end of the procedure. In cases of well-controlled cystic fibrosis this may be unnecessary. Table 4.4 lists the demographic data for the children together with preoperative hemoglobin and American Society of Anesthesiology classifications and duration of the procedures.

PREMEDICATION

Although this is a matter of personal preference, it must be remembered that these children are likely to undergo a large number of procedures spanning many years (>10). One bad experience at induction is likely to affect subsequent procedures, and may result in serious difficulties for the anesthetist, child *and* parents! Of the 76 procedures, 29 cases received trimeprazine elixir

Table 4.4 *Demographic data for 50 patients undergoing OGD with or without dilatation and injection of varices*

Demographic data	Results: mean values (± SD and ranges)
Age (years)	7.2 (3.75, 1–15)
Sex	24 M, 26 F
Weight (kg)	26 (13.9, 6.9–66)
ASA class	2 (2–3)
Hb (g/dL)	11.1 (1.1, 8.6–14.2)
Duration of procedure (hours)	0.4 (0.15, 0.15–0.97)

(3 mg/kg) orally 2 hours beforehand, 23 cases received no premedication (usually on request), 18 cases were given temazepam and the remainder received an opioid premedication. The eutectic mixture of prilocaine and lignocaine (EMLA cream) has been applied to both hands in the majority of patients and has been very successful in preventing venepuncture pain. These children are veterans of needlesticks and require a lot of persuasion that a needle is not going to hurt! Anticholinergics are avoided in the premedication, as they are given intravenously at induction.

INDUCTION

Induction of anesthesia is usually by the intravenous route. Endoscopy requires profound muscular relaxation unless deep inhalational anesthesia is to be employed for the procedure. Suxamethonium can be used both for intubation and for maintenance of relaxation (the latter by intermittent boluses). Although a longer-acting agent such as atracurium may be employed, the duration of the procedure is frequently too short (e.g. less than 10 minutes from induction) and could produce difficulty with reversal. The need for repeated suxamethonium injections means that precautions *must* be taken to prevent bradycardia. Only a full intravenous vagolytic dose of either atropine (20 µg/kg) or glycopyrrolate (10 µg/kg) at induction will guarantee prevention of bradycardia in all cases. An incidence of serious bradycardia (< 50 beats/minute) of 50% following repeated suxamethonium has been noted in the absence of anticholinergic medication (Green *et al.*, 1984). More recently, mivacurium has been used successfully in these patients, despite the potential for a prolonged effect due to reduced levels of pseudocholinesterase in such cases. Reversal of neuromuscular blockade is rarely necessary (Green *et al.*, 1998).

A nasogastric tube should be carefully inserted into the stomach via the nasal route in all children who weigh less than 15 kg. This is to prevent excessive gastric distension during gastroscopy, which in smaller infants can be sufficiently severe to completely prevent lung inflation. A rapid sequence induction will be necessary if the procedure is performed as an emergency, particularly during active bleeding. Although tracheal intubation is possible with a Sengstaken–Blakemore tube *in situ* (it also prevents regurgitation), it may be easier to remove it immediately prior to induction.

A normal endotracheal tube or an RAE-type pattern may be employed (cuffed or uncuffed, depending on the size of the child). In either case a very close watch must be kept on it in order to avoid accidental displacement during instrumentation and movement of the gastroscope.

MAINTENANCE

Routine monitoring is employed, including ECG, automatic non-invasive blood pressure, pulse oximetry and capnography. A low-rate alarm should be set, particularly if full vagolytic doses of anticholinergics have not been administered. Appropriate maintenance is by IPPV and isoflurane or desflurane supplementation. If suxamethonium is used, repeated boluses of 0.5 mg/kg are given on first return of muscle twitch, as monitored with a nerve stimulator. Repeat doses of mivacurium are rarely needed. In this way, anesthesia can be kept relatively light while at the same time avoiding coughing and bucking due to inadequate neuromuscular blockade.

As mentioned above, a close eye must be kept on the possible occurrence of excessive gastric distension, especially in infants. It is easily overcome by asking the surgeon to stop inflation and then by aspiration through the gastroscope.

RECOVERY

At the end of the procedure, neuromuscular function is allowed to recover and the patient is extubated on the side in a head-down position following the return of adequate respiration. Opioids are rarely required during maintenance, but they may be required postoperatively. Oxygen is administered until the patient is fully awake. The intravenous cannula should be left in place for several hours postoperatively if injection of varices has taken place. Otherwise it is removed when the patient is ready to return to the ward. Any dead space of the cannula must be flushed with saline to avoid the patient receiving an inadvertent dose of suxamethonium later on the ward. In a small patient, this can produce apnea of about 30–60 seconds if undiluted suxamethonium has been used during the operation.

Portosystemic shunting: central splenorenal shunt and mesocaval shunt

Since the introduction of sclerotherapy for the treatment of bleeding esophageal varices, the number of surgical procedures has decreased sharply. However, until the early 1980s the treatment of choice for bleeding esophageal varices was based on different variations of two main types of open surgery, namely devascularization and transection operations and portosystemic shunts (Maksoud and Goncalves, 1994).

OPERATIVE AND ANESTHETIC CONSIDERATIONS

The distal splenorenal shunt has been found to be of particular value, especially in children with extrahepatic PHT (Maksoud and Goncalves, 1994; Hasegawa *et al.*, 1999). Shunts are never used to control emergency bleeding, and may result in decompensation of hepatic function due to reduction of blood flow, even in patients with 'normal' liver function preoperatively.

Shunting is rarely performed in infants, so technical

aspects of intravenous and arterial access are not so problematic. As with any procedure where major blood loss is anticipated, adequate monitoring must be instituted. The anesthetic and postoperative management is as for hepatic resection. Following induction of anesthesia, the patient is positioned supine with the left shoulder and buttock elevated by 10 degrees with pads. The left arm is extended and attached to the anesthetic screen. Surgery may take 4 hours or more.

Transesophageal ligation of varices

This procedure is used to control acute bleeding in cases where medical management and injection sclerotherapy have failed (and thus is rarely needed for this indication), or more commonly to reduce recurrent bleeding in patients who do not have suitable vessels for shunting.

OPERATIVE AND ANESTHETIC CONSIDERATIONS

The procedure is performed in a lateral position, with the left side up in preparation for transverse thoracotomy. The incision is made just inferior to the tip of the scapula. The lung is retracted and the esophagus is mobilized and encircled. There is no need for endobronchial intubation, as lung deflation is assisted by temporary disconnection of the breathing circuit whilst the lung is simultaneously retracted by the surgeon. IPPV is then reinstituted. The esophagus is entered longitudinally after withdrawal of the nasogastric tube, and is opened for a length of 5–6 cm, down to the esophagogastric junction. The tortuous and dilated veins are identified and oversewn and the esophagus is then closed. Chest drainage is continued into the postoperative period, with a chest X-ray performed to check for optimal lung inflation. Operation can also be performed through an abdominal approach, thereby avoiding thoracotomy and chest drainage. In either case, blood loss may be massive and adequate facilities for rapid transfusion must be available.

Anesthesia for pediatric liver transplantation

Newer surgical techniques and immunosuppressive therapies have resulted in pediatric liver transplantation being available for most children with end-stage liver disease. Survival rates at 1 year for patients with chronic liver disease approach 90%. Survival of critically ill patients transplanted for acute liver failure approach 80% at 1 year, whereas mortality rates without transplantation are 70–80% (Cottam and Jenkins, 1999). The commonest indications for pediatric liver transplantation are biliary atresia (43%), metabolic disease (13%) and acute hepatic necrosis (11%). For approximately 75% of children with acute hepatic failure, the cause is

unknown. The timing of liver transplantation not only affects survival rate, but may also influence neurodevelopmental outcome. Fortunately, numerous types of donors, such as reduced sized, living related or unrelated and blood-type mismatched, have reduced the mortality of children who are waiting for liver transplantation. However, the mortality and morbidity before and after liver transplantation remain high for children who have fulminant hepatic failure or who are less than 5 months of age at the time of transplantation. The principal medical complications after liver transplantation are rejection, infection and multiple system organ failure (Starzl et al., 1987; Chardot et al., 1999; Cottam and Jenkins, 1999; Cox et al., 1999) (see Chapters 27 and 29).

ANESTHETIC MANAGEMENT

Preoperative assessment
Cardiopulmonary and renal problems may occur with the presence of hypoxemia and renal failure, as described earlier. The patient is often in end-stage liver disease in intensive care, in which case he or she may be receiving respiratory, cardiac and renal support (intubated and ventilated, on inotropes and undergoing peritoneal dialysis). However, in some series the majority of patients transplanted are non-urgent, and are thus fitter candidates for this procedure (Kalayoglu et al., 1989).

Prediction of intraoperative blood loss
The coagulopathy of end-stage liver disease involves deficiencies not only of those coagulation factors which are produced by the liver, but also of those factors which control coagulation and fibrinolysis. This imbalance between coagulation and fibrinolysis can lead to unpredictable coagulation changes, especially during the anhepatic and reperfusion phases of the operation.

Since blood loss may reach 10 times the EBV, at least 5 times EBV should be cross-matched together with adequate supplies of FFP, cryoprecipitate and platelets. The use of autotransfusion equipment peroperatively has become a standard method for reducing requirements for autologous blood products (Van Voorst et al., 1985; Rettke et al., 1989). Factors which can be used to predict blood loss would obviously be useful and would ease the burden of the transfusion laboratory (Lichtor et al., 1988).

As the technical skills have developed, some of these factors have become less important. In general, blood loss is greater in the following circumstances:

- the presence of portal vein hypoplasia or thrombosis, inpatient medical support, and use of a reduced-size liver graft (Ozier et al., 1995);
- those patients who have had a previous portoenterostomy due to the presence of (and shunting through) extensive adhesions, and those patients who have previously undergone portocaval shunting (Brems et al., 1987). More recent studies have failed

to demonstrate the prognostic significance of previous abdominal surgery (Ozier *et al.*, 1995);

- age < 2.5 years with associated PT >15, encephalopathy, bleeding varices, acute liver disease, planned segmental transplant (RLT) and being in an intensive-care unit prior to transplantation (Lichtor *et al.*, 1988).

Abnormalities of coagulation

Important differences exist between coagulation in pediatric and adult liver transplant patients (Abengochea *et al.*, 1995). Normal adult levels of vitamin-K-dependent clotting factors may not be reached for several weeks in the normal neonate. During the first few days of life, the already decreased levels of factors VII, IX and X and prothrombin become progressively lower, and this decrease can be prevented by administering vitamin K. Other vitamin-K-dependent proteins synthesized by the liver include proteins C and S. Protein C inhibits the function of factors VIII and V and enhances fibrinolysis; these properties are enhanced by protein S. Levels of protein C are significantly reduced in plasma from healthy, full-term, newborn infants, and remain below the levels found in serum from adults for at least 6 months. Protein S concentrations are reduced, but increase to within the range found in normal adult plasma by 3 months of age. After liver transplantation in children, a decrease in the plasma concentrations of both protein C and antithrombin III occur to below 50% of normal values, and this persists for 10 days, producing a hypercoagulable state. A similar but less prolonged decrease is seen in adults. Immediately after surgery, a 10-fold increase in plasminogen-activator inhibitor occurs, with a further increase 6–9 days later. Therefore between days 4 and 10 in the immediate postoperative period, children are at increased risk of thrombosis, especially of the hepatic artery. An attempt to minimize this risk may require anticoagulation therapy involving intravenous heparin, aspirin and antithrombin III.

Intraoperative care

It is absolutely essential for a team approach to be closely and carefully organized. This involves not only the intraoperative team of surgeons, nurses, anesthetists and technicians, but also support services such as porters, laboratory staff, transfusion laboratory services, and so on. The timing of the operation should be coordinated with the donor procurement team such that operation on the recipient commences when the donor organ is deemed to be satisfactory, and recipient hepatectomy does not begin until the donor liver arrives in the operating-room.

ANESTHETIC TECHNIQUE

This follows the scheme for hepatic resection. However, an additional triple-lumen cannula (specifically for infusion of dopamine and other drugs) and arterial line are necessary. The latter allows one line for monitoring blood pressure and one line for arterial sampling. A thermistor-tipped, flow-directed pulmonary artery catheter can be used in selected cases although, unlike the situation in adults, the wedge pressure has not proved superior to central venous pressure (Borland *et al.*, 1985). More recent methods of measuring cardiac output, such as suprasternal aortovelography, pulse contour methods and CO_2 breathing are less invasive than conventional thermodilution techniques, and show promise for the future. The operation has three major phases, which produce profoundly different physiological changes and should be noted by the anesthetic team. These phases are described below.

Phase 1: preparation for recipient hepatectomy

Operation is performed through a bilateral subcostal incision with xiphoid excision. Dense adhesions will be present if a Kasai procedure or portocaval shunt has been performed previously. Blood loss may therefore be excessive at this stage, as the surgeon attempts to identify structures in the porta hepatis, which has been altered by previous surgery. The bile duct and hepatic artery are divided and the supra- and infrahepatic venae cavae and portal vein are identified, mobilized and encircled. It is essential to optimize blood volume and cardiovascular status during this stage in order to avoid unnecessary hypotension in phase 2.

Phase 2: the anhepatic phase

This commences when the vena caval and portal veins are clamped and divided. It produces a significant reduction in venous return to the heart, and may result in a profound fall in blood pressure. In adults and children over 25 kg, this may be severe enough to require venovenous bypass in which the femoral and portal veins are cannulated and blood is returned to the axillary vein using heparin-bonded Gott shunts and a Biomedicus pump. Systemic heparinization is not needed provided that flow exceeds 1 L/minute. Cardiovascular hemostasis is preserved and portal venous distension is reduced. Technical difficulties with regard to shunt size and flow maintenance are encountered in children under 25 kg. However, they seem to tolerate cross-clamping well due to their greater cardiac reserve. For this reason, venovenous bypass is rarely employed.

Increasingly, a 'piggyback' technique is used whereby the recipient's liver is filleted off the inferior vena cava and a temporary portocaval shunt is inserted to decompress the splanchnic circulation. The advantage of this technique is that the anhepatic phase can be completed without major interruption to the caval flow, avoiding the need for either volume loading or the complexity of an extracorporeal circuit. Cross-clamping is reserved for small children, and bypass for cases in which the additional dissection required is impossible (Cottam and Jenkins, 1999).

During this stage the suprahepatic vena cava is anastomosed to the donor organ which is being flushed out via the portal vein with cold normal saline. The infrahepatic vena cava is left partially open to allow the flush (containing hyperkalemic preservative) to exit. Once the liver has been flushed, the portal vein anastomosis is made and the infrahepatic anastomosis is completed in preparation for reperfusion of the donor liver.

Phase 3: reperfusion of the donor liver

Once the portal vein clamp has been released, the liver is reperfused and the clamps on the supra- and infrahepatic venae cavae are removed. Venous return to the heart is re-established and cardiac output increases. However, depending on the adequacy of flushing, the patient may become severely hyperkalemic during this stage (occasionally necessitating treatment with calcium chloride and sodium bicarbonate) and then, when the liver begins to function, severely hypokalemic. Once hemostasis has been achieved, the hepatic artery and bile duct anastomoses are completed.

Hepatic venous oxygen saturation can provide a simple index of the initial graft status and be useful for a rapid etiological diagnosis of early postoperative graft dysfunction, and for estimating the graft outcome after liver transplantation (Shimizu et al., 1996).

Profound disturbances of coagulation may occur, and these must be closely monitored and treated. The thromboelastograph (TEG) is often used alongside conventional tests to detect clotting abnormalities intraoperatively during liver transplantation (Mallett and Cox, 1992). Major changes in clotting occur during reperfusion, including prolongation of PT, APTT and thrombocytopenia, correction being achieved in most instances by administration of FFP, platelets and cryoprecipitate. Excessive fibrinolytic activity may occasionally require treatment with ε-aminocaproic acid (EACA), tranexamic acid or aprotinin. A heparin effect has been demonstrated post reperfusion (Kang et al., 1989) and detected using heparinase- coated sample pots in the TEG (Harding et al., 1997).

Aprotinin, a broad-spectrum serine protease inhibitor, has been used to inhibit plasminogen-activator-mediated fibrinolysis (Cottam et al., 1991). Although some success has been reported (Grosse et al., 1991), and it appeared to show benefit and superiority over EACA (Llamas et al., 1998; Scudamore et al., 1995), a randomized trial in liver transplant recipients showed no significant reduction in intraoperative bleeding (Garcia-Huete et al., 1997). Despite the use of warming blankets, heated humidifiers, a warm environment and heated intravenous fluids, core temperature may fall during the procedure.

Both dopamine (2–3 µg/kg/minute) and mannitol (0.5–1 g/kg) have been used to help to maintain urine output and renal function. There is little direct evidence to support their use in the pediatric population.

INTRAOPERATIVE COMPLICATIONS

The following complications have been reported:

- air embolism in venovenous bypass or inadequate flushing of the implanted liver;
- hemodynamic instability due to bleeding, coagulopathies, hyperkalemia and hypokalemia, and myocardial depression due to acidosis or hypocalcemia;
- metabolic abnormalities such as hypoglycemia (common in children), hypocalcemia and citrate intoxication and acidosis;
- pulmonary complications, including pneumothorax, pleural effusion and atelectasis;
- difficulty in closure with large organs (this has been reduced with increasing use of RLT).

POSTOPERATIVE COURSE IN INTENSIVE CARE

The intensive-care course following pediatric liver transplantation has been reported in 16 patients (average age 9.5 years) from London, Ontario (Sommerauer et al., 1988). In total, 11 of the 16 patients survived, with one intraoperative death in a retransplant. The remaining deaths occurred late in the post-transplant period. All patients required IPPV and assisted respiration, 10 of the 16 patients for about 3 days, and longer for the rest. Three patients required continuing catecholamine support with dopamine. Kalayoglu and colleagues (Kalayoglu et al., 1989) reported an average duration of ICU stay of 3 to 4 days, and average duration of hospital stay of 38 days.

Immunosuppressive regimens and the treatment of acute rejection episodes in the immediate postoperative period are discussed in Chapter 29.

Problems encountered postoperatively in the ICU include the following:

- persistent hypertension (not common in adults) despite good pain relief and sedation and normal filling pressure (Sommerauer et al., 1988). The mechanism is unknown, but may be associated with hypomagnesemia (c.f. eclampsia and essential hypertension). It responds to sodium nitroprusside or hydralazine;
- bradydysrhythmias, presumably resulting from metabolic derangement. If, as is usual, it is not associated with hypotension, then treatment is unnecessary;
- metabolic problems, including hyperglycemia, hypocalcemia and hypokalemia. Hypomagnesemia requires oral and intravenous supplementation (Sommerauer et al., 1988). Hypophosphatemia was noted to be a serious problem in 70% of patients in the Dallas series (Andrews et al., 1989);
- despite a low rate of intravenous line sepsis, the main postoperative problem is still persistent infection in the immunosuppressed patient;
- re-exploration for surgical problems, such as hepatic artery thrombosis, may be required (see Chapter 30).

CONCLUSION

This chapter has covered aspects of anesthesia and perioperative care of patients undergoing surgery for pediatric liver disease. Provided that due consideration is given to the points mentioned, these patients tolerate surgery and anesthesia extremely well.

Key references

Green DW, Howard ER, Davenport M. Anaesthesia, perioperative management and outcome of correction of extrahepatic biliary atresia in the infant: a review of 50 cases in the King's College Hospital series. *Paediatric Anaesthesia* 2000; **10**: 581–9.

Most work on anesthesia for patients with liver disease has concentrated on adult patients. This is one of the few review papers to consider the problems of perioperative management of children with liver disease who are undergoing major abdominal surgery.

Lloyd-Thomas AR. Pain management in paediatric patients. *British Journal of Anaesthesia* 1990; **64**: 85–104.

This review was one of the first to draw attention to the differences in postoperative pain management in children compared with adults, a subject which had hitherto been virtually ignored. Many of the questions raised in the review remain unanswered!

O'Riordan J, O'Beirne HA, Young Y, Bellamy MC. Effects of desflurane and isoflurane on splanchnic microcirculation during major surgery. *British Journal of Anaesthesia* 1997; **78**: 95–6.

This is a report of one of the few randomized, single-blind, crossover studies that have been able to delineate differences in splanchnic microcirculatory blood flow between anesthetics in humans during surgery. In this case, desflurane proved to be superior to isoflurane.

Van Obbergh LJ, Carlier M, De Kock M, Otte JB, Moulin D, Veyckemans F. Hepatopulmonary syndrome and liver transplantation: a review of the peroperative management of seven paediatric cases. *Paediatric Anaesthesia* 1998; **8**: 59–64.

This is a fascinating study of a group of patients previously thought to be unsuitable for transplantation. All seven patients reversed their hepatopulmonary syndrome, showing that liver transplantation can be successfully achieved in severely hypoxemic children, and that postoperative correction of the right to left shunt is then obtained.

REFERENCES

Abengochea A, Vila JJ, Jimenez J *et al*. Pediatric liver transplantation (letter). *Anesthesia and Analgesia* 1995; **80**: 851–2.

Andrews WS, Wanek E, Fyock B, Gray S, Benser M. Pediatric liver transplantation: a 3-year experience. *Journal of Pediatric Surgery* 1989; **24**: 77–82.

Arden JR, Lynam DP, Castagnoli KP, Canfell PC, Cannon JC, Miller RD. Vecuronium in alcoholic liver disease: a pharmacokinetic and pharmacodynamic analysis. *Anesthesiology* 1988; **68**: 771–6.

Armbruster K, Noldge-Schomburg GF, Dressler IM, Fittkau AJ, Haberstroh J, Geiger K. The effects of desflurane on splanchnic hemodynamics and oxygenation in the anesthetized pig. *Anesthesia and Analgesia* 1997; **84**: 271–7.

Bacher A, Burton AW, Uchida T, Zornow MH. Sevoflurane or halothane anesthesia: can we tell the difference? *Anesthesia and Analgesia* 1997; **85**: 1203–6.

Borland LM, Roule M, Cook DR. Anesthesia for pediatric orthotopic liver transplantation. *Anesthesia and Analgesia* 1985; **64**: 117–24.

Bottiger LE, Dalen E, Hallen B. Halothane-induced liver damage: an analysis of the material reported to the Swedish Adverse Drug Reaction Committee, 1966–1973. *Acta Anaesthesiologica Scandinavica* 1976; **20**: 40–6.

Brems JJ, Hiatt JR, Colonna JOD *et al*. Variables influencing the outcome following orthotopic liver transplantation. *Archives of Surgery* 1987; **122**: 1109–11.

Carton EG, Rettke SR, Plevak DJ, Geiger HJ, Kranner PW, Coursin DB. Perioperative care of the liver transplant patient. Part 1. *Anesthesia and Analgesia* 1994; **78**: 120–33.

Chardot C, Branchereau S, de Dreuzy O *et al*. Paediatric liver transplantation with a split graft: experience at Bicetre. *European Journal of Pediatric Surgery* 1999; **9**: 146–52.

Chauvin M, Ferrier C, Haberer JP *et al*. Sufentanil pharmacokinetics in patients with cirrhosis. *Anesthesia and Analgesia* 1989; **68**: 1–4.

Colli A, Buccino G, Cocciolo M, Parravicini R, Scaltrini G. Disposition of a flow-limited drug (lidocaine) and a metabolic capacity-limited drug (theophylline) in liver cirrhosis. *Clinical Pharmacology and Therapeutics* 1988; **44**: 642–9.

Cottam S, Jenkins S. Anaesthetic principles in liver transplantation. *Current Anaesthesia and Critical Care* 1999; **10**: 291–8.

Cottam S, Hunt B, Segal H, Ginsburg R, Potter D. Aprotinin inhibits tissue plasminogen activator-mediated fibrinolysis during orthotopic liver transplantation. *Transplantation Proceedings* 1991; **23**: 1933–7.

Cox KL, Berquist WE, Castillo RO. Paediatric liver transplantation: indications, timing and medical complications. *Journal of Gastroenterology and Hepatology* 1999; **14(Supplement 1)**: S61–6.

Crotty B, Watson KJ, Desmond PV *et al*. Hepatic extraction of morphine is impaired in cirrhosis. *European Journal of Clinical Pharmacology* 1989; **36**: 501–6.

Debaene B, Goldfarb G, Braillon A, Jolis P, Lebrec D. Effects of ketamine, halothane, enflurane, and isoflurane on systemic and splanchnic hemodynamics in normovolemic and hypovolemic cirrhotic rats. *Anesthesiology* 1990; **73**: 118–24.

De Wolf AM, Freeman JA, Scott VL *et al*. Pharmacokinetics and pharmacodynamics of cisatracurium in patients with end-stage liver disease undergoing liver transplantation. *British Journal of Anaesthesia* 1996; **76**: 624–8.

Didolkar MS, Fitzpatrick JL, Elias EG *et al*. Risk factors before hepatectomy, hepatic function after hepatectomy and computed tomographic changes as indicators of mortality from hepatic failure. *Surgery, Gynecology and Obstetrics* 1989; **169**: 17–26.

Ebert TJ, Frink EJ Jr, Kharasch ED. Absence of biochemical evidence for renal and hepatic dysfunction after 8 hours of 1.25 minimum alveolar concentration sevoflurane anesthesia in volunteers. *Anesthesiology* 1998a; **88**: 601–10.

Ebert TJ, Messana LD, Uhrich TD, Staacke TS. Absence of renal and hepatic toxicity after 4 hours of 1.25 minimum alveolar concentration sevoflurane anesthesia in volunteers. *Anesthesia and Analgesia* 1998b; **86**: 662–7.

Garcia-Huete L, Domenech P, Sabate A, Martinez-Brotons F, Jaurrieta E, Figueras J. The prophylactic effect of aprotinin on intraoperative bleeding in liver transplantation: a randomized clinical study. *Hepatology* 1997; **26**: 1143–8.

Ghantous HN, Fernando J, Gandolfi AJ, Brendel K. Minimal biotransformation and toxicity of desflurane in guinea pig liver slices. *Anesthesia and Analgesia* 1991; **72**: 796–800.

Green DW. Comparison of isoflurane and halothane on recovery time from neuromuscular blockade using atracurium in infants with hepatic dysfunction undergoing major abdominal surgery. *Paediatric Anaesthesia* 1991; **1**: 125–8.

Green DW, Bristow AS, Fisher M. Comparison of i.v. glycopyrrolate and atropine in the prevention of bradycardia and arrhythmias following repeated doses of suxamethonium in children. *British Journal of Anaesthesia* 1984; **56**: 981–5.

Green DW, Fisher M, Sockalingham I. Mivacurium compared with succinylcholine in children with liver disease. *British Journal of Anaesthesia* 1998; **81**: 463–5.

Green DW, Howard ER, Davenport M. Anaesthesia, perioperative management and outcome of correction of extrahepatic biliary atresia in the infant: a review of 50 cases in the King's College Hospital series. *Paediatric Anaesthesia* 2000; **10**: 581–9.

Grosse H, Lobbes W, Frambach M, von Broen O, Ringe B, Barthels M. The use of high-dose aprotinin in liver transplantation: the influence on fibrinolysis and blood loss. *Thrombosis Research* 1991; **63**: 287–97.

Guay J, Gaudreault P, Tang A, Goulet B, Varin F. Pharmacokinetics of sufentanil in normal children. *Canadian Journal of Anaesthesia* 1992; **39**: 14–20.

Harding SA, Mallett SV, Peachey TD, Cox DJ. Use of heparinase-modified thrombelastography in liver transplantation. *British Journal of Anaesthesia* 1997; **78**: 175–9.

Hasegawa T, Tamada H, Fukui Y, Tanano H, Okada A. Distal splenorenal shunt with splenopancreatic disconnection for portal hypertension in biliary atresia. *Pediatric Surgery International* 1999; **15**: 92–6.

Hertzka RE, Gauntlett IS, Fisher DM, Spellman MJ. Fentanyl-induced ventilatory depression: effects of age. *Anesthesiology* 1989; **70**: 213–18.

Howard ER. Aetiology of portal hypertension and anomalies of the portal venous system. In: Howard ER (ed.) *Surgery of liver disease in children*. Oxford: Butterworth-Heinemann, 1991: 151–6.

Jacob L, Boudaoud S, Payen D *et al*. Isoflurane, and not halothane, increases mesenteric blood flow supplying esophageal ileocoloplasty. *Anesthesiology* 1991; **74**: 699–704.

Jaramillo JL, de la Mata M, Mino G, Costan G, Gomez-Camacho F. Somatostatin versus Sengstaken balloon tamponade for primary haemostasis of bleeding esophageal varices. A randomized pilot study. *Journal of Hepatology* 1991; **12**: 100–5.

Kalayoglu M, Stratta RJ, Sollinger HW *et al*. Liver transplantation in infants and children. *Journal of Pediatric Surgery* 1989; **24**: 70–6.

Kanaya N, Iwasaki H, Namiki A. Noninvasive ICG clearance test for estimating hepatic blood flow during halothane and isoflurane anaesthesia. *Canadian Journal of Anaesthesia* 1995; **42**: 209–12.

Kang Y, Borland LM, Picone J, Martin LK. Intraoperative coagulation changes in children undergoing liver transplantation. *Anesthesiology* 1989; **71**: 44–7.

Kart T, Christrup LL, Rasmussen M. Recommended use of morphine in neonates, infants and children based on a literature review. Part 1. Pharmacokinetics. *Paediatric Anaesthesia* 1997; **7**: 5–11.

Koblin DD. Characteristics and implications of desflurane metabolism and toxicity. *Anesthesia and Analgesia* 1992; **75**(**Supplement 4**): S10–16.

Lichtor JL, Emond J, Chung MR, Thistlethwaite JR, Broelsch CE. Pediatric orthotopic liver transplantation: multifactorial predictions of blood loss. *Anesthesiology* 1988; **68**: 607–11.

Liu H, Lee SS. Cardiopulmonary dysfunction in cirrhosis. *Journal of Gastroenterology and Hepatology* 1999; **14**: 600–8.

Llamas P, Cabrera R, Gomez-Arnau J, Fernandez MN. Hemostasis and blood requirements in orthotopic liver transplantation with and without high-dose aprotinin. *Haematologica* 1998; **83**: 338–46.

Lloyd-Thomas A. Assessment and control of pain in children (editorial). *Anaesthesia* 1995; **50**: 753–5.

Lloyd-Thomas AR. Pain management in paediatric patients. *British Journal of Anaesthesia* 1990; **64**: 85–104.

Lynn A, Nespeca MK, Bratton SL, Strauss SG, Shen DD. Clearance of morphine in postoperative infants during intravenous infusion: the influence of age and surgery. *Anesthesia and Analgesia* 1998; **86**: 958–63.

McCloskey JJ, Schleien C, Schwarz K, Klein A, Colombani P. Severe hypoxemia and intrapulmonary shunting resulting from cirrhosis reversed by liver transplantation in a pediatric patient. *Journal of Pediatrics* 1991; **118**: 902–4.

Maksoud JG, Goncalves ME. Treatment of portal hypertension in children. *World Journal of Surgery* 1994; **18**: 251–8.

Mallett SV, Cox DJA. Thromboelastography. *British Journal of Anaesthesia* 1992; **69**: 307–13.

Mones RL, DeFelice AR, Preud'Homme D. Use of neomycin as the prophylaxis against recurrent cholangitis after Kasai portoenterostomy. *Journal of Pediatric Surgery* 1994; **29**: 422–4.

Murray JM, Rowlands BJ, Trinick TR. Indocyanine green clearance and hepatic function during and after prolonged anaesthesia: comparison of halothane with isoflurane. *British Journal of Anaesthesia* 1992; **68**: 168–71.

Nagasue N, Kohno H, Tachibana M, Yamanoi A, Ohmori H, El-Assal ON. Prognostic factors after hepatic resection for hepatocellular carcinoma associated with Child-Turcotte class B and C cirrhosis. *Annals of Surgery* 1999; **229**: 84–90.

Navapurkar VU, Archer S, Gupta SK, Muir KT, Frazer N, Park GR. Metabolism of remifentanil during liver transplantation. *British Journal of Anaesthesia* 1998; **81**: 881–6.

Nordt SP, Clark RF. Midazolam: a review of therapeutic uses and toxicity. *Journal of Emergency Medicine* 1997; **15**: 357–65.

Oellerich M, Burdelski M, Ringe B *et al*. Lignocaine metabolite formation as a measure of pretransplant liver function. *Lancet* 1989; **1**: 640–2.

O'Riordan J, O'Beirne HA, Young Y, Bellamy MC. Effects of desflurane and isoflurane on splanchnic microcirculation during major surgery. *British Journal of Anaesthesia* 1997; **78**: 95–6.

Orko R, Alila A, Rosenberg PH. Effect of biliary obstruction on muscle relaxation with vecuronium. *European Journal of Anaesthesiology* 1988; **5**: 9–14.

Ozier YM, Le Cam B, Chatellier G *et al*. Intraoperative blood loss in pediatric liver transplantation: analysis of preoperative risk factors. *Anesthesia and Analgesia* 1995; **81**: 1142–7.

Park GR, Manara AR, Dawling S. Extrahepatic metabolism of midazolam. *British Journal of Clinical Pharmacology* 1989; **27**: 634–7.

Price MR, Sartorelli KH, Karrer FM, Narkewicz MR, Sokol RJ, Lilly JR. Management of esophageal varices in children by endoscopic variceal ligation. *Journal of Pediatric Surgery* 1996; **31**: 1056–9.

Przybylo HJ, Stevenson GW, Backer C *et al*. Anesthetic management of children with intracardiac extension of abdominal tumors. *Anesthesia and Analgesia* 1994; **78**: 172–5.

Raucoules-Aime M, Kaidomar M, Levron JC *et al*. Hepatic disposition of alfentanil and sufentanil in patients undergoing orthotopic liver transplantation. *Anesthesia and Analgesia* 1997; **84**: 1019–24.

Rettke SR, Chantigian RC, Janossy TA *et al*. Anesthesia approach to hepatic transplantation. *Mayo Clinic Proceedings* 1989; **64**: 224–31.

Sarner JB, Levine M, Davis PJ, Lerman J, Cook DR, Motoyama EK. Clinical characteristics of sevoflurane in children. A comparison with halothane. *Anesthesiology* 1995; **82**: 38–46.

Sasaki T, Hasegawa T, Nakajima K *et al*. Endoscopic variceal ligation in the management of gastroesophageal varices in postoperative biliary atresia. *Journal of Pediatric Surgery* 1998; **33**: 1628–32.

Schindler E, Muller M, Zickmann B, Kraus H, Reuner KH, Hempelmann G. Untersuchungen zur Durchblutung der Leber beim Menschen nach 1 MAC Desfluran im Vergleich zu Isofluran und Halothan. *Anasthesiologie, Intensivmedizin, Notfallmedizin, Schmerztherapie* 1996; **31**: 344–8.

Scudamore CH, Randall TE, Jewesson PJ *et al*. Aprotinin reduces the need for blood products during liver transplantation. *American Journal of Surgery* 1995; **169**: 546–9.

Servin F, Cockshott ID, Farinotti R, Haberer JP, Winckler C, Desmonts JM. Pharmacokinetics of propofol infusions in patients with cirrhosis. *British Journal of Anaesthesia* 1990; **65**: 177–83.

Sesto ME, Vogt DP, Hermann RE. Hepatic resection in 128 patients: a 24-year experience. *Surgery* 1987; **102**: 846–51.

Shashidhar H, Langhans N, Grand RJ. Propranolol in prevention of portal hypertensive hemorrhage in children: a pilot study. *Journal of Pediatric Gastroenterology and Nutrition* 1999; **29**: 12–17.

Shimizu H, Miyazaki M, Ito H, Nakagawa K, Ambiru S, Nakajima N. Evaluation of early graft function by hepatic venous hemoglobin oxygen saturation following orthotopic liver transplantation in the rat. *Transplantation* 1996; **62**: 1499–501.

Short TG, Aun CS, Tan P, Wong J, Tam YH, Oh TE. A prospective evaluation of pharmacokinetic model controlled infusion of propofol in paediatric patients. *British Journal of Anaesthesia* 1994; **72**: 302–6.

Simpson DA, Green DW. Use of atracurium during major abdominal surgery in infants with hepatic dysfunction from biliary atresia. *British Journal of Anaesthesia* 1986; **58**: 1214–17.

Singleton MA, Rosen JI, Fisher DM. Plasma concentrations of fentanyl in infants, children and adults. *Canadian Journal of Anaesthesia* 1987; **34**: 152–5.

Sommerauer J, Gayle M, Frewen T *et al*. Intensive-care course following liver transplantation in children. *Journal of Pediatric Surgery* 1988; **23**: 705–8.

Starzl TE, Esquivel C, Gordon R, Todo S. Pediatric liver transplantation. *Transplantation Proceedings* 1987; **19**: 3230–5.

Storck BH, Rutgers EJ, Gortzak E, Zoetmulder FA. The impact of the CUSA ultrasonic dissection device on major liver resections. *Netherlands Journal of Surgery* 1991; **43**: 99–101.

Stringer MD, Howard ER. The role of endoscopic sclerotherapy in the management of portal hypertension in children. In: Howard ER (ed.) *Surgery of liver disease in children*. Oxford: Butterworth-Heinemann, 1991: 157–70.

Thomson SR, Francel TJ, Youngson GG. Cavitron-assisted liver resection in a child. *Journal of Pediatric Surgery* 1987; **22**: 363–4.

Trouvin JH, Farinotti R, Haberer JP, Servin F, Chauvin M, Duvaldestin P. Pharmacokinetics of midazolam in anaesthetized cirrhotic patients. *British Journal of Anaesthesia* 1988; **60**: 762–7.

Van Obbergh LJ, Carlier M, De Kock M, Otte JB, Moulin D, Veyckemans F. Hepatopulmonary syndrome and liver transplantation: a review of the peroperative management of seven paediatric cases. *Paediatric Anaesthesia* 1998; **8**: 59–64.

Van Voorst SJ, Peters TG, Williams JW, Vera SR, Britt LG. Autotransfusion in hepatic transplantation. *American Surgeon* 1985; **51**: 623–6.

Vila R, Miguel E, Montferrer N *et al*. Respiratory depression following epidural morphine in an infant of three months of age. *Paediatric Anaesthesia* 1997; **7**: 61–4.

Walton B. Halothane hepatitis in children (editorial). *Anaesthesia* 1986; **41**: 575–8.

Wandel C, Bocker R, Bohrer H, Browne A, Rugheimer E, Martin E. Midazolam is metabolized by at least three different cytochrome P-450 enzymes. *British Journal of Anaesthesia* 1994; **73**: 658–61.

Wark H, Earl J, Chau DD, Overton J. Halothane metabolism in children. *British Journal of Anaesthesia* 1990; **64**: 474–81.

Wark HJ. Postoperative jaundice in children. The influence of halothane. *Anaesthesia* 1983; **38**: 237–42.

Weiskopf RB, Eger EID, Ionescu P *et al*. Desflurane does not produce hepatic or renal injury in human volunteers. *Anesthesia and Analgesia* 1992; **74**: 570–4.

Welborn LG, Hannallah RS, Norden JM, Ruttimann UE, Callan CM. Comparison of emergence and recovery characteristics of sevoflurane, desflurane and halothane in pediatric ambulatory patients. *Anesthesia and Analgesia* 1996; **83**: 917–20.

Yamamoto Y, Ikai I, Kume M *et al*. New simple technique for hepatic parenchymal resection using a Cavitron Ultrasonic Surgical Aspirator and bipolar cautery equipped with a channel for water dripping. *World Journal of Surgery* 1999; **23**: 1032–7.

Yanofsky RA, Jackson VG, Lilly JR, Stellin G, Klingensmith WCD, Hathaway WE. The multiple coagulopathies of biliary atresia. *American Journal of Hematology* 1984; **16**: 171–80.

Zaleski L, Abello D, Gold MI. Desflurane versus isoflurane in patients with chronic hepatic and renal disease. *Anesthesia and Analgesia* 1993; **76**: 353–6.

5

Nutritional care

PATRICIA McCLEAN

Malnutrition can accompany chronic liver disease of any etiology, and is associated with an increased morbidity and mortality. Infants are particularly susceptible (Roggero et al., 1997). In a recent study, standard deviation scores for weight of all infants under 12 months of age awaiting liver transplantation were depressed despite additional nutritional support (Van Mourik et al., 2000). Malnutrition increases susceptibility to infection, delays wound healing and is associated with poor mobilization postoperatively (Moukarzel et al., 1990; Shepherd et al., 1991). In the longer term, children may not achieve their full potential in terms of growth and development if nutritional problems are not tackled at an early stage. Improving the nutritional status of a child prior to liver transplantation is a well-recognized factor accounting for better survival (Moukarzel et al., 1990; Shepherd et al., 1991). Nutritional rehabilitation also improves liver function in patients with decompensated cirrhosis, ascites and bleeding esophageal varices (Kondrup and Muller, 1997).

FACTORS RESULTING IN MALNUTRITION IN LIVER DISEASE

The children most at risk of nutritional problems are those with chronic cholestasis (e.g. after a failed Kasai portoenterostomy), or those with cirrhosis and end-stage liver disease who are awaiting liver transplantation. Often intake is decreased due to anorexia, vomiting, unpalatable feeds, or fluid restriction because of the development of ascites. Maldigestion and malabsorption of dietary fat, which is a major source of calories in children, is secondary to a decreased bile salt pool in the duodenum (Glasgow et al., 1973). Pancreatic dysfunction in conditions such as cystic fibrosis, progressive familial intrahepatic cholestasis and Alagille's syndrome (Chong et al., 1989) also contributes to fat maldigestion. Diarrhea and malabsorption may occur due to bacterial overgrowth in a Roux loop, or in association with a severe portal enteropathy.

Low glycogen stores in liver and muscle result in the utilization of fat and protein as alternative fuels, causing further weight loss, muscle wasting and hypoproteinemia (McCullough et al., 1989). Plasma levels of branched-chain amino acids (BCAA), leucine, isoleucine and valine are low in patients with advanced cirrhosis, due to an increase in BCAA tissue uptake and/or catabolism and decreased BCAA production from proteins (Blonde-Cynober et al., 1999). There is an increase in circulating levels of aromatic amino acids, namely phenylalanine, tyrosine and tryptophan. These abnormalities of protein metabolism may promote hepatic encephalopathy by causing the production of false neurotransmitters (Fischer and Baldessarini, 1971). However, the evidence for a beneficial effect of supplementation with BCAA on hepatic encephalopathy in adults is equivocal (Fabbri et al., 1996).

Finally, resting energy expenditure is increased in chronic liver disease. The factors implicated include portosystemic shunting, gastrointestinal bleeding, ascites and infection (Pierro et al., 1989).

ASSESSMENT OF NUTRITIONAL STATUS

The abnormal body composition of children with advanced liver disease means that routine assessment of nutritional status can be misleading. Weight gain is influenced by organomegaly, ascites and edema. Rapid increases in weight should always suggest fluid retention. A fall in height velocity is a more reliable but late indicator of chronic malnutrition. Measurements of mid upper arm circumference and triceps skinfold thickness are less affected by peripheral edema, and serial measurements by the same trained observer can indicate early loss of fat stores (Sokal and Stall, 1990). All of these measurements can be plotted on centile charts at each clinic visit. Deviation from a previous pattern of growth or weight gain is obvious. Chronic illness and malnutrition can delay the onset of puberty. Physical examination in order to stage puberty is important during adolescence.

An accurate history of food intake and losses via vomiting or diarrhea/steatorrhea is essential. A 3-day weighed record of food intake is the most accurate method of assessing diet, especially in children whose eating habits vary from day to day. Semiquantitative evaluation of stool fats can be helpful. A low stool chymotrypsin level indicates that pancreatic enzyme supplementation may improve steatorrhea. Regular monitoring for asymptomatic deficiency of fat-soluble vitamins allows tailored supplementation (see later).

MANAGEMENT

The aims of nutritional therapy are to achieve normal growth and development and to avoid specific nutritional deficiencies. Energy requirements of 140–200% of the estimated average requirement (EAR) for age are usually necessary. Increasing protein intake up to 4 g/kg/day has been tolerated in infants with severe liver disease (Charlton et al., 1992) and may depress the catabolism of endogenous protein. In adults who cannot tolerate protein supplementation, nitrogen retention may be improved by increasing the intake of BCAA

(Horst et al., 1984). Chin et al. (1992) demonstrated an improvement in lean body mass in children awaiting liver transplantation, as a result of using a feed enriched with BCAA.

Long-chain triglycerides and fatty acids are malabsorbed in cholestasis, but medium-chain triglycerides (MCT) can be digested and absorbed in the absence of bile salts. Thus replacing approximately 50% of the dietary fat with MCT results in optimum weight gain and improvement of steatorrhea (Beath et al., 1993). It is important to ensure an adequate intake of the essential fatty acids, namely linoleic and linolenic acids. This should be achieved by providing 10% of the total energy intake as essential fatty acids (Aggett et al., 1991). Small quantities of walnut oil can be added to feeds in order to increase the essential fatty acid content if necessary. In health, elongation and desaturation of essential fatty acids produces long-chain polyunsaturated fatty acids (PUFA) such as arachadonic acid and docosahexanoic acid, which are important for visual and neurological development, eicosanoid synthesis and growth in infancy (Koletzko et al., 1998). In infancy in general, and in children with chronic liver disease in particular, the enzymes responsible for this process are immature or depressed, and long-chain PUFA become essential nutrients (Lapillonne et al., 2000). Further studies are needed to examine the benefits of supplementation with long-chain PUFA in infants with chronic liver disease.

In practice, for infants several nutritionally complete formulae are available containing 35–75% MCT and providing 0.66–1 kcal/mL (Table 5.1). With dietetic supervision, feeds can be concentrated or glucose polymers added to increase the calorific density of milk feeds to 2 kcal/mL. These modifications increase the osmolality of the feed, which can induce an osmotic diarrhea. Hydrolysed protein feeds have an unpleasant smell and taste, but young infants usually adapt to them within 48 hours. For older infants, whole-protein feeds are more likely to be accepted. Modular feeds, in which each component of the feed is prescribed, have the advantage of greater flexibility and can be modified to the requirements of the individual child. However, they are more complicated for parents to administer at home. In older

Table 5.1 *Complete formula feeds used in children with liver disease*

Feed	Manufacturer	Type of protein	MCT content (%)	Energy (kcal/mL)
Pregestamil	Mead Johnston	Totally hydrolyzed	55	0.68
Pepti-Junior	Cow & Gate	Partially hydrolyzed	50	0.66
Caprilon	SHS	Whole	75	0.75 (17% w/v)
Generaid Plus	SHS	Whole – BCAA	35	0.75 (17% w/v)

MCT, medium-chain triglyceride; SHS, Scientific Hospital Supplies; BCAA, branched-chain amino acids.

children, the diet can be supplemented with high-calorie drinks or the addition of glucose polymers or MCT emulsions to normal foods.

Nasogastric feeding

If anorexia or vomiting prevent adequate intake, or if weight gain remains poor, nasogastric (or occasionally nasojejunal) tube feeding needs to be implemented. Bolus tube feeding may be adequate if anorexia is the main problem, but more often a period of continuous nasogastric feeding, usually overnight, is necessary to prevent vomiting and diarrhea and improve growth (Kaufman et al., 1987; Moreno et al., 1991). The presence of esophageal varices is not a contraindication to nasogastric tube feeding. It is important to try to continue normal oral feeding with liquids and solids even when a child is on continuous tube feeding, otherwise normal feeding skills will be lost. Children with end-stage liver disease who are awaiting a liver transplant may become hypoglycemic if nasogastric feeding is stopped abruptly (e.g. if the tube becomes dislodged). Parents should be able to pass the tube themselves if the child is to be managed at home.

Gastrostomy feeding

Gastrostomy feeding is well established in many groups of children with chronic disease. The percutaneous endoscopic gastrostomy (PEG) is easily placed and usually well tolerated. It avoids the repeated discomfort of passing nasogastric tubes, the nasal irritation of the tube, and is more esthetically acceptable to parents and children. Reluctance to use PEG feeding in children with liver disease is due to concerns about placing the tube in the presence of hepatosplenomegaly, and the risks of infected ascites or development of peristomal varices. Duche et al. (1999), reported PEG feeding in five children awaiting liver transplantation. They concluded that PEG feeding may have a role in children with liver disease that progresses slowly to portal hypertension (e.g. Alagille's syndrome or progressive familial intrahepatic cholestasis), but should be avoided in patients with established portal hypertension.

Parenteral nutrition

As liver disease advances, enteral feeding alone may fail to achieve adequate growth. Indeed, feeding may be limited by episodes of variceal hemorrhage, diarrhea and sepsis. Instigation of parenteral nutrition (PN) while awaiting a liver transplant can maintain growth in these circumstances, although it may worsen cholestasis (Guimber et al., 1999). Consideration must be given to the volume of fluid administered via PN to avoid wors-

ening ascites and edema. High concentrations of dextrose stimulate insulin secretion, and hyperinsulinemia coupled with poor glycogen stores in the liver can cause profound hypoglycemia if PN is stopped suddenly.

Nutritional management post liver transplant

After a successful liver transplant, bile flow should be restored. In many children the donor bile duct will drain into a Roux loop, and therefore enteral feeding is delayed until gut motility returns. It may be necessary to use total parenteral nutrition (TPN) to maintain nutritional status, especially in children who were significantly undernourished prior to transplant. Once enteral feeding has commenced, normal milk formulae and foods are used. If cholestasis returns due to chronic rejection or biliary complications, MCT-based feeds will be needed again. Infants who have been tube fed for prolonged periods may be slow to learn oral feeding skills post transplant. The appetite of older children may be much improved after a transplant, although immunosuppressive drugs alter their taste perception. The many drugs used in the immediate post-transplant period may be responsible for symptoms of nausea, vomiting and diarrhea. Adjustments to dosage, timing and even changes of medication may be necessary if these symptoms do not settle. Children who suffer post-transplant complications are once again susceptible to the confounding factor of malnutrition, and this aspect of their care must be constantly reviewed.

PARENTERAL NUTRITION-ASSOCIATED CHOLESTASIS

While most of this chapter emphasizes the importance of nutritional rehabilitation in liver disease, this section will consider hepatobiliary dysfunction caused by a nutritional intervention. Parenteral nutrition transformed the prognosis of infants with primary intestinal failure or short gut syndrome secondary to surgical conditions and their treatment. Reports of liver disease associated with PN started to appear in the 1970s. In children the main pathology is cholestasis – hence the term PN-associated cholestasis (PNAC). The incidence of this condition is in the region of 40–60% of patients treated (Kelly, 1998).

Clinically, PNAC presents with jaundice which may appear after only 2–3 weeks of PN. Other liver function tests show impairment, and eventually signs of portal hypertension develop. Gallbladder disease, biliary sludge and gallstones are also well documented, and their incidence rises in parallel with the duration of PN (Messing et al., 1983). Histological changes in the liver commence with biliary stasis, progressing through periportal inflammation with ductular proliferation and fibrosis to biliary cirrhosis (Moss *et al.*, 1993). Steatosis, which is a major feature of PN-associated liver disease in adults, is rarely seen in children.

Recognized risk factors for the development of PNAC are listed in Box 5.1. However, the etiology remains elusive and is probably multifactorial. During an enteral fast, bile acid secretion and gallbladder contractility are decreased (Hofmann, 1995). This may be mediated via decreased levels of circulating gut hormones (Greenberg *et al.*, 1981; Aynsley-Green, 1983). Lack of oral feeding also causes intestinal stasis and reduced gallbladder emptying, which interrupt the enterohepatic recirculation of bile salts. In combination, these factors result in hepatotoxic bile (Palmer and Hruban, 1964).

The most effective way of improving bile flow is to recommence enteral feeding. Bile acid secretion is directly proportional to oral calorie intake (Brunner *et al.*, 1974). Pharmacological attempts to promote bile flow have included the use of intravenous cholecystokinin, which increases gallbladder contractility and small bowel motility (Teitelbaum *et al.*, 1995; Rintala *et al.*, 1997), or ursodeoxycholic acid, a hydrophilic bile acid which is not toxic to hepatocytes (Spagnuolo *et al.*, 1996). Improvement in bilirubin levels was observed in all three studies, but the numbers of cases were small and these were not randomized controlled trials.

Recent studies examining the factors associated with PNAC have emphasized the role of sepsis (Beath *et al.*, 1996; Sondheimer *et al.*, 1998). Sources of sepsis are central venous catheter infections and bacterial translocation from the gut due to underlying gut disease and/or fasting-induced intestinal stasis and mucosal atrophy. The association between sepsis and cholestasis has long been recognized (Rooney *et al.*, 1971). The mechanism may be decreased bile secretion due to bacterial endotoxin production (Utili *et al.*, 1976). Fastidious care of intravenous catheters by experienced personnel can decrease the frequency of line infections (Puntis *et al.*, 1991). Enteral feeding aids recovery of the mucosal architecture and stimulates gut motility, decreasing bacterial overgrowth and translocation.

The fact that PNAC can progress to fibrosis despite partial enteral feeding may implicate the constituents of the PN solution as an etiological factor. The evidence to date suggests that amino acids are more likely culprits than dextrose or current lipid solutions. Intravenous infusions of amino acids have been shown to decrease bile flow in animals (Graham *et al.*, 1984). Moss and Amii (1999) proposed an argument for methionine toxicity. Other constituents implicated have included phytosterols (plant sterol contaminants of commercial lipid emulsions) (Iyer *et al.*, 1998) and manganese. High circulating levels of manganese are more likely to be found in patients with PNAC (Fell *et al.*, 1996). However, convincing evidence of a cause-and-effect relationship between any specific constituent of PN and cholestasis is not available.

In summary, the only effective treatment for PNAC is to stop PN and resume full enteral feeding. If this is not possible, instigation of partial enteral feeding and policies to avoid sepsis improve outcome. Cycling of PN for 12 hours a day may be helpful (Collier *et al.*, 1994). The benefits of drugs to improve bile flow and decrease hepatotoxicity (e.g. ursodeoxycholic acid) have yet to be evaluated fully.

FAT-SOLUBLE VITAMINS, MINERALS AND TRACE ELEMENTS

Deficiency of the fat-soluble vitamins, namely vitamins A, D, E and K, occurs in children with chronic cholestasis (Argao and Heubi, 1993). The most immediate danger is bleeding due to malabsorption of vitamin K. Unfortunately, infants with undiagnosed cholestatic liver disease may present within a few weeks of birth with hemorrhagic disease of the newborn, with devastating consequences (Hope *et al.*, 1982). Clotting studies should be performed on all cholestatic children at presentation and about every 4–8 weeks thereafter. They should receive a maintenance dose of oral vitamin K. If the prothrombin time is prolonged or there is active bleeding, parenteral vitamin K should be administered. Vitamin K is also necessary for the production of osteocalcin, which has a role in bone formation. Early intervention trials suggest that vitamin K supplementation improves bone mineral density (Weber, 1997).

Rickets due to vitamin D deficiency is also fairly common, particularly in children with pigmented skin and unremitting cholestasis. Supplementation with vitamin D, calcium and phosphate will be considered in more detail later in the chapter.

Nowadays, clinical features of vitamin A or E deficiency are rarely apparent before diagnosis of liver disease and instigation of vitamin supplementation (Table 5.2). Alpha-tocopherol acetate is a water-soluble form of vitamin E. The conversion to α-tocopheryl occurs in the liver, but this process may be incomplete. An alternative formulation, D-α-tocopheryl polyethylene glycol-1000

Box 5.1 *Recognized risk factors for parenteral nutrition-associated cholestasis (PNAC)*

Prematurity
Low birth weight
Longer duration of total parenteral nutrition
Sepsis
Abdominal surgery
Lack of enteral feeding

Table 5.2 *Signs of deficiency, methods of monitoring and recommended doses of fat-soluble vitamins in children with liver disease*

	Signs of deficiency	Monitoring	Treatment
Vitamin A	Night blindness Xerophthalmia Follicular hyperkeratosis	Blood levels Dark adaptation tests in older children	5000–20 000 IU/day orally Beware of vitamin A hepatotoxicity in high doses
Vitamin D	Rickets, fractures Delayed eruption of teeth Proximal muscle weakness	Calcium, phosphate Alkaline phosphatase Parathormone 25-Hydroxy vitamin D X-ray wrist	Ergocalciferol: starting at 400–1200 IU/day (calciferol, vitamin D_2) Alphacalcidol: starting at 50–150 ng/kg/day (1α-hydroxycholecalciferol) Calcitriol: starting at 250 ng/day (1,25-dihydroxycholecalciferol)
Vitamin E	Hemolytic anemia Retinal dysfunction Loss of reflexes, vibration and proprioception, ataxia Ophthalmoplegia	Blood levels Vitamin E/lipid ratio	α-Tocopherol acetate, 15–200 mg/kg/day D-α-Tocopheryl polyethylene glycol-1000 succinate (TPGS), 15–25 IU/kg/day
Vitamin K	Bleeding diathesis	Prothrombin time	Menadiol phosphate or phytomenadione, 300 μg/kg/day

succinate (TPGS), is widely used in the USA. The α-tocopheryl is absorbed passively with the polyethylene glycol. The absorption of other fat-soluble vitamins can be enhanced by giving them simultaneously with TPGS (Argao *et al.*, 1992).

Usually vitamin deficiencies can be avoided by adequate oral supplementation. In severe ongoing cholestasis, regular intramuscular doses may be necessary.

Iron deficiency may occur due to poor intake or increased losses via gastrointestinal hemorrhage. Low hemoglobin and microcytic hypochromic indices suggest the diagnosis. Serum ferritin should be low, but may be raised as an acute phase reactant.

Cirrhosis is associated with depressed blood levels of zinc and selenium (Loguercio *et al.*, 1997). It is important to ensure that adequate quantities of these trace elements are added to modular feeds or PN solutions. Post liver transplant, low serum magnesium levels are described in association with the immunosuppressant drugs cyclosporine and tacrolimus (McDiarmid *et al.*, 1993). In addition to the recognized effects of magnesium deficiency listed in Table 5.3, low serum magnesium levels also potentiate the toxic effects of these drugs.

High blood levels of manganese are associated with chronic liver disease of various etiologies, including PNAC, as noted earlier in the chapter. Some patients have neurological symptoms, and magnetic resonance imaging has shown abnormalities in the basal ganglia (Devenyi *et al.*, 1994). It is recommended that manganese concentrations in PN solutions should be kept low (Fell *et al.*, 1996). Accumulation of copper occurs in the liver in chronic cholestasis, and additional copper should not be added to PN solutions.

METABOLIC BONE DISEASE

Throughout life, bone tissue is constantly being remodeled, and the balance between bone formation and bone resorption is affected by many factors. In the growing child, bone formation predominates and peak bone mass is reached some time in the third decade. Thereafter it declines. In children with chronic cholestatic liver disease, bone mineral content falls below the mean for age early in infancy, and worsens with increasing age and hepatic dysfunction (Argao *et al.*, 1993). In one study, bone mineral content did not correlate with serum levels of vitamin D, reflecting the fact that hepatic osteodystrophy has two main components, namely decreased bone mass (osteopenia, osteoporosis) and vitamin D defi-

Table 5.3 *Signs of deficiency, methods of monitoring and recommended doses of minerals and trace elements in children with liver disease*

	Signs of deficiency	Monitoring	Treatment
Iron	Tiredness, pallor, anorexia, growth failure	Hemoglobin, red cell indices Blood level	Various iron preparations
Zinc	Acrodermatitis, diarrhea	Low alkaline phosphatase	Zinc salt, 1 mg/kg/day of elemental zinc
Selenium	Muscle pain, cardiomyopathy, Weakness, white nailbeds	Blood level	RNI 10–45 µg/day (0–14 years)
Magnesium	Seizures, arrhythmias, tetany Gastrointestinal disturbances	Blood level	Magnesium glycerophosphate Start at 0.5–1 mmol/kg/day

RNI, recommended nutrient intake.

ciency (rickets, osteomalacia) (Argao *et al.*, 1993). Osteomalacia is rarely described in adults with chronic liver disease, but rickets is more common in children. Risk factors include severe cholestasis, pigmented skin, poor diet and lack of exposure to sunlight. Maintenance of vitamin D levels can be difficult in these children, and may require monthly intramuscular injections. Vitamin D insufficiency will not produce radiological or biochemical rickets, but the secondary hyperparathyroidism decreases bone turnover, resulting in osteopenia/osteoporosis. Other factors that increase the incidence of osteoporosis in general, namely low body mass index, inactivity and prolonged use of corticosteroids, are also present in children with chronic liver disease.

Severe hepatic osteodystrophy with recurrent fractures is now an indication for liver transplantation. However, adult and pediatric studies have shown that bone mineral density decreases in the first 6 months post transplant and there is still a high risk of fractures. Thereafter the bone mineral density increases (Argao *et al.*, 1994; Hill *et al.*, 1995; Feller *et al.*, 1999).

Management of hepatic osteodystrophy involves decreasing the risk factors by improving general nutrition, encouraging physical exercise and using as little corticosteroid therapy as possible. Treatment with adequate doses of vitamin D, using the intramuscular route if necessary, should prevent frank rickets. Oral alphacalcidol is often used instead of ergocalciferol because it has a shorter half-life and hypercalcemia due to excessive dosage will be transient. 1,25-Dihydroxycholecalciferol may be absorbed better in patients with cholestasis, but the conversion of vitamin D to 25-hydroxy vitamin D seems to be well preserved in patients with cirrhosis (Danielsson *et al.*, 1982; Sitrin and Bengoa, 1987). Serum calcium, magnesium, phosphate, alkaline phosphatase, parathyroid hormone and vitamin D levels can be monitored to detect vitamin D insufficiency. Calcium, magnesium and phosphate supplements may also be required. Increasingly, dual-energy X-ray absorptiometry (DEXA scan) is used to measure bone mineral density. Bisphosphonates, which inhibit osteoclast bone resorp-

tion, have been shown to improve bone mineral density in patients with primary biliary cirrhosis treated with steroids, and to decrease the incidence of atraumatic spinal fractures in the peritransplant period (Wolfhagen *et al.*, 1997; Reeves *et al.*, 1998). Concern about the safety of bisphosphonates in the growing skeleton has delayed their widespread use in the pediatric age group. However, they have been used in children with juvenile arthritis, osteogenesis imperfecta and idiopathic osteoporosis for up to 8 years, resulting in improved bone mineral density and minimal side-effects (Brumsen *et al.*, 1997).

GROWTH

Even with aggressive nutritional therapy many patients with liver disease remain malnourished and stunted. Growth hormone is an anabolic hormone that promotes growth and nitrogen retention via stimulation of insulin-like growth factor 1 (IGF-1), predominantly in the liver (Russell, 1985). IGF-1 transport to the tissues is in turn modulated by carrier-binding proteins, of which IGFBP-3 is the most important (Cohen *et al.*, 1991; Blum *et al.*, 1993). This is produced in the Kupffer cells of the liver (Arnay *et al.*, 1995). In healthy individuals, increased circulating growth hormone results in increased levels of IGF-1 and IGFBP-3. However, in children with cirrhosis, growth hormone levels are high but IGF-1 and IGFBP-3 levels are low and do not respond to standard doses of recombinant growth hormone, suggesting growth hormone insensitivity (Bucuvalas *et al.*, 1996). This may explain ongoing growth failure despite aggressive nutritional rehabilitation. Whether this insensitivity is just a manifestation of malnutrition or is due to a lack of growth hormone receptors in the cirrhotic liver is still unclear. Recent studies have shown that growth hormone resistance worsens with progression of liver disease, especially the development of portal hypertension, but that supraphysiological doses of growth hormone increase IGF-1 levels in some children

(Maghnie *et al.*, 1998; Holt *et al.*, 1999). Interestingly, when nasogastric feeding results in improved body composition in children with cirrhosis, circulating IGF-1 and IGFBP-3 levels remain abnormal and do not play a major role in mediating the changes (Holt *et al.*, 2000).

After a liver transplant 80% of children show good evidence of catch-up growth (Codoner-Franch *et al.*, 1994; Holt *et al.*, 1997). In general children who are most severely malnourished at the time of transplant show the greatest catch-up growth afterwards (Sarna *et al.*, 1994; Holt *et al.*, 1997). Improvement in body fat stores and weight gain occur within the first 6 months (Holt *et al.*, 1997), but linear growth is delayed by up to 24 months depending on post-transplant complications and the use of corticosteroids (Codoner-Franch *et al.*, 1994; Rodeck *et al.*, 1994). Several studies have shown that height velocity improves further when steroids are reduced to alternate-day regimens (Codoner-Franch *et al.*, 1994) or stopped altogether (Andrews *et al.*, 1994).

After liver transplantation there is a marked improvement in the IGF-IGFBP axis, but there are still persistent abnormalities which may explain some aspects of ongoing growth failure (Holt *et al.*, 1998). Sarna *et al.* (1996) induced an increase in height velocity using recombinant growth hormone in eight children with growth retardation post transplant. IGF-1 and IGFBP-3 levels increased during treatment. It is not known whether this treatment will affect final adult height, and there is a risk of growth hormone treatment inducing rejection of the graft, which needs to be evaluated further.

Key references

Kelly DA. Liver complications of pediatric parenteral nutrition – epidemiology. *Nutrition* 1998; **14**: 153–4.

Moss RL, Amii LA. New approaches to understanding the etiology and treatment of total parenteral nutrition-associated cholestasis. *Seminars in Pediatric Surgery* 1999; **8**: 140–7.

Two critical overviews of parenteral nutrition-associated cholestasis with complementary emphasis.

Shepherd RW, Chin SE, Cleghorn GJ *et al.* Malnutrition in children with chronic liver disease accepted for liver transplantation: clinical profile and effect on outcome. *Journal of Paediatric Child Health* 1991; **27**: 295–9.

Moukarzel AA, Najm I, Vargas J, McDiarmid SV, Busuttil RW, Ament ME. Effects of nutritional status on outcome of orthotopic liver transplantation in pediatric patients. *Transplantation Proceedings* 1990; **22**: 1560–3.

Two early papers highlighting the relationship between poor nutritional status prior to transplant and significantly worse outcome after liver transplantation.

REFERENCES

Aggett PJ, Haschke F, Heine W *et al*. Comment on the content and composition of lipids in infant formulas. ESPGAN Committee on Nutrition. *Acta Paediatrica Scandinavica* 1991; **80**: 887–96.

Andrews WS, Shimaoka S, Sommerauer J *et al*. Steroid withdrawal after paediatric liver transplantation. *Transplantation Proceedings* 1994; **26**: 159–60.

Argao EA, Heubi JE. Fat-soluble vitamin deficiency in infants and children. *Current Opinion in Pediatrics* 1993; **5**: 562–6.

Argao EA, Heubi JE, Hollis BW. D-Alpha-tocopheryl polyethylene glycol-1000 succinate enhances the absorption of vitamin D in chronic cholestasis of infancy and childhood. *Pediatric Research* 1992; **31**: 146–50.

Argao EA, Specker BL, Heubi JE. Bone mineral content in infants and children with chronic cholestatic liver disease. *Pediatrics* 1993; **91**: 1151–4.

Argao EA, Balistreri WF, Hollis BW, Ryckman FC, Heubi JE. Effect of orthotopic liver transplantation on bone mineral content and serum vitamin D metabolites in infants and children with chronic cholestasis. *Hepatology* 1994; **20**: 598–603.

Arnay E, Afford S, Strain AJ *et al*. Differential cellular synthesis of insulin-like growth factor binding protein-1 (IGFBP-1) and IGFBP-3 within the liver. *Journal of Clinical Endocrinology and Metabolism* 1995; **79**: 1871–6.

Aynsley-Green A. Plasma hormone concentrations during enteral and parenteral nutrition in the human newborn. *Journal of Pediatric Gastroenterology and Nutrition* 1983; **2**: S108–12.

Beath S, Hooley I, Willis K *et al*. Long-chain triacylglycerol malabsorption and pancreatic function in children with protein energy malnutrition complicating severe liver disease. *Proceedings of the Nutrition Society* 1993; **52**: 252A.

Beath SV, Davies P, Papadopoulou A *et al*. Parenteral nutrition-related cholestasis in postsurgical neonates: multivariate analysis of risk factors. *Journal of Pediatric Surgery* 1996; **31**: 604–6.

Blonde-Cynober F, Aussel C, Cynober L. Abnormalities in branched-chain amino acid metabolism in cirrhosis: influence of hormonal and nutritional factors and directions for future research. *Clinical Nutrition* 1999; **18**: 5–13.

Blum WF, Albertsson-Wikland K, Rosberg S *et al*. Serum levels of insulin-like growth factor 1 (IGF-1) and IGF binding protein 3 reflect spontaneous GH secretion. *Journal of Clinical Endocrinology and Metabolism* 1993; **76**: 1610–16.

Brumsen C, Hamdy NAT, Papapoulos SE. Long-term effects of biphosphonates on the growing skeleton. Studies of young patients with severe osteoporosis. *Medicine* 1997; **76**: 266–83.

Brunner H, Northfield TC, Hofman AF, Go VLW, Summerskill

WHJ. Gastric emptying and secretion of bile acids, cholesterol, and pancreatic enzymes during digestion: duodenal perfusion studies in healthy subjects. *Mayo Clinic Proceedings* 1974; **49**: 851–60.

Bucuvalas JC, Horn JA, Slusher J, Alfaro MP, Chernausek SD. Growth hormone insensitivity in children with biliary atresia. *Journal of Pediatric Gastroenterology and Nutrition* 1996; **23**: 135–40.

Charlton CPJ, Buchanan E, Holden C *et al*. The use of enteral feeding in the dietary management of children with chronic liver disease. *Archives of Disease in Childhood* 1992; **67**: 603–7.

Chin SE, Shepherd RW, Thomas BJ *et al*. Nutritional support in children with end-stage liver disease: a randomized crossover trial of a branched-chain amino acid supplement. *American Journal of Clinical Nutrition* 1992; **56**: 158–63.

Chong SKF, Lindridge J, Moniz C, Mowat A. Exocrine pancreatic insufficiency in syndromic paucity of interlobular bile ducts. *Journal of Pediatric Gastroenterology and Nutrition* 1989; **9**: 445–9.

Codoner-Franch P, Bernard O, Alvarez F. Long-term follow-up of growth in height after successful liver transplantation. *Journal of Pediatrics* 1994; **124**: 368–73.

Cohen P, Fielder PJ, Hasegawa Y *et al*. Clinical aspects of IGF binding proteins. *Acta Endocrinologica* 1991; **124**: 74–85.

Collier S, Crough J, Hendricks K, Caballero B. Use of cyclic parenteral nutrition in infants less than 6 months of age. *Nutrition in Clinical Practice* 1994; **9**: 65–8.

Danielsson A, Lorentzon R, Larsson SE. Intestinal absorption and 25-hydroxylation of vitamin D in patients with primary biliary cirrhosis. *Scandinavian Journal of Gastroenterology* 1982; **17**: 349–55.

Devenyi AG, Barron TF, Mamourian AC. Dystonia, hyperintense basal ganglia, and high whole blood manganese levels in Alagille's syndrome. *Gastroenterology* 1994; **106**: 1068–71.

Duche M, Habes D, Lababidi A, Chardot C, Wenz J, Bernard O. Percutaneous endoscopic gastrostomy for continuous feeding in children with chronic cholestasis. *Journal of Pediatric Gastroenterology and Nutrition* 1999; **29**: 42–5.

Fabbri A, Magrini N, Bianchi G, Zoli M, Marchesini G. Overview of randomized clinical trials of oral branched-chain amino acid treatment in chronic hepatic encephalopathy. *Journal of Parenteral and Enteral Nutrition* 1996; **20**: 159–64.

Fell JM, Reynolds AP, Meadows N *et al*. Manganese toxicity in children receiving long-term parenteral nutrition. *Lancet* 1996; **347**: 1218–21.

Feller RB, McDonald JA, Sherbon KJ, McCaughan GW. Evidence of continuing bone recovery at a mean of 7 years after liver transplantation. *Liver Transplantation and Surgery* 1999; **5**: 407–13.

Fischer JE, Baldessarini RJ. False neurotransmitters and hepatic failure. *Lancet* 1971; **2**: 75–80.

Glasgow JFT, Hamilton JR, Sass-Kortsak A. Fat absorption in congenital obstructive liver disease. *Archives of Disease in Childhood* 1973; **48**: 601–7.

Graham MF, Tavill AS, Halpin TC, Louis LN. Inhibition of bile flow in the isolated perfused rat liver by a synthetic parenteral amino acid mixture: associated net amino acid fluxes. *Hepatology* 1984; **4**: 69–73.

Greenberg G, Walman S, Christofides N *et al*. Effect of total parenteral nutrition on gut hormone release in humans. *Gastroenterology* 1981; **80**: 988.

Guimber D, Michaud L, Ategbo S, Turck D, Gottrand F. Experience of parenteral nutrition for nutritional rescue in children with severe liver disease following failure of enteral nutrition. *Pediatric Transplantation* 1999; **3**: 139–45.

Hill SA, Kelly DA, John PR. Bone fractures in children undergoing orthotopic liver transplantation. *Pediatric Radiology* 1995; **25 (Supplement 1)**: S112–17.

Hofmann AF. Defective biliary secretion during total parenteral nutrition: probable mechanisms and possible solutions. *Journal of Pediatric Gastroenterology and Nutrition* 1995; **20**: 376–90.

Holt RI, Broide E, Buchanan CR *et al*. Orthotopic liver transplantation reverses the adverse nutritional changes of end-stage liver disease in children. *American Journal of Clinical Nutrition* 1997; **65**: 534–42.

Holt RI, Baker AJ, Jones JS, Miell JP. The insulin-like growth factor and binding protein axis in children with end-stage liver disease before and after orthotopic liver transplantation. *Pediatric Transplantation* 1998; **2**: 76–84.

Holt RI, Jones JS, Baker AJ, Buchanan CR, Miell JP. The effect of short stature, portal hypertension and cholestasis on growth hormone resistance in children with liver disease. *Journal of Clinical Endocrinology and Metabolism* 1999; **84**: 3277–82.

Holt RI, Meill JP, Jones JS, Mieli-Vergani G, Baker AJ. Nasogastric feeding enhances nutritional status in paediatric liver disease but does not alter circulating levels of IGF-1 and IGF binding proteins. *Clinical Endocrinology* 2000; **52**: 217–24.

Hope PL, Hall MA, Millward-Sadler GH. α-1-antitrypsin deficiency presenting as a bleeding diathesis in the newborn. *Archives of Disease in Childhood* 1982; **57**: 69–79.

Horst D, Grace ND, Conn HO *et al*. Comparison of dietary protein with an oral, branched chain-enriched amino acid supplement in chronic portal-systemic encephalopathy: a randomized controlled trial. *Hepatology* 1984; **4**: 279–87.

Iyer KR, Spitz L, Clayton P. New insight into mechanisms of parenteral nutrition-associated cholestasis: role of plant sterols. *Journal of Pediatric Surgery* 1998; **33**: 1–6.

Kaufman SS, Murray ND, Wood RP, Shaw BW Jr, Vanderhoof JA. Nutritional support for the infant with extrahepatic biliary atresia. *Journal of Pediatrics* 1987; **110**: 679–86.

Kelly DA. Liver complications of pediatric parenteral nutrition – epidemiology. *Nutrition* 1998; **14**: 153–4.

Koletzko B, Demmelmair H, Socha P. Nutritional support of infants and children: supply and metabolism of lipids. *Baillière's Clinical Gastroenterology* 1998; **12**: 671–96.

Kondrup J, Muller MJ. Energy and protein requirements of patients with chronic liver disease. *Nutrition Reviews* 1997; **55**: 17–20.

Lapillonne A, Hakme C, Mamoux V *et al*. Effects of liver transplantation on long-chain polyunsaturated fatty acid status in infants with biliary atresia. *Journal of Pediatric Gastroenterology and Nutrition* 2000; **30**: 528–32.

Loguercio C, De Girolamo V, Federico A *et al*. Trace elements and chronic liver diseases. *Journal of Trace Elements in Medicine and Biology* 1997; **11**: 158–61.

McCullough AJ, Mullen KD, Smanik EJ, Tabbaa M, Szauter K. Nutritional therapy and liver disease. *Gastroenterology Clinics of North America* 1989; **18**: 619–43.

McDiarmid SV, Colonna JO II, Shaked A, Ament ME, Busuttil RW. A comparison of renal function in cyclosporine- and FK506-treated patients after primary orthotopic liver transplantation. *Transplantation* 1993; **56**: 847–53.

Maghnie M, Barreca A, Ventura M *et al*. Failure to increase insulin-like growth factor-1 synthesis is involved in the mechanisms of growth retardation of children with inherited liver disorders. *Clinical Endocrinology* 1998; **48**: 747–55.

Messing B, Bories C, Kunstlinger F, Bernier JJ. Does total parenteral nutrition induce gallbladder sludge formation and lithiasis? *Gastroenterology* 1983; **84**: 1012.

Moreno LA, Gottrand F, Hoden S, Turck D, Loeuille GA, Farriaux JP. Improvement of nutritional status in cholestatic children with supplemental nocturnal enteral nutrition. *Journal of Pediatric Gastroenterology and Nutrition* 1991; **12**: 213–16.

Moss RL, Amii LA. New approaches to understanding the etiology and treatment of total parenteral nutrition-associated cholestasis. *Seminars in Pediatric Surgery* 1999; **8**: 140–7.

Moss RL, Das JB, Raffensberger JG. Total parenteral nutrition-associated cholestasis: clinical and histopathologic correlation. *Journal of Pediatric Surgery* 1993; **28**: 1270–5.

Moukarzel AA, Najm I, Vargas J, McDiarmid SV, Busuttil RW, Ament ME. Effects of nutritional status on outcome of orthotopic liver transplantation in pediatric patients. *Transplantation Proceedings* 1990; **22**: 1560–3.

Palmer RH, Hruban Z. Production of bile duct hyperplasia and gallstones by lithocholic acid. *Journal of Clinical Investigation* 1964; **45**: 1255.

Pierro A, Koletzko B, Carnielli V *et al*. Resting energy expenditure is increased in infants and children with extrahepatic biliary atresia. *Journal of Pediatric Surgery* 1989; **24**: 534–8.

Puntis JWL, Holden CE, Smallman S *et al*. Staff training: a key factor in reducing intravascular catheter sepsis. *Archives of Disease in Childhood* 1991; **66**: 335–7.

Reeves HL, Francis RM, Manas DM, Hudson M, Day CP. Intravenous bisphosphonate prevents symptomatic osteoporotic vertebral collapse in patients after liver transplantation. *Liver Transplantation and Surgery* 1998; **4**: 404–9.

Rintala RJ, Lindahl H, Pohjavuori M. Use of cholecystokinin to prevent the development of parenteral nutrition-associated cholestasis. *Journal of Parenteral and Enteral Nutrition* 1997; **21**: 100–3.

Rodeck B, Melter M, Hoyer PF, Ringe B, Brodehl J. Growth in long-term survivors after orthotopic liver transplantation in childhood. *Transplantation Proceedings* 1994; **26**: 165–6.

Roggero P, Cataliotti E, Ulla L *et al*. Factors influencing malnutrition in children waiting for liver transplants. *American Journal of Clinical Nutrition* 1997; **65**: 1852–7.

Rooney JC, Hill DJ, Danks DM. Jaundice associated with bacterial infection in the newborn. *American Journal of Diseases in Childhood* 1971; **122**: 39.

Russell WE. GH, somatomedins and the liver. *Seminars in Liver Disease* 1985; **5**: 46–58.

Sarna S, Sipila I, Jalanko H, Laine J, Holmberg C. Factors affecting growth after pediatric liver transplantation. *Transplantation Proceedings* 1994; **26**: 161–4.

Sarna S, Sipila I, Ronnholm K, Koistinen R, Holmberg C. Recombinant human growth hormone improves growth in children receiving glucocorticoid treatment after liver transplantation. *Journal of Clinical Endocrinology and Metabolism* 1996; **81**: 1476–82.

Shepherd RW, Chin SE, Cleghorn GJ *et al*. Malnutrition in children with chronic liver disease accepted for liver transplantation: clinical profile and effect on outcome. *Journal of Paediatrics and Child Health* 1991; **27**: 295–9.

Sitrin MD, Bengoa JM. Intestinal absorption of cholecalciferol and 25-hydroxycholecalciferol in chronic cholestatic liver disease. *American Journal of Clinical Nutrition* 1987; **46**: 1011–15.

Sokal RJ, Stall C. Anthropometric evaluation of children with chronic liver disease. *American Journal of Clinical Nutrition* 1990; **52**: 203–8.

Sondheimer JM, Asturias E, Cadnapaphornchai M. Infection and cholestasis in neonates with intestinal resection and long-term parenteral nutrition. *Journal of Pediatric Gastroenterology and Nutrition* 1998; **27**: 131–7.

Spagnuolo MI, Iorio R, Vegnente A, Guarino A. Ursodeoxycholic acid for treatment of cholestasis in children on long-term total parenteral nutrition: a pilot study. *Gastroenterology* 1996; **111**: 716–19.

Teitelbaum DH, Han-Markey T, Schumacher RE. Treatment of parenteral nutrition-associated cholestasis with cholecystokinin-octapeptide. *Journal of Pediatric Surgery* 1995; **30**: 1082–5.

Utili R, Abernathy CO, Zimmerman HJ. Cholestatic effects of *Escherichia coli* endotoxin on the isolated perfused rat liver. *Gastroenterology* 1976; **70**: 248.

Van Mourik IDM, Beath SV, Brook GA *et al*. Long-term nutritional outcome and neurodevelopmental outcome of liver transplantation in infants aged less than 12 months. *Journal of Pediatric Gastroenterology and Nutrition* 2000; **30**: 269–75.

Weber P. Management of osteoporosis: is there a role for vitamin K? *International Journal for Vitamin and Nutrition Research* 1997; **67**: 350–6.

Wolfhagen FH, van Buuren HR, den Ouden JW *et al*. Cyclical etidronate in the prevention of bone loss in corticosteroid-treated primary biliary cirrhosis. A prospective controlled pilot study. *Journal of Hepatology* 1997; **26**: 325–30.

6

Psychosocial aspects of liver disease

SARAH HELPS

INTRODUCTION

Many children and families rise successfully to the challenge of coping with the debilitating, unpleasant symptoms of liver disease. However, liver disease can lead to tremendous stress, requiring practical and psychosocial adjustment both for the child and for their family (Mastroyannopoulou et al., 1998). Surgery is often viewed as one of the most challenging events in the lives of children with liver disease and their families. This chapter addresses the psychological effects of chronic liver disease and surgery on children and their families, and ways in which health care professionals can help them to manage.[1]

CHILDREN, FAMILIES AND CHRONIC ILLNESS

The effect of their child being diagnosed with a chronic health condition can have varying effects on parents, depending on several factors, including the nature and severity of the condition, age at diagnosis, the presence of handicap or functional limitation of the child, the intrusion of the condition into family life, personality and previous experience of parents, the temperament of the child, and the level and quality of social and professional support that is available. Parents' reactions to diagnosis

commonly follow stages akin to a grief reaction (Drotar, 1975) and parents may need to grieve the loss of the healthy child they were expecting. Initial shock and numbness are followed by extreme anxiety, when it is difficult to absorb the detailed information that is being supplied about their child's condition. A period of denial, when the family tries to carry on as if nothing has happened, may lead to sadness and anger, with rage against the diagnosis. Eventually the stage of adaptation to the new situation is reached, when the family develops coping strategies to deal with their child's condition. Not all parents go through all of these stages, and the stages may not take place in a linear manner.

RISK AND RESILIENCE

Pediatric chronic illnesses such as liver disease are often conceptualized as involving sources of chronic strain for both the child and the family, which affect psychological adjustment. Adjustment to the chronic strains depends on the balance of risk and resilience factors (Wallender and Varni, 1992, 1998). Risk factors include illness-related factors such as disease severity, functional independence and its limitations, and psychosocial stressors which may or may not be directly connected to the illness. Resistance factors include personal characteristics

---

[1] Throughout this chapter the term 'parent' is used to refer to the child's primary caregiver.

(e.g. temperament and problem-solving abilities), socioecological factors (e.g. family environment, social support and economic resources) and cognitive appraisal and coping strategies.

Coping refers to any response which has the function of reducing the stressful nature of a situation. Coping has been divided into two main types (Lazarus and Folkman, 1984). Problem-focused coping refers to behavioral and cognitive attempts to deal directly with the problem, and it includes trying to find out more about the problem, rehearsal and self-talk. Emotion-focused coping refers to attempts to manage the emotional aspects of the problem, including relaxation, ignoring the problem and distracting oneself. It also includes denial – an unconscious attempt to protect oneself from the emotional challenge associated with illness. The strategies used at different times by children and their families will vary depending on the individuals' appraisal of the demands of the situation compared with their perceived coping resources.

Different situational demands necessitate the use of different coping strategies. For example, in a situation where there is uncontrollable stress, emotion-focused strategies can be helpful. When one has control over a situation, (e.g. deciding whether and where to have a Portacath fitted), problem-focused strategies may be more appropriate (e.g. asking many questions, and seeking out other people who have been in the same situation). It has been suggested that children who use more problem-focused coping strategies may have more adaptive responses to hospitalization and surgery than those whose coping style is more passive and emotion focused (Harbeck-Webber and McKee, 1995).

Interventions based on the risk and resilience model aim to reduce modifiable risk factors and promote modifiable resistance factors (e.g. by teaching the child and the family problem-solving skills, enhancing social support and promoting autonomy of the family).

PSYCHOLOGICAL ADJUSTMENT OF CHILDREN WITH CHRONIC LIVER DISEASE AND THEIR FAMILIES

Children with liver disease have been identified as being at risk for psychological difficulties (House et al., 1983). Potentially life-threatening disorders such as biliary atresia, involving surgical procedures that take place very early on in the life of a child, impose particular strains on children and their families and can result in high levels of psychological distress. For example, in one study approximately 40% of children with biliary atresia were reported to show significant signs of emotional and behavioral difficulties, and 36% of mothers reported significant mental health difficulties (Bradford, 1994). These results are consistent with rates of disorder found in other chronic life-threatening conditions (Pless and

Nolan, 1991; Thompson et al., 1992). Children who manifest significant symptoms of liver disease within the first year of life are most likely to be at risk of developmental delay and cognitive impairment. Different patterns of cognitive impairment are found in children with different types of liver disease (for review see Stewart and Kennard, 1998). In both wider research on pediatric chronic illness and that specifically focusing on liver disease, families have been found to have a moderating effect in attenuating the negative effects of liver disease (e.g. families characterized by higher levels of emotional closeness and support appear to provide the most opportunities for enhancement of social development in children) (Hoffmann et al., 1995).

CHILDREN'S UNDERSTANDING OF ILLNESS

The development of a child's concept of illness is determined by both cognitive maturation and experience of or exposure to illness (Bibace and Walsh, 1979; Bibace et al., 1994). Before 3 years of age, children describe illness in terms of a single symptom and see the cause of illness as external and remote. Between 3 and 5 years of age, illness is still regarded as a single symptom, but the concept of contagion is used to explain the illness (e.g. by standing next to someone who has tummy ache, you get a tummy ache). Magical thinking may also occur (e.g. conceiving of illness as a punishment for doing something wrong). Magical thinking may persist until well into the teenage years. By 5 years of age, children begin to have a grasp of the concept of death and its finality. Between 5 and 7 years, illness starts to be construed by most children as involving multiple symptoms and being caused by internal processes such as eating germs. As children approach their teenage years they start to be able to give detailed physiological explanations of illnesses. Teenagers can show a detailed understanding of how many processes link together in disease, and they can explain the functions of the liver and what happens when it is diseased in a very sophisticated way.

Children with specific conditions may show a better than average understanding of the particular organs and processes involved in their condition. For example, children between 6 and 15 years of age who had liver disease or who had undergone transplantation were found to have higher levels of understanding of the functioning of the liver than their healthy peers (Mastroyannopoulou et al., 1998).

DECISION-MAKING AND INFORMED CONSENT TO SURGERY

As medical and surgical interventions become increasingly complex, so do the decisions faced by children and their families. Involving children in decision-making improves communication between doctors, parents and children, may facilitate children's cooperation with treatment, may promote a sense of control, and demonstrates respect for children's capacities (McCabe, 1996). As well as cognitive ability and understanding of illness, social and identity development, previous experience in taking responsibility for decisions, family factors (e.g. cultural background, religious beliefs, parents' values and beliefs, differences of opinion between two or more members of a family) and situational factors (e.g. time constraints) are also important in determining a child's capacity to participate in the decision-making process (McCabe, 1996). Factors such as the physical state of the child (including pain level and medications taken) will influence attention span and ability to concentrate. A child's emotional state will further affect their reasoning and information-processing ability.

Children aged 14 years have been shown to be able to demonstrate the same level of competency as adults in their understanding and reasoning about a hypothetical medical situation (Weithorn and Campbell, 1982). Alderson (1993) found that children wanted to be involved in – but rarely solely responsible for – decision-making. Children as young as 5–6 years were found to be able to make complex, wise decisions about proposed interventions.

THE CONCEPT OF PAIN IN CHILDREN

Pain is an unpleasant sensory and emotional experience associated with actual or potential tissue damage, or described in terms of such damage (Merskey, 1986). Like the development of illness concepts, the concept of pain is affected both by maturation and by experience (McGrath and McAlpine, 1993; McGrath, 1995) (Box 6.1). For children with liver disease, most pain experiences are associated with surgical procedures, although clinical experience suggests that they often experience chronic discomfort due to an enlarged spleen, abdominal distension and other physical manifestations of their condition.

Assessing pain in children

While children should always if possible be the main reporters of pain, when they are unable to report on their own pain, due to age or cognitive impairment, parental ratings are helpful and have been found to be accurate (McGrath, 1990).

In order for pain to be treated accurately it needs to be assessed accurately. Rating scales are generally held to be the most accurate assessment method. For preverbal children, many behavioral observational scales exist, such as the Children's Hospital of Eastern Ontario Pain Scale (CHEOPS) (McGrath et al., 1985) and the

---

Box 6.1 *Development of children's concept of pain and coping strategies*

0–3 months – no apparent understanding of pain, but pain is felt and needs treatment

Up to 6 months – clear memory of pain, demonstrated by anticipatory fear, sadness and anger responses shown when pain is inflicted

Up to 18 months – crying or simple verbalizations to indicate pain, but unable to verbalize level and intensity of pain

By 18 months – sophisticated avoidance behavior can be observed from pain stimuli (e.g. a needle)

By 24 months – children can say that a pain 'hurts' and can localize it. They may also show rudimentary efforts to cope with pain, seeking hugs and comfort from carers

By 2–3 years – children can clearly describe pain and attribute it to external causes

By 3–4 years – children can describe different intensities and qualities of pain and can verbalize these, and can spontaneously use coping techniques such as distraction to help them to cope

Between 5 and 7 years – children become increasingly proficient at describing pain, and can indicate fluctuations in pain intensity

Between 7 and 10 years – children become able to describe why pain hurts

By adolescence – teenagers can describe the adaptive value of pain in protecting people from harm

---

Neonatal Facial Action Coding System (Grunau and Craig, 1987).

Many self-report measures exist for children of 3 years and over, such as Hester's poker chips, where children are asked to describe their pain in terms of how many 'pieces of hurt' the pain is (Hester et al., 1990). More abstract measures, such as faces showing different expressions of pain intensity, are suitable for use with children of around 5 years and older (Kuttner and LePage, 1989; Bieri et al., 1990). For children of 7 years and over, visual analog scales and numerical rating scales (e.g. drawn out scales of 1–10 where 1 signifies no pain and 10 signifies worst possible pain) are useful.

Psychological aspects of pain management

Pain in children is surrounded by many myths that can lead to inadequate pain management (McGrath, 1995). The perceptions of health care professionals about pain are influenced by their personal beliefs, experiences, attitudes and values. Comprehensive education about the variety of children's pain behaviors, and the reasons why children may not express pain in expected ways, is needed, as is consideration of cultural, gender and societal expectations of a child in pain.

A variety of cognitive and behavioral interventions can be used alongside pharmacological interventions to help children either to alter their perception of pain or to alter their pain behavior or, through contingency management, to modify the social and environmental factors that influence pain expression.

Pain perception is commonly addressed through psychological education and self-regulatory techniques (e.g. deep muscle relaxation, distraction by engaging in competing activities, guided imagery, reframing, positive self-instructions in which the child is taught to repeat statements such as 'I am doing well, I am brave', and breathing exercises) (McGrath, 1995; Carr, 2000). To be effective, the distracting stimulus must be captivating enough to focus the child's attention fully before the procedure is attempted. Distraction should occur in the context of other behavioral methods, such as ignoring unwanted behavior and praising appropriate behavior.

PSYCHOLOGICAL PREPARATION FOR SURGERY

Psychological support from all members of the medical and surgical team throughout the process of surgery is vital. Listening to the child and the family, being unhurried, giving the child as much control as possible, explaining what is being done and being confident, in the context of an emotionally supportive and caring milieu, all appear to be effective and reflect good clinical practice (Box 6.2) (McGrath, 1995). Honesty is another key factor (e.g. telling a child that an injection will not hurt is clearly untrue, but telling them that it will not feel very nice is honest and likely to enhance trust).

Psychological preparation for surgery has been shown to be effective in reducing children's anticipatory anxiety and behavioral distress. Exposure to videos portraying a boy experiencing pre-surgery procedures, surgery recovery and discharge who demonstrated adaptive behavioral reactions to these procedures was found to reduce physiological and self-reported ratings of anxiety and observable behavioral distress in children who watched it (Melamed and Siegel, 1975). Taking an active role in preparation, rather than passively watching a video, was found to increase the magnitude of the preparation's impact (Saile et al., 1988).

Careful assessment of children's habitual coping styles is vital prior to preparation for any procedure. For example, children who have passive, avoidant coping styles may be more sensitized to pain as a result of brief psychological education, and may therefore require more intensive exposure to procedural information both to desensitize them to it and to equip them to use more

---

Box 6.2 *Preparation of children and families for surgical procedures*

Communicate with the child in honest, realistic, developmentally appropriate terms

Assess the understanding of all family members, and correct any misperceptions

Depending on the developmental level of the child, demonstrate the procedure by means of dolls, drawing or videotapes

Allow the child to practice the procedure on a doll

Provide written information for older children, siblings and parents

Teach relaxation and coping skills to the child and the parents

Allow the child control over certain aspects of the procedure

Take the child on a tour of the operating-theatre, recovery-room and intensive-care unit to see the environment and meet staff

Provide parents with specific instructions with regard to their role

Give the child permission to cry and be upset

Allow sufficient time for questions from the child and the parents

---

active coping styles when they face a painful procedure (Sarafino, 1994).

In assessing the effects of different methods of preparation of children undergoing minor surgical procedures (using filmed modeling, coping skills, or filmed modeling plus coping skills), children who had been prepared showed less fear, called the nurses less often, were given fewer doses of sedatives and slept better after the operation compared with non-prepared controls. Preparation programs that included coping skills training were associated with the greatest benefits in the post-surgical recovery phase (Ortigosa Quiles et al., 1998).

Previous experience of hospitalization

Melamed and Siegel (1980) investigated the role of previous hospital experience in terms of its effect on the efficacy of procedural preparation. Children who had previous experience of hospitalization did not show a reduction in distress behaviors, as was found in children who had no previous experience of surgery. It was proposed that a second hospitalization was more anxiety-provoking for children, and it was suggested that exposure to a preparation film may have further sensitized them. Therefore children who have had repeated hospital admissions may need more detailed evaluation in order to determine their memories and beliefs about previous experiences, and they may need more extensive preparation.

The role of parents in preparation for surgical procedures

Parents have been found to be useful co-therapists for pain and distress reduction during painful procedures (e.g. Blount et al., 1991; Barrera, 2000), but parental anxiety may contribute to the child's anxiety and interfere with the child's ability to cope (Dahlquist et al., 1994). Calm parents and those who have received stress management training or education prior to the child's surgery were found to make a valuable contribution in supporting their children. Children with anxious parents were found to be significantly less upset if their parents were not present during the induction (Harbeck-Weber and McKee, 1996). Parents should not be expected to participate in actively restraining a child or in doing anything that conflicts with their supportive role.

Preparation for emergency surgery

Ideally all children and families should have access to unrushed, detailed psychological preparation, but sometimes this is not possible. Studies that have evaluated preparation for emergency surgery have shown mixed results. Preparation on the same day as surgery may increase knowledge about procedures but has not been shown to be effective in reducing fear and distress (Harbeck-Webber and McKee, 1995). More research is needed to determine the best type of preparation for children undergoing emergency or same-day surgery.

A SPECIAL CASE: LIVER TRANSPLANTATION

As technical aspects of organ transplantation improve and high rates of survival following transplantation become commonplace, attention is turning to psychosocial and quality-of-life issues for children and their families.

Pretransplantation assessment

Although pretransplant psychological interviews are routinely conducted with adults undergoing transplantation, this is not the case in pediatric programs (Shaw and Taussig, 1999). This is surprising, since studies have documented the presence of significant psychological difficulty and family dysfunction in pretransplant recipients (Whitehead et al., 1991; DeMaso et al., 1995) (for further discussion see Shaw and Taussig, 1999). At King's College Hospital, London, the purpose of the assessment is to provide a space in which families can reflect on the information they have been given by the multitude of professionals involved in the 3-day assessment, to discuss worries or concerns, to mobilize the coping resources of the child and their family and to identify any need for ongoing psychological support (e.g. with regard to desensitization to needles, or family work) (Helps et al., 2000a).

Effects of liver transplantation on the child

Although psychological adaptation following transplantation is generally considered to be good (e.g. Zitelli et al., 1988; Zamberlan, 1989), increased rates of anxiety (Mastroyannopoulou et al., 1998), depressive experiences (Windsorova et al., 1991), peer relationship concerns, social competence difficulties, scholastic deficits (DeBolt et al., 1995) and developmental delay (Wayman et al., 1997) have been noted. From the child's perspective, many children post transplantation regard themselves as healthy rather than sick, and use similar coping strategies to those employed by a chronically ill comparison group (Mastroyannopoulou et al., 1998).

Walker et al. (1999) reported on 18 children aged 7–16 years who had undergone a liver transplant. Children who had a liver transplant were found to have significantly more symptoms of post-traumatic stress than children with chronic illness or those who had undergone routine ENT procedures. It was found that 11% of children who had undergone a liver transplant had severe symptoms of post-traumatic stress disorder, and it was suggested that this was linked to the acute life threat involved in the liver transplantation. This figure is comparable to that found in groups of children undergoing treatment for other life-threatening illnesses.

Age of onset of liver disease and mental delay prior to transplant are important predictors of intellectual ability at follow-up of 5 years or more (Bannister et al., 1995). Earlier transplantation (i.e. before 4 years of age may be beneficial to cognitive development (Stewart et al., 1989, 1994). There is little evidence that significant catch-up of cognitive ability occurs after transplantation, and around 30% of children who receive a transplant may show significant development/learning difficulties (for a review, see Stewart and Kennard, 1998).

Effects of liver transplantation on the family

Families adopt different coping strategies at different phases during the pre-transplant waiting time, the operation itself, and after discharge (Noble-Jamieson et al., 1996). Many families rise to the challenge of their child having a transplant. However, the practical demands are immense. Stressors include financial demands, arranging time away from one's job, organizing care for other children, parents being separated for weeks at a time, and single parents being separated from their usual support systems. High levels of parental psychological distress have been reported both before and after liver transplantation (Tarbell and Kosmach, 1998). Parents need to be kept regularly informed of their child's condition throughout the various phases of transplantation. Mothers have been shown to need most information in the pre-transplant and recovery phases, including knowledge of laboratory values, indications of rejection and infection, and ways to support their children emotionally (Weichler, 1990). It is important to consider how the whole family is affected by transplantation. For example, siblings of children awaiting liver transplantation were found not to have elevated rates of maladjustment in general compared with normative data, but those who did show behavioral maladjustment were the offspring of mothers who reported significantly greater personal strain than did other parents in the study (Stewart et al., 1993). Clinical experience suggests that families often feel more able to cope with the demands of the transplant compared with those of the Kasai procedure, which occurs early in the life of the newborn, when the parents have little time to prepare and mobilize their coping resources.

Living-related donation and transplantation

Psychological aspects of living-related transplantation in liver disease have not been well documented in the literature. Experience suggests that living-related transplantation can have a tremendous impact on family relationships in both positive and negative ways. Very few donors report that there is a true decision to be made, in the sense of there being a choice not to donate (Shaw and Taussig, 1999). Living-related donation involves practical limitations on the ability of parents who donate to support their child in the postoperative period, and to care for other children in the family. In one of the few studies to have addressed this issue, Goldman (1993) reported that three out of 20 living donors to infants experienced significant adjustment problems in the immediate postoperative period.

Psychological adjustment in the longer term: adherence

Failure to adhere to complex treatment regimens has been a significant and longstanding problem in health care. Not all transplant recipients adhere to their medication regimens, which can lead to graft loss and possibly death (Newton, 1999). Although much has been written about adherence in many types of pediatric transplantation, little has been published with regard to children who undergo liver transplantation.

Many factors contribute to adherence, and non-adherence takes a variety of forms (LaGreca and Schuman, 1995). It may occur when patients have failed to understand or remember what is expected of them, or when there is a practical reason why the regimen cannot be adhered to. Non-adherence may also be due to a conscious decision not to follow the guidance of the medical or surgical team, which can be for a variety of reasons.

The assessment of adherence is very difficult, as verbal reports are often unreliable (LaGreca, 1990). Written diaries and 'smart' pill boxes are just two of the approaches that have been used to try to measure adherence, but all methods have their weaknesses.

In younger children it is usually the parents who are responsible for the administration of medication. When non-adherence occurs here it may be a reflection of a broader issue of child management, and psychological input may be viewed in the context of helping the parents to gain more control over their child's behavior. In young people, non-adherence may reflect parent–adolescent conflict about autonomy-related issues as part of the normative tasks of adolescence.

Promotion of adherence

Any assessment of adherence should encompass an assessment of the child's and family's general health beliefs and beliefs about the medication regimen. In any intervention relating to adherence, immediate and delayed effects of non-adherence should be addressed (e.g. that in the short term one may be rid of the side-effects associated with a particular drug, but in the longer term one's health is likely to suffer if the drug is not being taken regularly). In the short term, education, supervision, audiotapes of discussions of the regimen, written schedules and frequent opportunities to discuss it can be beneficial. In the longer term, reinforcement of adherent behaviors has been found to be effective (e.g. token reward systems, verbal praise and monetary reinforcement) (for a review, see LaGreca and Schuman, 1995). With any form of non-adherence, it is most appropriate to start with just one part of the regimen and slowly build on adherent behaviors, rather than attempting to promote adherence to the whole regimen all at once.

DEATH AND BEREAVEMENT

Due to the sophisticated nature of treatment of children with many forms of liver disease, it is often extremely hard for the parent, child and health care team to address the possible imminent death of a child while actively and aggressively continuing with treatment. Children with chronic illnesses are often more aware of their situation than adults think, and teenagers frequently report being very frightened of death and dying (Helps *et al.*, 2000b). Failure to acknowledge impending death may leave children and their families bewildered, and may disallow them the opportunity for anticipatory grief (LeBaron and Zeltner, 1985).

Children and their families should be informed of their prognosis in an age-appropriate and factual way that allows room for realistic optimism (for a review, see Spinetta, 1980). Children frequently have many questions about their mortality, but are concerned about voicing these for fear of upsetting those close to them. Children may also have specific wishes about the practicalities of their death (e.g. where they would like to be and who they would like to have around them). Following the death of a child, appropriate grief counselling and therapy should be offered to parents, siblings and the wider family network, and this offer should be kept open for some time. Surviving children in the hospital or friends of the child who has died may need opportunities to discuss the death, as it may raise issues about their own mortality for them (Reynolds *et al.*, 1995). The health care team may also benefit from a structured debriefing session and the offer of confidential ongoing counselling after the death of a child in their care.

Key references

McCabe H. Involving children and adolescents in medical decision making: developmental and clinical considerations. *Journal of Pediatric Psychology* 1996; **21**: 505–16.

A useful paper that considers a variety of aspects on how to involve children in the decision-making process.

McGrath P. Aspects of pain in children and adolescents. *Journal of Child Psychology and Psychiatry* 1995; **36**: 717–31.

A thorough summary of all aspects of the development of the concept of pain, and of pain management strategies in children.

Walker AM, Harris G, Baker A, Kelly D, Houghton J. Post-traumatic stress responses following liver transplantation in older children. *Journal of Child Psychology and Psychiatry and Allied Disciplines* 1999; **40**: 363–74.

An important paper detailing the potential serious psychological impact that transplantation can have on some children.

Wallender J, Varni J. Effects of pediatric chronic physical disorders on child and family adjustment. *Journal of Child Psychology and Psychiatry* 1998; **39**: 29–48.

An important review paper detailing what is known about risk and resilience in children and families facing chronic illness.

SUMMARY

Advances in liver surgery have led to increased longevity for children with previously fatal conditions. These children can grow up to lead productive, happy lives, and although many families are resilient to the stressors that they face, some are vulnerable to a variety of psychological difficulties. Psychological adjustment of children and their families is inextricably linked, and the child should always be viewed in the context of the family system. An appreciation of the children's understanding of their condition is vital if one is to be able to communicate effectively with them about their condition and proposed surgical interventions. Behavioral and cognitive strategies have been shown to promote the coping abilities of children and their families when faced with stressors such as surgery. Psychological education, modeling and rehearsal, giving control to the child, distraction, relaxation and desensitization are among the strategies which can be utilized effectively in preparing children and their families for such procedures. These techniques are not the sole domain of psychology professionals, and should be incorporated into the standard clinical care of children who undergo surgery.

REFERENCES

Alderson P. *Children's consent to surgery*. Buckingham: Open University Press, 1993.

Bannister M, Stewart SM, Kennard BD, Benser M, Andrews WS, Moore PE. Developmental and physical growth status of pediatric liver transplantation patients at least 5 years after surgery. Paper presented at the Joint Congress on Liver Transplantation, London, September 1995.

Barrera M. Brief clinical report: procedural pain and anxiety management with mother and siblings and co-therapists. *Journal of Pediatric Psychology* 2000; **25**: 117–21.

Bibace R, Walsh M. Developmental stages in children's conceptions of illness. In: Stone G, Cohen F, Adler N (eds) *Health psychology: a handbook*. San Francisco, CA: Jossey Bass, 1979.

Bibace R, Schmidt LR, Walsh ME. Children's perceptions of illness. In: Penny GN, Bennett P, Herbert M (eds) *Health psychology: a lifespan perspective*. Amsterdam: Harwood, 1994: 13–30.

Bieri D, Reeve R, Champion G, Addicpat L. The faces pain scale for the self-assessment of the pain experienced by children: development, initial validation and preliminary investigation for ratio-scale properties. *Pain* 1990; **41**: 139–50.

Blount RL, Landolf-Fritsche B, Powers SW, Sturges JW. Differences between high and low coping children and between parent and staff behaviours during painful medical procedures. *Journal of Pediatric Psychology* 1991; **16**: 795–809.

Bradford R. *Children, families and chronic illness*. London: Routledge, 1994.

Carr A. *Handbook of child and adolescent clinical psychology*. London: Routledge, 2000.

Dahlquist LM, Powers TG, Cox CN, Fernbach DJ. Parenting and child distress during cancer procedures. *Children's Health Care* 1994; **23**: 149–66.

DeBolt A, Stewart SM, Kennard BD *et al*. A survey of psychosocial adaptation in long-term survivors of pediatric liver transplants. *Children's Health Care* 1995; **24**: 79–96.

DeMaso DR, Twente AW, Spratt EG, O'Brien P. Impact of psychologic functioning, medical severity and family functioning in pediatric heart transplantation. *Journal of Heart and Lung Transplantation* 1995; **14**: 1102–8.

Drotar D, Bastiewicz A, Irvin N, Kendell J, Klaus M. The adaptation of parents to the birth of an infant with a congenital malformation: a hypothetical model. *Pediatrics* 1975; **56**: 710–17.

Goldman LS. Liver transplantation using living donors: preliminary donor psychiatric outcomes. *Psychosomatics* 1993; **34**: 235–40.

Grunau RVE, Craig KD. Pain expression in neonates: facial action and cry. *Pain* 1987; **28**: 395–410.

Harbeck-Webber C, McKee DH. Prevention of emotional and behavioral distress in children experiencing hospitalization and chronic illness. In: Roberts MC (ed.) *Handbook of pediatric psychology*. New York: Guilford, 1995: 167–84.

Helps SL, Wilford G, McCutheon R, Singer J, Dare J. Psychosocial assessment prior to pediatric liver transplantation. Paper presented at World Congress of Pediatric Gastroenterology, Hepatology and Nutrition, Boston, August 2000a.

Helps SL, Dignan J, Wyatt H, Price J, Ruiz G. The Strengths and Difficulties Questionnaire is a useful psychological screening tool for use with children and young people with cystic fibrosis. Thirteenth International Cystic Fibrosis Congress, Stockholm, June 2000b.

Hester N, Foster R, Kristensen K. Measurement of pain in children: generalisabilty and validity of the pain ladder and poker chip tool. In: Tyler D, Krane E (eds) *Paediatric pain: advances in pain research and therapy. Vol. 15*. New York: Raven, 1990, 79–84.

Hoffmann RG, Rodrigue JR, Andres JM, Novak DA. Moderating effects of family functioning on the social adjustment of children with liver disease. *Children's Health Care* 1995; **24**: 107–17.

House R, Dubovsky S, Penn L. Psychiatric aspects of hepatic transplantation. *Transplantation* 1983; **36**: 146–50.

Kuttner L, LePage T. Face scales for the assessment of pediatric pain: a critical review. *Canadian Journal of Behavioural Science* 1989; **21**: 198–209.

LaGreca AM. Issues of adherence with pediatric regimes. *Journal of Pediatric Psychology* 1990; **15**: 285–308.

LaGreca AM, Schuman WB. Adherence to prescribed medical regimes. In: Roberts MC (ed.) *Handbook of pediatric psychology*. New York: Guilford, 1995: 55–83.

Lazarus RS, Folkman S. *Stress, appraisal and coping*. New York: Springer, 1984.

LeBaron S, Zeltner L. The role of imagery in the treatment of dying children and adolescents. *Journal of Developmental and Behavioral Pediatrics* 1985; **6**: 252–8.

McCabe H. Involving children and adolescents in medical decision making: developmental and clinical considerations. *Journal of Pediatric Psychology* 1996; **21**: 505–16.

McGrath P. *Pain in children: nature, assessment and treatment*. New York: Guilford, 1990.

McGrath P. Aspects of pain in children and adolescents. *Journal of Child Psychology and Psychiatry* 1995; **36**: 717–31.

McGrath P, McAlpine LM. Psychological perspectives on pediatric pain. *Journal of Pediatrics* 1993; **122**: S2–8.

McGrath P, Johnson G, Goodman J, Schillinger J, Dunn J, Chapman J. CHEOPS: a behavioral scale for rating postoperative pain in children. In: Fields H, Dubner R, Cerveero F (eds) *Advances in pain research and therapy. Vol. 9*. New York: Raven, 1985: 395–401.

Mastroyannopoulou K, Sclare I, Baker A, Mowat AP. Psychological effects of liver disease and transplantation. *European Journal of Pediatrics* 1998; **57**: 856–60.

Melamed BG, Siegel LJ. Reduction in anxiety in children facing hospitalisation and surgery by use of filmed modelling. *Journal of Consulting and Clinical Psychology* 1975; **43**: 511–21.

Melamed BG, Siegel LJ. *Behavioral medicine: practical applications in health care*. New York: Springer, 1980.

Merskey H (ed.) Classification of chronic pain: descriptions of chronic pain syndromes and definitions of pain terms. *Pain* 1986; **Supplement 3**.

Newton SE. Promoting adherence to transplant medication regimes: a review of behavioral analysis. *Journal of Transplant Coordination* 1999; **9**: 13–16.

Noble-Jamieson G, Cook P, Parkinson G, Barnes N. Coping strategies of parents of children receiving liver transplants. *Clinical Child Psychology and Psychiatry* 1996; **1**: 563–73.

Ortigosa Quiles JM, Mendez Carrillo FX, Vargas Torcal F. The impact of psychological preparation for pediatric surgery on postoperative recovery. *Anales Espanoles de Pediatria* 1998; **49**: 369–74.

Pless I, Nolan T. Revision, replication and neglect in research on maladjustment in chronic illness. *Journal of Child Psychology and Psychiatry* 1991; **82**: 347–65.

Reynolds LA, Miller DL, Jelalian E, Spirito A. Anticipatory grief and bereavement. In: Roberts MC (ed.) *Handbook of pediatric psychology*. New York: Guilford, 1995: 142–66.

Saile H, Burgmeier R, Schmidt LR. A meta-analysis of studies on psychological preparation of children facing medical procedures. *Psychology and Health* 1988; **2**: 107–32.

Sarafino E. *Health psychology: biopsychosocial interactions*, 2nd edn. New York: John Wiley & Sons, 1994.

Shaw RJ, Taussig HN. Pediatric psychiatric pretransplant evaluation. *Clinical Child Psychology and Psychiatry* 1999; **4**: 353–65.

Spinetta J. Disease-related communication: how to tell. In: Kellerman J (ed.) *Psychosocial aspects of childhood cancer*. Springfield, IL: Charles C Thomas, 1980: 257–69.

Stewart SM, Kennard B. Organ transplantation. In: Brown RT (ed.) *Cognitive aspects of chronic disease in children*. New York: Guilford Press, 1998.

Stewart SM, Uauy R, Waller D, Kennard B, Benser M, Andrews W. Mental and motor development, social competence and growth one year after successful pediatric liver transplantation. *Journal of Pediatrics* 1989; **114**: 574–81.

Stewart SM, Kennard B, DeBolt A, Petrik K, Waller DA, Andrews WS. Adaptation of siblings of children awaiting liver transplantation. *Children's Health Care* 1993; **22**: 205–15.

Stewart SM, Kennard BD, Waller DA, Fixler D. Cognitive function in children who receive organ transplants. *Health Psychology* 1994; **13**: 3–13.

Tarbell SE, Kosmach B. Parental psychosocial outcomes in pediatric liver and/or intestinal transplantation: pretransplantation and the early postoperative period. *Liver Transplantation and Surgery* 1998; **4**: 378–87.

Thompson J. Stress, coping and family functioning in psychological adjustment in mothers of children and adolescents. *Journal of Pediatric Psychology* 1992; **17**: 573–86.

Walker AM, Harris G, Baker A, Kelly D, Houghton J. Post-traumatic stress responses following liver transplantation in older children. *Journal of Child Psychology and Psychiatry and Allied Disciplines* 1999; **40**: 363–74.

Wallender J, Varni J. Adjustment in children with chronic physical disorders: programmatic research on a disability–stress–coping model. In: LaGreca L, Siegel J, Wallender C (eds) *Stress and coping in child health*. New York: Guilford, 1992: 279–98.

Wallender J, Varni J. Effects of pediatric chronic physical disorders on child and family adjustment. *Journal of Child Psychology and Psychiatry* 1998; **39**: 29–48.

Wayman KI, Cox KL, Esquivel CO. Neurodevelopmental outcome of young children with extrahepatic biliary atresia 1 year after liver transplantation. *Journal of Pediatrics* 1997; **131**: 894–8.

Weichler NK. Information needs of mothers of children who have had liver transplants. *Journal of Pediatric Nursing* 1990; **5**: 88–96.

Weithorn LA, Campbell SB. The competency of children and adolescents to make informed treatment decisions. *Child Development* 1982; **53**: 1589–99.

Whitehead B, Helms P, Goodwin M *et al*. Heart–lung transplantation for cystic fibrosis. 1. Assessment. *Archives of Disease in Childhood* 1991; **66**: 1018–21.

Windsorova D, Stewart SM, Lovitt R, Waller DA, Andrews WS. Emotional adaptation in children after liver transplantation. *Journal of Pediatrics* 1991; **119**: 884–7.

Zamberlan KE. Quality of life in school-age children following liver transplantation. *Dissertation Abstracts International* 1989; **50**: 1860.

Zitelli BJ, Miller JW, Gartner JC *et al*. Changes in lifestyle after liver transplantation. *Pediatrics* 1988; **82**: 173–80.

PART 3

Biliary disorders

7

Embryology of the liver and bile ducts

PATRICIA COLLINS

THE TIMING OF DEVELOPMENT

Accurate and consistent timing of development is vital if the many articles on human development are to be used comparatively (Streeter, 1942; O'Rahilly and Müller, 1987). The limitations of the systems for staging human development are described in the chapter on the embryology of the pancreas (see Chapter 32).

MORPHOGENESIS OF THE LIVER

The main morphological features of the early development of the liver are presented in Figures 7.1 and 7.2 (see also Figure 32.1 in Chapter 32, on the embryology of the pancreas, which illustrates the elongation of the extrahepatic ducts). Liver development in the human is similar to that in the rat (Godlewski *et al.*, 1992, 1997a, b, 1998). An evagination from the foregut, known as the hepatic diverticulum, proliferates and grows into the septum transversum. The caudal epithelium of the hepatic diverticulum retains its basal lamina and enlarges to form the gallbladder and cystic duct. The cranial epithelium loses its basal lamina, and lines of endodermal cells proliferate and migrate individually into the mesenchyme of the septum transversum. These primitive hepatocytes initially allocate their daughter cells as zigzag-shaped or branching cords (Shiojiri *et al.*, 2000).

There are many confusing descriptions of liver development which use a variety of undefined terms. The migrating and proliferating *hepatic endodermal epithelial cells* are also referred to as hepatic trabeculae and sometimes as hepatic parenchyma (a term to be avoided). *Hepatic mesenchyme* is also referred to as septum transversum mesenchyme and later in development as stroma (see also below). Accounts which specify the two tissue types within the liver are less confusing.

MORPHOGENESIS OF THE HEPATIC CIRCULATION

The liver develops precociously in the embryo. Its development is intimately related to that of the celomic cavities, the heart and the inferior vena cava, as well as the foregut. In the stage 11 embryo the heart begins to beat. The pulsations cause an ebb and flow in the early vessels and within the celomic pericardial cavity and pericardioperitoneal canals (Figures 7.1b and c). Endothelial vitelline plexuses form around the yolk sac, and vitelline veins (also termed omphalomesenteric veins) arising from these plexuses drain into the sinus venosus. Similarly, the umbilical veins returning from the placenta also drain into the sinus venosus (Figures 7.3a and b). By stage 12 a hepatic endothelial plexus has formed as a result of the interaction between the ingrowing hepatic endoderm and the hepatic mesenchyme. The hepatic

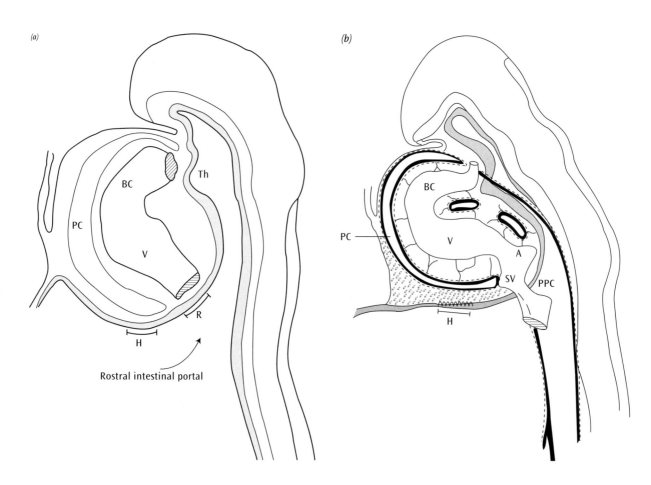

(a)

BC

PC

V

Th

R

H

Rostral intestinal portal

(b)

PC

BC

V

A

SV

PPC

H

(c)

Cranial

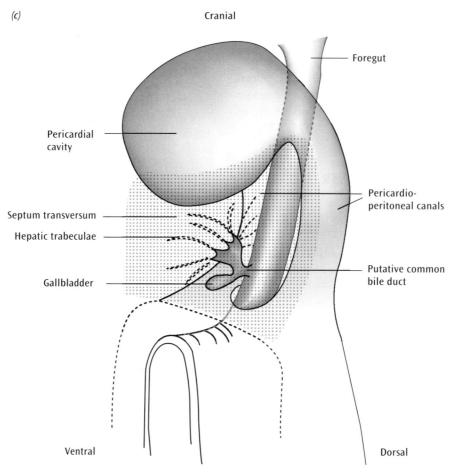

Foregut

Pericardial
cavity

Pericardio-
peritoneal canals

Septum transversum

Hepatic trabeculae

Putative common
bile duct

Gallbladder

Ventral

Dorsal

plexus is asymmetrical at this stage, and it forms anasto-motic connections on each side with the vitelline veins. Dorsally the hepatic plexus, within the right and left horns of the liver, empties on each side into an enlarged endothelial vessel, the hepatocardiac channel or vein, which then passes to the sinus venosus and the heart (Figures 7.2b and c and Figures 7.3c and d). Each hepa-tocardiac channel is surrounded by a pericardio-peri-toneal canal, separated from it by only a thin layer of celomic wall epithelium (Figure 7.2c). It is suggested that this region of the developing circulation may provide a site and mechanism for filling the rapidly expanding cardiovascular system with plasma, achieved by the movement of fluid from the celomic space to the vascu-lar space across a region of specialized celomic wall (O'Rahilly and Müller, 1987). The hepatocardiac chan-nel on the right side is more developed, whereas on the left side it is more plexiform, with only a transitory con-nection to the sinus venosus (Figure 7.3d).

At stage 13 all of the blood from the vitelline (omphalomesenteric) veins passes through the hepatic plexus, and this is the only blood supply that the early developing liver receives. The right and left vitelline veins form three transverse anastomoses around the develop-ing duodenum (Figures 7.3e and f). The relationship of these anastomoses alternates – the upper and lower anas-tomoses are ventral, whereas the intermediate one is dor-sal. They form a figure-of-eight around the duodenum. From the top (dorsal) vessel a midline branch grows cra-nially and anastomoses with a subdiaphragmatic anasto-mosis above (Figure 7.3f). This vessel is the primitive median ductus venosus, and it is dorsal to the expanding liver but ventral to the gut.

Blood from the umbilical veins continues to bypass the liver and enters the sinus venosus directly at stage 13 (Figure 7.3e). Subsequently, the cranial portions of both umbilical veins are also subsumed by the developing liver and their direct connection to the sinus venosus

ceases (Figure 7.3f). Both discharge placental blood into the hepatic sinusoids via venae advehentes (also known as venae afferentes hepatis). At late stage 14 and early stage 15 the right umbilical vein regresses completely. The left umbilical vein retains some branches which dis-charge blood directly into the hepatic sinusoids. However, new enlarging connections with the left half of the vitelline (omphalomesenteric) veins as they enter the hepatic sinusoids give rise to a bypass channel (Figure 7.3f) which connects to the midline ductus venosus and finally to the right half of the subdiaphragmatic anasto-moses to reach the termination of the inferior vena cava (Figure 7.3g).

Although it has traditionally been believed that most of the umbilical blood bypasses the liver sinusoids and is delivered directly to the right atrium, recent studies have shown that the average fraction of umbilical blood shunted through the ductus venosus is 28–32% at 20 weeks' gestation, decreasing to 22% at 25 weeks and 18% at 32 weeks (Kiserud, 2000; Kiserud et al., 2000). The degree of shunting seems to depend on both the resistance of the developing portal vascula-ture in the liver and the resistance of the ductus veno-sus itself.

The ductus venosus closes in 76% of term neonates before day 7, and in all infants before day 18 (Fugelseth et al., 1997). Absence of the ductus venosus is a rare vas-cular anomaly which may be associated with portal cir-culation disturbances and hydrops fetalis (Siven et al., 1995). However, other studies have found that the hepatic veins may assume the function of the ductus venosus without compromising the portal circulation or causing hydrops (Gembruch et al., 1998). Adult patent ductus venosus is often only diagnosed in cases of portal hypertension. A study which shows the presence of this vascular anomaly in three siblings suggests that a reces-sive genetic trait may be the underlying cause of patent ductus venosus (Jacob et al., 1999).

Figure 7.1 *Sagittal sections of early embryos. Reproduced from O'Rahilly and Müller (1987).*

(a) Stage 10 embryo. The rostral intestinal portal is still widely open to the yolk sac in this stage and the next. The neural tube is not yet completely closed. Specific regions of ventral foregut endoderm are indicated. The parietal wall of the pericardial cavity, the 'precardiac area', can be identified.

(b) Stage 11 embryo. Sagittal section with the left pericardio-peritoneal canal added. This covers the foregut. The left horn of the sinus venosus is curving over the canal to enter the sinus venosus. 'Cardiac mesenchyme' is proliferating from the parietal pericardial celom wall. The endoderm in contact with this mesenchyme thickens and becomes hepatic endoderm. PC, pericardial cavity; PPC, pericardio-peritoneal canal; SV, sinus venosus; A, atrium; V, ventricle; BC, bulbus cordis; Th, region of thyroid gland evagination; R, region of res-piratory evagination; H, region of hepatic evagination.

(c) Diagram of the pericardial cavity and pericardio-peritoneal canals viewed from the ventral left side. The foregut passes dorsal to the pericardial cavity and medial to the pericardio-peritoneal canals. From the distal foregut the hepatic endodermal epithelium evaginates ventrally. It forms cranial and caudal portions. The cranial portion proliferates as hepatic trabeculae and the caudal portion becomes the gallbladder. The cardiac mesenchyme into which the hepatic endoderm grows is now termed the septum transversum. Adapted from Collins P. Embryology: a user-friendly guide to embryology. Southampton: University of Southampton, 1998, with the kind permission of the University of Southampton.

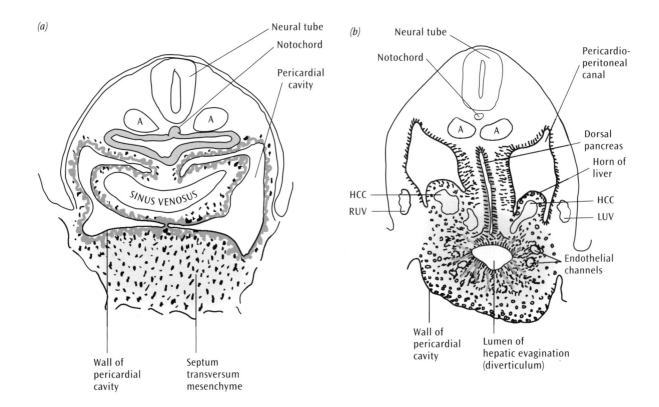

(a)

Neural tube

Notochord

Pericardial
cavity

A   A

SINUS VENOSUS

Wall of
pericardial
cavity

Septum
transversum
mesenchyme

(b)

Neural tube

Notochord

A   A

Pericardio-
peritoneal
canal

Dorsal
pancreas

Horn of
liver

HCC

LUV

HCC

RUV

Endothelial
channels

Wall of
pericardial
cavity

Lumen of
hepatic evagination
(diverticulum)

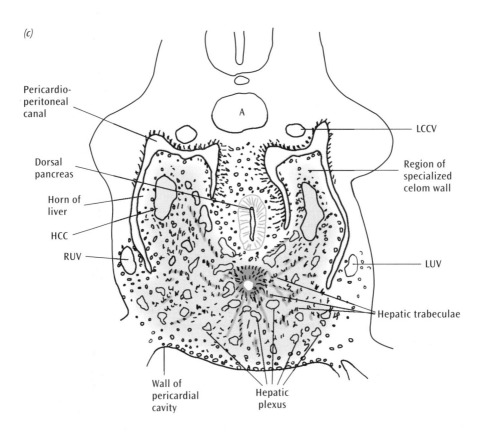

(c)

Pericardio-
peritoneal
canal

Dorsal
pancreas

Horn of
liver

HCC

RUV

A

LCCV

Region of
specialized
celom wall

LUV

Hepatic trabeculae

Wall of
pericardial
cavity

Hepatic
plexus

ORIGIN OF LIVER ENDODERM

Endoderm which will give rise to the hepatic primordium invaginates through the primitive or Hensen's node and the most rostral end of the primitive streak. From the 1-somite to the 8-somite stage in chick embryos, putative hepatic endoderm is rostral to the level of the third somite (Fukuda-Taira, 1981a). In the stage 11 human embryo, hepatic endoderm is induced to proliferate by the adjacent 'cardiac mesenchyme' (Figure 7.1a, b). At this stage the rostral intestinal portal is widely open and this region of endoderm faces caudally. By stage 12, the connection to the yolk sac is narrower and the hepatic endodermal primordium is directed ventrally into the septum transversum. Septum transversum mesenchyme then stimulates the proliferation and later differentiation of these cells, which commence expression of liver-specific molecular markers, including alpha-fetoprotein, albumin, urea cycle enzymes such as carbamoylphosphate synthetase I (CPSI) and glycogen storage (Koike and Shiojiri, 1996; Shiojiri, 1997) (Figure 7.4). The primitive hepatocytes have two developmental fates – they may differentiate into either biliary duct wall cells or mature hepatocytes (Shiojiri, 1981, 1997; Shiojiri and Mizuno, 1993) (Figure 7.5). Bile pigments can be detected within epithelial cells of the ductal plate and adjacent hepatocytes from week 12 (Tan and Moscoso, 1994a, b).

ORIGIN OF LIVER MESENCHYME

Hepatic mesenchyme originates from cells which invaginate through the middle part of the primitive streak during the early short-streak stage to early headfolding stage (Fukuda-Taira, 1981b). This population of cells migrates from the streak and comes to lie rostral to the buccopharyngeal membrane, where the cells will form the epithelial wall of the pericardial celom and the myocardium of the heart (Figures 7.1a and b and Figure 7.2a). The earliest

description of hepatic mesenchyme terms it 'precardiac' or 'cardiac' mesenchyme. Experimental studies have demonstrated that precardiac and cardiac mesenchyme from embryos from the headfolding stage to the 11-somite stage can induce proliferation of hepatic endodermal epithelium. In fact, all portions of the heart tube, truncus arteriosus, ventricle and atria, and both layers – endocardium and myocardium – have hepatic induction potency which is tissue specific but not species specific (Fukuda-Taira, 1981a). Later, as the heart and foregut are separated by accumulation of this mesenchyme, it is termed septum transversum. Thus during early development a succession of mesenchymal populations which are termed (from early to late) precardiac mesenchyme, cardiac mesenchyme and septum transversum mesenchyme will become hepatic mesenchyme. In the stage 11 human embryo the septum transversum forms a ventral mass caudal to the heart separating the endodermal layer from the celom (Figure 7.1b and Figure 7.2a). Dorsally the septum transversum impinges on the pericardio-pericardial canals laterally on each side (Figure 7.2b).

Hepatic mesenchyme contains a mixed population of cells with endothelial/angiogenic and connective tissue lineages. It has been suggested that the blood vessels and cells of the liver arise in situ from the proliferating mesoblastic cells of the celom wall (Rahilly and Müller, 1987). Circumstantial evidence has been offered to support a monoclonal hypothesis for human embryonic hematopoiesis, based on migration of stem and early progenitor cells from a generation site in the yolk sac to a colonization site in the liver via circulating blood (Migliaccio et al., 1986). The observation that yolk sac-derived hematopoietic stem cells seed the liver at about 6 weeks of development (Huyhn et al., 1995) is not consistent with the development of the hepatic plexus and blood cells in the stage 12 and 13 embryos at 26 and 28 days' gestation, respectively. However, chick/quail chimera experiments have shown that fetal hepatic hematopoiesis depends on migration of hematopoietic cells to the liver at the 28–30-somite stage. In culture of

Figure 7.2 *Transverse sections of embryos at the level of the developing liver. Reproduced from O'Rahilly and Müller (1987).*

(a) Stage 11 embryo. 'Cardiac' (septum transversum) mesenchyme is proliferating from the parietal wall of the pericardial cavity. This is the midline portion of the intra-embryonic celom. Compare this diagram with the sagittal section of a stage 11 embryo shown in Figure 7.1b.

(b) Stage 12 embryo. The hepatic endodermal epithelium has formed the hepatic evagination (diverticulum). Hepatic endodermal epithelial cells proliferate and migrate in columns into the septum transversum mesenchyme as hepatic trabeculae. Thus the proliferation of hepatic epithelium and hepatic mesenchyme is arising in opposite directions. Where they come into contact, the hepatic mesenchyme (also termed hepatic stroma) forms the endothelial channels of the hepatic plexus. The right and left horns of the developing liver project dorsally into the pericardio-peritoneal canals. A large vessel in each horn, the hepatocardial channel, is well placed to provide a region of specialized celom wall for the movement of celomic fluid into the developing cardiovascular system.

(c) Stage 13 embryo. The hepatocardiac channels have enlarged and the right and left lobes of the liver project fully into the pericardio-peritoneal canals. Hepatic trabeculae extend to the periphery of the developing liver. Hepatic mesenchyme (stroma) converts to endothelium and blood-forming cells on contact with the hepatic epithelium. A, aorta; LCCV, left caudal cardinal vein; HCC, hepatocardiac channel; RUV, right umbilical vein, LUV, left umbilical vein.

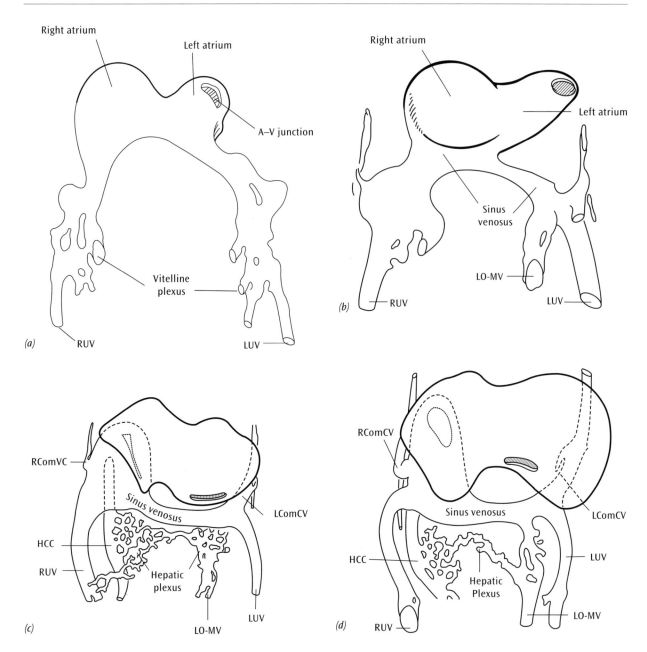

Figure 7.3 *Sequence of development of the main venous channels in the fetal liver. This diagram should be studied with reference to the text. Adapted from O'Rahilly and Müller (1987).*

(a) Diagram of a reconstruction of an early stage 11 embryo.

(b) Diagram of a reconstruction of a late stage 11 embryo.

(c) Diagram of a reconstruction of a stage 12 embryo.

(d) Diagram of a reconstruction of a stage 13 embryo.

hepatic primordium prior to this time, hepatocyte differentiation was normal but hematopoiesis did not occur (Houssaint, 1981). This aspect of liver developmental research is ongoing (Tavassoli, 1991).

Macrophages are found in loose aggregates in the sinusoids, and Kupffer cells, in contact with the endothelium, have been identified from about 6–7 weeks' gestation when hematopoiesis is inconspicuous in the liver (Enzan

et al., 1983). At this time the Kupffer cells actively engulf erythroblasts and erythocytes thought to be derived from the yolk sac. Kupffer cell activity increases in weeks 9–12, and erythroblasts and erythrocytes that are engulfed at this time are of hepatic origin (Enzan et al., 1983). The transformation of mesenchyme cells into endothelium produces a sinusoidal lining which is continuous without gaps or fenestrae. Erythroblasts and megakaryocytes are

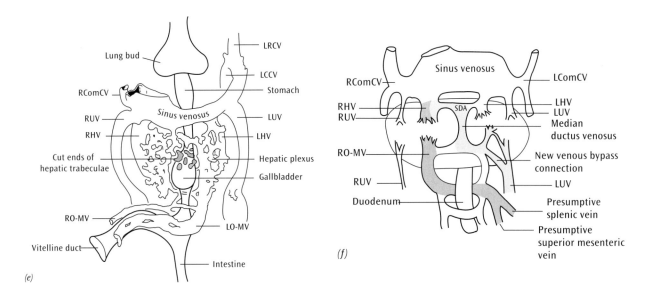

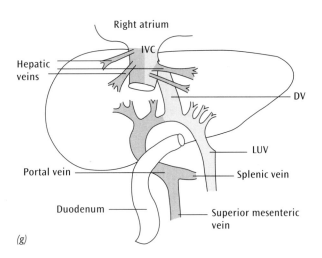

Figure 7.3 *(continued)*

(e) Diagram showing the developing venous channels relative to the gut.

(f) Diagram of a later stage showing the anastomoses within the fetal liver contributing to the development of the ductus venosus.

(g) Diagram of the venous arrangement of the liver in the fetus.

In all of the diagrams the following abbreviations apply: RUV, right umbilical vein; RO-MV, right omphalomesenteric vein (also termed right vitelline vein); RComCV, right common cardinal vein; HCC, hepatocardiac channel; RHV, right hepatocardiac vein; SDA, subdiaphragmatic anastomosis; LUV, left umbilical vein; LO-MV, left omphalomesenteric vein (also termed left vitelline vein); LRCV, left rostral cardinal vein; LComCV, left common cardinal vein; LCCV, left caudal cardinal vein; LHV, left hepatocardiac vein; DV, ductus venosus; IVC, inferior vena cava.

frequently observed migrating from their production sites through the sinusoidal wall into the sinusoids, but granulocytes are less frequently observed in this process (Enzan *et al.*, 1983).

Ito cells become trapped in the perisinusoidal spaces from 6 weeks. They are characterized by cytoplasmic fat droplets surrounded by glycogen granules. Between 9 and 12 weeks they are more numerous than in the adult,

and they lose their fat droplets as development advances. Fetal Ito cells are morphologically similar to fibroblasts in adult liver (Enzan *et al.*, 1983).

As development proceeds, mesenchyme cells differentiating into fibroblasts are found close to the portal triads and in the scant connective tissue of the liver capsule. This connective tissue seems to be specific for intrahepatic bile duct formation, as other gastrointestinal tract connective

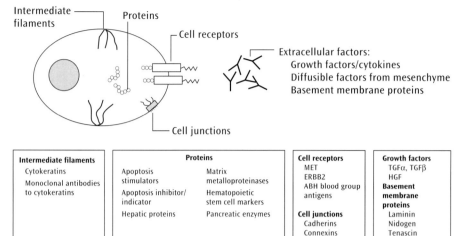

Figure 7.4 *Factors that influence liver development, and their location at the cellular level (Baloch* et al., *1992; Quondamatteo* et al., *1999a,b).*

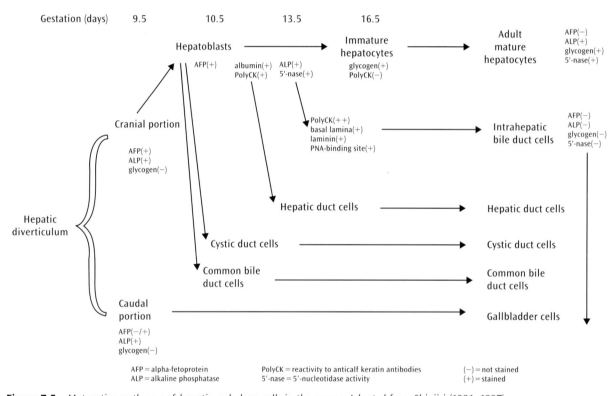

Figure 7.5 *Maturation pathways of hepatic endoderm cells in the mouse. Adapted from Shiojiri (1981, 1997).*

tissue will not induce biliary epithelial development in immature hepatocytes (Shiojiri and Mizuno, 1993).

EPITHELIAL–MESENCHYMAL INTERACTIONS WHICH GIVE RISE TO THE LIVER

The classical interaction experiments on liver showed that whereas precardiac mesenchyme is necessary for the normal differentiation of hepatic endoderm, other types of mesenchyme will also support its development and

differentiation (Le Douarin, 1975). All derivatives of the lateral plate mesenchyme (i.e. splanchnopleuric mesenchyme derived from the walls of the pericardio-peritoneal canals) can replace hepatic mesenchyme. Lung mesenchyme (a splanchnic and midline ventral mesenchyme) not only supports development and differentiation of hepatic endoderm, but it also promotes branching duct formation which resembles that of lung (Koike and Shiojiri, 1996). Axial mesenchyme, particularly somites, does not support hepatic endoderm development (Le Douarin, 1975; Koike and Shiojiri, 1996),

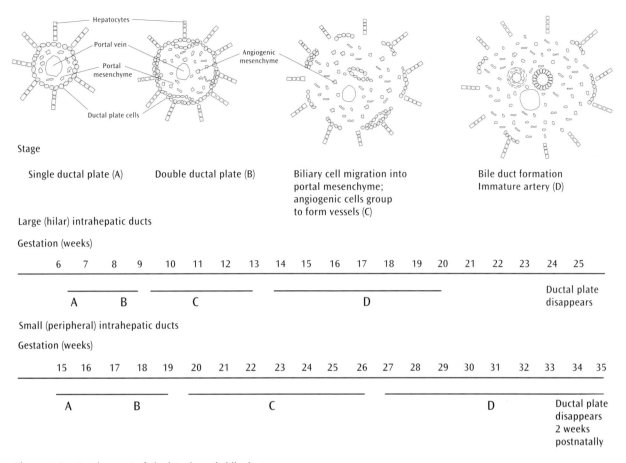

Figure 7.6 *Development of the intrahepatic bile ducts.*

nor does metanephric mesenchyme (Koike and Shiojiri, 1996).

The hepatic mesenchyme controls the specific pattern for liver morphogenesis. If a mechanical barrier is inserted across the hepatic mesenchyme just caudal to the endodermal evagination, normal liver tissue will develop cranial to the barrier where hepatic endoderm and mesenchyme are in contact. Caudal to the barrier the hepatic mesenchyme will form endothelium and hepatic lobes. However, no hepatocytes are present (Le Douarin, 1975).

DEVELOPMENT OF THE EXTRAHEPATIC BILIARY SYSTEM

The caudal portion of the early hepatic endodermal evagination of the foregut gives rise to the extrabiliary system consisting of the common hepatic duct, gallbladder, cystic duct and common bile duct (Figure 7.1c; also see Figure 32.1 in Chapter 32 on embryology of the pancreas). The right and left hepatic ducts develop from the cranial end of the common hepatic duct from 12 weeks' gestation (Nakanuma *et al.*, 1997). Extrahepatic biliary glands evaginate from the main ducts from about 11 weeks' gestation.

These branch and proliferate to become evenly distributed throughout the duct walls in childhood (Nakanuma *et al.*, 1997). The glands have an acinar structure.

DEVELOPMENT OF THE INTRAHEPATIC BILIARY SYSTEM

The development of the intrahepatic biliary ducts is intimately related to the branching pattern of the portal vein radicles. Portal veins and hepatic veins share a common origin from vitelline (omphalomesenteric) veins (Shiojiri, 1997). During the early stages of liver development the histology of both veins is similar. However, later on more hepatic mesenchyme is found around the portal veins compared to hepatic veins (Shiojiri and Nagai, 1992; Shiojiri, 1997). The condensation of mesenchyme around the portal veins seems to be a prerequisite for bile duct development.

The cranial portion of the early hepatic evagination of the foregut gives rise to all liver hepatocytes, the intrahepatic large bile ducts or hilar ducts (including the right and left hepatic ducts, segmental ducts, area ducts and their first branches) and the small bile ducts or peripheral bile ducts (including the septal bile ducts, interlobular bile ducts and bile ductules) (Nakanuma *et al.*, 1997).

Portal vein branches have been identified from 6 weeks, although no intrahepatic bile ducts are present during the first 7 weeks of gestation (Nakanuma *et al.*, 1997). The process of development progresses from the hilum to the periphery of the liver, from larger to smaller ducts during gestation, and remains immature at birth. Primitive hepatocytes form a sleeve around the portal vein branches and associated mesenchyme. This sleeve is termed the ductal plate (Figure 7.6a). Portions of the sleeve are duplicated, forming small linear tubules which move towards the portal vein and differentiate into bile ducts (Van Eyken *et al.*, 1988; Ruebner *et al.*, 1990; Nakanuma *et al.*, 1997; Shiojiri, 1997; Terada *et al.*, 1997; Vijayan and Tan, 1997, 1999; Godlewski *et al.*, 1998; Shah and Gerber, 1998) (Figure 7.6). The latter process is termed ductal plate remodeling. The newly formed bile ducts retain luminal continuity with ductal plate lumina through epithelial channels (future ductules). Incomplete remodeling of the ductal plate leaves rings of interrupted curved lumina around portal triad connective tissue (Desmet, 1998). Bile ducts have a patent lumen throughout development (Tan and Moscoso, 1994a, b; Vijayan and Tan, 1999). As bile ducts develop, angiogenic mesenchymal cells coalesce close by to form blood vessels which will become branches of the hepatic artery from 10 weeks' gestation. This mechanism for the formation of portal triads extends throughout the developing liver, with the most mature triads closer to the hilum and the most immature and smaller triads at the periphery (Costa *et al.*, 1998). Abnormalities of the portal triads are associated with abnormalities of the branching pattern of the portal vein, referred to as 'pollard-willow' pattern, which result in too many, too closely spaced small branches. In these regions several ductal plates may be seen around several hypoplastic or obliterated portal vein branches (Desmet, 1998).

Intrahepatic peribiliary glands develop as evaginations of the bile ducts. These glands form immature acinar structures close to the larger bile ducts prior to birth, and full maturation is completed at about 15 years of age (Nakanuma *et al.*, 1997). A peribiliary vascular plexus which will supply the biliary ducts develops concurrently with the intrahepatic biliary system. Progenitor vascular cells can be identified in the portal mesenchyme inside the ductal plate. At the bile duct stage, capillaries surround the bile ducts. These mature into the vascular plexus, mainly after birth (Terada and Nakanuma, 1993; Nakanuma *et al.*, 1997; Terada *et al.*, 1997).

FACTORS THAT REGULATE LIVER AND INTRAHEPATIC BILIARY SYSTEM DEVELOPMENT

Most of the studies on the development of the intrahepatic biliary system have utilized specific immunological

reactions of primitive hepatocytes to visualize the system. The range of cytoskeletal elements, intercellular proteins, cell adhesion molecules and extracellular growth factors (Baloch *et al.*, 1992; Quondamatteo *et al.*, 1999a, b) which have been shown to contribute to liver development is summarized in Figure 7.4. These factors are up-regulated and down-regulated within embryonic or fetal stages of development.

So far a range of genes necessary for liver development, as has been established for pancreatic development, has not been identified. The proteins expressed by adult liver, albumin and glycogen are expressed early in hepatocytes, and their differential expression has been used to trace the differentiation and maturation of the hepatic endodermal cells (Shiojiri, 1981, 1997; Koike and Shiojiri, 1996) (Figure 7.5). These cells also express pancreatic digestive enzymes (Terada *et al.*, 1997), blood group antigens (Terada *et al.*, 1997) and hematopoietic markers (Blakolmer *et al.*, 1995), making the study of liver development much more complex. This may be explained to some extent by the fetal hematopoietic function of the liver being set up early and then dismantled. This specific *in utero* purpose overlies the development of the postnatal functions of the liver, which may require contemporaneous exquisitely fine modulations of placental function.

Key references

Nakanuma Y, Hoso M, Sanzen T, Sasaki M. Microstructure and development of the normal and pathologic biliary tract in humans, including blood supply. *Microscopic Research and Technique* 1997; **38**: 552–70.

This paper gives a systematic description of biliary development.

Shiojiri N. Development and differentiation of bile ducts in the mammalian liver. *Microscopy Research and Technique* 1997; **39**: 328–35.

This paper describes bile duct maturation and the lineage of cells contributing to the ducts of the liver.

Terada T, Kitamura Y, Nakanuma Y. Normal and abnormal development of the human intrahepatic biliary system: a review. *Tohoku Journal of Experimental Medicine* 1997; **181**: 19–32.

This article explains the basis of the ductal plate.

Van Eyken P, Sciot R, Callea F, Van der Steen K, Moerman P, Desmet VJ. The development of the intrahepatic bile ducts in man: a keratin–immunohistochemical study. *Hepatology* 1988; **8**: 1586–95.

This paper provides a good illustration of ductal plate development.

REFERENCES

Baloch Z, Klapper J, Buchanan L, Schwartz M, Amenta PS. Ontogenesis of the murine hepatic extracellular matrix: an immunohistochemical study. *Differentiation* 1992; **51**: 209–18.

Blakolmer K, Jaskiewicz K, Dunsford HA, Robson SC. Hematopoietic stem cell markers are expressed by ductal plate and bile duct cells in developing human liver. *Hepatology* 1995; **21**: 1510–16.

Costa AM, Pegado CS, Porto LC. Quantification of the intrahepatic biliary tree during human fetal development. *Anatomical Record* 1998; **251**: 297–302.

Desmet VJ. Ludwig symposium on biliary disorders. Part I. Pathogenesis of ductal plate abnormalities. *Mayo Clinic Proceedings* 1998; **73**: 80–9.

Enzan H, Hara H, Yamshita Y, Ohkita T, Yamane T. Fine structure of hepatic sinusoids and their development in human embryos and fetuses. *Acta Pathologica Japonica* 1983; **33**: 447–66.

Fugelseth D, Lindemann R, Liestol K, Kiserud T, Langslet A. Ultrasonographic study of ductus venosus in healthy neonates. *Archives of Disease in Childhood, Foetal and Neonatal Edition* 1997; **77**: F131–4.

Fukuda-Taira S. Hepatic induction in the avian embryo: specificity of reactive endoderm and inductive mesoderm. *Journal of Embryology and Experimental Morphology* 1981a; **63**: 111–25.

Fukuda-Taira S. Location of prehepatic cells in the early developmental stages of quail embryos. *Journal of Embryology and Experimental Morphology* 1981b; **64**: 73–85.

Gembruch U, Baschat AA, Caliebe A, Gortner L. Prenatal diagnosis of ductus venosus: a report of two cases and review of the literature. *Ultrasound in Obstetrics and Gynecology* 1998; **11**: 185–9.

Godlewski G, Gaubert-Cristol R, Rouy S. Liver development in rats during the embryonic period (Carnegie stages 11–14). *Acta Anatomica (Basel)* 1992; **144**: 45–50.

Godlewski G, Gaubert-Cristol R, Rouy S, Prudhomme M. Liver development in the rat during the embryonic period (Carnegie stages 15–23). *Acta Anatomica (Basel)* 1997a; **160**: 172–8.

Godlewski G, Gaubert-Cristol R, Rouy S, Prudhomme M. Liver development in the rat and in man during the embryonic period (Carnegie stages 11–23). *Microscopy Research and Technique* 1997b; **39**: 314–27.

Godlewski G, Gaubert-Cristol R, Prudhomme M, Tang J, Rouy S. Comparison of the liver and biliary duct development in man and in the rat at the end of the embryonic period. *Morphologie: Bulletin de l'Association des Anatomistes* 1998; **82**: 11–14.

Houssaint E. Differentiation of the mouse hepatic primordium. II. Extrinsic origin of the haematopoietic cell line. *Cell Differentiation* 1981; **10**: 243–52.

Huyhn A, Dommergues M, Izac B *et al*. Characterization of hematopoietic progenitors from human yolk sacs and embryos. *Blood* 1995; **86**: 4474–85.

Jacob S, Farr G, De Vun D, Takiff H, Mason A. Hepatic manifestations of familial patent ductus venosus in adults. *Gut* 1999; **45**: 442–5.

Kiserud T. Fetal venous circulation – an update on hemodynamics. *Journal of Perinatal Medicine* 2000; **28**: 90–6.

Kiserud T, Rasmussen S, Skulstad S. Blood flow and the degree of shunting through the ductus venosus in the human fetus. *American Journal of Obstetrics and Gynecology* 2000; **182**: 147–53.

Koike T, Shiojiri N. Differentiation of the mouse hepatic primordium cultured *in vitro*. *Differentiation* 1996; **61**: 35–43.

Le Douarin NM. An experimental analysis of liver development. *Medicine and Biology* 1975; **53**: 427–55.

Migliaccio G, Migliaccio AR, Petti S *et al*. Human embryonic hemopoiesis. Kinetics of progenitors and precursors underlying the yolk sac–liver transition. *Journal of Clinical Investigation* 1986; **78**: 51–60.

Nakanuma Y, Hoso M, Sanzen T, Sasaki M. Microstructure and development of the normal and pathologic biliary tract in humans, including blood supply. *Microscopy Research and Technique* 1997; **38**: 552–70.

O'Rahilly R, Müller F. *Developmental stages in human embryos*. Washington, DC: Carnegie Institution of Washington, 1987.

Quondamatteo F, Knittel T, Mehde M, Ramadori G, Herken R. Matrix metalloproteinases in early human liver development. *Histochemistry and Cell Biology* 1999a; **112**: 277–82.

Quondamatteo F, Scherf C, Miosge N, Herken R. Immunohistochemical localization of laminin, nidogen and type IV collagen during the early development of human liver. *Histochemistry and Cell Biology* 1999b; **111**: 39–47.

Ruebner BH, Blankenberg TA, Burrows DA, SooHoo W, Lund JK. Development and transformation of the ductal plate in the developing human liver. *Pediatric Pathology* 1990; **10**: 55–68.

Shah KD, Gerber MA. Development of intrahepatic bile ducts in humans. Immunohistochemical study using monoclonal cytokeratin antibodies. *Archives of Pathology and Laboratory Medicine* 1998; **113**: 1135–8.

Shiojiri N. Enzymo- and immunocytochemical analyses of the differentiation of liver cells in the prenatal mouse. *Journal of Embryology and Experimental Morphology* 1981; **62**: 139–52.

Shiojiri N. Development and differentiation of bile ducts in the mammalian liver. *Microscopy Research and Technique* 1997; **39**: 328–35.

Shiojiri N, Nagai Y. Preferential differentiation of the bile ducts along the portal vein in the development of mouse liver. *Anatomy and Embryology (Berlin)* 1992; **185**: 17–24.

Shiojiri N, Mizuno T. Differentiation of functional hepatocytes and biliary epithelial cells from immature hepatocytes of the fetal mouse *in vitro*. *Anatomy and Embryology (Berlin)* 1993; **187**: 221–9.

Shiojiri N, Sano M, Inujima S, Nitou M, Kanazawa M, Mori M. Qualitative analysis of cell allocation during liver development, using the spf(ash)-heterozygous female mouse. *American Journal of Pathology* 2000; **156**: 65–75.

Siven M, Ley D, Hagerstrand I, Svenningsen N. Agenesis of the ductus venosus and its correlation to hydrops fetalis and the fetal hepatic circulation: case reports and review of the literature. *Pediatric Pathology and Laboratory Medicine* 1995; **15**: 39–50.

Streeter GL. *Developmental horizons in human embryos. Descriptions of age group XI, 13 to 20 somites, and age group XII, 21 to 29 somites*. Washington, DC: Carnegie Institution of Washington, 1942.

Tan CE, Moscoso GJ. The developing human biliary system at the porta hepatis level between 29 days and 8 weeks of gestation: a way to understanding biliary atresia. Part 1. *Pathology International* 1994a; **44**: 587–99.

Tan CE, Moscoso GJ. The developing human biliary system at the porta hepatis level between 11 and 25 weeks of gestation: a way to understanding biliary atresia. Part 2. *Pathology International* 1994b; **44**: 600–10.

Tavassoli M. Embryonic and fetal hemopoiesis: an overview. *Blood Cells* 1991; **17**: 269–81.

Terada T, Nakanuma Y. Development of human peribiliary capillary plexus: a lectin–histochemical and immunohistochemical study. *Hepatology* 1993; **18**: 529–36.

Terada T, Kitamura Y, Nakanuma Y. Normal and abnormal development of the human intrahepatic biliary system: a review. *Tohoku Journal of Experimental Medicine* 1997; **181**: 19–32.

Van Eyken P, Sciot R, Callea F, Van der Steen K, Moerman P, Desmet VJ. The development of the intrahepatic bile ducts in man: a keratin–immunohistochemical study. *Hepatology* 1988; **8**: 1586–95.

Vijayan V, Tan CE. Developing human biliary system in three dimensions. *Anatomical Record* 1997; **249**: 389–98.

Vijayan V, Tan CE. Development of the human intrahepatic biliary system. *Annals of the Academy of Medicine, Singapore* 1999; **28**: 105–8.

8

Biliary atresia: etiology, management and complications

EDWARD R HOWARD

Atresia of the extrahepatic bile ducts occurs in newborn infants and is the end-result of a destructive inflammatory process of unknown etiology. The extent of the atretic process varies from case to case, and this was clearly illustrated by Thomson as early as 1892 in a series of 29 cases which he collected from published case reports. Thomson's series was the first major review of biliary atresia, and it includes an excellent description of the natural history of the untreated condition. Thomson stated that:

> the children themselves are either jaundiced at birth, or they become so within the first week or two of life; otherwise they are healthy and well nourished. In some cases there is a discharge of normal meconium followed by colourless motions; in others the faeces are devoid of colour from the very first.

Most of the children in his report died within a few months as a result of spontaneous hemorrhage.

HISTORICAL ASPECTS

Single case reports of infants with biliary atresia were published in the nineteenth century (e.g. Home, 1813; Cursham, 1840), and were collected together by Thomson in 1892. In 1916 Holmes analyzed more than

100 reported cases and stated that the condition was more common than was supposed at that time. He made the important observation that occasionally a remnant of bile duct could be identified at postmortem, and he suggested that these cases might be suitable for a bile duct to bowel anastomosis. He recommended that laparotomy should be performed for definitive diagnosis in infants with suspected biliary atresia, and he believed that the condition could be divided into 'correctable' and 'non-correctable' types, depending on the presence or absence of a residual segment of bile duct.

The first reports of successful surgery were published by Ladd (1928), who described anastomotic procedures in six out of 11 cases who underwent laparotomy. Unfortunately, many of the early reports confused biliary atresia with other conditions, such as choledochal cyst, giant-cell hepatitis and inspissated bile syndrome, and the results of treatment of true biliary atresia remained extremely poor. Only 52 reported successes from surgery in biliary atresia were published between 1927 and 1970 (Bill, 1978). In a desperate attempt to achieve bile drainage, a variety of techniques were developed, including resection and anastomosis of portions of the liver (Longmire and Sandford, 1948), the implantation of intrahepatic tubes (Sterling and Lowenburg, 1963) and the anastomosis of hepatic lymphatics to the bowel (Fonkalsrud et al., 1966). The poor results obtained at that time were illustrated by Hays and Snyder (1963), who reported an average survival of only 19 months in 41 children treated at the Los Angeles Children's Hospital between 1947 and 1961.

The major advance in treatment followed the work of Morio Kasai in Sendai, Japan, who observed that dissection of the porta hepatis in a female infant with biliary atresia produced a flow of bile. He anastomosed an intestinal conduit to the exposed area in the porta hepatis and investigated the microscopic anatomy of the residual bile duct tissue in the porta hepatis. His operation was first published in 1959 (Kasai and Suzuki, 1959), and improvements in the technique followed rapidly.

Kasai described the presence of small channels in the porta hepatis, which varied in diameter up to 300 µm, and using reconstruction studies he showed that these communicated with intrahepatic ducts. Anastomosing a Roux-en-Y loop of jejunum to the porta hepatis is now known as the portoenterostomy procedure. The operation has been modified by many surgeons, but the basic technique of a radical excision of all remnants of bile duct tissue in the porta hepatis is unchanged. The benefits of the operation have been illustrated by many authors, and in an early series Lau and Ong (1983) reported that between 1955 and 1975 all infants with severe atresia had died, but that between 1975 and 1981 six out of 12 cases were successfully treated by a Kasai-type operation.

The operation of portoenterostomy has proved to be most effective when performed before 8 weeks of age, and an increasing number of patients are surviving into adult life after this operation. For those who do not respond satisfactorily or who develop complications after portoenterostomy, the likelihood of long-term survival has been improved by the development of liver transplantation, and a coordinated program of early portoenterostomy, and transplantation for those who fail with the initial operation, should now result in long-term survival in more than 90% of these patients.

ETIOLOGY

The etiology of biliary atresia remains unknown, although there is a wide range of hypotheses based on infective, embryological, metabolic and vascular studies. Surgical attempts to produce an experimental model have not been successful, and no etiological link has been demonstrated with either ionizing radiation (Brent, 1962) or teratogenic drugs (Gourevitch, 1971). Epidemiological studies are of interest, as they have suggested that the etiology may well be heterogenous. For example, Houwen et al. (1988) investigated the possibility of an infectious etiology, which should give rise to time–space clustering. They therefore analyzed 89 cases born in The Netherlands during a 10-year period, as well

as 130 cases born in West Germany. They found no evidence of clustering in any particular year or in any part of a year, and this result makes infection an unlikely factor. However, their results did suggest an etiological heterogeneity.

Chardot et al. (1999) investigated seasonality and clustering in 421 infants with biliary atresia born in France and 40 infants born in overseas territories between 1986 and 1996. Geographic distribution, seasonality and time clustering were analyzed. No regional variation in incidence was demonstrated in France, and there was no evidence of seasonality or time clustering. However, the incidence of biliary atresia was shown to be 5.7-fold higher in Polynesia than in France, where the incidence was 5.12 per 100 000 live births. The French incidence was very similar to the figure of 5.98 per 100 000 reported from a case study in the UK and Ireland (McKiernan et al., 2000).

Congenital factors

The association of biliary atresia with anomalies such as polysplenia, situs inversus, malrotation and absent inferior vena cava (Figure 8.1) and with cardiac defects is now well recognized, and in an early series from King's College Hospital approximately 20% of 237 cases fell within this group (Box 8.1). Associated abnormalities have been reported in up to 30% of biliary atresia patients (Lilly and Chandra, 1974; Miyamoto and Kajimoto, 1983; Silveira et al., 1993). A variety of splenic malformations have been reported, including double spleens and asplenia as well as polysplenia. The distinct syndromic association of situs inversus, polysplenia and portal vein anomalies (Figures 8.2 and 8.3) is now known as the polysplenia syndrome or *biliary atresia–splenic malformation (BASM)*. Davenport et al. (1993) reported a 7.5% incidence of the syndrome in 308 cases of atresia. Four of the infants were born to mothers with diabetes mellitus, and one infant with asplenia was shown, after investigation for chest infection, to have immotile respiratory tract cilia. Immotile cilia are recognized as part of the Kartegener syndrome (i.e. with situs inversus, paranasal sinusitis and bronchiectasis) but have also been described in association with polysplenia, situs inversus and biliary atresia (Gershoni-Baruch et al., 1989). It has been suggested that the BASM syndrome may be a subgroup, perhaps with a different etiology to the commoner isolated form of atresia, and that the disturbance in bile duct development might occur early in gestation, at the time of development of the spleen and rotation of the gut.

Mazziotti et al. (1999) have described histological studies in transgenic mice with a recessive deletion of the 'inversin' gene. The mice have situs inversus and jaundice secondary to a lack of continuity between the extrahepatic biliary tree and the small intestine. The authors

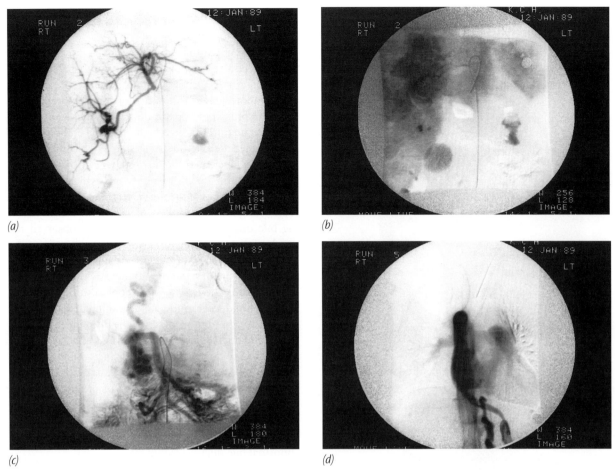

(a)

(b)

(c)

(d)

Figure 8.1 *Congenital abnormalities in biliary atresia demonstrated radiologically. (a) Celiac axis injection demonstrating situs inversus. (b) Right-sided polysplenia seen on the venous phase of an angiogram. (c) Congenital portosystemic shunt; portal vein joining with caval collaterals. (d) Congenital inferior vena caval interruption with azygos continuation.*

speculate that histological features of extrahepatic biliary obstruction and structural abnormalities of the bile ducts in these animals might suggest a role for the 'inversin' gene in normal bile duct development, and that alterations in 'inversin' could provide support for the hypothesis of a genetic basis for the BASM syndrome.

Other possible genetic influences in biliary atresia are indicated by the association with trisomy 17, 18 and 21 (Danks, 1965; Alpert *et al.*, 1969). However, twin studies do not suggest a simple genetic cause. For example, Strickland *et al.* (1985) reported a monozygotic pair and a dizygotic pair, only one child being affected with atresia in each case, and a review of 17 pairs of twins demonstrated concordance for biliary atresia in only one pair (Silveira *et al.*, 1991). This lack of concordance is in contrast to the pattern seen in twins with intrauterine infection, and Strickland *et al.* (1985) suggest that a defect in bile duct canalization or vascular supply might be implicated in the causation of biliary atresia. They quoted the embryological origin of stenotic and atretic congenital heart lesions in support of this hypothesis.

A survey of the literature by Cunningham and Sybert (1988) has revealed 11 instances of familial extrahepatic

biliary atresia, and the authors reported on two further families, each with two siblings affected. They concluded that a genetic susceptibility in combination with an environmental insult to the biliary tree may be responsible for the genesis of biliary atresia.

Box 8.1 *Congenital anomalies in 237 cases of biliary atresia investigated at King's College Hospital, London, during the period 1970–85 (expressed as percentage incidence)*

Cardiac	11.0%
Portal vein or inferior vena cava	8.5%
Splenic	8.0%
Malrotation	7.0%
Situs inversus	4.0%
Other gastrointestinal tract lesions (pyloric stenosis, atresia, etc.)	4.0%
Genitourinary	2.5%
Musculoskeletal (talipes, cleft palate, etc.)	2.0%

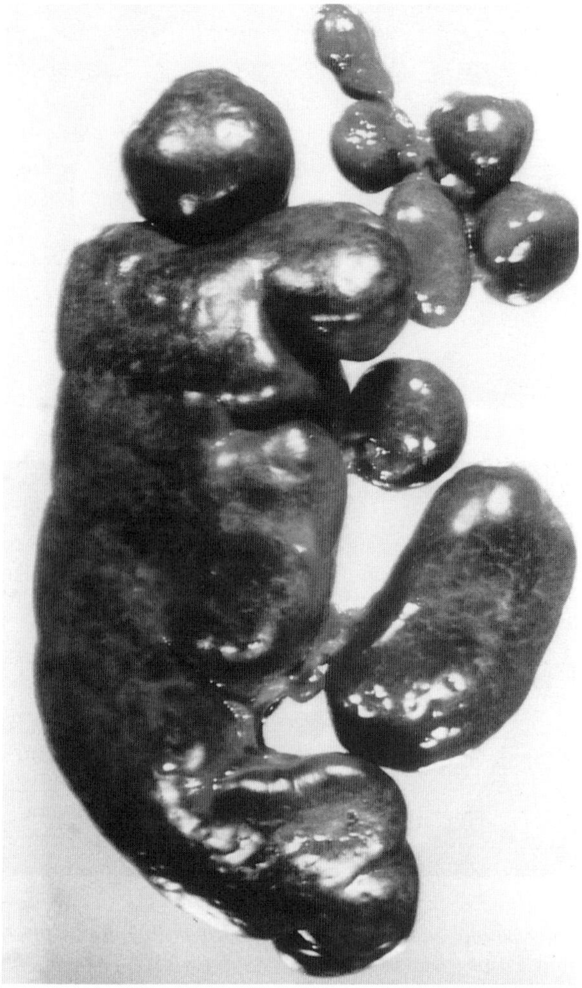

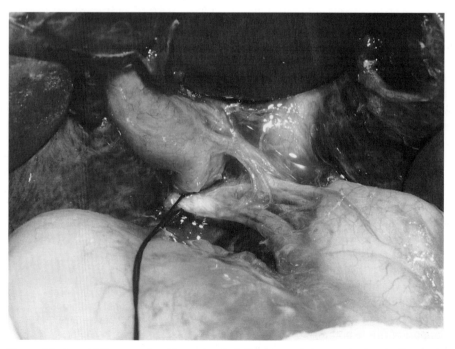

Figure 8.2 *An example of a right-sided polysplenia malformation.*

Embryological studies

Most intrahepatic bile ducts in biliary atresia have a mature tubular shape but show epithelial damage. However, 20–25% show features reminiscent of 'ductal plate malformation' with partial or complete persistence of embryonic intrahepatic ducts (Desmet and Callea, 1991; Desmet, 1992). Investigation of the embryology of the intrahepatic bile ducts (Desmet, 1992; Vijayan and Tan, 1999) elucidated the development of primitive biliary epithelium in the mesenchyme, which is situated along the branches of the portal vein, and the subsequent remodeling into the adult system of tubular anastomosing bile ducts. Tan *et al.* (1994a, b) also observed the development of the extrahepatic biliary tract from the hepatic diverticulum of the foregut and its luminal continuity with the developing intrahepatic ducts throughout gestation. These new embryological studies have not shown a 'solid stage' of ductal development as suggested previously. The authors describe the histological features of the fetal ductal plate in biliary atresia, and suggest that disruption of ductal plate remodeling could be implicated in the condition. This concept was examined again by Funaki *et al.* (1998) in a study of programmed cell death and apoptosis in biliary atresia. They demonstrated increased and disorganized cell turnover, which they also related to ductal plate malformation and abnormal bile duct development.

Atresia has been detected with antenatal ultrasound on at least five occasions between 19 and 32 weeks' gestation (Tsuchida *et al.*, 1995; Redkar *et al.*, 1998), and this

Figure 8.3 *Type 1 biliary atresia with a congenital cavernoma of the portal vein. The ligature is around the atretic bile duct.*

provides good evidence for the early onset of the condition in the fetus. Furthermore, levels of gamma-glutamyl transpeptidase (GGT), which is synthesized in the liver and then excreted through the bile ducts and the bowel into the amniotic fluid during pregnancy, were shown to be reduced in samples of amniotic fluid taken from mothers of infants born with biliary atresia (MacGillivray et al., 1994).

Infective factors

Much has been written about possible infective etiologies in biliary atresia, although the evidence is not conclusive. Strauss and Bernstein (1968) and Landing (1974) had suggested a viral origin, but attempts to identify or isolate viruses from the liver or bile ducts were unsuccessful (Jenner, 1978; Numazaki et al., 1980; Shiraki et al., 1980). Phillips et al. (1969) produced chronic liver disease and obstructive jaundice in 21-day-old weanling mice after inoculation with reo-3 virus. Moreover, Bangaru et al. (1980) and Morecki et al. (1983) showed that 3 to 6 weeks after infection there is occlusion of some of the proximal bile ducts and bile duct damage, including necrosis of the lining epithelium and inflammation of the walls. However, the infection does not produce total occlusion of the bile ducts. In a later study, Parashar et al. (1992) again demonstrated inflammatory lesions in the bile duct epithelium of mice infected with reovirus type 3, although hepatocyte necrosis was not observed. The mice recovered from the inflammation, and chronic liver disease did not follow the infection.

However, similar experiments performed with rhesus rotavirus did result in complete obstruction of the extrahepatic bile duct, accompanied by intrahepatic changes of necrosis and proliferation of small bile ducts (Riepenhoff-Talty et al., 1993; Petersen et al., 1997). The production of reversible and irreversible changes in these experiments reflected the original hypothesis of Landing (1974), in which he postulated a single etiology for neonatal hepatitis and biliary atresia.

Morecki et al. (1983) did demonstrate antibodies to reovirus in 68% of infants with biliary atresia, compared with 8% of controls, but Dussaix et al. (1984) and Brown et al. (1988) have been unable to repeat this finding. The latter authors investigated 23 infants with biliary atresia and 12 infants with neonatal hepatitis, and compared them with 30 patients with other liver diseases and with 55 controls. Antireo-3 antibodies showed no difference between the groups, and no reo-3 antigen was detected in the hepatobiliary tissues. There are no reports of the isolation of viral particles from affected infants (Strauss and Bernstein, 1968), except for a preliminary report of polymerase chain reaction (PCR) amplification of group C rotavirus sequences (Riepenhoff-Talty et al., 1992).

Metabolic factors

Intraperitoneal infusion of the amino acid L-proline in mice does cause bile duct abnormalities (Vacanti and Folkman, 1979), and abnormally low levels of this amino acid and high levels of its precursor, L-glutamic acid, were measured in a small number of infants with biliary atresia, suggesting an enzymatic block. A toxic effect of monohydroxy bile acids on the hepatobiliary system has also been proposed, and injection of lithocholic acid into pregnant rabbits was associated with obstructive lesions in the biliary tract in two of the offspring (Jenner and Howard, 1975).

Anatomical factors

An abnormally long common channel at the junction of the bile and pancreatic ducts in infants with atresia, similar to the abnormality found in more than 70% of patients with choledochal cyst, was reported by Miyano et al. (1979) from postmortem studies. This has now been confirmed by Takahashi et al. (1987) and Chiba et al. (1990). The latter authors performed retrograde cholangiography in 28 cases of biliary atresia, and compared the results in seven infants with hepatitis and eight infants with hypoplasia of the bile ducts. The results show that common channels could be identified in both biliary atresia and hypoplasia, which were 5.1 and 4.7 mm (mean value) in length, respectively, compared with 1.3 mm in hepatitis. The etiological significance of these observations is not yet clear.

Animal observations

Occasional reports have described biliary atresia in animals such as the pig, horse and lamb (Van Der Luer and Kroneman, 1982; Lofstedt et al. 1988). Harper et al. (1990) described an outbreak of the disease in 300 crossbred lambs and 9 crossbred calves in New South Wales, Australia. Histological examination of the liver and bile ducts showed appearances typical of human biliary atresia. A study of the animals showed no evidence either of an inherited defect or of infection, and epidemiological analysis suggested the possibility of a toxic insult on the affected fetuses. A common factor in this outbreak in 1988 and similar outbreaks of atresia in previous years was the restriction of grazing to particular areas of land when the animals were in the early stages of pregnancy. In previous years the animals had been unrestricted and could graze over a wide area, but in 1988 they had been restricted to a flat area on the foreshore of a dam. This area is intermittently under water, and the authors suggested that perhaps a plant toxin such as a phytotoxin or mycotoxin might be involved in the etiology of the atresia. The flora of the region was investigated, but no specific plant toxin could be implicated in the outbreak.

Acquired biliary atresia

Davenport *et al.* (1996) described three cases of acquired occlusion of the bile duct. Two infants showed evidence of previous perforation of the bile duct, and one had a history of surgery for duodenal atresia. All three cases presented with late-onset jaundice at between 10 and 24 weeks of age, and the histological features of liver biopsies could not be distinguished from congenital atresia. However, ultrasonography showed dilated intrahepatic ducts, which are not a feature of congenital biliary atresia. The results of resection of the atretic segments were excellent at follow-up between 15 months and 5 years after surgery.

PATHOLOGY

Biliary atresia occurs with an incidence of 0.8–1.0 per 10 000 live births throughout the world. The intra-hepatic histology is similar to that of any bile duct obstruction in this age group, with widening of the portal tracts by edema and fibrosis, and proliferation of bile ductules. There is bile stasis within canaliculi and hepatocytes. Multinucleate giant-cell formation, more frequent within the first 4 to 5 weeks of life, is not uncommon. Progressive disease leads to increasing hepatocellular damage in the neonatal period.

Hepatocellular necrosis, giant-cell formation and inflammatory-cell infiltrate are also typical features of neonatal hepatitis, and this limits the accuracy of percutaneous liver biopsy in biliary atresia to approximately 82% of cases (Manolaki *et al.*, 1983). Hepatic changes in alpha-1 antitrypsin deficiency may also mimic biliary atresia in early infancy, and alpha-1-antitrypsin phenotyping is essential in the investigation of infants with conjugated hyperbilirubinemia. Similar histological changes are observed in cases of intrahepatic biliary hypoplasia (arteriohepatic dysplasia or Alagille's syndrome), a condition that is characterized by facial appearance, pulmonary stenosis, vertebral anomalies,

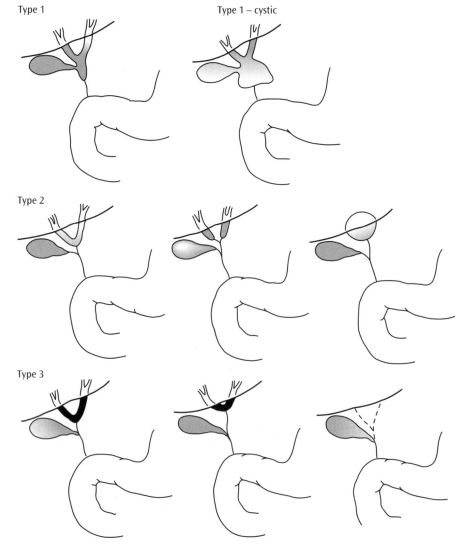

Figure 8.4 *Diagram of the main types of extrahepatic bile duct obstruction in biliary atresia. The type 1 lesion was originally known as 'correctable' atresia.*

hypogonadism and other abnormalities (Alagille *et al.*, 1975).

The historical division of biliary atresia into 'correctable' or 'non-correctable' types, depending on the presence or absence of a patent segment of bile duct, has now been replaced by the classification of the Japanese Society of Pediatric Surgeons. This classification describes the following three major patterns of disease (Figure 8.4):

- type 1 – atresia confined to the common bile duct; this type may be associated with a bile-containing cyst in the porta hepatis;
- type 2 – atresia of the common hepatic duct with residual patency of the right and left hepatic ducts;
- type 3 – atresia of the whole of the extrahepatic duct system.

The Japanese classification includes many subdivisions, depending on patency or occlusion of the distal common bile duct or gallbladder, as well as the morphological features of the porta hepatis, but these subdivisions have not been shown to be of prognostic significance. It is important to recognize that non-communicating cystic dilatations may occur in any segment of the extrahepatic bile ducts, and may lead an erroneous diagnosis of type 1 atresia or choledochal cyst during surgery. Unless the lumen of any dilated segment contains bile, it must be regarded as non-communicating and must be resected. In a Japanese survey of 643 cases, 566 (88%) were type 3, 64 (10%) were type 1 and only 13 cases (2%) were type 2 lesions (Ohi *et al.*, 1987).

Kasai *et al.* (1980) demonstrated that during the first few weeks of life patients with biliary atresia possess patent intrahepatic bile ducts which extend into the fibrous tissue of the porta hepatis. In type 3 disease, these extensions are represented by microscopic ductules. With increasing age the major intrahepatic ducts disappear, and this process is accompanied by a proliferation of ductules in the portal tracts of the liver. Kasai's studies suggested that attempts to establish bile drainage would be most successful before the ages of 6 or 8 weeks.

Residual extrahepatic bile duct tissue excised during surgery was studied in detail by Gautier and Eliot (1981), who confirmed the presence of duct-like structures with epithelial linings in the majority of cases. They classified their cases into three types as follows:

1 no visible ductal tissue and minimal inflammatory reaction in the surrounding tissue;
2 some duct lumina present, usually less than 50 µm in diameter and lined by cuboidal epithelium;
3 residual bile ducts lined by columnar epithelium and with a diameter of 150 µm or greater.

The duct-like structures do not all communicate with the intrahepatic ducts. They may represent blind-ending biliary glands, collecting ductules or residual lumina of true bile ducts (Ohi *et al.*, 1984). Figure 8.5 illustrates the typical histological findings at the porta hepatis in a severe case of type 2 atresia. Bile flow may be anticipated after portoenterostomy if the residual bile ducts measure more than 150 µm in diameter (Altman *et al.*, 1975; Ohi *et al.*, 1984), but this is not a strict rule, and bile flow has been documented with much smaller duct remnants (Odievre *et al.*, 1976; Lawrence *et al.*, 1981). It is likely that intrahepatic inflammation and fibrosis, as well as ductular size, are also important factors in determining bile flow.

The prognosis of intrahepatic pathology after surgery is variable, and Haas (1978) suggested that cirrhosis might be caused by both residual bile duct obstruction and a cholangiopathic process similar to that seen in neonatal hepatitis. The morphology of the intrahepatic ducts may change after surgery performed for type 1 atresia, and an investigation of six cases of biliary atresia with both operative and percutaneous cholangiography showed that the preoperative appearance of ill-defined ducts changed after successful surgery, when the intrahepatic ducts became more sharply defined. In failed cases the intrahepatic ducts at the porta hepatis tended to become cystic. In type 3 atresia (five cases) intrahepatic ducts did not become normal after surgery, even in the presence of good bile flow, and large ducts did not develop, even with a rapid flow of contrast medium to the Roux loop (Ito *et al.*, 1983).

Successful biliary drainage after portoenterostomy may also be associated with a decrease in hepatic fibrosis and inflammatory cell infiltrate (Dessanti *et al.*, 1985).

Davenport and Howard (1996) investigated a possible relationship between the macroscopic appearance of the liver and portal venous system at the time of surgery with the clinical outcome of portoenterostomy in 30 infants. A scoring system was applied to observations on liver consistency, size of portal remnant, degree of portal hypertension and any associated extrahepatic abnormalities such as polysplenia (the MAP (macroscopic appearance at portoenterostomy) score). At the end of the follow-up period, 20 infants who had a successful result from the surgery were compared with the 10 failures. Statistical analysis showed that the only significant observation to correlate with successful surgical outcome was the size of the portal remnant.

Tan *et al.* (1994) classified the size and number of residual ducts, and the degree of inflammation at the porta hepatis, in 205 cases of atresia. In addition, the pattern and extent of the obliteration of the extrahepatic bile ducts was classified into seven types. These observations were then related to age at the time of surgery and to survival. Age at surgery showed no correlation with bile duct morphology or portal histology, and there was no correlation between prognosis and pattern of bile duct obliteration. The authors concluded that the severity of intrahepatic bile duct inflammation and liver damage might be the more important factors in prognosis after surgery.

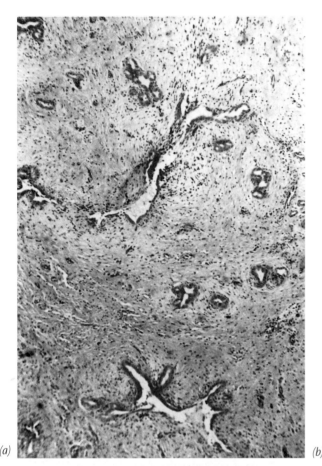

(a)

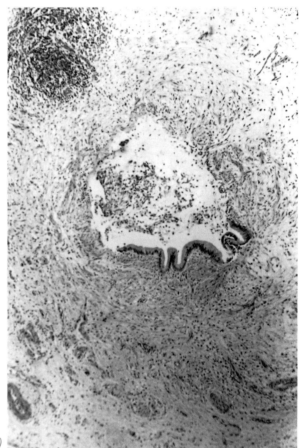

(b)

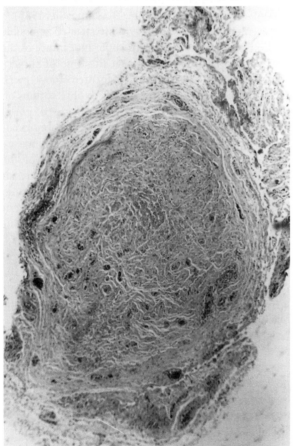

(c)

Figure 8.5 *Histological sections from a child aged 8 weeks with type 2 biliary atresia. (a) Section from the porta hepatis showing two medium-sized ducts lined by hyperplastic epithelium surrounded by cellular fibrous tissue. There is active chronic inflammation and small ducts are seen. The lumen of each of the two ducts shows partial obliteration (× 48). (b) An adjacent section showing a single duct with partial destruction of the lining epithelium and surrounding active chronic inflammation (× 48). (c) Section of the sclerosed distal hepatic duct (× 48).*

Immunohistochemistry

It has been suggested that macrophages, whose cytokines may perpetuate cellular injury and promote collagen synthesis, play a key role in the production of the fibrosis which accompanies chronic liver disease. In biliary atresia, Dillon *et al.* (1994) have shown an increased expression of the cell adhesion molecules ICAM and VCAM, upon which the recruitment and maintenance of inflammatory cells are dependent (ICAM and VCAM expression is not seen in normal liver tissue).

These observations were later extended to an examination of the macrophage receptor markers CD68 and CD14 in a study which confirmed that there was a proliferation of macrophages in association with cholestasis. The observations also suggested that the presence of the CD14-lipopolysaccharide receptor on periportal cells might be a potential source of cytokines responsible for the inflammatory reaction in biliary atresia (Tracy *et al.*, 1996). A further study of major histocompatibility complex (MHC) class II antigens and macrophage-associated antigens (CD68) again showed increased HLA-DR antigen expression, as well as CD68-positive macrophage infiltrates within the portal tracts and hepatic lobules of infants with biliary atresia (Kobayashi *et al.*, 1997). This study also indicated that the strongest expressions of hepatic antigen were observed in patients with the poorest prognosis after surgery.

Increased numbers of CD4 lymphocytes and CD56 cells were observed within the livers of 28 cases of biliary atresia during an investigation of a wide range of antigens. This report also suggested that there was a reduction in the expression of the macrophage marker CD68 within the liver and the excised biliary tract, as well as a reduction in ICAM expression on infiltrating cells in the biliary remnants, in the cases with a better prognosis (Davenport *et al.*, 2001). These observations were not dissimilar to those of Kobayashi *et al.* (1997).

Immunohistochemical observations therefore suggest that immune-mediated or immune-modulated damage to the intra- and extrahepatic bile ducts could have a role in the etiology of biliary atresia, and might explain the progressive liver damage observed in some of the cases who have achieved very satisfactory bile drainage after portoenterostomy.

CLINICAL PRESENTATION

Most large series of cases of biliary atresia show a preponderance of female infants. Of 617 patients collected in the Japanese biliary atresia registry between 1989 and 1994, 390 were female and 227 were male, giving a sex ratio of 1:0.58 (Ibrahim *et al.*, 1997). The majority of the infants in this collected series had a gestational age of 36 to 41 weeks and birth weights in the range 2500–4000 g. Only 19 cases (3%) weighed less than 2500 g at birth.

There are usually no abnormal factors related to the prenatal history of these infants, and the first indication of bile duct occlusion is often prolonged jaundice following the not infrequent period of neonatal physiological jaundice. In most instances the jaundice starts in this way, but occasionally this only becomes apparent after 2–3 weeks. Non-pigmented stools and dark urine are of course characteristic, but the infant usually thrives and feeds normally in the early stages of the condition. After 3 to 4 months, the child's general condition begins to deteriorate (Figure 8.6). The satisfactory general health

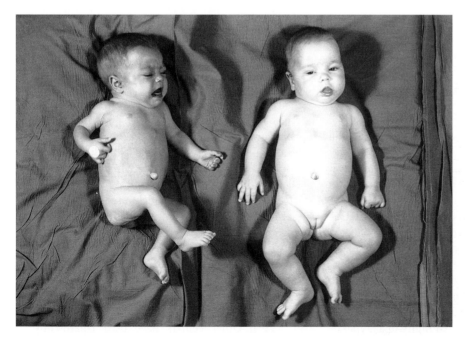

Figure 8.6 *The metabolic effect of biliary atresia on general development is clearly seen in the twin on the left of the picture, who presented at 6 months of age with a history of persistent jaundice. Her sister was completely well. (Reproduced by kind permission of Dr Colin Ball.)*

of the infant and the mild appearance of the jaundice during the first few weeks of life often deceive the child's medical advisers into making a late diagnosis. Early surgery, before 8 weeks of age, is now recognized as an important factor in determining the prognosis, but in a survey of 50 consecutive patients (Mieli-Vergani et al., 1989) the median age at referral was 8 weeks. Operations were performed at approximately 10 weeks, the interval between referral and surgery being necessary to exclude medical conditions which might cause jaundice. Reasons for the delayed referral were mainly concerned with failures to identify the fact that the hyperbilirubinemia was conjugated. There was also a lack of urgency in the referral of many of the children, even when the diagnosis of obstructive jaundice had been confirmed.

Apart from the jaundice, the physical signs at this age may be minimal and consist only of slight enlargement of the liver. The spleen may or may not be palpable. However, it should be emphasized that white stools and jaundice in a young infant should raise a very strong suspicion of biliary atresia. Ascites is unusual unless the baby is over 10 weeks of age.

An occasional reason for error in diagnosis is caused by a left-sided liver (situs inversus) which is mistaken for an enlarged spleen, and this may lead to investigations for splenomegaly rather than for specific hepatic diseases.

Persistent jaundice may eventually be associated with a vitamin K-responsive hemorrhagic diathesis which may present as bruising or overt bleeding. Neonatal bleeding occurred in 50 (8%) of the 626 patients in the Japanese registry (Ibrahim et al., 1997).

INVESTIGATIONS

There are many causes of conjugated hyperbilirubinemia in the neonatal period (see Chapter 3), and those most likely to be confused with biliary atresia include alpha-1-antitrypsin deficiency, cystic fibrosis and the neonatal hepatitis syndrome. Early diagnosis is crucial to the management of these children, and investigations must therefore be performed as rapidly as possible. Unfortunately, there is no single definitive test and the diagnosis therefore depends on a battery of investigations, the availability of which will depend on local expertise. For example, 7–10% of liver biopsies cause difficulty with diagnosis (Adelman, 1978), and failure to visualize extrahepatic bile ducts with endoscopic retrograde cholangiopancreatography (ERCP) is sometimes due to technical problems in cannulating the ampulla.

Investigation starts with a series of blood investigations which will exclude infections, metabolic disease and genetic disorders, particularly alpha-1-antitrypsin deficiency. Liver function tests are usually unhelpful, as there is an element of hepatocellular injury in all types of infantile cholestasis which is recognized by elevated serum transaminases, alkaline phosphatase and GGT. GGT levels in biliary atresia may be elevated to 10 times the normal value, but low levels may also occur.

Ultrasonography is useful in order to exclude choledochal cyst as a cause of jaundice, but it is not very specific for the diagnosis of biliary atresia. For example, although the gallbladder is thickened and shrunken in the majority of cases, it may be visualized as a relatively normal structure in up to 25% of affected infants. Occluded bile ducts may also be interpreted as 'normal'. Recently an ultrasonographic sign known as the 'triangular cord sign' has been introduced into diagnosis. The triangular cord is defined as a triangular or tubular echogenic density that is seen immediately cranial to the portal vein bifurcation. It represents the fibrotic remnant of the obliterated bile ducts. A positive diagnosis of atresia was made from the sign in 10 out of 12 affected infants (Tan Kendrick et al., 2000). Diminished gallbladder length was also recorded, in the range 0–1.45 cm, with a mean length of 0.52 cm, compared with a mean length of 2.39 cm in non-biliary cases which were used as controls.

Reference has already been made to the diagnosis of biliary atresia on at least five occasions with antenatal ultrasound (Greenholz et al., 1986; Tsuchida et al., 1995), but these observations depend on the presence of a prominent residuum of tissue in the porta hepatis, and this only applies to a small number of cases of biliary atresia.

Diagnostic percutaneous liver biopsy is very reliable in the majority of cases (Manolaki et al., 1983), and the main histological features are periportal edema and fibrosis, bile duct proliferation and bile pigment in the portal bile ducts. The histologist may be deceived by giant-cell hepatitis, which can show features similar to those of biliary atresia, and vice versa. Unfortunately, the earlier the liver biopsy is performed the more difficult it may be to separate the two conditions.

Hepatobiliary excretion scans employing technetium-labeled agents, which are excreted by hepatocytes into the biliary tracts, are widely used. Visualization of the small bowel with the isotope excludes biliary atresia. The value of the test is potentiated by using a 3-day course of phenobarbitone, and a correct diagnosis was made with this technique in 28 of 32 infants using the isotope technetium-99m-DISIDA (di-isopropyl iminodiacetic acid) (Dick and Mowat, 1986).

Duodenal aspiration is widely used as the definitive test in Japan (Hays and Kimura, 1980) and China (Hung and Su, 1987), but severe cases of hepatitis syndrome may also result in the absence of bilirubin from the aspirate. However, an accuracy of 98% has been achieved by adding a radioisotope marker to the technique and testing the aspirate for radioactivity as well as color. Liver imaging can be performed at the same time (Hung and Su, 1987). Other centers have used laparoscopy to inspect the gallbladder and bile ducts and to perform percutaneous cholecystography and liver biopsy (Leape and Ramenofsky, 1977) (Figure 8.7).

The recent introduction of pediatric side-viewing endoscopes (PJF endoscope Olympus KeyMed, UK) now allows ERCP examination in the smallest infants. Heyman et al. (1988) investigated 12 patients and demonstrated atresia of the hepatic ducts in two cases, hypoplasia of the ducts in one case and a satisfactory bil-

iary–enteric anastomosis in one postoperative case. There was no visualization of the ducts in eight infants, six of whom were later shown to have biliary atresia and two of whom were found to have neonatal hepatitis syndrome. Two out of 12 cases (16.5%) were therefore misdiagnosed using this technique. Similarly, Takahashi et al. (1987) and Iinuma et al. (2000) claimed 87% and 86% success rates, respectively. The latter authors completed 43 out of 50 ERCPs without complication, and six

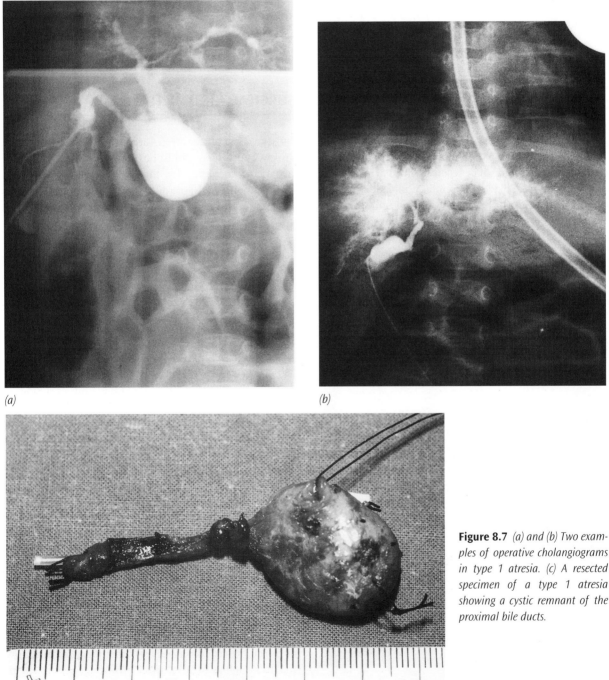

(a)

(b)

(c)

Figure 8.7 (a) and (b) Two examples of operative cholangiograms in type 1 atresia. (c) A resected specimen of a type 1 atresia showing a cystic remnant of the proximal bile ducts.

of the seven failed examinations were diagnosed as cases of biliary atresia at laparotomy. Visualization restricted to the pancreatic duct alone or a small segment of bile duct, after successful cannulation of the ampulla, was recorded in 29 infants with biliary atresia. Complete biliary tract visualization was achieved in 14 infants who had neonatal hepatitis, biliary hypoplasia or choledochal cysts.

The majority of infants with biliary atresia can now be correctly diagnosed using a combination of the above investigations, but surgery should not be unduly delayed in the minority of infants whose investigations remain equivocal even after ERCP. Historically, a two-stage operative procedure of liver biopsy and operative cholangiography, followed within a few days by definitive surgery, was recommended for the diagnosis of biliary atresia (Clatworthy and MacDonald, 1956). However, operative cholangiography is not possible in many cases of biliary atresia because of occlusion of the cystic and common bile ducts. Furthermore, atresia can often be diagnosed from the macroscopic appearance of the gallbladder and extrahepatic bile ducts. The two-stage approach is therefore only recommended when bile is identified in a gallbladder aspirate. Gallbladder aspiration produces clear or opalescent mucoid fluid in all but the rare type 1 cases of biliary atresia, and if there is any suspicion of bile within the gallbladder, a cholecystostomy is performed to allow the performance of detailed radiological studies in the X-ray department.

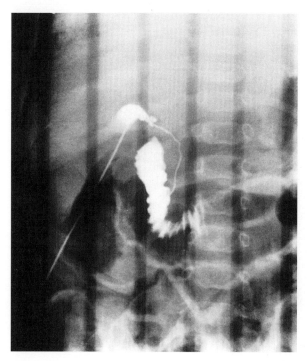

Figure 8.8 *An operative cholangiogram in a case of type 3 atresia. The cystic and distal segments of the common bile duct are patent.*

This approach, after the recognition of gallbladder bile, is recommended because the patency of bile ducts cannot always be recognized even with the most careful intraoperative cholangiography (Mason *et al.*, 1966), and this technical error may lead to erroneous diagnoses of biliary atresia and thus to unnecessary surgery (Kahn and Daum, 1983).

On the other hand, in at least 10% of children with biliary atresia the gallbladder communicates with the duodenum via a patent cystic duct and distal segment of bile duct (Figure 8.8). In these cases it is difficult to know whether the proximal bile ducts are atretic or whether they have not filled for technical reasons (Lilly and Altman, 1979), and meticulous dissection is required to determine the state of the proximal bile ducts.

SURGICAL TREATMENT

Most cases of biliary atresia are now diagnosed preoperatively, and surgeons must be prepared to perform either hepaticojejunostomy for the uncommon type 1 cystic disease found in 10–15% of cases, or the more radical portoenterostomy procedure for the remainder. The anatomical anomalies described previously must be expected in more than 10% of cases.

Preoperative preparation

Adequate vitamin K is given before surgery (1.0 mg/day for 4 days), as it is essential that the prothrombin time is normalized. Bowel preparation varies from one unit to another, but a typical regimen includes oral neomycin (50 mg/kg/day in six divided doses for 24 hours) and metronidazole (21 mg/kg/day). One unit of blood is cross-matched.

The infant is placed in a supine position on a heated operating-table with facilities for intraoperative cholangiography. An adequate intravenous line is set up, a rectal temperature probe is positioned and an intravenous dose of a broad-spectrum antibiotic (cephalosporin) is administered at the induction of anesthesia.

Hepaticojejunostomy for cystic type 1 atresia (FIGURE 8.9)

A laparotomy is performed through a transverse upper abdominal incision extending across both rectus muscles. A note is made of the size and texture of the liver, the size of the spleen, the presence or absence of ascites or portal hypertension and any other anatomical abnormalities, such as situs inversus, preduodenal portal vein, etc. The diagnosis of biliary atresia is confirmed. The gallbladder may be well hidden in the liver between segment 5 and the quadrate lobe. In many cases the

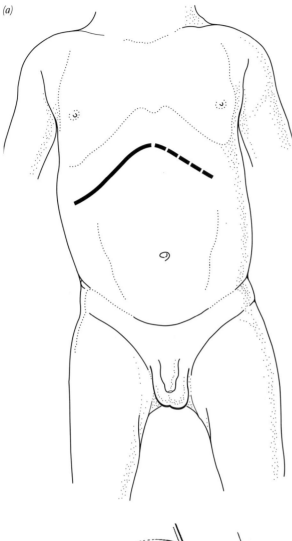

(a)

gallbladder is shrunken and fibrotic and cholangiography is not possible. Aspiration of any patent gallbladder is performed in order to exclude the presence of bile, but if bile is found then the operation is concluded by the insertion of a cholecystostomy tube for detailed cholangiography in the radiology department. Operative cholangiography may be necessary if other anomalies are detected, such as choledochal cyst or the very rare bile duct tumors, or for the confirmation of intrahepatic bile duct communication with a type 1 cystic atresia (Figure 8.7 above).

The confirmation of a rare type 1 cystic lesion with a satisfactory residual segment of proximal bile duct is followed by the operation of hepaticojejunostomy. The liver is mobilized completely to allow adequate exposure of the porta hepatis (Figure 8.9). Traction on the dissected gallbladder aids the identification of the atretic distal common bile duct, which is divided. The cystic remnant is mobilized from the hepatic artery and portal vein and transected. Anastomosis with a retrocolic, 50-cm Roux-en-Y loop of jejunum concludes the operation. Transanastomotic tubes are not used. A liver biopsy is taken, a drain is placed in the subhepatic space and the abdominal wound is closed in layers.

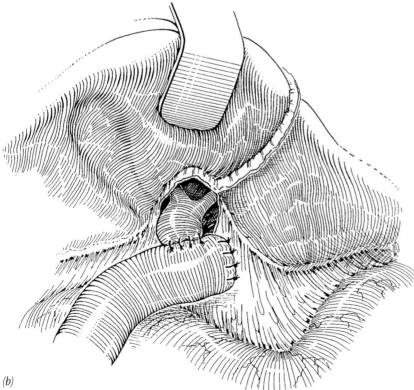

Figure 8.9 *(a) Abdominal incision used for the surgery of biliary atresia. (b) Hepaticojejunostomy. Reproduced with permission from* Rob *and* Smiths operative surgery, *5th edn, published by Chapman & Hall.*

(b)

Portoenterostomy (FIGURE 8.10)

This operation, which was devised by Kasai, is used in the majority of cases of biliary atresia when the ductal occlusion extends into the porta hepatis. The principle of the operation is to expose minute channels in the porta hepatis which communicate with intrahepatic ducts. The initial stages of the operation are similar to those used in the hepaticojejunostomy procedure, and it starts with gallbladder mobilization, which is used as a guide to the fibrous remnant of the common hepatic duct. The residual tissue in the porta hepatis may be obscured by thickened peritoneum and enlarged lymph nodes, and the dissection is helped by the use of magnifying lenses. The crucial part of this dissection is the excision of all tissue lying above the bifurcation of the portal vein, and it is necessary to mobilize both the right and left branches of the portal vein completely, tying and dividing any small tributaries which may run towards the caudate lobe. All lymphatics are ligated to prevent postoperative lymphatic ascites. The bile duct tissue is removed by a transection parallel to the liver capsule, and this extends to the right and to the left as far as the entry of the hepatic vessels into the liver parenchyma (Figure 8.11). This excision is aided by the use of angled scissors designed specifically for this purpose (Figure 8.12). Deeper dissection into liver substance is not advised, as it results in rapid obliteration of bile channels with fibrous tissue (Kimura *et al.*, 1979). Intraoperative examination of frozen sections of the tissue in the porta hepatis has been suggested as a method of confirming the adequacy of the resection of residual bile duct tissue (Altman, 1978), but this has not gained general acceptance. The tissue in the porta hepatis is simply resected as widely as possible.

Biliary tract continuity is established with a 50-cm retrocolic Roux loop of jejunum which is anastomosed

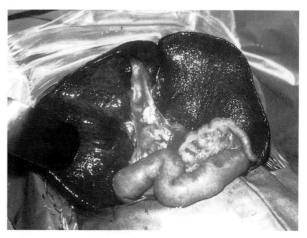

(a)

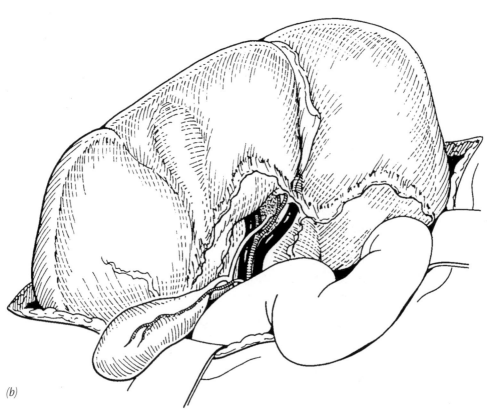

(b)

Figure 8.10 *The portoenterostomy operation. (a) Photograph of the initial mobilization of the gallbladder and atretic bile ducts. (b) Diagrammatic representation of liver mobilization. (continued)*

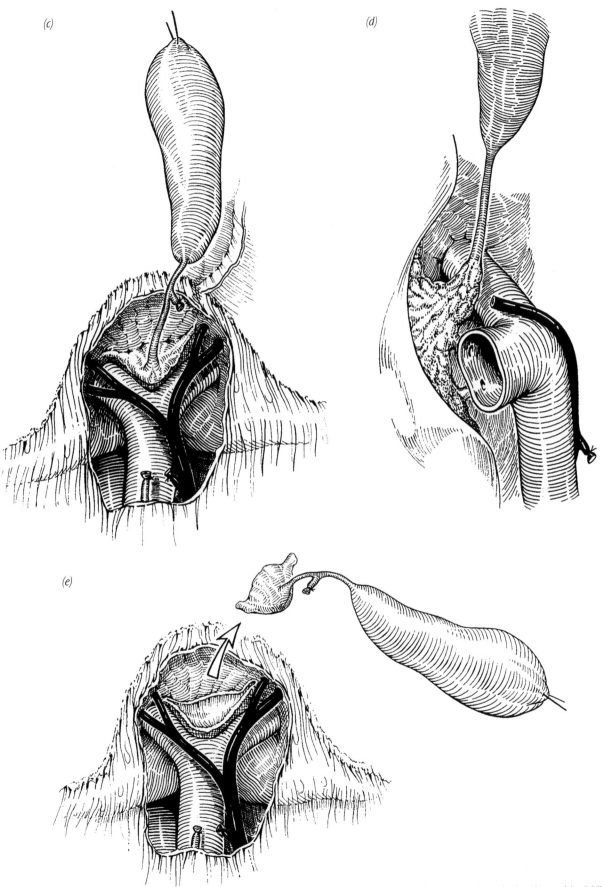

Figure 8.10 *(continued) (c) Dissection and exposure of the porta hepatis. (d) Lateral view of the porta hepatis showing residual bile duct tissue posterior to the portal vein. (e) Transection of bile duct tissue flush with the liver capsule. (Continued.)*

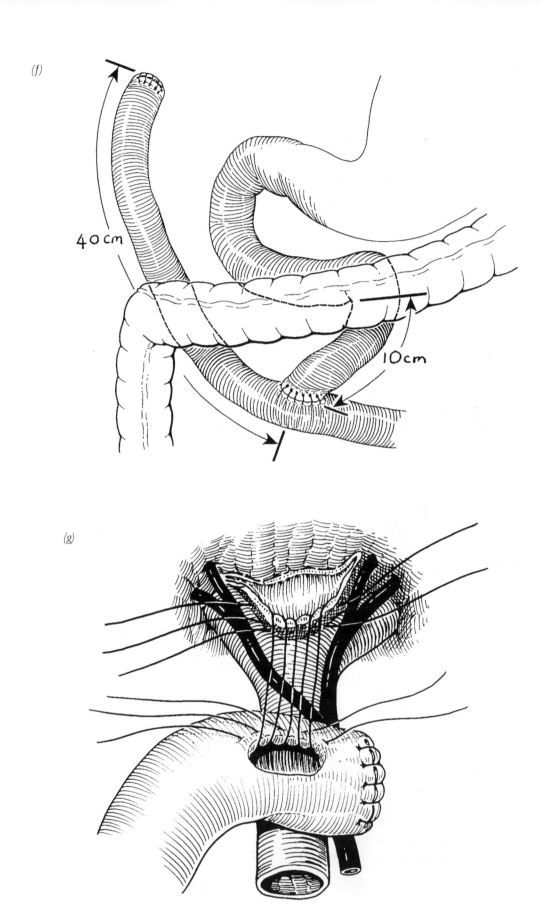

Figure 8.10 *(continued) (f) Preparation of a 40-cm Roux loop of jejunum. (g) Placement of posterior row of sutures between the edge of the transected tissue in the porta hepatis and the side of a 40-cm Roux-en-Y loop of jejunum. (Continued.)*

(h)

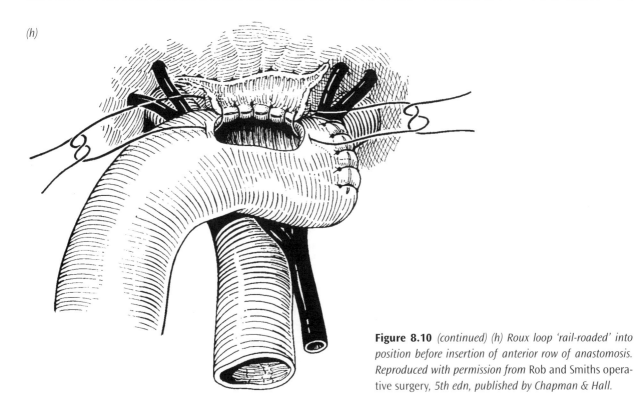

Figure 8.10 *(continued) (h) Roux loop 'rail-roaded' into position before insertion of anterior row of anastomosis. Reproduced with permission from* Rob and Smiths operative surgery, *5th edn, published by Chapman & Hall.*

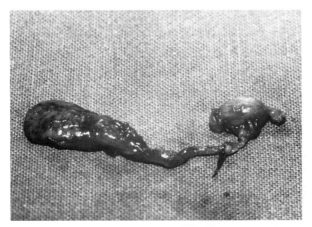

Figure 8.11 *A typical specimen of excised gallbladder and residual atretic bile ducts.*

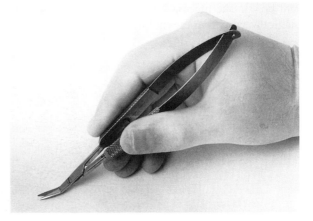

Figure 8.12 *Scissors with angled blades designed for dissection of the porta hepatis.*

to the transected edges of the porta hepatis using 5/0 polydioxanone (PDS). All of the sutures of the posterior row are placed in position before the loop is 'rail-roaded' into position. The sutures are tied and the anterior row is completed. A drain is then placed in the subhepatic space and the wound is closed in layers (Howard, 1994, 1997).

Cutaneous enterostomy

Episodes of ascending bacterial cholangitis are not uncommon after surgery (see below), and surgical techniques designed to reduce this complication have included a variety of biliary diversions (Kaufman *et al.*, 1981; Endo *et al.*, 1983; Shim and Zhang, 1985; Howard, 1997). However, their beneficial effects have not been confirmed (Altman, 1983). There was no reduction in the incidence of cholangitis in a personal series of cases, and the cutaneous enterostomies were complicated by episodes of dehydration, hyponatremia (Miyano *et al.*, 1985) and frequent bleeds from the stomas (Burnweit and Coln, 1986; Smith *et al.*, 1988) (Box 8.2). The stomas can also complicate a transplantation which may be required at a later date, and for these reasons their routine use is no longer recommended.

Box 8.2 Complications of cutaneous enterostomies in 12 patients (Burnweit and Coln, 1986)

	n
Death	2 (volvulus, sepsis)
Retraction	1
Bleeding	2
Prolapse	1

Modifications of portoenterostomy – the anti-reflux valve

Many modifications of the Roux loop conduit have been devised in an attempt to reduce the incidence of cholangitis after the portoenterostomy procedure (Ohi, 1991). However, retrospective reviews have failed to confirm the value of these procedures (see below), and they have been found to complicate any future liver transplantation. Surgeons who wish to modify the Roux loop now confine any modification to the construction of a mucosal intussusception type of anti-reflux valve. Yeh et al. (1990) constructed a 3-cm valve in dogs by stripping away the seromuscular layer for 6 cm in the midportion of a Roux loop anastomosed between the gallbladder and bowel. The mucosa was then invaginated isoperistaltically away from the cholecystojejunostomy to form the 3-cm valve, and the serosa was closed with interrupted sutures. The experiments confirmed that the valve protected the gallbladder against reflux from the lower jejunum, and from infection by organisms introduced into the gastrointestinal tract. Nakajo et al. (1990) described the results of the technique in 17 newly diagnosed infants with biliary atresia. Ascending cholangitis was not observed in any of these cases. However, a recent retrospective study of three groups of patients with a conventional portoenterostomy, a valved conduit or a long Roux loop showed no significant difference in the incidence of cholangitis. The incidence was 50% in the conventional group, 50% in the valved group and 33% in the long loop group. It was concluded that neither bacterial growth in the liver nor cholangitis were affected by the type of biliary reconstruction (Chuang et al., 2000).

Portocholecystostomy (FIGURE 8.13)

In a few cases the gallbladder and distal bile duct appear to be unaffected by the atretic process, and an anastomosis can be constructed between the gallbladder and the transected area in the porta hepatis (Lilly, 1979). Several authors have reported a reduced incidence of cholangitis after this operation, although there are technical problems which have included bile leaks, gallbladder conduit obstruction and cholelithiasis (Freitas et al.,

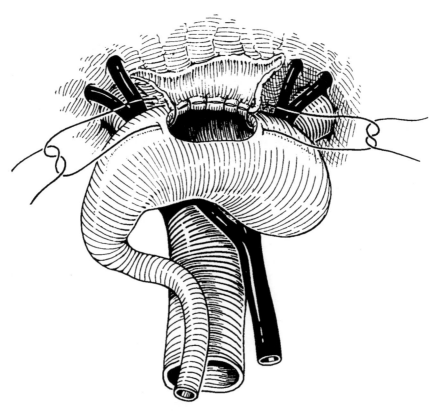

Figure 8.13 *Portocholecystostomy.*

1987). However, there does appear to be a reduction in postoperative cholangitis compared with the portoenterostomy operation. A survey of 670 children, in which data were collected from more than 100 institutions in the North American Biliary Atresia Registry, reported a 35% incidence of cholangitis after portocholecystostomy, compared with 55% after other types of reconstruction ($P = 0.02$) (Karrer et al., 1990). Ohi et al. (1987) suggested that the size of the cystic duct is a critical factor, and improved results have been claimed for stenting of the cystic duct (Lilly et al., 1987).

Revision procedures for the 'failed' portoenterostomy

Re-exploration of the porta hepatis has been recommended for patients who either remain jaundiced after portoenterostomy, or who become jaundiced again after a period of satisfactory bile flow (Altman, 1979; Suruga et al., 1982; Ohi et al., 1985). However, the results of this procedure have been poor unless an obvious mechanical cause, such as an obstructed Roux loop, has been identified before surgery (Figure 8.14). Freitas et al. (1987), in a review of 21 reoperations, found good results in patients with a mechanical cause of biliary obstruction and in those with an early recurrence of jaundice after a period of satisfactory bile flow. In a larger series of 210

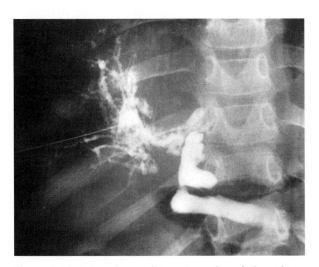

Figure 8.14 A Roux-loop stricture. Correction of the stricture cured the cholangitis.

reoperations, jaundice cleared in less than 30% of cases (Ohi et al., 1987).

Repeated attempts at dissection or curettage in the porta hepatis have been suggested in the past for patients who fail to develop satisfactory bile flow. The long-term outcome of these operations is unclear. However, a study of such early revision procedures was reported by Saito (1983), and this showed that only minimal benefit was gained from most of the operations (Box 8.3). Liver transplantation rather than re-exploration is now recommended for patients who fail a primary portoenterostomy operation.

Box 8.3 Results of secondary revisions of portoenterostomy procedures (after Saito, 1983)

Group 1 – resection of anastomosis at the porta hepatis
　　　　8 cases – improvement in 3 cases

Group 2 – deep curettage of anastomosis at the porta hepatis
　　　　22 cases – no improvement

Postoperative care

Intravenous fluid with antibiotic administration and nasogastric aspiration is continued until bowel activity resumes. The antibiotics are continued for a further week and then replaced by oral prophylaxis for a further month. Cholestyramine, phenobarbitone and vitamins A, B, D, E and K are given for at least one year after surgery. Choleretics may reduce the incidence of cholangitis (Kasai, 1974) by increasing bile flow, but no significant benefit was found with either cholestyramine or phenobarbitone in a randomized prospective trial (Vajro et al., 1986; Nittono et al., 1988) (Table 8.1). There is a single report of increased bile flow after the administration of prostaglandin E2 (Hirsig et al., 1983), which has not been confirmed by other studies.

Steroids have been used in an empirical manner in the belief that they might produce scar tissue formation at the anastomosis, but there are no controlled trials available. Karrer and Lilly (1985) used pulsed steroids in an attempt to combat cholangitis that was resistant to

---

Table 8.1 Effects of two choleretic agents (phenobarbital and cholestyramine) on bile flow in 80 patients after surgery for biliary atresia (Vajro et al., 1986)

	Phenobarbital	Cholestyramine	No drugs
Bile drainage	16	12	10
No drainage	11	15	16
	—	—	—
Total	27	27	26

antibiotic regimens, particularly in those cases with a decrease or cessation of bile flow. This report was a comparison of two groups of 16 patients who were treated with or without steroids. Steroids caused increased volumes of bile drainage, but the total excretion of bilirubin remained constant and the authors concluded that steroids had little or no effect on the decrease in bilirubin levels after portoenterostomy operations.

COMPLICATIONS OF TREATMENT

Bacterial cholangitis

This is a serious and not infrequent complication of portoenterostomy, and most reports show an incidence of 40–45% (Odievre et al., 1976; Psacharopoulos et al., 1980). Most of the attacks occur within the first year after surgery, and this may be related to the observation that bile flow may not become maximal until one year after surgery (Barkin and Lilly, 1980). During this time bile salts are excreted preferentially to cholesterol, and serum phospholipid concentrations may not normalize for several months (Lilly and Javitt, 1976). The attacks of cholangitis are characterized by the onset of fever and a rise in bilirubin over the following days, and repeated attacks cause a progressive deterioration in hepatic function. This is illustrated by the report of Houwen et al. (1989), who found a 5-year survival in 54% of their portoenterostomy patients who experienced cholangitis, compared with 91% of those who remained infection-free.

The etiology of ascending cholangitis is not entirely clear. It probably arises by direct infection from the bowel, but other suggestions include infection via the portal venous system (Danks et al., 1974) and the hilar lymphatics (Hirsig et al., 1978). The underlying cause is a partially obstructed biliary tree (Lilly, 1978). A diagnosis of intrahepatic infection is made from blood cultures or from percutaneous liver biopsy. A wide range of organisms may be involved, particularly E. coli, Proteus and Klebsiella species. Treatment is empirical in the first instance, and includes the prompt use of cephalosporin and gentamicin. The antibiotics are modified according to the cultures.

Prophylactic antibiotics have had little effect on the incidence of cholangitis. For example, cholangitis occurred in 9 out of 41 patients, five of whom received prophylactic antibiotics while four received no prophylaxis (Lilly et al., 1989). However, Chaudhary and Turner (1981) successfully treated four children for repeated cholangitis with a trimethoprim–sulfamethoxazole combination, and recommended that it should be used for one year after portoenterostomy in all cases. The length of Roux loop may be critical, and Lilly et al. (1989) reported cholangitis in three out of five patients with a

Roux loop less than 40 cm in length, but in only two out of 19 patients with a Roux loop longer than 40 cm. They concluded in their paper that early surgery and long Roux loops were the most important factors in reducing the incidence of cholangitis. The failure of cutaneous enterostomies to prevent cholangitis has been mentioned previously, and there is now good evidence that the frequency is not reduced by surgical maneuvers but more related to volumes of bile flow (Sawaguchi et al., 1980; Burnweit and Coln, 1986; Ecoffey et al., 1987; Ohi, 1991) (Tables 8.2, 8.3 and 8.4).

In summary, cholangitis occurs most commonly as an early complication of surgery, and treatment should be vigorous. Rothenberg et al. (1989) suggested a complete plan of management in a review of 28 postoperative patients, only two of whom did not suffer any episodes of infection. Their treatment started with a cephalosporin, and was changed to an aminoglycoside if there was no early response. Failure at this stage was treated with imipenem–cilastatin. Only patients who were refractory to this antibiotic regimen were given steroids, 60% of whom showed a satisfactory response.

Table 8.2 *Deleterious effects of biliary diversion on the incidence of cholangitis after portoenterostomy (Burnweit and Coln, 1986)*

	Diversion	No diversion
Patients	12.0	19.0
Cholangitis	4.0 (33%)	6.0 (32%)
Episodes per patient	2.5	1.7
Two-year survival	7.0 (58%)	14.0 (82%)

Table 8.3 *Relationship of bile flow to episodes of cholangitis after portoenterostomy (Ecoffey* et al.*, 1987)*

Flow	Number	Cholangitis
Good	27	29 (70%)
Partial	19	17 (89%)
None	55	7 (13%)
Total	101	53

Table 8.4 *Incidence of cholangitis after some types of modified portoenterostomy (modified from Ohi, 1991)*

Drainage modification	Incidence of cholangitis
Roux-en-Y	45%
Long Roux-en-Y	40%
Double Roux-en-Y	40%
End stoma of Roux	67%
Complete diversion	60%
Portocholecystostomy	20%
Gastric tube	44%

Portal hypertension

Hepatic fibrosis or cirrhosis is always present at the time of the primary operation for biliary atresia, and measurements of portal pressure have revealed portal hypertension in the majority of cases, even at 8 weeks of age (Valayer, 1983). The progression of liver disease, even after the establishment of good bile drainage, can lead to a progressive rise in portal pressure, and recordings in children who have suffered attacks of cholangitis have shown mean pressures of more than 20 cmH$_2$O (Kasai *et al.*, 1981). In contrast, 16 jaundice-free survivors showed pressures in the range 4–14 cmH$_2$O.

Variceal hemorrhage (Table 8.5) has been a problem in many series of long-term survivors (Howard *et al.*, 1982; Lilly and Stellin, 1984). Stringer *et al.* (1989) observed the development of esophageal varices in 67% of 61 children during endoscopic examination 2.5 years or more after portoenterostomy. Variceal bleeding had occurred in 17 children (28%). Portal hypertension was more frequent in children with persistent jaundice than in those who were anicteric (86% vs. 62%), and it was also more frequent in those who had suffered attacks of cholangitis. The latter observation confirmed the report of Ohi *et al.* (1986), and also confirmed the effectiveness of injection sclerotherapy in all children who completed a course of treatment.

Concern about the complications of injection sclerotherapy, such as esophageal stricture formation, stimulated the development of the technique of variceal banding. Hall *et al.* (1988) applied this to six children, two of whom had biliary atresia. Karrer *et al.* (1994) reported the long-term results after 31 episodes of banding in seven children with portal vein thrombosis who had been followed for 3 to 12 years. There were no deaths and no complications, and this now appears to be the procedure of choice for any child with esophageal varices.

Odievre (1978) has described a diminution in signs of portal hypertension with growth, but others have not observed this phenomenon.

Table 8.5 *The incidence of bleeding from esophageal varices more than 5 years after portoenterostomy (modified from Howard and Davenport, 1997)*

	Number of patients	Bleeding from varices
Kobayashi *et al.* (1984)	35	7 (20%)
Laurent *et al.* (1990)	40	15 (37%)
Tagge *et al.* (1991)	34	6 (18%)
Valayer (1996)	80	19 (24%)
Karrer *et al.* (1996)	35	20 (55%)
Howard and Davenport (1997)	51	8 (16%)
Total	275	75 (27%)

Portosystemic shunting has also been used in the management of portal hypertension in biliary atresia patients. Shunting is most useful in patients with ectopic varices in regions of the gut other than the esophagus, such as the stomach or at the sites of surgical anastomoses.

The formation of a percutaneous intrahepatic portosystemic shunt by creating a passage between the hepatic and portal veins was made possible by the introduction of expandable metal stents. The procedure, which is known as a transjugular intrahepatic portosystemic shunt (TIPS), may be complicated by shunt thrombosis, encephalopathy and damage to the portal vein, and shunt occlusion related to intimal proliferation within the lumen may be as high as 50% at 12 months. The technique has now been used in children with biliary atresia, and Schweizer *et al.* (1995) described the results in seven cases. However, long-term results are not yet available.

Transplantation is now generally regarded as the most effective way of treating recurrent variceal bleeding which is refractory to sclerotherapy and which is associated with progressive deterioration in liver function.

Splenomegaly secondary to portal hypertension is observed in the majority of long-term survivors after portoenterostomy, and is associated with complications that include moderate to severe abdominal pain, abdominal distension, thrombocytopenia and leucopenia. Low platelet counts are a problem in many long-term survivors, and the prevalence after 2 and 10 years has been recorded as 43% and 25%, respectively (Chiba *et al.*, 1991). The platelet count may be low enough to cause severe spontaneous bruising, particularly in the lower limbs.

Stellin *et al.* (1982) treated a 6.5-year-old girl with splenic embolization using a percutaneous femoral artery catheter to introduce gelfoam particles into the splenic artery. The procedure was complicated by abdominal pain, ileus and fever, but the platelet and white blood cell counts rapidly returned to normal. Chiba *et al.* (1991) confirmed the effectiveness of the procedure in 19 post-portoenterostomy pediatric patients aged between 3 and 13 years, in whom the platelet counts ranged from 26 000 to 110 000/mm^3. Between 45% and 90% of the splenic tissue was embolized, with no serious morbidity. Nine of the children were restudied 4 years after treatment by means of scintigraphic scans and measurements of platelet counts. The results showed that in some patients considerable regeneration of splenic tissue had occurred. In seven patients the regeneration ranged from 23% to 76%, with a mean of 41%, while in two cases there was no restoration of splenic volume. The platelet count increased more than fourfold in seven patients, but two children showed signs of hypersplenism which required further embolization.

In summary, portal hypertension is a problem in a proportion of survivors of the portoenterostomy operation. Sclerotherapy and banding are excellent methods for the control of esophageal varices, although portosystemic shunting may very occasionally be required for ectopic varices which have occurred at anastomotic sites within the gut. Hypersplenism remains a problem, and may be controlled by embolization rather than by splenectomy or portosystemic shunting.

Portal hypertension has caused major problems with regard to bleeding from the edges of cutaneous stomas, and this was highlighted by Smith *et al.* (1988), who reported the results of patient evaluation for liver transplant after failed portoenterostomy. A total of 22 patients with stomas all required transfusion for at least one bleed. A variety of treatments were used, including suture ligation of the bleeding points and stoma closure, but 57% of those treated by local suture re-bled. Repeated bleeding from the stoma is an indication for stoma closure. This should be a formal procedure, and preperitoneal techniques should be avoided because of the risk of further hemorrhage. Three out of four patients with preperitoneal closure developed occult gastrointestinal bleeding in Smith's series (1988).

Metabolic problems

A variety of metabolic problems (see Chapter 5) may occur after portoenterostomy, which may involve the metabolism of fat and protein and the absorption of vitamins, iron, calcium, zinc and copper (Greene, 1983). Malabsorption is a common finding after portoenterostomy, but it gradually resolves over a period of 9 months if surgery is effective. The abnormalities of metabolism are related to the magnitude of bile flow (Howard and Mowat, 1984), but even with good bile flow bile salts may be excreted in preference to cholesterol and phospholipids (Lilly and Javitt, 1976). Weight gain after surgery may be retarded if liver function remains grossly abnormal. Lipid absorption may be aided by the administration of milk containing fat in the form of medium-chain triglycerides.

Optimal care also includes the regular administration of fat-soluble vitamins, particularly vitamins D and K, and a multivitamin preparation which includes thiamin, riboflavin, pyridoxine, ascorbic acid and folic acid. Poor intestinal absorption may result in low vitamin D levels, which can be corrected with regular vitamin D supplements. Vitamin E levels are also monitored, as it is not uncommon for young children with cholestatic disease to show signs of neurological deficit (Nelson *et al.*, 1983). These signs include loss of tendon reflexes, reduction in proprioception, abnormal eye movements and intellectual deterioration. Peripheral nerve biopsy may show abnormalities, particularly in large-caliber sensory axons.

Intrahepatic cyst formation

Large intrahepatic cysts may occasionally occur in long-term survivors after portoenterostomy, and these may be associated with attacks of cholangitis. The cysts contain normal-looking bile, and may be treated either by aspiration (Saito *et al.*, 1984) or by cystogastrostomy (Howard, 1994). Smaller cysts may also be observed in non-draining areas of the liver.

Tsuchida *et al.* (1994) reported 29 well-documented cases, of whom there were 12 males and 17 females. The cysts were located near to the hepatic hilum in 20 cases and at the periphery of the liver in 8 cases.

A suggested classification of the recorded types of cystic change included the following three categories:

- type A – non-communicating;
- type B – communicating with the Roux-en-Y loop at the porta hepatis (Figure 8.15);
- type C – multiple cystic dilatations of irregular bile ducts.

Treatment included antibiotic therapy and percutaneous drainage. Cysto-enterostomy was possible in six cases.

Clinical symptoms caused by the cysts included cholangitis and jaundice, and in 66% of the patients these occurred within 4 years after the portoenterostomy operation. However, five of the six cases of type C disease devel-

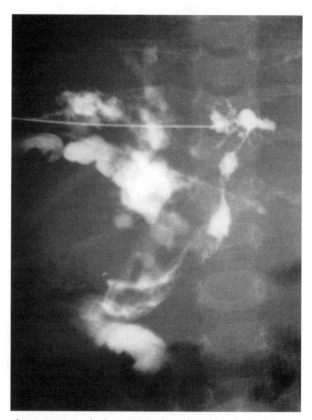

Figure 8.15 *Cystic change in the intrahepatic ducts despite excellent bile drainage.*

oped symptoms between 10 and 28 years after surgery, and the prognosis of this group was poor because of repeated infection. The development of this type of cystic change is probably an indication for liver transplantation.

Hepatopulmonary syndrome and pulmonary hypertension

In common with other forms of chronic liver disease, hypoxia with cyanosis on standing and exertion, dyspnea and finger clubbing may result from diffuse intrapulmonary shunting and intrapulmonary vascular dilatation in patients with biliary atresia. Valayer (1996) has pointed out that this complication, which is known as hepatopulmonary syndrome, is seen most frequently in the group of patients with an associated polysplenia syndrome, and that the condition can be reversed by liver transplantation.

Pulmonary arterial hypertension, which is recognized as a complication of cirrhosis in adults, may also occur in long-term survivors with biliary atresia. Possible etiological factors include vasoactive substances such as endothelin or prostaglandin F2, which are either not metabolized by the liver, or are secreted by endothelial cells. Soh et al. (1999) reported two cases of biliary atresia in whom pulmonary hypertension had developed on long-term follow-up. The first female patient died of right heart failure at 20 years of age, and postmortem showed severe thickening of the pulmonary artery. The second case, a boy aged 17 years, developed exertional dyspnea and pulmonary hypertension unresponsive to vasodilators. He has been considered for liver-lung transplantation. In view of the asymptomatic nature of early pulmonary hypertension, children with chronic liver disease such as biliary atresia should be followed up with assessments of pulmonary function and pulmonary hemodynamics, as liver transplantation might be an option for those who show increasing vascular resistance in the pulmonary arteries.

Malignant change in the liver

Malignant change in the cirrhotic livers of patients with biliary atresia has been reported on at least 10 occasions. Malignancies have included both cholangiocarcinomas and hepatomas associated with biliary cirrhosis (Kulkarni and Beatty, 1977). Small incidental hepatomas have been recognized during transplant procedures (Starzl, 1983; Valayer, 1996). It is likely that more cases will occur as the number of long-term survivors increases.

RESULTS

It remains impossible to predict the outcome of a portoenterostomy operation at the time of surgery. Factors

reported as favorable have included surgery before 8 weeks of age, and a satisfactory number of ductules in the porta hepatis. However, not all surgeons agree with these predictions. The complexity of the current situation is summarized in Box 8.4. The long-term results of portoenterostomy are discussed in the next chapter, and they may be compared with the results of surgical procedures performed between 1965 and 1975, which were analyzed by Carcassonne and Bensoussan (1977). A survey of 539 cases from 11 centers in Australia, Europe, Japan and the USA revealed that corrective surgery had been performed in 381 children, and that there were only 67 survivors (17.7%) at the time of the report. However, even in this early series there was a significant

---

Box 8.4 *Summary of studies on favorable and unfavorable factors in the outcome of surgery for biliary atresia*

Age at time of surgery (early surgery)
Favorable

        Hitch *et al.* (1979)
        Mieli-Vergani *et al.* (1989)
        Lally *et al.* (1989)
        Grosfeld *et al.* (1989)
        Karrer *et al.* (1990)
        Howard *et al.* (1991)
No relationship

        Suruga *et al.* (1985)
        Tagge *et al.* (1991)
        Miyano *et al.* (1993)

Histology of liver
Increased hepatic fibrosis
   – unfavorable

        Vasquez-Estevez *et al.* (1989)
        Karrer *et al.* (1990)
        Miyano *et al.* (1993)
Giant-cell transformation
   – unfavorable

        Hitch *et al.* (1979)
        Trivedi *et al.* (1984)
        Mieli-Vergani *et al.* (1989)
Number of biliary ductules at porta hepatis
   – favorable

        Hitch *et al.* (1979)
        Gautier and Eliot (1981)
   – no relationship
        Tagge *et al.* (1991)
        Miyano *et al.* (1993)
Serum factors (procollagen and laminin)
   – no relationship
        Trivedi *et al.* (1986)
        Sasaki *et al.* (1992)
Extrahepatic abnormalities
   – unfavorable

        Karrer *et al.* (1991)
        Davenport *et al.* (1993)

improvement in the results of those operated before 3 months of age and those operated later. Portoenterostomy revolutionized the management, and recent results (Kasai *et al.*, 1989) show early bile drainage in the majority of cases after portoenterostomy (Mieli-Vergani *et al.*, 1989). Kasai's group have clearly documented the gradual improvement in results since portoenterostomy was first described. They reported success rates of 13% during the first 18 years, 44% during the next 7 years, and an overall 50% success rate in the next 6 years (Ohi *et al.*, 1985). The factors that contribute to long-term success are not clear, although Vasquez-Estevez *et al.* (1989) found that infants with poor bilirubin excretion rates after operation tended to have severe giant-cell transformation and parenchymal degeneration on their liver biopsies. Fibrosis, ductular proliferation and bile stasis, on the other hand, were not related to postoperative progress. Approximately 28% of their patients did experience long-term survival with near normal liver function, and it is of interest that 13 severely fibrotic patients were alive 5 years after operation. Many groups have reported the relationship between bile flow and age at surgery. For example, Mieli-Vergani *et al.* (1989), in an analysis of cases from King's College Hospital, reported bile flow in 86% of infants treated before 8 weeks of age, compared with 36% of older children.

The influence of cholangitis on survival has been mentioned previously, and Houwen *et al.* (1989) achieved a 5-year survival rate of 91% in infection-free cases, but only 54% in those with attacks of cholangitis.

There are now significant numbers of patients who have lived for 10 years after portoenterostomy, and Saeki *et al.* (1987) described 26 long-term survivors, of whom 14 patients were over 15 years of age. About 40% of these survivors do have abnormal liver function tests, and all of them show abnormal intrahepatic bile ducts on cholangiography (Figure 8.16). Despite these observations, many of these patients live a virtually normal life. In a personal series of 147 portoenterostomies there was a 60% probability of survival at 5 years. The survival rate is of course higher when the results of hepatic transplantation are taken into account. However, it is now generally accepted that portoenterostomy and transplantation are complementary procedures, transplantation being reserved for children who do not achieve satisfactory bile drainage or who develop chronic liver failure at a later age. Davenport *et al.* (1997) concluded that portoenterostomy is an effective long-term procedure for biliary atresia in 40–50% of cases, but that the remainder will require transplantation, mostly within 2 years of age. They also pointed out that although age at the time of primary surgery is an important predictor of survival, it should not be used to dictate primary treatment, and portoenterostomy should remain the primary form of therapy.

In summary, portoenterostomy can result in very satisfactory bile drainage (Figure 8.17), and it is

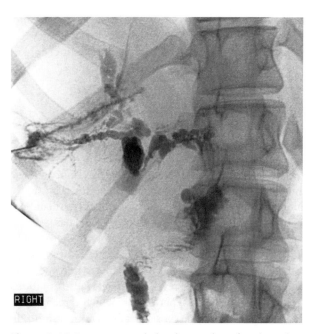

Figure 8.16 *Percutaneous cholangiogram in a female patient who presented with a transient episode of jaundice 20 years after a portoenterostomy operation for type 3 biliary atresia. Note the bizarre pattern of the intrahepatic bile ducts. There is prompt drainage of contrast material into the Roux loop.*

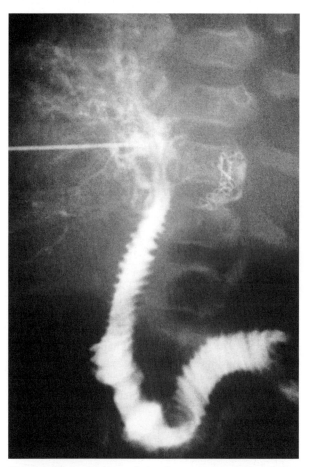

Figure 8.17 *Percutaneous cholangiogram performed in an infant 3 months after portoenterostomy. The drainage of contrast from the intrahepatic bile ducts is very satisfactory.*

recommended as the first-choice operation for extrahepatic biliary atresia. Current experience suggests that portoenterostomy procedures do not compromise liver transplantation, although complex loops and enterostomies are best avoided. Early diagnosis and treatment of these infants, preferably before 6 weeks of age, should be the aim, and transplantation should only be considered in an infant who fails to drain bile after portoenterostomy, or in a long-term survivor who shows signs of deteriorating liver function or life-threatening portal hypertension.

Key references

Hays DM, Kimura K. *Biliary atresia: the Japanese experience.* Cambridge, MA: Harvard University Press, 1980.

A comprehensive survey of the original Japanese development of treatment of biliary atresia. Any historical review of the subject should include reference to this text.

Karrer FM, Lilly JR, Stewart BA, Hall RJ. Biliary atresia registry, 1976–1989. *Journal of Pediatric Surgery* 1990; **25**: 1076–81.

This paper includes information on 904 children from more than 100 institutions in the USA. Factors associated with poor prognosis are analyzed and related to early referral for transplantation.

Mieli-Vergani G, Howard ER, Portmann B, Mowat AP. Late referral for biliary atresia – missed opportunities for effective surgery. *Lancet* 1989; **1**: 421–3.

A clear analysis of the relationship between age at the time of portoenterostomy and postoperative prognosis.

Tan CEL, Driver M, Howard ER, Moscoso GJ. Extrahepatic biliary atresia: a first-trimester event? Clues from light microscopy and immunohistochemistry. *Journal of Pediatric Surgery* 1994; **29**: 808–14.

An embryological study of the normal development of the biliary tract. A comparison with histological observations in biliary atresia suggests that an early embryological event might be implicated in the etiology of at least some cases of the condition.

Valayer J. Conventional treatment of biliary atresia: long-term results. *Journal of Pediatric Surgery* 1996; **31**: 1546–51.

A survey of 271 patients treated before 1983, representing the largest European series of long-term follow-ups. The prognosis and long-term problems in these patients are clearly defined.

REFERENCES

Adelman S. Prognosis of uncorrectable biliary atresia: an update. *Journal of Pediatric Surgery* 1978; **13**: 389–91.

Alagille D, Odievre M, Gautier M, Dommergues JP. Hepatic ductular hypoplasia associated with characteristic facies, vertebral malformation, retarded physical, mental and sexual development and cardiac murmur. *Journal of Pediatrics* 1975; **86**: 63–71.

Alpert LI, Strauss L, Hirschhorn K. Neonatal hepatitis and biliary atresia associated with trisomy 17–18 syndrome. *New England Journal of Medicine* 1969; **280**: 16–20.

Altman RP. The portoenterostomy procedure for biliary atresia. *Annals of Surgery* 1978; **188**: 357–61.

Altman RP. Results of reoperation for correction of extrahepatic biliary atresia. *Journal of Pediatric Surgery* 1979; **14**: 305–9.

Altman RP. Long-term results after the Kasai procedure. In: Daum F (ed.) *Extrahepatic biliary atresia*. New York: Marcel Dekker, 1983: 91–8.

Altman RP, Chandra R, Lilly JR. Ongoing cirrhosis after successful porticoenterostomy in infants with biliary atresia. *Journal of Pediatric Surgery* 1975; **10**: 685–9.

Bangaru B, Morecki R, Glaser JH, Gartner LM, Horwitz MS. Comparative studies of biliary atresia in the human newborn and reovirus-induced cholangitis in weanling mice. *Laboratory Investigations* 1980; **43**: 456–62.

Barkin RM, Lilly JR. Biliary atresia and the Kasai operation: continuing care. *Journal of Pediatrics* 1980; **96**: 1015–19.

Bill AH. Biliary atresia. *World Journal of Surgery* 1978; **2**: 557–9.

Brent RL. persistent jaundice in infancy. *Journal of Pediatrics* 1962; **61**: 111–44.

Brown WR, Sokol RJ, Levin MR *et al.* Lack of correlation between infection with reovirus 3 and extrahepatic biliary atresia or neonatal hepatitis. *Journal of Pediatrics* 1988; **113**: 670–6.

Burnweit CA, Coln D. Influence of diversion on the development of cholangitis after hepatoportoenterostomy for biliary atresia. *Journal of Pediatric Surgery* 1986; **21**: 1143–6.

Carcassonne M, Bensoussan A. Long-term results in treatment of biliary atresia. In: Rickham PP, Hecker WC, Prevot J (eds) *Progress in pediatric surgery*. Baltimore, MD: Urban & Schwarzenberg, 1977: 151–60.

Chardot C, Carton M, Spire-Bendelac N, Le Pommelet C, Golmard JL, Auvert B. Epidemiology of biliary atresia in France: a national study, 1986–96. *Journal of Hepatology* 1999; **31**: 1006–13.

Chaudhary S, Turner RB. Trimethoprim–sulfamethoxazole for cholangitis following hepatic portoenterostomy for biliary atresia. *Journal of Pediatrics* 1981; **99**: 656–8.

Chiba T, Ohi R, Mochizuki I. Cholangiographic study of the pancreaticobiliary ductal junction in biliary atresia. *Journal of Pediatric Surgery* 1990; **25**: 609–12.

Chiba T, Ohi R, Yaoita M, Goto M, Nio M, Hayashi Y *et al.* Partial splenic embolization for hypersplenism in pediatric patients with special reference to its long-term efficacy. In: Ohi R (ed.) *Biliary atresia*. Tokyo: ICOM Associates Inc., 1991: 154–8.

Chuang JH, Lee SY, Shieh CS, Chen WJ, Chang NK. Reappraisal of the role of the bilioenteric conduit in the pathogenesis of postoperative cholangitis. *Pediatric Surgery International* 2000; **16**: 29–34.

Clatworthy HW, MacDonald VG. The diagnostic laparotomy in obstructive jaundice in infants. *Surgical Clinics of North America* 1956; **36**: 1545.

Cunningham ML, Sybert VP. Idiopathic extrahepatic biliary atresia: recurrence in sibs in two families. *American Journal of Medical Genetics* 1988; **31**: 421–6.

Cursham G. Case of atrophy of the gall bladder with obliteration of the bile ducts. *London Medical Gazette* 1840; **26**: 388–9.

Danks DM. Prolonged neonatal obstructive jaundice. A survey of modern concepts. *Clinical Pediatrics* 1965; **4**: 499–510.

Danks DM, Campbell PE, Clarke AM, Jones PG, Solomon JR. Extrahepatic biliary atresia. *American Journal of Diseases of Children* 1974; **128**: 684–6.

Davenport M, Howard ER. Macroscopic appearance at portoenterostomy – a prognostic variable in biliary atresia. *Journal of Pediatric Surgery* 1996; **31**: 1387–90.

Davenport M, Savage M, Mowat AP, Howard ER. Biliary atresia splenic malformation syndrome: an etiologic and prognostic subgroup. *Surgery* 1993; **113**: 662–8.

Davenport M, Saxena R, Howard ER. Acquired biliary atresia. *Journal of Pediatric Surgery* 1996; **31**: 1721–3.

Davenport M, Kerkar N, Mieli-Vergani G, Mowat AP, Howard ER. Biliary atresia: the King's College Hospital experience (1974–1995). *Journal of Pediatric Surgery* 1997; **32**: 479–85.

Davenport M, Gonde C, Redkar R *et al.* Immuno-histochemistry of the liver and biliary tree in extrahepatic biliary atresia. *Journal of Pediatric Surgery* 2001; **36**: 1017–25.

Desmet VJ. Congenital diseases of intrahepatic bile ducts: variation on the theme 'ductal plate malformation'. *Hepatology* 1992; **16**: 1069–83.

Desmet V, Callea F. Ductal plate malformation (DPM) in extrahepatic biliary atresia (EHBDA). In: Ohi R (ed.) *Biliary atresia*. Tokyo: ICOM Associates Inc., 1991: 27–31.

Dessanti A, Ohi R, Hanamatsu M, Mochizuchi I, Chiba T, Kasai M. Short-term histological liver changes in extrahepatic biliary atresia with good postoperative bile drainage. *Archives of Disease in Childhood* 1985; **60**: 739–42.

Dick M, Mowat AP. Biliary scintigraphy with DISIDA. A simpler way of showing bile duct patency in suspected biliary atresia. *Archives of Disease in Childhood* 1986; **61**: 191–2.

Dillon PW, Belchis DB, Tracy TT, Cilley RE, Hafer L, Krumel TM. Increased expression of intercellular adhesion molecules in biliary atresia. *American Journal of Pathology* 1994; **145**: 263–7.

Dussaix E, Hadchouel M, Tardieu M, Alagille D. Biliary atresia and Reo virus type 3 infection. *New England Journal of Medicine* 1984; **311**: 658–61.

Ecoffey C, Rothman E, Bernard O, Hadchouel M, Valayer J, Alagille D. Bacterial cholangitis after surgery for biliary atresia. *Journal of Pediatrics* 1987; **111**: 824–9.

Endo M, Katsumata K, Yokoyama J, Morikawa Y, Ikawa H, Kamagata S. Extended dissection of the porta hepatis and creation of an intussuscepted ileocaecal conduit for biliary atresia. *Journal of Pediatric Surgery* 1983; **18**: 784–93.

Fonkalsrud EW, Kitagawa S, Longmire WP. Hepatic lymphatic drainage to the jejunum for congenital biliary atresia. *American Journal of Surgery* 1966; **112**: 188–94.

Freitas L, Gauthier F, Valayer J. Second operation for repair of biliary atresia. *Journal of Pediatric Surgery* 1987; **22**: 857–60.

Funaki N, Sasano H, Shizawa S *et al.* Apoptosis and cell proliferation in biliary atresia. *Journal of Pathology* 1998; **186**: 429–33.

Gautier M, Eliot N. Extrahepatic biliary atresia: morphological study of 98 biliary remnants. *Archives of Pathology and Laboratory Medicine* 1981; **105**: 397–402.

Gershoni-Baruch R, Gottfried E, Pery M, Sahin A, Etzioni A. Immotile cilia syndrome including polysplenia, situs inversus and extrahepatic biliary atresia. *American Journal of Medical Genetics* 1989; **33**: 390–3.

Gourevitch A. Duodenal atresia in the newborn. *Annals of the Royal College of Surgeons of England* 1971; **48**: 141–58.

Greene HL. Nutritional aspects in the management of biliary atresia. In: Daum F (ed.) *Extrahepatic biliary atresia*. New York: Marcel Dekker, 1983: 133–43.

Greenholz SK, Lilly JR, Shikes RH, Hall RJ. Biliary atresia in the newborn. *Journal of Pediatric Surgery* 1986; **12**: 1147–8.

Grosfeld JL, Fitzgerald JF, Predaina R, West KW, Vane DW, Rescorla FJ. The efficacy of hepatoportoenterostomy in biliary atresia. *Surgery* 1989; **106**: 692–700.

Haas JE. Bile duct and liver pathology in biliary atresia. *World Journal of Surgery* 1978; **2**: 561–9.

Hall RJ, Lilly JR, Stiegmann GV. Endoscopic esophageal varix ligation: technique and preliminary results in children. *Journal of Pediatric Surgery* 1988; **23**: 1222–3.

Harper PAW, Plant JW, Unger DB. Congenital biliary atresia and jaundice in lambs and calves. *Australian Veterinary Journal* 1990; **67**: 18–22.

Hays DM, Snyder WH. Life-span in untreated biliary atresia. *Surgery* 1963; **64**: 373–5.

Hays DM, Kimura K. *Biliary atresia: the Japanese experience*. Cambridge, MA: Harvard University Press, 1980.

Heyman MB, Shapiro HA, Thaler MM. Endoscopic retrograde cholangiography in the diagnosis of biliary malformations in infants. *Gastrointestinal Endoscopy* 1988; **34**: 449–53.

Hirsig J, Kara O, Rickham PP. Experimental investigations into the etiology of cholangitis following operation for biliary atresia. *Journal of Pediatric Surgery* 1978; **13**: 55–7.

Hirsig J, Bircher A, Rickham PP. Choleretic therapy for biliary atresia patients. In: Kasai M (ed.) *Biliary atresia and its related disorders*. Amsterdam: Excerpta Medica, 1983: 197–204.

Hitch DC, Shikes RH, Lilly JR. Determinants of survival after Kasai's operation for biliary atresia using actuarial analysis. *Journal of Pediatric Surgery* 1979; **14**: 310–4.

Holmes JB. Cogenital obliteration of the bile duct: diagnosis and suggestions for treatment. *American Journal of Diseases of Children* 1916; **11**: 405–31.

Home E. On the formation of fat in the intestine of living animals. *Philosophical Transactions of the Royal Society* 1813; **103**: 156–7.

Houwen RHJ, Kerremans II, van-Steensel-Moll HA, van-Romunde LK, Bijleveld CM, Schweizer P. Time–space distribution of extrahepatic biliary atresia in The Netherlands and West Germany. *Zeitschrift für Kinderchirurgie* 1988; **43**: 68–71.

Houwen RHJ, Zwierstra RP, Severijnen RS *et al*. Prognosis of extrahepatic biliary atresia. *Archives of Disease in Childhood* 1989; **64**: 214–18.

Howard ER. Biliary atresia. In: Blumgart L (ed.) *Surgery of the liver and biliary tract*, 2nd edn. Edinburgh: Churchill Livingstone, 1994: 835–52.

Howard ER. Extrahepatic biliary atresia. In: Schwartz SI, Ellis H (eds) *Maingot's abdominal operations*, 10th edn. Norwalk, CT: Appleton & Lange, 1997: 2117–30.

Howard ER, Mowat AP. Hepatobiliary disorders in infancy: hepatitis, extrahepatic biliary atresia, intrahepatic biliary hypoplasia. In: Thomas HC, McSween RNM (eds) *Recent advances in hepatology*. London: Churchill Livingstone, 1984: 153–69.

Howard ER, Davenport M. The treatment of biliary atresia in Europe, 1969–1995. *Tohoku Journal of Experimental Medicine* 1997; **181**: 75–83.

Howard ER, Driver M, McClement J, Mowat AP. Results of surgery in 88 consecutive cases of extrahepatic biliary atresia. *Journal of the Royal Society of Medicine* 1982; **75**: 408–13.

Howard ER, Davenport M, Mowat AP. Portoenterostomy in the eighties: the King's College Hospital experience. In: Ohi R (ed.) *Biliary atresia. Proceedings of the Fifth International Sendai Symposium on Biliary Atresia*. Tokyo: ICOM Associates, 1991: 111–15.

Hung WT, Su CT. Analysis of duodenal juice for diagnosis of atretic prolonged obstructive jaundice (radioactive excretion study, second report). In: Ohi R (ed.) *Biliary atresia*. Tokyo: Professional Postgraduate Services, 1987: 114–17.

Ibrahim M, Miyano T, Ohi R *et al*. Japanese biliary atresia registry, 1989 to 1994. *Tohoku Journal of Experimental Medicine* 1997; **181**: 85–95.

Iinuma Y, Narisawa R, Iwafuchi M *et al*. The role of endoscopic retrograde cholangiopancreatography in infants with cholestasis. *Journal of Pediatric Surgery* 2000; **35**: 545–9.

Ito T, Horisawa M, Ando H. Intrahepatic bile ducts in biliary atresia: a possible factor determining the prognosis. *Journal of Pediatric Surgery* 1983; **18**: 124–30.

Jenner RE. New perspectives on biliary atresia. *Annals of the Royal College of Surgeons of England* 1978; **60**: 367–74.

Jenner RE, Howard ER. Unsaturated monohydroxy bile acids as a cause of idiopathic obstructive cholangiopathy. *Lancet* 1975; **2**: 1073–4.

Kahn EI, Daum F. Arterio-hepatic dysplasia: evaluation of the extrahepatic biliary tract, porta hepatis and hepatic parenchyma. In: Daum F (ed.) *Extrahepatic biliary atresia*. New York: Marcel Dekker, 1983: 193–202.

Karrer FM, Lilly JR. Corticosteroid therapy in biliary atresia. *Journal of Pediatric Surgery* 1985; **20**: 693–5.

Karrer FM, Lilly JR, Stewart BA, Hall RJ. Biliary atresia registry, 1976–1989. *Journal of Pediatric Surgery* 1990; **25**: 1076–81.

Karrer FM, Hall RJ, Lilly JR. Biliary atresia and the polysplenia syndrome. *Journal of Pediatric Surgery* 1991; **26**: 524–7.

Karrer FM, Holland RM, Allshouse MJ, Lilly JR. Portal vein thrombosis: treatment of variceal haemorrhage by endoscopic variceal ligation. *Journal of Pediatric Surgery* 1994; **29**: 1149–51.

Karrer FM, Price MR, Bensard DD *et al*. Long-term results with the Kasai operation for biliary atresia. *Archives of Surgery* 1996; **131**: 493–6.

Kasai M. Treatment of biliary atresia with special reference to hepatic portoenterostomy and its modifications. *Progress in Pediatric Surgery* 1974; **6**: 5–52.

Kasai M, Suzuki S. A new operation for 'non-correctable' biliary atresia: hepatic portoenterostomy. *Shujitsu* 1959; **13**: 733–9.

Kasai M, Ohi R, Chiba T. Intrahepatic bile ducts in biliary atresia. In: Kasai M, Shiraki K (eds) *Cholestasis in infancy*. Baltimore, MD: University Park Press, 1980: 181–8.

Kasai M, Okamoto A, Ohi R, Yabe K, Matsumura Y. Changes of portal vein pressure and intrahepatic blood vessels after surgery for biliary atresia. *Journal of Pediatric Surgery* 1981; **16**: 152–9.

Kasai M, Mochizuki I, Ohkohchi N, Chiba T, Ohi R. Surgical limitations for biliary atresia: indications for liver transplantation. *Journal of Pediatric Surgery* 1989; **24**: 851–4.

Kaufman BH, Luck SR, Raffensberger JG. The evolution of a valved hepatoduodenal intestinal conduit. *Journal of Pediatric Surgery* 1981; **16**: 279–83.

Kimura K, Tsugawa C, Kubo M, Matsumoto Y, Itoh H. Technical aspects of hepatic portal dissection in biliary atresia. *Journal of Pediatric Surgery* 1979; **14**: 27–32.

Kobayashi A, Itabashi F, Ohbe Y. Long-term prognosis in biliary atresia after hepatic portoenterostomy: analysis of 35 patients who survived beyond 5 years of age. *Journal of Pediatrics* 1984; **105**: 243–6.

Kobayashi H, Puri P, O'Briain S, Surana R, Miyano T. Hepatic overexpression of MHC class II antigens and macrophage-associated antigens (CD68) in patients with biliary atresia of poor prognosis. *Journal of Pediatric Surgery* 1997; **32**: 590–3.

Kulkarni PB, Beatty EC. Cholangiocarcinoma associated with biliary cirrhosis due to congenital biliary atresia. *American Journal of Diseases of Children* 1977; **131**: 441–4.

Ladd WE. Congenital atresia and stenosis of the bile duct. *Journal of the American Medical Association* 1928; **91**: 1082–4.

Lally KP, Kenegaye J, Matsumura M, Rosenthal P, Sinatra F, Atkinson JB. Perioperative factors affecting the outcome following repair of biliary atresia. *Pediatrics* 1989; **83**: 723–6.

Landing BH. Considerations of the pathogenesis of neonatal hepatitis, biliary atresia and choledochal cyst: the concept of infantile obstructive cholangiopathy. *Progress in Pediatric Surgery* 1974; **6**: 113–39.

Lau JT, Ong GB. Biliary atresia before and after the introduction of the Kasai-type procedure. *Australian and New Zealand Journal of Surgery* 1983; **53**: 129–31.

Laurent J, Gauthier F, Bernard O *et al.* Long-term outcome after surgery for biliary atresia: study of 40 patients surviving for more than 10 years. *Gastroenterology* 1990; **99**: 1793–6.

Lawrence D, Howard ER, Tzanatos C, Mowat AP. Hepatic portoenterostomy for biliary atresia. *Archives of Disease in Childhood* 1981; **56**: 460–63.

Leape LL, Ramenofsky ML. Laparoscopy in infants and children. *Journal of Pediatric Surgery* 1977; **12**: 921–37.

Lilly JR. Etiology of cholangitis following operation for biliary atresia. *Journal of Pediatric Surgery* 1978; **13**: 559–60.

Lilly JR. Hepatic portocholecystostomy for biliary atresia. *Journal of Pediatric Surgery* 1979; **14**: 301–4.

Lilly JR, Chandra RS. Surgical hazards of coexisting anomalies in biliary atresia. *Surgery, Gynecology and Obstetrics* 1974; **139**: 49–54.

Lilly JR, Javitt NB. Biliary lipid excretion after hepatic portoenterostomy. *Annals of Surgery* 1976; **184**: 369–75.

Lilly JR, Altman RP. The biliary tree. In: Ravitch MM, Welch KJ, Benson CD (eds) *Pediatric surgery*, 3rd edn. Chicago: Year Book Publishers, 1979: 827–38.

Lilly JR, Stellin G. Variceal haemorrhage in biliary atresia. *Journal of Pediatric Surgery* 1984; **19**: 476–9.

Lilly JR, Hall RJ, Vasquez-Estevez J, Ohi R, Shikes RH. Hepatic portocholecystostomy: the Denver experience. In: Ohi R (ed.) *Biliary atresia*. Tokyo: Professional Postgraduate Services, 1987; 173–6.

Lilly JR, Karrer FM, Hall RJ *et al.* The surgery of biliary atresia. *Annals of Surgery* 1989; **210**: 289–96.

Lofstedt J, Koblik D, Jakowski DVM, McMillan MC, Engelking LR. Use of hepatobiliary scintigraphy to diagnose bile duct atresia in a lamb. *Journal of the American Veterinary Medical Association* 1988; **193**: 95–8.

Longmire WP, Sandford MC. Intrahepatic cholangiojejunostomy for biliary obstruction. *Surgery* 1948; **24**: 264–76.

MacGillivray TE, Scott Adzick N. Biliary atresia begins before birth. *Pediatric Surgery International* 1994; **9**: 116–17.

McKiernan PJ, Baker AJ, Kelly DA. The frequency and outcome of biliary atresia in the UK and Ireland. *Lancet* 2000; **355**: 25–9.

Manolaki AG, Larcher VF, Mowat AP, Barrett JJ, Portmann B, Howard ER. The prelaparotomy diagnosis of extrahepatic biliary atresia. *Archives of Disease in Childhood* 1983; **58**: 591–4.

Mason GR, Northway W, Cohn RB. Difficulties in the operative diagnosis of congenital atresia of the biliary ductal system. *American Journal of Surgery* 1966; **112**: 183–7.

Mazziotti MV, Willis LK, Heuckeroth RO *et al.* Anomalous development of the hepatobiliary system in the Inv mouse. *Hepatology* 1999; **30**: 372–8.

Mieli-Vergani G, Howard ER, Portmann B, Mowat AP. Late referral for biliary atresia – missed opportunities for effective surgery. *Lancet* 1989; **1**: 421–3.

Miyamoto M, Kajimoto T. Associated anomalies in biliary atresia patients. In: Kasai M (ed.) *Biliary atresia and its related disorders*. Amsterdam: Excerpta Medica, 1983: 13–19.

Miyano T, Suruga K, Suda K. Abnormal choledocho-pancreatico ductal junction related to the etiology of infantile obstructive jaundice diseases. *Journal of Pediatric Surgery* 1979; **14**: 16–26.

Miyano T, Suruga K, Kimura K. Postoperative management of biliary atresia with the Suruga II enterostomy. *Japanese Journal of Pediatric Surgery* 1985; **17**: 33–40.

Miyano T, Fujimoto T, Ohya T, Shimomura H. Current concept of the treatment of biliary atresia. *World Journal of Surgery* 1993; **17**: 332–6.

Morecki R, Glaser JH, Horwitz MS. Etiology of biliary atresia: the role of reo 3 virus. In: Daum F (ed.) *Extrahepatic biliary atresia*. New York: Marcel Dekker, 1983: 1–9.

Nakajo T, Hashizume K, Saeki M, Tsuchida Y. Intussusception-type antireflux valve in the Roux-en-Y loop to prevent ascending cholangitis after hepatic portojejunostomy. *Journal of Pediatric Surgery* 1990; **25**: 311–14.

Nelson JS, Rosenblum JL, Keating JP, Prensky AL. Neuropathological complications of childhood cholestatic disease. In: Daum F (ed.) *Extrahepatic biliary atresia*. New York: Marcel Dekker, 1983: 153–7.

Nittono H, Tokita A, Hayashi M, Nakatsu N, Obinata K, Watanabe T. Ursodeoxycholic acid in biliary atresia. *Lancet* 1988; **1**: 528.

Numazaki Y, Oshima T, Tanaka A *et al.* Neonatal liver disease and cytomegalovirus infection. In: Kasai M, Shiraki K (eds) *Cholestasis in infancy*. Tokyo: University of Tokyo Press, 1980: 61–6.

Odievre H. Long-term results of surgical treatment of biliary atresia. *World Journal of Surgery* 1978; **2**: 589–94.

Odievre M, Valayer J, Razemon-Pinta M, Habib EC, Alagille D. Hepatic portoenterostomy or cholecystostomy in the treatment of extrahepatic biliary atresia. *Journal of Pediatric Surgery* 1976; **88**: 774–9.

Ohi R. Biliary atresia: modification to the original portoenterostomy operation. In: Howard ER (ed.) *Surgery of liver disease in children*. Oxford: Butterworth–Heinemann, 1991: 72–7.

Ohi R, Shikes RH, Stellin GP, Lilly JR. In biliary atresia duct histology correlates with bile flow. *Journal of Pediatric Surgery* 1984; **19**: 467–70.

Ohi R, Hanamatsu M, Mochizuki I, Chiba T, Kasai M. Progress in the treatment of biliary atresia. *World Journal of Surgery* 1985; **9**: 285–93.

Ohi R, Mochizuki I, Komatsu K *et al*. Portal hypertension after successful hepatic portoenterostomy in biliary atresia. *Journal of Pediatric Surgery* 1986; **21**: 271–4.

Ohi R, Chiba T, Ohkochi N *et al*. The present status of surgical treatment for biliary atresia: report of the questionnaire for the main institutions in Japan. In: Ohi R (ed.) *Biliary atresia*. Tokyo: Professional Postgraduate Services, 1987: 125–30.

Parashar K, Taplow MJ, McCrae MA. Experimental Reovirus type 3-induced murine biliary tract disease. *Journal of Pediatric Surgery* 1992; **27**: 843–7.

Petersen D, Biermanns D, Kuske M, Schakel K, Meyer-Junghanel L, Mildenberger H. New aspects in a murine model for extrahepatic biliary atresia. *Journal of Pediatric Surgery* 1997; **32**: 1190–5.

Phillips PA, Keast D, Papadimitriou JM, Walters MNI, Stanley NF. Chronic obstructive jaundice induced by reovirus type 3 in weanling mice. *Pathology* 1969; **1**: 193–203.

Psacharopoulos HT, Howard ER, Portmann B, Mowat AP. Extrahepatic biliary atresia: preoperative assessment and surgical results in 47 consecutive cases. *Archives of Disease in Childhood* 1980; **55**: 851–6.

Redkar R, Davenport M, Howard ER. Antenatal diagnosis of congenital anomalies of the biliary tree. *Journal of Pediatric Surgery* 1998; **33**: 700–4.

Riepenhoff–Talty M, Gouvea V, Ruffin D, Barrett H, Rossi T. Group C rotavirus: one possible cause of extrahepatic biliary atresia in human infants (abstract). *Pediatric Research* 1992; **31**: 115A.

Riepenhoff–Talty M, Schaekel K, Clark HF *et al*. Group A rotaviruses produce extrahepatic biliary obstruction in orally inoculated newborn mice. *Pediatric Research* 1993; **33**: 394–9.

Rothenberg SS, Schroter PJ, Karrer FM, Lilly JR. Cholangitis after the Kasai operation for biliary atresia. *Journal of Pediatric Surgery* 1989; **24**: 729–32.

Saeki M, Ogata T, Nakano M. Problems in long-term survivors of biliary atresia. In: Ohi R (ed.) *Biliary atresia*. Tokyo: Professional Postgraduate Services, 1987: 287–93.

Saito S. Reoperation for biliary atresia after hepatic portoenterostomy. In: Kasai M (ed.) *Biliary atresia and its related disorders*. Amsterdam: Excerpta Medica, 1983: 224–7.

Saito S, Nishina T, Tsuchida Y. Intrahepatic cysts in biliary atresia after successful hepatoportoenterostomy. *Archives of Disease in Childhood* 1984; **59**: 274–5.

Sasaki F, Hata Y, Hamada H, Takahashi H, Uchino J. Laminin and procollagen III peptide as a serum marker for hepatic fibrosis in congenital biliary atresia. *Journal of Pediatric Surgery* 1992; **27**: 700–3.

Sawaguchi S, Akiyama H, Nakajo T. Long-term follow-up after radical operation for biliary atresia. In: Kasai M, Shiraki K (eds) *Cholestasis in infancy*. Tokyo: University of Tokyo Press, 1980: 371–9.

Schweizer P, Brambs HJ, Schweizer M, Astfalk W. TIPS: a new therapy for esophageal variceal bleeding caused by EHBA. *European Journal of Pediatric Surgery* 1995; **5**: 211–15.

Shim WKT, Zhang JZ. Antirefluxing Roux-en-Y biliary drainage valve for hepatic portoenterostomy: animal experiments and clinical experience. *Journal of Pediatric Surgery* 1985; **20**: 689–92.

Shiraki K, Sakurai M, Yoshihara N, Kawana T, Yasui H. Vertical transmission of HB virus and neonatal hepatitis. In: Kasai M, Shiraki K (eds) *Cholestasis in infancy*. Tokyo: University of Tokyo Press, 1980: 67–74.

Silveira TR, Salzano FM, Howard ER, Mowat AP. Congenital structural abnormalities in biliary atresia: evidence for etiopathogenic heterogeneity and therapeutic implications. *Acta Paediatrica Scandinavica* 1991; **80**: 1192–9.

Silveira TR, Salzano FM, Donaldson PT, Mieli-Vergani G, Howard ER, Mowat AP. Association between HLA and extrahepatic biliary atresia. *Journal of Pediatric Gastroenterology and Nutrition* 1993; **16**: 114–17.

Smith S, Wiener ES, Starzl TE, Rowe MI. Stoma-related variceal bleeding: an under-recognized complication of biliary atresia. *Journal of Pediatric Surgery* 1988; **23**: 243–5.

Soh H, Hasegawa T, Sasaki T *et al*. Pulmonary hypertension associated with postoperative biliary atresia: report of two cases. *Journal of Pediatric Surgery* 1999; **34**: 1779–81.

Starzl TE. Liver transplantation for biliary atresia. In: Daum F (ed.) *Extrahepatic biliary atresia*. New York: Marcel Dekker, 1983: 111–17.

Stellin G, Kumpe DA, Lilly JR. Splenic embolization in a child with hypersplenism. *Journal of Pediatric Surgery* 1982; **17**: 892–3.

Sterling JA, Lowenburg K. Increased longevity in congenital biliary atresia. *Annals of the New York Academy of Sciences* 1963; **111**: 483–503.

Strauss L, Bernstein J. Neonatal hepatitis in congenital rubella; a histopathological study. *Archives of Pathology* 1968; **86**: 317–27.

Strickland AD, Shannon K, Coln CD. Biliary atresia in two sets of twins. *Journal of Pediatrics* 1985; **107**: 418–19.

Stringer M, Howard ER, Mowat AP. Endoscopic sclerotherapy in the management of esophageal varices in 61 children with biliary atresia. *Journal of Pediatric Surgery* 1989; **24**: 438–42.

Suruga K, Miyano T, Kimura A, Arai T, Kojima Y. Reoperation in the treatment of biliary atresia. *Journal of Pediatric Surgery* 1982; **17**: 1–6.

Suruga K, Miyano T, Arai T, Ogawa T, Sasaki K, Deguchi E. A study of patients with long-term bile flow after hepatic portoenterostomy for biliary atresia. *Journal of Pediatric Surgery* 1985; **20**: 252–5.

Tagge DU, Tagge EP, Drongowski RA, Oldham KT, Coran AG. A long-term experience with biliary atresia. *Annals of Surgery* 1991; **214**: 590–8.

Takahashi H, Kuriyama Y, Maiae M, Ohnoma N, Eto T. ERCP in jaundiced infants. In: Ohi R (ed.) *Biliary atresia*. Tokyo: Professional Postgraduate Services, 1987: 110–13.

Tan CEL, Davenport M, Driver M, Howard ER. Does the morphology of the extrahepatic biliary remnants in biliary atresia influence survival? A review of 205 cases. *Journal of Pediatric Surgery* 1994a; **29**: 1459–64.

Tan CEL, Driver M, Howard ER, Moscoso GJ. Extrahepatic biliary atresia: a first-trimester event? Clues from light microscopy and immunohistochemistry. *Journal of Pediatric Surgery* 1994b; **29**: 808–14.

Tan Kendrick AP, Phua KB, Ooi BC, Subramaniam R, Tan CE, Goh AS. Making the diagnosis of biliary atresia using the triangular cord sign and gallbladder length. *Pediatric Radiology* 2000; **30**: 69–73.

Thomson J. *Congenital obliteration of the bile ducts*. Edinburgh: Oliver and Boyd, 1892.

Tracy TT, Dillon PW, Fox ES, Minnick K, Vogler C. The inflammatory response in pediatric biliary disease: macrophage phenotype and distribution. *Journal of Pediatric Surgery* 1996; **31**: 121–6.

Trivedi P, Tanner S, Portmann B, Mowat AP. Hepatic peptidyl prolyl hydroxylase activity and liver fibrosis – a propective study of 94 infants and children with hepatobiliary disorders. *Hepatology* 1984; **4**: 436–41.

Trivedi P, Cheeseman P, Portmann B, Mowat AP. Serum type III procollagen peptide as a non-invasive marker of liver damage during infancy and childhood in extrahepatic biliary atresia, idiopathic hepatitis of infancy and alpha-1-antitrypsin deficiency. *Clinica Chimica Acta* 1986; **161**: 137–46.

Tsuchida Y, Honna T, Kawarasaki H. Cystic dilatation of the intrahepatic biliary system in biliary atresia after hepatic portoenterostomy. *Journal of Pediatric Surgery* 1994; **29**: 630–4.

Tsuchida Y, Kawarsaki H, Iwanaka T, Uchida H, Nakanishi H, Uno K. Antenatal diagnosis of biliary atresia (type 1 cyst) at 19 weeks' gestation: differential diagnosis and etiologic implications. *Journal of Pediatric Surgery* 1995; **30**: 697–9.

Vacanti JP, Folkman J. Bile duct enlargement by infusion of L-proline: potential significance in biliary atresia. *Journal of Pediatric Surgery* 1979; **14**: 814–18.

Vajro P, Couterier M, Lemmonier F, Odievre M. Effects of postoperative cholestyramine and phenobarbital administration on bile flow restoration in infants with extrahepatic biliary atresia. *Journal of Pediatric Surgery* 1986; **21**: 362–5.

Valayer J. Biliary atresia and portal hypertension. In: Daum F (ed.) *Extrahepatic biliary atresia*. New York: Marcel Dekker, 1983: 105–8.

Valayer J. Conventional treatment of biliary atresia: long-term results. *Journal of Pediatric Surgery* 1996; **31**: 1546–51.

Van Der Luer RJT, Kroneman J. Biliary atresia in a foal. *Equine Veterinary Journal* 1982; **14**: 91–3.

Vasquez-Estevez J, Stewart B, Shikes RH, Hall RJ, Lilly JR. Biliary atresia: determination of the prognosis. *Journal of Pediatric Surgery* 1989; **24**: 48–51.

Vijayan V, Tan CE. Development of the human intrahepatic biliary system. *Annals of Academic Medicine, Singapore* 1999; **28**: 105–8.

Yeh TJ, Chin TW, Tsai WC, Wei CF. Mucosal intussusception to avoid ascending cholangitis. *British Journal of Surgery* 1990; **77**: 989–91.

9

Biliary atresia: long-term outcomes

RYOJI OHI

INTRODUCTION

The long-term outcomes of hepatic portoenterostomy for biliary atresia are now becoming clearer, but many clinical and histopathological questions remain unanswered. The so-called 'correctable type' of biliary atresia, in which there is a residual proximal segment of patent bile duct, was recognized and treated by Ladd as early as 1928. Eight of 11 patients were amenable to surgical treatment, of whom six patients recovered. Successful treatment for 'non-correctable-type' atresia was not available until Kasai and Suzuki (1959) described the operation of hepatic portoenterostomy (Ohi, 1988). The surgical results gradually improved, and recent results from several institutions worldwide have reported 70–80% of patients to be jaundice-free after the 'initial' hepatic portoenterostomy. However, many authors believe that liver disease will inevitably progress, even if good biliary drainage has been achieved with the operation, and that all patients with biliary atresia will eventually require liver replacement. The current strategy in management is a combination of initial hepatic portoenterostomy with later cadaveric or living-related transplantation if necessary. Living-related transplantation has been pioneered in particular in Japan (Ozawa et al., 1992; Tanaka et al., 1993).

The role of hepatic portoenterostomy can now be evaluated from reported long-term results, and the data from recent publications will be reviewed and discussed in this chapter.

IMPORTANCE OF EARLY OPERATION

The importance of early operation is now generally accepted as a major factor in the achievement of both early and late success with portoenterostomy. This is illustrated by the long-term survival of the Sendai series of patients shown in Table 9.1. The 10-year survival rate for the patients who were operated before 50 days of age was 75%, and it decreased with increasing age at the time of surgery. Only two out of nine (22.2%) of the patients who had undergone corrective surgery between the ages of 111 and 130 days, and a single case who was treated after the age of 131 days, survived for more than 10 years.

Although some investigators (Tagge et al., 1991; Maksoud et al., 1998; Carceller et al., 2000) state that surgical results are not always influenced by age at the time

Table 9.1 *Age at operation and 10-year survival of patients with biliary atresia during the period 1953–89 (Tohoku University Hospital)*

Days	n	Survivors	%
≤50	24	18	75.0
51–70	95	51	53.7
71–90	64	23	35.9
91–110	36	10	27.8
111–130	9	2	22.2
≥131	31	1	3.2
Total	259	105	40.2

of surgery, our results continue to show the reverse, and the series reported by Karrer *et al.* (1996) indicated that there were no long-term survivors who were over 90 days of age at the time of operation. As in our series, those who underwent surgery before 60 days of age achieved the best long-term outcome.

Schweizer and Lunzmann (1998) reported that in their experience there was a clear influence of age at surgery on the severity of hepatic fibrosis, as well as on life expectancy. Of 32 patients who underwent operation before 7 weeks of age, 26 individuals (81%) have lived for 5 years or more. The survival rate in children who were operated after week 7 was reduced to 47%. The experience in France between 1986 and 1996 (Chardot *et al.*, 1999) was similar, with 10-year survival rates of 80% and 66% in children who had undergone surgery before and after 45 days of age, respectively. Altman *et al.* (1997) reported that there was little difference in the comparative survival figures between the intermediate group (50–70 days) and those who were operated on before 49 days (*P* = 0.38). However, the older patients (≥ 71 days) had a significantly increased risk of failure compared with either of the other patient cohorts (*P* = 0.0077).

MULTICENTER SURVEYS OF LONG-TERM OUTCOMES

Several early reports provide baselines for any comparison of untreated patients with those who have undergone a Kasai operation. Hays and Snyder (1963) found that the average age of survival of 39 untreated patients was 19 months, and Adelman (1978) reported that the average age at death in untreated patients was 12 months (range 2 months to 4 years). Karrer *et al.* (1990) also reported that the 3-year survival rate for untreated cases was less than 10%.

The results of portoenterostomy, expressed as 'freedom from jaundice', have varied widely (Table 9.2). Howard and Davenport (1997) reported the surgical results achieved in Europe between 1969 and 1995, and showed that the 5- and 10-year jaundice-free survival rates after operation were 37% and 18%, respectively. Schweizer and Lunzmann (1998) also reported that of 108 children who were operated on between 1972 and 1992, 62 individuals (57%) were still alive and 58 (54%) were icterus-free at the time of the analysis. There was no progression of fibrosis in 25 cases, and 46 of 82 cases who were initially cirrhosis-free had no cirrhosis at the time of the report. The authors emphasized that the efficacy of hepatic portoenterostomy appeared to depend on the severity of hepatic fibrosis at the time of surgery, and the morphology of the porta hepatis, as well as the frequency of episodes of cholangitis episodes.

Altman *et al.* (1997) investigated possible risk factors for failure after the Kasai operation in 266 patients treated between 1972 and 1996. Age at surgery, surgical experience and anatomy of the atretic bile ducts were identified as independent risk factors. The 5-year survival rate was 49% and the median survival period was 15 years when bile drainage was achieved. The French National Study (Chardot *et al.*, 1999) calculated 5- and 10-year actuarial survival rates in 440 patients who had retained their native livers to be 32% and 27%, respectively.

All of these reports concluded that the Kasai portoenterostomy operation should remain the first-line treatment for biliary atresia. Early performance of the Kasai operation and treatment in an experienced center appeared to reduce the need for liver transplantation.

Our personal experience at Tohoku University Hospital after the introduction of a modified procedure for the prevention of postoperative cholangitis in 1972 has shown 5- and 10-year survival rates without transplantation of 61% and 54%, respectively (Table 9.2). The

Table 9.2 *Surgical results in patients with biliary atresia: actuarial survival with native liver*

	Period	Total number of cases	Five-year survival (%)	Ten-year survival (%)
New York and Denver (Altmann *et al.*, 1997)	1972–96	266	49	35
Europe (UK, The Netherlands, France and Italy) (Howard and Davenport, 1997)	1969–95	324	37	34
London, UK (Howard and Davenport, 1997)	1973–89	223	39	43
Paris, France (Chardot *et al.*, 1999)	1986–96	440	32	27
Tubingen, Germany (Schweizer and Lunzmann, 1998)	1972–97	151	57	—
Sendai, Japan (Author's experience)	1972–99	209	61	54

earlier 10-year survival rate of our patients who were treated between 1953 and 1971 was 16.3%. The operative results have continued to improve since 1972 when the operative technique and postoperative management were well optimized. Between 1982 and 1989 the rate improved still further to 59.4% (Table 9.3).

A total of 51 patients have survived more than 20 years in the Tohoku series, and the oldest patient is a 45-year-old woman. Four patients have undergone liver transplantation.

SUMMARY OF THE AUTHOR'S SERIES

Between 1953 and 1998, a total of 307 patients with biliary atresia underwent surgery in our hospital, of whom 197 were female (64%) and 110 (36%) were male. Complete obliteration of the extrahepatic bile ducts (type 3) was observed in 216 cases (70%). 'Correctable' (type 1) atresia with a patent segment of proximal common bile duct was present in 50 cases (16%). Some degree of patency of the hepatic ducts (type 2) was present in 41 cases (13%) (Ohi and Nio, 1998). The results of these 307 patients were analyzed according to the periods defined by the surgical modifications introduced for prevention of postoperative cholangitis. During the first period, from 1953 to 1971, a total of 104 patients underwent hepatic portoenterostomy using the original Roux-en-Y method described by Kasai. In the second period, from 1972 to 1981, a double Roux-en-Y method of drainage was used in 91 cases, and in the last period, from 1982 to 1998, an intussuscepted valve was added. The choleretic agent dehydrocholic acid and prednisolone were routinely administered to all postoperative cases.

An additional factor in the second period of our series was the appreciation of early diagnosis and operation, whilst in the third period we refined the transection level of the fibrous remnants of the bile ducts in the porta hepatis. After the introduction of liver transplantation, the indications for reoperative portoenterostomy were limited to patients who had shown definite bile drainage after the initial operation, but who later developed an abrupt cessation of bile flow (Ibrahim et al., 1991). Endoscopic injection sclerotherapy of esophageal varices and partial splenic embolization have improved

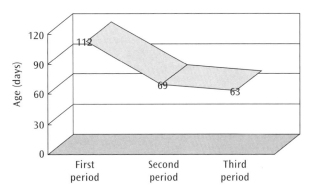

Figure 9.1 *Change in mean age of patients at the time of surgery at Tohoku University Hospital over three periods of time. First period: 1953 to 1971; second period: 1972 to 1981; third period: 1982 to 1998.*

both the surgical results and the quality of life of these patients.

Figure 9.1 shows the change in mean age at the time of corrective surgery during the three periods described above. The trend towards earlier referral is apparent between the first and second periods, although there has been no significant change between the second and third periods. Bile excretion after surgery was obtained in 65% of cases in the first period, in 74% of cases in the second period, and in 93% of cases in the third period, and jaundice cleared in 24%, 66% and 75% of cases, respectively. The incidence of postoperative cholangitis was 34% in the original Kasai group, 60% after the introduction of the double Roux-en-Y method, and 48% in the later valved procedure. Of the cases treated in the third period, 54% are still alive without jaundice after portoenterostomy alone, and 20% are alive after liver transplantation (Figure 9.2).

Transplantation has played an increasing role in the management of biliary atresia, and Figure 9.3 shows the cumulative survival curves of patients, including those with liver transplants, in each period. The stepwise improvement is clear. The overall 10-year survival rates

Table 9.3 *Period of surgery and 10-year survival rates (Tohoku University Hospital, 1953–89)*

Period	n	Survivors	%
1953–71	104	17	16.3
1972–81	91	49	53.8
1982–89	64	38	59.4
Total	259	104	40.2

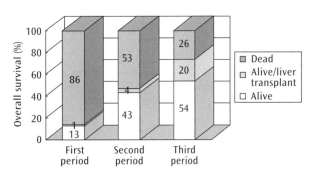

Figure 9.2 *Overall survival of patients after surgery at Tohoku University Hospital in each of the three time periods illustrated in Figure 9.1 (including patients who had undergone liver transplantation).*

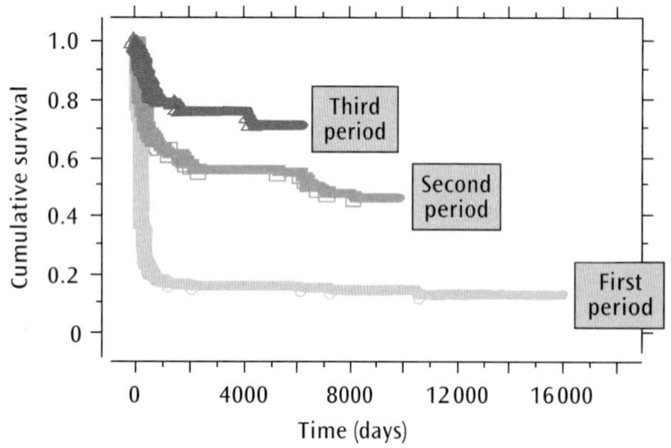

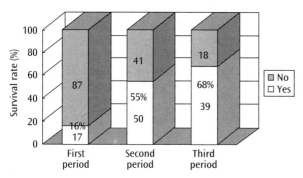

Figure 9.3 *Cumulative survival curves for patients at Tohoku University Hospital in each of the three time periods illustrated in Figure 9.1 (including patients who had undergone liver transplantation).*

DETAILED EVALUATION OF LONG-TERM RESULTS

Ascending bacterial cholangitis, disturbances of nutrition and growth, complications of portal hypertension and social and psychiatric difficulties are some of the sequelae of surgery for biliary atresia (Barkin and Lilly, 1980).

The long-term results of our series of portoenterostomy operations include 92 patients who have survived for more than 10 years, of whom 58 patients are female and 34 are male. In total, 62 patients were classified at the initial operation as type 3 disease, six were type 2 and 24 patients were type 1. Two patients are now more than 40 years of age, five are in their thirties and 37 patients are in their twenties (Figure 9.5). The heights and weights of most of the long-term survivors are comparable to those of normal, healthy Japanese, except for one 40-year-old woman who has shown poor growth related to repeated episodes of ileus and blind loop syndrome (Figure 9.6). Most patients have normal or moderately elevated liver function tests (serum total bilirubin, alkaline phosphatase, AST and ALT), but approximately one-third of the patients show abnormally high levels of alkaline phosphatase (Figure 9.7).

were 16%, 55% and 68%, respectively (Figure 9.4). A total of 32 patients underwent liver transplantation, most of these within the third period, and 19 recipients (60%) were under 5 years of age.

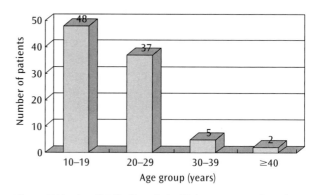

Figure 9.4 *Ten-year survival rate of patients after portoenterostomy surgery at Tohoku University Hospital in each time period. First period: 1953 to 1971; second period: 1972 to 1981; third period: 1982 to 1988.*

Figure 9.5 *Age distribution of the 92 long-term survivors from Tohoku University Hospital.*

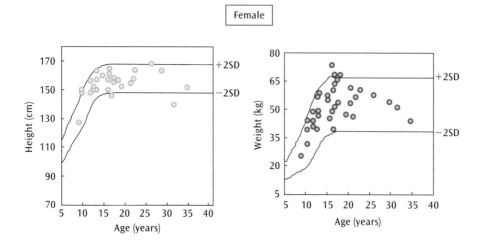

Figure 9.6 *Height and weight in the long-term survivors (female) after portoenterostomy surgery at Tohoku University Hospital. Normative ranges are illustrated by the continuous lines.*

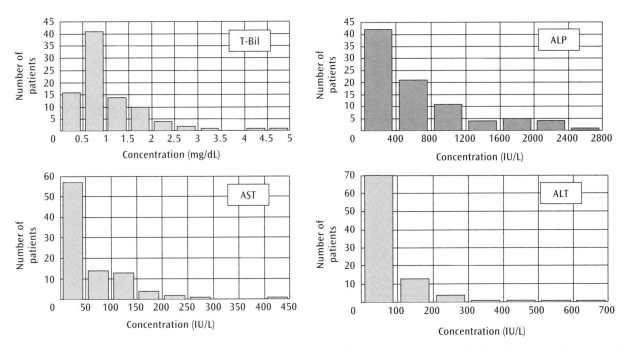

Figure 9.7 *Liver function tests in long-term survivors of biliary atresia after portoenterostomy at Tohoku University Hospital. Normal ranges: total bilirubin (T-Bil), 0.2–1.2 mg/dL; alkaline phosphatase (ALP), 112–330 IU/L; aspartate transaminase (AST), 12–30 IU/L; alanine transaminase (ALT), 8–35 IU/L.*

Investigation of amino acid metabolism in 42 long-term patients revealed that approximately 60% of the cases have a mild hyperacidemia and low branched/aromatic ratios (Matsumoto *et al.*, 1987) (Figure 9.8).

Plasma fatty acid components were abnormal in the majority of 36 patients with biliary atresia, but did show improvement after 2 years (Sawa *et al.*, 1984) (Figure 9.9). The concentrations of plasma fat-soluble vitamins were studied in 20 patients (Matsumoto and Ohi, 1987) (Figure 9.10). Although patients with jaundice tended to have low levels of vitamin A, a large number of long-term survivors showed normal levels. The data for vita-

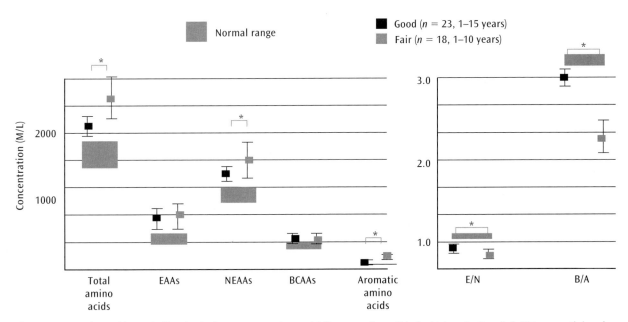

Figure 9.8 *Amino acid metabolism in the long-term survivors of biliary atresia at Tohoku University Hospital. EAAs, essential amino acids; NEAAs, non-essential amino acids; BCAAs, branched-chain amino acids, E/N, essential/non-essential; B/A, branched/aromatic. Mean values ± SD are shown. *P < 0.01.*

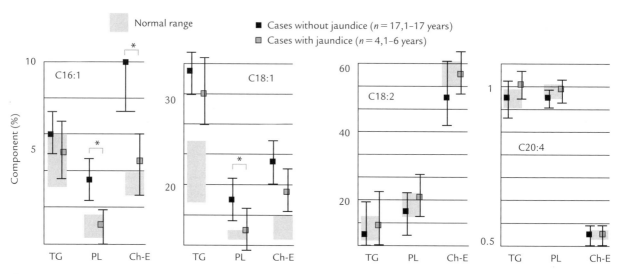

Figure 9.9 *Plasma fatty acid components in the long-term survivors of biliary atresia at Tohoku University Hospital. TG, triglyceride; PL, phospholipid; Ch-E, cholesterol ester. Mean values ± SD are shown. *P < 0.01.*

min E are similar to those for vitamin A. However, vitamin D levels were found to be lower than normal in the majority of cases, although they did not develop clinical signs of vitamin D deficiency, despite the fact that they did not receive vitamin D supplementation.

General nutritional status was assessed in 45 patients whose ages ranged from 0.5 to 38 years (mean age 9 years). Although the triceps skinfold (TSF) was not significantly different between patients with and without hepatic dysfunction, the mid-arm muscle area (MAMA) and albumin level were significantly lower in patients compared with controls (Shiga *et al.*, 1997).

Toyosaka *et al.* (1993) reported the outcome of 21 patients who had survived for more than 10 years after surgery. In total, 20 patients were leading almost normal lives. However, 13 patients (61.9%) did have a history of

complications, which included hemorrhage from esophageal varices in 10 cases, from gastric ulcers or erosions in three cases, and from duodenal ulcers in two cases. Three patients had suffered further biliary obstruction, and multiple pulmonary arteriovenous fistulae had occurred in two patients. Liver function tests were nearly normal in six out of eight patients who did not have complications, but two showed evidence of liver dysfunction with hypersplenism. Only alkaline phosphatase levels were abnormal in all patients. Of the 12 living survivors who experienced complications, liver function was almost normal in three cases, whilst nine patients had mild-to-moderate liver dysfunction with mild hypersplenism. None of the patients showed any evidence of mental retardation, and physical growth was almost within the normal range. Matsuo *et al.* (1998)

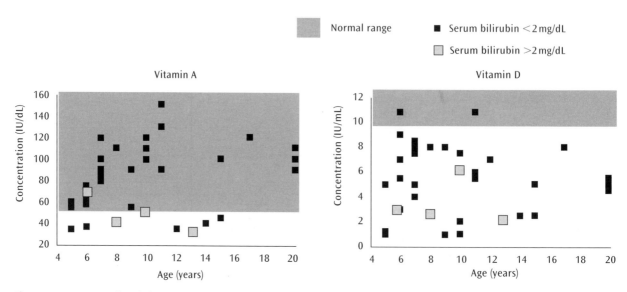

Figure 9.10 *Serum vitamin levels in the long-term survivors of biliary atresia at Tohoku University Hospital.*

reported that 14 (22.5%) of 71 patients treated between 1962 and 1986 had survived for more than 10 years. Six had suffered no severe complications, and total bilirubin levels were less than 20 µmol/L. In contrast, eight patients whose serum total bilirubin was more than 20 µmol/L demonstrated several clinical problems, including esophageal varices, hypersplenism and recurrent jaundice after cholangitis. The authors emphasized that a close and careful follow-up is essential after the correction of biliary atresia, especially for patients whose serum bilirubin concentration is more than 20 µmol/L.

Karrer *et al.* (1996) evaluated a consecutive series of 104 infants diagnosed with biliary atresia and treated more than 10 years previously. In total, 35 children (13 boys and 22 girls) survived for 10 years or more after surgery, and portoenterostomy was the only mode of treatment in 23 patients (24%). The heights of 30 children who had survived for more than 10 years were compared with standard nomograms. A total of 25 heights fell within the 10th to 90th percentile of expected height for age range, and five were below the 10th percentile.

Ten of the female patients began menstruation as teenagers, and one patient was pregnant. In total, 75% of the 10-year survivors were attending age-appropriate school or were gainfully employed, but two were having psychological treatment for clinical depression.

In 18 (78%) of the 23 long-term survivors without transplantation, serum bilirubin and serum albumin concentrations and prothrombin time were normal. Five patients showed mild elevations of bilirubin levels less than 51 µmol/L or mild hypoalbuminemia (30–35 g/L), but none had coagulopathy demonstrable by prolonged prothrombin time.

Valayer (1996) reported on 271 children with biliary atresia who underwent surgery during the period 1968–1983. Of these, 80 patients survived for at least 10 years without the need for liver transplantation. However, 13 children did subsequently require transplantation. Six patients died, and three of these deaths were due to complications of liver transplantation. Thus of the overall series of 271 patients, 64 patients with a mean follow-up period of 14 years survived for 10 years or longer without liver transplantation. The oldest is now 24 years of age, and 25 patients are over 15 years of age. Growth has been normal in all but three of the 38 long-term survivors, with normal serum bilirubin levels (< 18 µmol/L) recorded in all 38 patients. Near-normal serum bilirubin levels (18–36 µmol/L) were found in 14 cases, and high levels (> 36 µmol/L) were found in 12 cases. However, it was noted that serum bilirubin levels might be normal whilst other liver function tests remained abnormal. At a mean age of 12.5 years, the mean alkaline phosphatase value was 274 U/L (normal range 30–120 U/L). The mean value of alanine aminotransferase was 34.4 U/L (normal range 0–35 U/L), and the gamma-glutamyl transferase activity was 57.8 U/L (normal range 0–30 U/L). In a group of patients with near-normal serum bilirubin levels, the mean values of liver enzymes were very abnormal (e.g. alkaline phosphatase, 547.9 U/L; alanine aminotransferase, 256 U/L). The authors emphasized that a bilirubin level alone is not an accurate measure of 'cure'.

Four of the patients aged 2 to 4 years with normal to near-normal serum bilirubin levels underwent liver biopsy at the time of jejunostomy closure. A moderate to severe degree of fibrosis was found in all cases. Shimizu *et al.* (1997) evaluated the clinical status of six biliary atresia patients surviving more than 20 years after the Kasai procedure. None of them was receiving hospital care, but three had experienced complications. Two patients required partial splenic embolization, endoscopic injection sclerotherapy or devascularization surgery for portal hypertension and/or hypersplenism, and one required hospital care for recurrent cholangitis. Laboratory investigations showed a serum total bilirubin concentration of less than 20 µmol/L in three patients, a value between 20 and 40 µmol/L in one patient, and values higher than this in the remaining case. The ALT level was within the normal range in only one case, and was mildly to moderately elevated in four cases. The white blood cell count was less than 3×10^9/L and the platelet count was less than 10×10^9/L in one patient, and within normal ranges in the other four patients.

Toki *et al.* (1997) reported data from bone mineral analysis in eight patients with biliary atresia after successful Kasai procedures. The follow-up periods in these patients ranged from 3 to 27 years after operation. The bone mineral content of the lumbar spine was assessed by dual-energy X-ray absorptiometry. Plasma levels of 1,25-dihydroxy vitamin D $(1,25\text{-}(OH)_2\text{-}D3)$, calcium and phosphate were normal in all patients. Bone mineral density levels were normal in six patients, but low in two who had undergone partial splenic embolization and splenectomy, respectively. It was suggested that measurement of bone mineral density in long-term survivors of the Kasai procedure may detect bone mineral deficiency earlier than measurements of serum levels of vitamin D, calcium and phosphate.

Alagille *et al.* (1983) reported that high serum bile acid levels are the most frequent and persistent abnormality in long-term survivors. However, in our series, in more than 50% of the long-term survivors serum bile acid levels were below 10 µg/mL, although the levels in three cases with jaundice were severely elevated.

GROSS AND HISTOLOGICAL CHANGES IN THE LIVER

Progressive changes in liver histology are of considerable importance in the assessment of long-term survivors. Watanabe *et al.* (1997) reported changes in hepatic volume measured by CT scan in 19 patients 3 to 27 years after successful Kasai operations. The size of the liver increased at first to between 1.7 and 1.9 times the normal volume, and then decreased to normal size at approximately 5 years of age. After 12 years of age the hepatic volume decreased to below the normal expected volume. Segmental hypertrophy accompanying atrophy in other hepatic segments was observed in 9 out of 10 patients. This occurred as right lobe hypertrophy in six cases, medial segment hypertrophy in two cases and lateral segment hypertrophy in one case. Takahashi et al. (1997) reported MRI findings in the liver in biliary atresia patients 2 to 11 years after surgery. An atrophic change was found in 10 of 16 patients in at least one liver lobe.

Kimura et al. (1980) emphasized that the histological changes in biliary atresia patients after surgery were not uniform throughout the liver. The authors suggested that the observations might be the result of strictures between the intrahepatic bile ducts and the anastomosed bowel at the porta hepatis.

Ohi et al. (1983) reported the results of histometrical studies on 26 liver specimens taken at the time of repeat laparotomy, mostly during stoma closure, between the ages of 1 and 9 years. Hepatic fibrosis had progressed in 11 children, remained unchanged in 8 children and decreased in 7 cases. Nine out of 11 patients who showed progressive hepatic fibrosis had suffered complications with severe cholangitis during their postoperative course. Several pessimistic reports on the follow-up of liver histology have had a depressing influence on evaluation of the hepatic portoenterostomy operation. For example, Altman et al. (1975) observed that portal fibrosis progressed in eight of their 11 patients in whom needle biopsies were repeated during the first two years postoperatively. Gautier et al. (1984) evaluated liver specimens obtained by surgical biopsy in 20 patients who had survived for at least 5 years after surgery. They found definite biliary cirrhosis in all but two cases. Callea et al. (1987) reported that 12 of the 16 patients who were jaundice-free during 4- to 7-year follow-ups after surgery showed a severe degree of architectural disturbance with fully developed or early biliary cirrhosis, and that seven of the 16 cases showed complete absence of interlobular bile ducts. Alagille et al. (1983) evaluated the changes in liver histology by wedge biopsies taken from 20 children aged 5–8 years. There was complete clearing of cholestasis with micronodular cirrhosis in 13 cases and with macronodular cirrhosis in seven cases. Apart from the cirrhosis, atypical ductular proliferation was observed in 16 cases.

Schweizer and Lunzmann (1998) reported the persistence or progression of the histological changes in the liver in 108 patients who had undergone surgery 5 or more years previously. All seven children who had an initial level 2 fibrosis developed progressive fibrosis, to level 3 in five cases and to level 4 in two cases. The 43 children who initially showed level 3 fibrosis underwent no change in 18 cases (44%), showed progression to a level

4 fibrosis in 14 cases (33%) and cirrhosis in 19 cases (23%). Of 32 children with an initial level 4 fibrosis, there was no change in six cases (19%), but cirrhosis developed in 26 cases (81%). The rate of cirrhotic change was therefore extremely high in the group of patients with an initial level 4 fibrosis, whereas only 23% of the children with an initial level 2 or 3 fibrosis at portoenterostomy developed cirrhosis. The difference is statistically significant. Most of the children with an initial level 2 or level 3 fibrosis were considered to be 'stable' because their fibrosis persisted for several years without progression. The authors proposed a 'point of no return' between an initial level 3 fibrosis and a level 4 fibrosis, and they suggested that the former tends to persist, whereas the latter tends to progress to cirrhosis.

COMPLICATIONS AND SEQUELAE OF LONG-TERM SURVIVORS

In our series of 92 long-term survivors (surviving more than 10 years) the postoperative complications included cholangitis in 58 cases, esophageal varices in 30 cases, hypersplenism in 18 cases, ileus in 13 cases and hepatopulmonary syndrome in two cases.

Valayer (1996) reported splenomegaly and/or esophageal varices and/or abdominal ultrasound signs of portal hypertension in 21 of the 52 long-term survivors who showed normal and near-normal serum bilirubin levels. Esophageal variceal bleeding episodes occurred in 19 of the 10-year survivors, and the age at the first episode ranged from 1 to 11 years (in 10 cases it occurred before the age of 5 years).

The reported incidence of postoperative cholangitis after hepatic portoenterostomy is in the range 40–60% (Ohi et al., 1987). The attacks are manifested by fever, a decreased quantity and quality of bile, and a rise in serum bilirubin levels. Postoperative cholangitis within 3 months of surgery may be accompanied by a cessation of bile flow, and repeated attacks cause a progressive deterioration of hepatic function.

Although bacterial cholangitis is thought to be rare after 2 years of age, Gottrand et al. (1991) reported late cholangitis in four out of 76 patients who had been free of jaundice for more than 5 years after surgery. Cholangiography consistently demonstrated abnormalities in intrahepatic bile duct morphology, although there was no definite obstruction to the biliary–enteric anastomosis. Good hepatic function returned within 3 weeks to 4 years after episodes of cholangitis. These observations suggest that although cholangitis may occur several years after surgery, it does not necessarily alter the prognosis. Karrer et al. (1996) suggested that two-thirds of long-term survivors experienced one or more episodes of cholangitis.

Cholangitis occurs most frequently in the early postoperative years, although some of the 10-year survivors continue to experience sporadic attacks. In our series (Nio et al., 1996), 10 of the 21 patients who had survived for more than 20 years experienced cholangitis. Of these, five had mild to moderate cholangitis which had required hospitalization on at least one occasion during the last 5 years. Three patients still suffer repeated attacks almost every year.

Lunzmann and Schweizer (1999) assessed the effect of postoperative cholangitis on the prognosis of biliary atresia patients after Kasai operation. They reported that children with or without a history of cholangitis, who had level 2 or level 3 liver fibrosis, developed cirrhosis in 20% and 50% of cases, respectively.

A variable degree of hepatic fibrosis is already present in patients with biliary atresia at the time of initial operation. Moreover, intrahepatic disease is often progressive not only in failed portoenterostomies but also in 'successful' ones. Portal hypertension is therefore inevitable in many survivors. The reported incidence of portal hypertension has ranged from 34% to 76% (Akiyama et al., 1983; Lilly and Stellin, 1984; Ohi et al., 1986; Stringer et al., 1989), and postoperative cholangitis was recognized as a significant factor in its development (Lawrence et al., 1981). In our own experience of 106 jaundice-free survivors, significant esophageal varices developed in 26 cases (24.5%) and hypersplenism developed in 15 cases (14.1%). Esophageal varices were present in 7 out of 21 patients who had survived for more than 20 years (Nio et al., 1996), but none of these cases had suffered massive variceal bleeding or required endoscopic injection sclerotherapy. Of the four patients with significant splenomegaly and esophageal varices, three underwent splenectomy and proximal splenorenal shunting before 1986, and transitory shunt encephalopathy occurred postoperatively in one patient. Karrer et al. (1996) reported frequent complications from portal hypertension in 35 children who had survived for at least 10 years, and variceal bleeding occurred in 20 children (55%). The varices were treated endoscopically with either sclerotherapy or variceal band ligation. Significant hypersplenism occurred in seven of the patients who were treated with partial splenic embolization. Symptomatic ascites that was responsive to diuretic therapy and dietary manipulation developed in two patients.

Toyosaka et al. (1993) also reported that the commonest late complication in 21 long-term surviving patients was hemorrhage from esophageal varices, which occurred in 10 patients (47.6%). This complication has been reported in 20–60% of patients (Lilly and Stellin, 1984; Howard, 1991). A review of major European series concluded that esophageal varices were present in 48% and bleeding in 19% of 121 survivors (Howard and Davenport, 1997). Long-term follow-up with ultrasound and endoscopic investigation is recommended for these patients (Tanaka et al., 1992; Nakada et al., 1995; Kardorff et al., 1999). Although it is uncommon, intestinal hemorrhage from ectopic varices has also been reported in an increasing number of long-term survivors (Chiba et al., 1990).

Major interventional surgical procedures such as portal shunts and esophageal transection should be avoided in the initial management of portal hypertension in biliary atresia. Endoscopic injection sclerotherapy (EIS) or variceal ligation are recommended as the treatments of choice for esophageal varices (Howard et al., 1984, 1988; Hall et al., 1988; Paquet and Lazar, 1994).

The transjugular intrahepatic portosystemic shunt procedure (TIPS) has now been introduced for the treatment of recurrent bleeding in children (Astfalk et al., 1997; Heyman et al., 1997). Heyman et al. reported that 12 procedures were attempted in nine children with a mean age of 9 ± 3.9 years, including four biliary atresia patients. TIPS placement was successful in seven of the nine patients. It was concluded that the success rate was related to the vascular anatomy, and not to technical aspects such as the size of the vessels or the stents.

Hypersplenism can be a significant problem in long-term survivors, but this can be controlled with partial splenic embolization (PSE), which avoids the complication of overwhelming infection after splenectomy and of encephalopathy after shunt surgery. The beneficial effect on the platelet count was confirmed after 60–70% embolization of the spleen (Hayashi et al., 1987), although the patients commonly suffered from postprocedural pyrexia and abdominal pain. The latter was controlled with epidural spinal anesthesia.

Cystic dilatation of the intrahepatic bile ducts has been observed in increasing numbers of long-term survivors (Saito et al., 1984; Tsuchida et al., 1994). Kawarasaki et al. (1997) diagnosed 10 cases in 88 survivors using ultrasound examinations, and they suggested that the etiology might be related to peribiliary glands rather than to bile ducts. Nio et al. (1996) and Toyosaka et al. (1993) reported several cases of hemorrhage from peptic ulcer in long-term survivors. Several cases of hepatocellular carcinoma associated with biliary cirrhosis secondary to biliary atresia have been reported (Kohno et al., 1995).

Impaired bile flow and residual hepatic disease may be associated with a variety of problems related to the metabolism of fat and protein as well as the absorption of vitamins and trace minerals (Andrews et al., 1981; Greene, 1983; Shiga et al., 1997), and weight gain may be suboptimal.

Pulmonary arteriovenous shunting has been described in long-term survivors, and sudden death caused by pulmonary arterial hypertension was reported by Moscoso et al. (1991). Valayer (1996) reported five patients with either clinical signs such as dyspnea in the upright position that was relieved by lying down, or cyanosis precipitated by exertion, among 17 long-term survivors. Early recognition of these complications should lead to consideration of liver transplantation for these patients (see Chapters 22 and 27).

QUALITY OF LIFE (QoL) OF LONG-TERM SURVIVORS

In this section the current status of our 92 long-term survivors who have survived for more than 10 years is reported. Liver transplantation has been performed in 12 cases. In total, 74 patients are jaundice-free, while three have persistent jaundice. Other problems are present in 23 cases (26%), including easy fatigability in 20 cases, itching in 10 cases, episodes of abdominal pain in four cases, dyspnea mainly due to hepatopulmonary syndrome in three cases and recurrent pyrexia in two cases.

The occupations or academic status of the long-term survivors are listed in Table 9.4. A total of 70 out of 89 cases available for assessment are leading normal to near-normal lives, and the majority are able to participate in social events. Six patients have married, three women have two children each and one patient has one child.

The quality of life of the remaining nine patients is unsatisfactory, and several of these are considered as potential candidates for liver transplantation. None of the patients show evidence of brain dysfunction.

Schweizer and Lunzmann (1998) also evaluated the quality of life (QoL) of 108 patients who had survived for more than 5 years after surgery. Pruritus was a problem in 44 patients (41%) and physical fitness was partly or considerably reduced in 47 patients (43.5%). In total, 46 of 108 children were not able to attend school regularly because of recurrent symptoms, and 70 children (or their parents) reported social problems and difficulties when playing with children of the same age. It was not surprising that quality of life was related to the severity of hepatic fibrosis/cirrhosis.

Howard *et al.* (2001) compared detailed QoL measures in a cohort of Japanese patients (from Tohoku University Hospital) with an age-matched cohort from a hospital in the UK (King's College Hospital). Satisfactory QoL data were collected and analyzed for 25 Japanese and 21 English children. The QoL assessments were made using the 'Short Form 36' type of questionnaire containing assessments of bodily pain, general health, mental health, physical functioning, emotional role, physical role, social functioning and vitality. Interestingly, there were no significant differences between the Japanese and English patients, except for marginal differences in indices of general health and vitality ($P = 0.06$ and 0.04, respectively). The significant conclusion was that the QoL of long-term survivors was comparable in Japan and the UK.

Valayer (1996) could not demonstrate any specific problem in puberty in an analysis of 25 patients over 15 years of age, and sexual development was reported to be normal in all cases. Information on academic status was available for 26 long-term survivors with normal and near-normal serum bilirubin levels. School performance related to age had been normal in eight cases, 1 year below normal in 11 cases, and 2 or 3 years below normal in seven cases.

The professional status of those who had reached their twenties appeared to be satisfactory for age, but there were no instances of outstanding achievement. A survey of extracurricular activities revealed that 12 teenagers with normal serum bilirubin levels were good at sports. It was emphasized that QoL can be acceptable even in long-term survivors with abnormal serum bilirubin levels.

PREGNANCY AND DELIVERY

A questionnaire survey based on the Japanese Biliary Atresia Registry (Shimaoka *et al.*, 2001) revealed that 23 out of 1246 female patients were married. The age of menarche of these 23 cases ranged from 11 to 15 years (mean age 13.1 ± 1.2 years). In total, 14 patients (60.9%) had regular bleeding, 7 patients (30.4%) had irregular bleeding, and one had profuse bleeding.

A total of 18 patients have become pregnant. The pregnancies were uncomplicated in 14 cases (77.8%), but four patients experienced complications such as recurrent ascending cholangitis and portal hypertension. The 18 women gave birth 25 times, and there were two abortions, one of which was related to severe variceal bleeding. Nine patients delivered once and eight patients delivered twice, with Cesarean section being required in three cases. Other problems in three patients included a placental complication, fetal distress leading to Cesarean section, and deteriorating liver function. Problems experienced after delivery are summarized in Box 9.1. The patient who lost her first baby as a complication of severe

Table 9.4 *Occupations and school status of long-term survivors with native liver (Tohoku University, Sendai)*

Occupation or school grade	Number of cases
Housewife	4
Housekeeper	2
Teacher	3
Office worker	16
Factory worker	2
Salesman	2
Home-help	1
Industrial engineer	1
Self-defense force officer	1
Part-time worker	6
University student	3
Vocational school student	4
High-school student	12
Middle-high-school pupil	15
Primary-school pupil	10
Unknown	5

<hr>

> **Box 9.1**   *Problems in 25 pregnancies in 18 patients*
>
> **Problems during pregnancy**
> Abortion: $n = 2$
>   (hemorrhagic shock following bleeding from
>   esophageal varices in one case and severe atopic
>   dermatitis in one case)
> Increased portal hypertension: $n = 1$
> Placental abnormality: $n = 1$
> Fetal distress leading to Cesarean section: $n = 1$
> Aggravation of hepatic dysfunction: $n = 1$
>
> **Problems after delivery**
> Deterioration of liver function: $n = 6$
> Ascending cholangitis: $n = 4$
> Liver transplantation: $n = 1$

esophageal variceal bleeding is the same case who underwent liver transplantation after delivery of a second baby.

The mean gestational age of 23 babies was 37.5 ± 3.9 weeks (range 31–41 weeks) and the mean birth body weight was 2898 ± 652 g (range 980–3600 g). No congenital abnormalities were observed in the newborn infants, although one had a very low birth weight, one had infant respiratory distress syndrome, and one was treated with phototherapy.

McMichens and Robichaux (1992) reported the successful delivery of an infant of 36.5 weeks' gestation in a patient with biliary atresia who had experienced antenatal complications from bleeding esophageal varices and hypersplenism. There is a risk of worsening portal hypertension and bleeding during pregnancy, and these patients require close antenatal monitoring.

The National Transplant Pregnancy Registry (Radomski *et al.*, 1995) analyzed the outcomes of 48 pregnancies in 34 female liver transplant recipients and concluded that there is a high rate of premature and low-birth-weight births. It was suggested that the pregnancies should be considered high risk and that there should be close antenatal monitoring of liver function.

INDICATIONS FOR LIVER TRANSPLANTATION

Liver transplantation is not indicated in non-jaundiced patients who have neither serious complications nor progressive hepatic dysfunction. It should be considered in patients who fail to establish bile drainage after portoenterostomy, and for those who develop uncontrollable complications of cirrhosis (see Chapter 27). Liver transplantation in small infants does not appear to be associated with an increased risk compared with older children (Beath *et al.*, 1993; Dunn *et al.*, 1993; Vasquez *et al.*, 1993; Inomata *et al.*, 1995).

It is generally agreed that a portoenterostomy is a reasonable first-choice operation, and that it should be performed at an early stage in the disease, preferably within the first 2 months of life. The advantages of an initial Kasai procedure as opposed to primary liver transplantation are as follows.

- Approximately 50% of patients achieve adequate liver function after portoenterostomy.
- Further refinement of the portoenterostomy operation, including universal early diagnosis, might increase the overall success rate to 60–70%.
- The native organ is preferred to a donated liver.
- Successful portoenterostomy reduces the pressures on the waiting-list for suitable donors.
- Liver transplantation is not without complications, which include the risk of serious infections and malignant disease.

The timing of liver transplantation is critical. We employ a scintigraphic method of assessing liver function, using the radiopharmaceutical agent 99mTcGSA. This compound binds to asialoglycoprotein receptors on hepatocytes (Shimaoka *et al.*, 1997). The calculation of blood clearance (HH15) and hepatic accumulation (LHL15) indices provides a measure of liver function and a guide to the timing of transplantation (Figure 9.11).

A method of assessing the prognosis after portoenterostomy would be extremely valuable. Doppler ultrasound (Wanek *et al.*, 1990), urinary excretion of D-glucaric acid (Fujimoto *et al.*, 1994), the macroscopic appearance at portoenterostomy (Davenport and Howard, 1996) and evaluation of needle biopsy of the liver (Azarow *et al.*, 1997) have all been proposed as preoperative and/or intraoperative predictors. Unfortunately, none of these methods is capable of providing predictive information in all cases.

THE DEFINITION OF CURE IN BILIARY ATRESIA

Alagille *et al.* (1983) defined cure as 'an objective improvement after the construction of a functional enterobiliary anastomosis, which leads to regression in the size of the liver, return of liver function to normal, and regression or stabilization of histological changes of the liver'. Tsunoda *et al.* (1987) also suggested certain guidelines for the term 'cure' in survivors. These criteria consisted of the absence of jaundice, a serum bilirubin level of less than 20 μmol/L, the absence of portal hypertension and the absence of hepatosplenomegaly. One-third of their cases who survived for more than 5 years after surgery were classified as 'cured'.

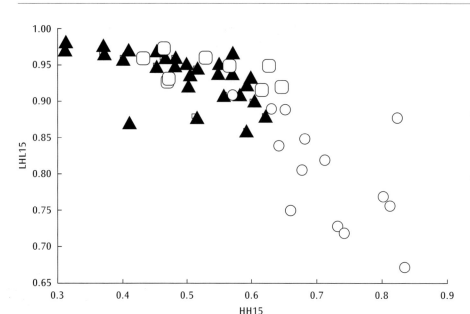

Figure 9.11 *The relationship between blood clearance of radioisotope (HH15) and hepatic accumulation of isotope (LHL15) and indication for liver transplantation.* ▲, *group with almost normal liver function;* ☐, *group with severe portal hypertension;* ○, *indications for liver transplantation.*

Key references

Karrer FM, Price MR, Bensard DD *et al*. Long-term results with the Kasai operation for biliary atresia. *Archives of Surgery* 1996; **131**: 493–6.

This paper evaluates in detail a consecutive series of 104 infants with biliary atresia diagnosed more than 10 years previously.

Kasai M, Suzuki M. A new operation for 'non-correctable' biliary atresia: hepatic portoenterostomy [in Japanese]. *Shujyutsu* 1959; **13**: 733–9.

This is the first and original report of hepatic portoenterostomy (the Kasai procedure).

Nio M, Ohi R, Hayashi Y *et al*. Current status of 21 patients who have survived more than 20 years since undergoing surgery for biliary atresia. *Journal of Pediatric Surgery* 1996; **31**: 381–4.

This is a report of the long-term results from the largest series of patients surviving for more than 20 years after the Kasai operation.

Schweizer P, Lunzmann K. Extrahepatic bile duct atresia: how efficient is the hepatoporto-enterostomy? *European Journal of Pediatric Surgery* 1998; **8**: 150–4.

This paper analyzes the findings in 151 children with biliary atresia who were operated on during the period 1972–1997. Of particular interest are the 108 patients who underwent operation 5 or more years ago.

Valayer J. Conventional treatment of biliary atresia: long-term results. *Journal of Pediatric Surgery* 1996; **31**: 1546–51.

This paper evaluates in detail 80 children with biliary atresia who had survived for more than 10 years after a portoenterostomy operation, without the need for liver transplantation.

REFERENCES

Adelman S. Prognosis of uncorrected biliary atresia: an update. *Journal of Pediatric Surgery* 1978; **13**: 389–91.

Akiyama H, Saeki M, Ogata T. Portal hypertension after successful surgery for biliary atresia. In: Kasai M (ed.) *Biliary atresia and its related disorders*. Amsterdam: Excerpta Medica, 1983: 276–82.

Alagille J, Vlayer J, Odievre M, Hadchouel M. Long-term follow-up in children operated on by corrective surgery for extrahepatic biliary atresia. In: Kasai M (ed.) *Biliary atresia and its related disorders*. Amsterdam: Excerpta Medica, 1983: 233–8.

Altman RP, Chandre R, Lilly JR. Ongoing cirrhosis after successful porticoenterostomy. *Journal of Pediatric Surgery* 1975; **10**: 685–91.

Altman RP, Lilly JR, Greenfeld J *et al*. A multivariable risk factor analysis of the portoenterostomy (Kasai) procedure for biliary atresia. *Annals of Surgery* 1997; **226**: 348–55.

Andrews WS, Pau CML, Chase HP, Foley LC, Lilly JR. Fat-soluble vitamin deficiency in biliary atresia. *Journal of Pediatric Surgery* 1981; **16**: 284–90.

Astfalk W, Huppert PE, Schweizer P, Plinta-Zgrabczynski A. Recurrent intestinal bleeding from jejuno-jejunostomy caused by portal hypertension following hepatoportojejunostomy in extrahepatic biliary atresia (EHBA) – successful treatment by transjugular intrahepatic portosystemic shunt (TIPS). *European Journal of Pediatric Surgery* 1997; **7**: 147–8.

Azarow KS, Phillips MJ, Sandler AD, Hagerstrand I, Superina RA. Biliary atresia: should all patients undergo a portoenterostomy? *Journal of Pediatric Surgery* 1997; **32**: 168–74.

Barkin RM, Lilly JR. Biliary atresia and the Kasai operation: continuing care. *Journal of Pediatrics* 1980; **96**: 1015–19.

Beath S, Pearmain D, Kelly P et al. Liver transplantation in babies and children with extrahepatic biliary atresia. *Journal of Pediatric Surgery* 1993; **28**: 1044–7.

Callea F, Facchetti F, Lucini L et al. Liver morphology in anicteric patients at long-term follow-up after Kasai operation: a study of 16 cases. In: Ohi R (ed.) *Biliary atresia*. Tokyo: Professional Postgraduate Services, 1987: 304–10.

Carceller A, Blanchard H, Alvarez F et al. Past and future of biliary atresia. *Journal of Pediatric Surgery* 2000; **35**: 717–20.

Chardot C, Carton M, Spire-Bendelac N et al. Prognosis of biliary atresia in the era of liver transplantation: French National Study from 1986 to 1996. *Hepatology* 1999; **30**: 606–11.

Chiba T, Mochizuki I, Ohi R. Postoperative gastrointestinal hemorrhage in biliary atresia. *Tohoku Journal of Experimental Medicine* 1990; **152**: 255–9.

Davenport M, Howard ER. Macroscopic appearance at portoenterostomy – a prognostic variable in biliary atresia. *Journal of Pediatric Surgery* 1996; **31**: 1387–90.

Dunn SP, Weintraub W, Vinocur CD, Billmire DF, Falkenstein K. Is age less than 1 year a high-risk category for orthotopic liver transplantation? *Journal of Pediatric Surgery* 1993; **28**: 1048–50.

Fujimoto T, Ohya T, Miyano T. A new clinical prognostic predictor for patients with biliary atresia. *Journal of Pediatric Surgery* 1994; **29**: 757–60.

Gautier M, Vaqlayer J, Odievre M, Alagille D. Histological liver evaluation 5 years after surgery for extrahepatic biliary atresia: a study of 20 cases. *Journal of Pediatric Surgery* 1984; **19**: 263–8.

Gottrand F, Bernard O, Hadchouel M et al. Late cholangitis after successful surgical repair of biliary atresia. *American Journal of Diseases in Children* 1991; **145**: 213–15.

Greene HL. Nutritional aspects of the management of biliary atresia. In: Daum F (ed.) *Extrahepatic biliary atresia*. New York: Dekker, 1983: 133–43.

Hall RJ, Lilly JR, Stiegman GV. Endoscopic esophageal varix ligation: technique and preliminary results in children. *Journal of Pediatric Surgery* 1988; **23**: 1222–3.

Hayashi Y, Ohi R, Chiba T et al. Effect of partial splenic embolization on hypersplenism in patients with biliary atresia. In: Ohi R (ed.) *Biliary atresia*. Tokyo: Professional Postgraduate Services, 1987: 268–71.

Hays DM, Synder WH. Life-span in untreated biliary atresia. *Surgery* 1963; **64**: 373–5.

Heyman MB, LaBerge JM, Somberg KA et al. Transjugular intrahepatic portosystemic shunts (TIPS) in children. *Journal of Pediatrics* 1997; **131**: 914–19.

Howard ER. Biliary atresia: aetiology, management and complications. In: Howard ER (ed.) *Surgery of liver disease in children*. London: Butterworth, 1991: 39–59.

Howard ER, Davenport M. The treatment of biliary atresia in Europe 1969–1995. *Tohoku Journal of Experimental Medicine* 1997; **181**: 75–83.

Howard ER, Stamatakis JQ, Mowat AP. Management of esophageal varices in children by injection sclerotherapy. *Journal of Pediatric Surgery* 1984; **19**: 2–5.

Howard ER, Stringer MD, Mowat AP. Assessment of injection sclerotherapy in the management of 152 children with esophageal varices. *British Journal of Surgery* 1988; **75**: 404–8.

Howard ER, MacClean G, Nio M, Donaldson N, Singer J, Ohi R. Biliary atresia: survival patterns after portoenterostomy and comparison of a Japanese with a UK cohort of long-term survivors. *Journal of Pediatric Surgery* 2001; **36**: 892–7.

Ibrahim M, Ohi R, Chiba T, Nio M. Indications and results of reoperation for biliary atresia. In: Ohi R (ed.) *Biliary atresia*. Tokyo: Icom Associates, 1991: 96–100.

Inomata Y, Tanaka K, Okajima H et al. Living related liver transplantation for children younger than one year old. *European Journal of Pediatric Surgery* 1995; **6**: 148–51.

Kardorff K, Klotz M, Melter M, Rodeck B, Hoyer PF. Prediction of survival in extrahepatic biliary atresia by hepatic duplex sonography. *Journal of Pediatric Gastroenterology and Nutrition* 1999; **28**: 411–17.

Karrer FM, Lilly JR, Stewart BA, Hall RJ. Biliary atresia registry, 1976–1989. *Journal of Pediatric Surgery* 1990; **25**: 1076–81.

Karrer FM, Price MR, Bensard DD, Sokol RJ, Narkewicz MR. Long-term results with the Kasai operation for biliary atresia. *Archives of Surgery* 1996; **131**: 493–6.

Kasai M, Suzuki M. A new operation for 'non-correctable' biliary atresia: hepatic portoenterostomy [in Japanese]. *Shujyutsu* 1959; **13**: 733–9.

Kawarasaki H, Itoh M, Mizuta K, Tanaka H, Makuuchi M. Further observations on cystic dilatation of the intrahepatic biliary system in biliary atresia after hepatic portoenterostomy: report on 10 cases. *Tohoku Journal of Experimental Medicine* 1997; **181**: 175–83.

Kimura S, Tomomatsu T, Jodo Y, Togon H. Studies on the postoperative changes in the liver tissue of long-term survivors after successful surgery for biliary atresia. *Zeitschrift für Kinderchirurgie* 1980; **31**: 228–38.

Kohno M, Kitatani H, Wada H et al. Hepatocellular carcinoma complicating biliary cirrhosis caused by biliary atresia: report of a case. *Japanese Journal of Surgery* 1995; **30**: 1713–18.

Ladd WE. Congenital atresia and stenosis of the bile duct. *Journal of the American Medical Association* 1928; **91**: 1082–5.

Lawrence D, Howard ER, Tzannatos C, Mowat AP. Hepatic portoenterostomy for biliary atresia; a comparative study of histology and prognosis after surgery. *Archives of Disease in Childhood* 1981; **56**: 460–3.

Lilly JR, Stellin G. Variceal hemorrhage in biliary atresia. *Journal of Pediatric Surgery* 1984; **19**: 476–9.

Lunzmann K, Schweizer P. The influence of cholangitis on the prognosis of extrahepatic biliary atresia. *European Journal of Pediatric Surgery* 1999; **9**: 19–23.

McMichens TT, Robichaux AG III, Smith JBB. Successful pregnancy outcome in a patient with congenital biliary atresia. *Obstetrics and Gynecology* 1992; **80**: 492–4.

Maksoud JG, Fauza DO, Silva MM *et al.* Management of biliary atresia in the transplantation era: a 15 years, single center experience (1974–1995). *Journal of Pediatric Surgery* 1998; **33**: 115–18.

Matsumoto Y, Ohi R. Fat-soluble vitamin status in children with biliary atresia [in Japanese]. *Japanese Journal of Pediatric Surgery* 1987; **19**: 1069–75.

Matsumoto Y, Ohi R, Chiba T, Uchida T. Amino acid metabolism in patients with biliary atresia. In: Ohi R (ed.) *Biliary atresia*. Tokyo: Professional Postgraduate Services, 1987: 226–33.

Matsuo S, Suita S, Kubota M, Shono K. Long-term results and clinical problems after portoenterostomy in patients with biliary atresia. *European Journal of Pediatric Surgery* 1998; **8**: 142–5.

Moscoso G, Mieli-Vergani G, Mowat AP, Portmann B. Sudden death caused by unsuspected pulmonary arterial hypertension, 10 years after surgery for extrahepatic biliary atresia. *Journal of Pediatric Gastroenterology and Nutrition* 1991; **12**: 388–93.

Nakada M, Nakada K, Fujioka T *et al.* Doppler ultrasonographic evaluation of hepatic circulation in patients following Kasai's operation for biliary atresia. *Japanese Journal of Surgery* 1995; **25**: 1023–6.

Nio M, Ohi R, Hayashi Y *et al.* Current status of 21 patients who have survived more than 20 years since undergoing surgery for biliary atresia. *Journal of Pediatric Surgery* 1996; **31**: 381–4.

Ohi R. A history of the Kasai operation: hepatic porto-enterostomy for biliary atresia. *World Journal of Surgery* 1988; **12**: 871–4.

Ohi R, Nio M. The jaundiced infants: biliary atresia and other obstructions. In: O'Neill JA Jr (ed.) *Pediatric surgery*, 5th edn. St Louis, MO: Mosby, 1998: 1465–81.

Ohi R, Shikes RH, Stellin GP, Lilly JR. Histological studies of the liver in biliary atresia – further observation. In: Kasai M (ed.) *Biliary atresia and its related disorders*. Amsterdam: Excerpta Medica, 1983: 71–82.

Ohi R, Mochizuki I, Komatsu K, Kasai M. Portal hypertension after successful hepatic portoenterostomy. *Journal of Pediatric Surgery* 1986; **21**: 271–4.

Ohi R, Chiba T, Ohkohchi N *et al.* The present status of surgical treatment for biliary atresia: report of the questionnaire for the main institutions in Japan. In: Ohi R (ed.) *Biliary atresia*. Tokyo: Professional Postgraduate Services, 1987: 125–30.

Ozawa K, Uemoto S, Tanaka K *et al.* An appraisal of pediatric liver transplantation from living relatives: initial clinical experiences in 20 liver transplantations from living relatives as donors. *Annals of Surgery* 1992; **216**: 547–53.

Paquet KJ, Lazar A. Current therapeutic strategy in bleeding esophageal varices in babies and children and long-term results of endoscopic paravariceal sclerotherapy over twenty years. *European Journal of Pediatric Surgery* 1994; **4**: 165–72.

Radomski JS, Moritz MJ, Munos SJ *et al.* National Transplantation Pregnancy Registry: analysis of pregnancy outcomes in female liver transplant recipients. *Liver Transplantation and Surgery* 1995; **1**: 281–4.

Saito S, Nishina T, Tsuchida Y. Intrahepatic cysts in biliary atresia after successful hepatoportoenterostomy. *Archives of Disease in Childhood* 1984; **59**: 274–5.

Sawa N, Mochizuki I, Uchida T *et al.* Absorption disturbance and intermittent administration of fat in biliary atresia [in Japanese]. *Japanese Journal of Parenteral and Enteral Nutrition* 1984; **16**: 383–7.

Schweizer P, Lunzmann K. Extrahepatic bile duct atresia: how efficient is the hepatoporto-enterostomy? *European Journal of Pediatric Surgery* 1998; **8**: 150–4.

Shiga C, Ohi R, Chiba T *et al.* Assessment of nutritional status of postoperative patients with biliary atresia. *Tohoku Journal of Experimental Medicine* 1997; **181**: 217–23.

Shimaoka S, Ohi R, Nio M, Iwami D, Sano N. Clinical significance of 99mTc-DTPA galactosyl human serum albumin scintigram in follow-up after Kasai operation. *Tohoku Journal of Experimental Medicine* 1997; **81**: 201–3.

Shimaoka S, Ohi R, Saeki M *et al.* Problems during and after pregnancy of former biliary atresia patients treated successfully by the Kasai procedure. *Journal of Pediatric Surgery* 2001; **36**: 349–51.

Shimizu Y, Hashimoto T, Otobe Y *et al.* Long-term survivors in biliary atresia – findings for a 20-year survival group. *Tohoku Journal of Experimental Medicine* 1997; **181**: 225–33.

Stringer MD, Howard ER, Mowat AP. Endoscopic sclerotherapy in the management of esophageal varices in 61 children with biliary atresia. *Journal of Pediatric Surgery* 1989; **24**: 438–42.

Tagge DU, Tagge EP, Drongowski RA, Oldham KT, Coran AG. A long-term experience with biliary atresia. Reassessment of prognostic factors. *Annals of Surgery* 1991; **214**: 590–8.

Takahashi A, Hatakeyama S, Suzuki N *et al.* MRI findings in the liver in biliary atresia patients after the Kasai operation. *Tohoku Journal of Experimental Medicine* 1997; **181**: 193–202.

Tanaka K, Shirahase I, Uemoto S *et al.* Changes in portal vein hemodynamics after hepatic portoenterostomy in biliary atresia. *Pediatric Surgery International* 1992; **7**: 260–4.

Tanaka K, Uemoto S, Tokunaga Y *et al.* Surgical techniques and innovations in living related liver transplantation. *Annals of Surgery* 1993; **217**: 82–91.

Toki A, Todani T, Watanabe Y *et al.* Bone mineral analysis in patients with biliary atresia after successful Kasai procedure. *Tohoku Journal of Experimental Medicine* 1997; **181**: 213–16.

Toyosaka A, Okamoto E, Okasora T, Nose K, Tomimoto Y. Outcome of 21 patients with biliary atresia living more than 10 years. *Journal of Pediatric Surgery* 1993; **28**: 1498–501.

Tsuchida Y, Honna T, Kawarasaki H. Cystic dilatation of the intrahepatic biliary system in biliary atresia after hepatic portoenterostomy. *Journal of Pediatric Surgery* 1994; **29**: 630–4.

Tsunoda A, Nishi T, Yamada R, Yamamoto H, Ohama Y, Masaki D. Criteria for cure state in survivors of biliary atresia. In: Ohi R (ed.) *Biliary atresia*. Tokyo: Professional Postgraduate Services, 1987: 294–8.

Valayer J. Conventional treatment of biliary atresia: long-term results. *Journal of Pediatric Surgery* 1996; **31**: 1546–51.

Vasquez J, Gamez ML, Santamaria J *et al*. Liver transplantation in small babies. *Journal of Pediatric Surgery* 1993; **28**: 1051–3.

Wanek EA, Horgan JG, Karrer FM *et al*. Portal venous velocity in biliary atresia. *Journal of Pediatric Surgery* 1990; **25**: 146–8.

Watanabe Y, Todani T, Toki A *et al*. Changes of hepatic volume after successful Kasai operation. *Tohoku Journal of Experimental Medicine* 1997; **181**: 185–91.

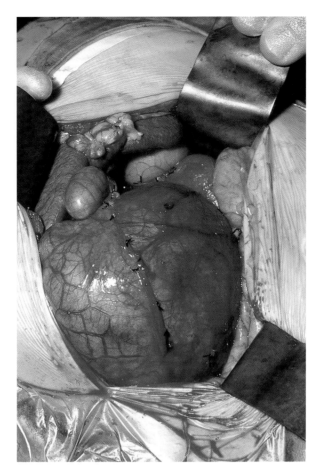

Plate 1 *Operative appearance of a large type I cystic choledochal dilatation. (Reproduced courtesy of ER Howard.)*

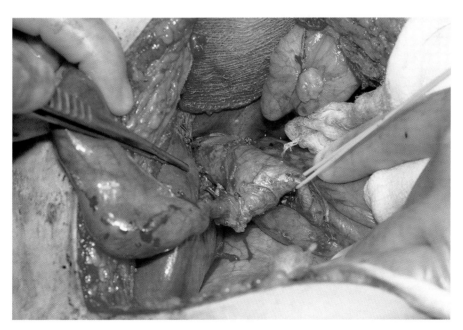

Plate 2 *Intraoperative dissection of a choledochal cyst in a 15-year-old girl. A sling has been placed around the distal common bile duct.*

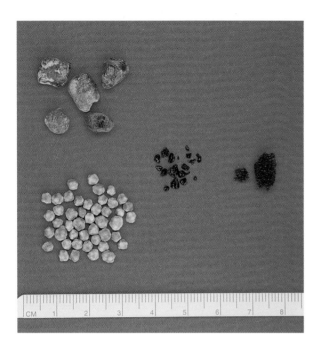

Plate 3 *Varieties of gallstones in children. Mixed cholesterol stones (left), black pigment stones (middle) and brown pigment stones (right).*

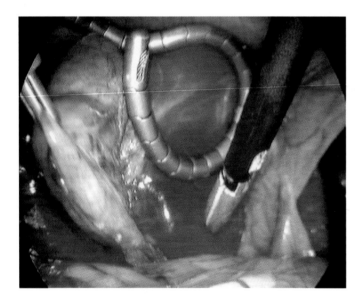

Plate 4 *Laparoscopic cholecystectomy in a 9-year-old boy with symptomatic gallstones. A liver retractor has been inserted. Lateral retraction of Hartmann's pouch opens up Calot's triangle.*

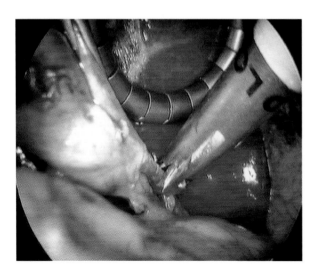

Plate 5 *Clip ligation of the cystic artery close to the gallbladder after clear identification of the cystic duct and artery.*

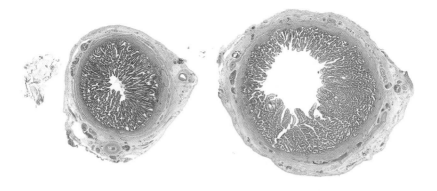

Plate 6 *Transverse section through gallbladder neck demonstrating mucosal papillary hyperplasia and thickening of the muscularis (hematoxylin and eosin).*

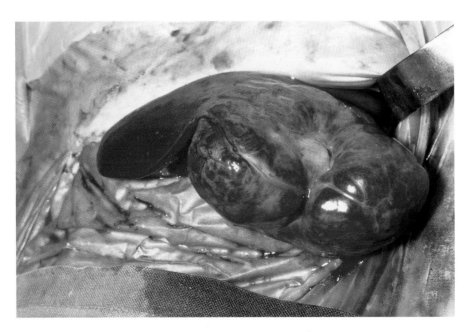

Plate 7 *Operative appearance of a mesenchymal hamartoma in a neonate.*

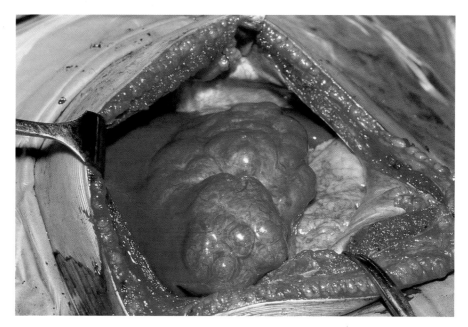

Plate 8 *Operative appearance of focal nodular hyperplasia affecting the right lobe of the liver in a 7-year-old girl.*

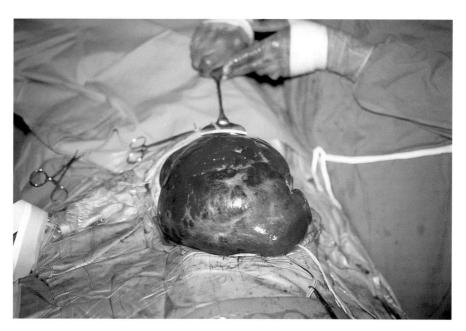

Plate 9 *Operative appearance of vascular liver tumor in a 4-year-old girl (see Figure 19.1 and Plate 10). The tumor was resected leaving only segment 4.*

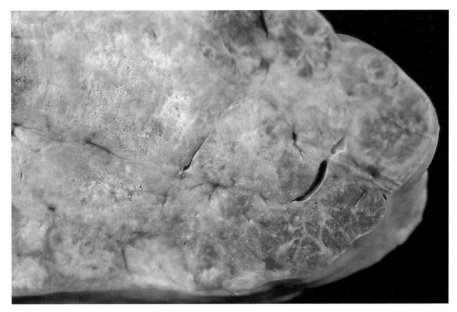

Plate 10 *Hemangioendothelioma in a 4-year-old girl (see Figure 19.1). An extensive vascular tumor was revealed on cut section of the resected specimen and, despite the clinical picture, histology again showed a benign hemangioendothelioma. Five months later the patient developed fatal multiple pulmonary metastases and recurrent tumor. (Reproduced courtesy of Professor ER Howard.)*

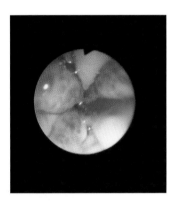

Plate 11 *Endoscopic appearance of grade 4 esophageal varices with 'red color signs'.*

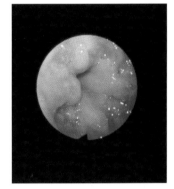

Plate 12 *Early post-sclerotherapy appearance of the same varices after successful obliteration.*

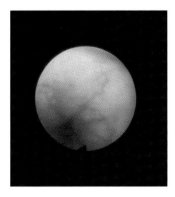

Plate 13 *Late appearance of distal esophagus at surveillance endoscopy. Some mucosal tags persist, whilst others, as in this case, gradually resolve.*

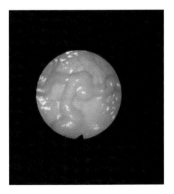

Plate 14 *Endoscopic view of gastric fundal varices.*

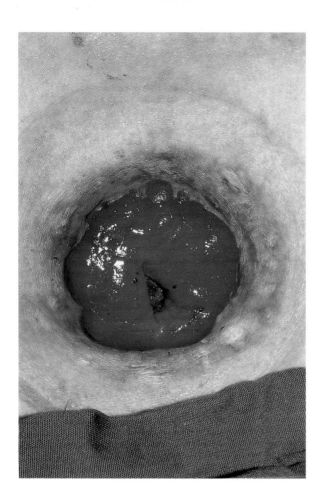

Plate 15 *Peristomal varices. This 13-year-old boy with cirrhosis and portal hypertension had required a defunctioning sigmoid colostomy after a road traffic accident in which he sustained a pelvic fracture and rectal injury. (Reproduced courtesy of MD Stringer.)*

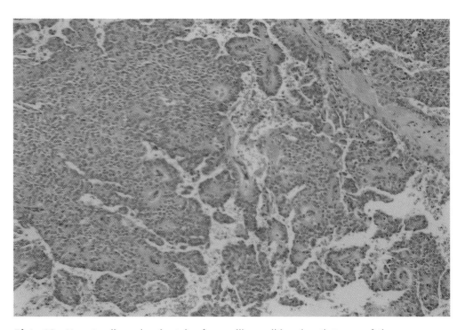

Plate 16 *Hematoxylin and eosin stain of a papillary solid and cystic tumor of the pancreas (same patient as Figure 37.2).*

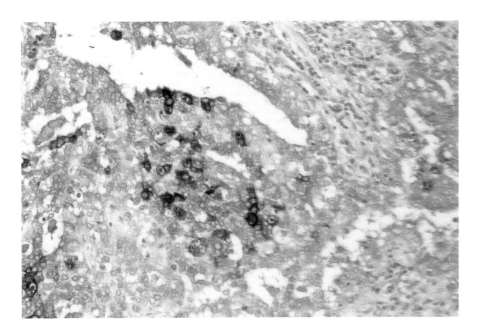

Plate 17 *Immunohistochemical stain for alpha-1-antitrypsin. This palliary solid and cystic tumor of the pancreas shows scattered strongly staining cells characteristic of this tumor. (Reproduced courtesy of Dr Caroline Verbeke.)*

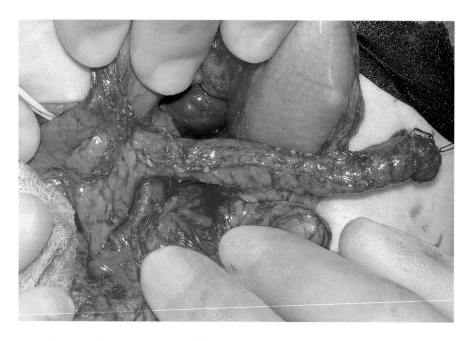

Plate 18 *Operative photograph of a 95% pancreatic resection for hyperinsulinemic hypoglycemia of infancy in progress. Bipolar diathermy hemostasis maintains a dry operative field. Reproduced from Cade and Stringer (1998) with kind permission of W.B. Saunders & Co.*

Choledochal cysts

MARK D STRINGER

Cystic dilatation of the biliary tree is a rare congenital abnormality of unknown etiology. It is frequently associated with an anatomically abnormal union between the pancreatic and common bile ducts. Choledochal cysts (Greek: *chole*, bile + *dochus*, containing or receiving) may cause symptoms at any age, but typically present with obstructive jaundice and/or abdominal pain in infants and children. Recognized complications include pancreatitis, cholangitis, cholelithiasis, secondary liver disease and malignant degeneration. Outcome studies have established that radical cyst excision and biliary reconstruction is the optimum treatment.

HISTORICAL ASPECTS

The German anatomist Abraham Vater is credited with one of the earliest descriptions of pathological common bile duct dilatation (Vater, 1720). Choledochal cysts were documented in subsequent reports (Todd, 1817), but the first detailed account of a patient with massive dilatation of the bile duct was provided by Halliday Douglas, an Edinburgh physician (Douglas, 1852). He described a girl aged 17 years who had a 3-year history of intermittent right-sided abdominal pain and recent onset of obstructive jaundice and fever. Clinical examination revealed a large, tender, cystic mass in the right side of her abdomen and signs of cholangitis. The cyst was treated by percutaneous aspiration of 900 mL of bile, and she died 1 month later. An autopsy confirmed the presence of a choledochal cyst and an undilated gallbladder. Douglas believed that the bile duct dilatation was due to an abnormality in its wall, possibly of tubercular origin.

The first successful operation was performed by William Swain, an English surgeon, in 1894. He anastomosed a loop of jejunum to a huge choledochal cyst in a 17-year-old girl who was still alive and jaundice-free 2 months later (Swain, 1895). Sporadic reports of choledochocystenterostomy followed, but it was not until 1922 that Golder McWhorter from Chicago successfully removed a choledochal cyst (McWhorter, 1924). His patient was a 49-year-old woman whose symptoms dated from infancy. She was reported to be well 1 year after hepaticoduodenostomy.

EPIDEMIOLOGY

Choledochal cysts are more common in females and in Oriental races. The hospital admission rate for choledochal cysts is highest in Japan (1 per 1000 admissions), whereas in the USA (1 per 13 000) and Australia (1 per

15 000) it is less common. Tsardakas and Robnett (1956) found only one case in 26 000 admissions to a London hospital. The true incidence in Western countries is unknown, but it has been estimated to be between 1 in 100 000 and 1 in 150 000 live births. In West Yorkshire, the prevalence in a mixed Caucasian and Asian community is about 1 in 50 000. More than two-thirds of cases are diagnosed in children under 10 years of age. The female:male ratio ranges between 3:1 and 4:1 in most series.

CYST CLASSIFICATION

Bile duct cysts have been categorized in various ways, but the scheme proposed by Alonso-Lej *et al.* (1959) and modified by Todani *et al.* (1977) is most commonly used (Figure 10.1). With slight modification, this is as follows:

- type I – cystic (I cystic) or fusiform (I fusiform);
- type II – diverticulum;
- type III – choledochocele (dilatation of the terminal common bile duct within the duodenal wall);
- type IV – multiple cysts of extra- and intra-hepatic ducts (IVa) or multiple extrahepatic duct cysts (IVb);
- type V – intrahepatic duct cyst (single or multiple).

Examples of these variants are shown in Figure 10.2. The frequency of different cyst types in recent larger pediatric series employing the Todani classification is shown in Table 10.1. Intrahepatic duct dilatation which resolves after successful treatment of an extra-hepatic cyst should be distinguished from true cystic dilatation of the intrahepatic ducts, which tends to persist, albeit after some regression. A congenital choledochal diverticulum (type II) is the rarest variety. Iuchtman *et al.* (1971) described a woman with a 25-cm-diameter diverticulum which was attached to the common bile duct by a channel 1 cm in diameter. The gallbladder was normal.

The King's College Hospital series of 78 children included 44 cases (56%) of type I cystic, 28 cases (36%) of type I fusiform, 4 cases (5%) of type IV and 2 cases (3%) of type V. In addition, there were two children who

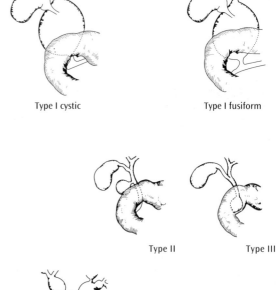

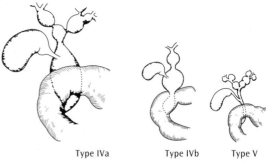

Figure 10.1 *Classification of choledochal cysts. Based on Todani* et al., *1977.*

presented with pancreatitis and long common channels above which were bile duct strictures, and a further child with dilatation of the pancreatic and common bile ducts caused by a stone impacted in a common channel. Pancreaticobiliary malunion without cystic biliary dilatation has been termed a 'forme fruste' of chole-dochal cyst (Lilly *et al.*, 1985) (Figure 10.3). Miyano *et al.* (1996a) identified eight cases from a series of 180 children with choledochal cysts. This abnormality should be treated by bile duct disconnection in a similar way to a choledochal cyst.

Table 10.1 *Distribution of choledochal cyst types in recent pediatric series*

Author and year	*n*	I cystic	I fusiform	II	III	IVa	IVb	V
Joseph (1990)	52	45		1	2	3	0	1
Stringer *et al.* (1995)	78	44	28	0	0	4	0	2
Rha *et al.* (1996)	16	13		0	1	2	0	0
Poddar *et al.* (1998)	23	20		0	0	3	0	0
Todani (1998)	103	31	18	0	0	54	0	0
Total	272	73%		0.4%	1.1%	24%	0%	1.1%

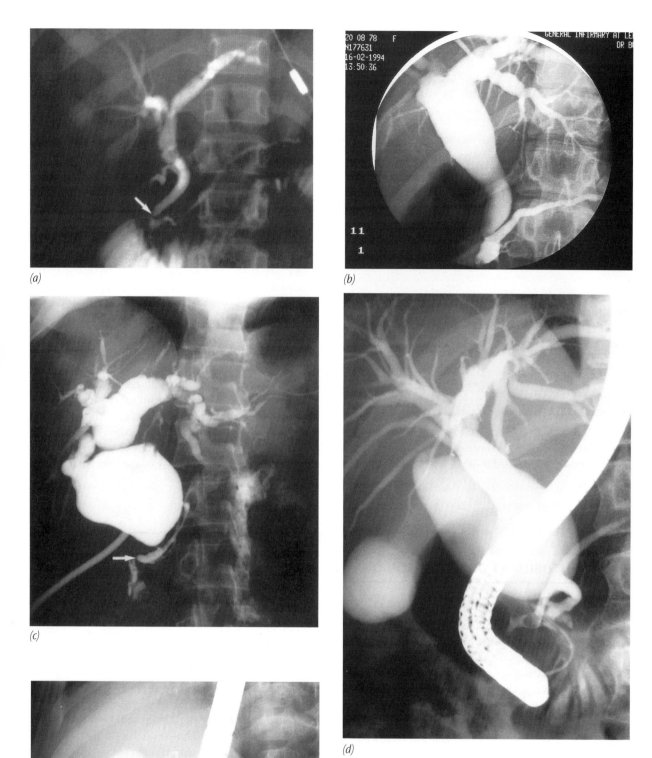

(a)

(b)

(c)

(d)

(e)

Figure 10.2 *Choledochal variants. (a) Type I fusiform. The common bile duct is only mildly dilated, and there is a distal stricture (arrow). There is a common pancreaticobiliary channel which drains into the third part of the duodenum. (b) Type I fusiform dilatation in a 15-year-old girl with recurrent pancreatitis. Note the dilated common pancreaticobiliary channel. (c) Type I Va cystic dilatation of the common bile duct. There is a hilar stricture and secondary cystic dilatation of the left hepatic duct, and a tight stricture of the distal common bile duct and a long common channel (arrow). (d) Choledochal cyst associated with relatively complex pancreaticobiliary malunion. (e) Type V intrahepatic choledochal cyst. The gallbladder is not filled, but a tortuous cystic duct is shown. (Reproduced courtesy of ER Howard.)*

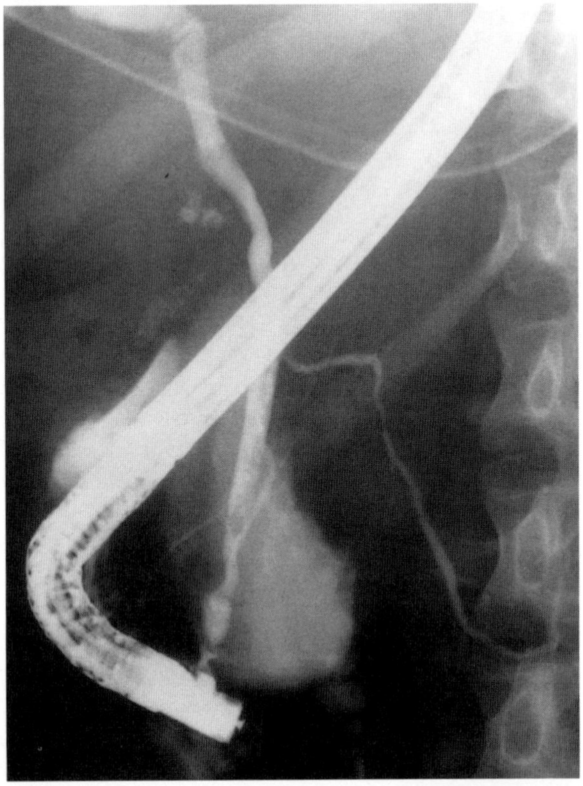

Figure 10.3 *Pancreaticobiliary malunion without common bile duct dilatation. There is an inspissated bile plug in the distal comon bile duct and radiopaque calculi in the gallbladder and cystic duct.*

PANCREATICOBILIARY DUCTAL MALUNION

Choledochal cysts are frequently associated with an anomalous junction between the terminal common bile duct and the pancreatic duct, whereby the ducts unite well outside the duodenal wall and are therefore not surrounded by the normal sphincter mechanism (Iwai *et al.*, 1992). This encourages reflux of pancreatic juice into the biliary tree, since the excretion pressure of the pancreatic duct normally exceeds that of the common bile duct. Occasionally, bile may reflux into the pancreatic duct. Pancreaticobiliary reflux has been confirmed by dynamic magnetic resonance cholangiopancreatography after secretin stimulation (Matos *et al.*, 1998). High concentrations of pancreatic enzymes are commonly found in the bile within cysts; beyond infancy biliary amylase levels often exceed several thousand units. A long common channel may be complicated not only by pancreatitis but also by protein plugs, calculi and, in adults, the development of gallbladder carcinoma (Gauthier *et al.*, 1986; Yamauchi *et al.*, 1987; Kawaguchi *et al.*, 1995). In a Japanese study of 1586 endoscopic retrograde cholangiopancreatography examinations, common channels

were detected in 24 patients (1.5%). Of these, 18 cases were associated with choledochal cysts; in six there was no cyst, but four of these patients had gallbladder cancer (Yamauchi *et al.*, 1987).

Pancreaticobiliary ductal malunion (PBM) results in a long common pancreaticobiliary channel, usually exceeding 10 mm in length, compared with the normal common channel length of up to 5 mm in children (Guelrud *et al.*, 1999). In most cases the common channel represents a simple union of the two ducts and may or may not be dilated, but in some cases this union is very complex (Todani *et al.*, 1984b). A study of human fetuses by Wong and Lister (1981) showed that the normal pancreaticobiliary junction lies outside the duodenal wall and sphincter of Oddi muscle complex before 8 weeks' gestation, and gradually migrates towards the duodenal lumen. Early arrest of this process may be the cause of PBM.

Pancreaticobiliary ductal malunion was identified in 76% of the King's College Hospital series (Stringer *et al.*, 1995), and has been reported even more frequently in Japanese children with choledochal cysts. It is particularly common in association with type I and IVa choledochal cysts but is rarely seen with other varieties. Since PBM is not present in all cases, Lilly (1979) has suggested that the abnormal common channel should be regarded as only one manifestation of a disordered embryology which affects the whole of the extrahepatic biliary tree.

PATHOLOGY

The wall of a choledochal cyst is thickened, and usually measures between 2.0 and 7.5 mm in width. It is typically composed of fibrous tissue with occasional elastic and smooth muscle fibers (Figure 10.4). The cyst may be accompanied by pancreaticobiliary malunion, intrahepatic bile duct dilatation and hepatic histology which ranges from normal to cirrhotic. Most commonly the dilatation of the common bile duct starts just above the duodenum and ends abruptly just below the bifurcation of the common hepatic duct. The gallbladder is usually of normal size or only slightly dilated, even though the cystic duct enters the choledochal cyst. The terminal common bile duct is absent in some patients and biliary drainage is via a complex arrangement of pancreatic ducts.

In many cases the histology of the bile duct shows that the cuboidal biliary epithelium is ulcerated, and occasionally only small patches of viable epithelium remain (Figure 10.4). Ectopic pancreatic tissue may rarely be found in the cyst wall. The number of ganglion cells in the choledochal wall is lower than normal, but this is probably a secondary phenomenon (Shimotake *et al.*, 1995). Histochemical studies in children and adults have revealed that the degree of histological damage to the

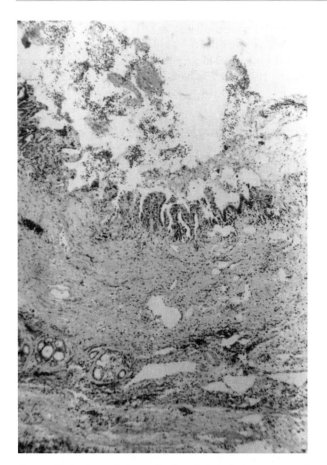

Figure 10.4 *Part of the wall of a choledochal cyst removed from a 13-year-old girl. The section shows a lining of hyperplastic columnar epithelium with areas of ulceration. The wall is composed of fibrovascular connective tissue in which there is acute and chronic inflammation (× 80). (Reproduced courtesy of ER Howard.)*

cyst wall can be directly correlated with age. In children under 2 years of age, Komi *et al.* (1986) found epithelial desquamation and fibrosis but little inflammation. In older children, an intact epithelial lining was uncommon. In young adults, there was marked acute and/or chronic inflammation with intramural glandular structures which contained gastrin and somatostatin-like immunoreactivity. In some older patients, malignancy was detected. Komi *et al.* (1986) concluded that there was an age-related increase in the rate of epithelial metaplasia and dysplasia in choledochal cysts.

Liver histology varies from mild inflammatory infiltration of the portal tracts and some periportal fibrosis through to cirrhosis. Portal hypertension may develop in association with portal vein obstruction from cyst compression, secondary biliary cirrhosis or intrahepatic cystic change and fibrosis (Caroli's disease).

ASSOCIATED ABNORMALITIES

Abnormalities of pancreaticobiliary duct union are common. In addition the papilla of Vater is frequently located distal to the mid-descending duodenum (Li *et al.*, 2001). Hilar duct strictures may be found in association with type IVa cysts. In a series of 55 patients with type IVa cysts, Todani *et al.* (1998) identified 18 cases with hilar duct strictures. Other associated biliary abnormalities are rare. In the King's College Hospital series of 78 children, one patient had a non-communicating multiseptate gallbladder (Tan *et al.*, 1993), and another multiple accessory bile ducts, which have also been described by others (Duh *et al.*, 1997; Todani *et al.*, 1998). A double common bile duct with cystic dilatation of one (Swartley and Weeder, 1935), duplicated gallbladder (Kazar, 1950) and gallbladder agenesis (Rheinlander and Bowens, 1957) have also been documented in association with choledochal cysts.

Malformations outside the biliary tree are rare in patients with choledochal cysts. There may be a higher prevalence of urinary tract anomalies and intestinal malrotation (Dudin *et al.*, 1995; Stringer *et al.*, 1995; Samuel and Spitz, 1996), and isolated examples of duodenal atresia, annular pancreas and digital abnormalities have been reported (Dudin *et al.*, 1995).

ETIOLOGY

Choledochal cysts are congenital lesions. Cysts have been detected by prenatal ultrasound scan as early as 15 weeks' gestation. There are several theories concerning the etiology and pathogenesis of choledochal cysts.

1 The extrahepatic biliary system develops from the hepatic diverticulum, an outgrowth from the foregut into the septum transversum (see Chapter 7). During embryogenesis, the lumen of the future duct system is transiently obstructed by cellular proliferation (around the fifth week). Disordered recanalization, leading to congenital weakness of the wall of the common bile duct, was an early hypothesis (Yotuyanagi, 1936).

2 Abnormality of innervation of the distal common bile duct resulting in functional obstruction and proximal dilatation was suggested by Saltz and Glaser (1956).

3 An acquired weakness of the wall of the bile duct associated with PBM was first proposed by Babbitt (1969), who described choledochal cysts with a common pancreaticobiliary channel, and suggested that reflux of pancreatic juice might damage the common bile duct and cause dilatation. Anastomosis of the pancreatic duct to the gallbladder in dogs results in common bile duct dilatation with destruction of epithelium and inflammation of the bile duct wall (Kato *et al.*, 1981). In addition,

progressive enlargement of a fusiform choledochal cyst has been observed in association with PBM (Han *et al.*, 1997). However, PBM is not found in all patients with a choledochal cyst, and it does occur in some patients without duct dilatation.

4 Obstruction of the distal common bile duct has been a popular theory for many years. Ligation of the distal bile duct in newborn lambs causes cystic dilatation of the proximal duct, whereas if this is performed in mature sheep the gallbladder distends selectively, suggesting that the timing of obstruction is critical (Spitz, 1977). A stenosis is often seen just below a type I cyst, but whether this is congenital or secondary to biliary inflammation is unclear (Ito *et al.*, 1984) (Figure 10.5). In one young infant with inspissated bile the diameter of the common bile duct increased from 4 mm to 3 cm during a 7-week period (Lai *et al.*, 1998). However, the role of obstruction in the etiology of choledochal cysts remains uncertain.

A genetic predisposition seems probable in view of the female preponderance and geographical distribution of the condition. Numerous examples of familial choledochal cysts have been reported (Lane *et al.*, 1999), but twin studies have not helped to unravel any genetic contribution. Both concordance (Urushihara *et al.*, 1988) and discordance (Uchida *et al.*, 1992) have been recorded in monozygotic twins. It would be interesting to know the prevalence of the condition in high-risk communities (e.g. Japanese) which have migrated to low-risk regions (e.g. North America).

CLINICAL PRESENTATION

The majority of choledochal cysts are diagnosed before 10 years of age, but they can present at any age, and cases have been reported as late as the eighth decade. In the

King's College Hospital series of 78 children (57 girls and 21 boys), more than two-thirds of patients presented by 5 years of age. The presenting features are shown in Figure 10.6, but are best considered according to age group.

Prenatal diagnosis

Choledochal cysts may be detected at routine prenatal ultrasound examinations as early as 15 weeks' gestation (Schroeder *et al.*, 1989; Bancroft *et al.*, 1994; Stringer *et al.*, 1995; Redkar *et al.*, 1998). They may be confused with duodenal atresia, ovarian cysts, duplication cysts and other fetal pathology. The cysts are typically but not exclusively type I cystic lesions (Table 10.2). It has been suggested that cystic dilatation of the common bile duct is a prenatal event, whereas fusiform dilatation begins after birth (Shimotake *et al.*, 1995).

Postnatally, affected infants who are otherwise well should be treated by early surgery, particularly if they are jaundiced. This is for several reasons:

1 to exclude (and treat) a cystic variant of biliary atresia. Early surgery provides the opportunity to definitively exclude biliary atresia in those with biliary obstruction (Greenholz *et al.*, 1986; Bancroft *et al.*, 1994; Redkar *et al.*, 1998). Distinguishing between a choledochal cyst and a cystic variant of biliary atresia can be difficult. Progressive enlargement of the fetal cyst during pregnancy is a pointer to a choledochal cyst (Matsubara *et al.*, 1997), and the demonstration of sonographic continuity of the cyst with a normal or distended

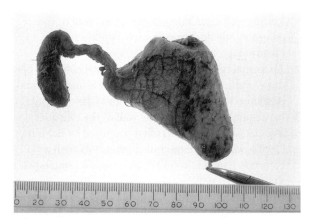

Figure 10.5 *Type I cystic choledochal dilatation removed by radical excision. Note the extremely narrow segment of distal common bile duct. (Reproduced courtesy of ER Howard.)*

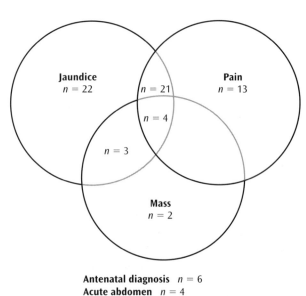

Antenatal diagnosis *n* = 6
Acute abdomen *n* = 4
Others *n* = 3

Figure 10.6 *Presenting features in 78 children with choledochal cysts (Stringer* et al., *1995).*

Table 10.2 *Clinical features of antenatally diagnosed choledochal cysts (n = 6) in the King's College Hospital series (Stringer et al., 1995)*

Number	Gestational age at detection (weeks)	Cyst type	Postnatal symptoms	Biliary amylase (IU/L)	Age at operation
1	28	V	Asymptomatic	—	—
2	16*	I cystic	Persistent jaundice	6	3 weeks
3	20	I cystic	Persistent jaundice	< 10	17 days
4	18	I cystic	Recurrent jaundice	7	3 weeks
5	17*	I cystic	Jaundice	50	7 days
6	16	I cystic	Asymptomatic	7000	9 months

* Initially considered to have a 'double-bubble' on prenatal ultrasound scan.

gallbladder or hepatic ducts or dilatation of the intrahepatic bile ducts strongly favors choledochal pathology (Kim *et al.*, 1998);

2 to avoid the risk of biliary or hepatic complications. Liver fibrosis may develop rapidly in prenatally detected cases with obstruction, and was found in 60% of 14 cases reviewed by Lugo-Vincente (1995). In another report, a laparotomy at 10 days of age confirmed a prenatally diagnosed choledochal cyst associated with extensive hepatic fibrosis (Dewbury *et al.*, 1980). Prompt surgical treatment can reverse the fibrosis. If left untreated, there is a risk of rapid progression to secondary biliary cirrhosis in infants with a cyst and obstructive jaundice; liver failure has been reported in a 5-month-old infant (Harris and Kahler, 1978). Early treatment also reduces the risk of cholangitis, the accumulation of biliary sludge and progressive obstructive jaundice (Howell *et al.*, 1983), as well as cyst perforation;

3 because the results of surgical treatment at this age are generally excellent (Stringer *et al.*, 1995; Redkar *et al.*, 1998; Suita *et al.*, 1999).

Infants

Infants typically present with obstructive jaundice. Vomiting, fever, failure to thrive and an abdominal mass may be noted. Even in the presence of PBM, hyperamylasemia is not found (Davenport *et al.*, 1995; Todani *et al.*, 1995a). This is because the amylase concentration in pancreatic juice at birth, and therefore the biliary amylase level in those with a common channel, is low due to pancreatic immaturity and only reaches significant levels at about 1–2 years of age (Todani *et al.*, 1995a). In contrast, biliary concentrations of pancreatic lipase, elastase and trypsin are significantly elevated in infants with a common channel (Todani *et al.*, 1995a; Urushihara *et al.*, 1995).

Older children

Abdominal pain is a more prominent symptom in older children. Of the 72 patients in the King's College Hospital series who presented after birth, 50 patients (69%) presented with jaundice, which was associated with abdominal pain in 25 cases and a palpable mass in seven cases. In small infants the jaundice was frequently persistent, but in older children it was almost always intermittent. In total, 13 patients (18%) presented only with abdominal pain, which was frequently recurrent, and two (3%) presented with a mass. The classic triad of jaundice, pain and a right hypochondrial mass was present in only four patients (6%) (Figure 10.6). This compares with 8% of 52 cases reported by Joseph (1990) from Singapore.

Plasma and/or biliary amylase values were elevated in almost all patients with abdominal pain, and some of these showed evidence of pancreatitis at operation. Four children aged 6 months to 3 years presented acutely following spontaneous perforation of a choledochal cyst; three developed biliary peritonitis and the other had an acute onset of abdominal pain and fever due to a retroperitoneal perforation. Two children presented with abdominal distension due to ascites, one of whom was in liver failure, and one child presented with melena from variceal bleeding.

Delayed referral and diagnosis

Diagnostic delay appears to be common and is largely avoidable. In 35 (52%) of the 67 patients who had not previously undergone surgery, symptoms had been present for more than 1 month, and in 14 of these patients for more than 1 year, before diagnosis. Reasons for delayed diagnosis and referral are shown in Box 10.1. A total of 12 patients with jaundice with or without pain were initially diagnosed as having hepatitis, yet none of them had serological confirmation. In four other children jaundice was wrongly attributed to other causes. In six children with repeated attacks of abdominal pain, all of whom had PBM, there were delays of up to 3 years before a plasma amylase level was checked. Five patients with acute or recurrent pancreatitis were not initially referred for further investigation, and in 10 patients with jaundice and/or pancreatitis the finding of a dilated

differential diagnosis of jaundice and pancreatitis. Both conditions require careful detailed anatomical investigation of the patient with fasting abdominal ultrasonography. The common bile duct diameter is less than 3.5 mm in healthy children and less than 2 mm in infants (Hernanz-Schulman *et al.*, 1995). The presence of sonographically dilated bile ducts is an indication for further imaging studies. Recurrent abdominal pain and pancreatitis have long been recognized as complications of choledochal cyst (Raffensperger *et al.*, 1973; Okada *et al.*, 1983). Children with severe, recurrent abdominal pain should have a plasma amylase level measured, even though the yield from this investigation in unselected children with recurrent abdominal pain is extremely low (Wheeler *et al.*, 1992). The hyperamylasemia associated with choledochal cysts and a common channel may be caused by acute pancreatitis as evidenced by typical findings on imaging and at surgery. However, most patients with hyperamylasemia show no evidence of clinical pancreatitis and have so-called 'biochemical pancreatitis' or 'pseudopancreatitis' (Todani *et al.*, 1995a; Urushihara *et al.*, 1995). The hyperamylasemia in these patients is considered to be due either to diffusion of pancreatic amylase through the denuded epithelium of the cyst wall (Stringel and Filler, 1982) or to cholangiovenous reflux of amylase-rich fluid induced by a high choledochal pressure (Urushihara *et al.*, 1995). Transient increases in biliary pressure may also be responsible for episodes of abdominal pain. Hyperamylasemia does not recur after cyst excision, provided that any associated common channel pathology has been adequately treated.

common bile duct at abdominal ultrasonography failed to prompt further investigation. Unexplained pancreatitis in children should be investigated in order to exclude anatomical abnormalities such as a common pancreaticobiliary channel, which may be found in the absence of significant bile duct dilatation (Miyano *et al.*, 1996a).

Choledochal cyst should always be considered in the

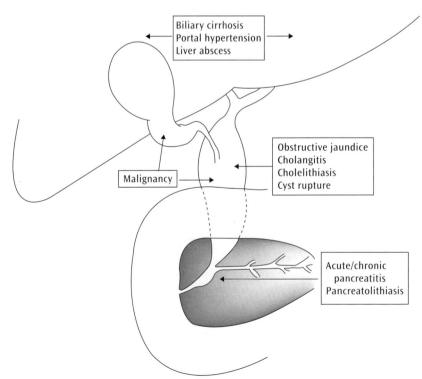

Figure 10.7 *Schematic representation of the potential complications of choledochal cysts.*

COMPLICATIONS

Choledochal cysts are prone to complications (Figure 10.7). In the King's College Hospital series of 67 children who had not previously undergone surgery, there were five cases with biliary calculi, two with pancreatic duct stones, four with evidence of portal hypertension and two with biliary cirrhosis. In contrast, of 11 children referred or re-presenting after cystenterostomy, five had gallstones, four had portal hypertension and two had biliary cirrhosis.

Rupture

This complication develops in up to 7% of children in larger series, and most cases are under 4 years of age (Stringer *et al.*, 1995; Ando *et al.*, 1998). Spontaneous perforation may affect any part of the cyst, or rarely the gallbladder. Intraperitoneal rupture causes biliary peritonitis, whereas retroperitoneal rupture is less dramatic (Ohkawa *et al.*, 1977; Ando *et al.*, 1998). Abdominal pain and distension, vomiting, fever, mild jaundice and progressive biliary ascites are the typical presenting features. Prior laparotomy for suspected appendicitis is not uncommon (Samuel and Spitz, 1996; Karnak *et al.*, 1997; Ando *et al.*, 1998). Perforations may be single or multiple (Ando *et al.*, 1998), and there is no relationship between cyst size and rupture. Biliary amylase levels were high in all 13 cases reported by Ando *et al.* (1998), highlighting the importance of PBM in pathogenesis. Perforation is probably due to inflammatory changes in the wall of the bile duct induced by refluxing pancreatic enzymes, but occasionally trauma or inspissated bile may precipitate rupture. Infection does not appear to be important. Cyst rupture during pregnancy has been described (Hewitt *et al.*, 1995).

At operation, a ruptured choledochal cyst must be distinguished from idiopathic perforation of the bile duct with an associated pseudocyst, and intraoperative cholangiography is advisable. Definitive surgery may be possible at the time of diagnosis (Karnak *et al.*, 1997), but temporary T-tube drainage of the choledochal cyst and delayed surgery once the inflammation has subsided and after the anatomy has been clarified is a safe alternative (Stringer *et al.*, 1995; Ando *et al.*, 1998).

Pancreatic disease

A dilated long common channel, most often seen in association with type I fusiform dilatation, may be complicated by recurrent acute pancreatitis, chronic pancreatitis, protein plugs and calculi (Figure 10.8). An association with pancreatic cancer has been suggested (Binks and Pauline, 1970; Wood and Baum, 1975), although this is very tenuous.

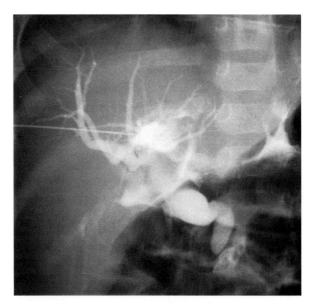

Figure 10.8 *Percutaneous transhepatic cholangiogram in a child demonstrating a type I fusiform choledochal dilatation associated with a common pancreaticobiliary channel. The dilated proximal pancreatic duct contains protein plugs and debris.*

Cholelithiasis

Gallstones are uncommon in bile duct cysts. Yamaguchi (1980) reported an 8% prevalence in 1433 Japanese cases, and a similar frequency was observed in children in the King's College Hospital series (Figure 10.9).

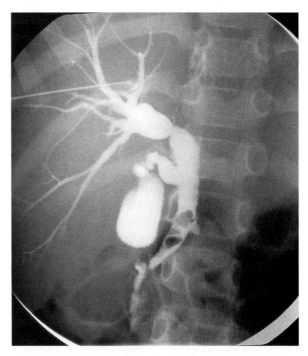

Figure 10.9 *A type I fusiform choledochal dilatation with a long common channel (the junction of the pancreatic duct with the distal common bile duct is just visible). There are multiple gallstones in the distal common bile duct.*

Portal hypertension

Secondary biliary cirrhosis, compression of the portal vein by the choledochal cyst or, rarely, portal vein thrombosis can cause portal hypertension. Occasionally, portal hypertension resolves after cyst excision as a result of relieving portal vein compression, or following significant improvements in liver architecture (Yeong et al., 1982).

Malignancy

Malignant change is a well-recognized complication of choledochal cysts, mainly affecting adults. However, teenagers are also at risk (Yamaguchi, 1980; Bismuth and Krissat, 1999). The age-related cancer risk has been estimated to be 0.7% in the first decade, 7% in the second decade and 14% after 20 years of age (Voyles et al., 1983). Iwai et al. (1990) reported the case of a 12-year-old girl who presented with jaundice, and investigations revealed a type IVa cyst with a long common channel. There was extensive carcinomatous change in the extrahepatic biliary system, with invasion of the inferior vena cava and portal vein. The biliary amylase level was approximately 400 000 units. The authors suggested that chronic inflammation might be one of the factors predisposing to malignant change. Other potential carcinogens include other refluxed pancreatic enzymes (trypsin, elastase and phospholipase) and their products, and secondary bile acids (Reville et al., 1990).

Diagnosis of malignancy associated with a choledochal cyst is often delayed. Symptoms other than weight loss are easily attributed to the choledochal cyst, and malignant lesions are not always obvious at operation (Voyles et al., 1983; Nagorney et al., 1984). The prognosis of malignant choledochal cyst tumors is poor. The 5-year survival rate in cases detected at the time of surgery is generally less than 10% (Rossi et al., 1987; Bismuth and Krissat, 1999).

The risk of malignancy is greatest in patients who have been treated by internal drainage of a choledochal cyst (cystenterostomy). The mean age of affected patients (35 years) is approximately a decade less than the mean age of patients who develop malignancy in an unoperated cyst (Todani et al., 1987). Teenagers are also at risk of cancer after cystenterostomy (Fujiwara et al., 1976a). Even after cyst excision, malignancy may affect incompletely excised extrahepatic ducts or dilated intrahepatic ducts, indicating the need for lifelong surveillance (Nagorney et al., 1984; Yoshikawa et al., 1986; Coyle and Bradley, 1992). In particular, type IVa cysts need careful observation (Kobayashi et al., 1999).

In type I cystic dilatations, malignancy may develop in the cyst wall or gallbladder, whereas in type I fusiform dilatations, the gallbladder is the dominant site. Pancreaticobiliary ductal malunion is now an accepted factor predisposing to malignancy. Malunion is found in approximately 10% of patients with gallbladder cancer (Todani et al., 1994). Clinical and experimental studies have established that PBM increases biliary epithelial turnover (Kaneko et al., 2000).

Histology usually shows adenocarcinoma or cholangiocarcinoma, but squamous-cell cancer has been described (Voyles et al., 1983; Nagorney et al., 1984; Bismuth and Krissat, 1999). Reports of rhabdomyosarcoma are potentially misleading, since this malignancy tends to be misdiagnosed as a choledochal cyst unless the intraductal biliary tumor is recognized on preoperative imaging (Sanz et al., 1997; Spunt et al., 2000).

INVESTIGATIONS (FIGURE 10.10A–E)

Biochemical liver function tests may be completely normal or show evidence of biliary obstruction in jaundiced patients. Plasma amylase levels are often elevated during episodes of abdominal pain. Clotting studies may be abnormal in patients with a history of cholestasis. A plain abdominal radiograph may show displacement of the stomach and duodenum and occasionally calculi in the biliary tract or pancreas.

Modern imaging methods are highly accurate in the diagnosis of choledochal cysts (Box 10.2). Ultrasonography is the initial investigation of choice, as the size, contour and position of the cyst, the proximal ducts, vascular anatomy and hepatic echotexture can all be accurately assessed. Complications such as cholelithiasis, portal hypertension and biliary ascites may be noted. Percutaneous transhepatic cholangiography and endoscopic retrograde cholangiopancreatography (ERCP) give excellent visualization of the cyst and duct anatomy. ERCP best visualizes the pancreaticobiliary junction. However, both investigations are invasive and are associated with a

---

Box 10.2 *Investigations used in the diagnosis of choledochal cysts*

Commonly used
  Ultrasonography
  Endoscopic retrograde cholangiopancreatography (ERCP)
  Intraoperative cholangiography
Occasionally used
  Plain abdominal X-ray
  Hepatobiliary scintigraphy
  Computed tomography with or without intravenous cholangiography
  Percutaneous transhepatic cholangiography (PTC)
  Magnetic resonance cholangiopancreatography (MRCP)
Rarely used
  Laparoscopy
  Angiography

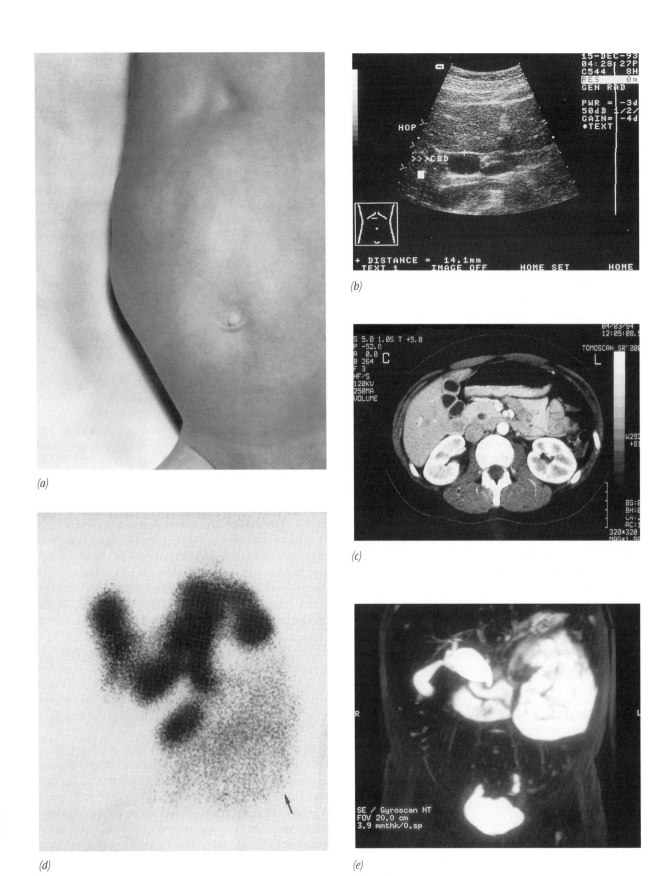

Figure 10.10 *Investigation of a choledochal cyst. (a) An infant with a right upper quadrant abdominal mass and jaundice. (b) An abdominal ultrasound scan demonstrating a fusiform choledochal cyst. CBD, common bile duct (c) CT scan showing intrahepatic duct dilatation in a type IVa choledochal cyst. (d) A radioisotope scan confirming biliary dilatation with diluted tracer in the cyst (arrow). The gallbladder and main hepatic ducts are densely opacified. (e) Magnetic resonance scan of a type I cystic choledochal dilatation in an infant.*

small risk of complications such as iatrogenic pancreatitis and biliary sepsis, and both are best performed under general anesthesia in children. ERCP should be avoided during episodes of acute pancreatitis.

Magnetic resonance cholangiopancreatography (MRCP) is non-invasive and can be performed under sedation in children without the use of contrast agents or irradiation (Matos *et al.*, 1998). Fluids such as bile and pancreatic secretions have a high signal intensity on T2-weighted images. However, definition of the pancreatic duct and common channel may be suboptimal, and calculi may be overlooked (Lam *et al.*, 1999). This is particularly likely in infants and small children using non-breath-holding magnetic resonance cholangiography. Recent advances in magnetic resonance technology have reduced the time for image acquisition to a few seconds, making MRCP much more reliable in this age group (Kim *et al.*, 2000).

Intraoperative cholangiography is often best performed by injection of contrast directly into the lower end of the common bile duct and into the common hepatic duct. Injection into the cyst itself may fail to fill the intrahepatic ducts, and may obscure any filling of the distal duct. In most patients a detailed ultrasound scan supplemented by intraoperative cholangiography provides sufficient anatomical information. ERCP or MRCP is useful in selected cases.

Hepatobiliary scintigraphy with technetium-99m iminodiacetic acid is widely available. A typical scan shows a filling defect in the liver followed by an increase in radioactivity in the cyst. A 24-hour post-injection scan may be necessary in the jaundiced patient. Radioisotope scanning can also be useful for assessing biliary drainage after surgery.

Computed tomography (CT) with contrast clearly demonstrates the cyst and intrahepatic bile ducts, and may be extremely useful in patients with pancreatitis. It is also valuable when an associated malignancy is suspected. Laparoscopy and angiography are rarely necessary.

DIFFERENTIAL DIAGNOSIS

In the newborn, a choledochal cyst needs to be distinguished from cystic varieties of biliary atresia and other intra-abdominal cysts. In infants and older children, rhabdomyosarcoma of the extrahepatic bile ducts, mucocele of the gallbladder, hepatic tumors, duplication cysts and cystic lesions of the pancreas, adrenal gland and kidney also need to be considered.

SURGICAL MANAGEMENT

Radical cyst excision and reconstruction by hepaticoenterostomy is the optimum treatment for most types of

choledochal cyst (Tan and Howard, 1988; Miyano *et al.*, 1996b; Todani, 1998). In experienced centers, the procedure can be performed safely at all ages with no mortality and minimal morbidity. Consequently, many of the potential complications of choledochal cysts can be avoided. Disease regression has been recorded after surgery in a patient with biliary cirrhosis and portal hypertension (Yeong *et al.*, 1982).

Cystenterostomy should rarely, if ever, be undertaken. Symptomatic control may be achieved in the short term, but there is an unacceptable long-term morbidity (due to cholangitis, cholelithiasis, pancreatolithiasis, anastomotic stricture, biliary cirrhosis and malignancy) necessitating reoperation. Cases treated previously by cystenterostomy should undergo further surgery with cyst excision, although this can be a demanding procedure (Kaneko *et al.*, 1999).

Radical cyst excision and hepaticoenterostomy (FIGURE 10.11A–C)

All type I and IV choledochal cysts can be treated in this way. Preoperatively, vitamin K is given to correct any coagulopathy. Lactulose, oral metronidazole and neomycin are given for 24 hours preoperatively to decontaminate the gut. Prophylactic intravenous broad-spectrum antibiotics (e.g. ampicillin and gentamicin) are given on induction and continued postoperatively for 5 days if there is a history of cholangitis.

A high transverse or oblique incision gives excellent exposure. The gallbladder may or may not be distended, and the duodenum and pancreas may be displaced forward over the cyst (Plate 1). The appearance of the liver, spleen and pancreas is noted. If the anatomy of the choledochal cyst is not clear from preoperative imaging studies, an operative cholangiogram should be performed to delineate the choledochal dilatation, the pancreaticobiliary junction and the intrahepatic ducts. A sample of bile is aspirated from the cyst for culture and estimation of pancreatic enzyme concentrations. A high concentration of biliary amylase indicates a common pancreaticobiliary channel.

A plane is developed between the overlying peritoneum and the anterior wall of the cyst. The dissection extends downwards between the duodenum and the cyst and laterally, keeping adjacent to the cyst wall, using bipolar diathermy to provide safe and accurate hemostasis. Larger cysts can be decompressed to facilitate exposure. The gallbladder and cystic duct are mobilized, care being taken to avoid damaging an aberrant right hepatic artery, which can be very adherent to the wall of the cyst. The bile duct is then dissected circumferentially and encircled where it narrows down, either at its inferior margin or at the junction with the common hepatic duct (Plate 2). The cyst and gallbladder can then be lifted forward. The most difficult part of the dissection is in

Figure 10.11 *(a–c) Main operative steps in radical excision and biliary reconstruction for a type I cystic choledochal cyst.*

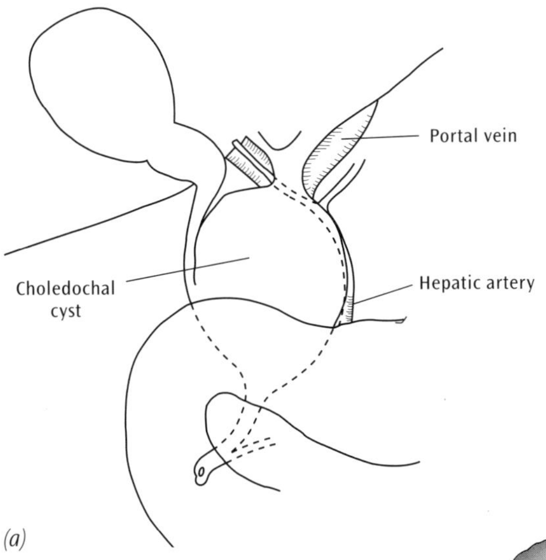

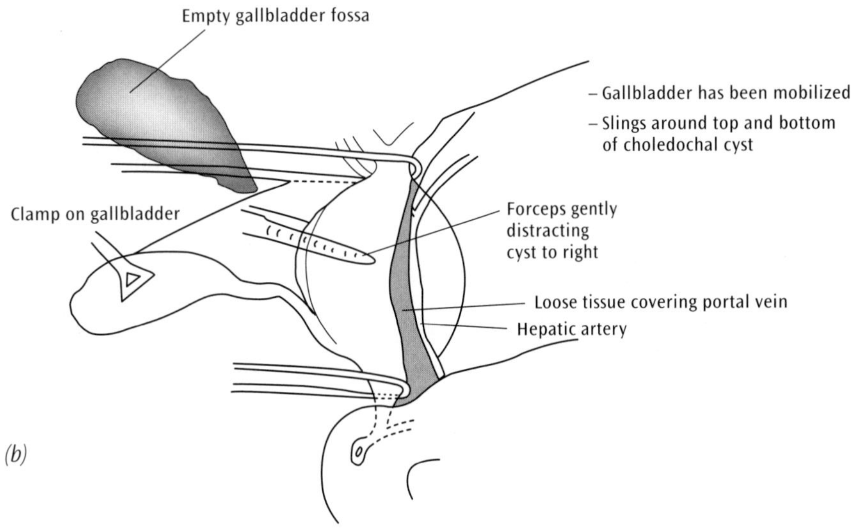

(a)

Portal vein

Choledochal cyst

Hepatic artery

Empty gallbladder fossa

– Gallbladder has been mobilized
– Slings around top and bottom of choledochal cyst

Clamp on gallbladder

Forceps gently distracting cyst to right

Loose tissue covering portal vein
Hepatic artery

(b)

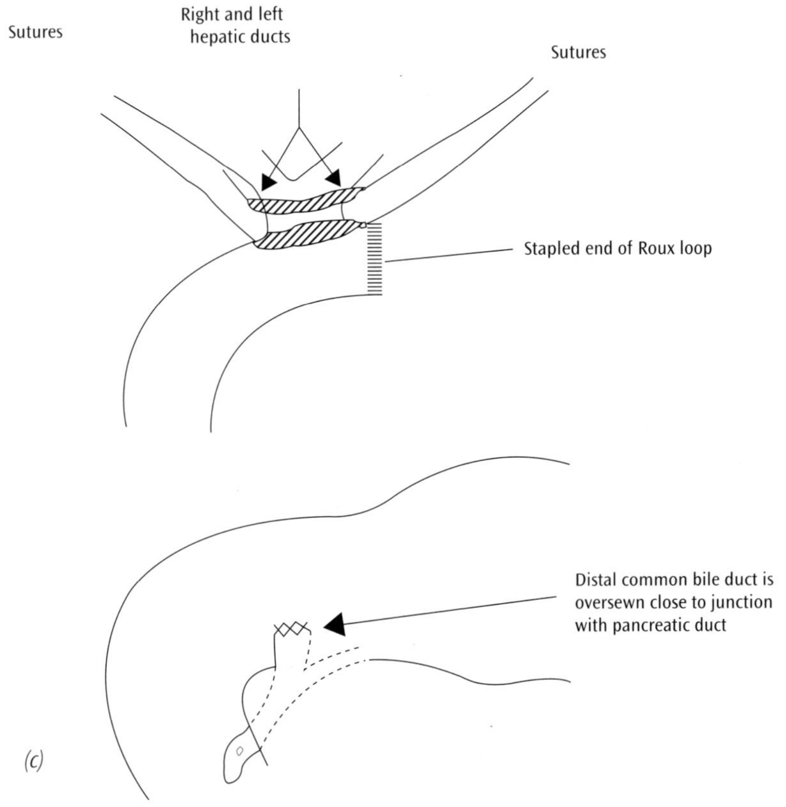

Sutures

Right and left hepatic ducts

Sutures

Stapled end of Roux loop

Distal common bile duct is oversewn close to junction with pancreatic duct

(c)

the region of the distal bile duct, where many small vessels arise from the pancreas. The common hepatic duct is divided at the level of the bifurcation, where it should be healthy and well vascularized. Any dilated proximal intrahepatic ducts should be cleared of debris using irrigation and, in larger ducts, biliary balloon catheters or choledochoscopy. The distal duct is dissected to just within the head of the pancreas and oversewn with monofilament absorbable sutures (e.g. polydioxanone). Operative cholangiography gives a useful guide to the distal limit of bile duct transection. Todani (1998) recommends the use of a surgical clip on the edge of the distal bile duct at the time of cholangiography to demonstrate the proximity of the pancreaticobiliary duct junction. Protein plugs or calculi within a common channel should be removed using a combination of saline irrigation, balloon catheters and intraoperative endoscopy (Yamataka *et al.*, 2000). Transduodenal sphincteroplasty should be considered if the common channel is particularly dilated and contains debris.

A 40-cm retrocolic Roux-loop of jejunum is widely anastomosed to the hepatic duct bifurcation at the hilum of the liver using fine interrupted monofilament absorbable sutures. The anastomosis to the Roux should be performed near the end of the jejunal limb to avoid the development of a sump with future growth of the bowel. Alternatively, an end-to-end hilar hepaticojejunostomy can be performed (Todani *et al.*, 1995b). Anastomosis to the narrow common hepatic duct should be avoided because of the long-term risk of stricture (Todani *et al.*, 1995b). Occasionally, hilar ductal anomalies necessitate a modified anastomosis by incorporation of aberrant ducts or inclusion of some form of ductoplasty for narrowed ducts (Todani, 1998). A liver biopsy is performed at the conclusion of the operation in order to document hepatic histology. In straightforward cases, abdominal drainage is unnecessary.

Todani has advocated hepaticoduodenostomy in preference to hepaticojejunostomy. It is argued that this is more physiological, associated with a smaller risk of adhesive small bowel obstruction, minimizes the loss of absorptive mucosa and is perhaps less prone to late stricturing (Todani *et al.*, 1981; Todani, 1998). There is also potentially an increased risk of peptic ulceration after Roux-en-Y hepaticojejunostomy (Nielsen *et al.*, 1980). However, good results can be achieved with hepaticojejunostomy (Stringer *et al.*, 1995; Miyano *et al.*, 1996b), and provided that a wide anastomosis is constructed there is likely to be little difference in outcome. The incidence of cholangitis is similar with both anastomotic techniques (Todani *et al.*, 1995b). Other techniques of biliary reconstruction include hepatico-appendico-duodenostomy (Crombleholme *et al.*, 1989) and hepatico-jejuno-duodenostomy (Oweida and Ricketts, 1989), but the long-term outcome of these alternatives is poorly documented. A high incidence of late biliary obstruction requiring revisional surgery has recently been reported

after hepatico-appendico-duodenostomy (Delarue *et al.*, 2000). In some infants the hilar ducts are so small that a precise mucosal biliary–enteric anastomosis is extremely demanding. In such cases, the hilar ducts may be incised and everted by sutures to the hilar plate and a Kasai-type portoenterostomy performed (Morotomi *et al.*, 1995).

Temporary external drainage

Temporary drainage via a T-tube is occasionally required for complex cases, such as patients with cyst rupture or uncontrolled cholangitis. Cyst excision can then be performed when the patient is fit. The bile drainage may be recycled. Electrolyte replacement and nutritional/vitamin supplements are required if the bile is discarded.

Occasionally, portal hypertension or dense inflammation from previous infection or surgery makes radical excision hazardous. Intramural resection of the posterior wall of the cyst (excising only the mucosa and the inner wall of the cyst) can help to avoid damage to the portal vein and hepatic arteries (Lilly, 1978). In adults, preliminary portal decompression has been recommended for patients with a choledochal cyst complicated by portal hypertension (Nagorney *et al.*, 1984). Patients with advanced biliary cirrhosis are candidates for liver transplantation.

Variations in surgical treatment have been reported for the following types of choledochal dilatation.

TYPE I FUSIFORM DILATATION

Endoscopic sphincterotomy or transduodenal sphincteroplasty have been reported to provide effective short-term control of symptoms, but this approach cannot be recommended for the majority of these patients because of the presence of a common pancreaticobiliary channel. Persistent PBM results in an ongoing risk of recurrent pancreatitis and later biliary tract malignancy (Miyano *et al.*, 1996a). For the same reason, resection of a fusiform cyst and reanastomosis of the bile duct is inappropriate.

TYPE II DIVERTICULUM

Excision of the diverticulum and reconstruction of the common bile duct is a satisfactory procedure for this very rare type of choledochal cyst (Iuchtman *et al.*, 1971; Powell *et al.*, 1981).

TYPE III CHOLEDOCHOCELE

Large choledochoceles can be removed transduodenally (Powell *et al.*, 1981). This may sometimes require hepaticoenterostomy and pancreatic sphincteroplasty. Smaller choledochoceles can be treated by sphincteroplasty or endoscopic sphincterotomy (O'Neill *et al.*, 1987; Dohmoto *et al.*, 1996). Concomitant cholecystectomy is advisable.

TYPE IV COMBINED CYSTS

Biliary drainage is improved by excision of the extrahepatic ductal system and a wide Roux-loop anastomosis to the hepatic duct bifurcation. Debris and calculi should be removed from dilated intrahepatic ducts, and the biliary–enteric anastomosis may need to be extended to incorporate hilar duct strictures (Lilly, 1979; Todani *et al.*, 1984a).

TYPE V INTRAHEPATIC CYSTS

Occasionally the cystic dilatation is confined to one side of the liver, when a hepatic lobectomy may be curative (Watts *et al.*, 1974). In more diffuse varieties, recurrent cholangitis and stone formation are common despite surgery, and liver transplantation may need to be considered.

RESULTS AND EARLY COMPLICATIONS OF SURGERY

Radical cyst excision and hepaticoenterostomy achieves consistently good results, even in small infants (Joseph, 1990; Stringer *et al.*, 1995; Miyano *et al.*, 1996b; Todani, 1998). Successful treatment is associated with reversal of hepatic fibrosis and, in rare cases, regression of early biliary cirrhosis. Postoperatively, patients should be followed with annual biochemical liver function tests and ultrasound scans because of potential long-term complications.

Early postoperative complications such as anastomotic leakage, bleeding, acute pancreatitis and intestinal obstruction are rare. Hilar hepaticoduodenostomy may cause transient duodenal obstruction/ileus, making temporary nasojejunal enteral feeding necessary (Todani, 1998). Anastomotic leakage is rare and resolves with local drainage, parenteral nutrition and nasogastric decompression.

LATE COMPLICATIONS

Choledochocystenterostomy is almost always associated with long-term complications. Late complications after radical cyst excision and biliary–enteric anastomosis are uncommon. Nevertheless, an anastomotic stricture may develop up to 10 or more years postoperatively (Saing *et al.*, 1997) (Figure 10.12). Todani reported a 10% reoperation rate after primary cyst excision in 103 children followed up for a median of 14 years (Todani, 1998). Revisional surgery was necessary between 3 and 21 years after the initial operation because of cholangitis due to anastomotic or ductal strictures. These complications

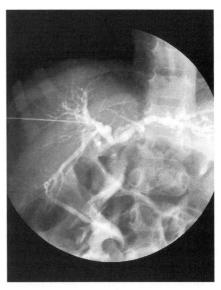

Figure 10.12 *This 2-year-old girl was referred for biliary reconstruction after previous surgery for a type I choledochal cyst complicated by an anastomotic stricture. She had evidence of obstructive jaundice, and dilated intrahepatic bile ducts were shown on the percutaneous transhepatic cholangiogram.*

were more likely with type IVa cysts (seven cases) or after biliary anastomosis to the common hepatic duct (three cases). Reoperation was not required after hilar hepaticojejunostomy or hepaticoduodenostomy for type I choledochal cysts.

In another large Japanese series of 200 children with type I or IVa cysts followed up for a mean period of 11 years after cyst excision and hepaticoenterostomy (principally Roux-en-Y hepaticojejunostomy) there were 25 late complications in 18 children (9%) (Yamataka *et al.*, 1997). These included ascending cholangitis, intrahepatic and common channel calculi, anastomotic stricture, pancreatitis and adhesive bowel obstruction. There were no instances of malignancy. No calculi or anastomotic strictures developed in children undergoing surgery before 5 years of age. This may be because anastomotic strictures are related to fibrosis and inflammation at the site of the biliary–enteric anastomosis, which is much more likely in older children. A wide hilar anastomosis should help to prevent this complication.

Cholangitis may signify an anastomotic stricture, an intrahepatic ductal stricture, Roux-loop obstruction, or calculi within the redundant blind pouch of an end-to-side Roux loop (Todani, 1998). Type IVa cysts are particularly prone to developing intrahepatic calculi (Lipsett *et al.*, 1994). Standard imaging methods supplemented by biliary scintigraphy and percutaneous transhepatic cholangiography (with antibiotic prophylaxis) will demonstrate the site of the problem. Although interventional radiological techniques may be able to clear stones and dilate strictures, surgery is usually required to revise a biliary–enteric anastomotic stricture. Liver resection may be needed for complicated intrahepatic duct strictures.

Pancreatitis may develop many years after cyst excision in patients with a dilated or complex common channel containing protein plugs or calculi, or in those with a substantial segment of retained terminal common bile duct. This complication is usually preventable by appropriate primary surgery. ERCP is useful for the investigation of such patients, who usually present with recurrent abdominal pain after choledochal cyst excision. Endoscopic sphincterotomy may be curative.

Malignancy has been reported at several sites after choledochal cyst excision. The intrahepatic bile ducts, the biliary–enteric anastomosis and the terminal common bile duct have been affected, the latter following choledochal excision at 14 years of age (Chaudhuri et al., 1982; Nagorney et al., 1984; Yoshikawa et al., 1986; Yamamoto et al., 1996).

CAROLI'S DISEASE (SEE CHAPTER 16)

Caroli's disease is a congenital segmental saccular dilatation of the intrahepatic bile ducts with intervening normal or near-normal ducts (Figure 10.13). The condition overlaps with type V choledochal cyst. It may affect the liver diffusely or be localized to one lobe, more often the left. The condition typically causes recurrent cholangitis, which may present with any combination of fever, jaundice or abdominal pain. The frequency and severity of attacks vary. Hepatosplenomegaly is common, and intrahepatic abscess and/or stone formation may complicate the disease. Most cases present as young adults, but pediatric examples have been reported (Fujiwara et al., 1976b; Keane et al., 1997; Pinto et al., 1998). The condition is best evaluated by ERCP together with cross-sectional imaging and liver biopsy.

Caroli (1968) classified intrahepatic cysts into type 1, which is rarer and presents with recurrent cholangitis alone, and type 2 (sometimes called Caroli's syndrome), where cholangitis is associated with congenital hepatic fibrosis, portal hypertension and renal disease (e.g. renal cysts, renal tubular ectasia or medullary sponge kidney). However, with increasing experience of the disease, these two subtypes have become less distinct. Most patients in both groups demonstrate histological features of a ductal plate malformation on liver biopsy (Tsuchida et al., 1995), and a large proportion of pediatric cases have renal pathology (Pinto et al., 1998). Caroli's disease can have features of either an autosomal-recessive or, less commonly, an autosomal-dominant pattern of inheritance in different kindreds.

Prophylactic antibiotics may help to prevent attacks of cholangitis (Tsuchida et al., 1995). The value of

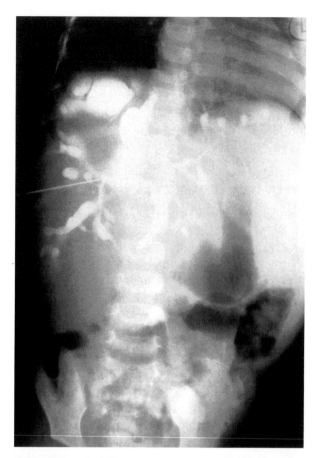

Figure 10.13 *Caroli's disease in a child. Percutaneous transhepatic cholangiography demonstrates cystic dilatation of the intrahepatic ducts, but the extrahepatic ducts were normal. (Reproduced courtesy of ER Howard.)*

ursodeoxycholic acid is unknown. Liver abscesses require drainage. Intrahepatic calculi and biliary malignancy may complicate Caroli's disease, particularly in adults. Localized forms of the disease can be treated by hepatic resection, whereas liver transplantation is an option for more diffuse varieties associated with complications.

CONCLUSION

Choledochal cysts require careful assessment to characterize the type of biliary dilatation and associated abnormalities of the pancreaticobiliary junction, the intrahepatic bile ducts and the liver. Most choledochal cysts are best treated by radical excision and hepaticoenterostomy, which yields excellent results even in small infants. Cystenterostomy should be avoided. All patients require long-term surveillance because of the risk of late complications, which include anastomotic stricture, pancreatic disease and malignancy.

Key references

Miyano T, Yamataka A, Kato Y *et al.* Hepaticoenterostomy after excision of choledochal cyst in children: a 30-year experience with 180 cases. *Journal of Pediatric Surgery* 1996; **31**: 1417–21.

Todani T, Watanabe Y, Toki A, Ogura K, Wang Z-Q. Coexisting biliary anomalies and anatomical variants in choledochal cyst. *British Journal of Surgery* 1998; **85**: 760–3.

Yamataka A, Ohshiro K, Okada Y *et al.* Complications after cyst excision with hepaticoenterostomy for choledochal cysts and their surgical management in children versus adults. *Journal of Pediatric Surgery* 1997; **32**: 1097–102.

These three papers from authoritative Japanese centers detail large series of children undergoing choledochal cyst excision and hepaticoenterostomy. Long-term outcome and complications are carefully documented.

Wong KC, Lister J. Human fetal development of the hepato-pancreatic duct junction – a possible explanation of congenital dilation of the biliary tract. *Journal of Pediatric Surgery* 1981; **16**: 139–45.

A useful account of the embryological and fetal development of the pancreaticobiliary junction.

Ando K, Miyano T, Kohno S *et al.* Spontaneous perforation of choledochal cyst: a study of 13 cases. *European Journal of Pediatric Surgery* 1998; **8**: 23–5.

Bismuth H, Krissat J. Choledochal cystic malignancies. *Annals of Oncology* 1999; **10(Supplement 4)**: S94–8.

These studies document two important complications of choledochal cysts, namely rupture and malignant change. Both accounts include institutional experience and a review of the literature.

REFERENCES

Alonso-Lej F, Rever WB, Pessagno DJ. Congenital choledochal cyst with a report of 2, and an analysis of 94 cases. *International Abstracts of Surgery* 1959; **108**: 1–30.

Ando K, Miyano T, Kohno S *et al.* Spontaneous perforation of choledochal cyst: a study of 13 cases. *European Journal of Pediatric Surgery* 1998; **8**: 23–5.

Babbitt DP. Congenital choledochal cysts: new etiological concept based on anomalous relationships of common bile duct and pancreatic bulb. *Annals of Radiology* 1969; **12**: 231–40.

Bancroft JD, Bucuvalas JC, Ryckman FC, Dudgeon DL, Saunders RC, Schwarz KB. Antenatal diagnosis of choledochal cyst. *Journal of Pediatric Gastroenterology and Nutrition* 1994; **18**: 142–5.

Binks JB, Pauline GJ. Choledochal cyst and carcinoma of the pancreas in a boy of 15 years. *Australian and New Zealand Journal of Surgery* 1970; **40**: 42–4.

Bismuth H, Krissat J. Choledochal cystic malignancies. *Annals of Oncology* 1999; **10(Supplement 4)**: S94–8.

Caroli J. Diseases of intrahepatic bile ducts. *Israel Journal of Medical Science* 1968; **4**: 21–35.

Chaudhuri PK, Chaudhuri B, Schuler JJ *et al.* Carcinoma associated with congenital cystic dilatation of bile duct. *Archives of Surgery* 1982; **117**: 1349–51.

Coyle KA, Bradley EL. Cholangiocarcinoma developing after simple excision of a type II choledochal cyst. *Southern Medical Journal* 1992; **85**: 540–44.

Crombleholme TM, Harrison MR, Langer JC, Longaker MT. Biliary appendico-duodenostomy: a non-refluxing conduit for biliary reconstruction. *Journal of Pediatric Surgery* 1989; **24**: 665–7.

Davenport M, Stringer MD, Howard ER. Biliary amylase and congenital choledochal dilatation. *Journal of Pediatric Surgery* 1995; **30**: 474–7.

Delarue A, Chappuis JS, Esposito C *et al.* Is the appendix graft suitable for routine biliary surgery in children? *Journal of Pediatric Surgery* 2000; **35**: 1312–16.

Dewbury KC, Aluwihare APR, Birch SJ, Freeman NV. Prenatal ultrasound demonstration of a choledochal cyst. *British Journal of Radiology* 1980; **53**: 906–7.

Dohmoto M, Kamiya T, Hunerbein M *et al.* Endoscopic treatment of a choledochocele in a 2-year-old child. *Surgical Endoscopy* 1996; **10**: 1016–18.

Douglas AH. Case of dilatation of the common bile duct. *Monthly Journal of Medical Science* 1852; **14**: 97–101.

Dudin A, Abdelshafi M, Ramband-Cousson A. Choledochal cyst associated with rare hand malformation. *American Journal of Medical Genetics* 1995; **56**: 161–3.

Duh Y-C, Lai H-S, Chen W-J. Accessory hepatic duct associated with a choledochal cyst. *Pediatric Surgery International* 1997; **12**: 54–6.

Fujiwara Y, Ohizumi T, Kakizaki G *et al.* A case of congenital choledochal cyst associated with carcinoma. *Journal of Pediatric Surgery* 1976a; **11**: 587–8.

Fujiwara Y, Ohizumi T, Kakizaki G, Fujiwara T. Congenital dilatation of intrahepatic and common bile ducts with congenital hepatic fibrosis. *Journal of Pediatric Surgery* 1976b; **11**: 273–4.

Gauthier F, Brunelle F, Valayer J. Common channel for bile and pancreatic ducts. Presentation of 12 cases and discussion. *Chirurgie Pediatrique* 1986; **27**: 148–52.

Greenholz SK, Lilly JR, Shikes RH, Hall RJ. Biliary atresia in the newborn. *Journal of Pediatric Surgery* 1986; **21**: 1147–8.

Guelrud M, Morera C, Rodriguez M, Prados JG, Jaen D. Normal and anomalous pancreaticobiliary union in children and adolescents. *Gastrointestinal Endoscopy* 1999; **50**: 189–93.

Han SJ, Hwang EH, Chung KS *et al.* Acquired choledochal cyst from an anomalous pancreatobiliary duct union. *Journal of Pediatric Surgery* 1997; **32**: 1735–8.

Harris VJ, Kahler J. Choledochal cyst. Delayed diagnosis in a jaundiced infant. *Pediatrics* 1978; **62**: 235–7.

Hernanz-Schulman M, Ambrosino MM, Freeman PC, Quinn CB. Common bile duct in children: sonographic dimensions. *Radiology* 1995; **195**: 193–5.

Hewitt PM, Krige JE, Bornman PC, Terblanche J. Choledochal cyst in pregnancy: a therapeutic dilemma. *Journal of the American College of Surgeons* 1995; **181**: 237–40.

Howell CG, Templeton JM, Weiner S *et al*. Antenatal diagnosis and early surgery for choledochal cyst. *Journal of Pediatric Surgery* 1983; **18**: 387–93.

Ito T, Ando H, Nagaya M, Sugito T. Congenital dilatation of the common bile duct in children. The etiologic significance of the narrow segment distal to the dilated common bile duct. *Zeitschrift für Kinderchirurgie* 1984; **39**: 40–5.

Iuchtman M, Martins MS, Scheidemantel RE. Congenital diverticulum of the choledochus: report of a case. *International Surgery* 1971; **55**: 280–82.

Iwai N, Deguchi E, Yanagihara J *et al*. Cancer arising in a choledochal cyst in a 12-year-old girl. *Journal of Pediatric Surgery* 1990; **12**: 1261–3.

Iwai N, Yanagihara J, Tokiwa K *et al*. Congenital choledochal dilatation with emphasis on pathophysiology of the biliary tract. *Annals of Surgery* 1992; **215**: 27–30.

Joseph VT. Surgical techniques and long-term results in the treatment of choledochal cyst. *Journal of Pediatric Surgery* 1990; **25**: 782–7.

Kaneko K, Ando H, Watanabe Y *et al*. Secondary excision of choledochal cysts after previous cystenterostomies. *Hepatogastroenterology* 1999; **46**: 2772–5.

Kaneko K, Ando H, Watanabe Y, Seo T, Harada T. Pathologic changes in the common bile duct of an experimental model with pancreaticobiliary maljunction without biliary dilatation. *Pediatric Surgery International* 2000; **16**: 26–8.

Karnak I, Tanyel FC, Buyukpamukcu N, Hicsonmez A. Spontaneous rupture of choledochal cyst: an unusual cause of acute abdomen in children. *Journal of Pediatric Surgery* 1997; **32**: 736–8.

Kato T, Hebiguchi T, Matsuda K, Yoshino H. Action of pancreatic juice on the bile duct: pathogenesis of congenital choledochal cyst. *Journal of Pediatric Surgery* 1981; **16**: 146–51.

Kawaguchi F, Nakada K, Fujioka T, Nakada M. Pancreatitis as a late complication after total excisional surgery for congenital biliary dilatation. *Japanese Journal of Pediatric Surgery* 1995; **27**: 304–10.

Kazar G. Kettos epeholyag es choledochyscysta. *Magyar Sebesz* 1950; **3**: 298–301.

Keane F, Hadzic N, Wilkinson ML *et al*. Neonatal presentation of Caroli's disease. *Archives of Disease in Childhood* 1997; **77**: F145–6.

Kim SH, Lim JH, Yoon HK *et al*. Choledochal cyst: comparison of MR and conventional cholangiography. *Clinical Radiology* 2000; **55**: 378–83.

Kim WS, Kim IO, Yeon KM *et al*. Choledochal cyst with or without biliary atresia in neonates and young infants: US differentiation. *Radiology* 1998; **209**: 465–9.

Kobayashi S, Asano T, Yamasaki M *et al*. Risk of bile duct carcinogenesis after excision of extrahepatic bile ducts in pancreaticobiliary maljunction. *Surgery* 1999; **126**: 939–44.

Komi N, Tamura T, Tsuge S, Miyosh Y, Udaka H, Takehara H. Relation of patient age to premalignant alterations in choledochal cyst epithelium: histochemical and immunohistochemical studies. *Journal of Pediatric Surgery* 1986; **21**: 430–3.

Lai H-S, Duh Y-C, Chen WJ. Inspissated bile syndrome followed by choledochal cyst formation. *Surgery* 1998; **123**: 706–8.

Lam WWM, Lam TPW, Saing H, Chan FL, Chan KL. MR cholangiography and CT cholangiography of pediatric patients with choledochal cysts. *American Journal of Roentgenology* 1999; **173**: 401–5.

Lane GJ, Yamataka A, Kobayashi H *et al*. Different types of congenital biliary dilatation in dizygotic twins. *Pediatric Surgery International* 1999; **15**: 403–4.

Li L, Yamataka A, Yian-Xia W *et al*. Ectopic distal location of the papilla of Vater in congenital biliary dilatation: implications for pathogenesis. *Journal of Pediatric Surgery* 2001; **36**: 1617–22.

Lilly JR. Total excision of choledochal cyst. *Surgical Gynecology and Obstetrics* 1978; **146**: 254–6.

Lilly JR. Surgery of coexisting biliary malformations in choledochal cyst. *Journal of Pediatric Surgery* 1979; **14**: 643–7.

Lilly JR, Stellin GP, Karrer FM. Formefruste choledochal cyst. *Journal of Pediatric Surgery* 1985; **20**: 449–51.

Lipsett PA, Pitt HA, Colombani PM *et al*. Choledochal cyst disease. A changing pattern of presentation. *Annals of Surgery* 1994; **220**: 644–52.

Lugo-Vincente HL. Prenatally diagnosed choledochal cysts: observation or early surgery? *Journal of Pediatric Surgery* 1995; **30**: 1288–90.

McWhorter GL. Congenital cystic dilatation of the common bile duct. Report of a case, with cure. *Archives of Surgery* 1924; **8**: 604–26.

Matos C, Nicaise N, Deviere J *et al*. Choledochal cysts: comparison of findings at MR cholangiopancreatography and endoscopic retrograde cholangiopancreatography in eight patients. *Radiology* 1998; **209**: 443–8.

Matsubara H, Oya N, Suzuki Y *et al*. Is it possible to differentiate between choledochal cyst and congenital biliary atresia (type I cyst) by antenatal ultrasonography? *Fetal Diagnosis and Therapy* 1997; **12**: 306–8.

Miyano T, Ando K, Yamataka A *et al*. Pancreatobiliary maljunction associated with non-dilatation or minimal dilatation of the common bile duct in children: diagnosis and treatment. *European Journal of Pediatric Surgery* 1996a; **6**: 334–7.

Miyano T, Yamataka A, Kato Y *et al*. Hepaticoenterostomy after excision of choledochal cyst in children: a 30-year experience with 180 cases. *Journal of Pediatric Surgery* 1996b; **31**: 1417–21.

Morotomi Y, Todani T, Watanabe Y *et al*. Modified Kasai's procedure for a choledochal cyst with a very narrow hilar duct. *Pediatric Surgery International* 1995; **11**: 58–9.

Nagorney DM, McIlrath DC, Adson MA. Choledochal cysts in adults: clinical management. *Surgery* 1984; **96**: 656–63.

Nielsen ML, Jensen SL, Malmstrom J, Nielsen OV. Gastrin and gastric acid secretion in hepaticojejunostomy Roux-en-Y. *Surgery, Gynecology and Obstetrics* 1980; **150**: 61–4.

Ohkawa H, Takahashi H, Maie M. A malformation of the pancreatico-biliary system as a cause of perforation of the biliary tract in childhood. *Journal of Pediatric Surgery* 1977; **12**: 541–6.

Okada A, Oguchi Y, Kamata S, Ikeda Y, Kawashima Y, Saito R. Common channel syndrome – diagnosis with endoscopic retrograde cholangiopancreatography and surgical management. *Surgery* 1983; **93**: 634–42.

O'Neill JA, Templeton JM, Schnaufer L *et al.* Recent experience with choledochal cyst. *Annals of Surgery* 1987; **205**: 533–40.

Oweida SW, Ricketts RR. Hepatico-jejuno-duodenostomy reconstruction following excision of choledochal cysts in children. *American Surgeon* 1989; **55**: 2–6.

Pinto RB, Lima JP, da Silveira TR *et al.* Caroli's disease: report of 10 cases in children and adolescents in Southern Brazil. *Journal of Pediatric Surgery* 1998; **33**: 1531–5.

Poddar U, Thapa BR, Chhabra M *et al.* Choledochal cysts in infants and children. *Indian Pediatrics* 1998; **35**: 613–18.

Powell CS, Sawyers JL, Reynolds VH. Management of adult choledochal cysts. *Annals of Surgery* 1981; **193**: 666–76.

Raffensperger JG, Given GZ, Warrner RA. Fusiform dilatation of the common bile duct with pancreatitis. *Journal of Pediatric Surgery* 1973; **8**: 907–10.

Redkar R, Davenport M, Howard ER. Antenatal diagnosis of congenital anomalies of the biliary tract. *Journal of Pediatric Surgery* 1998; **33**: 700–4.

Reville RM, van Stiegmann ML, Everson GT. Increased secondary bile acids in a choledochal cyst. Possible role in biliary metaplasia and carcinoma. *Gastroenterology* 1990; **99**: 525–7.

Rha SY, Stovroff MC, Glick PL, Allen JE, Ricketts RR. Choledochal cysts: a ten-year experience. *American Surgeon* 1996; **62**: 30–4.

Rheinlander HF, Bowens OL. Congenital absence of the gallbladder with cystic dilatation of the common bile duct. *New England Journal of Medicine* 1957; **256**: 557–9.

Rossi RL, Silverman ML, Braasch JW *et al.* Carcinoma arising in cystic conditions of the bile ducts: a clinical and pathological study. *Annals of Surgery* 1987; **205**: 377–84.

Saing H, Han H, Chan K *et al.* Early and late results of excision of choledochal cysts. *Journal of Pediatric Surgery* 1997; **32**: 1563–6.

Saltz NJ, Glaser K. Congenital cystic dilatation of the common bile duct. *American Journal of Surgery* 1956; **91**: 56–9.

Samuel M, Spitz L. Choledochal cyst: varied clinical presentations and long-term results of surgery. *European Journal of Pediatric Surgery* 1996; **6**: 78–81.

Sanz N, de Mingo L, Florez F, Rollan V. Rhabdomyosarcoma of the biliary tree. *Pediatric Surgery International* 1997; **12**: 200–1.

Schroeder D, Smith L, Prain HC. Antenatal diagnosis of choledochal cyst at 15 weeks' gestation: etiologic implications and management. *Journal of Pediatric Surgery* 1989; **24**: 936–8.

Shimotake T, Iwai N, Yanagihara J *et al.* Innervation patterns in congenital biliary dilatation. *European Journal of Pediatric Surgery* 1995; **5**: 265–70.

Spitz L. Experimental production of cystic dilatation of the common bile duct in neonatal lambs. *Journal of Pediatric Surgery* 1977; **12**: 39–42.

Spunt SL, Lobe TE, Pappo AS *et al.* Aggressive surgery is unwarranted for biliary tract rhabdomyosarcoma. *Journal of Pediatric Surgery* 2000; **35**: 309–16.

Stringel G, Filler RM. Fictitious pancreatitis in choledochal cyst. *Journal of Pediatric Surgery* 1982; **17**: 359–61.

Stringer MD, Dhawan A, Davenport M, Mieli-Vergani G, Mowat AP, Howard ER. Choledochal cysts: lessons from a 20-year experience. *Archives of Disease in Childhood* 1995; **73**: 528–31.

Suita S, Shono K, Kinugasa Y *et al.* Influence of age on the presentation and outcome of choledochal cyst. *Journal of Pediatric Surgery* 1999; **34**: 1765–8.

Swain WP. A case of cholecystenterostomy with the use of Murphy's button. *Lancet* 1895; **1**: 743–4.

Swartley WB, Weeder SD. Choledochus cyst with a double common bile duct. *Annals of Surgery* 1935; **101**: 912–20.

Tan CEL, Howard ER, Driver M, Murray-Lyon IM. Non-communicating multiseptate gallbladder and choledochal cyst: a case report and review of publications. *Gut* 1993; **34**: 853–6.

Tan KC, Howard ER. Choledochal cyst: a 14-year surgical experience with 36 patients. *British Journal of Surgery* 1988; **75**: 892–5.

Todani T. Choledochal cysts. In: Stringer MD, Oldham KT, Mouriquand PDE, Howard ER (eds) *Pediatric surgery and urology: long-term outcomes.* Philadelphia, PA: WB Saunders Co., 1998: 417–29.

Todani T, Watanabe Y, Narusue M, Tabuchi K, Okajima K. Classification, operative procedures and review of 37 cases including cancer arising from choledochal cyst. *American Journal of Surgery* 1977; **134**: 263–9.

Todani T, Watanabe Y, Mizuguchi T, Fujii T, Toki A. Hepaticoduodenostomy at the hepatic hilum after excision of choledochal cyst. *American Journal of Surgery* 1981; **142**: 584–7.

Todani T, Watanabe Y, Fujii T *et al.* Congenital choledochal cyst with intrahepatic involvement. *Archives of Surgery* 1984a; **119**: 1038–43.

Todani T, Watanabe Y, Fujii T, Uemura S. Anomalous arrangement of the pancreatobiliary ductal system in patients with a choledochal cyst. *American Journal of Surgery* 1984b; **147**: 672–6.

Todani T, Watanabe Y, Toki A, Urushihara N. Carcinoma

related to choledochal cysts with internal drainage operations. *Surgery, Gynecology and Obstetrics* 1987; **164**: 61–4.

Todani T, Watanabe Y, Urushihara N, Morotomi Y, Maeba T. Choledochal cyst, pancreatobiliary malunion and cancer. *Journal of Hepato-Biliary-Pancreatic Surgery* 1994; **1**: 247–51.

Todani T, Urushihara N, Morotomi Y *et al.* Characteristics of choledochal cysts in neonates and early infants. *European Journal of Pediatric Surgery* 1995a; **5**: 143–5.

Todani T, Watanabe Y, Urushihara N *et al.* Biliary complications after excisional procedure for choledochal cyst. *Journal of Pediatric Surgery* 1995b; **30**: 478–81.

Todani T, Watanabe Y, Toki A, Ogura K, Wang Z-Q. Co-existing biliary anomalies and anatomical variants in choledochal cyst. *British Journal of Surgery* 1998; **85**: 760–3.

Todd CH. History of a remarkable enlargement of the biliary duct. *Dublin Hospital Reports* 1817; **1**: 325–30.

Tsardakas E, Robnett AH. Congenital cystic dilation of the common bile duct: report of 3 cases, analysis of 57 cases and review of the literature. *Archives of Surgery* 1956; **72**: 311–27.

Tsuchida Y, Sato T, Sanjo K *et al.* Evaluation of long-term results of Caroli's disease: 21 years' observation of a family with autosomal-dominant inheritance, and review of the literature. *Hepatogastroenterology* 1995; **42**: 175–81.

Uchida M, Tsukahara M, Fuji T *et al.* Discordance for anomalous pancreaticobiliary ductal junction and congenital biliary dilatation in a set of monozygotic twins. *Journal of Pediatric Surgery* 1992; **27**: 1563–4.

Urushihara N, Todani T, Watanabe Y, Toki A. Choledochal cyst in an identical twin. *Pediatric Surgery International* 1988; **3**: 189–92.

Urushihara N, Todani T, Watanabe Y *et al.* Does hyperamylasemia in choledochal cyst indicate true pancreatitis? An experimental study. *European Journal of Pediatric Surgery* 1995; **5**: 139–42.

Vater A. *Dissertatio anatomica qua novum bilis diverticulum circa orificium ductus cholidochi ut et valvulosam colli vesicae felleae constructionem ad disceptandum proponit.* Wittenbergae: Lit. Gerdesianus, 1720.

Voyles CR, Smadja C, Shands WC, Blumgart LH. Carcinoma in choledochal cysts: age-related incidence. *Archives of Surgery* 1983; **118**: 986–8.

Watts DR, Lorenzo GA, Beal JM. Congenital dilation of the intrahepatic biliary ducts. *Archives of Surgery* 1974; **108**: 592–4.

Wheeler RA, Colquhoun-Flannery WA, Johnson CD. Plasma amylase estimation in recurrent abdominal pain in children. *Annals of the Royal College of Surgeons of England* 1992; **74**: 335–6.

Wong KC, Lister J. Human fetal development of the hepato-pancreatic duct junction – a possible explanation of congenital dilation of the biliary tract. *Journal of Pediatric Surgery* 1981; **16**: 139–45.

Wood CB, Baum M. Carcinoma of the head of the pancreas developing in a young woman with a choledochal cyst. *British Journal of Clinical Practice* 1975; **29**: 160–2.

Yamaguchi M. Congenital choledochal cyst. Analysis of 1433 patients in the Japanese literature. *American Journal of Surgery* 1980; **140**: 653–7.

Yamamoto J, Shimamura Y, Ohtani I *et al.* Bile duct carcinoma arising from the anastomotic site of hepaticojejunostomy after the excision of congenital biliary dilatation: a case report. *Surgery* 1996; **119**: 476–9.

Yamataka A, Ohshiro K, Okada Y *et al.* Complications after cyst excision with hepaticoenterostomy for choledochal cysts and their surgical management in children versus adults. *Journal of Pediatric Surgery* 1997; **32**: 1097–102.

Yamataka A, Segawa O, Kobayashi H *et al.* Intraoperative pancreatoscopy for pancreatic duct stone debris distal to the common channel in choledochal cyst. *Journal of Pediatric Surgery* 2000; **35**: 1–4.

Yamauchi S, Koga A, Matsumoto S, Tanaka M, Nakayama F. Anomalous junction of pancreaticobiliary duct without congenital choledochal cyst: a possible risk factor for gallbladder cancer. *American Journal of Gastroenterology* 1987; **82**: 20–4.

Yeong ML, Nicholson GI, Lee SP. Regression of biliary cirrhosis following choledochal cyst drainage. *Gastroenterology* 1982; **82**: 332–5.

Yoshikawa K, Yoshida K, Shirai Y *et al.* A case of carcinoma arising in the intrahepatic terminal choledochus 12 years after primary excision of a giant choledochal cyst. *American Journal of Gastroenterology* 1986; **81**: 378–84.

Yotuyanagi S. Contributions to the aetiology and pathogeny of idiopathic cystic dilatation of the common bile duct with report of three cases. *Gann* 1936; **30**: 601–5.

11

Spontaneous biliary perforation

EDWARD R HOWARD

INTRODUCTION

Spontaneous perforation of the extrahepatic bile ducts is the commonest surgical cause of jaundice in infants, after biliary atresia. The surgical differential diagnosis also includes choledochal cysts, which may themselves present with peritonitis secondary to perforation, and inspissated bile plug syndrome.

Approximately 100 cases of spontaneous perforation of the bile ducts in young infants have been reported since the first description in English was published by Caulfield (1936). He reported two cases who had presented at 7 and 10 weeks of age, respectively. The first infant, who underwent laparotomy and simple drainage of the perforation, survived. The second infant died without surgical intervention. Lilly et al. (1974) reviewed 53 cases reported up to 1974, and added two of their own. Twelve (22%) of the infants died, including all five who did not undergo laparotomy. Seven infants died after a variety of procedures which included simple drainage ($n = 3$), cholecystectomy ($n = 2$) and bile duct–bowel anastomoses ($n = 2$).

Lilly et al. (1974) concluded from their review that, in the management of spontaneous perforation of the bile ducts in infancy, complex surgical procedures were unnecessary and that simple drainage was the procedure of choice. However, it is noteworthy that one of their two cases who was treated with cholecystostomy and simple drainage developed a prolonged bile leak and died after a second operation. Prolonged postoperative bile leaks after simple drainage procedures have also been described in other case reports (Megison and Votteler, 1992; Spigland et al., 1996).

PATHOLOGY OF PERFORATION OF THE BILE DUCT

Etiology

Spontaneous perforation commonly presents without previous signs of biliary tract disease. It must be differentiated from other causes of bile duct perforation, which include trauma (Narasimhan et al., 1993), choledochal cyst (Ohkawa et al., 1977; Ando et al., 1995), necrotizing enterocolitis (Dolgin et al., 1991; Ibanez et al., 1999) and Ascaris infestation of the bile duct (Witcombe, 1978). Spontaneous perforation of the bile duct has also been associated with a multiple organ disorder, known as the Ivemark syndrome (Prabakaran et al., 2000), which consists of splenic abnormalities, cardiac pathology and abnormalities of the gastrointestinal tract.

The clinical presentation of a perforated choledochal cyst may be indistinguishable from that of spontaneous perforation of a normal bile duct, except that infants with cysts are usually over 1 year of age, and ultrasound will demonstrate a dilated common bile duct. Perforated choledochal cysts are also associated with anomalous pancreaticobiliary junctions (common channels) which allow reflux of pancreatic juice into the common bile duct. Leaking bile from a congenital cyst may therefore contain high levels of amylase and lipase, and blood levels of these enzymes may also be elevated. Ohkawa et al. (1977) described three infants with perforated choledochal cysts, aged between 11 months and 3 years, and provided very clear diagrams of the long common channels found in each case. The common bile ducts entered the main pancreatic ducts almost at right angles.

The typical age at presentation of infants with spontaneous perforation of an undilated duct is between 1 week and 2 months after birth. Jaundice and biliary ascites are the most frequent signs, and perforations are identified at surgery either in the cystic duct or at the junction of the cystic and common hepatic bile ducts.

Pathology

Although the site of the perforation is so constant, there is no obvious local cause in the duct wall. Pettersson (1955) and Johnston (1961) postulated a developmental weakness in the bile duct wall, but recent embryological studies of the biliary tract have not suggested any reason for such a weakness (Tan and Moscoso, 1994). Johnston (1961) also suggested that necrosis secondary to pancreatic reflux might be a possible factor. However, reflux from common pancreaticobiliary channels is not, by definition, present in infants with spontaneous perforation. Moore (1975) suggested an etiological role for viral infections, but this remains unproven.

A rise in intraluminal pressure may precede the perforation, and intraoperative cholangiography demonstrates biliary obstruction due to inspissated bile within the lower third of the common bile duct in many cases. Similar bile plugs have also been demonstrated within the common channels of perforated choledochal cysts (Ando et al., 1995), and rises in ductal pressure from intraductal stones have been implicated in spontaneous perforations of bile ducts in adults (Donald and Ozent, 1977).

Stenosis of the ampulla of Vater (Donahoe and Hendren, 1976; Spigland et al., 1996) may also occur in association with ductal perforations, but this can be very difficult to assess when there is significant inflammatory change around the bile duct. Stenotic lesions may be clearly delineated only on post-laparotomy cholangiography.

In summary, current evidence suggests that perforation in an otherwise normal biliary tract is associated with an obstruction at the distal end of the common bile duct, secondary either to inspissated bile which may clear spontaneously, or to a stenosis of the ampulla of Vater. The reason for the common site of perforation at the junction of the cystic and common bile ducts is still unknown.

CLINICAL PRESENTATION

Spontaneous perforation of the bile duct is a very rare condition, although it is recognized as the second most frequent cause of obstructive jaundice in infancy after biliary atresia (Lilly et al., 1974; Hammoudi and Alauddin, 1988). Most of the published reports, including those from specialist referral centres, describe only one or two cases (Pettersson, 1955; Lilly et al., 1974; Fitzgerald et al., 1978). The patients usually have uncomplicated birth histories and develop normally until either the acute onset of generalized peritonitis or a more chronic onset of painless jaundice, acholic stools and dark urine. The variable clinical signs have been described by Chardot et al. (1996) who suggested, from their experience of 11 cases, that three types of presentation could be recognized, namely with acute peritonitis, with localized peritonitis or with bile duct stenosis.

Generalized peritonitis

An acute presentation with generalized biliary peritonitis has been described by Stringal and Mercer (1983) and by Carubelli and Abramo (1999). The latter authors described an infant who presented as an acute emergency with abdominal distension, ascites, rectal bleeding and shock. Perforation of the bile duct was diagnosed at laparotomy, and the authors pointed out that this diagnosis was often overlooked in the differential diagnosis of the acute abdomen in infancy.

Localized biliary peritonitis

This is the commonest type of presentation. The signs are commonly noted within the first 8 weeks of life, but have been seen as late as 30 months (Hindmarsh, 1947; Lees and Mitchell, 1966). Pyrexia is usually absent, and signs of peritoneal inflammation are rarely present on abdominal examination. Progressive abdominal distension and failure to thrive are noted, and ascites becomes gradually more prominent. The accumulation of ascites may be accompanied by vomiting, perhaps due to compression of the second part of the duodenum. The ascites can also cause inguinal swellings and hydroceles due to fluid collections within the peritoneal sacs of the processi vaginales. Bile staining of the inguinal and scrotal regions is pathognomonic of biliary ascites. This sign may also be seen around the umbilicus (Figure 11.1).

Secondary bile duct stenosis

Intraperitoneal bile causes a severe inflammatory reaction in the porta hepatis which can result in stenosis or complete occlusion of the bile duct. Chardot et al. (1996) described five cases in which stenotic lesions of the bile ducts were associated with perforations, and which required biliary tract reconstruction. Davenport et al. (1996) also described two infants who presented at 10 weeks and 24 weeks of age, respectively, with obstructive jaundice and dilatation of the intrahepatic ducts.

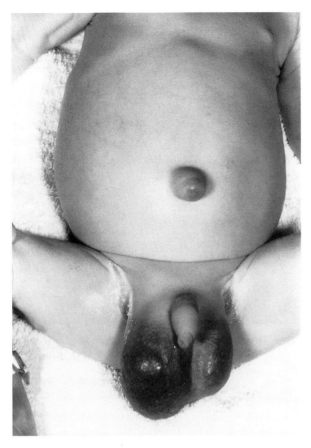

Figure 11.1 *A 5-week-old infant with bile staining of the umbilicus and scrotum. Biliary ascites had accumulated within hydrocele sacs. (Reproduced from Howard et al. (1976) with the permission of the publisher.)*

mal range (Lilly *et al.*, 1974) or moderately elevated. A neutrophil leukocytosis is usual.

The stability of most infants, apart from the uncommon cases who present with generalized peritonitis, allows time for investigation. This should include abdominal ultrasonography, which may demonstrate loculated collections of bile as complex echogenic masses around the common bile duct and within the lesser sac (Figure 11.2). Ascites may also be identified by

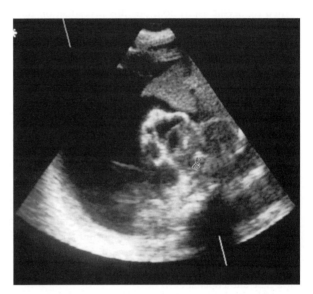

Figure 11.2 *Ultrasound image of 16-week-old infant showing a complex cystic collection of fluid around the common bile duct caused by a spontaneous perforation of the bile duct.*

Laparotomy in both cases revealed collections of inspissated bile surrounding occluded segments of the common bile ducts. The bile had leaked from the typical site of bile duct perforation at the junction of the cystic and common bile ducts. Both cases had an uncomplicated postoperative course after primary reconstruction with hepaticojejunostomies.

Antenatal diagnosis

A fourth presentation should be added to the Chardot classification. Chilukuri *et al.* (1990) described an ultrasonographic observation of ascites at 25 weeks of pregnancy. A hepatic excretion nuclide scan soon after birth, at 32 weeks' gestation, demonstrated a bile leak into the peritoneal cavity which was confirmed at laparotomy. Recovery followed a simple drainage procedure.

DIAGNOSIS

Jaundice is of the conjugated type, with pale stools and dark urine. Liver enzymes may be either within the nor-

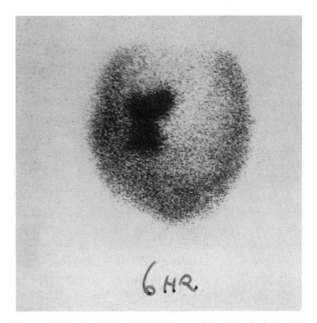

Figure 11.3 *An abdominal scintiscan of the infant illustrated in Figure 11.2 6 hours after an intravenous injection of radionuclide (DISIDA). There is a dense area of radioactivity below the liver (region of the common bile duct). Radioactivity throughout the abdomen confirms the diagnosis of a bile duct perforation.*

means of ultrasound scanning. Radionuclide hepatobiliary scanning using agents such as technetium-99m-labeled di-isopropyl iminodiacetic acid (DISIDA) demonstrate zones of persistent radioactivity around the common bile duct, as well as generalized abdominal radioactivity caused by leakage of bile into the general peritoneal cavity (Figure 11.3). The radionuclide investigation is extremely useful for confirming the diagnosis (Haller *et al.*, 1989).

The biliary nature of any ascites may also be confirmed by needle aspiration, but this investigation does have the risk of introducing infection into the peritoneal cavity.

MANAGEMENT

Laparotomy is mandatory as soon as a diagnosis of bile duct perforation has been confirmed. All cases of non-surgical management have resulted in death of the patients (Lilly *et al.*, 1974).

The perforation may be immediately apparent at laparotomy, but it may be hidden by an inflammatory mass extending from the top of the porta hepatis to the duodenum, which can form a type of pseudocyst. The thin capsule of such a pseudocyst must not be mistaken for a true choledochal cyst.

Careful dissection into the mass allows identification of the common bile duct and a biliary leak from either the cystic duct or the common bile duct (Figure 11.4). An 'on-table' cholangiogram via the gallbladder, which may be thick-walled from secondary inflammation, will help in this identification, and will also demonstrate patency or occlusion of the distal common bile duct.

Distal bile duct obstruction is caused by inspissated bile, and in many cases the obstruction will clear spontaneously a variable time after the episode of bile duct perforation. Bile duct obstruction was demonstrated in 15 of the 53 cases collected by Lilly *et al.* (1974), but normal drainage was eventually established without surgical exploration of the distal bile duct. The authors concluded from this data that simple drainage and antibiotics might be the treatment of choice, and that 'more complicated procedures such as t-tube drainage, common duct exploration and dilatation, suture repair, or intestinal anastomoses are unnecessary and probably foolhardy'. However, as was mentioned above, one of their own cases who was treated with cholecystostomy and simple drainage of the subhepatic space developed a prolonged bile leak and died after a second operation, and a further case who was treated with simple drainage developed a bile leak which lasted for 5 weeks (Megison and Votteler, 1992).

Spigland *et al.* (1996) reported a case of perforation in whom there was a relative narrowing of the distal bile duct which resulted in a persistent bile leak. A Roux-

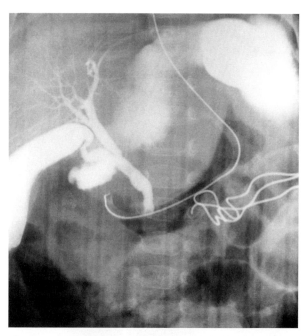

Figure 11.4 *Operative cholangiogram of the infant illustrated in Figure 11.1, showing perforation at the cystic duct insertion, with contrast leaking into the lesser sac.*

en-Y reconstruction was necessary at a second operation, and the authors emphasized the dangers of using simple drainage as the definitive treatment for all cases of spontaneous perforation. They advised that simple drainage should only be used when there is no distal bile duct obstruction, and that hepaticojejunostomy should be considered if a stricture is demonstrated.

The reports of spontaneous bile duct perforation describe a varied surgical approach to the problem, although the rationale for the choice of procedure is not always clear. Chardot *et al.* (1996), with a relatively wide experience of 10 cases, performed cholecystectomy for cystic duct perforation in two infants, simple drainage of the common bile duct in three cases, and biliary reconstruction in five cases. Despite this selective approach, two of the infants died and four developed complications which included cholangitis, prolonged bile leaks and portal vein thrombosis. Five infants underwent secondary surgery on the biliary tract, including three major reconstructions. Portal vein thrombosis as a complication of bile duct perforation has also been reported by Moore (1975).

Suggested plan of management

It is now clear that spontaneous perforation of the biliary tract is not always the benign condition suggested in some single case reports, and the following plan of management is suggested.

INITIAL PROCEDURES

- Laparotomy in all cases.
- Intraoperative cholangiogram through gallbladder.
- Confirmation of site of perforation.
- Confirmation of either free flow of contrast into duodenum or obstruction of distal bile duct.

DEFINITIVE SURGERY

Patent duct with free flow to duodenum

- Cholecystectomy for cystic duct perforation.
- Suture of small perforations in bile duct or cholecystostomy and simple drainage.
- T-tube insertion into large perforations of the common bile duct (Figure 11.5).

Obstructed bile duct

- Passage of fine catheter into obstructed bile duct with flushing to remove bile plug.
- Bile duct suture and/or simple drainage after cholangiographic confirmation of clearance of the obstruction.
- Cholecystostomy if duct remains obstructed.

Bile duct stricture

- Primary hepaticojejunostomy for chronic strictures and minimal inflammatory change.
- Secondary hepaticojejunostomy for strictures demonstrated after preliminary cholecystostomy.

SUMMARY

Perforation of the common bile duct should always be considered in a young infant who develops jaundice after an initial anicteric period of good health, or who presents with ascites and peritonitis. Surgery is mandatory after appropriate investigations, and the technique should take into account the obstructed or unobstructed condition of the bile duct.

Key references

Chardot C, Iskandarani F, De Dreuzy O *et al.* Spontaneous perforation of the biliary tract in infancy: a series of 11 cases. *European Journal of Paediatric Surgery* 1996; **6**: 341–6.

A total of 11 patients, 10 of whom underwent surgery, are reviewed. This paper is useful for its illustration of the wide range of clinical presentations which may be encountered in this condition, and the rationale and complications of surgery.

Johnston JH. Spontaneous perforation of the common bile duct in infancy. *British Journal of Surgery* 1961; **48**: 532–3.

This is a very clear early report of the typical site of perforation at the junction of the cystic and common bile ducts. The author describes the typical clinical presentation, comments on the low mortality rate after surgical intervention, and discusses the possible role of raised pressure in the biliary tract in etiology.

Lilly JR, Weintraub WH, Altman RP. Spontaneous perforation of the extrahepatic bile ducts and bile peritonitis in infancy. *Surgery* 1974; **75**: 664–73.

This is a major review of 53 reported cases recorded up until 1974. The case details are summarized and provide useful details of treatment and outcome. Most perforations occurred between 4 and 17 weeks of life.

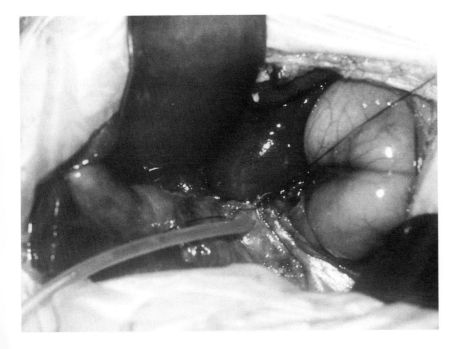

Figure 11.5 *Operative photograph of a large perforation in the common bile duct which has been intubated with a T-tube.*

REFERENCES

Ando H, Ito T, Watanabe Y, Seo T, Kaneko K, Nagaya M. Spontaneous perforation of choledochal cyst. *Journal of the American College of Surgeons* 1995; **181**: 125–8.

Carubelli CM, Abramo TJ. Abdominal distension and shock in an infant. *American Journal of Emergency Medicine* 1999; **17**: 342–4.

Caulfield E. Bile peritonitis in infancy. *American Journal of Diseases in Children* 1936; **52**: 1348–60.

Chardot C, Iskandarani F, De Dreuzy O *et al.* Spontaneous perforation of the biliary tract in infancy: a series of 11 cases. *European Journal of Pediatric Surgery* 1996; **6**: 341–6.

Chilukuri S, Bonet V, Cobb M. Antenatal spontaneous perforation of the extrahepatic biliary tree. *American Journal of Obstetrics and Gynecology* 1990; **163**: 1201–2.

Davenport M, Saxena R, Howard ER. Acquired biliary atresia. *Journal of Pediatric Surgery* 1996; **31**: 1721–3.

Dolgin SE, Levine RL, Norton KI, Marolda JR, Parles JG, LeLeiko NS. Complete spontaneous disruption of the common bile duct: a late complication of necrotizing enterocolitis? *Journal of Pediatric Gastroenterology and Nutrition* 1991; **12**: 379–82.

Donahoe PK, Hendren WH. Bile duct perforation in a newborn with stenosis of the ampulla. *Journal of Pediatric Surgery* 1976; **11**: 823–5.

Donald JW, Ozent ED. Spontaneous perforation of bile ducts. *American Surgeon* 1977; **43**: 524–7.

Fitzgerald RJ, Parbhoo K, Guiney EJ. Spontaneous perforation of the bile ducts in neonates. *Surgery* 1978; **83**: 303–5.

Haller JO, Condon VR, Berdon WE *et al.* Spontaneous perforation of the common bile duct in children. *Radiology* 1989; **172**: 621–4.

Hammoudi SM, Alauddin A. Idiopathic perforation of the biliary tract in infancy and childhood. *Journal of Pediatric Surgery* 1988; **23**: 185–7.

Hindmarsh FD. Bile peritonitis in infancy. *British Medical Journal* 1947; **2**: 131.

Howard ER, Johnston DI, Mowat AP. Spontaneous perforation of common bile duct in infants. *Archives of Disease in Childhood* 1976; **51**: 883–6.

Ibanez DV, Vila JJ, Fernandez MS, Guemes I, Gutierrez C, Garcia-Sala C. Spontaneous biliary perforation and necrotizing enterocolitis. *Pediatric Surgery International* 1999; **15**: 401–2.

Johnston JH. Spontaneous perforation of the common bile duct in infancy. *British Journal of Surgery* 1961; **48**: 532–3.

Lees W, Mitchell JE. Bile peritonitis in infancy. *Archives of Disease in Childhood* 1966; **41**: 188–92.

Lilly JR, Weintraub WH, Altman RP. Spontaneous perforation of the extrahepatic bile ducts and bile peritonitis in infancy. *Surgery* 1974; **75**: 664–73.

Megison SM, Votteler TP. Management of common bile duct obstruction associated with spontaneous perforation of the biliary tree. *Surgery* 1992; **111**: 237–9.

Moore TC. Massive bile peritonitis in infancy due to spontaneous perforation with portal vein occlusion. *Journal of Pediatric Surgery* 1975; **10**: 537–8.

Narasimhan KL, Shailinderjit S, Katariya S, Rao KLN, Mitra SK. Repair of bile duct perforation by omental onlay. *Pediatric Surgery International* 1993; **8**: 507–8.

Ohkawa H, Takahashi H, Maie M. A malformation of the pancreatico-biliary system as a cause of perforation of the biliary tract in childhood. *Journal of Pediatric Surgery* 1977; **12**: 541–6.

Pettersson G. Spontaneous perforation of the common bile duct in infants. *Acta Chirurgica Scandinavica* 1955; **60**: 192–201.

Prabakaran S, Kumaran N, Regunanthan SR, Prasad N, Sridharan S. Spontaneous biliary perforation in a child with features of Ivemark syndrome. *Pediatric Surgery International* 2000; **16**: 109–10.

Spigland N, Greco R, Rosenfeld D. Spontaneous biliary perforation: does external drainage constitute adequate therapy? *Journal of Pediatric Surgery* 1996; **31**: 782–4.

Stringal G, Mercer S. Idiopathic perforation of the biliary tract in infancy. *Journal of Pediatrics* 1983; **18**: 546–50.

Tan CEL, Moscoso GJ. The developing human biliary system at the porta hepatis level between 29 days and 8 weeks of gestation: a way to understanding biliary atresia. Part 1. *Pathology International* 1994; **44**: 587–99.

Witcombe JB. *Ascaris* perforation of the common bile duct demonstrated by intravenous cholangiography. *Pediatric Radiology* 1978; **19**: 124–5.

12

Benign extrahepatic bile duct obstruction and cholestatic syndromes

EDWARD R HOWARD

Inspissated bile within the lower third of the common bile duct presents as obstructive jaundice in infants, either within or just beyond the neonatal period. It is the commonest of the many causes of pediatric bile duct obstruction, and is also known as the bile plug syndrome. Older children may present with biliary obstruction from a variety of benign strictures, or from compression by extraductal pathology such as lymph node enlargement.

The majority of the many causes of bile duct obstruction reported in infants and children are summarized in Box 12.1 (the list excludes biliary atresia, which is considered in Chapter 8).

EMBRYOLOGICAL MALFORMATIONS

Cholecystohepatic duct represents a rare variant of bile duct anatomy in which the common hepatic duct drains directly into the cystic duct or the gallbladder. The common bile duct is therefore absent and the gallbladder drains to the duodenum via a relatively small and inefficient cystic duct (Figure 12.1). The abnormality has been described in two children (one male and one female) who presented with obstructive jaundice at 3 and 4 years of age, respectively. Both of the children had previously undergone successful correction of esophageal atresia. The obstructive jaundice was relieved by hepaticojejunostomy after gallbladder excision (Redkar *et al.*,

1999). Another variant of this type of abnormality was described by Schorlemmer *et al.* (1984) in a 5-year-old girl who was shown to have multiple irregular cholecystohepatic communications from the undersurface of the liver draining directly into the gallbladder. The right and left hepatic ducts were absent in this case.

A non-symptomatic and commoner abnormality consists of accessory cholecystohepatic ductules (of Luschka) which drain a portion of the liver parenchyma directly into the gallbladder (Foster and Wayson, 1962). The abnormality was found in 0.9% of 1410 cholecystectomies in adults in whom the hepatic and bile ducts were normal (Champetier *et al.*, 1991).

These embryological abnormalities may be the result of a disordered pattern of growth of the gallbladder and the extrahepatic bile ducts when they develop from the foregut diverticulum.

INTRALUMINAL OBSTRUCTION

Inspissated bile plug syndrome (FIGURE 12.2)

Early reports included that of Ladd (1935), who described five infants with obstructive jaundice. At laparotomy they were found to have a mechanical obstruction caused by plugs of thickened bile. Ladd suggested that the condition was secondary to distal common bile duct stenosis. Hsia *et al.* (1952) investigated

Box 12.1 *Causes of extrahepatic bile duct obstruction in pediatric practice*

Embryological malformation
   Cholecystohepatic duct

Intraluminal obstruction
   Inspissated bile plug syndrome
   Ascariasis

Inflammatory strictures
   Common pancreaticobiliary channels
   Idiopathic
   Post-radiotherapy
   Sclerosing cholangitis
   Recurrent pyogenic cholangitis
   Association with gastroschisis
   Following spontaneous perforation
   Gastric heterotopy

Traumatic strictures
   Blunt abdominal trauma
   Liver transplantation

Extramural compression
   Lymph nodes
   Duodenal malformation
   Pancreatic tumors
   Hydronephrosis
   Neuroblastoma
   Duodenal polyps
   Peritoneal (Ladd's) bands

Miscellaneous
   Foreign body (nasoenteric tube)
   Periportal varices
   Bile duct ischemia
   Cystic fibrosis

156 infants with obstructive jaundice, of whom 60% had biliary atresia. Inspissated bile plug syndrome was diagnosed in 15% of the cases in association with erythroblastosis fetalis and in a further 19% with no obvious etiological factor. The authors suggested that the syndrome was caused by a combination of factors which included small bile ducts, hepatic immaturity and dehydration.

In early reports, inspissated bile within the common bile duct in early infancy was particularly associated with hemolysis secondary to blood group incompatibility (Oppe and Valaes, 1959; Dunn, 1963; Lightwood and Bodian, 1973), and it was more common before the introduction of exchange transfusion.

Recent reports suggest a relationship between neonatal gallstone formation and diuretic therapy (Whitington and Black, 1980), parenteral nutrition (Matos *et al.*, 1987), bowel dysfunction (Benjamin, 1982), disseminated intravascular coagulopathy (Gur *et al.*, 1986) and cystic fibrosis (Davies *et al.*, 1986). Parenteral nutrition has been a causative factor and has been implicated in cholestasis (Rodgers *et al.*, 1976), bile plug syndrome (Enzenauer *et al.*, 1985), biliary sludge (Bowen, 1984) and gallstones (Roslyn *et al.*, 1983). A prospective ultrasound study of neonates receiving total parenteral nutrition identified biliary sludge in 44% of cases and discrete stones in 5% (Schirmer *et al.*, 1989). Viscid bile may also be produced by an increase in bilirubin load after multiple transfusions, dehydration and impaired hepatic bile secretion (Bernstein *et al.*, 1969). Lilly and Sokol (1985) considered that neonatal common bile duct obstruction in the absence of any of these factors was unusual. Congenital cystic dilatations of the common bile duct may also become obstructed with inspissated bile. Germiller *et al.* (1997) reported a neonatal case of choledochal cyst which presented with obstructive jaundice secondary to bile duct obstruction. Ultrasound showed a

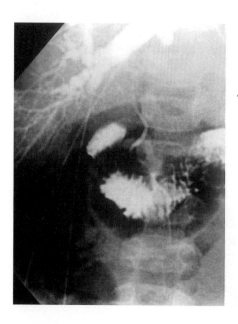 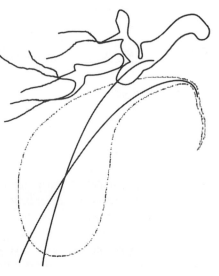

Figure 12.1 *Cholecystohepatic duct. Intraoperative cholangiogram in a 3-year-old boy who presented with obstructive jaundice. The diagram illustrates the manner in which two catheters were inserted into the biliary tract. One catheter passes through a cholecystohepatic duct into the proximal bile ducts, which are filled with contrast. The second catheter passes through the cystic duct to opacify the duodenum.*

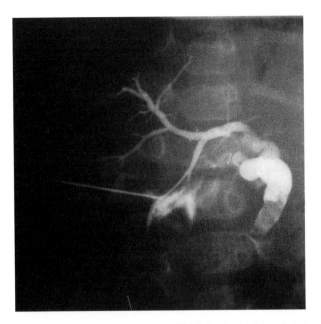

Figure 12.2 *Fine-needle cholangiography in a 3-month-old infant showing inspissated bile in the lower common bile duct.*

mass of material within a 2.0-cm cyst which cleared spontaneously within 5 days. Occasionally it may be difficult to differentiate congenital bile duct dilatation from simple dilatation secondary to an obstruction. Follow-up scans are essential in these cases after removal of the obstructing material.

Heaton *et al.* (1991) described nine male infants who presented with obstructive jaundice at between 2 weeks and 6 months of age. Seven cases were affected by viscid bile and two had gallstones.

DIAGNOSIS

Inspissated bile syndrome or the rarer gallstone obstruction in the neonatal period may be difficult to differentiate from the commoner condition of biliary atresia. Jaundice and acholic stools are typical of both conditions, and liver function tests show an obstructive picture with raised levels of conjugated bilirubin, alkaline phosphatase and gamma-glutamyl transferase.

When severe inspissated bile obstruction is present, radionuclide scans may show an absence of hepatic excretion, leading to further confusion with atresia. However, the diagnosis can be confirmed with ultrasonography which reveals a dilated proximal biliary tree in association with biliary sludge or stones. Endoscopic retrograde cholangiopancreatography (ERCP) is now possible in the youngest infants and is very useful for confirmation of the diagnosis of inspissated bile syndrome. Occasionally, however, patients with suspected biliary atresia are found to have inspissated bile syndrome at laparotomy. The diagnosis is confirmed with an operative cholangiogram performed via the gallbladder, which is dilated with thick bile.

TREATMENT

Inspissated bile may disappear spontaneously in the neonatal period (Keller *et al.*, 1985), and some dilatation of the gallbladder with bile-sludging has been recorded in up to 30% of sick neonates on ultrasound scans. Milder forms of obstruction may be cleared by percutaneous, transhepatic irrigation of the bile ducts or by retrograde irrigation during an ERCP examination. Brown (1990) has described successful irrigation of the bile duct at surgery with the mucolytic agent *N*-acetylcysteine, which has been used for 25 years to reduce the viscosity of pulmonary mucus. Persistent bile duct obstruction is treated surgically with either saline irrigation of the common bile duct or, occasionally, with duodenotomy, ampullary sphincterotomy and removal of any impacted mass of pigment (Lilly, 1980). The range of treatments described in the report by Heaton *et al.* (1991) is summarized in Table 12.1.

Parasitic obstruction – ascariasis

Infection with the roundworm, *Ascaris lumbricoides*, is a worldwide problem and is particularly common in Africa, Asia and Central America. Poor environment and heavy contamination of soil in rural areas can result in infestation in 60–70% of the pediatric population (Louw, 1966).

Adult roundworms live within the small bowel, where the fertilized female produces several thousand eggs each day. The eggs are passed in the feces and continue their

Table 12.1 *Operative findings and treatment of 9 cases of inspissated bile syndrome (Heaton et al., 1991)*

Case	Operative findings	Procedure
1	Nil	Spontaneous resolution
2	Dilated common bile duct + cholecystitis	Cholecystectomy + T-tube
3	Dilated common bile duct	Cholecystectomy, sphincteroplasty + T-tube
4	Dilated common bile duct	T-tube
5	Dilated common bile duct	Cholecystectomy + saline flush
6	Hepatic hemangioma and dilated bile duct	Cholecystostomy + saline flush
7	Dilated common bile duct	Choledochoduodenostomy + sphincteroplasty
8	Stones in gallbladder and common bile duct	Cholecystectomy + sphincteroplasty
9	Stones in common bile duct	Cholecystectomy+ T-tube + sphincteroplasty

maturation in the soil. Poor hygiene is responsible for onward transmission by swallowing. The ova hatch in the duodenum of the new host to produce larvae which penetrate the gut wall. They reach the pulmonary circulation via the portal venous system and the liver. Further maturation in the lungs is followed by larval migration into the trachea and the esophagus before further maturation in the small bowel. The adult worm lives approximately 2 years and reaches up to 30 cm in length. Invasion of the common bile duct may occur in patients who have large numbers of worms within the duodenum. However, only a portion of a worm may lie within the biliary tract, with the remainder protruding into the duodenum and obstructing the ampulla of Vater. A review of more than 1000 pediatric cases (Davies and Rode, 1982) revealed biliary ascariasis in 424 cases, and the authors recommended that all children presenting with pain in association with intestinal ascariasis should have investigations of the biliary tract. Approximately 5% of the children developed complications, which included pyogenic cholangitis, perforation of the bile duct, cholecystitis and pancreatitis.

An intrahepatic abscess may arise after impaction of a worm within the intrahepatic ducts (Lloyd, 1982). The abscess may eventually rupture into the peritoneal cavity or through the diaphragm (Chang and Han, 1966; Lloyd, 1981).

A diagnosis of ascariasis can always be confirmed by examination of the stools. There may also be a history of vomiting worms or of passing the parasites in the stools.

Biliary symptoms include upper abdominal pain with localized signs of peritonitis in the right hypochondrium. Jaundice is not usually present in uncomplicated cases, although the gallbladder may be palpable.

Ultrasound confirms the gallbladder distension, and endoscopy may show worms within the duodenum and across the ampulla. However, the symptoms may settle spontaneously and endoscopy is therefore not usually advised unless the child fails to respond to more conservative treatment (Khuroo et al., 1993).

The onset of acute suppurative cholangitis is recognized by the onset of high fever, jaundice and tender hepatomegaly. Investigations show a leukocytosis and deranged liver function tests typical of obstructive jaundice. Pain referred to the back is suggestive of acute pancreatitis, and was reported in many of the pediatric cases described by Louw (1966).

The conservative management of uncomplicated cases consists of analgesics, antispasmodics, intravenous fluids and nasogastric decompression. This treatment will result in worms returning to the duodenum in 98% of affected children (Chang and Han, 1966; Louw, 1966). Anthelmintics (e.g. piperazine below 2 years of age and mebendazole for older children) are prescribed, and are repeated at 2-monthly intervals to prevent reinfestation. Endoscopy with ERCP is recommended if symptoms persist beyond 2 weeks.

Surgical extraction of worms via a choledochotomy has been reported in approximately 20% of cases (Wani and Chrungoo, 1992). All worms are identified by intraoperative cholangiography, and after worm extraction the bile duct is closed around a T-tube which allows postoperative cholangiography and irrigation to remove any residual fragments of worms.

In a series of 500 ascariasis patients of all ages, 171 cases had biliary, 40 cases had hepatic, eight had gallbladder and seven had pancreatic infestation. Five clinical presentations were recognized, namely cholecystitis, cholangitis, biliary colic, pancreatitis and hepatic abscess. Endoscopic removal of worms from the ampullary orifice led to rapid relief from biliary colic and pancreatitis. During a follow-up period of 48 months, 76 patients had worm reinvasion of the biliary tract (Khuroo et al., 1990).

BENIGN STRICTURES

As in adults, a wide variety of pathological processes can affect the wall of the extrahepatic bile ducts and result in stricture formation. These are mostly traumatic and inflammatory processes, but occasionally the bile duct may be compressed or infiltrated by tumor.

Inflammatory strictures

COMMON PANCREATICOBILIARY CHANNELS

The association of common pancreaticobiliary channels with stricture formation in the bile duct has been discussed in relation to choledochal cyst in Chapter 10. The strictures occur just proximal to the junction of the pancreatic and common bile ducts, and are associated with high concentrations of pancreatic enzymes in the bile. Amylase concentrations in these cases are often greater than 100 000 U/L (Tan and Howard, 1988). The diagnosis is usually clear on ERCP, and the recommended treatment is disconnection of the bile duct and hepaticojejunostomy. The gallbladder is often thickened in these cases, and cholecystectomy is also advised.

IDIOPATHIC

Standfield et al. (1989) described 12 patients with benign non-traumatic strictures of the extrahepatic bile ducts, which were mostly misdiagnosed as bile duct tumors before surgery. Four of these cases occurred in children aged 1.5, 6, 13 and 15 years, and all of them underwent Roux-en-Y reconstruction hepaticojejunostomy (Figures 12.3 and 12.4). Bowles et al. (2001) reported the long-term results of treatment in seven children (six girls and one boy) who were aged from 2.5 to 15 years. Two of the cases had been included in the earlier paper of Standfield et al. (1989). All of the children underwent

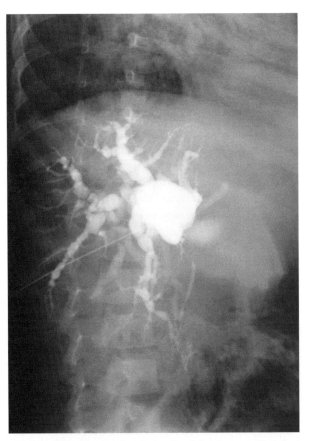

Figure 12.3 *Fine-needle cholangiography in a male infant aged 2.5 years with conjugated hyperbilirubinemia. The cholangiogram shows a tight common hepatic duct stricture which was histologically benign. Hepaticojejunostomy was curative.*

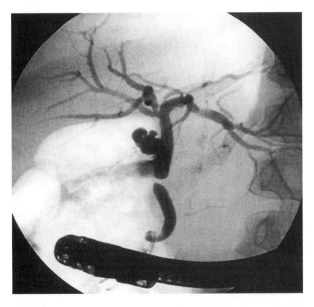

Figure 12.4 *ERCP in a 4.5-year-old girl who presented with obstructive jaundice. A short stricture is seen in the mid common bile duct. Histology of the resected stricture showed an inflammatory stricture with fibrosis in the wall of the duct. This is an example of a benign inflammatory stricture of unknown origin (described as 'idiopathic').*

biliary–enteric anastomosis, and five had resection of the stricture. All of the patients were well 1 to 17 years after the initial referral.

The etiology of the lesions remains unknown, but they are characterized by four histological features, namely chronic inflammation of the bile duct wall, loss of epithelium (sometimes with extensive ulceration), fibrosis immediately below the bile duct epithelium, and changes in the epithelium (which show hyperplastic and regenerative features).

Of these four main features, at least three were present in each case in both the paper by Standfield *et al.* (1989) and that by Bowles *et al.* (2001).

The mucosal ulceration suggests an etiology distinct from sclerosing cholangitis, a condition in which the epithelium remains intact. Sclerosing cholangitis is also associated with multiple strictures, which were not seen in these cases. Long-term follow-up of the patients showed that they remained well, without any evidence of recurrent stricture formation. Verbeek *et al.* (1992) described a further nine cases of idiopathic bile duct stricturing with ulceration in patients aged 23 to 72 years.

In summary, isolated benign inflammatory bile duct strictures of unknown etiology appear to represent a definite entity, which can affect both adults and children, and the long-term outcome after surgical excision appears to be excellent.

RADIOTHERAPY

Late irradiation injury resulting in strictures of the common bile duct has been described in two cases 10 years after abdominal radiotherapy for malignant lymphoma (Cherqui *et al.*, 1994). Both patients underwent successful hepaticojejunostomy, and histology confirmed late irradiation injury.

A further child was referred to King's College Hospital at the age of 5 years with a history of severe jaundice for 2 months. She had been treated previously for acute leukemia with cytotoxic therapy, with a good response, but had since relapsed and showed evidence of disease in the central nervous system. She was therefore given a course of radiotherapy which included the spinal column. Soon after completion of this treatment she became jaundiced. Investigations showed complete obstruction of the common bile duct, and at surgery there was severe inflammatory change around the extrahepatic bile ducts, with complete destruction of the distal two-thirds of the common bile duct. Treatment with hepaticojejunostomy resulted in complete resolution of the jaundice. The onset of jaundice coincided with the radiotherapy treatment, and no other cause of the bile duct destruction could be identified.

SCLEROSING CHOLANGITIS

Spivak *et al.* (1982) reported a 4-year-old boy who presented with a common bile duct stricture which required a cholecystjejunostomy for relief of jaundice. One year after surgery, an ERCP confirmed further changes suggestive of primary sclerosing cholangitis with multiple segmental dilatations and constrictions of the biliary tree. It was noted that the patient did not show any evidence of inflammatory bowel disease, and the authors compared this with a previous case report of a child aged 10 years who had developed sclerosing cholangitis in association with Crohn's disease (Werlin et al., 1980). Surgery may be used to bypass the extrahepatic bile duct strictures, but it has little influence on the course of the disease.

El-Shabrawi et al. (1987) described 13 children with sclerosing cholangitis, only nine of whom had clinical features of chronic inflammatory bowel disease. One of the children developed a localized stricture of the distal common bile duct, but none of them underwent surgery. The lack of an association with inflammatory bowel disease was also noted in 24% of 78 cases reviewed by Sisto et al. (1987), although ulcerative colitis was diagnosed in 47% of the series.

Neither liver function tests nor histology is a reliable diagnostic predictors, and cholangiography is essential for establishing the diagnosis.

RECURRENT PYOGENIC CHOLANGITIS (ORIENTAL CHOLANGIO-HEPATITIS)

This condition, which has a wide distribution in South-East Asia (see Chapter 24), affects patients of all ages, and 3% of those affected are teenagers. Enteric organisms are responsible for cholangitis within intrahepatic cholangioles, and this eventually leads to the secondary formation of bilirubinate stones within the bile ducts. The patients may also develop strictures of the extrahepatic bile duct. Saing et al. (1988), in a review of 10 children aged 3 to 12 years, described one or more strictures in the right, left and common hepatic ducts. The authors emphasized that stricture formation is an important feature of pyogenic cholangitis, and that surgical treatment ranging from emergency choledochotomy and T-tube drainage to stricture resection and hepaticojejunostomy may be required for the relief of biliary obstruction. Intraoperative choledochoscopy is a useful aid to the complete removal of all intraductal stones. The effects of periampullary strictures may be relieved by transduodenal sphincteroplasty.

STRICTURE ASSOCIATED WITH GASTROSCHISIS

A single case report describes obstructive jaundice in a 3-week-old female child (Hancock et al., 1989). Ultrasound at 14 weeks of age showed biliary dilatation, and a percutaneous cholangiogram demonstrated complete occlusion of the common bile duct just distal to the insertion of the cystic duct. The child had previously been treated for a gastroschisis complicated by intestinal fistulae. The etiology of the stricture was unknown, and it was treated by percutaneous dilatation, which included three episodes of

balloon dilatation, and an indwelling catheter was left *in situ* for 8 months. The stricture resolved and at 2 years of age the patient was reported to be well and free of jaundice. Percutaneous cholangiography is a well-established technique of investigation in children (Howard and Nunnerley, 1979), and the value of extending this to the performance of biliary tract dilatation has been emphasized by Gallacher et al. (1985), who reported balloon dilatation and percutaneous stenting of a 4-year-old child who had suffered an injury to the common hepatic duct during surgery. They also reported dilatation of a hepaticojejunostomy stricture in an 11-year-old girl who had previously undergone surgery for choledochal cyst.

STRICTURE FOLLOWING SPONTANEOUS PERFORATION

Complete obliteration of the lumen of the common bile duct following spontaneous perforation (two cases) and surgical correction of duodenal atresia has been described in three infants aged between 8 and 24 weeks (Davenport et al., 1996). All three cases had uncomplicated recoveries after reconstruction of their biliary tracts, and their liver function tests rapidly returned to normal.

GASTRIC HETEROTOPY

Martinez-Urrutia et al. (1990) described the case of a 12-year-old girl who was admitted with jaundice, hepatomegaly and tenderness in the right hypochondrium. Percutaneous cholangiography showed an obstruction at the junction of the cystic and common bile ducts, and laparotomy revealed extensive fibrosis around the biliary tract. Hepaticoduodenostomy was performed and the gallbladder was removed. Histology showed heterotopic gastric epithelium in the gallbladder neck and adjacent bile duct, with fibrosis of the latter. At least three previous reports of this condition have been recorded (Whitaker et al., 1967; Curtis and Sheaham, 1969; Keramidis et al., 1977).

ISCHEMIA

Ischemic damage to the bile duct, resulting in stricture formation, was reported in a 19-month-old boy who had undergone right hepatectomy for a mesenchymal hamartoma of the liver (Takehara et al., 1992). The child presented with signs of stricture formation 10 months after the original operation.

TRAUMATIC STRICTURES

Blunt abdominal trauma (FIGURE 12.5)

Extrahepatic bile duct damage following blunt abdominal trauma in childhood is rare. It may occur in association with lacerations of the liver (Ahmed, 1976; Moulton et al.,

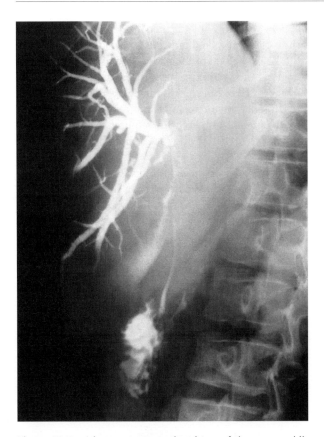

Figure 12.5 *A long post-traumatic stricture of the common bile duct in a 14-year-old girl who had sustained hepatobiliary trauma. The right duct system is obstructed above the stricture. The left hepatic duct is occluded.*

1993) or as an isolated injury (Rohatgi and Gupta, 1987). The latter case concerned a 10-year-old boy who fell on to the handlebars of a bicycle. Signs of generalized abdominal tenderness developed over the next 24 hours, but abdominal distension was not noted until the fifth day post injury. The onset of physical signs was insidious, but laparotomy 12 days after injury revealed complete transection of the bile duct, which was successfully treated by choledochojejunostomy. The first description of bile duct transection after blunt trauma in a child was probably given by Battle (1894) in a report of a 6-year-old boy. Bourque *et al.* (1989) reviewed 13 other cases of bile duct injury collected from the pediatric literature, and added a new case involving a complete transection of the common bile duct in a 3-year-old boy who had sustained an abdominal injury during a sledging accident. The authors emphasized that diagnosis may be difficult and that the presentation includes both free bile in the abdomen (Pandit *et al.*, 2000) and loculated collections. The average age at presentation in the series was 5 years, and the lesion (which occurred four times more frequently in boys than in girls) was usually secondary to a crush injury of the abdomen. Around 60% of the injuries were in the retroduodenal area, which reflects the experience in adults.

Non-infective bile is innocuous, and the clinical progress of the patient is often as chronic as it is in spontaneous perforation of the bile ducts in infancy (see Chapter 11). The patient develops a mild jaundice and low-grade fever, and abdominal examination may reveal free intraperitoneal fluid. Endoscopic cholangiography, ultrasonography and excretion radionuclide scintigraphy are useful for diagnosis.

The mortality rate of the series was 40%, but many of the patients had had either external drainage or primary end-to-end anastomosis of the damaged bile duct. The general acceptance of choledochoenterostomy has improved the results dramatically, and mortality from isolated injuries is now very rare.

Liver transplantation

Strictures of donor–recipient biliary anastomoses are not uncommon after transplantation, and occur in approximately 10% of pediatric patients. Strictures may not be recognized until more than a year after surgery, although the majority present with jaundice or cholangitis within a few months. Many are ischemic in origin and may be associated with hepatic artery thrombosis. Treatment may be achieved with percutaneous dilatation or revisional surgery. The complications of liver transplantation and their management are described in Chapter 30.

EXTRAMURAL BILE DUCT COMPRESSION

Extrahepatic bile ducts may be compressed by enlargement of adjacent lymph nodes, and there are reports of obstructive jaundice secondary to reactive lymphadenitis (Cacciaguerra *et al.*, 1996) and to tuberculous infection (Delanoe *et al.*, 1993).

Obstruction of the extrahepatic bile ducts has also been reported in association with duodenal malformations (Reid, 1973), pancreatic hemangioendothelioma and hydronephrosis (Cook and Rickham, 1978), neuroblastoma (Gow *et al.*, 1995), intussusception from duodenal polyps (Gentile *et al.*, 1994), and Ladd's bands in chronic malrotation of the mid-gut (Spitz *et al.*, 1983). The latter patient, a 5-month-old girl, was treated by division of the compressing bands which allowed the common bile duct to dilate. The malrotation was corrected by a standard Ladd's procedure (Figure 12.6).

A duodenal fibrosarcoma (Shearman *et al.*, 1975), a carcinoma of the pancreas (Beck, 1957) and a hemangioendothelioma of the pancreas (Chappell, 1973) have been reported in infants, and all were treated with pancreaticoduodenectomy. Tunell (1976) described an alternative approach for hemangioma in a 3-month-old infant who presented with common bile duct and gastric obstruction. The lesion was managed with bypass

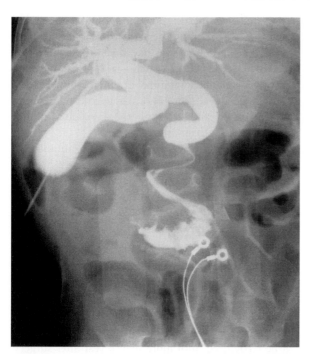

Figure 12.6   *Operative cholangiogram in a young infant with obstructive jaundice showing extrinsic compression and distortion of the common bile duct by peritoneal bands (Ladd's bands). Reproduced from Spitz* et al. *(1983) with kind permission of the author and the publisher.*

surgery accompanied by steroid therapy and radiotherapy. The mass had disappeared by 3 years of age, at which time the bypass was disconnected. A similar obstruction in a neonate caused by a hemolymphangioma has been treated at King's College Hospital. The mass and symptoms resolved spontaneously after a diagnostic laparotomy.

MISCELLANEOUS CAUSES OF STRICTURE FORMATION

Very rare causes of obstruction to the flow of bile in the common bile duct include a case of coiling of a nasoenteric feeding tube in the duodenum of a 4-year-old boy who had undergone cardiac surgery. The tube caused acute biliary tract obstruction and dilatation, with a rapid rise in bilirubin levels. The signs of obstruction resolved and the bilirubin level fell rapidly to normal after removal of the tube (Rinker *et al.*, 2000). Bile duct compression by periductal varices has also been reported in association with extrahepatic portal vein occlusion (Takehara *et al.*, 1992).

Gaskin *et al.* (1988) reported a high incidence of common bile duct strictures in patients who showed signs of liver disease associated with cystic fibrosis. Investigation with hepatobiliary scanning and cholangiography showed evidence of biliary tract obstruction in 96% of 50 cases who had obvious hepatomegaly, and strictures of the common bile duct were reported in the majority of these cases. Two of the patients had severe inflammatory strictures reminiscent of sclerosing cholangitis. A further case of severe stricturing, with histologically proven inflammatory change, was reported in a 17-year-old with cystic fibrosis who required hepaticojejunostomy for the relief of obstructive jaundice (Bilton *et al.*, 1990).

On the basis of these findings, Gaskin *et al.* (1988) suggested that the onset of cirrhosis in patients with cystic fibrosis might be related to bile duct stenosis, but this has not been confirmed in other reported cases with apparent bile duct narrowing (Strandvick *et al.*, 1988). Furthermore, a later investigation of 20 patients with cystic fibrosis and liver disease showed intrahepatic changes similar to those seen in sclerosing cholangitis, but no evidence of an abnormality in the extrahepatic bile ducts (O'Brien *et al.*, 1992).

In summary, it is apparent that a few patients with cystic fibrosis may develop inflammatory strictures of the bile duct. However, progressive intrahepatic cholestasis does not appear to be related to extrahepatic bile duct disease in the majority of cases.

SURGERY FOR CHOLESTATIC SYNDROMES

Conventional surgery has nothing to contribute to the relief of symptoms in the more common forms of infantile intrahepatic hepatocellular cholestasis, such as idiopathic neonatal hepatitis, alpha-1-antitrypsin deficiency, inborn errors of bile acid synthesis, sclerosing cholangitis, drugs or parenteral nutrition. However, prolonged biliary drainage has been shown to be effective in at least a proportion of children suffering from the form of persistent cholestasis known as Byler's disease, or progressive familial intrahepatic cholestasis (PFIC). Partial symptomatic relief has also been achieved with biliary diversion in a smaller number of cases of persistent cholestasis secondary to arteriohepatic dysplasia, or Alagille's syndrome (Gauderer and Boyle, 1997), although the latter application remains controversial (see Chapter 27).

Progressive familial intrahepatic cholestasis (PFIC)

Clayton *et al.* (1965) originally described this condition in Amish families who were descended from Jacob Byler – hence the term 'Byler's disease'. The condition is a severe intrahepatic cholestasis which commonly begins in the first few months of life and progresses to cirrhosis within the next 10–20 years.

The dominant clinical features include severe pruritus (which may lead to self-mutilation), jaundice, hepatomegaly and growth failure. Adolescent patients commonly show evidence of delayed sexual development. Secondary complications from the persistent cholestasis include fat-soluble vitamin deficiencies with rickets, osteopenia and hypoprothrombinemia, and neuropathy may be associated with vitamin E deficiency.

The progression from cholestasis within the first 12 months of life to fibrosis and cirrhosis results in death from liver failure. Death from hepatocellular carcinoma and from complications of liver transplantation has also been recorded (Whitington et al., 1992).

The underlying defect in PFIC is believed to be a defect in bile acid secretion. The condition is inherited in an autosomal-recessive pattern, and specific defects in the FIC1, BSEP and MDR3 genes have been identified as being responsible for distinct PFIC phenotypes of varying severity (Jacquemin, 2000).

DIAGNOSIS

A strikingly low serum gamma-glutamyl transpeptidase level differentiates PFIC from other cholestatic disorders of infancy (Whitington et al., 1994), although the levels of serum bilirubin and other liver enzymes are similar. Serum cholesterol levels also tend to be lower in PFIC than in other disorders, such as Alagille's syndrome and sclerosing cholangitis.

TREATMENT

The clinical features of pruritus and progressive liver disease are unresponsive to medical therapy with choleretic agents of bile-acid-binding substances such as cholestyramine. However, liver transplantation (see Chapter 27) has been used successfully since the 1980s to treat patients with progressive disease or established cirrhosis (Whitington and Balistreri, 1991), and has not been followed by recurrent disease.

A lesser procedure of permanent biliary diversion was suggested on the basis of the observation that retention of bile salts may lead to secondary hepatocyte damage and progressive liver damage. It was therefore proposed that diversion of bile from the gut might be effective in reducing the level of the bile acid pool, thereby reducing the clinical signs and preventing the progression of pathological change in the liver.

SURGICAL TECHNIQUES OF PARTIAL BILIARY DIVERSION

Jejunal conduit

The first cases to be treated by biliary diversion underwent a preliminary cholecystostomy to assess the effects of biliary drainage before proceeding to the more complex and permanent procedure (Emond and Whitington, 1995). This step is no longer considered to be necessary.

The current most widely accepted procedure for permanent partial drainage of bile consists of the placement of a conduit of small bowel between the gallbladder and

the skin surface of the right lower quadrant of the abdomen (jejunostomy). The conduit is fashioned in the following manner:

1 A vascularized, 10-cm segment of jejunum, the proximal end of which is 15 cm from the ligament of Treiz, is isolated and the small bowel reconstituted with an end-to-end anastomosis.
2 The isolated segment of jejunum is placed in an antecolic position and the proximal end anastomosed to the most dependent portion of the gallbladder.
3 The distal end of the conduit is brought to the skin surface as a standard jejunostomy in the right iliac fossa.

The patients are followed up with regular measurements of serum bilirubin and total serum bile salt concentrations.

Surgical complications of the procedure have been reported by Emond and Whitington (1995). They included hemoperitoneum, stomal herniation and intestinal obstruction.

Cholecystoappendicostomy
Gauderer and Boyle (1997) suggested the use of the appendix as a conduit between the gallbladder and the skin of the abdominal wall. The reasons advanced by the authors for their choice of the appendix as the biliary conduit included the small diameter of the lumen, which they believed would not accumulate or resorb significant amounts of bile. The technique also leaves the small bowel undisturbed, and avoids the necessity of a small bowel anastomosis and possible interference with any future liver transplant operation. The case report of the technique concerned a patient with arteriohepatic dysplasia (Alagille's syndrome), who showed a postoperative fall in bilirubin levels from 16.2 to 2.2 mg/dL, and a moderate improvement in liver enzyme values. However, the child continued to require ursodeoxycholic acid therapy for mild pruritus.

Limited ileal diversion
This alternative method of decreasing the bile acid pool has been used in patients who have previously undergone cholecystectomy. The rationale of the operation is based on the observation that exclusion of the terminal ileum creates a degree of malabsorption. This results in a reduced bile acid pool by decreasing the enterohepatic circulation of bile salts. Whitington et al. (1992) described the excision of more than 100 cm of distal ileum at a distance of 110–150 cm proximal to the ileocecal valve. The distal bowel was closed at the resection line to form a self-emptying loop, and the proximal ileum was re-anastomosed to the ileum 3–4 cm proximal to the ileocecal valve. The procedure was performed in two children, both of whom obtained relief from their symptoms of PFIC. However, both suffered from 'modest' postoperative diarrhea.

Terminal ileal exclusion

Hollands et al. (1998) recommend complete exclusion of the terminal ileum. They measure a 15% length of terminal ileum back from the ileocecal valve. The ileum is divided at this point with a linear stapling device. Intestinal continuity is re-established with a side-to-side anastomosis between the proximal ileum and the cecum, thus effectively bypassing the whole of the terminal ileum.

This 'standardized' technique was reported in two children aged 15 months and 4 years, respectively. The younger child did not respond, but the second child had complete relief of symptoms and a fall in serum bilirubin from 9.2 to 0.9 mg/dL.

The advantages claimed for this 'standardized' type of ileal exclusion include the avoidance of complications associated with long-term stomas and the wearing of bile-collecting bags on the abdominal wall. It also avoids the problem of parental reluctance to consent to their child undergoing stoma formation, and it reduces the incidence of diarrhea, which was a complication of 'limited ileal diversion'.

RESULTS OF BILIARY DIVERSION

Jejunal conduit

Emond and Whitington (1995) reported the cases of eight children with PFIC but no evidence of cirrhosis. The mean age at operation was 10.5 years, and the follow-up was between 2.3 and 4.9 years.

Six children responded to external biliary diversion with complete resolution of pruritus and improvement in liver function, and four of them showed improvement in growth. Transplantation was necessary for progressive disease in two cases.

The authors suggested that the beneficial results observed in this group of children, who had not progressed to cirrhosis at a mean age of 10.5 years, might have indicated a milder from of PFIC. In contrast, the mean age of the 11 severely affected patients in the series who were treated with transplantation was only 4.6 years. Melter et al. (2000) reported a further series of six non-cirrhotic children, all of whom improved after surgery, with a loss of pruritus and an improvement in liver function. Growth retardation was reversed in all six cases.

A third series of 16 cases (Ismail et al., 1999) also showed an 80% success rate in the relief of symptoms. In summary, there is now good evidence for the effectiveness of external biliary diversion using the jejunal conduit technique, particularly in the relief of disabling pruritus. The follow-up periods are still relatively short, and the long-term effects on liver pathology are awaited with interest.

Cholecystoappendicostomy

The long-term effectiveness of this operation, which was proposed by Gauderer and Boyle (1997), is not known in patients with PFIC.

Limited ileal diversion

Whitington et al. (1992) described two teenage patients who had previously undergone cholecystectomies. The gallbladders were therefore not available for an external biliary diversion procedure. Both patients obtained complete postoperative relief from pruritus, and their serum bilirubin levels returned to normal. However, they both suffered from postoperative diarrhea. The length of follow-up is not known.

Terminal ileal exclusion

Hollands et al. (1998) used this technique to treat five children aged 1.5, 4, 5, 11 and 17 years, respectively. Relief from pruritus was complete in four cases, and bilirubin levels were reduced to between 0.9 and 4.5 mg/dL. The length of follow-up was 6 to 22 months (mean value 16 months).

In conclusion, there is good evidence that a reduction in the bile acid pool can be achieved in the short term after either external biliary diversion or ileal bypass operations. Pruritus can be abolished and liver function improved in the majority of non-cirrhotic patients with PFIC. The long-term results of these procedures, particularly with regard to liver histology, are awaited with interest.

Key references

Bilton D, Fox R, Webb AK, Lawler W, McMahon RFT, Howat JMT. Pathology of common bile duct stenosis in cystic fibrosis. *Gut* 1990; **31**: 236–8.

This case is a clear illustration of an example of the occasional occurrence of an inflammatory stricture in association with cystic fibrosis. A short review of the literature is included.

Davies MR, Rode H. Biliary ascariasis in children. *Progress in Pediatric Surgery* 1982; **15**: 55–74.

Biliary ascariasis in children is a major problem in many areas of the world. This paper reports 424 cases from the Cape Town Children's Hospital. The frequent invasion of the ampulla of Vater is discussed, together with the typical signs of biliary colic. Complications of biliary ascariasis are dealt with in detail.

Emond JC, Whitington PF. Selective surgical management of progressive familial intrahepatic cholestasis (Byler's disease). *Journal of Pediatric Surgery* 1995; **30**: 1635–41.

This was the first major report of the beneficial effects of biliary diversion in Byler's disease. The operative technique is illustrated and the selection criteria for diversion are presented. This paper established biliary diversion as an alternative to transplantation in non-cirrhotic children with persistent cholestasis.

Heaton ND, Davenport M, Howard ER. Intraluminal biliary obstruction. *Archives of Disease in Childhood* 1991; **66**: 1395–8.

Intraluminal bile duct obstruction in infancy may be related either to biliary sludge or to gallstones. The paper includes a description of the possible etiologies in nine cases, and their management. The discussion reviews the large number of etiological associations reported in the literature.

Saing H, Tam PK, Choi TK, Wong J. Childhood recurrent pyogenic cholangitis. *Journal of Pediatric Surgery* 1988; **23**: 424–9.

This report is based on the management of 10 children in Queen Mary Hospital, Hong Kong. The role of ERCP and intraoperative choledochoscopy is discussed, together with the range of operative procedures employed by the authors.

REFERENCES

Ahmed S. Bile duct injuries from non-penetrating trauma in childhood. *Australian and New Zealand Journal of Surgery* 1976; **46**: 209–12.

Battle WH. Traumatic rupture of the common bile duct. *Transactions of the Clinical Society of London* 1894; **27**: 144–8.

Beck WF. Pancreaticoduodenectomy for carcinoma of the pancreas in an infant. *Annals of Surgery* 1957; **145**: 864–70.

Benjamin DR. Cholelithiasis in infants: the role of parenteral nutrition and gastrointestinal dysfunction. *Journal of Pediatric Surgery* 1982; **17**: 386–9.

Bernstein J, Braylan R, Brough AJ. Bile plug syndrome: a correctable cause of obstructive jaundice in infants. *Pediatrics* 1969; **43**: 273–6.

Bilton D, Fox R, Webb AK, Lawler W, McMahon RFT, Howat JMT. Pathology of common bile duct stenosis in cystic fibrosis. *Gut* 1990; **31**: 236–8.

Bourque MD, Spigland N, Bensoussan AL, Garel L, Blanchard H. Isolated complete transection of the common bile duct due to blunt trauma in a child, and review of the literature. *Journal of Pediatric Surgery* 1989; **24**: 1068–70.

Bowles MJ, Salisbury JR, Howard ER. Localized, benign, non-traumatic strictures of the extrahepatic biliary tree in children. *Surgery* 2001; **130**: 55–9.

Bowen A. Ultrasound of the normal neonatal gallbladder. *Diagnostic Imaging in Clinical Medicine* 1984; **52**: 231–6.

Brown DM. Bile plug syndrome: successful management with a mucolytic agent. *Journal of Pediatric Surgery* 1990; **25**: 351–2.

Cacciaguerra S, Barone P, Villa Trujillo GI *et al.* Obstructive jaundice caused by lymph node compression in a child. *European Journal of Surgery* 1996; **6**: 367–8.

Champetier J, Letoublon C, Alnaasan I, Charvin B. The cystohepatic ducts: surgical implications. *Surgical and Radiologic Anatomy* 1991; **13**: 203–11.

Chang CC, Han CT. Biliary ascariasis in childhood. *Chinese Medical Journal* 1966; **85**: 167–71.

Chappell JS. Benign haemangioendothelioma of the head of the pancreas treated by pancreaticoduodenectomy. *Journal of Pediatric Surgery* 1973; **8**: 431–2.

Cherqui D, Palazzo L, Piedbois P *et al.* Common bile duct stricture as a late complication of upper abdominal radiotherapy. *Journal of Hepatology* 1994; **20**: 693–7.

Clayton RJ, Iber FL, Ruebner BH, McKusick VA. Fatal familial intrahepatic cholestasis in an Amish kindred. *Journal of Pediatrics* 1965; **67**: 1025–8.

Cook RCM, Rickham PP. The liver and biliary tract. In: Rickham PP, Lister J, Irving IM (eds) *Neonatal surgery*, 2nd edn. London: Butterworths, 1978: 483.

Curtis LE, Sheaham DG. Heterotopic tissues in the gallbladder. *Archives of Pathology* 1969; **88**: 677–83.

Davenport M, Saxena R, Howard ER. Acquired biliary atresia. *Journal of Pediatric Surgery* 1996; **31**: 1721–3.

Davies C, Daneman A, Stringer DA. Inspissated bile in a neonate with cystic fibrosis. *Journal of Ultrasound in Medicine* 1986; **5**: 335–7.

Davies MRQ, Rode H. Biliary ascariasis in children. *Progress in Pediatric Surgery* 1982; **15**: 55–74.

Delanoe C, Pararnau JM, Raabe JJ, Arbogast J. Icterus caused by tuberculous adenopathies. *Gastroenterologie Clinique et Biologique* 1993; **7**: 765–6.

Dunn PM. Obstructive jaundice and haemolytic disease of the newborn. *Archives of Disease in Childhood* 1963; **38**: 54–61.

El-Shabrawi M, Wilkinson ML, Portmann B *et al.* Primary sclerosing cholangitis in childhood. *Gastroenterology* 1987; **92**: 1226–35.

Emond JC, Whitington PF. Selective surgical management of progressive familial intrahepatic cholestasis (Byler's disease). *Journal of Pediatric Surgery* 1995; **30**: 1635–41.

Enzenauer RW, Montrey JS, Barcia PJ, Woods J. Total parenteral nutrition cholestasis: a case of mechanical biliary obstruction. *Pediatrics* 1985; **76**: 905–8.

Foster JH, Wayson EE. Surgical significance of aberrant bile ducts. *American Journal of Surgery* 1962; **104**: 14–19.

Gallacher DJ, Kadir S, Kaufman SL, Mitchell SE, Kinisson ML, Chang R. Non-operative management of benign postoperative biliary strictures. *Radiology* 1985; **156**: 625–9.

Gaskin KJ, Waters DL, Howman-Giles R *et al.* Liver disease and common-bile-duct stenosis in cystic fibrosis. *New England Journal of Medicine* 1988; **318**: 340–6.

Gauderer MWL, Boyle JT. Cholecystappendicostomy in a child with Alagille syndrome. *Journal of Pediatric Surgery* 1997; **32**: 166–7.

Gentile AT, Bickler SW, Harrison MW, Campbell JR. Common bile duct obstruction related to intestinal polyposis in a child with Peutz–Jeghers' syndrome. *Journal of Pediatric Surgery* 1994; **29**: 1584–7.

Germiller GA, Strouse PJ, Golladay ES, DiPietro MA. Early presentation of choledochal cyst transiently obstructed by an inspissated bile plug. *Journal of Pediatric Surgery* 1997; **32**: 1522–5.

Gow KW, Blair GK, Phillips R *et al.* Obstructive jaundice caused by neuroblastoma managed with temporary cholecystostomy tube. *Journal of Pediatric Surgery* 1995; **30**: 878–82.

Gur I, Vinograd I, Dgani Y, Arad I. Jaundice due to inspissated bile following disseminated intravascular coagulation. *Israel Journal of Medical Sciences* 1986; **22**: 448–50.

Hancock BJ, Wiseman NE, Rusnak BW. Bile duct stricture in an infant with gastroschisis treated by percutaneous transhepatic drainage, biliary stenting and balloon dilatation. *Journal of Pediatric Surgery* 1989; **24**: 1071–3.

Heaton ND, Davenport M, Howard ER. Intraluminal biliary obstruction. *Archives of Disease in Childhood* 1991; **66**: 1395–8.

Hollands CM, Rivera-Pedrogo FJ, Gonzalez-Vallina R, Loret-de-Mola O, Nahmad M, Burnweit CA. Ileal exclusion for Byler's disease: an alternative surgical approach with promising early results for pruritus. *Journal of Pediatric Surgery* 1998; **33**: 220–4.

Howard ER, Nunnerley HB. Percutaneous cholangiography in prolonged jaundice of childhood. *Journal of the Royal Society of Medicine* 1979; **72**: 495–508.

Hsia DY, Patterson P, Allen FH, Diamond LK, Gellis SS. Prolonged obstructive jaundice in infancy: general survey of 156 cases. *Pediatrics* 1952; **10**: 243–51.

Ismail H, Kalicinski P, Markiewicz M *et al.* Treatment of progressive familial intrahepatic cholestasis: liver transplantation or partial external biliary diversion. *Pediatric Transplantation* 1999; **3**: 219–24.

Jacquemin E. Progressive familial intrahepatic cholestasis. Genetic basis and treatment. *Clinics in Liver Disease* 2000; **4**: 753–63.

Keller MS, Markle BM, Laffey PA, Chawla HS, Jacir N, Frank JL. Spontaneous resolution of cholelithiasis in infants. *Radiology* 1985; **157**: 345–8.

Keramidis DC, Anagostou D, Doulas N. Gastric heterotopia in the gallbladder. *Journal of Pediatric Surgery* 1977; **12**: 759–62.

Khuroo MS, Zargar SA, Mahajan R. Hepatobiliary and pancreatic ascariasis in India. *Lancet* 1990; **335**: 1503–6.

Khuroo MS, Zargar SA, Yattoo GN *et al.* Worm extraction and biliary drainage in hepatobiliary and pancreatic ascariasis. *Gastrointestinal Endoscopy* 1993; **39**: 680–5.

Ladd WE. Congenital obstruction of the bile ducts. *Annals of Surgery* 1935; **102**: 742–51.

Lightwood R, Bodian M. Biliary obstruction associated with icterus gravis neonatorum. *Archives of Disease in Childhood* 1973; **21**: 209–17.

Lilly JR. Common bile duct calculi in infants and children. *Journal of Pediatric Surgery* 1980; **15**: 577–80.

Lilly JR, Sokol RJ. On the bile sludge syndrome, or is total parenteral nutrition cholestasis a surgical disease? *Pediatrics* 1985; **76**: 992–3.

Lloyd DA. Massive hepatobiliary ascariasis in childhood. *British Journal of Surgery* 1981; **68**: 468–73.

Lloyd DA. Hepatobiliary ascariasis in children. *Surgery Annual* 1982; **14**: 277–97.

Louw JH. Abdominal complications of *Ascaris lumbricoides* infestation in children. *British Journal of Surgery* 1966; **53**: 510–21.

Martinez-Urrutia MJ, Vasquez Estevez J, Larrauri J, Diez Pardo JA. Gastric heterotopy of the biliary tract. *Journal of Pediatric Surgery* 1990; **25**: 356–7.

Matos C, Avni EF, Van Gansbeke D *et al.* Total parenteral nutrition (TPN) and gallbladder diseases in neonates. *Journal of Ultrasound Medicine* 1987; **6**: 243–8.

Melter M, Rodeck B, Kardorff R *et al.* Progressive familial intrahepatic cholestasis: partial biliary diversion normalizes serum lipids and improves growth in non-cirrhotic patients. *American Journal of Gastroenterology* 2000; **95**: 3522–8.

Moulton SL, Downey EC, Anderson DS, Lynch FP. Blunt bile duct injuries in children. *Journal of Pediatric Surgery* 1993; **28**: 795–7.

O'Brien S, Keogan M, Casy M *et al.* Biliary complications of cystic fibrosis. *Gut* 1992; **33**: 387–91.

Oppe TE, Valaes T. Obstructive jaundice and haemolytic disease of the newborn. *Lancet* 1959; **1**: 536–9.

Pandit SK, Budhiraja S, Rattan KN. Post-traumatic bile ascites. *Indian Journal of Pediatrics* 2000; **67**: 72–3.

Redkar RG, Davenport M, Myers N, Howard ER. Association of oesophageal atresia and cholecystohepatic duct. *Pediatric Surgery International* 1999; **15**: 21–3.

Reid IS. Biliary tract abnormalities associated with duodenal atresia. *Archives of Disease in Childhood* 1973; **48**: 952–7.

Rinker B, Ginsburg HB, Genieser NB, Gittes GK. Obstructive jaundice caused by placement of a nasoenteric tube. *Journal of Pediatric Surgery* 2000; **35**: 619–20.

Rodgers BM, Hollenbeck JI, Donelly WH, Talbert JL. Intrahepatic cholestasis with parenteral alimentation. *American Journal of Surgery* 1976; **131**: 149–55.

Rohatgi M, Gupta DK. Isolated complete transection of common bile duct following blunt bicycle handlebar injury. *Journal of Pediatric Surgery* 1987; **22**: 1029–30.

Roslyn JJ, Berguist WE, Pitt HA *et al.* Increased risk of gallstones in children receiving total parenteral nutrition. *Pediatrics* 1983; **71**: 784–9.

Saing H, Tam PKH, Choi TK, Wong J. Childhood recurrent pyogenic cholangitis. *Journal of Pediatric Surgery* 1988; **23**: 424–9.

Schirmer WJ, Grisoni ER, Ganderer MWL. The spectrum of cholelithiasis in the first year of life. *Journal of Pediatric Surgery* 1989; **24**: 1064–7.

Schorlemmer GR, Wild RE, Manndell V, Newsome JF. Cholecystohepatic connections in a case of extrahepatic biliary atresia. A 27-year follow-up. *Journal of the American Medical Association* 1984; **252**: 1319–20.

Shearman EW, Teja K, Botero LM, Shaw A. Pancreaticoduodenectomy in the treatment of congenital fibrosarcoma of the duodenum. *Journal of Pediatric Surgery* 1975; **10**: 801–6.

Sisto A, Feldman P, Garel L *et al.* Primary sclerosing cholangitis in children: study of five cases and review of the literature. *Pediatrics* 1987; **80**: 918–23.

Spitz L, Orr JD, Harries JT. Obstructive jaundice secondary to chronic mid-gut volvulus. *Archives of Disease in Childhood* 1983; **58**: 383–5.

Spivak W, Grand RJ, Eraklis A. A case of primary sclerosing cholangitis in childhood. *Gastroenterology* 1982; **82**: 129–32.

Standfield NJ, Salisbury JR, Howard ER. Benign non-traumatic inflammatory strictures of the extrahepatic biliary system. *British Journal of Surgery* 1989; **76**: 849–52.

Strandvick B, Hjelte L, Gabrielsson N, Glaumann H. Sclerosing cholangitis in cystic fibrosis. *Scandinavian Journal of Enterology* 1988; **23 (Supplement 143)**: 121–4.

Takehara H, Komi N, Okada A *et al.* Unusual cases of benign stricture of the biliary tract. *Tokushima Journal of Experimental Medicine* 1992; **39**: 135–43.

Tan KC, Howard ER. Choledochal cyst: a 14-year surgical experience with 36 patients. *British Journal of Surgery* 1988; **75**: 892–5.

Tunell WP. Haemangioendothelioma of the pancreas obstructing the common bile duct and duodenum. *Journal of Pediatric Surgery* 1976; **11**: 827–30.

Verbeek PCM, van Leeuwen DJ, de Wit LT *et al.* Benign fibrosing disease at the hepatic confluence mimicking Klatskin tumors. *Surgery* 1992; **112**: 866–71.

Wani NA, Chrungoo RK. Biliary ascariasis – surgical aspects. *World Journal of Surgery* 1992; **16**: 976–9.

Werlin SL, Glichlich M, Jona J, Starshak RJ. Sclerosing cholangitis in childhood. *Journal of Pediatrics* 1980; **96**: 433–5.

Whitaker LD, Lynn HB, Dockert MB. Heterotopic gastric mucosa in the wall of the cystic duct: report of a case. *Surgery* 1967; **62**: 382–5.

Whitington PF, Black DD. Cholelithiasis in premature infants treated with parenteral nutrition and frusemide. *Journal of Pediatrics* 1980; **97**: 647–9.

Whitington PF, Balistreri WF. Liver transplantation in pediatrics: indications, contraindications, and pretransplant management. *Journal of Pediatrics* 1991; **118**: 169–77.

Whitington PF, Freese DK, Alonso EM, Fishbein MH, Emond JC. Progressive familial intrahepatic cholestasis (Byler's disease). In: Lentze M, Reichen J (eds) *Paediatric cholestasis*. Dordrecht: Kluwer Academic Publishers, 1992: 165–80.

Whitington PF, Freese DK, Alonso EM, Schwarzenberg SJ, Sharp HL. Clinical and biochemical findings in progressive familial intrahepatic cholestasis. *Journal of Pediatric Gatroenterology* 1994; **18**: 134–4.

13

Gallbladder disease and cholelithiasis

MARK D STRINGER

The main function of the gallbladder is to store and concentrate hepatic bile. The motility and absorptive capacity of the organ are influenced by circulating hormones such as cholecystokinin, secretin, gastrin and pancreatic polypeptide, and by the enteric nervous system. The gallbladder mucosa also secretes proteins, including mucin, and electrolytes. The gallbladder is not essential to human digestion, and many animals (e.g. horses and rats) manage perfectly well without one. It is the presence of stones in the gallbladder that accounts for most of the pathology of this organ.

CONGENITAL ANOMALIES OF THE GALLBLADDER

Gallbladder development begins as an outgrowth from the caudal part of the hepatic endodermal evagination of the foregut from the fourth week of gestation onwards (see Chapter 7). Various developmental anomalies of the gallbladder have been recorded, most of which are incidental findings. These include abnormalities of number, shape, position and mucosal lining.

Agenesis

Excluding those cases associated with biliary atresia, most other instances of gallbladder agenesis are discovered at autopsy or at laparotomy. The estimated incidence at autopsy is about 1 in 3–6000 (Turkel *et al.*, 1983; Bennion *et al.*, 1988). Agenesis of the gallbladder may be an isolated anomaly, when it is sometimes familial, or it may be associated with multiple congenital anomalies (principally cardiac, genitourinary and gastrointestinal).

Occasionally, the gallbladder is found to be absent at operation for a presumed non-functioning gallbladder associated with apparent cholelithiasis, but this rarely occurs with modern preoperative imaging. Failure to identify the gallbladder at operation is not proof of its absence, since it may be intrahepatic (when it is rarely covered entirely by hepatic parenchyma), but a detailed ultrasound scan usually suggests this possibility.

Duplication

Although rare, this congenital anomaly is well described (Gross, 1936; Harlaftis *et al.*, 1977). From an extensive autopsy study, Boyden (1926) estimated the frequency of gallbladder duplication to be 1 in 3800. Renewed interest in the condition has been stimulated by the advent of laparoscopic cholecystectomy. Duplication encompasses a spectrum of anatomical variations which include septate, bilobed and completely duplicated gallbladders. A gallbladder diverticulum may be a variant of bilobar gallbladder. Triple gallbladders have also been reported.

Completely duplicated gallbladders have either a Y-shaped cystic duct or two separate cystic ducts. The latter usually drain directly into the common bile duct, but the gallbladder nearest the liver sometimes drains into the right hepatic duct. The two gallbladders may be invested by a common peritoneal coat, or they may lie in separate but adjacent fossae. Cholelithiasis is a relatively common complication of gallbladder duplication in adults, but it is uncertain whether duplication significantly predisposes to gallstone formation (Harlaftis *et al.*, 1977). Symptomatic patients should have both gallbladders removed, but only after biliary anatomy has been confirmed by intraoperative cholangiography (Figure 13.1).

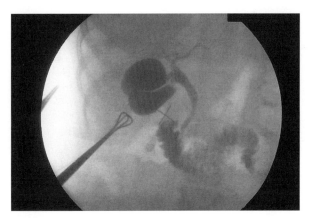

Figure 13.1 *A double gallbladder with two separate cystic ducts outlined by intraoperative cholangiography in an 8-year-old girl (Bailie* et al., *2002).*

Septation

Gallbladder septae may be congenital or acquired, longitudinal or transverse, and single or multiple. Some are composed of fibrous tissue alone, whilst others contain smooth muscle fibers that are continuous with the gallbladder wall (Harlaftis *et al.*, 1977). When there are communicating chambers in the gallbladder, bile stasis may lead to cholelithiasis (Esper *et al.*, 1992).

Cystic duct atresia

This causes a congenital mucocele of the gallbladder. A prenatal vascular accident affecting the cystic artery has been suggested as a possible cause (Deshmukh *et al.*, 1999).

Left-sided gallbladder

The gallbladder lies under the left lobe of the liver to the left of the falciform ligament, with the cystic duct either joining the hepatic duct from the left or, more commonly, entering the common duct on its right side (Newcombe and Henley, 1964). Gross (1936) suggested two possible mechanisms of development – either that the embryonic gallbladder bud from the hepatic diverticulum migrates to the left rather than the right, or that the left-sided gallbladder arises directly from the left hepatic duct whilst the normal gallbladder fails to develop. The condition is not usually clinically significant.

Heterotopic gastric mucosa

There are numerous reports in both adults and children of ectopic gastric mucosa within the extrahepatic biliary system. The gallbladder is more often affected than the bile ducts (Evans *et al.*, 1990; Lamont *et al.*, 1991). In most cases, gastric heterotopia is an incidental finding in older patients undergoing cholecystectomy for cholelithiasis, although rarely it may cause chronic intermittent abdominal pain, acute cholecystitis, hemobilia and/or obstructive jaundice. The mucosa is typically fundic in type with both parietal and chief cells. Imaging studies may reveal a persistently contracted or non-functioning gallbladder or, in older patients, a polypoid lesion, but frequently there are no clues to this pathology.

CHOLELITHIASIS

Epidemiology

Few studies have addressed the epidemiology of gallstones in children. Palasciano *et al.* (1989) undertook an ultrasonographic survey of nearly 1500 Italian students aged between 6 and 19 years. Those with a history of hepatobiliary disease were excluded. Two girls with gallstones were identified, giving an overall prevalence of cholelithiasis of 0.13%. This compares with 0.1% in previous pediatric autopsy studies (Newman *et al.*, 1968) and 0.5% in neonates (Wendtland-Born *et al.*, 1997). Racial variations in the incidence of cholelithiasis are well documented in adults.

Cholelithiasis in childhood appears to have a bimodal distribution, with a small peak in infancy and a steadily rising incidence from early adolescence onwards. Most series show a similar sex distribution, or even a predominance of males in infancy and early childhood, but a clear female predisposition emerges during adolescence.

Numerous studies indicate that there has been a steady increase in the frequency of cholecystectomy for cholelithiasis in children during the last three decades (Takiff and Fonkalsrud, 1984; Bailey *et al.*, 1989; Waldhausen and Benjamin, 1999; Kumar *et al.*, 2000). This may be related to several factors, such as widespread availability of superior diagnostic techniques (principally ultrasonography), surgical enthusiasm in the era of laparoscopic cholecystectomy, and a genuine increase in the prevalence of cholelithiasis from multiple causes, including parenteral nutrition, obesity, the complications of prematurity, etc.

Pathogenesis

There are four major types of gallstone (Table 13.1 and Plate 3). Mixed cholesterol stones are the commonest variety in adults, and are typically found in obese adolescents. They develop from cholesterol supersaturation of bile (because of either excess cholesterol or insufficient bile salts and phosphatidylcholine to allow complete micellar solubilization of cholesterol in bile) in combination with factors that promote nucleation and bile stasis. Non-cholesterol components of such calculi include calcium salts (bilirubinate, carbonate, phosphate, fatty

Table 13.1 *Major varieties of gallstone; adapted from Lafont and Ostrow (2000)*

Type	Mixed cholesterol	Pure cholesterol	Black pigment	Brown pigment
Composition	Cholesterol, calcium salts	Cholesterol	Pigment polymer, calcium bilirubinate	Calcium bilirubinate, calcium salts of fatty acids
Shape	Round or faceted	Round, smooth	Spiky or faceted	Ovoid or irregular
Color	Brown pigment in rings or specks	Yellow-white, pigmented center	Black, shiny or dull	Brown, soft, laminated
Number	Multiple	Usually single	Multiple	Single or multiple
Microbiology	Sterile	Sterile	Sterile	Infected
Major risk factors	Female, obesity	Female, obesity	Hemolysis	Cholangitis, strictures

acids) and proteins. In children all stone types may occur, but black pigment stones are relatively more common. Supersaturation of bile with calcium bilirubinate, the calcium salt of unconjugated bilirubin, together with inorganic salts (calcium carbonate and phosphate) causes the formation of black pigment stones. These are typically seen in hemolytic disorders, but are also found in association with total parenteral nutrition (Takiff and Fonkalsrud, 1984; O'Brien *et al.*, 1986). Biliary stasis and infection are associated with brown pigment stones, which occur more often in the bile ducts than in the gall-

bladder. Rarely, calculi are composed of pure calcium carbonate crystals, when the bile typically appears milky and radiopaque (Wu *et al.*, 2001).

Biliary sludge is a sonographically echogenic substance that gravitates to the dependent part of the gallbladder or bile duct and does not cast an acoustic shadow (Ko *et al.*, 1999). It is composed of mucin, calcium bilirubinate and cholesterol crystals. Gallbladder sludge is typically found in association with total parenteral nutrition/fasting, pregnancy, sickle-cell disease, treatment with ceftriaxone or octreotide, and after bone-marrow

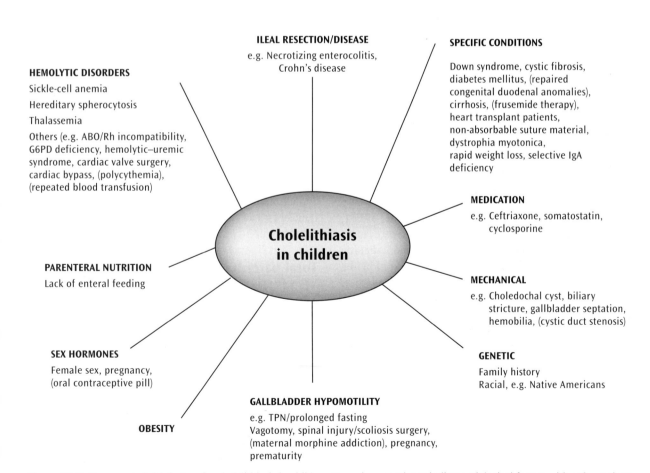

Figure 13.2 *Documented risk factors for cholelithiasis in children. Items in parentheses indicate etiological factors with only weak or anecdotal evidence.*

transplantation. The natural history of biliary sludge varies, and spontaneous resolution, a waxing and waning course and progression to gallstones are all possible. Sludge itself may cause biliary colic, obstructive jaundice, acute cholecystitis or pancreatitis.

Many etiological factors have been associated with cholelithiasis in children (Figure 13.2) and various pathogenic mechanisms, often working in combination, have been identified (Afdhal, 2000). The dominant factors are as follows:

- biliary stasis;
- excess bilirubin pigment;
- lithogenic bile.

The importance of different etiological factors in published series of children with cholelithiasis varies with time and is dependent on institutional referral patterns (Table 13.2). These large retrospective studies, most of which have excluded children with choledochal cysts, highlight the variable contribution of risk factors in different centers.

Hemolytic disorders

The major hemolytic diseases which produce pigment stones in children are sickle-cell disease, hereditary spherocytosis and thalassemia major. The incidence of gallstones increases with age in all conditions.

Children with sickle-cell anemia, hemoglobin sickle-cell disease and hemoglobin S beta-thalassemia are all at risk of cholelithiasis. The prevalence of pigment stones in sickle-cell anemia is approximately 10–15% in children under 10 years of age, and up to 40% or more in those aged 10–18 years (Sarnaik et al., 1980; Bond et al., 1987; Webb et al., 1989). About 10–20% of children with hereditary spherocytosis show evidence of cholelithiasis (Croom et al., 1986). In thalassemia, gallstones are rare before 5 years of age, but thereafter 4–14% of affected children develop this complication (Borgna-Pignatti et al., 1981; Chittmittrapap et al., 1990; Kalayci et al., 1999). Some authors have suggested that hypertransfusion therapy which suppresses thalassemic red-cell production by the bone marrow and/or splenectomy reduce the degree of hemolysis and the tendency to pigment stone formation.

Hemolysis due to hemolytic–uremic syndrome (Brandt et al., 1998), ABO or Rhesus incompatibility or cardiac valve replacement (Williams and Johnson, 1984) may also be complicated by pigment stones. Non-hemolytic disorders resulting in an excessive bilirubin load in the presence of an immature bilirubin excretion mechanism have been linked to pigment stone formation in some reports. Thus polycythemia (Tay and Werlin, 1987), multiple blood transfusions (Jeffrey et al., 1984) and phototherapy (which stimulates the biliary excretion of unconjugated bilirubin) (McDonagh, 1981) have been implicated as etiological factors in the newborn.

Ileal resection/disease

Ileal resection or disease is an unequivocal risk factor for cholelithiasis (Pellerin et al., 1975; Roslyn et al., 1983; Davies et al., 1999). Even limited ileal resection in the neonate, particularly when combined with parenteral nutrition, predisposes to cholelithiasis. Davies et al. (1999) studied 24 children at a median age of 7.4 years following limited ileal resection (< 50 cm) in infancy for necrotizing enterocolitis (NEC) or intussusception. Seven control subjects who had developed neonatal NEC but recovered without surgery were also evaluated. Four children had cholelithiasis, all of whom had previously undergone limited ileal resection for NEC. No biliary abnormalities were noted either in the intussusception group or in the NEC control group. The prevalence of cholelithasis after limited ileal resection for NEC was 24% at a median age of 7.0 years.

Other studies have shown that symptomatic gallstones occur in 10–20% of children with short bowel syndrome (Georgeson and Brown, 1998). Children with Crohn's disease affecting the terminal ileum are similarly at risk of cholelithiasis. The traditional explanation for such gallstones is that the normal reabsorption of bile salts in the terminal ileum is impaired, leading to depletion of the bile salt pool in the enterohepatic circulation. This promotes the formation of lithogenic bile, which becomes oversaturated with cholesterol. In support of this theory, Pellerin et al. (1975) described four children with calcium carbonate and cholesterol calculi after ileal resection. However, pediatric gallstones associated with ileal resection in infants who have received total parenteral nutrition tend to be pigmented (Roslyn et al., 1983). Moreover, analysis of bile from patients with ileal dysfunction/resection demonstrates a significantly reduced cholesterol saturation and a significantly higher bilirubin concentration (Heubi et al., 1982; Lapidus and Einarsson, 1998). Thus an alternative explanation for the pathogenesis of cholelithiasis after ileal resection/disease is that bile salt deficiency leads to incomplete solubilization of unconjugated bilirubin, which can then form calcium bilrubinate.

Total parenteral nutrition (TPN)

The association between TPN and biliary sludge/cholelithiasis has been recognized for many years (Whitington and Black, 1980; Benjamin, 1982; Suita et al., 1984). The pathogenesis is complex because of associated pathologies in patients receiving TPN and the inextricable link between TPN and lack of enteral feeding. Fasting and TPN are known to promote biliary stasis by impairing both the enterohepatic circulation of bile acids and cholecystokinin-induced gallbladder contraction (Jawaheer et al., 1995). In animal studies, TPN without oral feeding results in gallbladder bile that is less acidified (Dawes et al., 1999). Acidification of bile helps to protect against the precipitation of calcium salts

Table 13.2 *Distribution of etiological factors in larger series of cholelithiasis in children*

Author(s)	Origin	Study period	n	Female (%)	Infants (%)	Hematological (%)	TPN (%)	Ileal resection or disease (%)	Obesity (%)	Cystic fibrosis (%)	Idiopathic (%)	Comment
Takiff and Fonkalsrud (1984)	California, USA	1970–82	44 (0–18 years)	73	?	7	25	16	23	0	48	Only patients undergoing cholecystectomy
Bailey et al. (1989)	Missouri, USA	1970–88	47 (0–17 years)	55	13 (< 2 years)	23	9	2	13	0	?	Only patients undergoing cholecystectomy
Reif et al. (1991)	New York, USA	1979–89	50 (0–20 years)	58	8	36	16	8	6	2	20	All patients with gallstones
Kumar et al. (2000)	New South Wales, Australia	1979–96	102 (0–14 years)	42	9	23	?	3	?	4	55	All patients with sonographically determined cholelithiasis
Miltenburg et al. (2000)	Texas, USA	1980–96	128 (0–18 years)	53	6	41	8	2	6	5	23	Only patients undergoing cholecystectomy
Waldhausen and Benjamin (1999)	Washington, USA	1984–96	121 (0–18 years)	54	?	26	13	?	10	0	40	Only patients undergoing cholecystectomy

TPN, total parenteral nutrition.

which promote gallstone formation. Limited data suggest that TPN-associated calculi are pigment stones with a high calcium bilirubinate content (Roslyn *et al.*, 1983; O'Brien *et al.*, 1986).

Premature infants are particularly susceptible to this complication, and gallstones have been documented after only 2 weeks of TPN (Boyle *et al.*, 1983). Matos *et al.* (1987) undertook a prospective sonographic study of 41 neonates receiving TPN. Gallbladder sludge developed in 18 infants (44%) after a mean period of 10 days of TPN, and was more common in premature infants. Sludge cleared in 12 infants during the first week of enteral feeding, but two of the remaining patients went on to develop asymptomatic gallstones.

Other risk factors

Adolescents with cholelithiasis usually have cholesterol stones associated with an adult pattern of risk factors, namely female gender, obesity and pregnancy (Nilsson, 1966; Honore, 1980; Reif *et al.*, 1991). Estrogens increase cholesterol secretion and progesterone reduces bile acid secretion and slows gallbladder emptying (Afdhal, 2000). Rapid weight loss is also a risk factor in adults. Biliary stasis is a major factor predisposing to stone formation. Mechanical causes include choledochal cysts and abnormalities of pancreaticobiliary union (see Chapter 10), septate gallbladder (Esper *et al.*, 1992) and gallbladder diverticulum (Soderlund and Zetterstrom, 1962). Cystic duct stenosis has been suggested as another cause (Forshall and Rickham, 1955), but it is not clear whether such cases are acquired secondary to calculous gallbladder disease. Functional causes of biliary stasis include vagotomy, which results in gallbladder hypotonia and an increased resting gallbladder volume, and possibly maternal morphine addiction (Figueroa-Colon *et al.*, 1990).

Specific disorders associated with cholelithiasis

A variety of specific medical conditions have been associated with an increased incidence of cholelithiasis in children (Table 13.3).

Clinical features

The clinical features of cholelithiasis are dependent on the age at presentation.

THE FETUS

Fetal gallstones were first described by Beretsky and Lankin in 1983, and several other case reports have subsequently been published (Table 13.4 and Figure 13.3). Analysis of these patients reveals the following:

- a male predominance;
- almost all cases were detected after 30 weeks' gestation following previously normal sonograms (although fetal gallbladder sludge has been detected at 28 weeks' gestation);
- known predisposing factors to cholelithiasis were notably absent;
- a family history of gallstones was present in only a few cases.

The etiology of fetal cholelithiasis is unknown, but differences in the lithogenicity of human fetal bile and biliary stasis may be important (Setchell *et al.*, 1988).

Sonographically diagnosed fetal cholelithiasis usually resolves spontaneously during infancy, often within a few months, without evidence of biliary complications (Stringer *et al.*, 1996). Resolution probably occurs as a result of dissolution and then passage through the biliary tree.

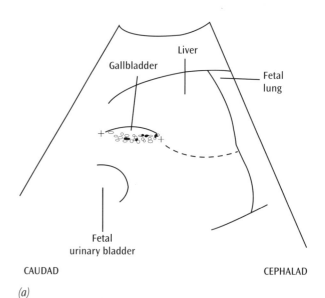

(a)

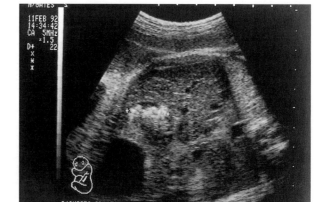

(b)

Figure 13.3 *(a) and (b) Coronal ultrasound section through fetal abdomen at 32 weeks' gestational age. The gallbladder contains multiple echogenic foci consistent with calculi (Stringer et al., 1996)*

Table 13.3 *Specific conditions associated with pediatric cholelithiasis*

Condition	Etiological factors	Comment	Author(s)
Cystic fibrosis	Abnormalities of biliary lipid and mucin composition; common bile duct stenosis	A small but definite increased incidence	Stern et al., 1986; Anagnostopoulos et al., 1993
Down syndrome	Prenatal factors may be important because calculi have been detected soon after birth	Most calculi diagnosed in first 2 years. Potential confounding variables in those with congenital heart disease (e.g. frusemide therapy and polycythemia)	Aughton et al., 1992; Llerena et al., 1993; Toxano et al., 2001
Cardiac transplantation	Multifactorial (hemolysis, cyclosporine-induced changes in bile and lipid metabolism, gallbladder stasis, frusemide therapy)	Noted in adults and children	Milas et al., 1996
Childhood cancer	Multifactorial (ileal conduit, parenteral nutrition, abdominal surgery, repeated blood transfusions and abdominal radiation therapy)	Small cumulative risk of 0.42% at 10 years and 1.03% at 18 years after diagnosis	Mahmoud et al., 1991
Bone-marrow transplantation	Blood transfusions (highest risk in bone-marrow failure patients)	Prevalence of cholelithiasis $\geq 3.5\%$ in children receiving bone-marrow transplants	Safford et al., 2001
Spinal surgery/injury	Immobilization and disturbed calcium hemostasis combined with bilirubin load secondary to blood transfusion	Cholelithiasis in 20% of 92 children who had undergone surgery for scoliosis up to 10 years previously	Teele et al., 1987
Hepatobiliary trauma	6–12 months after blunt liver trauma complicated by hemobilia	Sporadic cases only	Luzuy et al., 1987; Reif et al., 1991
Selective IgA deficiency	May predispose to gallbladder infection or a decreased bile acid pool from intestinal losses		Danon et al., 1983
Dystrophia myotonica	Impaired gallbladder emptying secondary to smooth muscle insensitivity to cholecystokinin		Schwindt et al., 1969
Chronic intestinal pseudo-obstruction	Impaired gallbladder motility associated with intestinal hypoganglionosis	Gallbladder neuropathology identified but TPN, ileostomy and sepsis often coexist in these patients	Shimotake et al., 1993
Congenital duodenal anomalies	Fibrosis around the distal common bile duct after repair of duodenal atresia/stenosis	Anecdotal evidence only. Potential confounding etiological factors	Tchirkow et al., 1980

Table 13.4   *Collected case reports of fetal gallstones*

Author(s)	*n*	Sex	Gestation at detection (weeks)	Prenatal sonogram	Postnatal sonogram	Outcome
Beretsky and Lankin (1983)	1	?	36	Multiple foci	Multiple at < 1 week	Resolution within 1 month
Heijne and Ednay (1985)	1	F	34	Multiple foci	Multiple at < 4 weeks	Resolution within 6 months
Klingensmith and Cioffi-Ragan (1988)	1	M	37	Multiple foci	Multiple at < 1 week	Resolution within 6 weeks
Abbitt and McIlhenny (1990)	1	M	33	Multiple foci	Multiple at < 1 week	Resolution within 10 months
Broussin and Daube (1990)	3	M	33	Two foci	Two at < 1 week	Unknown
		M	38	Multiple foci	Multiple at < 1 week	Resolution within 6 months
		M	36	Multiple foci	Multiple at < 1 week	Resolution within 6 weeks
Stringer *et al.* (1996)	3	M	32	Multiple foci	Single stone at 1 week	Resolution within 1 month
		M	35	Multiple foci	Normal at 6 weeks	Resolution within 6 weeks
		M	32	Multiple foci	Single stone at 6 months	Asymptomatic stone at 9 months

INFANCY

In an extensive literature search, Brill *et al.* (1982) collected only 12 cases of children under 2 months of age. In recent years, the number of reports of infants with gallstones has increased dramatically in parallel with the widespread use of diagnostic ultrasonography and an increase in neonatal risk factors such as total parenteral nutrition. Premature infants are particularly prone to cholelithiasis for several reasons. Extreme prematurity (< 32 weeks' gestation) is associated with poor gallbladder contractility in response to enteral feeding (Lehtonen *et al.*, 1993). Other potential predisposing factors include ileal resection or disease, repeated blood transfusions, frusemide therapy, phototherapy, decreased bile acid output (Watkins *et al.*, 1973; Halpern *et al.*, 1996), and systemic or biliary infection (Jonas *et al.*, 1990; Debray *et al.*, 1993). Treem *et al.* (1989) analyzed bile from two infants with pigment stones and obstructive jaundice, and both cases showed a heavy growth of bacteria in the bile. They suggested that this is the cause of pigment stones in at least some infants. Bacterial β-glucuronidase is capable of hydrolyzing bilirubin diglucuronide to unconjugated bilirubin, which encourages the formation of calcium bilirubinate calculi. Despite this list of potential risk factors, gallstones are idiopathic in many infants (St-Vil *et al.*, 1992; Debray *et al.*, 1993).

The presentation of cholelithiasis in infants is very variable. Gallstones are frequently asymptomatic, but they may cause non-specific symptoms such as poor feeding, vomiting and irritability, or give rise to acute cholecystitis, choledocholithiasis with obstructive jaundice and/or cholangitis, or rarely biliary perforation (of the gallbladder or common bile duct) (Jonas *et al.*, 1990; Heaton *et al.*, 1991; St-Vil *et al.*, 1992; Debray *et al.*, 1993). The overall incidence of common duct stones is higher in infants.

CHILDHOOD

Hemolytic disorders, ileal resection, total parenteral nutrition and a variety of other conditions contribute to cholelithiasis in this age group (Grosfeld *et al.*, 1994). Rarer problems account for some cases, documented examples of which include cyclosporine therapy in transplant recipients (Weinsten *et al.*, 1995; Cao *et al.*, 1997) (Table 13.3), severe cervical spine anomalies (Kose *et al.*, 1993) and ceftriaxone therapy. Ceftriaxone, a parenteral third-generation cephalosporin antibiotic, can cause sludge or pseudolithiasis (sonographically echogenic debris with acoustic shadowing) in the gallbladder (Palanduz *et al.*, 2000). This is related to high antibiotic concentrations that crystallize in gallbladder bile. The echogenic material usually dissolves spontaneously within 2 weeks of stopping therapy, but may progress to stone formation.

Older children are much better at localizing pain, and they more often report abdominal pain located in the right upper quadrant or epigastrium, nausea and vomiting, and fatty food intolerance with symptomatic gallstones. Thus biliary colic and acute or chronic cholecystitis are more readily diagnosed in this age group. Occasionally presentation is with obstructive jaundice or pancreatitis.

ADOLESCENCE

Typically these patients are adolescent girls with risk factors such as obesity, pregnancy or a positive family history (Grosfeld *et al.*, 1994), but cholelithiasis is also seen in association with hemolytic disorders, ileal disease or resection (including resection for reconstructive surgery) and other recognized etiologies (Filston and Ware, 1998). Several studies have shown no evidence of a link between cholelithiasis and the oral contraceptive pill (Vessey and Painter, 1994).

Fatty food intolerance, biliary colic and acute or chronic cholecystitis are well described in most cases with symptomatic stones. In acute cholecystitis there may be fever, localized tenderness in the right upper quadrant, and sometimes a palpable mass. In chronic cases, physical examination may be normal. Jaundice may be seen in children with hemolytic disorders and in those with a common duct stone.

Diagnosis

Clinical suspicion of cholelithiasis is readily confirmed by an ultrasound scan (US) in fasting patients. Gallstones typically cast an acoustic shadow, are usually mobile, and may be solitary or multiple. Stone size and not calcium content determines the presence or absence of acoustic shadowing (Good et al., 1979). Stones as small as 1.5 mm in diameter can be detected by US, but acoustic shadowing is usually seen with larger calculi measuring 4 mm or more in diameter (Figure 13.4). Biliary sludge produces internal echoes without a sonic shadow. Morphological abnormalities of the gallbladder such as wall thickening and the diameter of the common bile duct can also be assessed by US, but the latter may be difficult to visualize in the presence of duodenal gas. Common bile duct dilatation is frequently noted with choledocholithiasis. Color Doppler imaging has expanded the role of US by allowing the evaluation of vascular anatomy and physiology. The sensitivity and specificity of US are 98% and more than 95%, respectively, for gallbladder cholelithiasis (Cooperberg and Burhenne, 1980), but only about 50–75% of common bile duct stones are detected. Sensitivity is increased by repeated scanning.

The incidence of radiopaque stones in children ranges from 20% to 47% (Holcomb et al., 1980; Takiff and Fonkalsrud, 1984; Robertson et al., 1988; Kumar et al.,

2000). As many as 50% of pigment stones associated with hemolytic disorders are calcified (Stephens and Scott, 1980). This is a much higher proportion than in adults, in whom about 15% of mixed cholesterol stones are calcified.

Radioisotope studies using technetium-99m-di-iso-propyl iminodiacetic acid (DISIDA) or technetium-99m-mebrofenin represent an extremely sensitive and highly specific investigation in the diagnosis of acute cholecystitis, even in the presence of jaundice. Non-visualization of the gallbladder in an otherwise patent biliary system usually indicates acute cholecystitis. False-positive results have been reported in severely ill patients receiving TPN. Computed tomography (especially helical CT) can be useful in the assessment of choledocholithiasis and gallstone pancreatitis, but small gallstones or those that are as isodense as bile may be overlooked. Magnetic resonance cholangiography is being increasingly employed, since it is non-invasive and does not require radiation or the administration of contrast materials.

Both endoscopic retrograde cholangiopancreatography (ERCP) (see Chapter 35) and operative cholangiography are invaluable in the management of common duct stones.

Management of cholelithiasis

NON-OPERATIVE MANAGEMENT

Infants with spontaneously resolving cholelithiasis have been reported by many authors (Keller et al., 1985; Jacir et al., 1986; St-Vil et al., 1992; Debray et al., 1993; Miltenburg et al., 2000). Resolution presumably occurs as a result of dissolution and/or passage through the biliary tree, and both increased bile flow and changes in its composition are likely to be significant postnatal factors. There is only one report of natural resolution of a calcified stone (Debray et al., 1993). For the asymptomatic infant with gallbladder calculi, early surgery should be avoided because of this possibility of spontaneous cure. Clinical and sonographic monitoring is sufficient provided that the infant has no other evidence of biliary tract disease. Calculous cholecystitis in infancy should generally be treated surgically, although in the newborn a brief trial of non-operative management may be warranted, provided that the infant is closely monitored, since this can be rewarded by complete resolution (Ghose and Stringer, 1999) (Figure 13.5).

In older children, management of asymptomatic gallbladder calculi is controversial because the natural history in some situations is not well defined. Bruch et al. (2000) followed 41 older children with gallstones of non-hemolytic origin for a mean period of 21 months. Eight of these were truly asymptomatic, but symptoms in the remainder were considered to be unrelated to gallstones. The children were treated with a low-fat, high-fiber diet. The truly asymptomatic patients

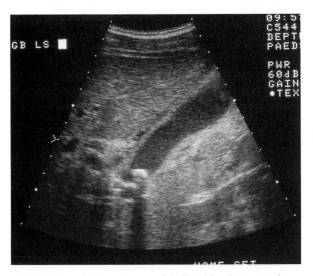

Figure 13.4 Ultrasound scan of gallbladder demonstrating a single stone with acoustic shadow.

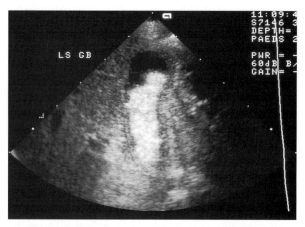

Figure 13.5 *Abdominal ultrasound scan demonstrating acute calculous cholecystitis in a neonate which resolved with non-operative management. The gallbladder contains echogenic sludge and small-calculi, and its wall is edematous.*

remained well, and 80% of the remainder experienced symptomatic improvement. None of the children developed biliary tract complications. Only three children required cholecystectomy for continued symptoms during the study period, prompting the authors to advocate a conservative approach. Nevertheless, cholecystectomy for asymptomatic gallstones is common practice, and this may be the correct policy outside infancy, first because cholecystectomy in experienced pediatric surgical centers is a safe procedure, second because the likelihood of spontaneous resolution of cholelithiasis in older children is small (particularly when stones are calcified), and third because the child is at risk of complications of cholelithiasis for life. Moreover, there are subgroups of children in whom the case for elective cholecystectomy for cholelithiasis is stronger because they are particularly prone to subsequent biliary complications and the hazards of emergency surgery are greater. These include individuals with sickle-cell disease and heart transplant recipients.

Gallbladder sludge frequently resolves spontaneously. For example, biliary sludge associated with TPN is usually transient provided that enteral feeding can be resumed. For infants who remain dependent on TPN, cholecystokinin or ursodeoxycholic acid can be effective in clearing sludge (Komura *et al.*, 1988; Rintala *et al.*, 1995). Ursodeoxycholic acid also encourages bile flow and renders the bile less hepatotoxic.

Dissolution therapy for gallstones in children is of limited value. Despite prolonged treatment, low dissolution rates and high recurrence rates have been observed in adults with cholesterol stones. Calcified and pigment stones and those within a non-functioning gallbladder are not amenable to treatment. Limited success has been reported with ursodeoxycholic acid in TPN-related cholelithiasis (Komura *et al.*, 1988), but this therapy is ineffective in children with calculi complicating cystic

fibrosis (Colombo *et al.*, 1993) and other conditions (Gamba *et al.*, 1997).

Extracorporeal shock-wave lithotripsy for gallstones has rarely been described in children. Sokal *et al.* (1994) reported successful treatment in a child without gallbladder calculi and a single obstructing 7-mm-diameter stone in the distal common bile duct.

SURGICAL MANAGEMENT

Surgery is generally necessary for *symptomatic* or *complicated* gallstone disease. Cholecystectomy is the standard treatment for gallbladder cholelithiasis, but rarely cholecystostomy may be appropriate in a severely ill patient. Acute calculous cholecystitis can be treated either by emergency cholecystectomy or by delayed surgery once the acute episode has settled with medical management. In the hemolytic disorders, *asymptomatic* calculi merit special consideration.

- In hereditary spherocytosis, cholecystectomy is indicated for patients with asymptomatic calculi who are undergoing splenectomy for hematological reasons (Lawrie and Ham, 1974; Croom *et al.*, 1986). A less successful alternative is cholecystotomy with stone removal at the time of splenectomy. Robertson *et al.* (1988) reported five children who were treated in this way and followed up for 1 to 2 years. One of these children had evidence of persistent cholelithiasis. Cholecystolithotomy has also been shown to be inferior to cholecystectomy in other groups of children with gallstones (De Caluwé *et al.*, 2001). Prophylactic cholecystectomy at the time of splenectomy is not indicated in children with hereditary spherocytosis who do not have gallstones (Sandler *et al.*, 1999).
- In sickle-cell anemia, gallstones are frequently asymptomatic in children under 15 years of age, but there is a rising incidence of symptomatic disease thereafter (Bond *et al.*, 1987; Webb *et al.*, 1989). Opinion on the management of asymptomatic stones is divided, but many authors favor elective cholecystectomy (Malone and Werlin, 1988; Alexander-Reindorf *et al.*, 1990; Winter *et al.*, 1994). Reasons include the increasing risk of complications with age (Lachman *et al.*, 1979), the increased morbidity of emergency surgery for gallstone complications (Stephens and Scott, 1980), and the difficulty of distinguishing between cholecystitis and a sickle-cell abdominal crisis (Ariyan *et al.*, 1976). Winter *et al.* (1994) also recommended prophylactic cholecystectomy in sickle-cell patients with gallbladder sludge, because all such patients in their series subsequently developed gallstones. Alexander-Reindorf *et al.* (1990) noted that sickle-cell patients with gallstones had twice as many admissions and clinic visits as those without stones. Preoperative blood transfusion to achieve a hemoglobin

concentration of > 9.0 g/dL and to reduce the proportion of hemoglobin S to less than 40% together with avoidance of acidosis, hypovolemia and hypothermia, help to minimize the risk of perioperative hematological complications (Malone and Werlin, 1988; Ware *et al.*, 1988). Laparoscopic cholecystectomy appears to be advantageous in these patients (Tagge *et al.*, 1994), and using this approach a selective preoperative transfusion policy may be sufficient (McDermott *et al.*, 1993).

- In thalassemia major, cholecystectomy is recommended for children with asymptomatic cholelithiasis who are undergoing splenectomy (Pappis *et al.*, 1989).

Cholecystectomy

Preparation for surgery should include a recent biliary tract ultrasound scan, a full blood count and clotting profile, biochemical liver function tests and blood grouping and saving of serum, in addition to any specific preoperative measures related to background disease. Conventional open cholecystectomy via a small right upper quadrant incision or laparoscopic cholecystectomy are both associated with minimal morbidity. In recent years, laparoscopic cholecystectomy has emerged as the preferred approach in most cases. As with all biliary tract surgery, a thorough understanding of normal anatomical variants is important.

The following technique of laparoscopic cholecystectomy is used by the author.

- General anesthesia, a temporary orogastric tube, preliminary bladder expression and a slight head-up tilt facilitate safe peritoneal access and exposure.
- Antibiotic prophylaxis (usually a single dose of a cephalosporin).
- Subumbilical cut-down and open Hasson technique for primary port (10 mm) insertion. A pursestring suture at this site ensures a gas seal and aids subsequent closure.
- A pneumoperitoneum maintained at 7–8 mmHg provides good exposure and minimizes hemodynamic disturbances and postoperative discomfort.
- Secondary ports are introduced under direct vision with a camera in the primary port. Exact port positioning varies with age (Holcomb, 1993), but in older children three secondary 5-mm ports are inserted (Figure 13.6).
- A malleable retractor is inserted in the most lateral subcostal port, and a grasping forceps is inserted in the medial port. The epigastric port is used for dissecting forceps, scissors and clip applicators.
- As an alternative to the Reddick–Olsen technique, in which the fundus of the gallbladder is retracted superiorly over the liver, thereby stretching the cystic duct in a parallel direction to the common bile duct

(Reddick and Olsen, 1989), a liver retractor is used and Hartmann's pouch is retracted *laterally*, thereby opening up Calot's triangle (Ainslie *et al.*, 2000) (Plate 4).

- Gallbladder dissection begins close to Hartmann's pouch, and a window is created above and behind the cystic duct and artery prior to ligation of any structures (Plate 5). In this way, the two structures entering the gallbladder can only be the cystic duct and artery.
- An operative cholangiogram may be used to clarify anatomy and/or to identify common bile duct stones, but the latter are unlikely in the presence of a normal-caliber common duct (on preoperative US imaging) and in the absence of a history of jaundice, pancreatitis or disturbed liver function. Cholangiography can be performed either through a catheter inserted into a partially divided cystic duct (secured with a temporary clip) or with a Kumar clamp and sclerotherapy needle (Holzman *et al.*, 1994). Intraoperative cholangiography may not be possible if a stone is impacted in the cystic duct (but a common duct stone is unlikely in such cases).
- Once the anatomy is clear, the cystic duct is 'milked' towards the gallbladder, and the cystic duct and artery are doubly clipped and divided. It is not necessary to define the junction of the cystic and common bile ducts provided that the cystic duct close to Hartmann's pouch is adequately defined.

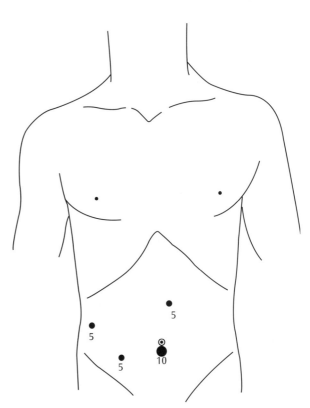

Figure 13.6 *Laparoscopic port positions for an older child undergoing cholecystectomy.*

- The gallbladder is removed by retrograde dissection using electrocautery. Prior to its complete detachment from the liver, the gallbladder bed is inspected for hemostasis. The operative site is irrigated to remove any blood or bile. The gallbladder is then removed via graspers inserted through the umbilical port and viewed from the epigastric port with a 5-mm camera.
- Conversion to open cholecystectomy may rarely be necessary in the event of bleeding, if the anatomy is uncertain or if there is severe inflammation.
- Choledocholithiasis can be treated by conversion to open exploration of the common bile duct, stone retrieval via the cystic duct, laparoscopic common duct exploration, or postoperative ERCP and extraction.
- The ports are removed under direct vision to exclude significant bleeding, and the umbilical 10-mm port site is closed with the pursestring suture.
- A temporary subhepatic drain can be inserted, and removed a few hours later if there is no evidence of a bile leak.

Compared with open cholecystectomy, studies have consistently demonstrated the need for less analgesia, a reduced stress response, more rapid recovery, earlier discharge and better cosmesis after laparoscopic cholecystectomy (Kim et al., 1995). Many children can be safely discharged home 24 hours after elective laparoscopic cholecystectomy. In adults, there is a slightly higher incidence of common bile duct injury in laparoscopic (0.2–0.5%) vs. open techniques (0.1–0.2%) (Terpstra, 1996), and judging from reports from legal societies and insurance companies in the UK and the USA, this problem is probably under-reported in the literature. Bile duct injury is more common in a surgeon's early experience of laparoscopic cholecystectomy. To date, there have been no published cases in children.

Other local complications of laparoscopic cholecystectomy include bile leaks, a missed common duct stone, bleeding, hepatic arterial injury, infection, and wound complications. In a consecutive series of 50 laparoscopic cholecystectomies in children, Tagge et al. (1995) reported conversion to open cholecystectomy in one case, postoperative hemorrhage in two cases, respiratory complications in three cases, and one readmission with gallstone pancreatitis. Miltenburg et al. (2000) drew attention to the higher complication rate in emergency cholecystectomy (open or laparoscopic), and a 2% risk of mortality in children undergoing urgent surgery with congenital heart disease. Holcomb et al. (1999) recorded no major complications and no conversions in 100 laparoscopic operations; the smallest patient weighed 10 kg, and intraoperative cholangiography was attempted in 57 cases (and was successful in 85%). Minor bile leaks usually settle after a brief period of external drainage, but more significant leaks require investigation by ERCP. Prasad et al.

(2000) described a cystic duct stump leak diagnosed by ERCP and treated successfully by external drainage, antibiotics and endoscopic insertion of a nasobiliary drain.

Choledocholithiasis

Common bile duct stones are relatively uncommon overall, although there are specific patient subgroups who have a much higher incidence. In one series of 131 children undergoing laparoscopic cholecystectomy, 14 cases (11%) were suspected preoperatively of having choledocholithiasis (a dilated common bile duct, clinical or laboratory evidence of obstructive jaundice or gallstone pancreatitis). In six children no stones were visualized at preoperative ERCP, and eight had stones which were extracted with the aid of endoscopic sphincterotomy or sphincter dilatation (Newman et al., 1997). Two-thirds of the remaining 117 children underwent intraoperative cholangiography, and only one of these was found to have evidence of a common duct stone. However, approximately 25% of children with cholelithiasis and sickle-cell disease will have choledocholithiasis (Ware et al., 1988; Bhattacharyya et al., 1993; Al-Salem et al., 1997). Infants also have a higher incidence of common bile duct stones (St-Vil et al., 1992; Debray et al., 1993; Kumar et al., 2000).

Obstructive jaundice and/or cholangitis are the usual presenting features, but acute pancreatitis occurs in some cases (Sutton and Cheslyn-Curtis 2001). Ultrasound scanning will frequently demonstrate a dilated common bile duct, but only detects about 50–75% of common duct stones. Without preoperative ERCP, some common duct stones are only confirmed by intraoperative cholangiography (Figure 13.7). The diagnosis of choledocholithiasis in children with sickle-cell disease is particularly difficult (Serafini et al., 1987). These patients develop recurrent jaundice, fever and leukocytosis in relation to sickling crises, and the common bile duct may be difficult to visualize with US. Although CT scanning and magnetic resonance cholangiography may be helpful in diagnosis, ERCP is the definitive investigation in most cases.

There are several approaches to the management of choledocholithiasis. If the expertise is available, ERCP and sphincterotomy with stone retrieval can be undertaken before or after laparoscopic cholecystectomy, even in small infants (Guelrud et al., 1992; Gholson et al., 1995). Similarly, gallstone pancreatitis can be successfully managed by preoperative ERCP and sphincterotomy and subsequent semi-elective cholecystectomy. Alternatively, laparoscopic cholecystectomy with intraoperative cholangiography can be undertaken a few weeks after the episode of gallstone pancreatitis, since the common duct stone has often passed spontaneously (Holcomb et al., 1999). Surgical approaches include cholecystotomy and irrigation in small infants or, in

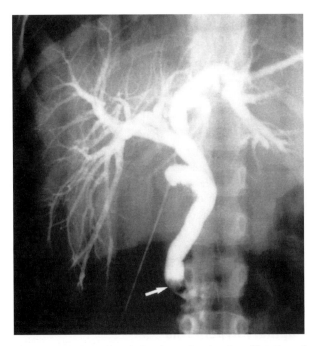

Figure 13.7 *Operative cholangiography showing dilatation of the biliary system proximal to an 8-mm stone in the distal common bile duct in a 7-year-old boy.*

older children, cholecystectomy, choledochotomy and stone removal or transduodenal sphincteroplasty (Heaton *et al.*, 1991). Laparoscopic common bile duct exploration is possible in older children, but requires considerable expertise (Holcomb *et al.*, 1999). In some centers, percutaneous techniques are used. Direct puncture of the gallbladder or insertion of a catheter into a dilated intrahepatic duct with irrigation of the biliary tract and/or removal of stones has been described (Pariente *et al.*, 1989; Debray *et al.*, 1993).

In infants with obstructive jaundice, stones may pass spontaneously with resolution of symptoms (Keller *et al.*, 1985; Jonas *et al.*, 1990; St-Vil *et al.*, 1992), and thus a period of a few weeks' observation in an otherwise well infant without evidence of sepsis or progressive obstruction may be warranted. A decreasing diameter of intrahepatic bile ducts on serial US scans often parallels resolution.

Outcome after cholecystectomy

Post-cholecystectomy syndrome is a poorly characterized entity which occurs in a small but significant proportion of adults after cholecystectomy for cholelithiasis (Shaffer, 2000). Symptoms range from the trivial and non-specific to severe attacks of abdominal pain. The frequency of this problem in children is unknown. Filston and Ware (1998) followed up 25 children with sickle hemoglobinopathies who had undergone cholecystectomy at a mean age of 13 years. After a median

interval of 30 months, residual symptoms were largely related to sickle-cell disease. No children developed recurrent stones, but 20% had frequent loose stools. Further studies are required to determine whether the post-cholecystectomy syndrome is a significant problem in children. Cholecystectomy is associated with a transient tendency to looser stools and a slightly increased incidence of duodenogastric reflux, but no serious adverse sequelae have been reported. There may be a weak association between gallstones and right-sided colon cancer in women, but there is no convincing link with cholecystectomy *per se* (Filston and Ware, 1998).

ACQUIRED GALLBLADDER DISORDERS

Torsion

The gallbladder is at risk of torsion when the peritoneum around it continues as a suspensory fold or mesentery on to the undersurface of the liver (Gross, 1936). Torsion is usually described in elderly patients, but is occasionally seen in children. Nine cases were reviewed by Iwanaka *et al.* (1982), and a further case was reported by Levard *et al.* (1994). Presentation is with acute abdominal pain and vomiting, and there may be a mobile tender mass in the right hypochondrium. The diagnosis is usually made at laparotomy, and the treatment is cholecystectomy.

Acute hydrops and acalculous cholecystitis

Severe acute distension of the gallbladder in the absence of any other disease of the biliary tract is a rare but well-documented condition. Acute hydrops may progress to cholecystitis if infection, ischemia or chemical irritation supervene. Acute hydrops and acalculous cholecystitis may occur in isolation (Mukamel *et al.*, 1981), but are most often seen in severely ill children with other conditions (Box 13.1).

Box 13.1 *Conditions associated with acute gallbladder hydrops and acalculous cholecystitis*

- Sepsis (Robinson *et al.*, 1977)
- Hypotension (Orlando *et al.*, 1983)
- Burns (Ternberg and Keating, 1975)
- Trauma (Rice *et al.*, 1980)
- Gastroenteritis (Ternbeg and Keating, 1975)
- TPN (Petersen and Sheldon, 1979)
- Kawasaki disease (Wheeler *et al.*, 1990; Bishop and Kao, 1991)
- Prematurity (Fernandes *et al.*, 1989)
- Typhoid fever

Chamberlain and Hight (1970) reviewed 29 cases of acute hydrops in whom there was no obvious inflammatory disease, calculi or congenital anomaly. They found that there was a male preponderance, and that the average age at presentation was just over 5 years. A multifactorial etiology is likely, involving dehydration, biliary stasis, infection and gallbladder ischemia. In Western countries, acute acalculous cholecystitis may occur in association with shock, trauma, cardiac surgery, burns, systemic sepsis, *Salmonella* infection and parenteral nutrition (Tsakayannis *et al.*, 1996). In the tropics, *Salmonella typhi* infection and ascariasis should be considered, although no known etiological factors are identifiable in some cases (Ameh, 1999).

Clinical features include abdominal pain, vomiting, fever, localized tenderness and, in 50% of cases, a palpable right upper quadrant mass. Laboratory investigations reveal a leukocytosis, raised acute phase reactants, hyperbilirubinemia and mild hyperamylasemia. Differential diagnosis includes appendicitis and intussusception (Ternberg and Keating, 1975; Crankson *et al.*, 1992), but these are readily distinguished by US, which shows a markedly distended gallbladder. Initial management is non-operative with antibiotics, intravenous fluids and bowel rest. Cholecystectomy is indicated if there is progressive clinical deterioration, a persistent tender mass and/or increasing gallbladder distension on US. Tube cholecystostomy is a good alternative if there has been no progression to gallbladder necrosis.

Xanthogranulomatous cholecystitis

This is a rare focal or diffuse destructive inflammatory disease of the gallbladder that is assumed to be a variant of conventional chronic cholecystitis. It is most often seen in adults, frequently in association with cholelithiasis. There is full-thickness inflammation of the gallbladder wall, with dense surrounding adhesions and local extension into adjacent tissues. On cut section the gallbladder wall reveals multiple yellow nodular lesions, and on microscopy there are collections of foamy histiocytes containing abundant lipid. Clinically and radiologically the condition can be confused with malignancy. Inflammation may progress to fistula formation, as in the 6-year-old boy with a cholecystoduodenal fistula reported by Byard *et al.* (1990). There is only one report of an infant with xanthogranulomatous cholecystitis (Kawana *et al.*, 1990).

Gallbladder dyskinesia

Impaired gallbladder contractility in the absence of cholelithiasis has been identified as a cause of chronic abdominal pain in adults. Two recent studies have suggested that a similar disorder exists in children (Dumont and Caniano, 1999; Gollin *et al.*, 1999). In a child with upper abdominal pain and no evidence of cholelithiasis, diagnosis relies on the demonstration of significantly impaired gallbladder contraction during a technetium-99m-di-isopropyl iminodiacetic acid (DISIDA) scan in response to an injection of cholecystokinin (ejection fraction of < 40%). Ultrasound scans show an anatomically normal gallbladder. Dumont and Caniano (1999) reported an excellent response to cholecystectomy in such patients, half of whom were shown to have histological evidence of chronic cholecystitis. Gollin *et al.* (1999) recorded resolution of symptoms in 79% of their patients. These patients must be carefully evaluated prior to cholecystectomy in an attempt to exclude other causes of their symptoms, such as gastro-esophageal reflux and irritable bowel syndrome.

Papillary hyperplasia

A variety of metaplastic and hyperplastic changes may affect the gallbladder mucosa in association with calculous cholecystitis or other inflammatory conditions. Primary papillary hyperplasia of the gallbladder, also known as adenomatous hyperplasia, is a rare and poorly defined clinicopathological entity which occurs in the absence of gallbladder cholelithiasis or cholesterolosis. It is recognized in adults, and has been reported as a cause of biliary colic in a child (Plate 6) (Stringer *et al.*, 2001). Rare associations include ulcerative colitis with primary sclerosing cholangitis, childhood metachromatic leukodystrophy, and anomalous pancreaticobiliary ductal union (Oak *et al.*, 1997; Tanno *et al.*, 1997). Polypoid lesions of the gallbladder may be caused by a variety of pathogies, including papillary hyperplasia, cholesterol polyps, adenoma, gastric heterotopia and hamartomatous lesions.

Porcelain gallbladder

Calcification of the gallbladder wall, otherwise known as porcelain gallbladder, is relatively rare in adults and is frequently asymptomatic. Up to 0.8% of adult gallbladders removed at cholecystectomy show some calcification in the wall, probably related to chronic inflammation. Casteel *et al.* (1990) reported the case of a 10-year-old girl in whom gallbladder calcification was noted during investigation of a urinary tract infection. She was treated by cholecystectomy. She did not have gallstones, but histology of the gallbladder showed chronic cholecystitis. The authors of the report pointed out the association in adults between calcification, gallstones and carcinoma of the gallbladder.

Key references

Grosfeld JL, Rescorla FJ, Skinner MA, West KW, Scherer LR III. The spectrum of biliary tract disorders in infants and children: experience with 300 cases. *Archives of Surgery* 1994; **129**: 513–20.

A review of 300 infants and children with biliary tract disease treated between 1972 and 1993 at the Whitcomb Riley Hospital for Children, Indianapolis. Included in the series were 169 children (106 girls) with cholelithiasis treated mainly by open cholecystectomy. There were eight postoperative complications and one death (0.6% mortality).

Holcomb GW III, Morgan WM III, Neblett WW III *et al.* Laparoscopic cholecystectomy in children: lessons learned from the first 100 patients. *Journal of Pediatric Surgery* 1999; **34**: 1236–40.

A retrospective review of 100 consecutive infants and children undergoing laparoscopic cholecystectomy between 1990 and 1998 at Vanderbilt Children's Hospital, Nashville. The series highlights the advantages and safety of laparoscopic techniques in children with simple and complicated cholelithiasis.

Matos C, Avni EF, Van Gansbeke D *et al.* Total parenteral nutrition (TPN) and gallbladder diseases in neonates. Sonographic assessment. *Journal of Ultrasound in Medicine* 1987; **6**: 243–8.

A prospective ultrasound study of the biliary tract in 41 neonates receiving total parenteral nutrition. The study documented the development of gallbladder sludge and gallstones, and demonstrated spontaneous resolution of cholelithiasis after reinstituting enteral feeding.

St-Vil D, Yazbeck S, Luks FI, Hancock BJ, Filiatrault D, Youssef S. Cholelithiasis in newborns and infants. *Journal of Pediatric Surgery* 1992; **27**: 1305–7.

An analysis of 13 infants with cholelithiasis from the University of Montreal, Quebec. The authors reviewed predisposing factors and highlighted the frequency of spontaneous resolution of cholelithiasis in this age group.

Tsakayannis DE, Kozakewich HP, Lillehei CW. Acalculous cholecystitis in children. *Journal of Pediatric Surgery* 1996; **31**: 127–30.

A review of 25 children with acalculous cholecystitis during a 25-year period at the Children's Hospital, Boston. The paper gives details of etiology, symptoms, laboratory findings and management.

REFERENCES

Abbitt PL, McIlhenny J. Prenatal detection of gallstones. *Journal of Clinical Ultrasound* 1990; **18**: 202–4.

Afdhal NH. Epidemiology, risk factors, and pathogenesis of gallstones. In: Afdhal NH (ed.) *Gallbladder and biliary tract diseases*. New York: Marcel Dekker Inc., 2000: 127–46.

Ainslie WB, Larvin M, Martin IG, McMahon MJ. Liver retraction techniques for laparoscopic cholecystectomy. *Surgical Endoscopy* 2000; **14**: 311.

Alexander-Reindorf C, Nwaneri RU, Worrell RG. The significance of gallstones in children with sickle-cell anemia. *Journal of the National Medical Association* 1990; **82**: 645–50.

Al-Salem AH, Qaisaruddin S, Al-Abkari H *et al.* Laparoscopic versus open cholecystectomy in children. *Pediatric Surgery International* 1997; **12**: 587–90.

Ameh EA. Cholecystitis in children in Zaria, Nigeria. *Annals of Tropical Paediatrics* 1999; **19**: 205–9.

Anagnostopoulos D, Tsagari N, Noussia-Arvanitaki S *et al.* Gallbladder disease in patients with cystic fibrosis. *European Journal of Pediatric Surgery* 1993; **3**: 348–51.

Ariyan S, Shessel FS, Pickett LK. Cholecystitis and cholelithiasis masking as abdominal crises in sickle-cell disease. *Pediatrics* 1976; **58**: 252–8.

Aughton DJ, Gibson P, Cacciarelli A. Cholelithiasis in infants with Down syndrome. Three cases and literature review. *Clinical Pediatrics* 1992; **31**: 650–2.

Bailie AG, Wyatt JI, Sheridan MB, Stringer MD. Heterotopic gastric mucosa in a duplicate gallbladder. *Journal of Pediatric Surgery* (in press).

Bailey PV, Connors RH, Tracy TF Jr *et al.* Changing spectrum of cholelithiasis and cholecystitis in infants and children. *American Journal of Surgery* 1989; **158**: 585–8.

Benjamin DR. Cholelithiasis in infants: the role of total parenteral nutrition and gastrointestinal dysfunction. *Journal of Pediatric Surgery* 1982; **17**: 386–9.

Bennion RS, Thompson JE, Tompkins RK. Agenesis of the gallbladder without extrahepatic biliary atresia. *Archives of Surgery* 1988; **123**: 1257–60.

Beretsky I, Lankin DH. Diagnosis of fetal cholelithiasis using real-time high-resolution imaging employing digital detection. *Journal of Ultrasound in Medicine* 1983; **2**: 381–3.

Bhattacharyya N, Wayne AS, Kevy SV *et al.* Perioperative management for cholecystectomy in sickle-cell disease. *Journal of Pediatric Surgery* 1993; **28**: 72–5.

Bishop WP, Kao SC. Prolonged postprandial abdominal pain following Kawasaki syndrome with acute gallbladder hydrops: association with impaired gallbladder emptying. *Journal of Pediatric Gastroenterology and Nutrition* 1991; **13**: 307–11.

Bond LR, Hatty SR, Horn MEC *et al.* Gallstones in sickle-cell disease in the United Kingdom. *British Medical Journal* 1987; **295**: 234–6.

Borgna-Pignatti C, De Stefano P, Pajno D *et al.* Cholelithiasis in children with thalassemia major: an ultrasonographic study. *Journal of Pediatrics* 1981; **99**: 243–4.

Boyden EA. The accessory gallbladder: an embryological and comparative study of aberrant biliary vesicles occurring in man and the domestic mammals. *American Journal of Anatomy* 1926; **38**: 177–87.

Boyle RJ, Sumner TE, Volberg FM *et al.* Cholelithiasis in a 3-week-old small premature infant. *Pediatrics* 1983; **71**: 967–9.

Brandt JR, Joseph MW, Fouser LS *et al.* Cholelithiasis following *Escherichia coli* O157:H7-associated hemolytic uremic syndrome. *Pediatric Nephrology* 1998; **12**: 222–5.

Brill PW, Winchester P, Rosen MS. Neonatal cholelithiasis. *Pediatric Radiology* 1982; **12**: 285–8.

Broussin B, Daube E. La lithiase vesiculaire foetale. *Journal de Gynecologie, Obstetrique et Biologie de la Reproduction* 1990; **19**: 90–5.

Bruch SW, Ein SH, Rocchi C, Kim PC. The management of non-pigmented gallstones in children. *Journal of Pediatric Surgery* 2000; **35**: 729–32.

Byard RW, Thorner PS, Cutz E, Filler RM, Durie P. Xanthogranulomatous cholecystitis and cholecystoduodenal fistula formation associated with total parenteral nutrition in a six-year-old child. *Pathology* 1990; **22**: 239–41.

Cao S, Cox K, So SS *et al.* Potential effect of cyclosporin A in formation of cholesterol gallstones in pediatric liver transplant recipients. *Digestive Diseases and Sciences* 1997; **42**: 1409–15.

Casteel HB, Williamson SL, Golladay ES, Fiedorek SC. Porcelain gallbladder in a child: a case report and review. *Journal of Pediatric Surgery* 1990; **25**: 1302–3.

Chamberlain JW, Hight DW. Acute hydrops of the gallbladder in childhood. *Surgery* 1970; **68**: 899–905.

Chittmittrapap S, Buachum V, Dharmklong-at A. Cholelithiasis in thalassemic children. *Pediatric Surgery International* 1990; **5**: 114–17.

Colombo C, Bertolini E, Assaisso ML *et al.* Failure of ursodeoxycholic acid to dissolve radiolucent gallstones in patients with cystic fibrosis. *Acta Pediatrica* 1993; **82**: 562–5.

Cooperberg PL, Burhenne HJ. Real-time ultrasonography. Diagnostic technique of choice in calculous gallbladder disease. *New England Journal of Medicine* 1980; **302**: 1277–9.

Crankson S, Nazer H, Jacobsson B. Acute hydrops of the gallbladder in childhood. *European Journal of Pediatrics* 1992; **151**: 318–20.

Croom RD III, McMillan CW, Sheldon GF, Orringer EP. Hereditary spherocytosis. Recent experience and current concepts of pathophysiology. *Annals of Surgery* 1986; **203**: 34–9.

Danon YL, Dinari G, Garty BZ *et al.* Cholelithiasis in children with immunoglobulin A deficiency: a new gastroenterologic syndrome *Journal of Pediatric Gastroenterology and Nutrition* 1983; **2**: 663–6.

Davies BW, Abel G, Puntis JWL *et al.* Limited ileal resection in infancy; the long-term consequences. *Journal of Pediatric Surgery* 1999; **34**: 583–7.

Dawes LG, Greiner M, Joehl RJ. Altered gallbladder bile acidification with long-term total parenteral nutrition. *Journal of Surgical Research* 1999; **81**: 21–6.

Debray D, Pariente D, Gauthier F *et al.* Cholelithiasis in infancy: a study of 40 cases. *Journal of Pediatrics* 1993; **122**: 385–91.

De Caluwé D, Aki A, Corbally M. Cholecystectomy versus cholecystolothotomy for cholelithiasis in childhood: long-term outcome. *Journal of Pediatric Surgery* 2001; **36**: 1518–21.

Deshmukh SS, Gandhi RK, Patel RV *et al.* Cystic duct atresia with cholecystocele. *Australian and New Zealand Journal of Surgery* 1999; **69**: 889–90.

Dumont RC, Caniano DA. Hypokinetic gallbladder disease: a cause of chronic abdominal pain in children and adolescents. *Journal of Pediatric Surgery* 1999; **34**: 858–62.

Esper E, Kaufman DB, Crary GS, Snover DC, Leonard AS. Septate gallbladder with cholelithiasis: a cause of chronic abdominal pain in a 6-year-old child. *Journal of Pediatric Surgery* 1992; **27**: 1560–2.

Evans MM, Nagorney DM, Pernicone PJ, Perrault J. Heterotopic gastric mucosa in the common bile duct. *Surgery* 1990; **108**: 96–100.

Fernandes ET, Hollabaugh RS, Boulden TF, Angel C. Gangrenous acalculous cholecystitis in a premature infant. *Journal of Pediatric Surgery* 1989; **24**: 608–9.

Figueroa-Colon R, Tolaymat N, Kao SC. Gallbladder sludge and lithiasis in an infant born to a morphine-user mother. *Journal of Pediatric Gastroenterology and Nutrition* 1990; **10**: 234–8.

Filston HC, Ware RE. Biliary stone disease. In: Stringer MD, Oldham KT, Mouriquand PDE, Howard ER (eds) *Pediatric surgery and urology: long-term outcomes*. Philadelphia, PA: WB Saunders Co., 1998; 454–64.

Forshall I, Rickham PP. Cholecystitis and cholelithiasis in childhood. *British Journal of Surgery* 1955; **42**: 161–4.

Gamba PG, Zancan L, Midrio P *et al.* Is there a place for medical treatment in children with gallstones? *Journal of Pediatric Surgery* 1997; **32**: 476–8.

Georgeson K, Brown P. Short bowel syndrome. In: Stringer MD, Oldham KT, Mouriquand PDE, Howard ER (eds) *Pediatric surgery and urology: long-term outcomes* Philadelphia, PA: WB Saunders Co., 1998: 237–42.

Gholson CF, Grier JF, Ibach MB *et al.* Sequential endoscopic/laparoscopic management of sickle hemoglobinopathy-associated cholelithiasis and suspected choledocholithiasis. *Southern Medical Journal* 1995; **88**: 1131–5.

Ghose SI, Stringer MD. Successful non-operative management of neonatal acute calculous cholecystitis. *Journal of Pediatric Surgery* 1999; **34**: 1029–30.

Gollin G, Raschbaum GR, Moorthy C, Santos L. Cholecystectomy for suspected biliary dyskinesia in children with chronic abdominal pain. *Journal of Pediatric Surgery* 1999; **34**: 854–7.

Good LI, Edell SL, Soloway RD *et al.* Ultrasonic properties of gallstones. Effect of stone size and composition. *Gastroenterology* 1979; **77**: 258–63.

Grosfeld JL, Rescorla FJ, Skinner MA, West KW, Scherer LR III. The spectrum of biliary tract disorders in infants and children: experience with 300 cases. *Archives of Surgery* 1994; **129**: 513–20.

Gross RE. Congenital anomalies of the gallbladder. A review of 148 cases, with report of a double gallbladder. *Archives of Surgery* 1936; **32**: 131–62.

Guelrud M, Mendoza S, Jaen D *et al.* ERCP and endoscopic sphincterotomy in infants and children with jaundice due to common bile duct stones. *Gastrointestinal Endoscopy* 1992; **38**: 450–3.

Halpern Z, Vinograd Z, Laufer H *et al.* Characteristics of gallbladder bile of infants and children. *Journal of Pediatric Gastroenterology and Nutrition* 1996; **23**: 147–50.

Harlaftis N, Gray SW, Skandalakis JE. Multiple gallbladders. *Surgery, Gynecology and Obstetrics* 1977; **45**: 928–34.

Heaton ND, Davenport M, Howard ER. Intraluminal biliary obstruction. *Archives of Disease in Childhood* 1991; **66**: 1395–8.

Heijne L, Ednay D. The development of fetal gallstones demonstrated by ultrasound. *Radiography* 1985; **51**: 155–6.

Heubi JE, Soloway RD, Balistreri WF. Biliary lipid composition in healthy and diseased infants, children and young adults. *Gastroenterology* 1982; **82**: 1295–9.

Holcomb GW Jr, O'Neill JA Jr, Holcomb GW III. Cholecystitis, cholelithiasis and common duct stenosis in children and adolescents. *Annals of Surgery* 1980; **191**: 626–35.

Holcomb GW III. Laparoscopic cholecystectomy. *Seminars in Pediatric Surgery* 1993; **2**: 159–67.

Holcomb GW III, Morgan WM III, Neblett WW III *et al.* Laparoscopic cholecystectomy in children: lessons learned from the first 100 patients. *Journal of Pediatric Surgery* 1999; **34**: 1236–40.

Holzman MD, Sharp K, Holcomb GW *et al.* An alternative technique for laparoscopic cholangiography. *Surgical Endoscopy* 1994; **8**: 927–30.

Honore LH. Cholesterol cholelithiasis in adolescent females. *Archives of Surgery* 1980; **115**: 62–4.

Iwanaka R, Kohda Y, Beppu T. Torsion of the gallbladder. *Japanese Journal of Pediatric Surgery* 1982; **14**: 129–33.

Jacir NN, Anderson KD, Eichelberger M *et al.* Cholelithiasis in infancy: resolution of gallstones in three of four infants. *Journal of Pediatric Surgery* 1986; **21**: 567–9.

Jawaheer G, Pierro A, Lloyd DA, Shaw NJ. Gallbladder contractility in neonates: effects of parenteral and enteral feeding. *Archives of Disease in Childhood* 1995; **72**: F200–2.

Jeffrey I, Lund RJ, Whitelaw A. Cholelithiasis in a preterm infant. *Pediatric Pathology* 1984; **2**: 207–13.

Jonas A, Yahav J, Fradkin A *et al.* Choledocholithiasis in infants: diagnostic and therapeutic problems. *Journal of Pediatric Gastroenterology and Nutrition* 1990; **11**: 513–17.

Kalayci AG, Albayrak D, Gunes M, Incesu L, Agac R. The incidence of gallbladder stones and gallbladder function in beta-thalassemic children. *Acta Radiologica* 1999; **40**: 440–3.

Kawana T, Suita S, Arima T *et al.* Xanthogranulomatous cholecystitis in an infant with obstructive jaundice. *European Journal of Pediatrics* 1990; **149**: 765–7.

Keller MS, Markle BM, Laffey PA *et al.* Spontaneous resolution of cholelithiasis in infants. *Radiology* 1985; **157**: 345–8.

Kim PC, Wesson D, Superina R, Filler R. Laparoscopic cholecystectomy versus open cholecystectomy in children: which is better? *Journal of Pediatric Surgery* 1995; **30**: 971–3.

Klingensmith WC, Cioffi-Ragan DT. Fetal gallstones. *Radiology* 1988; **167**: 143–4.

Ko CW, Sekijima JH, Lee SP. Biliary sludge. *Annals of Internal Medicine* 1999; **130**: 301–11.

Komura J, Yano H, Tomita T *et al.* Gallbladder stone and sludge formation with total parenteral nutrition in childhood – an experience of eight cases. *Japanese Journal of Surgical Metabolism and Nutrition* 1988; **22**: 296–305.

Kose G, Ozkan H, Ozdamar F *et al.* Cholelithiasis in cervico-oculo-acoustic (Wildervanck's) syndrome. *Acta Paediatrica* 1993; **82**: 890–1.

Kumar R, Nguyen K, Shun A. Gallstones and common bile duct calculi in infancy and childhood. *Australian and New Zealand Journal of Surgery* 2000; **70**: 188–91.

Lachman BS, Lazerson J, Starshak RJ, Vaughters FM, Werlin SL. The prevalence of cholelithiasis in sickle-cell disease as diagnosed by ultrasound and cholecystography. *Pediatrics* 1979; **64**: 601–3.

Lafont H, Ostrow JD. Calcium salt precipitation in bile and biomineralization of gallstones. In: Afdhal NH (ed.) *Gallbladder and biliary tract diseases*. New York: Marcel Dekker Inc., 2000: 317–60.

Lamont N, Winthrop AL, Cole FM *et al.* Heterotopic gastric mucosa in the gallbladder: a cause of chronic abdominal pain in a child. *Journal of Pediatric Surgery* 1991; **26**: 1293–5.

Lapidus A, Einarsson C. Bile composition in patients with ileal resection due to Crohn's disease. *Inflammatory Bowel Disease* 1998; **4**: 89–94.

Lawrie GM, Ham JM. The surgical treatment of hereditary spherocytosis. *Surgery, Gynecology and Obstetrics* 1974; **139**: 208–10.

Lehtonen L, Svedstrom E, Kero P, Korvenranta H. Gallbladder contractility in preterm infants. *Archives of Disease in Childhood* 1993; **68**: 43–5.

Levard G, Weil D, Barret D *et al.* Torsion of the gallbladder in children. *Journal of Pediatric Surgery* 1994; **29**: 569–70.

Llerena JC, Boy R, Neto JB *et al.* Abdominal ultrasound scan in Down syndrome patients: high frequency of non-symptomatic biliary tract disease. *American Journal of Medical Genetics* 1993; **46**: 612.

Luzuy F, Reinberg O, Kauszlaric D *et al*. Biliary calculi caused by hemobilia. *Surgery* 1987; **102**: 886–9.

McDermott EWM, AlKhalifa K, Murphy JJ. Laparoscopic cholecystectomy without exchange transfusion in sickle-cell disease. *Lancet* 1993; **342**: 1181.

McDonagh AF. Phototherapy: a new twist to bilirubin. *Journal of Pediatrics* 1981; **99**: 909–11.

Mahmoud H, Schell M, Pui CH. Cholelithiasis after treatment for childhood cancer. *Cancer* 1991; **67**: 1439–42.

Malone BS, Werlin SI. Cholecystectomy and cholelithiasis in sickle-cell anemia. *American Journal of Diseases in Childhood* 1988; **142**: 799–800.

Matos C, Avni EF, Van Gansbeke D *et al*. Total parenteral nutrition (TPN) and gallbladder diseases in neonates. Sonographic assessment. *Journal of Ultrasound in Medicine* 1987; **6**: 243–8.

Milas M, Ricketts RR, Amerson JR, Kanter K. Management of biliary tract stones in heart transplant patients. *Annals of Surgery* 1996; **223**: 747–53.

Miltenburg DM, Schaffer R, Breslin T, Brandt ML. Changing indications for pediatric cholecystectomy. *Pediatrics* 2000; **105**: 1250–3.

Mukamel E, Zer M, Avidor I *et al*. Acute acalculous cholecystitis in an infant; a case report. *Journal of Pediatric Surgery* 1981; **16**: 521–2.

Newcombe JF, Henley FA. Left-sided gallbladder. *Archives of Surgery* 1964; **88**: 494–7.

Newman HF, Northup JD, Rosenblum M, Abrams H. Complications of cholelithiasis. *American Journal of Gastroenterology* 1968; **50**: 476–96.

Newman KD, Powell DM, Holcomb GW III. The management of choledocholithiasis in children in the era of laparoscopic cholecystectomy. *Journal of Pediatric Surgery* 1997; **32**: 1116–19.

Nilsson S. Gallbladder disease and sex hormones. A statistical study. *Acta Chirurgica Scandinavica* 1966; **132**: 275–9.

Oak S, Rao S, Karmarkar S *et al*. Papillomatosis of the gallbladder in metachromatic leukodystrophy. *Pediatric Surgery International* 1997; **12**: 424–5.

O'Brien CB, Berman JM, Fleming CR, Malet PF, Soloway RD. Total parenteral nutrition gallstones contain more calcium bilirubinate than sickle-cell gallstones. *Gastroenterology* 1986; **90**: 1752.

Orlando R, Gleason E, Drezner AD. Acute acalculous cholecystitis in the critically ill patient. *American Journal of Surgery* 1983; **145**: 472–6.

Palanduz A, Yalcin I, Tonguc E *et al*. Sonographic assessment of ceftriaxone-associated biliary pseudolithiasis in children. *Journal of Clinical Ultrasound* 2000; **28**: 166–8.

Palasciano G, Portincasa P, Vinciguerra V *et al*. Gallstone prevalence and gallbladder volume in children and adolescents: an epidemiological ultrasonographic survey and relationship to body mass index. *American Journal of Gastroenterology* 1989; **84**: 1378–82.

Pappis CH, Galanakis S, Moussatos G. Experience of splenectomy and cholecystectomy in children with chronic hemolytic anemia. *Journal of Pediatric Surgery* 1989; **24**: 543–6.

Pariente D, Bernard O, Gauthier F *et al*. Radiological treatment of common bile duct lithiasis in infancy. *Pediatric Radiology* 1989; **19**: 104–7.

Pellerin D, Bertin P, Nihoul-Fekete CI, Ricour CI. Cholelithiasis and ileal pathology in childhood. *Journal of Pediatric Surgery* 1975; **10**: 35–41.

Petersen SR, Sheldon GF. Acute acalculous cholecystitis: a complication of hyperalimentation. *American Journal of Surgery* 1979; **138**: 814–17.

Prasad H, Poddar U, Thapa BR *et al*. Endoscopic management of post-laparoscopic cholecystectomy bile leak in a child. *Gastrointestinal Endoscopy* 2000; **61**: 506–7.

Reddick EJ, Olsen DO. Laparoscopic laser cholecystectomy: a comparison with mini-lap cholecystectomy. *Surgical Endoscopy* 1989; **3**: 131–3.

Reif S, Sloven DG, Lebenthal E. Gallstones in children. Characterization by age, etiology and outcome. *American Journal of Disease in Childhood* 1991; **145**: 105–8.

Rice J, Williams HC, Flint LM *et al*. Post-traumatic acalculous cholecystitis. *Southern Medical Journal* 1980; **73**: 14–17.

Rintala RJ, Lindahl H, Pohjavuori M. Total parenteral nutrition-associated cholestasis in surgical neonates may be reversed by intravenous cholecystokinin: a preliminary report. *Journal of Pediatric Surgery* 1995; **30**: 827–30.

Robertson JFR, Carachi R, Sweet EM, Raine PAM. Cholelithiasis in childhood: a follow-up study. *Journal of Pediatric Surgery* 1988; **23**: 246–9.

Robinson AE, Erwin JE, Wiseman HJ, Kodroff MB. Cholecystitis and hydrops of the gallbladder in the newborn. *Pediatric Radiology* 1977; **122**: 749–51.

Roslyn JJ, Berquist WE, Pitt HA *et al*. Increased risk of gallstones in children receiving total parenteral nutrition. *Pediatrics* 1983; **71**: 784–9.

Safford SD, Safford KM, Martin P, Rice H, Kurtzberg J, Skinner MA. Management of cholelithiasis in pediatric patients who undergo bone-marrow transplantation. *Journal of Pediatric Surgery* 2001; **36**: 86–90.

Sandler A, Winkel G, Kimura K, Soper R. The role of prophylactic cholecystectomy during splenectomy in children with hereditary spherocytosis. *Journal of Pediatric Surgery* 1999; **34**: 1077–8.

Sarnaik S, Slovis TL, Corbett DP *et al*. Incidence of cholelithiasis in sickle-cell anemia using the ultrasonic gray-scale technique. *Journal of Pediatrics* 1980; **96**: 1005–8.

Schwindt WD, Bernhardt LC, Peters HA. Cholelithiasis and associated complications of myotonia dystrophica. *Postgraduate Medicine* 1969; **46**: 80–3.

Serafini AN, Spolianski G, Sfakianakis GN, Montalvano B, Jensen WN. Diagnostic studies in patients with sickle-cell anaemia and acute abdominal pain. *Archives of Internal Medicine* 1987; **147**: 1061–2.

Setchell KDR, Dumaswala R, Colombo C, Ronchi M. Hepatic bile acid metabolism during early development revealed from the analysis of human fetal gallbladder bile. *Journal of Biological Chemistry* 1988; **263**: 16637–44.

Shaffer EA. Morphine and biliary pain revisited. *Gut* 2000; **46**: 750–1.

Shimotake T, Iwai N, Yanagihara J, Tokiwa K, Fushiki S. Biliary tract complications in patients with hypoganglionosis and chronic idiopathic intestinal pseudo-obstruction syndrome. *Journal of Pediatric Surgery* 1993; **28**: 189–92.

Soderlund S, Zetterstrom B. Cholecystitis and cholelithiasis in children. *Archives of Disease in Childhood* 1962; **37**: 174–80.

Sokal EM, DeBilderling G, Clapuyt P *et al.* Extracorporeal shock-wave lithotripsy for calcified lower choledocholithiasis in an 18-month-old boy. *Journal of Pediatric Gastroenterology and Nutrition* 1994; **18**: 391–4.

Stephens CG, Scott RB. Cholelithiasis in sickle-cell anemia: surgical or medical management. *Archives of Internal Medicine* 1980; **140**: 648–51.

Stern RC, Rothstein FC, Doershuk CF. Treatment and prognosis of symptomatic gallbladder disease in patients with cystic fibrosis. *Journal of Pediatric Gastroenterology and Nutrition* 1986; **5**: 35–40.

Stringer MD, Lim P, Cave M, Martinez D, Lilford RJ. Fetal gallstones. *Journal of Pediatric Surgery* 1996; **31**: 1589–91.

Stringer MD, Abbott C, Arthur RJ, Lealman G. Primary papillary hyperplasia of the gallbladder: a rare cause of biliary colic. *Journal of Pediatric Surgery* 2001; **36**: 1584–6.

St-Vil D, Yazbeck S, Luks FI, Hancock BJ, Filiatrault D, Youssef S. Cholelithiasis in newborns and infants. *Journal of Pediatric Surgery* 1992; **27**: 1305–7.

Suita S, Ikeda K, Naito K *et al.* Cholelithiasis in infants: association with parenteral nutrition. *Journal of Parenteral and Enteral Nutrition* 1984; **8**: 568–70.

Sutton R, Cheslyn-Curtis S. Acute gallstone pancreatitis in childhood. *Annals of the Royal College of Surgeons of England* 2001; **83**: 406–8.

Tagge EP, Othersen HB, Jackson SM *et al.* Impact of laparoscopic cholecystectomy on the management of cholelithiasis in children with sickle-cell disease. *Journal of Pediatric Surgery* 1994; **29**: 209–13.

Tagge EP, Othersen HB Jr, Chandler JC, Smith CD. *Complications of laparoscopic cholecystectomy in children*. Paper presented at British Association of Paediatric Surgeons XLII Annual International Congress, Sheffield, July 1995.

Takiff H, Fonkalsrud EW. Gallbladder disease in childhood. *American Journal of Disease in Childhood* 1984; **138**: 565–8.

Tanno S, Obara T, Maguchi H *et al.* Thickened inner hypoechoic layer of the gallbladder wall in the diagnosis of anomalous pancreaticobiliary ductal union with endosonography. *Gastrointestinal Endoscopy* 1997; **46**: 520–6.

Tay JS, Werlin SL. Cholelithiasis in an infant with polycythemia. *Journal of Pediatric Gastroenterology and Nutrition* 1987; **6**: 311–12.

Tchirkow G, Highman LM, Shafer AD. Cholelithiasis and cholecystitis in children after repair of congenital duodenal anomalies. *Archives of Surgery* 1980; **115**: 85–6.

Teele RL, Nussbaum AR, Wyly JB, Allred EN, Emans J. Cholelithiasis after spinal fusion for scoliosis in children. *Journal of Pediatrics* 1987; **111**: 857–60.

Ternberg JL, Keating JP. Acute acalculous cholecystitis: complication of other illnesses in childhood. *Archives of Surgery* 1975; **110**: 543–7.

Terpstra OT. Laparoscopic cholecystectomy: the other side of the coin. *British Medical Journal* 1996; **312**: 1375–6.

Toscano E, Trivellini V, Andria G. Cholelithiasis in Down's Syndrome. *Archives of Disease in Childhood* 2001; **85**: 242–3.

Treem WR, Malet PF, Gourley GR, Hyams JS. Bile and stone analysis in two infants with brown pigment gallstones and infected bile. *Gastroenterology* 1989; **96**: 519–23.

Tsakayannis DE, Kozakewich HP, Lillehei CW. Acalculous cholecystitis in children. *Journal of Pediatric Surgery* 1996; **31**: 127–30.

Turkel SB, Swanson V, Chandrasoma P. Malformations associated with congenital absence of the gallbladder. *Journal of Medical Genetics* 1983; **20**: 445–9.

Vessey M, Painter R. Oral contraceptive use and benign gallbladder disease; revisited. *Contraception* 1994; **50**: 167–73.

Waldhausen JHT, Benjamin DR. Cholecystectomy is becoming an increasingly common operation in children. *American Journal of Surgery* 1999; **177**: 364–7.

Ware R, Filston HC, Schultz WH, Kinney TR. Elective cholecystectomy in children with sickle hemoglobinopathies: successful outcome using a preoperative transfusion regimen. *Annals of Surgery* 1988; **208**: 17–22.

Watkins JB, Ingall D, Szczepanik P *et al.* Bile salt metabolism in the newborn. *New England Journal of Medicine* 1973; **288**: 431–4.

Webb DK, Darby JS, Dunn DT, Terry SI, Serjeant GR. Gallstones in Jamaican children with homozygous sickle-cell disease. *Archives of Disease in Childhood* 1989; **64**: 693–6.

Weinsten S, Lipsitz EC, Addonizio L *et al.* Cholelithiasis in pediatric cardiac transplant patients on cyclosporine. *Journal of Pediatric Surgery* 1995; **30**: 60–4.

Wendtland-Born A, Wiewrodt B, Bender SW, Weitzel D. Prevalence of gallstones in the neonatal period. *Ultraschall Medizine* 1997; **18**: 80–3.

Wheeler RA, Najmaldin AS, Soubra M *et al.* Surgical presentation of Kawasaki disease (mucocutaneous lymph node syndrome). *British Journal of Surgery* 1990; **77**: 1273–4.

Whitington PF, Black DD. Cholelithiasis in premature infants treated with parenteral nutrition and furosemide. *Journal of Pediatrics* 1980; **97**: 647–9.

Williams HJ, Johnson KW. Cholelithiasis: a complication of cardiac valve surgery in children. *Pediatric Radiology* 1984; **14**: 146–7.

Winter SS, Kinney TR, Ware RE. Gallbladder sludge in children with sickle-cell disease. *Journal of Pediatrics* 1994; **125**: 747–9.

Wu SS, Casas AT, Abraham SK *et al.* Milk of calcium cholelithiasis in children. *Journal of Pediatric Surgery* 2001; **36**: 644–7.

14

Tumors of the extrahepatic bile ducts

EDWARD R HOWARD

INTRODUCTION

Tumors arising in the bile ducts of children (Box 14.1) are all extremely rare. The majority are rhabdomyosarcomata, and there are only approximately 10 reports of other tumorous lesions. Examples of benign lesions include three cases of 'inflammatory tumor' (Haith et al., 1964; Stamatakis et al., 1979; Bolla et al., 1988), one case of granular cell tumor (Reynolds et al., 2000) and two cases of villous adenomata (Leriche, 1934; Khan et al., 1996). Malignant lesions have included two carcinomata (Czaja et al., 1985; Liao et al., 1986), a liposarcoma of the porta hepatis (Soares et al., 1989) and a carcinoid tumor of the common bile duct in a 13-year-old girl (Carle et al., 1990).

Jaundice is the usual presenting sign of these lesions, and preoperative diagnosis depends on a combination of liver function tests showing conjugated hyperbilirubinemia and raised transaminase levels, ultrasonography and computed tomography. Differential diagnoses include choledochal cyst, cholelithiasis and hepatitis.

Box 14.1 *Tumors reported in the extrahepatic bile ducts of children*

Benign
  Inflammatory
  Villous adenoma
  Granular cell

Malignant
  Rhabdomyosarcoma
  Carcinoma
  Liposarcoma

BENIGN TUMORS

Inflammatory tumors

An inflammatory tumor (or 'pseudotumor') of the bile ducts was first reported in a child by Haith et al. in 1964. The 3-cm lesion, initially believed to be malignant, was situated in the distal portion of the common bile duct, and was excised by pancreaticoduodenectomy. Histology revealed a yellow-tan mass of collagen fibers and fibroblasts interspersed throughout with chronic inflammatory cells. There was a loss of epithelium within the narrowed segment of bile duct.

A second case occurred in a 13-year-old girl who presented with a history of obstructive jaundice for 12 weeks (Stamatakis et al., 1979). A 3-cm mass surrounded the junction of the cystic and common bile ducts and was completely excised (Figure 14.1a and b). Histology showed that the mass was completely encapsulated, mottled yellow-brown in color and with a soft centre. The encased bile duct showed loss of epithelium and, as in the first case, the lesion consisted of a mass of collagenous tissue with a mixed inflammatory cell infiltrate. Long-term follow-up of this patient showed no evidence of recurrence. A third pediatric case was reported in a 10-year-old child (Bolla et al., 1988).

Inflammatory 'pseudotumors' of the bile duct are not confined to children, and a typical case has been reported in a 58-year-old Japanese woman who underwent pancreaticoduodenectomy for a stricture of the lower common bile duct (Fukushima et al., 1997).

The etiology of these lesions remains obscure, although it has been suggested that the mass might develop in response to a local irritant (either chemical or

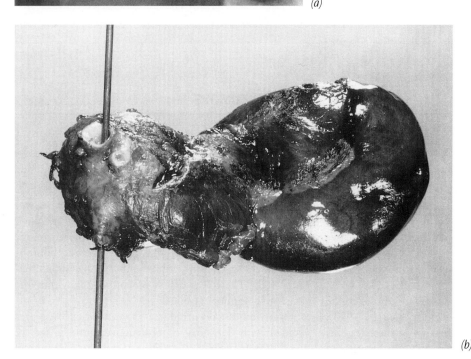

(a)

(b)

Figure 14.1 *Benign inflammatory tumor of the bile duct in a 13-year-old girl. Reproduced from Stamatakis* et al. *(1979) with the kind permission of the authors and publisher. (a) Fine-needle cholangiography shows dilatation of the main left and right hepatic ducts, with a stricture of the common hepatic duct with evidence of extrinsic compression of the bile duct lumen. (b) Surgical specimen of benign inflammatory tumor. This posterior view shows a distended gallbladder and a spherical tumor surrounding the common hepatic, cystic and common bile ducts. The probe passes through the common hepatic and common bile ducts.*

infective in origin). The prognosis after excisional surgery is excellent.

Villous adenoma

Papillomatous tumors of the bile duct have been described in children on two occasions. Jaundice caused by a large tumor weighing 750 g was reported in a 4-year-old (Leriche, 1934), and pancreatitis secondary to a lesion of the ampulla of Vater has been described in a 14-year-old (Figure 14.2) (Khan *et al.*, 1996). These tumors may contain areas of dysplasia and carcinoma, features which have been reported in three adult patients (Cattell *et al.*, 1962). Complete surgical excision is essential to abolish the risk of later malignant transformation.

Granular cell tumor

These benign tumors, which were first described as myoblastomas by Abrikosoff in 1926, have been reported in many areas of the body. There is now immunohisto-chemical evidence that they have a neural origin from Schwann cells (Cheslyn-Curtis *et al.*, 1986) rather than from myoblasts. Most of the tumors have been reported in young adult African-American girls, but there are now records of four cases under 15 years of age (Reynolds *et al.*, 2000). The clinical presentation is of a stricture in the bile duct, and histology shows cells with abundant granular eosinophilic cytoplasm. The tumors are also positive for S-100 protein immunoreactivity, which is usually associated with Schwann cells and autonomic ganglia. The lesions are not encapsulated and they may infiltrate

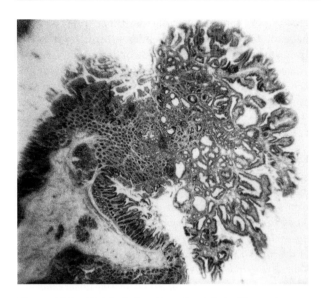

Figure 14.2 *Histological section of a tubulovillous adenoma arising within the ampulla of Vater in a 14-year-old boy. The lesion measured 5 mm in diameter and the epithelium was mildly dysplastic.*

adjacent structures, particularly when they arise in the retropancreatic bile duct. Pancreaticoduodenectomy may therefore be required for the curative resection of distal lesions.

MALIGNANT TUMORS

Rhabdomyosarcoma

Rhabdomyosarcoma is the commonest soft-tissue sarcoma in children, and it accounts for 10–15% of all pediatric solid tumors (Sutow *et al.*, 1970; Young and Miller, 1975). Although the occurrence of rhabdomyosarcoma in the biliary tree was first described in 1875 by Wilks and Moxon, it remains a rare tumor and represents only 0.8% of all rhabdomyosarcomas (Ruymann *et al.*, 1985). Approximately 100 cases have been reported in the world literature. However, Lack *et al.* (1981) emphasized that it is the commonest primary tumor of the extrahepatic biliary tree, and should be considered in the differential diagnosis of all cases of obstructive jaundice in childhood.

During the last two decades, the treatment of rhabdomyosarcomata in other sites has changed from primary radical surgery towards aggressive chemotherapy combined with some form of local tumor control using either radiotherapy or limited surgical excision. In sites such as the bladder neck, radical surgery remains an option for those who fail to respond or who have residual disease following chemo- and radiotherapy. Biliary

rhabdomyosarcomata are difficult to treat effectively, and until recently the overall outcome had been poor. However, recent experience has indicated that surgical resection (complete or partial) with adjuvant chemotherapy and radiotherapy can lead to prolonged survival.

Presentation

The median age at presentation is 3.4 years (Spunt *et al.*, 2000). There is no male preponderance as there is in genitourinary rhabdomyosarcoma. The children present with painless, fluctuating or progressive obstructive jaundice which may be complicated by fever, abdominal distension, weight loss, lethargy and irritability. The commonest preoperative diagnosis is of a congenital cystic abnormality of the bile ducts. However, with increasing awareness of the disease, preoperative diagnosis can be made by recognizing the appearance of solid material within dilated intra- and extrahepatic bile ducts on ultrasound or CT imaging (Mihara *et al.*, 1982; Ruyman *et al.*, 1985). Liver function tests confirm the pattern of obstructive jaundice and should raise suspicion of biliary rhabdomyosarcoma in young children (Ruymann *et al.*, 1985).

Ultrasound is the initial and possibly the most important investigation, and CT scanning and nuclear magnetic resonance (NMR) imaging have proved helpful in managing patients postoperatively to follow recurrent disease and any response to chemotherapy. Percutaneous transhepatic cholangiography (Figure 14.3a) has also been recommended as a helpful investigation in the preoperative diagnosis of patients who present with atypical clinical features (Cannon *et al.*, 1979).

Local or distant metastatic spread is found in 30–40% of affected children at the time of presentation (Ruymann *et al.*, 1985). Sites include the regional lymph nodes, omentum, peritoneum, lung, liver and bones (Taira *et al.*, 1976: Spunt *et al.*, 2000).

Pathology (FIGURE 14.3B, C, D AND E)

Microscopically these tumors are invariably embryonal rhabdomyosarcomata with botryoid features. This is in contrast to rhabdomyosarcomata at other sites, which frequently show alveolar or undifferentiated features. The tumors consist of mesenchymal cells with a myxomatous appearance and eosinophilic cytoplasm. Some of the mesenchymal cells show varying degrees of maturation towards rhabdomyoblasts, and occasional longitudinal cross-striations can be identified (Taira *et al.*, 1976). Botryoid polyps are often remarkably hypocellular, with edema of the superficial parts of the tumor.

The tumor is thought to arise from mesenchymal cell rests beneath the extrahepatic bile duct epithelium, and often arises from the common bile or hepatic ducts, close to their junction with the cystic duct (Lack *et al.*, 1981).

Macroscopically these tumors are polypoid in appearance with grape-like projections pushing into the bile duct lumen, and they are associated with obvious thickening of the common bile duct wall. The tumor spreads beneath the bile duct epithelium proximally into the liver substance. It may also invade or become adherent to adjacent structures such as the inferior vena cava, stomach and duodenum.

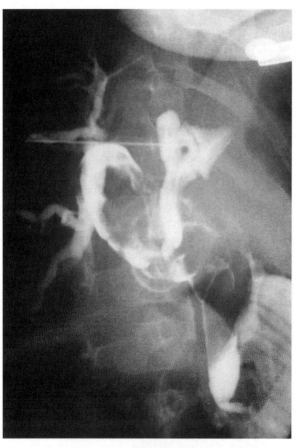

(a)

Figure 14.3 *A rhabdomyosarcoma of the bile ducts. (a) A 3-year-old child with obstructive jaundice. Cholangiography shows extensive intraluminal tumor expanding and infiltrating the common bile duct, with extension into the intrahepatic ducts. (b) Tumor removed from the common bile duct at surgery. Typical appearance of 'grape-like' polypoid masses. (c) Total excision of extrahepatic bile duct expanded with intraluminal tumor. (d) Transverse section of the excised bile duct containing rhabdomyosarcoma. (e) Histological section showing tumor composed of spindle-shaped cells with small round or oval nuclei in an abundant loose and myxoid stroma (× 80).*

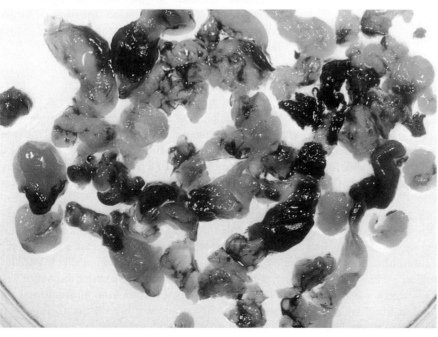

(b)

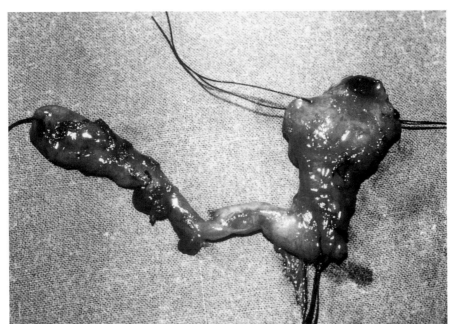

(c)

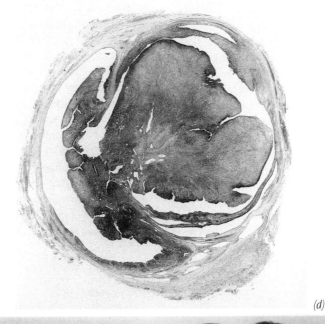

(d)

(e)

The staging suggested by the Intergroup Rhabdomyosarcoma Study Group was as follows.

- Group 1 – includes localized disease, either completely resected and confined to organ of origin (1a), or with contiguous involvement of tissues other than lymph nodes (1b).
- Group 2 – consists of complete macroscopic but incomplete microscopic resection of tumor.
- Group 3 – includes tumors that are incompletely resected, or simply biopsied, with gross residual disease.
- Group 4 – includes tumors that have metastatic disease at presentation (Maurer et al., 1977).

Treatment

The recommended treatment has been to resect as much of the tumor bulk and extrahepatic biliary tract as possible. If necessary, the technique has included a pancreaticoduodenectomy and restoration of biliary tract continuity with a hepaticojejunostomy. The surgery has often been technically demanding, but it has only rarely been possible to excise the tumor completely.

Chemotherapy now has a dominant role, and the more aggressive regimens designed for soft-tissue tumors in other sites appear to have increasing success (Spunt et al., 2000). The most commonly used drugs include actinomycin D, Adriamycin, vincristine and cyclophosphamide. The role of radiotherapy is less well defined, but it may confer immediate benefit on survival. One case of radiation hepatitis has been reported after treatment (Spunt et al., 2000).

Outcome

Because of the rarity of rhabdomyosarcomata of the bile duct, the total number of cases available for analysis is small. Until recently the average survival time was only 6 months, but the combination of surgery, chemotherapy and radiotherapy has resulted in an increase in the number of long-term survivors (Akers and Needham, 1971; Martinez et al., 1982; Ruymann et al., 1985). Spunt et al. (2000) have reported an estimated 5-year survival rate of 66% in a series of 25 children treated since 1972 with the protocols of the Intergroup Rhabdomyosarcoma Study Group (IRSG). After exclusion of patients with distant metastatic disease, all of whom died, the 5-year survival rate in this series rose to 78%. This was despite the fact that only 29% of the children had undergone complete tumor resection.

The results of various modalities of treatment reported up until 1987 are shown in Table 14.1, which demonstrates a possible benefit of combining radical surgery with chemotherapy. However, this conclusion has not been confirmed in the most recent analysis from the IRSG (Table 14.2) (Spunt et al., 2000), which includes survivors who did not undergo radical surgery but who received chemotherapy and radiotherapy. Furthermore, only two of the 17 surgical resections were shown to have clear surgical margins on histology. The role of radical surgery in the treatment of this tumor is therefore now in doubt, as is also the optimum form of treatment with chemotherapy and/or radiotherapy. The IRSG study confirms the possibility of cure without radical surgery, an observation that has been reported in previous single case reports (Perisic et al., 1991).

The prognosis for rhabdomyosarcoma in other parts of the body may depend on histological grading (Dodd et al., 1989), but so far this has not been confirmed in lesions of the bile duct. It has also been suggested (Anon., 1989) that the poor survival seen in patients with rhabdomyosarcoma may correlate with tumor aneuploidy, karyotypic abnormalities and n-myc amplification, but this hypothesis has yet to be confirmed.

Table 14.1 *Survival in 66 collected cases of rhabdomyosarcoma of the bile duct*

	n	Alive	Survival Mean	Range
No treatment	8	0	2 months	1 week – 6 months
T-tube biopsy	8	0	5 months	2 weeks – 18 months
Partial resection	11	0	4.5 months	1–9 months
Partial resection with or without RT or CT	17	6	9.5 months	1 week – 2 years
Radical resection with or without RT or CT	22	11	3 years	2 weeks – 14 years
Total	66			

RT, radiotherapy; CT, cytotoxic therapy.
Collected data from Akers et al., 1971; Arnaud et al., 1987; Babut et al., 1976; Cannon et al., 1979; Corbinaeud, 1973; Friedburg et al., 1984; Geoffrey et al., 1987; Gout et al., 1974; Hashimoto, 1980; Isaacson, 1978; Lack et al., 1981; Majmudar and Kumar, 1976; Martinez et al., 1982; Mihara et al., 1982; Mulet et al., 1982; Nagaraj et al., 1977; Neidhart, 1968; O'Meira, 1981; Phatak and Prabhu, 1982; Sarrazin et al., 1977; Shimada et al., 1987; Taira et al., 1976.

Table 14.2 *Analysis of 25 cases of bile duct rhabdomyosarcoma treated between 1972 and 1998 (Intergroup Rhabdomyosarcoma Study Group) (Spunt et al., 2000)*

	n	**Survivors**
CT + RT + surgical resection	14	10
CT + surgical resection	3	3
CT + RT + biopsy	5	4
CT + biopsy	3	0
Total	25	17 (68%)

CT, chemotherapy; RT, radiotherapy.

Carcinoma

Malignant change in the bile ducts usually presents in the sixth or seventh decade. However, it is well recognized in younger patients as a complication of untreated chole-dochal cysts. The clinical data for 23 patients who developed malignant change between 1 and 19 years after cyst excision were reviewed by Watanabe *et al.* (1999), who noted that the ages at which cyst excision had been performed ranged from 1 to 55 years. Malignant change may occur in any portion of the residual intrahepatic or extrahepatic biliary tract. For example, a 15-year-old girl underwent successful resection of a giant cyst but developed a carcinoma within the remaining intrapancreatic portion of the terminal bile duct 12 years later (Yoshikawa *et al.*, 1986).

Bile duct cancer has also been reported as a secondary phenomenon 20 years after external beam radiation for Wilms' tumor (Cunningham, 1990).

The youngest case of carcinoma reported in patients without any obvious predisposing factors occurred in a 17-year-old girl (Czaja *et al.*, 1985).

Liposarcoma

Liposarcoma is a very rare tumor of childhood, but one case has been reported in the hepatic hilum of a child aged 2 years 4 months who presented with jaundice and fever. The diagnosis was confirmed at autopsy (Soares *et al.*, 1989).

Key references

Martinez FLA, Haase GM, Koep LJ, Akers DR. Rhabdomyosarcoma of the biliary tree: the case for aggressive surgery. *Journal of Pediatric Surgery* 1982; **17**: 508–11.

The authors present three cases of bile duct rhabdomyosarcomata treated with aggressive resectional surgery, irradiation and chemotherapy. After a review of the management of 36 cases, they conclude that aggressive surgery is an essential part of the management of these rare tumors.

Spunt SL, Lobe TE, Pappo AS *et al.* Aggressive surgery is unwarranted for biliary tract rhabdomyosarcoma. *Journal of Pediatric Surgery* 2000; **35**: 309–16.

This recent report of the Intergroup Rhabdomyosarcoma Study Group is a very detailed analysis of the outcome of 25 cases. The estimated 5-year survival rate was 78% after exclusion of the cases presenting with distant metastases. However, histological analysis of resected specimens revealed that only two children had undergone complete ablation of tumor tissue, and the authors therefore conclude that the aggressive surgical approach proposed in the previous paper is not essential for the cure of bile duct rhabdomyosarcomata.

Stamatakis JD, Howard ER, Williams R. Benign inflammatory tumour of the common bile duct. *British Journal of Surgery* 1979; **66**: 257–8.

This short paper defines the presentation and illustrates the pathology of benign inflammatory tumors of the bile duct.

REFERENCES

Abrikosoff A. Uber myome, ausgehend von der quergestreiften willkurlichen muskulatur. *Virchows Archiv* 1926; **260**: 215–33.

Akers DR, Needham ME. Sarcoma botryoides (rhabdomyosarcoma) of the bile ducts with survival. *Journal of Pediatric Surgery* 1971; **6**: 474–9.

Anon. Prognostic factors in childhood rhabdomyosarcoma. *Lancet* 1989; **ii**: 959–60.

Arnaud O, Bosq M, Asquier E, Michel J. Embryonal rhabdomyosarcoma of the biliary tree in children: a case report. *Pediatric Radiology* 1987; **17**: 250–1.

Babut JM, Ferrand B, Bracq H, Feuillu J, Mention J, Lecrnu M. Rhabdomyosarcome hepatique chez enfant, á propos d'un cas. *Annales de Chirurgie (Paris)* 1976; **39**: 251–5.

Bolla G, Stracca-Pansa V, Cimaglia ML, Spata F, Guarise P. Inflammatory pseudotumour as a cause of obstructive jaundice. Report of a case in a child. *Pediatria Medica e Chirurgica (Vicenza)* 1988; **10**: 523–5.

Cannon PM, Legge DA, O'Donnell B. The use of percutaneous transhepatic cholangiography in a case of embryonal rhabdomyosarcoma. *British Journal of Radiology* 1979; **52**: 326–7.

Carle JP, Tarasco A, Daude M, Nayraud P, Gislon J. Carcinoide de la voie biliaire principale chez une fillette de 13 ans. *Presse Médicale* 1990; **19**: 1946–7.

Cattell RB, Braasch JW, Kahn F. Polypoid epithelial tumors of the bile ducts. *New England Journal of Medicine* 1962; **266**: 57–61.

Cheslyn-Curtis S, Russell RC, Rode J, Dhillon AP. Granular cell tumour of the common bile duct. *Postgraduate Medical Journal* 1986; **62**: 961–3.

Corbinaeud D. *Sarcome botryoide du choledoque chez enfant.* Angers: These Médicale, 1973.

Cunningham JJ. Cholangiocarcinoma occurring after childhood radiotherapy for Wilms' tumour. *Hepatogastroenterology* 1990; **37**: 395–7.

Czaja MJ, Goldfarb JP, Cho KC, Biempica L, Morehouse HT, Abelow A. Bile duct carcinoma in an adolescent. *American Journal of Gastroenterology* 1985; **80**: 486–9.

Dodd S, Malone M, McCullough W. Rhabdomyosarcoma in children: a histological and immunohistochemical study of 59 cases. *Journal of Pathology* 1989; **158**: 13–18.

Friedburg H, Kauffman GW, Bohm N, Fiedter L, Jobke A. Sonographic and computed tomographic features of embryonal rhabdomyosarcoma of the biliary tract. *Pediatric Radiology* 1984; **14**: 436–8.

Fukushima N, Suzuki M, Abe T, Fukuyama M. A case of inflammatory pseudotumour of the common bile duct. *Virchows Archiv* 1997; **431**: 219–24.

Geoffrey A, Couanet D, Montagne JP, Lectere J, Flamant F. Ultrasonography and computer tomography for diagnosis and follow-up of biliary duct rhabdomyosarcoma. *Pediatric Radiology* 1987; **17**: 127–31.

Gout JP, Pont J, Pasquier B, Sarrazin R, Rossignol AM, Roget J. Sarcome botryoide du choledoque. *Pediatrie* 1974; **29**: 689–702.

Haith EE, Kepes JJ, Holder TM. Inflammatory pseudotumour involving the common bile duct of a six-year-old: successful pancreatico-duodenectomy. Surgery 1964; **56**: 436–41.

Hashimoto S. Botryoid sarcoma of the bile ducts. *Rinsho Hoshasen* 1980; **25**: 507–10.

Isaacson C. Embryonal rhabdomyosarcoma of the ampulla of Vater. *Cancer* 1978; **41**: 365–8.

Khan MAM, Thomas DM, Howard ER. Pancreatitis in childhood associated with villous adenoma of the ampulla of Vater. *British Journal of Surgery* 1996; **83**: 1211.

Lack EE, Perez-Atayade AR, Shuster SR. Botryoid rhabdomyosarcoma of the biliary tree. *American Journal of Surgical Pathology* 1981; **5**: 643–52.

Leriche R. Volomineuse tumeur papillomateuse du choledoque chez un enfant. *Lyon Chirurgie* 1934; **31**: 598–602.

Liao XP, Han MT, Wang MM, Wang XW. Carcinoma of the extrahepatic bile duct in a young child: a case report. *Chung Hua Chung Liu Tsa Chih* 1986; **8**: 314–15.

Majmudar B, Kumar VS. Embryonal rhabdomyosarcoma (sarcoma botryoides) of the common bile duct: a case report. *Human Pathology* 1976; **7**: 705–8.

Martinez FLA, Haase GM, Koep LJ, Akers DR. Rhabdomyosarcoma of the biliary tree: the case for aggressive surgery. *Journal of Pediatric Surgery* 1982; **17**: 508–11.

Maurer HM, Moon T, Donalson M *et al*. The intergroup rhabdomyosarcoma study. A preliminary report. *Cancer* 1977; **40**: 2015–26.

Mihara S, Matsumoto H, Tokunaga F, Yamo H, Ota M, Yamashita S. Botryoid rhabdomyosarcoma of the gallbladder in a child. *Cancer* 1982; **49**: 812–18.

Mulet JF, Illa J, Mainon C, Ros J, Claret EI. Rhabdomyosarcoma of the biliary tract. *Anales Espanoles de Pediatria (Madrid)* 1982; **17**: 65–70.

Nagaraj HS, Kemetz DR, Leitner C. Rhabdomyosarcoma of the bile ducts. *Journal of Pediatric Surgery* 1977; **12**: 1070–4.

Neidhart M. Das embryonale (rhabdomyo-) sarkom. *Zeitschrift für Kinderheilkunde* 1968; **33**: 366–8.

O'Meira A. Rhabdomyosarcoma of the bile ducts. *Zeitschrift der Kinderchirurgie* 1981; **33**: 366–8.

Perisic VN, Howard ER, Mihailovic T, Vujanic G, Milovanovic P, Ivanovski P. Cholestasis caused by biliary botryoid sarcoma. *European Journal of Pediatric Surgery* 1991; **1**: 242–3.

Phatak AM, Prabhu SR. Sarcoma botryoides of the common bile duct: a case report. *Indian Journal of Cancer* 1982; **19**: 170–2.

Reynolds EM, Tsivis PA, Long JA. Granular cell tumour of the biliary tree in a pediatric patient. *Journal of Pediatric Surgery* 2000; **35**: 652–4.

Ruymann FB, Raney RB, Crist WM, Lawrence W, Lindberg RD, Soule EH. Rhabdomyosarcoma of the biliary tree in childhood. A report from the Intergroup Rhabdomyosarcoma Study. *Cancer* 1985; **56**: 575–81.

Sarrazin R, Dyon JF, Brabant A, Pont J, Gout JP. Sarcome botryoide du choledoque. *Médécin et Chirurgie Digestives (Paris)* 1977; **6**: 45–50.

Shimada H, Newton WA, Soule EH, Beltangady MS, Mauds HM. Pathology of fetal rhabdomyosarcoma. *Cancer* 1987; **59**: 459–65.

Soares FA, Landell GA, Peres LC, Oliveira MA, Vicente YA, Tone LG. Liposarcoma of hepatic hilum in childhood: report of a case and review of the literature. *Medical and Pediatric Oncology (New York)* 1989; **17**: 239–43.

Spunt SL, Lobe TE, Pappo AS *et al*. Aggressive surgery is unwarranted for biliary tract rhabdomyosarcoma. *Journal of Pediatric Surgery* 2000; **35**: 309–16.

Stamatakis JD, Howard ER, Williams R. Benign inflammatory tumour of the common bile duct. *British Journal of Surgery* 1979; **66**: 257–8.

Sutow WW, Sullivan MP, Reid HL, Taylor HG, Griffiths KM. Prognosis in childhood rhabdomyosarcomas. *Cancer* 1970; **25**: 1384–90.

Taira Y, Nakayama I, Moriuchi A, Takahara O. Sarcoma botryoides arising from the biliary tract of children – a case report with review of the literature. *Acta Pathologica Japonica* 1976; **26**: 709–18.

Watanabe Y, Toki A, Todani T. Bile duct cancer developed after cyst excision for choledochal cyst. *Journal of Hepatobiliary and Pancreatic Surgery* 1999; **6**: 207–12.

Wilks S, Moxon W. *Lectures on pathological anatomy*, 2nd edn. London: Longmans, Green and Co., 1875.

Yoshikawa K, Yoshida K, Shirai Y *et al*. A case of carcinoma arising in the intrapancreatic terminal choledochus 12 years after primary excision of a giant choledochal cyst. *American Journal of Gastroenterology* 1986; **81**: 378–84.

Young JL, Miller RW. Incidence of malignant tumours in US children. *Journal of Pediatrics* 1975; **86**: 254–8.

PART 4

Liver tumors

15

Hemangiomas and other vascular anomalies

MARK DAVENPORT

INTRODUCTION

Although the precise figure can never be known with certainty, perhaps 10% of all liver masses are of vascular origin. These are mostly benign vascular lesions termed *hemangiomas* or *hemangioendotheliomas*. These can present in many ways, ranging from entirely asymptomatic, incidental lesions to multiple tumors almost entirely replacing liver tissue and causing life-threatening cardiac failure. As with hemangiomas in other parts of the body, the natural history of most hemangiomas in the liver is an initial rapid proliferation within the first 6–12 months of life, followed by spontaneous involution over the next 5–10 years. Hepatic *angiosarcoma* is the rare malignant counterpart of hemangioma, which may present in childhood. The liver has a unique blood supply compared with other organs of the body, which consists of both systemic arterial and portal venous inflows. Venous drainage from the liver is predominantly via the hepatic veins and, to a lesser extent, the caudate veins. Abnormal vascular communications may occur involving any of these three elements. Thus *congenital hepatic arteriovenous fistulas* of the liver may occur with similar clinical features (typically cardiac failure) to the hemangiomatous lesions considered above. Hepatic *arterioportal fistulas* may be congenital or acquired, and are characterized by an arterial communication with the portal venous system and consequent portal hypertension. Anomalous portosystemic venous fistulas are nearly always congenital, and are characterized by portal venous diversion away from the liver. This diversion of portal blood may be associated with encephalopathy (see Chapter 20). There is no tendency with such structural vascular malformations to change over time.

Finally, *hepatic peliosis* is an acquired disorder, occasionally seen in children, where there is widespread breakdown of intrahepatic vascular integrity with the appearance of large intrahepatic blood-filled spaces or lakes.

Table 15.1 summarizes the relationship of all of the vascular abnormalities considered in this chapter.

HEMANGIOMAS AND HEMANGIOENDOTHELIOMAS

Historical aspects

Isolated case reports of lesions appearing in infancy, which were probably hemangioendotheliomas, appeared at the end of the nineteenth century (Parker, 1880), although at that time they were usually termed angiosarcomas. John Foote (1919), on describing his own findings in a 3-month-old boy with massive hepatomegaly due to multiple angiomatous lesions, first suggested that some were histologically benign and used the compromise term *hemangio-endotheliosarcoma*.

Table 15.1 *Classification of hepatic vascular tumors and malformations*

			Notes
Benign neoplastic lesions	Hemangioendothelioma	Type 1	
		Type 2	Malignant potential
	Cavernous hemangioma		
Malignant neoplastic lesions	Epithelioid hemangioendothelioma		
	Angiosarcoma		
Structural vascular malformations	Hepatic artery–venous fistulas	Syndromic (e.g. hereditary hemorrhagic telangiectasia)	
		Isolated	
	Arterioportal fistulas	Syndromic (e.g. Ehlers–Danlos syndrome)	
		Isolated	
		Acquired (e.g. trauma)	
	Portocaval shunts	Intrahepatic	
		Extrahepatic	
	Peliosis hepatis		Widespread sinusoidal breakdown

Later, Kundstadler reported a case, by now termed a hemangioendothelioma, and reviewed the literature up to 1933, identifying 14 other cases. There was still some confusion with regard to the malignant potential, as about one-third of cases reported 'metastases' in skin, lungs, etc., although we would now consider these manifestations to be part of a multiple hemangioma syndrome. All of the cases reported died within 1 month of presentation.

Anemia was frequently mentioned by early authors as a manifestation of hemangioendotheliomas. The association of thrombocytopenic purpura and a giant capillary hemangioma of the skin was first reported by Haig Kasabach and Katharine Merritt (1940), and was recognized by later authors in large liver hemangiomas.

Blaxland Levick and Rubie (1953) first described the relationship with cardiac failure in a description of a 1-month-old female infant who presented with severe cyanosis and cardiomegaly simulating a congenital cardiac lesion. At postmortem she was found to have multiple hemangiomas in an enlarged liver and a structurally normal heart.

Hemangiomas vs. hemangioendotheliomas

Although there is a broad histological division between the predominantly solitary cavernous hemangiomas and the often multifocal and bilobar hemangioendotheliomas, this may mean little in clinical practice. There can be histological overlap, and commonly hepatic tissue is not obtained for histological analysis. Most clinical authors use either term without implying histological precision. Both terms will be used in this review, depending on the original source of the data.

Histological and immunohistochemical features

Both hemangiomas and hemangioendotheliomas (HAEs) are histologically benign tumors arising from the hepatic mesenchyme. The cut surface varies from gray to reddish-brown, usually having a spongy consistency. There may be areas of fibrosis, calcification, cystic degeneration and hemorrhage.

'Cavernous' hemangiomas are usually small, solitary and confined to one lobe. They are of variable size, and lesions larger than 4 cm in diameter are termed 'giant hemangiomas'. Histologically, these tumors consist of large vascular channels lined by immature endothelial cells, separated by a pale, myxoid-like connective tissue containing fibroblasts and smooth muscle. There may be a pseudocapsule of compressed fibrous tissue, particularly in adults.

Hemangioendotheliomas may be isolated or multiple, and they tend to have smaller vascular spaces than cavernous hemangiomas. Confusingly, some authors (e.g. Stanley *et al.*, 1989) refer to HAEs as 'capillary hemangiomas'.

Dehner and Ishak (1971) subdivided hemangioendotheliomas into two histological types, with the most common, type 1, being composed of multiple small vascular channels lined by immature endothelial cells and separated by a fibrous stroma, which may contain biliary ductules. Type 2 HAEs are less common lesions in which the vascular spaces are lined by more pleomorphic and even frankly malignant-looking endothelial cells which may form papillary-like structures budding into the vascular spaces. Stromal bile ductules are absent. Type II tumors tend to present later, and there is a definite tendency for malignant transformation into overt angiosarcoma. The immunohistochemical characteristics of 91 HAEs have been reported by Selby *et al.* (1994). Of these, 19% were type 2. Immunohistochemical staining for factor VIII was present in 20 of 21 cases tested. Bile ducts, demonstrable by cytokeratin staining, were present in all cases, although they were largely confined to the periphery of the tumor. Flow cytometry was performed in 20 cases, of which 16 cases were normal (DNA diploid) and four were abnormal (three were DNA aneuploid).

Cerar *et al.* (1996) also studied the immunohistochemical characteristics of a single case of fatal infantile hemangioendothelioma. Endothelial cells strongly expressed Von Willebrand factor (factor VIII related), vimentin and CD31, while the underlying stromal cells expressed α-smooth-muscle actin (α-SMA) and vimentin but not desmin, having all the characteristics of pericytes. This finding was contrary to that of Selby *et al.* (1994), who could find no evidence of such cells in any case of their series. Vascular endothelial cadherin (VE-cadherin) is a calcium-dependent adhesion receptor that is specifically expressed by human endothelial tissue. Martin-Padura *et al.* (1995) studied its expression in a variety of vascular tumors (mostly extrahepatic) and showed that loss of expression was associated with increasingly malignant variants (e.g. angiosarcoma). Otherwise, there was moderate expression of intercellular adhesion molecule (ICAM-1) and PECAM/CD31, but not of vascular cell adhesion molecule (VCAM) or e-selectin on the endothelial lining cells.

Epidemiology and prevalence

Cavernous hemangiomas of the liver are considered to be the second commonest hepatic tumor in the general population, exceeded only by hepatic metastases. However, most of them are incidental, asymptomatic lesions that usually present in the fourth and fifth decades. There is a distinct female predominance in adults (Nichols *et al.*, 1989), although this seems to be less marked in infants and children (Dehner and Ishak, 1971; Selby *et al.*, 1994). Becker and Heitler (1989) noted that 62% of 95 infants presenting with HAE were female.

There is a single report of a possible genetic mutation (interstitial deletion of chromosome 6q) in a child with a small asymptomatic hepatic HAE (Ito *et al.*, 1989), who was also noted to have microcephaly, hypertelorism, atrial septal defect and thymic atrophy.

In one family there were three females in three generations who developed large symptomatic liver hemangiomas, and ultrasound screening revealed smaller liver hemangiomas in a further two female relatives (Moser *et al.*, 1998). Drigo *et al.* (1994) also reported a family with a multiple cavernous angioma syndrome, presenting principally with neurological symptoms, who were also found to have incidental liver hemangiomas.

Clinical features

ANTENATAL FEATURES

The antenatal diagnosis of liver hemangiomas is now well described (Samuel and Spitz, 1995). Dreyfus *et al.* (1996) identified a large, vascular, septated liver mass in a fetus. No intervention was necessary, and postnatal investigations showed spontaneous regression of the tumor. In contrast, Morris *et al.* (1999) reported a liver hemangioma in a fetus at 17 weeks' gestation. Repeat scanning later in pregnancy revealed evidence of heart failure. The hemangioma was treated with maternal, and later postnatal, corticosteroids with resolution. Hydrops fetalis has been described in association with large liver hemangiomas (Gonen *et al.*, 1989; Albano *et al.*, 1998). The infant died at 2 weeks in the former report, but successful postnatal treatment was reported in the latter.

Fetal liver hemangiomas may have effects on the mother. Associated vascular anomalies of the placenta, such as chorioangiomas, have been reported (Drut *et al.*, 1992; Kanai *et al.*, 1998; Meirowitz *et al.*, 2000). Abnormally elevated maternal alpha-fetoprotein levels have also been identified, and although the fetal tumor must be the source, the actual mechanism is obscure (Meirowitz *et al.*, 2000; Mhani *et al.*, 2000).

POSTNATAL FEATURES

Hemangiomas may remain asymptomatic, particularly if they are small. Increasing size and vascularity increase the likelihood of symptoms which include hepatomegaly, failure to thrive, respiratory distress, cardiac failure, jaundice, anemia, thrombocytopenia and disseminated intravascular coagulation (Figures 15.1 and 15.2). A diagnostic clue is provided by the presence of cutaneous hemangiomas, which have been described in up to 60% of cases (Davenport *et al.*, 1995; Samuel and Spitz, 1995).

Cardiac failure is high-output in nature, and is due to the large hepatic artery to hepatic vein shunt through the liver. This can account for up to 50% of cardiac output in some cases (Becker and Heitler, 1989), and is manifested as cardiomegaly, systolic cardiac murmurs, an abdominal bruit and marked aortic disparity above and below the origin of the relevant hepatic artery. It is not uncommon for the cardiac features to be so prominent that the true cause of the heart failure is not considered, resulting in a delay in diagnosis (Figures 15.3 and 15.4).

The hemodynamic changes which accompany the rapid enlargement of the lesions are usually postnatal phenomenona. This was suggested by Stanley *et al.* (1989), who noted that all of those infants who had angiography via the umbilical artery within the first week of life had no aortic disparity, whereas this was almost invariably observed in those who had percutaneous angiograms some weeks later. Nevertheless, there

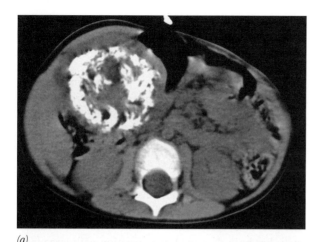

(a)

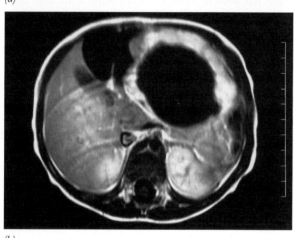

(b)

Figure 15.1 *Cystic degeneration of solitary hemangioendothelioma. Imaging of 4-year-old girl with asymptomatic abdominal mass. (a) CT scan shows right-sided tumor with dense peripheral calcification. (b) MRI scan shows left-sided cystic tumor. Operative findings confirmed highly mobile hemangioendothelioma arising from left lobe of liver with central cystic degeneration.*

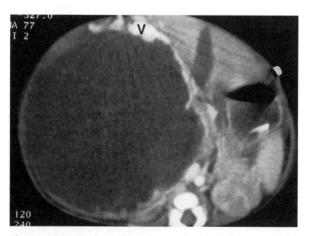

Figure 15.2 *Massive solitary hemangioendothelioma. CT (with intravenous contrast) scan of 4-week-old boy with cardiac failure and massive hepatomegaly showing huge hemangioma arising from right lobe of liver. Obvious peripheral vascular (V) enhancement with intravenous contrast. Found to be unresectable (involved left lobe) at operation, and treated with hepatic arterial ligation.*

are reports of prenatal cardiac failure (Morris *et al.*, 1999).

Rupture of a liver hemangioma and hemoperitoneum has been reported both in children and in adults, usually with fatal consequences (Ehren *et al.*, 1983; Samuel and Spitz, 1995).

Jaundice may occur in up to 50% of cases, and is multifactorial in origin. Commonly it is caused by increased hemolysis and a reduced erythrocyte lifespan consequent upon 'sumping' in the dilated tortuous vascular channels of the hemangioma. Occasionally, hemangiomas at the hilum appear to be a direct cause of

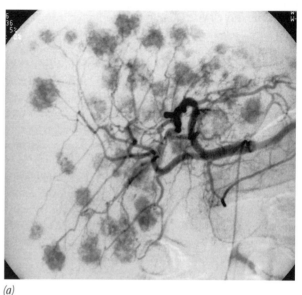

(a)

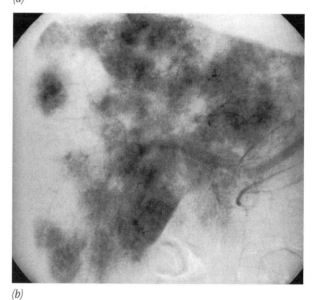

(b)

Figure 15.3 *Multiple bilobar hemangioendothelioma. Celiac angiogram of 8-month-old girl with high-output cardiac failure, erroneously believed to be cardiac in origin. Angiogram shows (a) immediate well-defined enhancement of multiple, bilobar hemangioendotheliomas with (b) delayed 'blush'. There was immediate control of the cardiac failure by hepatic arterial ligation.*

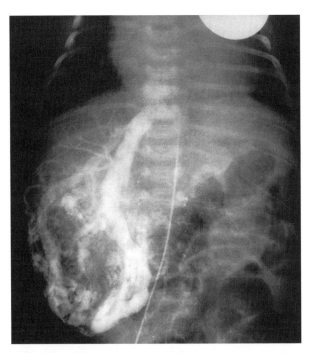

Figure 15.4 *Celiac angiogram of a large right-sided hemangioendothelioma. An 8-week-old male infant who had presented with cardiac failure. Note the massive venous drainage through the right hepatic vein and the enlarged heart. (Reproduced courtesy of ER Howard.)*

(Stanley *et al.*, 1989; Bar-Sever *et al.*, 1994). Other rarer sites have included the small bowel, larynx and trachea (Becker and Heitler, 1989; Iyer *et al.*, 1996), vertebral column (Holden and Alexander, 1970) and spleen (Samuel and Spitz, 1995). Table 15.2 gives examples of liver hemangiomas that have been reported as part of a recognized malformation syndrome. Isolated cases have also been observed in association with congenital heart defects (Davenport *et al.*, 1995).

Hemangiomatous tissue may also secrete protein, hormones or hormone-like substances, although clinical manifestations of this phenomenon are rare. The commonest example is the secretion of alpha-fetoprotein, and abnormally high serum levels may cause diagnostic confusion with hepatoblastomas (Dachman *et al.*, 1983; Holcomb *et al.*, 1988; Luks *et al.*, 1991; Davenport *et al.*, 1993).

Larcher *et al.* (1981) first observed a 7-week-old infant with multiple liver HAE, exophthalmos and raised thyroxine and thyroid-stimulating hormone (TSH) levels. Both the abnormalities in thyroid function and the exophthalmos resolved completely following successful treatment of the liver lesions (Davenport *et al.*, 1995). A recent analysis of the King's College Hospital series identified eight infants with multifocal liver HAE who had abnormal biochemical thyroid function (Ayling *et al.*, 2001). This series included raised TSH and variable plasma thyroxine levels in seven of the children. Autopsy liver material from one case showed positive immunohistochemical staining for TSH. This was thought to be evidence for secretion of a TSH-like substance by the hemangiomatous tissue causing inappropriate stimulation of the thyroid gland. An alternative view of thyroid dysfunction was reported by Huang *et al.* (2000). They reported a 3-month-old infant with multiple hepatic hemangiomas and severe hypothyroidism which was believed to be caused by an abnormal iodothyronine deiodinase activity in the hemangiomatous tissue. This may have caused increased breakdown of thyroxine and clinical hypothyroidism.

Ito *et al.* (1997) described an adult with a giant hepatic hemangioma who had evidence of immune dysfunction and grossly raised transforming growth factor (TGF-β) levels. Both reverted to normal following resection of the tumor, again implying active secretion of this cytokine.

obstructive jaundice. For instance, Hase *et al.* (1995) described a 4-month-old boy who presented with conjugated jaundice and who had a hemangioma 4 cm in diameter arising in the hepatoduodenal ligament. This extended to the hepatic hilum and caused biliary obstruction, which was successfully treated by internal biliary stenting. Spontaneous resolution of the tumor occurred by 20 months, allowing stent removal. Gastrointestinal symptoms such as diarrhea and malabsorption may occur, although the cause of these symptoms, in the absence of arterioportal hypertension, may be obscure (Samuel and Spitz, 1995).

Liver hemangiomas may be part of a multiple hemangioma syndrome. The commonest sites, apart from the skin, are the lungs (up to 10% of cases according to Samuel and Spitz, 1995) and the central nervous system

Table 15.2 *Reported associations of liver hemangiomas or HAE*

Association	Notes	Reference
Beckwith–Wiedemann syndrome	Also placental chorioangiomas	Stanley *et al.*, 1989; Drut *et al.*, 1992; Samuel and Spitz, 1995
Hemihypertrophy syndrome		Wood *et al.*, 1977; Stanley *et al.*, 1989; Davenport *et al.*, 1993; Miller *et al.*, 1999
Cornelia de Lange's syndrome	Also Wilms' tumors	Maruiwa *et al.*, 1988
Multiple cavernous angioma syndrome	Cerebral and retinal angiomas	Drigo *et al.*, 1994

Diagnosis

A combination of ultrasonography, Doppler flow studies and dynamic contrast CT scanning should be adequate for the diagnosis of most cases of hemangioma. Occasionally, plain radiographs may show hepatomegaly and intratumoral calcification, with features such as cardiac enlargement and pulmonary plethora due to cardiac failure (Stanley et al., 1989).

Ultrasonography and Doppler flow studies are not in themselves characteristic, and may show hypoechoic, complex or even hyperechoic lesions (Dachman et al., 1983; Stanley et al., 1993). Dilatation of the draining hepatic veins may be seen, and this is consistent evidence of increased vascularity and a high-flow shunt. However, even the most recent technical modifications, such as color flow and power Doppler imaging, lack sufficient discrimination when considered in isolation (Perkins et al., 2000), presumably reflecting the heterogeneous nature of these lesions.

The characteristic CT appearance of hemangiomas is of an area of low attenuation and an immediate, intense, peripheral enhancement following intravenous contrast administration (Paley et al., 1997). Delayed scans will show contrast retained within the periphery, although there may be sequential central enhancement.

Magnetic resonance imaging (MRI) shows a decreased signal on T1-weighted images and increased signal on T2-weighted images (Stanley et al., 1993; Paley et al., 1997). Functionally they exhibit fast flow, which is seen as flow voids on spin-echo images and high signal intensity on gradient-recalled echo images (Chung et al., 1996). Hepatic angiography has been used extensively to study the vascular nature of these tumors (Stanley et al., 1989; Fellows et al., 1991). The blood supply may be very variable, although it is predominantly from the hepatic arteries, which may be noted to be enlarged. Enlargement of both collaterals and accessory arteries (e.g. phrenic arteries) is also common. Most lesions exhibit a rapid homogenous capillary blush, while others show peripheral opacification. Some hemangiomas may have a predominantly portal venous rather than arterial blood supply (McLean et al., 1972; Burrows, 1991; Fellows et al., 1991) that is apparent on angiography as late re-opacification of hepatic lesions. Direct portal vein to hepatic vein communications may also be demonstrated with a minimal systemic arterial collateral circulation (McHugh and Burrows, 1992). Attempts at therapeutic embolization or arterial ligation will be completely ineffective for this latter type of hemangioma.

Radionuclide techniques are not often used for diagnosis, although some elements of the functionality of hemangiomas and HAEs may be demonstrated. Technetium-99m-labeled red cells have been suggested as a highly specific method of diagnosing small obscure hepatic lesions (Miller, 1987). Most scans show increased flow on immediate dynamic scintigraphy, and photopenic areas or voids within the parenchyma on delayed scintigrams. Single photon-emission computed tomography (SPECT) has been used principally in adults, and experience in pediatrics has been limited. Nevertheless, a prospective study in adults has shown a high diagnostic sensitivity (91%) for lesions smaller than 30 mm in diameter (Langsteger et al., 1989), and it may have a role in the investigation of isolated lesions.

Management (TABLES 15.3 AND 15.4)

The management of both symptomatic hemangiomas and HAEs is controversial, and there is widespread

Table 15.3 *Treatment options for symptomatic hemangioma/hemangioendothelioma of infancy*

Option	Notes	Reference
Corticosteroids	Prednisone, prednisolone	Jackson et al., 1977; Holcomb et al., 1988; Samuel and Spitz, 1995; Boon et al., 1996
Vincristine	Limited experience	Perez Payarols et al., 1995
Cyclophosphamide	"	Hurvitz et al., 1986; Fellows et al., 1991
Irradiation	Variable dose range	Jackson et al., 1977; Rotman et al., 1980; Holcomb et al., 1988
Surgical resection	Morbidity, especially in neonates. Indicated in solitary unilobar lesions	Luks et al., 1991
Alpha-interferon		Ezekowitz et al., 1992; Boon et al., 1996; Woltering et al., 1997
Hepatic artery ligation	Indicated in high-flow shunts	Moazam et al., 1983; Davenport et al., 1995
Hepatic artery embolization	"	Stanley et al., 1989; Daller et al., 1999
Excision and transplantation	Limited experience	Egawa et al., 1994; Daller et al., 1999

Table 15.4 *Recent single-center clinical experience with symptomatic hemangioma/hemangioendothelioma of infancy*

Reference (year)	Period	Number	Treatment	Survival	Notes
Nguyen *et al.* (1982)	1955–80	14	3	79%	No intervention (*n* = 5)
Ehren *et al.* (1983)*	1950–81	16	1, 3, 4, 5	73%	
Cohen and Myers (1986)	1962–82	12	1, 3, 4, 5	42%	
Holcomb *et al.* (1988)	1955–87	16	1, 3, 4, 5	80%	
Luks *et al.* (1991)	1965–89	16	1, 3	96%	No intervention (*n* = 4)
Stanley *et al.* (1989)*	1974–88	20	1, 2, 3, 4, 5	85%	
Davenport *et al.* (1995)	1970–90	11	3, 4	82%	
Samuel and Spitz (1995)	1982–93	16	1, 3, 4	94%	No intervention (*n* = 2)
Boon *et al.* (1996)	1968–95	39	1, 3, 4, 6	82%	No intervention (*n* = 5)
Iyer *et al.* (1996)*	1958–92	30	1, 3, 4, 5	80%	
Daller et al. (1999)	1989–97	13	1, 3, 4, 6	46%	

Key to treatment: 1 = steroids, 2 = chemotherapy, 3 = resection, 4 = hepatic artery ligation/embolization, 5 = irradiation, 6 = transplantation.
* Presumed to be same institutional series (Los Angeles, USA).

disagreement between authors with regard to the most appropriate choice of therapy. Figure 15.5 illustrates a suitable management algorithm used at King's College Hospital for hepatic hemangiomas.

Most asymptomatic lesions can simply be managed expectantly, perhaps using serial ultrasonography to document the expected pattern of resolution. However, infants who present with severe cardiac and respiratory failure will need urgent and effective therapy. This implies interventional strategies such as hepatic resection, hepatic arterial ligation or embolization.

The medical treatment for liver HAE and hemangiomas has not been standardized, but in addition to the specific agents detailed below, infants with clinical signs of cardiac failure will also require fluid restriction, digitalization and diuretics as supportive therapy. Occasionally, ε-aminocaproic acid has also been suggested as supportive therapy to counter the intravascular coagulation seen in multiple HAE (Luks *et al.*, 1991).

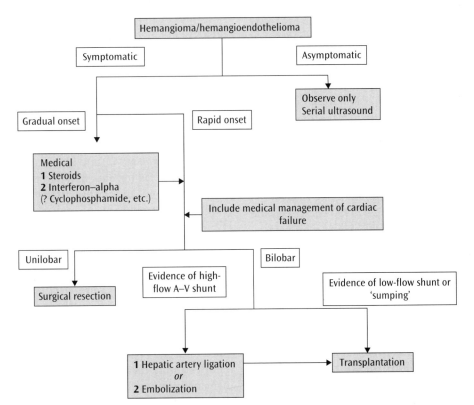

Figure 15.5 *Management algorithm for hemangioma/hemangioendothelioma of childhood. Algorithm for management of hemangioma/ HAE of infants and children derived from clinical experience at King's College Hospital, London. AV, arteriovenous.*

CORTICOSTEROIDS

Goldberg and Fonkalsrud in 1969 and Touloukian in 1970 first reported the use of corticosteroids in hemangiomas, and most pediatricians would administer these as first-line therapy. The usual suggested dose is 2 mg/kg/day of oral prednisone or prednisolone, perhaps following an initial regimen of intravenous methylprednisolone at 20 mg/kg/day. However, some authors have advocated higher doses. For instance, Samuel and Spitz (1995) suggested up to 5 mg/kg/day of prednisolone for 1 month.

As no randomized clinical trial data are available, publication bias and small numbers will distort any estimate of steroid effectiveness. The largest reported experience is the series from Boston, USA (Boon et al., 1996), which documented 22 infants with liver hemangiomas treated with steroids (2 mg/kg/day). 'Accelerated' regression was seen in only five cases (23%). We would concur with this fairly disappointing response, and we believe that it is probably typical of the experience in larger referral centres.

ALPHA$_{2A}$-INTERFERON

Alpha$_{2a}$-interferon has had a role in the treatment of life-threatening hemangiomas in sites other than the liver since 1989 (Orchard et al., 1989). However, its use in liver hemangiomas has been less clearly documented (Ezekowitz et al., 1992; Woltering et al., 1997). The largest experience is that of Boon et al. (1996), who reported the use of alpha-interferon in 13 infants, in six of whom steroid therapy had failed. The mean duration of therapy was about 8 months, and accelerated regression was shown in 11 of 13 cases (85%). There is certainly an effect on angiomatous tissue, although it requires a period of several weeks to induce involution, and this inevitably restricts its use to less severe cases. A variety of dosage schedules have been quoted (e.g. 1–3 mU/m^2/day) (Daller et al., 1999). Potential side-effects of alpha-interferon include diminished appetite, alopecia, hypothyroidism and (rarely) neurological sequelae such as spastic diplegia (Woltering et al., 1997; Barlow et al., 1998). Chung et al. (1996) described the progression of MRI features in five infants with hemangiomas who underwent treatment with interferon, all of whom showed resolution within 6 months.

MISCELLANEOUS MEDICAL TREATMENT

Perhaps surprisingly, experience of the use of antineoplastic agents in benign, albeit potentially life-threatening, vascular tumors such as HAE is limited. Individual cases have also been reported showing effective treatment of symptomatic HAE of infancy using vincristine (Perez Payarols et al., 1995) and cyclophosphamide (Holcomb et al., 1988; Manglani et al., 1994). Hurvitz et al. (1986) have also described the successful use of cyclophosphamide in two cases of extrahepatic hemangiomas involving the duodenum and small bowel mesentery, and a major proportion of the skin of the lower limbs.

Irradiation

There are many isolated reports of liver irradiation for HAE in infants and children. However, this has usually been in the context of its use as failed therapy (e.g. Stanley et al., 1983; Cohen and Myers, 1986). Nevertheless, some authors have documented effective tumor control and resolution. For instance, Park and Philips (1970) reported adequate control in three children and one infant with liver hemangiomas using 1200 to 1500 rads. Holcomb et al. (1988) described liver irradiation in five children who received from 350 to 2000 rads, with reasonable tumor control in three cases. They also noted that an early case died later, at the age of 12 years, of leukemia. Rotman et al. (1980) described successful radiation treatment (with a total of 400 rads) of a 6-month-old child with cardiac failure that was unresponsive to conservative measures. Similarly, Fellows et al. (1991) described an infant in severe cardiac failure due to HAE who had undergone steroid and cyclophosphamide therapy and multiple arterial embolization procedures, and who only responded following liver irradiation. Finally, Kantor et al. (1999) recently described successful irradiation therapy which was used as an emergency in a 6-week-old ventilated infant who had not responded to interferon or steroids. Although an embolization procedure was also subsequently performed, the authors attributed the resolution to the irradiation.

Hepatic arterial ligation

Reports of successful hepatic arterial ligation (HAL) by de Lorimier et al. (1967) and Rake et al. (1970) in infants with cardiac failure and multiple liver hemangiomas showed the value of selective arterial devascularization. Before the introduction of arterial ligation there was 80–90% mortality in infants presenting with heart failure. This was the first effective treatment for the high-output cardiac failure due to shunting through unresectable bilobar lesions, and further case reports by Mattioli et al. (1974), Laird et al. (1976), Vorse et al. (1983) and Moazam et al. (1983) confirmed its value.

The effectiveness of HAL depends on the observation that liver hemangiomas and HAE are preferentially supplied by hepatic arterial rather than portal venous blood. Dearterialization causes selective ischemia in abnormal hemangiomatous tissue with the sparing of normal hepatic parenchyma. In humans, hepatic necrosis is not a consequence of HAL provided that sepsis and shock are avoided.

The largest experience of HAL in symptomatic HAE is from King's College Hospital, London. The most recent report concerned the use of HAL in eight infants (Davenport *et al.*, 1995) who had presented at a median age of 4 weeks with symptomatic cardiac failure. This was successful in controlling the high-flow shunt and cardiac failure in six infants. In a 9-month-old infant who had arterioportal shunting, portal hypertension and had presented with bleeding varices, HAL was combined with porto-azygous disconnection and gastric transection. Only partial resolution of symptoms occurred, and the child died later at 22 months of age. The other exception was a 1-month-old boy who had the multiple hemangioma syndrome and who had initially shown an excellent response to HAL, but whose symptoms recurred later due to collateralization. He was then treated medically, and eventually his HAE resolved. At operation it is important to look for all possible arterial sources in order to dearterialize the liver effectively, including accessory arteries in the lesser omentum from the right gastric artery and any aberrant right hepatic artery from the superior mesenteric artery. A cholecystectomy should also be performed, as the cystic artery will be ligated. Bile duct ischemia due to devascularization is a possible sequel, and we have experience of one child who developed a spontaneous duodenobiliary fistula, manifested some years after HAL as recurrent cholangitis.

Rokitansky *et al.* (1998) described a modification of dearterialization. They reported a 2-month-old infant with multiple HAE and cardiac failure whose high-flow shunts were treated by transhepatic compression sutures. Intraoperative ultrasound and Doppler imaging were used to aid localization of the shunts.

Hepatic artery embolization

Transcatheter arterial embolization of the feeding vessels was introduced in the 1980s to control the high-output cardiac failure in infants with HAE (Burrows *et al.*, 1985). Numerous materials have since been used to achieve thrombosis, including gelatin sponge particles (Gelfoam), polyvinyl alcohol particles (Ivalon), silicone balloons, cyanoacrylate and coils. A variety of technique-related complications have been reported, including hepatic necrosis (Burrows *et al.*, 1985), renal infarction (Tegtmeyer *et al.*, 1977) and pulmonary embolism. Femoral artery damage may occur, but a good collateral blood supply usually prevents serious sequelae. However, a possible late manifestation of femoral artery damage is restriction of growth in the affected lower limb.

The effectiveness of dearterialization (either HAL or embolization) procedures will depend on the scale of the arterial input, the type of arteriovenous shunt and its contribution to the symptoms. If the blood supply to the hemangiomatous tissue is predominantly from the portal vein, then arterial embolization will not be helpful and is contraindicated (Holcomb *et al.*, 1988). Dearterialization is also unlikely to be of benefit in infants where the clinical manifestations are more characteristic of low-flow 'sumping' (e.g. consumption coagulopathy and anemia) rather than a high-flow arteriovenous shunt (e.g. cardiac failure) (Holcomb *et al.*, 1988; McHugh and Burrows, 1992).

Hepatic resection

Unilobar tumors may be excised by partial hepatectomy (right, left or non-anatomical). Nevertheless, resection of a large hemangioma can be formidable, as the liver is soft and friable in the early weeks of life, coupled with the difficult dissection that is necessary to control dilated hepatic veins. Resection is usually the most suitable treatment for the late-presenting solitary tumor, particularly if there is doubt about its histological nature. In some centers liver resection has been the only alternative to medical treatment. For instance, Luks *et al.* (1991) in Montreal described 7 of 16 cases where resection was performed without morbidity or mortality, the other cases being managed entirely medically.

Some novel techniques have been used to aid safe resectional surgery. For instance, Ranne *et al.* (1988) reported the use of hypothermic circulatory arrest and liver resection in two infants with cardiac failure and liver hemangiomas. The first, a 4-day-old infant, underwent closure of an atrial septal defect and a left partial hepatectomy for hemangioma and the second, a 12-day-old infant, underwent an extended right hepatectomy for HAE.

Transplantation

The option of complete liver excision and transplantation arrived with the advent of successful liver transplant programs in the early 1990s. However, real evidence of its value is still lacking, and there are considerable logistical problems related to lack of suitable size-matched donor organs and the urgency with which therapy is often needed.

The first successful liver excision and orthotopic liver transplantation (OLT) for HAE was reported by Egawa *et al.* (1994). At the time of transplant the child was 6 months old and had required ventilation due to the massive size of her tumor. Daller *et al.* (1999) reported their experience with 13 cases of infantile HAE who presented with a median age of 14 days. A variety of interventional techniques was used, including resection ($n = 5$), embolization ($n = 6$), HAL ($n = 2$) and OLT ($n = 3$). The overall results were disappointing and only six children (46%) survived. Of the three infants who underwent OLT, one case was for treatment of bilobar disease and the other two were for Budd–Chiari syndrome following attempted resections. Only one case remains alive, the others having died from transplant-related complications.

Calder *et al.* (1996) reported the case of a girl who presented at 30 months of age with gross hepatomegaly due to extensive bilobar HAEs (only in retrospect were they confirmed as type 2 lesions). Other modalities were considered to be unsuitable, and the patient underwent liver excision and OLT, later dying of metastatic disease at 3 years of age (Achilleos *et al.*, 1997).

New developments

Without doubt there will be further developments of anti-angiogenesis agents that are capable of reducing clinically significant hepatic vascular lesions. O'Reilly *et al.* (1995) described the use of the angiogenesis inhibitor AGM-1470 (a synthetic analog of fumagillin) in a mouse model of grafted hemangioendothelioma. This resulted in a 10-fold inhibition of tumor growth and increased survival, although there was no actual regression of the lesions. Similarly, Verheul *et al.* (1999) recently described the use of pegylated recombinant human megakaryocyte growth and development factor in a mouse model of HAE, and showed effective control of platelet consumption and even tumor regression.

CAVERNOUS HEMANGIOMAS IN ADOLESCENTS AND ADULTS

Although the majority of cavernous hemangiomas will be incidental findings, some of the larger lesions may become symptomatic, causing a dull ache or feelings of dragging in the abdomen. Cardiac failure is not a feature, and consumption coagulopathy is exceptional. A relation-ship with use of estrogens has been suggested, although in view of the female predominance this may well be incidental (Sinanan and Marchioro, 1989). Most surgical series have concentrated on lesions larger than 4 cm in diameter. For example, Trastek *et al.* (1983) reported the Mayo Clinic experience of 118 adult patients with cavernous hemangiomas. Of these, 49 hemangiomas (41%) were more than 4 cm in diameter and 12 (10%) were resected. No complications occurred in 35 cases who were followed expectantly for an average period of 5 years. Reading *et al.* (1988) reported 24 adults (of mean age 43 years) with cavernous hemangiomas, of whom 15 cases were symptomatic. Resection and/or gel-foam embolization was performed in 11 cases. The latter treatment was usually associated with a reduction in symptoms, but seldom with a reduction in size, and furthermore in two of the larger examples multiple liver abscesses occurred.

MALIGNANT VASCULAR TUMORS

Malignant vascular tumors of the liver are rare in children, less than 40 cases having been reported in the literature. Three histological variants are recognized, namely hepatic angiosarcoma, malignant epithelioid hemangioendothelioma and type 2 HAE (as defined by Dehner and Ishak, 1971). There may also be a relationship between type 2 HAE and later transformation into angiosarcoma as described by Kirchner *et al.* (1981), Awan *et al.* (1996) and Selby *et al.* (1992).

Angiosarcoma (TABLE 15.5)

The annual incidence of angiosarcoma in the UK has been estimated to be 1.4 per 10 million population (Elliot and Kleinschmidt, 1997), with most cases being

Table 15.5 *Recent reports of angiosarcoma in children*

Reference (year)	Number	Treatment	Outcome
Kirchner *et al.* (1981)	1	4-year-old: steroids, resection, irradiation and chemotherapy	Alive at 2 years
Noronha *et al.* (1984)	1	5-year-old female: resection and chemotherapy	Probable death from recurrence
Alt *et al.* (1985)	1	1-year-old male: chemotherapy	Died
Selby *et al.* (1992)*	10	Six males and four females: multiple, including resection, chemotherapy and irradiation	Single survivor at 3 years
Awan *et al.* (1996)	4	6-month-old female: malignant transformation. Multiple resections 3-year-old female: steroids, irradiation and OLT 3-year-old male: chemotherapy 6-year-old female: chemotherapy and irradiation	No survivors
Gunawardena *et al.* (1997)	1	4-year-old female: chemotherapy and resection	Alive at 4 years

* Pathological review series from the Armed Forces Institute, Washington, DC, USA.
† Possible variant of HAE rather than overt angiosarcoma.

linked to industrial exposure to vinyl chloride monomer. Exposure to the radiological contrast material Thorotrast (thorium dioxide) and environmental arsenic are also considered to be risk factors. However, in the pediatric literature there is only a single report of a possible link to arsenic exposure (Falk *et al.*, 1981).

In 1944, Andries and Kaump from Detroit, USA, first defined the histological criteria of malignancy, which included the absence of encapsulation and tumor infiltration with hypercellular whorls of spindle-shaped cells. However, their case was not at all typical of angiosarcoma, as it occurred in a 10-day-old infant who died of anemia and a hemoperitoneum and was shown to have a further hemangiomatous lesion in the adrenal gland. The largest histopathological review was by Selby *et al.* (1992), who reported the features of 10 cases. These typically involved almost complete replacement of the liver with multiple coalescing lesions and an absence of encapsulation. Hemorrhagic cavities and a variable amount of necrosis were also seen.

Histologically, the infiltrating spindle-shaped cells have an increased nuclear-to-cytoplasmic ratio and mitoses are evident. Cytoplasmic periodic acid-Schiff (PAS)-positive eosinophilic globules are often seen, and the cells are usually positive for both factor VIII and alpha-1-antitrypsin antigens. Nevertheless, histological confirmation of malignancy in vascular tumors may be difficult, and the diagnosis may only be confirmed some way into the course of the disease.

Clinical features

Most angiosarcomas in children present from 3 to 5 years of age with a painless abdominal mass due to hepatomegaly. Less common features include jaundice, abdominal pain, anemia and (rarely) spontaneous hemoperitoneum (Selby *et al.*, 1992). There may be a marginal female predominance. Most tumors are unresectable, and lung metastases are also not uncommonly seen from the outset (Noronha *et al.*, 1984; Alt *et al.*, 1985; Selby *et al.*, 1992; Awan *et al.*, 1996). Sometimes, the history is more complicated and there are a number of reports of probable malignant transformation from pre-existing HAE (Kirchner *et al.*, 1981; Awan *et al.*, 1996). Awan *et al.* (1996) described a girl who presented with typical clinical features of bilobar HAE at 6 months of age. Following steroid treatment of the lesions there was marked regression and resolution of all symptoms until she re-presented 3 years later with two recurrent lesions in each lobe (Figure 15.6a and b). These were resected by a staged procedure with histological features retrospectively suggestive of angiosarcomatous change. The tumor recurred in the residual liver, and fatal extrahepatic metastases appeared within 6 months.

Unfortunately, there are no clear radiographic features that can distinguish between benign and malignant vascular tumors. Angiographic findings are variable, show-

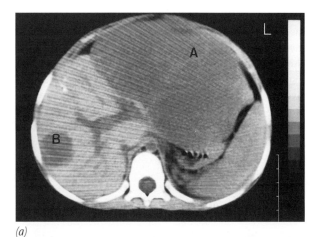

(a)

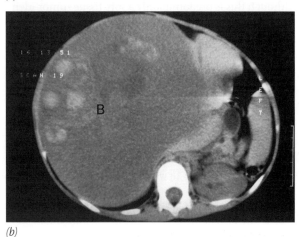

(b)

Figure 15.6 *Malignant transformation of treated hemangioendothelioma. (a) CT scan of 3-year-old girl who re-presented with hepatomegaly, following steroid treatment of multiple hemangioendothelioma as an infant. There is a huge vascular lesion in the left lobe (A), with a smaller lesion in the right lobe (B). (b) CT scan with intravascular contrast following left lobectomy and gross enlargement of residual right lobe vascular lesion. Reproduced with permission from Awan S, Davenport M, Portmann B, Howard ER. Angiosarcoma of the liver in children.* Journal of Pediatric Surgery 1996; **31**: 1729–32.

ing pooling of blood in abnormal vascular channels with (occasionally) overt infiltration of the portal vein. Laparotomy and an open-wedge biopsy should be considered early in the management strategy because of the difficulty in achieving an accurate histological diagnosis from needle biopsies.

The treatment of angiosarcoma has not been standardized. Complete surgical resection is desirable, and this may be facilitated by pre- and postoperative chemotherapy. The efficacy of various chemotherapeutic agents has not been established by controlled trials, although drugs such as Adriamycin, cisplatin, ifosfamide, etoposide, vincristine and actinomycin have been used (Gunawardena *et al.*, 1997).

Liver transplantation has been performed in this disease either inadvertently (Daller *et al.*, 1999) or where there was no evidence of extrahepatic involvement (Achilleos *et al.*, 1996; Awan *et al.*, 1996). However, the results have been disappointing, with no long-term survivors in the pediatric literature. Indeed, the adult experience with liver transplantation in angiosarcoma has also been extremely poor. Penn *et al.* (1991) reported 12 cases taken from an international registry with no long-term survivors, most of these cases dying of local recurrence within 2 years.

Malignant epithelioid hemangioendothelioma

Although this is predominantly a soft-tissue tumor identified in adults (Ishak *et al.*, 1984), cases involving the liver have been reported in older children (Dietze *et al.*, 1989; Taege *et al.*, 1999). It has diverse histological characteristics, including an infiltrative pleomorphic cellular component staining for factor VIII antigen, tuft-like projections into dilated sinusoids and a marked sclerosing tendency. The tumor appears to display biological behavior between that of overt angiosarcoma and type 2 HAE. Metastases can occur, although the primary tumor tends to be quite slowly growing.

HEPATIC ARTERY–PORTAL VEIN FISTULA (ARTERIOPORTAL HYPERTENSION)

Abnormal communications between the hepatic artery or its branches and the portal vein or its branches may lead to portal hypertension and an arterialized portal venous system. Arterioportal fistulas (APFs) may be congenital or acquired, and in children they usually present with symptoms such as failure to thrive and recurrent gastrointestinal bleeding. The first case of an APF was described by Sachs in 1892, in a 60-year-old man with esophageal varices secondary to a fistulous communication between the hepatic artery and portal vein.

Table 15.6 *Reported cases of congenital arterioportal fistula*

Reference (year)	Age and gender	Clinical features	Treatment	Outcome
Gryboski and Clemett (1967)	18 weeks M	Malabsorption, bloody diarrhea	Nil	Died
Helikson *et al.* (1977)	5 weeks F	Diarrhea, abdominal distension, failure to thrive	Embolization (failed) HAL	Well at 6 months
Inon and d'Agostino (1987)	12 months M	Diarrhea, failure to thrive	HAL	Well at 8 months
Fasching *et al.* (1993)	3 months F	Necrotizing enterocolitis, ascites	HAL Left hepatectomy	Portal vein thrombosis
Routh *et al.* (1992)	4 months F	Failure to thrive, gastrointestinal bleeding	Surgical dearterialization, embolization	Portal vein occlusion, portal hypertension
Meunier *et al.* (1993)	4 months	Melena	HAL, embolization (×2), left hepatectomy	Portal vein occlusion
Gorenflo *et al.* (1993)	4 months F	Diarrhea, failure to thrive	HAL and excision of local fistula	Well at 1 year
Hazebroek *et al.* (1995)	3 weeks	Abdominal distension, bloody diarrhea	HAL	Well at 4 years
Heaton *et al.* (1995)	8 months F	Atrial septal defect, ascites and melena, failure to thrive	Embolization (multiple), hepatic artery ligation, liver transplant	Recurrent gastrointestinal bleeding at 8 years
	14 months M	Anemia, gastrointestinal bleeding	Embolization, left hepatectomy, right hepatic artery ligation	Recurrent gastrointestinal bleeding at 7 years
Vauthey *et al.* (1997)	2 years	Von Willebrand's disease, fatigue, hepatomegaly	Embolization (×2)	Well
D'Agostino *et al.* (1998)	14 years M	Diarrhea, ascites, splenomegaly	Embolization (multiple), OLT	Well
Alkim C *et al.* (1999)	—	Variceal bleeding	HAL	Well
Marchand *et al.* (1999)	3 years M	Diarrhea	Embolization (×3)	Portal vein occlusion
Stringer *et al.* (1999)	9 weeks M	Biliary atresia, gastrointestinal bleeding	Embolization (multiple), OLT	Well
	10 weeks M	Biliary atresia, gastrointestinal bleeding	Embolization, OLT	Persistent portal hypertension

HAL, hepatic artery ligation; OLT, orthotopic liver transplant.

Isolated, congenital APFs are rare (Table 15.6). Sometimes there appears to be a definite localized arterial anomaly such as an aneurysm (Gryboski and Clemett, 1967) or other vascular anomaly (Helikson *et al.*, 1977; Routh *et al.*, 1992), while in other cases there is no obvious macroscopic arterial anomaly and the lesions are of a more generalized nature (Fasching *et al.*, 1993; Heaton *et al.*, 1995). Occasionally, APFs may be identified as part of the vascular anomalies within hemangiomas and HAEs (Davenport *et al.*, 1995; Boon *et al.*, 1996; Fishman *et al.*, 1998). In such cases the presenting clinical features are usually related to the high-flow arteriohepatic venous communication causing cardiac failure.

Arterioportal fistulas may also be symptomatic of more generalized connective tissue disorders such as Osler–Weber–Rendu, Ehlers–Danlos or Marfan's syndromes (Vauthey *et al.*, 1997). Interestingly, the clinical presentation of this congenital syndromic type may be delayed until well into adulthood. Marks *et al.* (1985) have also described APFs as a consequence of the Kawasaki or mucocutaneous lymph node syndrome, and hence of a possible infectious etiology.

Most acquired communications are traumatic in origin and can follow blunt or penetrating abdominal trauma, including percutaneous liver biopsy. It may be an under-appreciated complication of trauma. Tanaka *et al.* (1991) described five examples (8%) in 65 cases of blunt abdominal trauma in adults. Most of these were asymptomatic and closed spontaneously. Only one patient required intervention. Most reports of acquired APFs in the pediatric literature are described as complications of surgery. For example, Pashankar and Schreiber (1998) described a 21-month-old child who presented with melena following a Kasai operation for biliary atresia. An APF was demonstrated on angiography close to the site of portoenterostomy. We have also treated a child who developed an APF following partial hepatectomy as an infant (Davenport *et al.*, 1999). She re-presented at 6 years of age with variceal bleeding due to an arterialized portal venous system, which required fistula embolization to restore normal prograde portal venous flow (Figure 15.7).

Clinical features

Presenting symptoms may be vague and are predominantly gastrointestinal. Bleeding from esophageal or gastric varices (Marchand *et al.*, 1999) may be profuse and life-threatening, but occult bleeding also occurs. Ascites has been a common mode of presentation in adults but, although it has been described, this seems to be less frequent in children (Fasching *et al.*, 1993; Heaton *et al.*, 1995; D'Agostino *et al.*, 1998). Similarly, although intestinal ischemia secondary to an arterial 'steal' phenomenon has been described in adults (Vauthey *et al.*,

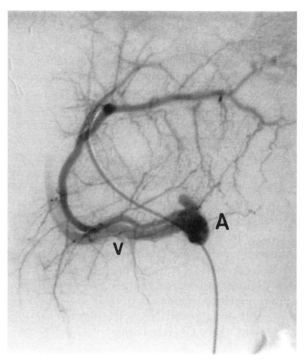

Figure 15.7 *Acquired arterioportal fistula. Arterioportal fistula in 6-year-old child following partial hepatectomy. Selective catheterization of left hepatic artery showing false aneurysm (A), arterioportal fistula and early venous filling (V). Reproduced with permission from Davenport M, Redkar R, Howard ER, Karani J. Arterioportal hypertension: a rare complication of partial hepatectomy.* Pediatric Surgery International *1999;* **15***: 543–5.*

1997), this also appears to be exceptional in pediatric reports. Specific clinical signs are unusual, although occasionally there may be a palpable thrill related to the intrahepatic fistula (Inon and D'Agostino, 1987; Routh *et al.*, 1992). At laparotomy, the portal vein may be tense and pulsatile and the intestine may be edematous (D'Agostino *et al.*, 1998). An unusual neovascularization appearance within the mesentery has also been observed (Heaton *et al.*, 1995). Most cases present after the neonatal period, and it has been suggested that the abnormally large flow through the ductus venosus maintains its patency for a more prolonged period after birth, and only when closure has occurred does the portal venous pressure rise.

The diagnosis may be made on the basis of hepatic ultrasound and Doppler flow studies of the portal vein and hepatic artery. Turbulent flow and hepatofugal flow into venous collaterals are observed in cases with a large fistula. Dynamic CT studies may also show early filling of the fistula with increased arterial flow. Liver segments supplied by the fistula have an early hyperdense attenuation relative to the rest of the liver. Mesenteric angiography is used to confirm the site of the fistula and early filling of the portal venous system. Liver biochemistry should be normal, as there is conservation of liver perfusion, albeit with arterialized blood.

The treatment of symptomatic APFs in children has varied. There is rarely a tendency to spontaneous improvement, and the current treatment of choice seems to be arterial embolization. This is not without risk, as late portal vein thrombosis has been described in up to half of all cases (Routh *et al.*, 1992; Vauthey *et al.*, 1997; Marchand *et al.*, 1999). Open surgical procedures have been described in children either as a primary option or following attempts at embolization (Helikson *et al.*, 1977; Hazebroek *et al.*, 1995; Heaton *et al.*, 1995). Arterial ligation is useful in cases where the APF is extrahepatic or hilar, and is usually successful. If the lesion is intrahepatic and localized, then partial hepatectomy may be the treatment of choice (Fasching *et al.*, 1993). The most difficult types to treat are those where the APFs are multiple and bilobar, and a range of procedures has been performed, including liver transplantation (D'Agostino *et al.*, 1998). The reported cases are summarized in Table 15.6.

The problems in the management of these cases were illustrated by Heaton *et al.* (1995), who described two cases of congenital intrahepatic APFs, both of whom presented in infancy with recurrent gastrointestinal bleeding, ascites and failure to thrive. Both had multiple small APFs that appeared to be localized initially within the left lobe in one case. The lesions in the second case were bilobar from the outset. Embolization was attempted in both children, but it was only helpful in the short term. Hepatic artery ligation was performed in the case with bilobar APFs, although there was subsequent recurrent bleeding due to portal hypertension. The child with localized left lobar lesions underwent partial hepatectomy but developed APFs within the right lobe after a few months. These were treated by right hepatic arterial ligation, but with only temporary effect. Total liver excision and transplantation were eventually performed in this case, but even this approach proved unsatisfactory, and the patient re-presented later with recurrent gastrointestinal bleeding and anemia requiring transfusion.

HEREDITARY HEMORRHAGIC TELANGIECTASIA (OSLER–WEBER–RENDU SYNDROME)

Hereditary hemorrhagic telangiectasia (HHT) is a condition of autosomal-dominant inheritance which consists of multiple vascular anomalies within a number of different organs caused by mutations in at least two genes, namely endoglin and ALK-1. Although the telangiectasia is usually manifested within the skin and mucous membranes of the gastrointestinal tract, liver involvement is not uncommon. This is usually in the form of multiple small arteriovenous shunts, although arterioportal shunts can also occur (Martini *et al.*, 1978; Buscarini *et al.*, 1997). The prevalence of liver involvement within affected families has been studied by Buscarini *et al.* (1997), who identified hepatic vascular malformations in 13 (32%) of 40 related patients with HHT. Interestingly, all of them were female.

The clinical manifestations of the liver lesions are not apparent in childhood, presumably because of the lack of significant arteriovenous shunting at this stage in the evolution of the disease. However, there have been reports both of arteriovenous shunting and hyperdynamic cardiac failure (Boillot *et al.*, 1999) and of arterioportal shunting leading to portal hypertension and variceal development (Zentler-Munroe *et al.*, 1989) in adults with HHT (Mukasa *et al.*, 1998). Most affected individuals present with mild cholestasis, although occasionally progression to fibrosis and cirrhosis leading to liver failure is also seen.

PELIOSIS HEPATIS (TABLE 15.7)

This condition was named by Schoenlank in 1916, although Wagner had described a typical case in 1861. The features are of multiple, irregularly shaped blood lakes, usually without an endothelial lining, scattered throughout the liver and giving a 'Swiss-cheese' type of appearance. The underlying etiology is not known, although most early examples were identified at autopsy in adults with tuberculosis. A relationship with hormone

Table 15.7   *Peliosis hepatis in children*

Author (year)	Number	Clinical features	Treatment	Outcome
Nuernberger and Ramos (1975)	1	15-month-old female: pyelonephritis, pneumonia	Nil specific	Died
Usatin and Wigger (1976)	1	10-year-old male: liver findings at autopsy, cystic fibrosis	Nil specific	Died
Jacquemin *et al.* (1999)	2	5-year-old female: fever and abdominal pain, intraperitoneal bleeding	Nil specific	Died
		2-year-old female: fever, hepatomegaly, intraperitoneal bleeding	Nil specific	Well at 3 years
Current case	1	Fever, hepatomegaly, intraperitoneal bleeding	Nil specific	Well at 1 year

usage, typically anabolic steroids, has been identified. Interestingly, a disease of cattle called 'St George disease' involves the same peliotic appearance of the liver and is also believed to be due to a hormonal imbalance.

Postmortem diagnoses of peliosis hepatis were reported in a 15-month-old child who had presented with pneumonia, pyelonephritis and hepatomegaly (Nuernberger and Ramos, 1975) and in a 10-year-old boy who had died of cystic fibrosis (Usatin and Wigger, 1976). Seven further pediatric cases were collected by Jacquemin *et al.* (1999).

Clinical features

Peliosis hepatis may present with a sudden onset of hepatomegaly, acute liver failure or intraperitoneal bleeding. The commonest precipitating feature in children appears to be bacterial sepsis (Nuernberger and Ramos, 1975; Jacquemin *et al.*, 1999), but other associations have included cystic fibrosis (Usatin and Wigger, 1976), human immunodeficiency syndrome (Scoazec *et al.*, 1988) and malnutrition (Simon *et al.*, 1988). There is an association with drugs, particularly steroid hormones, in adults, and there is a report of a child who developed peliosis in association with an androgen-secreting adrenal tumor (Bagheri and Boyer, 1974).

Radiographic imaging (either CT or MRI) shows the blood-filled spaces as multiple areas of decreased density scattered randomly through the liver. Most cases have bilobar involvement, although one lobe may be more extensively affected.

We have treated a single pediatric case of peliosis who presented at 6 years of age with intraperitoneal bleeding, anemia, jaundice and hepatomegaly (Figure 15.8). She underwent laparotomy, peritoneal lavage and local control of the surface bleeding and an open liver biopsy confirmed the diagnosis. The patient recovered, and imaging 6 months later showed complete restoration of hepatic architecture.

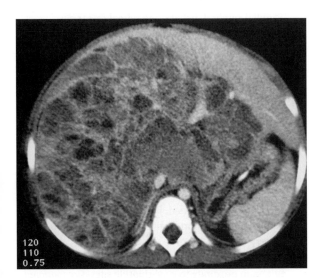

Figure 15.8 *Peliosis hepatis. CT scan of 6-year-old girl showing multiple blood-filled lakes of varying densities involving both lobes. There is minimal early enhancement with intravenous contrast.*

Key references

Awan S, Davenport M, Portmann B, Howard ER. Angiosarcoma of the liver in children. *Journal of Pediatric Surgery* 1996; **31**: 1729–32.

Large series and comprehensive review of possible strategies for this rare tumor.

Boon LM, Burrows PE, Palitiel HJ *et al.* Hepatic vascular anomalies in infancy: a 27-year experience. *Journal of Pediatrics* 1996; **129**: 346–54.

Large recent series with the emphasis on medical management of hemangiomas.

Davenport M, Hansen L, Heaton ND, Howard ER. Hemangioendothelioma of the liver in infants. *Journal of Pediatric Surgery* 1995; **30**: 44–8.

Large single-centre series with the emphasis on management by hepatic artery ligation.

Selby DM, Stocker JT, Waclawiw MA, Hitchcock CL, Ishak KG. Infantile hemangioendothelioma of the liver. *Hepatology* 1994; **20**: 39–45.

Definitive series of the pathological features of pediatric hepatic hemangiomatous lesions.

Vauthey J-N, Tomczak RJ, Helmberger T *et al.* The arterioportal fistula syndrome: clinicopathologic features, diagnosis and therapy. *Gastroenterology* 1997; **113**: 1390–401.

Extensive review of pathophysiology and clinical features.

REFERENCES

Achilleos OA, Buist LJ, Kelly DA, *et al.* Unresectable hepatic tumors in childhood and the role of liver transplantation. *Journal of Pediatric Surgery* 1996; **31**: 1563–7.

Albano G, Pugliese A, Stabile M, Sirimarco F, Arsieri R. Hydrops foetalis caused by hepatic hemangioma. *Acta Paediatrica* 1998; **87**: 1307–9.

Alkim C, Sahin T, Oguz P *et al.* A case report of congenital intrahepatic arterioportal fistula. *American Journal of Gastroenterology* 1999; **94**: 523–5.

Alt B, Hafez R, Trigg M, Shahidi NT, Gilbert EF. Angiosarcoma of the liver and spleen in an infant. *Pediatric Pathology* 1985; **4**: 331–9.

Andries GH, Kaump H. Multiple malignant hemangiomas of the liver. *American Journal of Clinical Pathology* 1944; **46**: 803–10.

Awan S, Davenport M, Portmann B, Howard ER. Angiosarcoma of the liver in children. *Journal of Pediatric Surgery* 1996; **31**: 1729–32.

Ayling RM, Davenport M, Hadzic N *et al.* Hepatic hemangioendothelioma associated with elevated thyroid-stimulating hormone. *Journal of Pediatrics* 2001; **138**: 932–5.

Bagheri SA, Boyer JL. Peliosis hepatis associated with androgenic–anabolic steroid therapy. A severe form of liver injury. *Annals of Internal Medicine* 1974; **81**: 610–18.

Barlow CF, Priebe C, Mulliken JB *et al.* Spastic diplegia as a complication of interferon alfa-2a treatment of hemangiomas of infancy. *Journal of Pediatrics* 1998; **132**: 527–30.

Bar-Sever Z, Horev G, Lubin E *et al.* A rare coexistence of a multicentric hepatic hemangioendothelioma with a large brain hemangioma in a preterm infant. *Pediatric Radiology* 1994; **24**: 1141–2.

Becker JM, Heitler MS. Hepatic hemangioendotheliomas in infancy. *Surgery, Obstetrics and Gynecology* 1989; **168**: 189–200.

Blaxland Levick C, Rubie J. Haemangioendothelioma of the liver simulating congenital heart disease in an infant. *Archives of Disease in Children* 1953; **28**: 49–51.

Boillot O, Bianco F, Viale JP *et al.* Liver transplantation resolves the hyperdynamic circulation in hereditary hemorrhagic telangiectasia with hepatic involvement. *Gastroenterology* 1999; **116**: 187–92.

Boon LM, Burrows PE, Palitiel HJ *et al.* Hepatic vascular anomalies in infancy: a 27-year experience. *Journal of Pediatrics* 1996; **129**: 346–354.

Burrows PE. Variations in the vascular supply to infantile hepatic hemangioendotheliomas (editorial). *Radiology* 1991; **181**: 631–2.

Burrows PE, Rosenberg HC, Chuang HS. Diffuse hepatic hemangiomas: percutaneous transcatheter embolization with detachable silicone balloons. *Radiology* 1985; **156**: 85–8.

Buscarini E, Buscarini L, Danesino C *et al.* Hepatic vascular malformations in hereditary hemorrhagic telangiectasia: Doppler sonographic screening in a large family. *Journal of Hepatology* 1997; **26**: 111–18.

Calder CJ, Raafat F, Buckels JAC, Kelly D. Orthotopic liver transplantation for type 2 infantile haemangio-endothelioma. *Histopathology* 1996; **28**: 271–3.

Cerar A, Doelnc-Strazar ZD, Bartenjev D. Infantile hemangioendothelioma of the liver in a neonate. Immunohistochemical observations. *American Journal of Surgical Pathology* 1996; **20**: 871–6.

Chung T, Hoffer FA, Burrows PE, Paltiel HJ. MR imaging of hepatic hemangiomas of infancy and changes seen with interferon alpha-2α treatment. *Pediatric Radiology* 1996; **26**: 341–8.

Cohen RC, Myers NA. Diagnosis and management of massive hepatic hemangiomas in childhood. *Journal of Pediatric Surgery* 1986; **21**: 6–9.

Dachman AH, Lichtenstein JE, Friedman AC, Hartman DS. Infantile hemangioendothelioma of the liver: a radiologic–pathologic–clinical correlation. *American Journal of Radiology* 1983; **140**: 1091–6.

D'Agostino D, Garcia Monaco R, Alonso V *et al.* Liver transplantation as treatment for arterioportal fistulae. *Journal of Pediatric Surgery* 1998; **33**: 938–40.

Daller JA, Bueno J, Gutierrez J *et al.* Hepatic hemangioendothelioma: clinical experience and management strategy. *Journal of Pediatric Surgery* 1999; **34**: 98–106.

Davenport M, Mieli-Vergani G, Howard ER. Hepatic haemangioendothelioma occurring in an infant with hemihypertrophy. *Pediatric Surgery International* 1993; **8**: 505–6.

Davenport M, Hansen L, Heaton ND, Howard ER. Hemangioendothelioma of the liver in infants. *Journal of Pediatric Surgery* 1995; **30**: 44–8.

Davenport M, Redkar R, Howard ER, Karani J. Arterioportal hypertension: a rare complication of partial hepatectomy. *Pediatric Surgery International* 1999; **15**: 543–5.

Dehner LP, Ishak KG. Vascular tumors of the liver in infants and children: a study of 30 cases and review of the literature. *Archives of Pathology* 1971; **92**: 101–11.

de Lorimier AA, Simpson EB, Baum RS *et al.* Hepatic artery ligation for hepatic hemangiomatosis. *New England Journal of Medicine* 1967; **277**: 333–7.

Dietze O, Davies SE, Williams R, Portmann B. Malignant epithelioid haemangioendothelioma of the liver: a clinicopathological and histochemical study of 12 cases. *Histopathology* 1989; **15**: 225–37.

Dreyfus M, Baldauf JJ, Dadoun K, Becmeur F, Berrut F, Ritter J. Prenatal diagnosis of hepatic hemangioma. *Fetal Diagnosis and Therapy* 1996; **11**: 57–60.

Drigo P, Mammi I, Battistella PA, Ricchieri G, Carollo C. Familial cerebral, hepatic and retinal cavernous angiomas: a new syndrome. *Childs Nervous System* 1994; **10**: 205–9.

Drut R, Drut RM, Toulouse JC. Hepatic hemangio-endothelioma, placental chorioangiomas and dysmorphic kidneys in Beckwith–Wiedemann syndrome. *Pediatric Pathology* 1992; **12**: 197–203.

Egawa H, Berquist W, Garcia-Kennedy R *et al.* Respiratory distress from benign liver tumors: a report of two unusual cases treated with hepatic transplantation. *Journal of Pediatric Gastroenterology and Nutrition* 1994; **19**: 114–17.

Ehren H, Mahour GH, Issacs H. Benign liver tumors in infancy and childhood: report of 48 cases. *American Journal of Surgery* 1983; **145**: 325–9.

Elliot P, Kleinschmidt I. Angiosarcoma of the liver in Great Britain in proximity to vinyl chloride sites. *Occupational and Environmental Medicine* 1997; **54**: 14–18.

Ezekowitz AB, Mulliken JB, Folkman J. Interferon alfa-2a therapy for life-threatening hemangiomas of infancy. *New England Journal of Medicine* 1992; **326**: 1456–63.

Falk H, Herbert JT, Edmonds L et al. Review of four cases of childhood hepatic angiosarcoma – elevated environmental arsenic exposure in one case. Cancer 1981; 47: 382–91.

Fasching G, Schimpl G, Sauer H et al. Necrotizing enterocolitis due to congenital arterioportal fistulas in an infant. Pediatric Surgery International 1993; 8: 264–7.

Fellows KE, Hoffer FA, Markowitz RI, O'Neil JA. Multiple collaterals to hepatic infantile hemangioendotheliomas and arteriovenous malformations: effect on embolization. Radiology 1991; 181: 813–18.

Fishman SJ, Burrows PE, Leichtner AM, Mulliken JB, Moir CR. Gastrointestinal manifestations of vascular anomalies in childhood. Journal of Pediatric Surgery 1998; 33: 1163–7.

Foote J. Hemangio-endotheliosarcoma of the liver: case report and review of the literature. Journal of the American Medical Association 1919; 73: 1042–5.

Goldberg SJ, Fonkalsrud E. Successful treatment of hepatic hemangioma with corticosteroids. Journal of the American Medical Association 1969; 208: 2473–4.

Gonen R, Fong K, Chiasson DA. Prenatal sonographic diagnosis of hepatic hemangioendothelioma with secondary non-immune hydrops fetalis. Obstetrics and Gynecology 1989; 73: 485–7.

Gorenflo M, Waldschmidt J, Bein G et al. Arterioportal fistula in infancy. Journal of Pediatric Gastroenterology and Nutrition 1993; 16: 87–9.

Gryboski JD, Clemett A. Congenital hepatic artery aneurysm with superior mesenteric artery insufficiency: a steal syndrome. Pediatrics 1967; 39: 344–7.

Gunawardena SW, Trautwein LM, Fineglod MJ, Ogden AK. Hepatic angiosarcoma in a child: successful treatment with surgery and adjuvant chemotherapy. Medical and Pediatric Oncology 1997; 28: 139–43.

Hase T, Kodama M, Kishada A et al. Successful management of infantile hepatic hilar hemangioendothelioma with obstructive jaundice and consumption coagulopathy. Journal of Pediatric Surgery 1995; 30: 1485–7.

Hazebroek FWJ, Tibboel D, Robben SGF et al. Hepatic artery ligation for hepatic vascular tumors with arteriovenous and arterioportal venous shunts in the newborn: successful management of two cases and review of the literature. Journal of Pediatric Surgery 1995; 30: 1127–30.

Heaton ND, Davenport M, Karani J, Mowat AP, Howard ER. Congenital hepatoportal arteriovenous fistula. Surgery 1995; 117: 170–4.

Helikson MA, Shapiro DL, Seashore JH. Hepatoportal arteriovenous fistula and portal hypertension in an infant. Pediatrics 1977; 60: 921–4.

Holcomb GW, O'Neil JA, Mahboubi S, Bishop HC. Experience with hepatic hemangioendothelioma in infancy and childhood. Journal of Pediatric Surgery 1988; 23: 661–6.

Holden KR, Alexander F. Diffuse neonatal hemangiomatosis. Pediatrics 1970; 46: 411–21.

Huang SA, Tu HM, Harney JW et al. Severe hypothyroidism caused by type 3 iodothyronine deiodinase in infantile hemangiomas. New England Journal of Medicine 2000; 343: 185–9.

Hurvitz CH, Alkalay AL, Sloninsky L et al. Cyclophosphamide therapy in life-threatening vascular tumors. Journal of Pediatrics 1986; 109: 360–3.

Inon AE, D'Agostino D. Portal hypertension secondary to congenital arterioportal fistula. Journal of Pediatric Gastroenterology and Nutrition 1987; 6: 471–3.

Ishak KG, Sesterhenn IA, Goodman MZD et al. Epithelioid hemangioendothelioma of the liver. Human Pathology 1984; 15: 839–52.

Ito H, Yamasaki T, Okamoto O, Tahara E. Infantile hemangioendothelioma of the liver in patient with interstitial deletion of chromosome 6q: report of an autopsy case. American Journal of Medical Genetics 1989; 34: 325–9.

Ito N, Kawata S, Tsushima H et al. Increased circulating transforming growth factor-beta in a patient with giant hepatic hemangioma: possible contribution to an impaired immune function. Hepatology 1997; 25: 93–6.

Iyer CP, Stanley P, Mahour GH. Hepatic hemangiomas in infants and children: a review of 30 cases. American Surgeon 1996; 62: 356–60.

Jackson C, Green HL, O'Neill J, Kirchner S. Hepatic hemangioendothelioma. American Journal of Diseases in Children 1977; 131: 74–7.

Jacquemin E, Pariente D, Fabre M, Huault G, Valayer J, Bernard O. Peliosis hepatis with initial presentation as acute hepatic failure and intraperitoneal hemorrhage in children. Journal of Hepatology 1999; 30: 1146–50.

Kanai N, Saito K, Homma Y, Makino S. Infantile hemangioendothelioma of the liver associated with anomalous dilated and tortuous vessels on the placental surface. Pediatric Surgery International 1998; 13: 175–6.

Kantor G, Huchet A, Remy S et al. Radiation treatment of a massive hepatic hemangioma for a six-week-old baby. Cancer Radiotherapie 1999; 3: 503–37.

Kasabach HA, Merritt KK. Capillary hemangioma with extensive purpura: report of a case. American Journal of Diseases in Children 1940; 59: 1063–70.

Kirchner SG, Heller RM, Kasselberg AG et al. Infantile hepatic hemangioendothelioma with subsequent malignant degeneration. Pediatric Radiology 1981; 11: 42–5.

Kundstadler RH. Hemangioendothelioma of the liver in infancy. American Journal of Diseases in Children 1933; 46: 803–10.

Laird WP, Friedman S, Koop CE, Schartz GJ. Hepatic hemangiomatosis: successful management by hepatic artery ligation. American Journal of Diseases in Children 1976; 130: 657–9.

Langsteger W, Lind P, Eber B, Koltringer P, Beham A, Eber O. Diagnosis of hepatic hemangioma with 99mTc-labelled red cells: single photon emission computed tomography (SPECT) versus planar imaging. Liver 1989; 9: 288–93.

Larcher VF, Howard ER, Mowat AP. Hepatic haemangiomata: diagnosis and management. Archives of Disease in Childhood 1981; 56: 7–14.

Luks FI, Yazbeck S, Brandt ML *et al.* Benign liver tumors in children: a 25-year experience. *Journal of Pediatric Surgery* 1991; **26**: 1326–30.

McHugh K, Burrows PE. Infantile hepatic hemangio-endotheliomas: significance of portal venous and systemic collateral arterial supply. *Journal of Vascular and Interventional Radiology* 1992; **3**: 337–44.

McLean RH, Moller JH, Warwick WJ, Satran L, Lucas RV. Multinodular hemangiomatosis of the liver in infancy. *Pediatrics* 1972; **49**: 563–73.

Manglani M, Chari G, Sharma U *et al.* Successful treatment with cyclophosphamide in a large hepatic hemangioendothelioma. *Indian Pediatrics* 1994; **31**: 875–7.

Marchand V, Uflacker R, Baker SS, Baker RD. Congenital hepatic arterioportal fistula in a 3-year-old. *Journal of Pediatric Gastroenterology and Nutrition* 1999; **28**: 435–41.

Marks WH, Coran AG, Wesley JR *et al.* Hepatic artery aneurysm associated with the mucocutaneous lymph node syndrome. *Surgery* 1985; **98**: 598–601.

Martini GA. The liver in haemorrhagic telangiectasia: an inborn error of vascular structure with multiple manifestations. *Gut* 1978; **19**: 531–7.

Martin-Padura I, De Castellarnau C, Uccini S *et al.* Expression of VE (vascular endothelial) cadherin and other endothelial-specific markers in haemangiomas. *Journal of Pathology* 1995; **175**: 51–7.

Maruiwa M, Nakamura Y, Motomura K, Murakami T *et al.* Cornelia de Lange syndrome associated with Wilms' tumor and infantile haemangioendothelioma: report of two autopsy cases. *Virchow's Archives (Pathological Anatomy and Histopathology)* 1988; **413**: 463–8.

Mattioli L, Lee KR, Holder TM. Hepatic artery ligation for cardiac failure due to hepatic hemangioma in the newborn. *Journal of Pediatric Surgery* 1974; **9**: 859–62.

Meirowitz NB, Guzman ER, Underberg-Davis SJ *et al.* Hepatic hemangioendothelioma: prenatal sonographic findings. *Journal of Clinical Ultrasound* 2000; **28**: 258–63.

Meunier C, Dabadie A, Darnault P *et al.* Congenital arterioportal fistula. Diagnostic and therapeutic aspects. *Pediatrie* 1993; **48**: 211–16.

Mhani AA, Chodirker BN, Evans JA *et al.* Fetal hepatic haemangioendothelioma: a new association with elevated maternal serum alpha-fetoprotein. *Prenatal Diagnosis* 2000; **20**: 433–5.

Miller JH. Technetium-99m-labelled red blood cells in the evaluation of hemangioma of the liver in infants and children. *Journal of Nuclear Medicine* 1987; **28**: 1412–18.

Miller JH, Gillet PM, Hendry GM, Wallace WH. Congenital hemihypertrophy and epithelioid haemangio-endothelioma in a 10-year-old boy: case report. *Pediatric Radiology* 1999; **29**: 613–16.

Moazam F, Rodgers BM, Talbert JL. Hepatic artery ligation for hepatic hemangiomatosis. *Journal of Pediatric Surgery* 1983; **18**: 120–3.

Morris J, Abbott J, Burrows P, Levine D. Antenatal diagnosis of fetal hepatic hemangioma treated with maternal corticosteroids. *Obstetrics and Gynecology* 1999; **94**: 813–15.

Moser C, Hany A, Spiegel R. Familial giant hemangiomas of the liver. *Schweizerische Rundschau für Medizin Praxis* 1998; **87**: 461–8.

Mukasa C, Nakamura K, Chijiiwa Y, Sakai H, Nawata H. Liver failure caused by hepatic angiodysplasia in hereditary hemorrhagic telangiectasia. *American Journal of Gastroenterology* 1998; **93**: 471–3.

Nguyen L, Shandling B, Ein S, Stephens C. Hepatic hemangiomas in childhood: medical management or surgical management? *Journal of Pediatric Surgery* 1982; **17**: 576–9.

Nichols FC, van Heerden, Weiland LH. Benign liver tumors. *Surgical Clinics of North America* 1989; **69**: 297–314.

Noronha R, Goanzalez-Crussi F. Hepatic angiosarcoma in childhood. A case report and review of the literature. *American Journal of Surgical Pathology* 1984; **8**: 863–71.

Nuernberger SP, Ramos CV. Peliosis hepatis in an infant. *Journal of Pediatrics* 1975; **87**: 424–6.

Orchard PJ, Smith CM, Woods WG *et al.* Treatment of haemangioendotheliomas with alpha interferon. *Lancet* 1989; **ii**: 565–7.

O'Reilly MS, Brem H, Folkman J. Treatment of murine hemangioendotheliomas with the angiogenesis inhibitor AGM-1470. *Journal of Pediatric Surgery* 1995; **30**: 325–9.

Paley MR, Farrant P, Kane P *et al.* Development intrahepatic shunts of childhood: radiological features and management. *European Radiology* 1997; **7**: 1377–82.

Park WC, Philips R. The role of radiation therapy in the management of hemangiomas of the liver. *Journal of the American Medical Association* 1970; **212**: 1496–8.

Parker RW. Diffuse sarcoma of the liver, probably congenital. *Transactions of the Pathological Society of London* 1880; **31**: 290.

Pashankar D, Schreiber RA. Arterioportal fistula in a child with biliary atresia (letter). *Gastroenterology* 1998; **114**: 862–3.

Penn I. Hepatic transplantation for primary and metastatic cancers of the liver. *Surgery* 1991; **110**: 726–35.

Perez Payarols P, Masferrer JP, Bellvert CG. Treatment of life-threatening infantile hemangioma with vincristine. *New England Journal of Medicine* 1995; **333**: 69.

Perkins AB, Imam K, Smith WJ, Cronan JJ. Color and power Doppler sonography of liver hemangiomas: a dream unfulfilled? *Journal of Clinical Ultrasound* 2000; **28**: 159–65.

Rake MO, Liberman MM, Dawson JL *et al.* Ligation of the hepatic artery in the treatment of heart failure due to hepatic haemangiomatosis. *Gut* 1970; **11**: 512–15.

Ranne RD, Ashcraft KW, Holder TM, Sharp RJ, Murphy JP. Hepatic hemangioma: resection using hypothermic circulatory arrest in the newborn. *Journal of Pediatric Surgery* 1988; **23**: 924–6.

Reading NG, Forbes A, Nunnerley HB, Williams R. Hepatic

haemangioma: a critical review of diagnosis and management. *Quarterly Journal of Medicine* 1988; **67**: 431–45.

Rokitansky AM, Jaki RJ, Gopfrich H *et al.* Special compression sutures: a new surgical technique to achieve a quick decrease in shunt volume caused by diffuse hemangiomatosis. *Pediatric Surgery International* 1998; **14**: 119–21.

Rotman M, John M, Stowe S, Inamdar S. Radiation treatment of pediatric hepatic hemangiomatosis and coexisting cardiac failure. *New England Journal of Medicine* 1980; **302**: 852.

Routh WD, Keller FS, Cain WS, Royal SA. Transcatheter embolization of a high-flow congenital intrahepatic arterial–portal venous malformation in an infant. *Journal of Pediatric Surgery* 1992; **27**: 511–14.

Sacks R. Casuistik der Gefaesserkrankugen. *Deutsche Medizininische Wochenschrift* 1892; **18**: 443–4.

Samuel M, Spitz L. Infantile hepatic haemangio-endothelioma: the role of surgery. *Journal of Pediatric Surgery* 1995; **30**: 1425–9.

Schoenlank W. Ein von Peliosis hepatis. *Virchows Archives of Pathology and Anatomy* 1916; **222**: 358–64.

Scoazec JY, Marche C, Giruad PM *et al.* Peliosis hepatis and sinusoidal dilatation during infection by the human immunodeficiency virus (HIV). *American Journal of Pathology* 1988; **131**: 38–47.

Selby DM, Stocker JT, Ishak KG. Angiosarcoma of the liver in childhood. *Pediatric Pathology* 1992; **12**: 485–98.

Selby DM, Stocker JT, Waclawiw MA, Hitchcock CL, Ishak KG. Infantile hemangioendothelioma of the liver. *Hepatology* 1994; **20**: 39–45.

Simon DM, Krause R, Galambos JT. Peliosis hepatis in a patient with marasmus. *Gastroenterology* 1988; **95**: 805–9.

Sinanan MN, Marchioro T. Management of cavernous hemangioma of the liver. *American Journal of Surgery* 1989; **157**: 519–22.

Stanley P, Grinnell VS, Stanton RE, Williams KO, Shore NA. Therapeutic embolization of infantile hepatic hemangioma with polyvinyl alcohol. *American Journal of Roentgenology* 1983; **141**: 1047–51.

Stanley P, Geer GD, Miller JH, Gilsanz V, Landing BH, Boechat IM. Infantile hepatic hemangiomas: clinical features, radiologic investigations and treatment of 20 patients. *Cancer* 1989; **64**: 936–49.

Stringer MD, McClean P, Heaton ND, Karani J, Mieli-Vergani G. Congenital hepatic arterioportal fistula. *Journal of*

Pediatric Gastroenterology and Nutrition 1999; **29**: 487–8.

Taege C, Holzhausen HJ, Gunter G, Flemming P, Rodeck B, Rath FW. Malignant epithelioid hemangioendothelioma of the liver – a very rare tumor in children. *Pathologie* 1999; **20**: 345–50.

Tanaka H, Iwai A, Sugimoto H, Yoshioka T, Sugimoto T. Intrahepatic arterioportal fistula after blunt abdominal trauma: case reports. *Journal of Trauma* 1991; **31**: 143–6.

Tegtmeyer CJ, Smith TH, Shaw A, Barwick KW, Kattwinkel J. Renal infarction: a complication of gelfoam embolisation of a hemangioendothelioma of the liver. *American Journal of Roentgenology* 1977; **128**: 305–7.

Touloukian RJ. Hepatic hemangioendothelioma during infancy: pathology, diagnosis and treatment with prednisone. *Pediatrics* 1970; **45**: 71–6.

Trastek VF, van Heerden JA, Sheedy PF, Adson MA. Cavernous hemangiomas of the liver: resect or observe? *American Journal of Surgery* 1983; **145**: 49–53.

Usatin MS, Wigger J. Peliosis hepatis in a child. *Archives of Pathology and Laboratory Medicine* 1976; **100**: 419–21.

Vauthey J-N, Tomczak RJ, Helmberger T *et al.* The arterioportal fistula syndrome: clinicopathologic features, diagnosis and therapy. *Gastroenterology* 1997; **113**: 1390–401.

Verheul HM, Panigraphy D, Flynn E, Pinedo HM, D'Amato RJ. Treatment of the Kasabach–Merrritt syndrome with pegylated recombinant human megakaryocyte growth and development factor in mice: elevated platelet counts, prolonged survival and tumor growth inhibition. *Pediatric Research* 1999; **46**: 562–5.

Vorse HB, Smith I, Luckstead EF, Fraser J. Hepatic hemangiomatosis of infancy. *American Journal of Diseases in Children* 1983; **137**: 672–3.

Wagner E. Fall von Blutcysten der Leber. *Archiv für Heilkunde* 1861; **2**: 369–70.

Woltering MC, Robben S, Egeler RM. Hepatic hemangio-endothelioma of infancy: treatment with interferon-alpha. *Journal of Pediatric Gastroenterology and Nutrition* 1997; **24**: 348–51.

Wood BP, Putnam TC, Chacko AK. Infantile hepatic hemangioendotheliomas associated with hemihypertrophy. *Pediatric Radiology* 1977; **5**: 242–5.

Zentler-Munroe PL, Howard ER, Karani J, Williams R. Variceal haemorrhage in hereditary haemorrhagic telangiectasia. *Gut* 1989; **30**: 1293–7.

Cysts

EDWARD R HOWARD

A summary of the more frequent causes of liver cysts in children is given in Box 16.1. Cystic dilatation of the biliary tract is discussed in Chapter 10, and neoplastic, parasitic and post-traumatic cysts are dealt with in Chapters 17, 24 and 26. Cysts secondary to biliary atresia and infection are discussed in Chapters 8 and 24.

SIMPLE NON-PARASITIC CYSTS

Congenital simple non-parasitic cysts, which may be uni- or multilocular, are uncommon in children, although they are being recognized with increasing frequency on ultrasound and CT examinations of the abdomen (Kays, 1992; Rypens *et al.*, 1993; Avni *et al.*, 1994; Donovan *et al.*, 1995; Ramesh *et al.*, 1995). The majority of the cysts that are discovered incidentally remain small, but a few continue to grow and eventually present as an abdominal mass. They may be completely intrahepatic, partially extrahepatic, or pedunculated from the edge of the liver. Most are not detected until the fourth to sixth decades of life, and there is a female preponderance of 4:1 (Geist, 1955).

It is believed that simple cysts originate early in development from aberrant bile ducts. This suggestion was originally made by Moschowitz (1906), who noted aberrant bile ducts in the walls of the cysts during a pathological study of 85 cases. The fluid within the cysts varies in color from clear to brown. The lining epithelium is extremely variable and may be cuboidal, columnar, ciliated, mucoid or squamous (Jones, 1994). The outer layer of the cyst wall, which is composed of collagen, muscle fibers, bile ducts and compressed liver cells, is separated

> **Box 16.1** *A classification of intrahepatic cysts*
>
> *Congenital liver cysts*
>   Non-parasitic, simple cysts
>   Polycystic disease
>   Autosomal-dominant polycystic kidney disease (ADPKD)
>   Autosomal-recessive polycystic kidney disease (ARPKD)
>   Congenital hepatic fibrosis (CHF)
>   Caroli's disease
>
> *Other intrahepatic biliary cysts*
>   Congenital choledochal cysts
>   Acquired (biliary atresia)
>
> *Parasitic cysts*
>   Hydatid (*Echinococcus*)
>
> *Tumors*
>   Mesenchymal hamartoma
>   Cystadenoma
>   Teratoma
>
> *Post-traumatic cysts*
>
> *Cysts secondary to infection*
>   Abscess formation (pyogenic or amebic)

from the epithelial lining by vascular tissue (Clark *et al.*, 1967).

Congenital liver cysts have been reported for at least 150 years, and it is believed that Brodie (1846) gave the first accurate description of the solitary type (Jones, 1994). Ten years later, Bristowe (1856) gave the first clear description of an association between multiple cysts in the liver and cystic disease of the kidneys in a report of a postmortem examination which he had performed on a man who was 53 years of age. The liver in this case weighed approximately 2 kg, and the kidneys each weighed 1 kg.

Atkinson (1885) provided one of the earliest reports of the surgical treatment of liver cysts in his description of a laparotomy performed on a 32-year-old woman who had presented with abdominal pain. The cyst, which arose from the quadrate lobe, was aspirated and found to contain altered blood.

The commonest finding in children is an asymptomatic abdominal swelling (Kays, 1992; Quillin and McAllister, 1992), in contrast with adults, who may complain of pain, weight loss and jaundice.

Massive enlargement can cause severe problems because of the compression of surrounding organs, and the report of Merine et al. (1990) illustrates this problem. A 3.42-kg neonate was born with a protuberant abdomen and a rapid onset of respiratory distress, which required intubation. The symptoms were secondary to a large, solitary cyst arising from the edge of the right lobe of the liver. The infant could not be weaned from ventilation, and at 5 days the cyst was resected. Recovery from the operation was uncomplicated.

Cysts can present at any age. Byrne and Fonkalsrud (1982) reported the presentation of a cyst as a rapidly enlarging abdominal mass in a 13-month-old child whose abdomen measured 60 cm in circumference at the umbilicus. The cyst was delineated on ultrasound and, at surgery, was found to arise from the inferior margin of the left lobe of the liver. The cyst was attached to the liver with a pedicle, which was easily resected from the liver. Histology showed the cyst to be lined with cuboidal epithelium, which was reminiscent in some areas of bile duct epithelium. The authors pointed out that, at the time of their report, approximately 400 cases of non-parasitic liver cysts had been reported but only 12 cases had been diagnosed in patients under 2 years of age. Unlike the lesions in polycystic disease, simple cysts are not associated with renal or pancreatic cysts.

The presentation of simple cysts can be unusual. For example, a left lobe cyst was mistaken for a congenital diaphragmatic hernia in a newborn infant. The cyst had herniated into the left thoracic cavity through a congenital defect in the tendinous portion of the diaphragm, causing compression of the lung and shifting of the mediastinum to the right. Respiratory distress necessitated ventilation, and at surgery the large multiloculated cyst was found to occupy almost the whole of the left thorax. The presentation of the cyst at birth suggested that the cyst arose very early in embryonic development (Chu et al., 1986).

Occasionally, liver cysts may present with other congenital abnormalities, and an association with right-sided hemihypertrophy was reported in an 8-month-old girl (Kyi et al., 1995).

Ultrasound or CT scanning defines the structure and position of liver cysts very clearly, and more complex investigations are rarely necessary. The majority are seen to be unilocular on scanning, but multilocular or septated cysts are identified in 10% of cases (Athey et al., 1986). They have now been diagnosed during antenatal ultrasound examinations (Brown et al., 1990; Shankar et al., 2000).

Complications of non-parasitic simple liver cysts include rupture, which may be either spontaneous or traumatic. Akriviadis et al. (1989) reported a case which was monitored with CT scanning and in which there were no serious sequelae from the rupture, and no signs of peritonitis. Occasional cases of intracystic bleeding, which have resolved satisfactorily with conservative management, have been reported in adults (Zanen and van Tilburg, 1995), and extrahepatic cysts attached to the liver by pedicles of variable length have presented with symptoms of torsion (Sinha and Prasad, 1983).

Malignant change within non-parasitic cysts has been described on a few occasions. For example, Pliskin et al. (1992) reported intracystic squamous-cell carcinoma in an 82-year-old patient and reviewed all adult cases reported up to the time of their publication. Weimann et al. (1996) described a patient with squamous-cell carcinoma in the wall of a cyst which had previously been treated by percutaneous drainage. Although malignant change should be considered in the differential diagnosis of a symptomatic adult patient, it has not been described in childhood.

Total excision was previously recommended as the treatment of choice, as lesser procedures had been followed by cyst recurrence. A review of 12 adult patients, in whom 83% of the cysts were located in the right lobe, revealed that simple aspiration was followed by recurrence in 100% of cases, and partial excision was followed by recurrence in 61% of cases (Sanchez et al., 1991). The only reliable treatment in the series was total cyst excision by either enucleation or liver resection. However, a formal partial hepatectomy is required to achieve total excision of a deeply placed cyst, and many surgeons would regard this as an unnecessarily severe operation for such a benign lesion. Total excision would therefore appear to be a satisfactory option for easily accessible lesions, and judicious wide fenestration for deeper cysts. However, it must be remembered that a cyst wall may impinge on major structures such as the retrohepatic vena cava or the hepatic veins, and that conservatism is advisable in these cases in order to minimise the risk of major complications during the surgery.

Aspiration of a cyst before resection has been advised in order to exclude the presence of bile-stained fluid. If bile is identified, then intraoperative cholangiography can be utilized to confirm the presence of a communication with the biliary tract (Roemer et al., 1981). Internal drainage via a cysto-enterostomy, rather than resection, is the operation of choice for rare communicating lesions of the biliary tract.

Recent reports have suggested that laparoscopic fenestration is an effective method of treatment for giant non-parasitic cysts in adults. Katkhouda *et al.* (1999) reported the laparoscopic management of 31 adult patients with no recurrence at a median time of 30 months. However, Diez *et al.* (1998) did report one recurrence in 10 patients, and the affected patient underwent a second laparoscopic fenestration. Nagorney (2000) reviewed 96 laparoscopic cases from 11 series. The recurrence rate after a mean follow-up period of 40 months was 9.5%. This approach is now technically possible in children, but previous experience of cyst recurrence after open operations suggests that long-term follow-up will be needed before the effectiveness of the technique can be assessed completely.

Simple cyst aspiration is a useful method for assessing symptoms. The persistence of symptoms after total aspiration suggests that the cyst is not the cause, and that an alternative diagnosis should be sought.

Cyst aspiration with sclerotherapy of the lining epithelium has been used in small numbers of patients. Kakizaki *et al.* (1998) and McCullough (1993) treated a total of six symptomatic adult cysts with aspiration and injection of absolute alcohol. The authors claimed that the cysts showed a decrease in size, with relief of symptoms, but long-term follow-up data are not available. Nagorney (2000) reviewed 130 cases from eight series. Relief from symptoms was experienced by 85% of the patients, but 17% required further treatment for recurrence. There are no similar reports in children.

CLASSIFICATION OF POLYCYSTIC ('FIBROPOLYCYSTIC') DISEASE

Hepatic surgical intervention in this group of disorders is rarely required in children, and in the majority of the patients the severity of associated renal disease dominated the clinical management.

The normal embryology of the bile ducts, including their development from the 'ductal plate', is discussed in Chapter 7. Based on these concepts, Desmet (1992) has provided a comprehensive theory of the etiology of a wide range of congenital liver disorders, including the group known as 'fibropolycystic disease'. The ductal plate is an early embryological stage in the development of the bile ducts, and is normally remodeled to form recognizable bile ducts at approximately 12 weeks' gestation. Jorgensen (1977) postulated that an interruption in this remodeling process results in the retention of embryonic duct structures, which he designated 'ductal plate malformation' (DPM). Desmet (1992) also suggested that DPM is the basic lesion in the various types of polycystic disease of the liver, and that this can affect any portion of the biliary tract (i.e. segmental, septal or interlobular ducts and bile ductules). The condition includes persistence of the ductal plate, an increased number of ductal structures, which tend to become cystic, and an increase in portal fibrous tissue, which can result in nodular change in the parenchyma.

The possible role of keratinocyte growth factor (KGF) in this process has been identified in transgenic mouse experiments which involved the expression of human KGF in mouse hepatocytes. The embryos of these animals developed epithelial hyperplasia within the bile ducts, hepatomegaly, and cystic change within the kidneys (Nguyen *et al.*, 1996). Recent classifications have divided the more common forms of these disorders into autosomal-dominant polycystic kidney disease (ADPKD), previously known as 'adult polycystic kidney disease', and autosomal-recessive polycystic kidney disease (ARPKD), previously known as 'infantile polycystic disease'. Other related conditions include congenital hepatic fibrosis (CHF) and Caroli's disease.

Autosomal-dominant polycystic kidney disease (ADPKD)

This disease, which is inherited via an autosomal-dominant trait, affects both sexes equally. It is the second commonest inherited monogenic disease after familial cholesterolemia (Uddin *et al.*, 1995), and it affects 12% of patients with end-stage renal disease in the USA (Vollmer *et al.*, 1983). The liver component is characterized by cysts throughout the organ, which are lined by biliary epithelium secreting serous fluid. Commonly they do not communicate with the biliary tree, although communicating cysts have now been recognized in the disorder, and a generalized dilatation of the intrahepatic bile ducts has also been described (Terada and Nakanuma, 1988). The cysts tend to enlarge with age.

Gabow *et al.* (1990) examined 239 ADPKD patients in order to define the factors that influence the presence and severity of liver cysts. They found that the frequency of occurrence of cysts was related to increased age and also to increased severity of kidney disease. The number and size of the cysts was related to a history of pregnancy and to female gender, as well as to increased age and a decline in kidney function. Large liver cysts are unusual in children who are affected by ADPKD, although cysts have been identified histologically on liver-biopsy specimens in infants as young as 8 months of age (Milutinovic *et al.*, 1989). Complications do not usually occur in children.

Additional cysts may occur in many other organs, including the pancreas, thyroid, spleen and epididymis, and other associated disorders that are recognized in adults include intracranial aneurysms, arachnoid cysts, aneurysms of the coronary arteries and abdominal wall herniae.

The typical clinical presentation consists of abdominal distension secondary to enlargement of the liver and kidneys. Abdominal pain may be a feature, but the commonest complications are the result of kidney disease and include urinary tract infection, hematuria, hypertension and renal failure.

Complications of liver cysts are less common, and include ascites, non-cirrhotic portal hypertension (Vauthey *et al.*, 1992), Budd–Chiari syndrome caused by compression of the retrohepatic vena cava (Clive *et al.*, 1993; Uddin *et al.*, 1995), cholangitis and biliary colic.

Much of the treatment of ADPKD is related to the management of declining renal function and hypertension, and these aspects will not be discussed here.

Surgical treatment of the liver cysts is only indicated if there is severe abdominal discomfort or pain, and this is mainly a problem of adulthood. Although percutaneous decompression may be effective in the short term, unfortunately the symptoms invariably return. Cyst fenestration or even partial hepatectomy is occasionally warranted, and although this operation is usually reserved for adults, Marcellini *et al.* (1986) reported a right hepatectomy performed in a child for cystic disease confined to the right half of the liver.

Transudative ascites is an occasional complication in ADPKD, which may be associated with portal hypertension secondary to hepatic fibrosis. Uddin *et al.* (1995) described exudative ascites in four adult patients secondary to hepatic venous outflow obstruction. The cause appeared to be a mechanical compression and thrombosis of the hepatic veins. Three of the patients underwent orthotopic liver transplantation, and the fourth was treated with a mesocaval shunt.

Occasional cases have now been treated successfully with combined liver and kidney transplantation (Taylor *et al.*, 1991).

Autosomal-recessive polycystic kidney disease (ARPKD)

This condition was previously known as 'infantile polycystic disease', but it is now well recognized that it may present in adult life, and the term ARPKD is therefore preferred. Presentation in early infancy is related to enlargement of the kidneys caused by a combination of cystic change within the terminal collecting tubules and interstitial fibrosis. Infantile presentation is associated with severe renal dysfunction and chronic renal failure.

Enlargement of the liver, caused by portal fibrosis and abnormal dilated bile ducts which communicate with the main biliary system, may also be noted in infancy. However, the complications of liver fibrosis are not usually problematic until later in childhood. Large macroscopic liver cysts are unusual in ARPKD.

Older children who survive with the milder forms of renal disease tend to develop the complications of increasing liver fibrosis, which may worsen with age. This variability in the dominance of the renal and liver manifestations of the condition at different ages has suggested a classification into perinatal, neonatal, infantile and juvenile types of ARPKD (Blyth and Ockenden, 1971).

The complications of the fibrotic liver disease in ARKPD are mainly related to the associated portal hypertension. Splenomegaly and the secondary changes of hypersplenism (thrombocytopenia and leucopenia) are always present, and hematemesis or melena from bleeding varices are common presenting signs (Kerr *et al.*, 1961; Boley *et al.*, 1963; Blyth and Ockenden, 1971; Alvarez *et al.*, 1981). Interestingly, hepatic fibrosis in ARPKD is not commonly associated with any severe alteration in hepatocellular function.

The initial treatment of symptomatic esophageal varices is by endoscopic sclerotherapy or by banding of the dilated veins (see Chapter 21). Failure to control intestinal bleeding by using these measures may necessitate a portosystemic decompressive operation such as a lienorenal shunt (see Chapter 22). McGonigle *et al.* (1981) described lienorenal shunting in two patients, aged 13 and 16 years, respectively, one of whom eventually underwent successful renal transplantation.

In summary, ARPKD may present at any age during childhood, with younger patients presenting with the complications of renal disease and older children presenting with the complications of portal hypertension. The relative importance of either the hepatic or renal manifestations in the older child is very variable.

Congenital hepatic fibrosis (CHF)

Kerr *et al.* (1978) were the first to describe the association between hepatomegaly secondary to periportal fibrosis and dilated intrahepatic bile ducts, which is now believed to be a manifestation of ductal plate malformation (Desmet, 1992). The kidneys are affected by cystic disease, but the early clinical presentation is dominated by the hepatic rather than renal complications. It is arguable whether CHF is simply a variant of ARPKD.

CHF has been described as an associated condition with a wide range of abnormalities. These have been summarized by Schwarz and Zellos (1999), and they include encephalocele and polydactyly (Meckel-Gruber's syndrome), pulmonary hypoplasia (Jeune's syndrome), pulmonary fibrosis and emphysema, and intestinal lymphangiectasia. The reader is referred to this article for a full list of references.

Unless associated with infection secondary to significant saccular dilatation of the intrahepatic ducts, the dominant presentation of CHF is hepatomegaly and bleeding from esophagogastric varices in the presence of satisfactory liver function tests. The age at presentation is commonly between 5 and 13 years, and Alvarez *et al.* (1981) reported that in 27 of their patients the mean age at the time of surgery for portal hypertension was approximately 9 years, with an age range of 3 to 16 years. No cases of encephalopathy were detected up to 8 years after portosystemic shunting. However, mental deterioration was reported in two out of eight children who were treated by end-to-side portacaval shunts in an earlier series of CHF (Kerr *et al.*, 1978).

Investigations for suspected CHF include liver and renal function tests, ultrasound scanning of liver and kidneys, and percutaneous liver biopsy. Esophagogastric endoscopy is used to assess variceal size, and mesentericoceliac angiography is used to image portal venous anatomy.

The management of portal hypertension has been summarized in the previous section on ARPKD. It is important to note that these patients may eventually require renal and/or liver transplantation at a later stage in their disease, and the choice of portosystemic shunt operations should take this into account. A lienorenal shunt avoids compromising either the vena cava or the portal vein, and is therefore recommended in cases of CHF.

The prognosis for CHF in childhood is good in the majority of cases, provided that the portal hypertension is adequately controlled. A few children will require renal transplantation as they approach adolescence.

Caroli's disease (SEE FIGURE 10.13)

Caroli *et al.* (1958b) were the first to describe a condition in which there are multiple strictures and dilatations of the intrahepatic ducts, and bile stasis which is responsible for recurrent infection and stone formation. They pointed out that this disease is not related to the noncommunicating cysts of polycystic liver disease.

Two types of intrahepatic duct dilatation were defined (Caroli, 1968). In the rarer form there is dilatation of the main right and left hepatic ducts, as well as the segmental bile ducts, and an association with medullary sponge kidneys and pancreatic cysts. However, portal hypertension is not a feature. This type of segmental bile duct dilatation may be confined to one part of the liver, which is more commonly the left lobe (Caroli *et al.*, 1958a), and it may also be associated with a choledochal cyst (Loubeau and Steichen, 1976).

In the more usual variant seen in children, the bile duct dilatation, which affects larger intrahepatic and interlobular bile ducts, is associated with congenital hepatic fibrosis and portal hypertension. Dilatation of the common bile duct may be present. As in ARPKD, the condition is inherited, in an autosomal-recessive manner, and it is also thought to be a variant of DPM (Desmet, 1992).

Caroli's disease presents with recurrent cholangitis, intrahepatic gallstone formation and abscess formation. Symptoms may not become apparent for the first 5 to 20 years of life, and there is usually no obvious cause of the first attack of infection. The first presentation may be as painless jaundice with fever, and occasionally this may be precipitated by an invasive procedure such as cholecystectomy or ERCP. Investigations include ultrasound, CT, nuclide-excretion scans (Waters *et al.*, 1995) and percutaneous liver biopsy. ERCP or percutaneous cholangiography will confirm the communicating nature of the ductal dilatations and exclude a differential diagnosis of polycystic liver disease.

The treatment of recurrent cholangitis is based on the intermittent use of antibiotics, and regular medication with ursodeoxycholic acid may help to prevent intrahepatic stone formation. Transhepatic intubation and drainage of the dilated bile ducts has been used in cases that are resistant to antibiotic treatment. For example, Witlin *et al.* (1982) presented two cases who had been treated by the insertion of transhepatic silicone stents. One of these patients became asymptomatic after suffering recurrent infections for 20 years.

Drainage or resectional surgery for recurrent cholangitis is disappointing except in patients with disease that is localized to one side of the liver (Caroli *et al.*, 1958a). Thus in a review of 84 patients, recurrent cholangitis was documented after all types of drainage procedures, including biliary–enteric anastomoses and endoscopic sphincterotomy (Watts *et al.*, 1974). Three patients showed improvement after partial hepatectomy, and three others developed cholangiocarcinoma – a well-recognized complication of the condition (Caroli *et al.*, 1958b). Nagasue (1984) reported hepatic resections in six patients with localized disease (right lobectomy in two cases, left lobectomy in three cases and left lateral segmentectomy in one case). All were reported to have obtained relief from their symptoms up to 13 years after surgery. Liver transplantation may be considered for the diffuse form of the disease affected by uncontrolled severe recurrent cholangitis, or for uncontrollable portal hypertension secondary to hepatic fibrosis.

Key references

Desmet VJ. Ludwig symposium on biliary disorders. Part 1. Pathogenesis of ductal plate abnormalities. *Mayo Clinic Proceedings* 1998; **73**: 80–9.

This review develops the theory that congenital diseases of the intrahepatic bile ducts are related to ductal plate malformation (DPM) in the embryo. The disorders are characterized by segmental dilatation of the ducts and periportal fibrosis, and it is suggested that autosomal-recessive polycystic kidney disease represents DPM of the interlobular ducts, and that Caroli's disease represents DPM of the larger ducts. The origin of congenital hepatic fibrosis is explained on the basis of a destructive type of cholangiopathy. Desmet suggests in the paper that other disease of the bile ducts can also be explained on the basis of DPM.

Farges O, Menu Y, Benhamou JP. Non-parasitic cystic diseases of the liver and intrahepatic biliary tree. In: Blumgart LH, Fong Y (eds) *Surgery of the liver and biliary tract*, 3rd edn. London: WB Saunders, 2000: 1245–60.

This is a comprehensive overview of the pathology, presentation and treatment of this varied group of disorders. The review of Caroli's syndrome is particularly clear, and the illustrations provide very good examples of the typical images in each condition. The reference list is very useful.

McGonigle JS, Mowat AP, Bewick M, Howard ER, Snowden SA, Parsons V. Congenital hepatic fibrosis and polycystic kidney disease: role of portacaval shunting and transplantation in three patients. *Quarterly Journal of Medicine* 1981; **50**: 269–78.

The prognosis of autosomal-recessive polycystic kidney disease (ARPKD) depends on the severity of portal hypertension and the degree of renal dysfunction. This report, which details the clinical progress of three children with ARPKD, illustrates the value of a combined management program of surgical portal decompression and renal transplantation in appropriate cases.

Nagasue N. Successful treatment of Caroli's disease by hepatic resection. *Annals of Surgery* 1984; **200**: 718–23.

This series of six patients with the 'simple' type of Caroli's disease was successfully treated with partial hepatectomy. The paper outlines the indications for surgical intervention and reviews the clinical presentation and complications of the disease.

REFERENCES

Akriviadis EA, Steindel H, Ralls P, Redeker AG. Spontaneous rupture of nonparasitic cyst of the liver. *Gastroenterology* 1989; **97**: 213–15.

Alvarez F, Bernard O, Brunelle F *et al*. Congenital fibrosis in children. *Journal of Pediatrics* 1981; **99**: 370–5.

Athey PA, Lauderman JA, King VE. Massive congenital solitary non-parasitic cyst of the liver in infancy. *Journal of Ultrasound Medicine* 1986; **5**: 585–7.

Atkinson E. Hepatic cysts with abdominal section and aspiration of cyst. *British Medical Journal* 1885; **2**: 873.

Avni EF, Rypens F, Donner C, Cuvelliez P, Rodesch F. Hepatic cysts and hyperechogenicities: perinatal assessment and unifying theory on their origin. *Pediatric Radiology* 1994; **24**: 569–72.

Blyth H, Ockenden BG. Polycystic kidneys and liver presenting in childhood. *Journal of Medical Genetics* 1971; **8**: 257.

Boley SJ, Arlen M, Mogilner LJ. Congenital hepatic fibrosis

causing portal hypertension in children. *Surgery* 1963; **54**: 356–60.

Bristowe F. Cystic disease of the liver, associated with similar disease of the kidneys. *Transactions of the Pathological Society of London* 1856; **7**: 229–34.

Brodie BC. *Lectures illustrative of various subjects in pathology and surgery. Lecture V*. London: Longman, 1846.

Brown DK, Kimura K, Sato Y, Pringle KC, Abu-Yousef MM, Sope RT. Solitary intrahepatic biliary cyst: diagnostic and therapeutic strategy. *Journal of Pediatric Surgery* 1990; **25**: 1248–9.

Byrne WJ, Fonkalsrud EW. Congenital non-parasitic cyst of the liver: a rare cause of a rapidly enlarging abdominal mass in infancy. *Journal of Pediatric Surgery* 1982; **17**: 316–17.

Caroli J. Disease of intrahepatic bile ducts. *Israel Journal of Medical Science* 1968; **4**: 21–35.

Caroli J, Couinaud C, Soupault R, Porcher P, Eteve J. Une affection nouvelle, sans doute congenitale, des voies biliaires: la dilatation kystique unilobaire des canaux hepatiques. *Semaine des Hopitaux de Paris* 1958a; **34**: 136–43.

Caroli J, Soupault R, Kassakowki J, Plocker L, Pardowska L. La dilatation polykystique congenitale des voies biliaires intrahepatiques. Essai de classification. *Semaine des Hopitaux de Paris* 1958b; **34**: 488–95.

Chu DY, Olson AL, Mishalany HG. Congenital liver cyst presenting as congenital diaphragmatic hernia. *Journal of Pediatric Surgery* 1986; **21**: 897–9.

Clark DD, Marks C, Bernhard VM. Solitary hepatic cysts. *Surgery* 1967; **61**: 687–93.

Clive D, Davidoff A, Schweizer R. Budd–Chiari syndrome in autosomal dominant polycystic kidney disease: a complication of nephrectomy in patients with liver cysts. *American Journal of Kidney Disease* 1993; **21**: 202–5.

Desmet V. Congenital disease of intrahepatic bile ducts: variations on the theme 'ductal plate malformation'. *Hepatology* 1992; **16**: 1069–83.

Diez J, Decoud J, Gutierrez L, Suhl A, Merello J. Laparoscopic treatment of symptomatic cysts of the liver. *British Journal of Surgery* 1998; **85**: 25–7.

Donovan MJ, Kozakewich H, Perez-Atayde A. Solitary non-parasitic cysts of the liver: Boston Children's Hospital experience. *Pediatric Pathology and Laboratory Medicine* 1995; **15**: 419–28.

Gabow PA, Johnson AM, Kaehny WD, Manco-Johnson ML, Duley IT, Everson GT. Risk factors for the development of hepatic cysts in autosomal dominant polycystic kidney disease. *Hepatology* 1990; **11**: 1033–7.

Geist DC. Solitary non-parasitic cyst of the liver. *Archives of Surgery* 1955; **71**: 867–80.

Jones RS. Surgical management of non-parasitic liver cysts. In: Blumgart LH (ed.) *Surgery of the liver and biliary tract*, 2nd edn. Edinburgh: Churchill Livingstone, 1994; 1211–18.

Jorgensen MJ. The ductal plate malformation. *Acta*

Pathologica Microbiologica Scandinavica Supplement 1977; **257**: 1–87.

Kakizaki K, Yamauchi H, Teshima S. Symptomatic liver cyst: special reference to surgical management. *Journal of Hepato-Biliary-Pancreatic Surgery* 1998; **5**: 192–5.

Katkhouda N, Hurwitz M, Gugenheim J *et al.* Laparoscopic management of benign solid and cystic lesions of the liver. *Annals of Surgery* 1999; **229**: 460–6.

Kays DW. Pediatric liver cysts and abscesses. *Seminars in Pediatric Surgery* 1992; **1**: 107–14.

Kerr DNS, Harrison CV, Sherlock S, Walker RM. Congenital hepatic fibrosis. *Quarterly Journal of Medicine* 1961; **30**: 91–117.

Kerr DNS, Okonkowo S, Choa RG. Congenital hepatic fibrosis. The long-term prognosis. *Gut* 1978; **19**: 514–20.

Kyi A, Mya GH, Saing H. Hemihypertrophy with a liver cyst: a case report. *European Journal of Pediatric Surgery* 1995; **5**: 363–4.

Loubeau JM, Steichen FM. Dilatation of intrahepatic bile ducts in choledochal cysts. Case report with follow-up and review of the literature. *Archives of Surgery* 1976; **111**: 1384–90.

McCullough KM. Alcohol sclerotherapy of simple parenchymal liver cysts. *Australasian Radiology* 1993; **37**: 177–81.

McGonigle RJS, Mowat AP, Bewick M, Howard ER, Snowden SA, Parsons VP. Congenital hepatic fibrosis and polycystic kidney disease: role of portacaval shunting and transplantation in three cases. *Quarterly Journal of Medicine* 1981; **50**: 269–78.

Marcellini M, Palumbo M, Caterino S *et al.* Adult polycystic liver disease in childhood. A case report. *Italian Journal of Surgical Sciences* 1989; **16**: 217–21.

Merine D, Nussbaum AR, Sanders RC. Solitary non-parasitic hepatic cyst causing abdominal distension and respiratory distress in a newborn. *Journal of Pediatric Surgery* 1990; **25**: 349–50.

Milutinovic J, Schabel S, Ainsworth S. Autosomal dominant polycystic kidney disease with liver and pancreatic involvement in early childhood. *American Journal of Kidney Disease* 1989; **13**: 340–4.

Moschowitz E. Non-parasitic cysts (congenital) of the liver with a study of aberrant bile ducts. *American Journal of the Medical Sciences* 1906; **131**: 676–99.

Nagasue N. Successful treatment of Caroli's disease by hepatic resection. *Annals of Surgery* 1984; **200**: 718–23.

Nagorney DM. Surgical management of cystic disease of the liver. In: Blumgart LH, Fong Y (eds) *Surgery of the liver and biliary tract*, 3rd edn. London: WB Saunders, 2000: 1261–74.

Nguyen H, Danilenko D, Bucay N *et al.* Expression of keratinocyte growth factor in embryonic liver of transgenic mice causes changes in epithelial growth and differentiation resulting in polycystic kidneys and other organ malformations. *Oncogene* 1996; **12**: 2109–19.

Pliskin A, Cualing H, Stenger RJ. Primary squamous-cell carcinoma originating in congenital cysts of the liver.

Archives of Pathology and Laboratory Medicine 1992; **116**: 105–7.

Quillin SP, McAllister WH. Congenital solitary non-parasitic cyst of the liver in a newborn. *Pediatric Radiology* 1992; **22**: 543–4.

Ramesh J, Walrond ER, Prussia PR, Williams K, St John MA. Congenital solitary non-parasitic cyst of the liver. *West Indian Medical Journal* 1995; **44**: 36–7.

Roemer CE, Ferrucci JT, Mueller PR, Simeone JF, van Sonnenberg E, Wittenberg J. Hepatic cysts: diagnosis and therapy by sonographic needle aspiration. *American Journal of Roentgenology* 1981; **136**: 1065–70.

Rypens F, Avni EF, Houben JJ, Struyven J. Large solitary non-parasitic cyst of the liver. *Journal Belge de Radiologie* 1993; **76**: 24–5.

Sanchez H, Gagner M, Rossi RL *et al.* Surgical management of nonparasitic cystic liver disease. *American Journal of Surgery* 1991; **161**: 113–18.

Schwarz KB, Zellos A. Congenital and structural abnormalities of the liver. In: Kelly DA (ed.) *Diseases of the liver and biliary system in children*. Oxford: Blackwell Science, 1999: 124–40.

Shankar SR, Parelkar SV, Das SA, Mathure AB. An antenatally diagnosed solitary, non-parasitic hepatic cyst with duodenal obstruction. *Pediatric Surgery International* 2000; **16**: 214–15.

Sinha MR, Prasad SB. Twisted solitary hepatic cyst. *Journal of the Indian Medical Association* 1983; **80**: 141–2.

Taylor J, Calne R, Stewart W. Massive cystic hepatomegaly in a female patient with polycystic kidney disease treated by combined hepatic and renal transplantation. *Quarterly Journal of Medicine* 1991; **80**: 771–5.

Terada T, Nakanuma Y. Congenital biliary dilatation in autosomal-dominant adult polycystic disease of the liver and kidneys. *Archives of Pathology and Laboratory Medicine* 1988; **112**: 1113–16.

Uddin W, Ramage JK, Portmann B *et al.* Hepatic venous outflow obstruction in patients with polycystic liver disease: pathogenesis and treatment. *Gut* 1995; **36**: 142–5.

Vauthey J, Maddern G, Kolbinger P, Baer H. Clinical experience with adult polycystic liver disease. *British Journal of Surgery* 1992; **79**: 562–5.

Vollmer W, Wahl P, Blagg C. Survival with dialysis and transplantation in patients with end-stage renal disease. *New England Journal of Medicine* 1983; **308**: 1553–8.

Waters K, Howman-Giles R, Rossleigh M, Lam A, Uren R, Knight J. Intrahepatic bile duct dilatation and cholestasis in autosomal recessive polycystic kidney disease. Demonstration with hepatobiliary scintigraphy. *Clinical Nuclear Medicine* 1995; **20**: 892–5.

Watts DR, Lorenzo GA, Beal JM. Congenital dilatation of the intrahepatic ducts. *Archives of Surgery* 1974; **108**: 592–8.

Weimann A, Klempnauer J, Gebel M *et al.* Squamous cell carcinoma of the liver originating from a non-parasitic cyst: case report and review of the literature. *HPB Surgery* 1996; **10**: 45–9.

Witlin LT, Gadacz TR, Zuidema GD, Kridelbough WW.
     Transhepatic decompression of the biliary tree in Caroli's
     disease. *Surgery* 1982; **91**: 205–9.

Zanen AL, van Tilburg AJ. Bleeding into a liver cyst can be
     treated conservatively. *European Journal of
     Gastroenterology and Hepatology* 1995; **7**: 91–3.

17

Benign tumors

MARK D STRINGER

INTRODUCTION

A broad spectrum of liver tumors has been described in children (Figure 17.1). This chapter is principally concerned with benign liver neoplasms. Although there are reliable data on the incidence of malignant liver tumors in Western children (Mann *et al.*, 1990), accurate information on the incidence and prevalence of benign tumors is lacking. Benign mesenchymal tumors such as hemangiomas and hamartomas are much more common than benign epithelial tumors such as hepatic adenomas, which is the opposite situation to that observed with malignant liver lesions.

Most liver tumors in children present with abdominal distension and/or a mass. Investigation with ultrasound imaging (US) will usually confirm whether the mass is hepatic, cystic or solid, and whether it is single or multiple, as well as providing information about its vascularity. Computed tomography (CT) and magnetic resonance imaging (MRI) provide further details about the nature, size and extent of the tumor. MR angiography is particularly useful when planning surgical resection. The level of serum alpha-fetoprotein (AFP) should be measured because it is a valuable tumor marker in hepatic malignancy.

For tumors that require resection, the aim of surgery is complete excision. Good operative access is achieved via a bilateral subcostal incision. Intraoperative US imaging is useful in selected cases to confirm the extent of the tumor and the proximity of major intrahepatic vascular structures. Standard techniques of liver resection are employed (Randolph *et al.*, 1978; Filler, 1995; Glick *et al.*, 2000), aided by ultrasonic surgical aspiration (Fasulo *et al.*, 1992; Hodgson *et al.*, 1992), argon-beam coagulation and fibrin sealant. Most hepatic resections are based on the segmental anatomy of the liver (Couinaud, 1957; Strasberg, 1997) (Figure 17.2), but benign tumors are occasionally excised non-anatomically because wide excision is rarely necessary. The surgeon must be aware of potential anatomical variations in vascular and biliary anatomy (see Chapter 1). Up to 85% of the liver may be safely resected in children provided that the remaining parenchyma is healthy. Intraoperative blood loss can be reduced by maintenance of a low central venous pressure during the phase of parenchymal transection. This is facilitated by a slight head-down tilt. Normothermic total vascular occlusion may be valuable for lesions adjacent to the hepatic veins or vena cava. This technique requires complete mobilization of the liver with vascular inflow control (the Pringle maneuver), supra- and infrahepatic caval clamping, and control of the right adrenal vein together with any accessory hepatic arteries. The non-cirrhotic liver will tolerate up to 1 hour of warm ischemia (Huguet *et al.*, 1978).

Major intraoperative complications include hemorrhage, air embolism and primary or secondary (ischemic) bile duct injury. Abdominal drainage is advisable after extended liver resections, but is not routinely necessary after lesser anatomical resections. Postoperatively, the patient is supported with albumin, dextrose, vitamin K and clotting factors for 2–3 days after a major resection. Postoperative complications include hemorrhage, bile

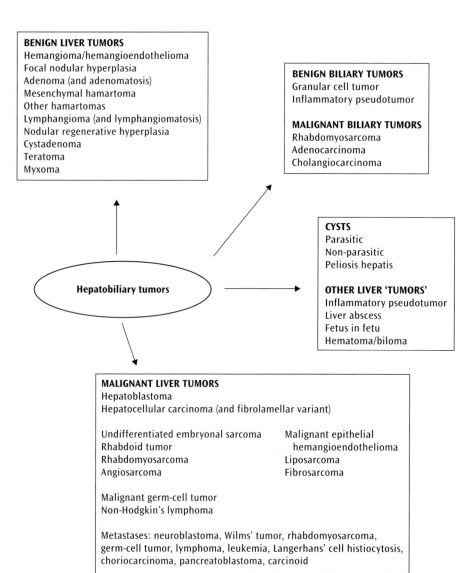

BENIGN LIVER TUMORS
Hemangioma/hemangioendothelioma
Focal nodular hyperplasia
Adenoma (and adenomatosis)
Mesenchymal hamartoma
Other hamartomas
Lymphangioma (and lymphangiomatosis)
Nodular regenerative hyperplasia
Cystadenoma
Teratoma
Myxoma

BENIGN BILIARY TUMORS
Granular cell tumor
Inflammatory pseudotumor

MALIGNANT BILIARY TUMORS
Rhabdomyosarcoma
Adenocarcinoma
Cholangiocarcinoma

Hepatobiliary tumors

CYSTS
Parasitic
Non-parasitic
Peliosis hepatis

OTHER LIVER 'TUMORS'
Inflammatory pseudotumor
Liver abscess
Fetus in fetu
Hematoma/biloma

MALIGNANT LIVER TUMORS
Hepatoblastoma
Hepatocellular carcinoma (and fibrolamellar variant)

Undifferentiated embryonal sarcoma   Malignant epithelial
Rhabdoid tumor   hemangioendothelioma
Rhabdomyosarcoma   Liposarcoma
Angiosarcoma   Fibrosarcoma

Malignant germ-cell tumor
Non-Hodgkin's lymphoma

Metastases: neuroblastoma, Wilms' tumor, rhabdomyosarcoma,
germ-cell tumor, lymphoma, leukemia, Langerhans' cell histiocytosis,
choriocarcinoma, pancreatoblastoma, carcinoid

Figure 17.1 *Classification of liver tumors.*

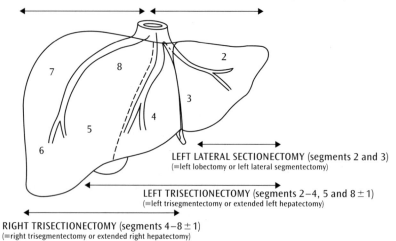

RIGHT HEMIHEPATECTOMY (segments 5–8 ± 1)   LEFT HEMIHEPATECTOMY (segments 2–4)

LEFT LATERAL SECTIONECTOMY (segments 2 and 3)
(≡left lobectomy or left lateral segmentectomy)

LEFT TRISECTIONECTOMY (segments 2–4, 5 and 8 ± 1)
(≡left trisegmentectomy or extended left hepatectomy)

RIGHT TRISECTIONECTOMY (segments 4–8 ± 1)
(≡right trisegmentectomy or extended right hepatectomy)

OTHER RESECTIONS: segmental or non-anatomical
   Note: the caudate lobe (segment 1) is not visible

Figure 17.2 *Current nomenclature for standard liver resections.*

leak (usually from the plane of parenchymal transection and resolving spontaneously with drainage), subphrenic abscess, adhesive bowel obstruction, and pulmonary and wound complications. Hepatic insufficiency is rare, except in patients with cirrhosis.

Rarely, orthotopic liver transplantation is the only therapeutic option for an extensive unresectable benign tumor (Tepetes et al., 1995).

MESENCHYMAL HAMARTOMA

These are large multicystic liver tumors that are usually found in infants and preschool children with an equal sex incidence (DeMaioribus et al., 1990; Otal et al., 1994). They occasionally occur in older children and young adults (Dooley et al., 1983; Stocker and Ishak, 1983; Murray and Ricketts, 1998). After hemangiomas, mesenchymal hamartomas are the second commonest benign hepatic tumor in children (Luks et al., 1991).

Tumors may be asymptomatic masses, but they often present with abdominal distension from progressive accumulation of serous or mucoid fluid within the cysts. Anorexia, vomiting and poor weight gain may be evident. Rarer presentations include respiratory distress or apnea in the newborn (Balmer et al., 1996), ascites (George et al., 1994) and obstructive jaundice from a centrally located tumor (Heller et al., 1992). In recent years, prenatal ultrasound diagnosis during the last trimester has been reported (Bartho et al., 1992; Bessho et al., 1996). In one of these cases the tumor was associated with mesenchymal stem villous hyperplasia of the placenta (Kitano et al., 2000).

Biochemical liver function tests are usually normal. The serum AFP concentration may be slightly elevated, in which case levels decrease to normal after resection (Srouji et al., 1978; Lack, 1986; Yandza and Valayer, 1986; Murray and Ricketts, 1998). Ultrasound scan and CT/MRI demonstrate a multiloculated cystic mass with variable amounts of solid (mesenchymal) tissue between the cysts. Solid areas and septae may be enhanced after intravenous contrast, although the mass is generally hypovascular (DeMaioribus et al., 1990). Nevertheless, large portal branches may supply the tumor (Okeda, 1976), and highly vascular peripheral areas may be present (Weinberg and Finegold, 1983).

Mesenchymal hamartomas must be distinguished from other cystic liver tumors such as cystic hepatoblastoma, biliary cystadenoma, parasitic and non-parasitic cysts and cystic malignant mesenchymal tumors.

Pathology and pathogenesis

Mesenchymal hamartomas are more frequently found in the right lobe of the liver, but they may occur in either lobe or bilaterally. They have solid and cystic components and may be pedunculated (Figure 17.3 and Plate 7). Tumors may be very large, occasionally reaching diameters of 20–30 cm and weighing up to 3 kg (DeMaioribus et al., 1990; Shuto et al., 1993; Otal et al., 1994; Murray and Ricketts, 1998). Significant necrosis or calcification is uncommon (Weinberg and Finegold, 1983), but hemorrhage into a cyst occasionally occurs. On cut section there are multiple cysts containing pale yellow serous fluid or mucoid material. The cysts are separated by fibrous septae and surrounded by loose mesenchymal tissue containing biliary ductules, blood vessels and small islands of liver parenchyma. A few large cysts may predominate (Figure 17.4).

Microscopically, larger cysts are frequently devoid of an epithelial lining, but smaller cysts are lined by biliary epithelium (Ishida et al., 1966), which suggests that tumors may arise as a developmental anomaly of the embryonal ductal plate. The absence of mesenchymal mitotic activity prompted Stocker and Ishak (1983) to suggest that most proliferative activity in mesenchymal hamartomas occurs before birth, whereas cyst enlargement is predominantly responsible for postnatal tumor growth.

Although a developmental origin is most likely, regional ischemia has been proposed as an alternative pathogenetic mechanism (Lennington et al., 1993). Furthermore, cytogenetic studies have reported instances of chromosomal abnormalities, in particular involving the chromosome 19q region, suggestive of neoplasia (Mascarello and Krous, 1992; Otal et al., 1994; Lauwers et al., 1997). In a review of archival material from eight mesenchymal hamartomas, Otal et al. (1994) found evidence of aneuploidy in two specimens.

Complications

Mesenchymal hamartomas are not traditionally considered to have malignant potential, but in recent years there have been several reports of an undifferentiated (embryonal) sarcoma arising within a mesenchymal hamartoma (Table 17.1) (Corbally and Spitz, 1992; De Chadarevian et al., 1994; Lauwers et al., 1997; Ramanujam et al., 1999). Two of these cases occurred years after incomplete excision of a mesenchymal hamartoma in early childhood.

Infective complications are also possible after misguided attempts to drain cysts or biopsy the tumor. Cysts may then become infected, leading to recurrent abscess and sinus formation (ER Howard, personal communication).

Treatment

Mesenchymal hamartomas are best treated by complete excision. This may be achieved by either conventional hepatic resection or non-anatomical excision with a rim

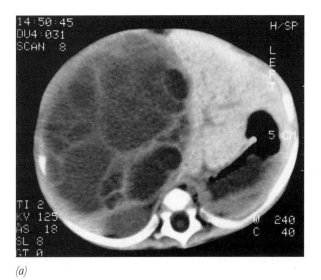

(a)

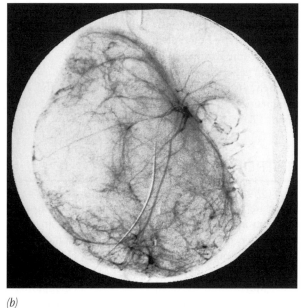

(b)

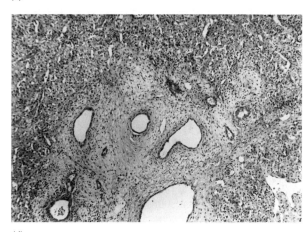

(d)

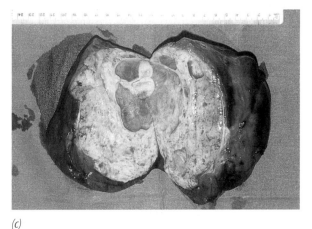

(c)

Figure 17.3 *Mesenchymal hamartoma. (a) CT scan demonstrating multiseptate cystic tumor replacing the right lobe, but with preservation of left lobe architecture. (b) Arteriography demonstrating an essentially avascular tumor, but with abnormal arteries related to the septae of the tumor. (c) Mesenchymal hamartoma from a child aged 20 months. The multicystic tumor was pedunculated and weighed 970 g. (d) Histology of a mesenchymal hamartoma showing cysts lined by columnar epithelium with surrounding loose cellular stroma. Numerous vascular channels are seen together with hepatocytes and a few small bile ducts (×80). (Reproduced courtesy of ER Howard.)*

of normal liver. Despite the relative hypovascularity of the lesions, resections often involve highly vascular hepatic parenchyma. An excellent prognosis can be anticipated after complete excision (DeMaioribus *et al.*, 1990). Incomplete resection should be avoided because of the long-term risk of malignancy and the propensity for symptomatic tumor recurrence, which has been documented up to 13 years later (Shuto *et al.*, 1993; Murray and Ricketts, 1998). In addition, marsupialization may lead to intractable local complications (Meinders *et al.*, 1998). Very rarely, mesenchymal hamartomas are unresectable and liver transplantation should

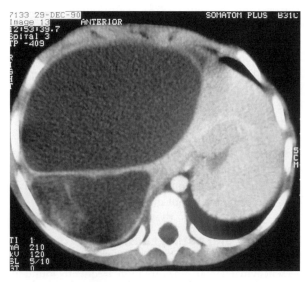

Figure 17.4 *CT scan of a mesenchymal hamartoma in a 7-year-old girl with two dominant cysts.*

Table 17.1 *Reports of undifferentiated sarcoma associated with mesenchymal hamartoma (MH) of the liver*

Author (year)	Age/sex	Comment
Corbally and Spitz (1992)	9 years/F	Malignancy after incomplete excision of MH in infancy
De Chadarevian *et al.* (1994)	12 years/F	Malignancy arising within an MH
Lauwers *et al.* (1997)	15 years/F	Malignancy arising within an MH
Ramanujam *et al.* (1999)	6 years/M	Malignancy after incomplete excision of an MH at 18 months

then be considered. In the Pittsburgh series, two 4-year-old boys with a mesenchymal hamartoma required transplantation for intractable pain and progressive liver failure (Tepetes *et al.*, 1995).

Spontaneous regression of mesenchymal hamartoma has been reported, prompting the suggestion that asymptomatic cases can be managed non-operatively (Barnhart *et al.*, 1997). Patients who are managed in this way require careful and regular long-term surveillance. However, in view of the significant risk of tumor recurrence (Meinders *et al.*, 1998) and other potential complications, a conservative approach is not recommended.

OTHER HEPATIC HAMARTOMAS

Hepatic hamartomas are also found in tuberous sclerosis, an autosomal-dominant disorder with variable clinical signs which may include seizures, developmental delay and various tumors. The commonest visceral lesion in this condition is the renal angiomyolipoma. The prevalence of asymptomatic hepatic hamartomas detected by US increases with age, reaching almost 50% in children over the age of 10 years (Jozwiak *et al.*, 1992). Lesions are frequently small (< 1 cm in diameter) and multiple, are more common in girls, and cause no disturbance of liver function. Histologically, they resemble angiomyolipomas. These tumors are benign and almost never require treatment.

FOCAL NODULAR HYPERPLASIA

This benign liver tumor is most often encountered in young women in association with use of the oral contraceptive pill (Pain *et al.*, 1991). Children account for approximately 7% of reported cases (Stocker and Ishak, 1981). Any age group may be affected, including the fetus (Petrikovsky *et al.*, 1994), and girls outnumber boys by a ratio of 4:1 (Stocker and Ishak, 1981).

Focal nodular hyperplasia (FNH) most commonly presents as an asymptomatic liver mass, but occasionally the lesion may be painful. FNH is usually a large, solitary lesion in children (Figure 17.5 and Plate 8), in contrast to the situation in adult females, in whom small multiple tumors may also occur. Biochemical liver function tests

and serum AFP are normal (Hutton *et al.*, 1993; Herman *et al.*, 2000; Leconte *et al.*, 2000). There is one report of polycythemia in a child secondary to erythropoietin production by the lesion (Sandler *et al.*, 1997).

US imaging reveals a well-demarcated, variably echogenic lesion. Large feeding vessels and a prominent celiac axis may be noted with color Doppler studies (Hutton *et al.*, 1993; Cheon *et al.*, 1998). Dynamic CT scan shows an iso- or low-attenuation lesion which typically enhances in the arterial phase after injection of intravenous contrast. A central scar may be demonstrated by CT or MRI, but is not visible in all cases (Cheon *et al.*, 1998). The surrounding liver parenchyma appears normal. With MRI, FNH is usually isointense in T1-weighted spin-echo images and slightly hyperintense in T2-weighted images (Figure 17.6) (Ohtomo *et al.*, 1991). Technological refinements in MRI are continuing to help to distinguish FNH from other focal liver lesions (Paley *et al.*, 2000). Overall, in about one-third of cases imaging studies demonstrate a typical central feeding artery. Angiography typically shows a hypervascular lesion with a centrifugal arterial supply. In scintigraphic studies, FNH displays a normal or increased uptake of technetium-99m-sulphur colloid because of contained Kupffer cells (Rogers *et al.*, 1981). Although this investigation has a specificity of more than 90%, it is relatively insensitive (Herman *et al.*, 2000), and is likely to become outmoded with further advances in MRI technology.

Pathology and pathogenesis

FNH shows no lobar predisposition. In children, lesions vary in diameter from 1 to 15 cm (Lack and Ornvold, 1986; Pain *et al.*, 1991; Hutton *et al.*, 1993; Cheon *et al.*, 1998). Individual tumors are well circumscribed, yellow or tan colored, but have no discrete capsule. They are composed of hyperplastic parenchyma with a characteristic central stellate fibrous scar which divides the mass into nodules of various sizes. They frequently arise just below Glisson's capsule, and are occasionally pedunculated. Fibrous pale gray septa containing blood vessels and biliary ductules radiate out from the center of the lesion. Typically there is no evidence of hemorrhage, necrosis or calcification.

Tumors are supplied exclusively by arterial blood which flows centrifugally from the central arteries to the

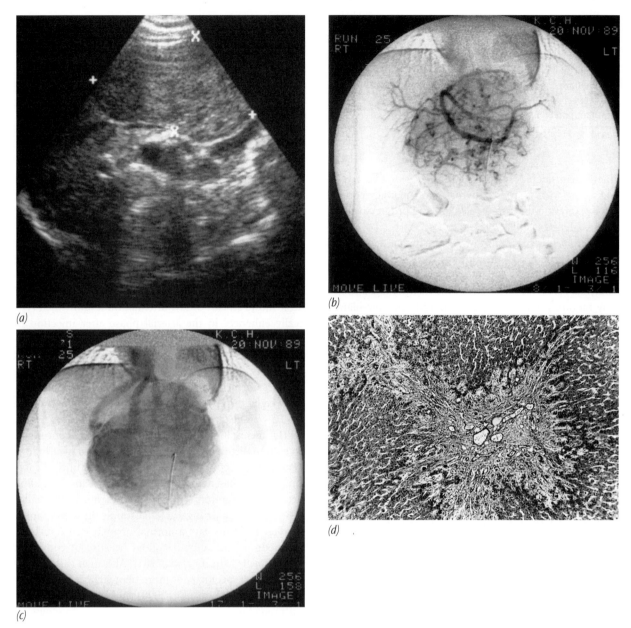

(a)

(b)

(c)

(d)

Figure 17.5 *Focal nodular hyperplasia. (a) Ultrasound scan – the appearances are not specific, but confirm a focal tumor within the liver. (b) Arterial phase of hepatic angiogram demonstrating a large central hepatic artery with the branches distributed peripherally. (c) Large draining hepatic veins are seen in the venous phase. (d) Histological section showing liver parenchyma transected by bands of fibrous connective tissue which expand portal tracts. These contain dilated vascular channels and numerous bile ductules (×80). (Reproduced courtesy of ER Howard.)*

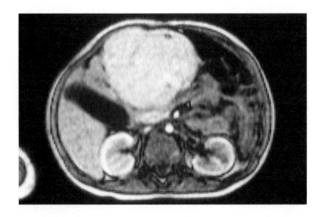

Figure 17.6 *Magnetic resonance image of focal nodular hyperplasia affecting the left hepatic lobe in a 4-year-old boy. No central scar is visible.*

periphery of the lesion (Wanless et al., 1985). The nodules are composed of histologically normal hepatocytes without central veins or portal tracts (Lack and Ornvold, 1986).

The pathogenesis of FNH is unknown, but there are several indications of an underlying vascular disturbance or anomaly. Differential blood flow leading to localized ischemia and scarring with hypervascular repair is one mechanism that has been suggested (Wanless et al., 1985). This is supported by recognized associations of FNH with hepatic hemangiomas, oral contraceptive steroids and sickle-cell disease. Whelan et al. (1973) suggested that turbulent blood flow caused platelet disruption, microvascular thrombosis and release of platelet-derived growth factor which may stimulate hepatocyte hyperplasia.

In contrast to hepatic adenoma, it is likely that female sex hormones (including the oral contraceptive pill) have a growth-promoting effect on FNH rather than a role in tumor genesis.

Associated conditions

FNH in children has been associated with numerous conditions (see Box 17.1), although some of these may be chance associations. Multiple lesions characteristically occur in a syndromic form associated with vascular malformations or cerebral neoplasms (Wanless et al., 1985; Haber et al., 1995).

Box 17.1 *Reported associations with focal nodular hyperplasia in childhood*

Hepatic hemangiomas
Congenital absence of portal vein and portocaval shunt
Patent ductus venosus
Biliary atresia

Congenital heart disease
Sickle-cell disease
Glycogen storage disease (type 1)
Klippel–Trenaunay–Weber syndrome

Oral contraceptive pill

Adrenal and cerebral tumors (glioblastoma/astrocytoma/meningioma)

References: Mathieu et al., 1989; Heaton et al., 1991; Ohtomo et al., 1991; Haber et al., 1995; Matsubara et al., 1996; Guariso et al., 1998; Grazioli et al., 2000; Kinjo et al., 2001.

Treatment

FNH must be distinguished from hepatic adenoma and other liver tumors, although this can be difficult (Mathieu et al., 1989). Rupture and hemorrhage are extremely uncommon in childhood lesions, and there are no confirmed cases of malignant transformation at any age. An expectant policy is therefore reasonable in *asymptomatic* patients with FNH. Ultrasound scan follow-up is advisable, and resection is indicated for progressive enlargement or symptoms. Although FNH itself is not premalignant, the lesion has been found in association with fibrolamellar carcinoma (Saul et al., 1987; Pain et al., 1991). Ideally, the diagnosis should be confirmed by biopsy, but there is a risk of hemorrhage from percutaneous needle biopsy, and intraoperative biopsy may be safer (Belghiti et al., 1993; Herman et al., 2000). The contraceptive pill should be avoided. In those who discontinue the pill, tumor regression is variable, and the lesion may increase in size during pregnancy (Pain et al., 1991).

The natural history of FNH in children is not well documented, and historically various treatment strategies have been adopted. Reymond et al. (1995) reviewed reports of 31 cases of pediatric FNH. Tumor resection was performed in 18 cases, operative biopsy alone in nine, arterial ligation in two and selective hepatic arterial embolization in two cases. Although progressive enlargement and increasing symptoms may rarely occur (Vivas Alegre et al., 2000), a large number of lesions remain asymptomatic for many years (Lack and Ornvold, 1986). In adults, outcome is also variable but many lesions show gradual regression. Leconte et al. (2000) followed 18 biopsy-proven FNH lesions in 14 adults for a mean period of 3 years with serial CT/MRI scans. Tumor volume remained stable in six lesions, decreased in 10, and only increased in two.

Resection, hepatic artery ligation and embolization have been used to treat *symptomatic* cases (Pain et al., 1991; Reymond et al., 1995). Resection is the most reliable option, and it is clearly the preferred treatment if there is diagnostic uncertainty.

ADENOMA

Although they are rare, hepatic adenomas may affect children of any age and either sex. They have also been described in the fetus (Lack and Ornvold, 1986; Resnick et al., 1995).

Adenomas commonly present with abdominal pain which may be acute. Some tumors are asymptomatic and are discovered incidentally. Serum AFP concentration and biochemical liver function tests are normal.

Imaging investigations reveal a solid mass on US, a hypodense heterogenous mass on CT which enhances in the arterial phase (sometimes with central hemorrhage), and a hyperintense heterogenous mass on MRI. In 50% of cases a peripheral rim may be seen with MRI, which is probably the most discriminating imaging modality (Herman et al., 2000). Both FNH and hepatic adenoma usually take up and retain isotope with technetium-99m-labeled DISIDA (di-isopropyl iminodiacetic acid) liver scintigraphy. In contrast to FNH, adenomas show a normal or decreased uptake with technetium-99m-sulphur colloid scintigraphy (Herman *et al.*, 2000).

Pathology and pathogenesis

Pediatric adenomas are usually single and may achieve diameters of up to 14 cm (Resnick *et al.*, 1995). Tumors are well circumscribed and often have a thin fibrous capsule. They show no lobar predisposition. Multiple lesions can be found in glycogen storage diseases, Hurler's mucopolysaccharidosis and in liver adenomatosis. The latter is characterized by the presence of more than 10 adenomas in an otherwise normal liver, and may affect adolescents as well as adults (Chiche *et al.*, 2000).

Histologically, adenomas are composed of benign hepatocytes arranged in trabeculae with intervening sinusoidal spaces. Portal and biliary structures are lacking (Figure 17.7), and Kupffer cells are not present.

In young women, there is a well-established association between hepatic adenomas and use of the estrogen/progesterone oral contraceptive pill. However, unlike FNH, these agents do not simply stimulate tumor growth, but they also cause tumors to develop. In children, hepatic adenomas may be idiopathic, associated with exogenous estrogen or androgen therapy, or associated with a variety of other disorders, including glycogen storage diseases (types I, III and IV), transfusion-induced hemosiderosis, Fanconi's anemia (probably as a result of androgen therapy), Hurler's disease, severe combined immunodeficiency, familial adenomatous polyposis, congenital absence of the portal vein, and

galactosemia (Dehner *et al.*, 1979; Resnick *et al.*, 1995; Bala *et al.*, 1997; Grazioli *et al.*, 2000). In addition, a familial variant associated with diabetes mellitus has been described (Foster *et al.*, 1978).

Complications

In adults, hepatic adenomas pose a small risk of malignant transformation into hepatocellular carcinoma (Belghiti *et al.*, 1993; Foster and Berman, 1994; Resnick *et al.*, 1995; Herman *et al.*, 2000). Hemorrhage into the tumor is well recognized, and this may cause pain or be complicated by tumor rupture and intraperitoneal bleeding (Dehner *et al.*, 1979). Some lesions can be difficult to distinguish from a well-differentiated hepatocellular cancer on biopsy (Lack and Ornvold, 1986).

Treatment

Hepatic adenomas generally require resection to control symptoms and avert potential complications. Some tumors regress after withdrawal of androgen or estrogen therapy, but this is an inconsistent response (Belghiti *et al.*, 1993; Resnick *et al.*, 1995) and, in adults, malignant degeneration has been reported in the adenoma 'scar' after such regression (Herman *et al.*, 2000). Dietary intervention in glycogen storage disorders does not prevent the development of hepatic adenomas (Rosh *et al.*, 1995) but it may reduce their incidence.

NODULAR REGENERATIVE HYPERPLASIA

Nodular regenerative hyperplasia (NRH) is characterized by the presence of regenerative nodules throughout a non-cirrhotic liver with little or no fibrosis. A total of 16 cases were reported by Moran *et al.* (1991) occurring at all ages throughout childhood with an equal sex incidence. A recent review by Trenschel *et al.* (2000) identified only 27 pediatric and two fetal cases. Although NRH is often asymptomatic over many years, it may present with hepatomegaly or splenomegaly and portal hypertension. Liver function is only minimally impaired.

In adults, NRH is associated with rheumatoid arthritis, myeloproliferative disorders and neoplasia. Rarely, it is familial (Dumortier *et al.*, 1999). In children, NRH may be idiopathic or associated with hematological disorders, autoimmune conditions, intra-abdominal tumors, azathioprine therapy or anticonvulsant drug treatment (Moran *et al.*, 1991; Pettei *et al.*, 1995). It has also been described in at least four children in association with congenital absence of the portal vein (with a congenital portosystemic shunt) (Grazioli *et al.*, 2000). It is interesting to note that this developmental anomaly

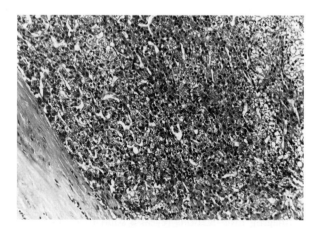

Figure 17.7 *Hepatic adenoma in a 10-year-old girl. The section is from a well-circumscribed nodule within the liver measuring 4.5 cm in diameter. The tumor was pale, yellow and homogeneous. The hepatocytes are small, uniform and arranged in a trabecular pattern. No bile ducts or fibrous septa are seen (×80). (Reproduced courtesy of ER Howard.)*

has also been linked with other intrahepatic tumors, both benign and malignant, including FNH, adenoma, hepatoblastoma and hepatocellular carcinoma. Whether this association is related to the absence of normal portal blood flow, compensatory hepatic arterialization, or both, is unknown.

Nodules are variable in size, hyperechoic on US and hypodense on CT in relation to the surrounding liver parenchyma. They tend not to enhance after intravenous contrast. MRI findings are variable and non-specific (Trenschel et al., 2000).

NRH may be confused clinically or radiologically with cirrhosis or neoplasia, but the condition is readily distinguished by biopsy. Histopathology reveals characteristic nodules composed of hyperplastic hepatocytes separated by thin fibrous septae. These architectural features are well demonstrated by reticulin stains. Tissue obtained by needle biopsy may be inadequate for diagnosis, and a wedge biopsy is recommended by some authors (Trenschel et al., 2000).

The natural history of pediatric cases is poorly understood. Specific treatment is not usually required, since complications (e.g. rupture of a nodule) are very rare. Any associated portal hypertension may require treatment. There is one report of NRH with portal hypertension causing severe hypoxemia as a result of intrapulmonary shunting (Pettei et al., 1995).

HEMANGIOMA

Hemangiomas are the commonest liver tumor in children, and are discussed in detail in Chapter 15.

LYMPHANGIOMA

Isolated asymptomatic small lymphangiomas are occasionally found in the liver. Larger discrete lesions are extremely rare (Koh and Sheu, 2000). Large diffuse lesions tend to form part of a generalized disorder in which lymphangiomas involve the skeletal system, liver, spleen and lungs in a multifocal manner (Asch et al., 1974). Hepatomegaly may be the presenting feature. Visceral involvement has been associated with a poor prognosis because of diffuse pulmonary or hepatic disease or complications of lytic bone lesions. Massive diffuse hepatic lymphangiomatosis has been treated by orthotopic liver transplantation (Tepetes et al., 1995).

INFLAMMATORY PSEUDOTUMOR

Inflammatory pseudotumors, also known as inflammatory myofibroblastic tumors, are proliferative inflammatory lesions that resemble but are distinct from a true neoplasm. They are of unknown etiology, can occur at any age, and can affect almost any organ (Stringer et al., 1992). Fewer than 20 cases involving the liver have been reported in children (Passalides et al., 1996; Hsiao et al., 1999; Lee and DuBoir, 2001).

Lesions are usually solitary, well circumscribed but rarely encapsulated, and have no lobar predisposition. They are of variable size (2–15 cm in diameter). Rarely these pseudotumors are small and multiple (Lee and DuBoir, 2001). Inflammatory pseudotumors are generally considered to be benign reactive lesions with no malignant potential, but they may spread locally and have a tendency to recur after incomplete excision. Histologically, they are composed of a fibrovascular stroma consisting of compact bundles of mature spindle cells (myofibroblasts) with an admixture of plasma cells, lymphocytes and histiocytes.

Fever, abdominal pain and vomiting are common presenting features. Obstructive jaundice and/or portal hypertension arising from local compression have rarely been described (Lee and DuBoir, 2001). Laboratory investigations frequently reveal a microcytic hypochromic anemia, a normal or slightly elevated erythrocyte sedimentation rate (ESR) or C-reactive protein concentration, minimally disturbed biochemical liver function and raised serum immunoglobulin levels. Serum AFP levels are normal. Imaging investigations suggest a solid lesion of relatively low attenuation on CT that enhances gradually after administration of intravenous contrast (Fukuya et al., 1994). A definitive diagnosis can be made by guided percutaneous needle biopsy or open biopsy. It is important to avoid misdiagnosing the lesion as a malignant neoplasm. DNA content assessed by flow cytometry may provide the opportunity to distinguish relatively benign pseudotumors with a diploid karyotype from more aggressive aneuploid lesions (Sakai et al., 2001).

In adults, inflammatory pseudotumors have occasionally been associated with primary sclerosing cholangitis and pyogenic cholangitis. Associated pathologies in children are uncommon, but include Papillon–Lefevre syndrome and severe congenital neutropenia (Czauderna et al., 1999; Hsiao et al., 1999). The former is an autosomal-recessive condition characterized by palmoplantar keratosis and severe periodontopathy. The disease is related to a defect in cell-mediated immunity and neutrophil function which is also responsible for infections at other sites, including liver abscesses. Numerous etiological theories have been suggested to explain the development of inflammatory pseudotumors (Hsiao et al., 1999). Some form of immunological pathogenesis appears to be likely (Stringer et al., 1992).

Most cases have been treated by resection. However, spontaneous regression may occur and an expectant policy is therefore reasonable, with resection reserved for tumor progression, diagnostic uncertainty, persistent symptoms or complications related to tumor location. The role of corticosteroids and antibiotics is uncertain.

Benign liver tumors in children also include *myxoma* (a benign mesenchymal tumor) (Weinberg and Finegold, 1983) and *teratoma*. The latter has mostly been found in girls under the age of 3 years, and may be benign or malignant (Todani *et al.*, 1977), but these tumors are exceptionally rare. Four children with *hepatobiliary cystadenoma* have been described (Williams *et al.*, 1990). These are multilocular, cystic tumors lined by columnar, mucin-secreting epithelium. Most of them are intrahepatic. They should be treated by complete excision because of the risks of recurrence and malignant transformation. Two cases of *intrahepatic fetus in fetu* have been reported, both in infants (Magnus *et al.*, 1999).

PELIOSIS HEPATIS

This unusual pathology is briefly included in this chapter because the imaging appearances may easily be mistaken for a benign, multicystic liver tumor (Figure 17.8). This condition is discussed in more detail in Chapter 15. Peliosis hepatis is characterized by the presence of multiple, blood-filled cystic areas of variable size within the liver, spleen, lungs and other organs. It may develop in association with bacterial infection, malnutrition, cystic fibrosis, renal transplantation or a rare congenital muscle disorder known as myotubular myopathy (Ahsan *et al.*, 1998; Jacquemin *et al.*, 1999; Wang *et al.*, 2001).

In the liver, hepatocyte necrosis and destruction of the reticulin framework allow cystic blood-filled spaces to form. This may be accompanied by a consumptive coagulopathy. Clinical presentation may be acute or chronic with hepatomegaly, liver failure, or rupture with intraperitoneal hemorrhage. Biochemical liver function may be minimally disturbed. Ultrasound scan shows multiple hypoechoic areas of different sizes, and CT typically reveals patchy low-attenuation areas. Angiography may demonstrate characteristic peliotic nodules (Tsukamoto *et al.*, 1984). Definitive diagnosis is histological, but percutaneous biopsy can be hazardous and transjugular or open liver biopsy may be preferable.

Treatment and outcome are variable. Any underlying bacterial sepsis should be treated. Liver resection is rarely indicated, and bleeding complications are best dealt with by embolization. In some children, the disease is transient with a good prognosis provided that the acute phase can be managed successfully. In adults, liver cirrhosis and portal hypertension have been described as a long-term consequence of peliosis.

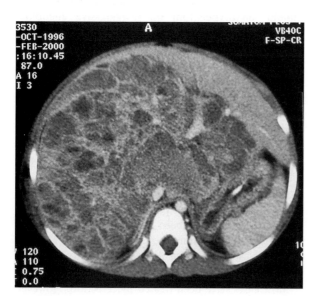

Figure 17.8 *CT scan of a 3-year-old child with peliosis hepatis. The patient had a severe coagulopathy but, despite the CT appearance, biochemical liver function was reasonably well preserved.*

Key references

Herman P, Pugliese V, Machado MA *et al*. Hepatic adenoma and focal nodular hyperplasia: differential diagnosis and treatment. *World Journal of Surgery* 2000; **24**: 372–6.

A contemporary account of these two pathologies (principally in adults) focusing on the difficulties of distinguishing these lesions using modern imaging techniques.

Murray JD, Ricketts RR. Mesenchymal hamartoma of the liver. *American Surgeon* 1998; **64**: 1097–103.

A review of eight patients (newborn to 23 years of age) with mesenchymal hamartoma seen during a 6-year period at Emory University, Atlanta, Georgia. There is a detailed analysis of clinical and pathological material. One tumor recurrence was reported after an initial incomplete resection.

Resnick MB, Kozakewich HP, Perez-Atayde AR. Hepatic adenoma in the pediatric age group. Clinicopathological observations and assessment of cell proliferative activity. *American Journal of Surgical Pathology* 1995; **19**: 1181–90.

A clinicopathological review of eight children with hepatic adenoma from the Children's Hospital, Boston. A detailed description is given of the pathology of hepatic adenoma in children.

Weinberg AG, Finegold MJ. Primary hepatic tumors of childhood. *Human Pathology* 1983; **14**: 512–37.

An authoritative review of benign and malignant pediatric liver tumors from a pathological perspective based on the authors' own series of 73 patients from Texas and a study of the literature.

REFERENCES

Ahsan N, Holman MJ, Riley TR *et al.* Peliosis hepatis due to *Bartonella henselae* in transplantation. *Transplantation* 1998; **65**: 1000–3.

Asch MJ, Cohen AH, Moore TC. Hepatic and splenic lymphangiomatosis with skeletal involvement: report of a case and review of the literature. *Surgery* 1974; **76**: 334–9.

Bala S, Wunsch PH, Ballhausen WG. Childhood hepatocellular adenoma in familial adenomatous polyposis: mutations in adenomatous polyposis coli gene and p53. *Gastroenterology* 1997; **112**: 919–22.

Balmer B, Le Coultre C, Feldges A, Hanimann B. Mesenchymal liver hamartoma in a newborn: case report. *European Journal of Pediatric Surgery* 1996; **6**: 303–5.

Barnhart DC, Hirschl RB, Garver KA *et al.* Conservative management of mesenchymal hamartoma of the liver. *Journal of Pediatric Surgery* 1997; **32**: 1495–8.

Bartho S, Schulz HJ, Bollman R, Specht U. Prenatally diagnosed mesenchymal hamartoma of the liver. *Zentralblatt Pathologie* 1992; **138**: 141–4.

Belghiti J, Pateron D, Panis Y *et al.* Resection of presumed benign liver tumors. *British Journal of Surgery* 1993; **80**: 380–3.

Bessho T, Kubota K, Komori S *et al.* Prenatally detected hepatic hamartoma: another cause of non-immune hydrops. *Prenatal Diagnosis* 1996; **16**: 337–41.

Cheon JE, Kim WS, Kim IO *et al.* Radiological features of focal nodular hyperplasia of the liver in children. *Pediatric Radiology* 1998; **28**: 878–83.

Chiche L, Dao T, Salame E *et al.* Liver adenomatosis: reappraisal, diagnosis and surgical management. *Annals of Surgery* 2000; **231**: 74–81.

Corbally MT, Spitz L, Malignant potential of mesenchymal hamartoma: an unrecognised risk. *Pediatric Surgery International* 1992; **7**: 321–2.

Couinaud C. *Le foie. Etudes anatomiques et chirurgicales.* Paris: Masson, 1957.

Czauderna P, Sznurkowska K, Korzon M, Roszkiewicz A, Stoba C. Association of inflammatory pseudotumor of the liver and Papillon-Lefevre syndrome – case report. *European Journal of Pediatric Surgery* 1999; **9**: 343–6.

De Chadarevian JP, Pawel BR, Faerber EN, Weintraub WH. Undifferentiated (embryonal) sarcoma arising in conjunction with mesenchymal hamartoma of the liver. *Modern Pathology* 1994; **7**: 490–3.

Dehner LP, Parker ME, Franciosi RA, Drake RM. Focal nodular hyperplasia and adenoma of the liver. A pediatric experience. *American Journal of Pediatric and Medical Oncology* 1979; **1**: 85–93.

DeMaioribus CA, Lally KP, Sim K, Isaacs H, Mahour GH. Mesenchymal hamartoma of the liver. A 35-year review. *Archives of Surgery* 1990; **125**: 598–600.

Dooley JS, Li AKC, Scheuer PJ, Hobbs KEF, Sherlock S. A giant cystic mesenchymal hamartoma of the liver: diagnosis, management and study of cyst fluid. *Gastroenterology* 1983; **85**: 958–61.

Dumortier J, Boillot O, Chevallier M *et al.* Familial occurrence of nodular regenerative hyperplasia of the liver: a report of three families. *Gut* 1999; **45**: 289–94.

Fasulo F, Giori A, Fissi S *et al.* Cavitron ultrasonic surgical aspirator (CUSA) in liver resection. *International Surgery* 1992; **77**: 64–6.

Filler RM. Liver resections. In: Spitz L, Coran AG (eds) *Pediatric surgery*. London: Chapman and Hall Medical, 1995: 579–89.

Foster JH, Berman MM. The malignant transformation of liver cell adenomas. *Archives of Surgery* 1994; **129**: 712–7.

Foster JH, Donohue TA, Berman MM. Familial liver-cell adenomas and diabetes mellitus. *New England Journal of Medicine* 1978; **299**: 239–41.

Fukuya T, Honda H, Matsumata T *et al.* Diagnosis of inflammatory pseudotumor of the liver: value of CT. *American Journal of Roentgenology* 1994; **163**: 1087–91.

George JC, Cohen MD, Tarver RD, Rosales RN. Ruptured cystic mesenchymal hamartoma: an unusual cause of neonatal ascites. *Pediatric Radiology* 1994; **24**: 304–5.

Glick RD, Nadler EP, Blumgart LH, LaQuaglia MP. Extended left hepatectomy (left hepatic trisegmentectomy) in childhood. *Journal of Pediatric Surgery* 2000; **35**: 303–8.

Grazioli L, Alberti D, Olivetti L *et al.* Congenital absence of portal vein with nodular regenerative hyperplasia of the liver. *European Journal of Radiology* 2000; **10**: 820–5.

Guariso G, Fiorio S, Altavilla G *et al.* Congenital absence of the portal vein associated with focal nodular hyperplasia of the liver and cystic dysplasia of the kidney. *European Journal of Pediatrics* 1998; **157**: 287–90.

Haber M, Reuben B, Burrell M *et al.* Multiple focal nodular hyperplasia of the liver associated with hemihypertrophy and vascular malformations. *Gastroenterology* 1995; **108**: 1256–62.

Heaton ND, Pain J, Cowan NC, Salisbury J, Howard ER. Focal nodular hyperplasia of the liver: a link with sickle-cell disease? *Archives of Disease in Childhood* 1991; **66**: 1073–4.

Heller K, Markus BH, Waag KL. Central hamartoma of the liver in a child. *European Journal of Pediatric Surgery* 1992; **2**: 108–9.

Herman P, Pugliese V, Machado MA *et al.* Hepatic adenoma and focal nodular hyperplasia: differential diagnosis and treatment. *World Journal of Surgery* 2000; **24**: 372–6.

Hodgson WJB, Morgan J, Byrne D *et al.* Hepatic resections for primary and metastatic tumors using the ultrasonic surgical dissector. *American Journal of Surgery* 1992; **163**: 246–50.

Hsiao C-C, Chen C-L, Eng H-L. Inflammatory pseudotumor of the liver in Kostmann's disease. *Pediatric Surgery International* 1999; **15**: 266–9.

Huguet CL, Nordlinger B, Bloch P et al. Tolerance of the human liver to prolonged normothermic ischaemia. *Archives of Surgery* 1978; **113**: 1448–51.

Hutton KAR, Spicer RD, Arthur RJ, Batcup G. Focal nodular hyperplasia of the liver in childhood. *European Journal of Pediatric Surgery* 1993; **3**: 370–2.

Ishida M, Tsuchida Y, Saito S, Sawaguchi S. Mesenchymal hamartoma of the liver: case report and literature review. *Annals of Surgery* 1966; **164**: 175–82.

Jacquemin E, Pariente D, Fabre M et al. Peliosis hepatis with initial presentation as acute hepatic failure and intraperitoneal hemorrhage in children. *Journal of Hepatology* 1999; **30**: 1146–50.

Jozwiak S, Pedich M, Rajszys P, Michalowicz R. Incidence of hepatic hamartomas in tuberous sclerosis. *Archives of Disease in Childhood* 1992; **67**: 1363–5.

Kinjo T, Aoki H, Sunagawa H, Kinjo S, Muto Y. Congenital absence of the protal vein associated with focal nodular hyperplasia of the liver and congenital choledochal cyst: a case report. *Journal of Pediatric Surgery* 2001; **36**: 622–5.

Kitano Y, Ruchelli E, Weiner S, Adzick NS. Hepatic mesenchymal hamartoma associated with mesenchymal stem villous hyperplasia of the placenta. *Fetal Diagnosis and Therapy* 2000; **15**: 134–8.

Koh CC, Sheu JC. Hepatic lymphangioma – a case report. *Pediatric Surgery International* 2000; **16**: 515–16.

Lack EE. Mesenchymal hamartoma of the liver. A clinical and pathologic study of nine cases. *American Journal of Pediatric Hematology and Oncology* 1986; **8**: 91–8.

Lack EE, Ornvold K. Focal nodular hyperplasia and hepatic adenoma: a review of eight cases in the pediatric age group. *Journal of Surgical Oncology* 1986; **33**: 129–35.

Lauwers GY, Grant LD, Donnelly WH et al. Hepatic undifferentiated (embryonal) sarcoma arising in a mesenchymal hamartoma. *American Journal of Surgical Pathology* 1997; **21**: 1248–54.

Leconte I, Van Beers BE, Lacrosse M et al. Focal nodular hyperplasia: natural course observed with CT and MRI. *Journal of Computer-Assisted Tomography* 2000; **24**: 61–6.

Lee SL, DuBoir JJ. Hepatic inflammatory pseudotumor: case report, review of the literature, and a proposal for morphologic classification. *Pediatric Surgery International* 2001; **17**: 555–9.

Lennington WJ, Gray GF, Page DL. Mesenchymal hamartoma of liver: a regional ischemic lesion of a sequestered lobe. *American Journal of Diseases in Children* 1993; **147**: 193–6.

Luks F, Yazbeck S, Brandt M et al. Benign liver tumors in children: a 25-year experience. *Journal of Pediatric Surgery* 1991; **26**: 1326–30.

Magnus KG, Millar AJW, Sinclair-Smith CC, Rode H. Intrahepatic fetus-in-fetu: a case report and review of the literature. *Journal of Pediatric Surgery* 1999; **34**: 1861–4.

Mann JR, Kasthuri N, Raafat F et al. Malignant hepatic tumors in children: incidence, clinical features and aetiology. *Paediatric and Perinatal Epidemiology* 1990; **4**: 276–89.

Mascarello JT, Krous HF. Second report of a translocation involving 19q13.4 in a mesenchymal hamartoma of the liver. *Cancer Genetics and Cytogenetics* 1992; **58**: 141–2.

Mathieu D, Zafrani ES, Anglade MC, Dhumeaux D. Association of focal nodular hyperplasia and hepatic hemangioma. *Gastroenterology* 1989; **97**: 154–7.

Matsubara T, Sumazaki R, Saitoh H et al. Patent ductus venosus associated with tumor-like lesions of the liver in a young girl. *Journal of Pediatric Gastroenterology and Nutrition* 1996; **22**: 107–11.

Meinders A, Simons M, Heij H et al. Mesenchymal hamartoma of the liver: failed management by marsupialization. *Journal of Pediatric Gastroenterology and Nutrition* 1998; **26**: 353–5.

Moran CA, Mullick FG, Ishak KG. Nodular regenerative hyperplasia of the liver in children. *American Journal of Surgical Pathology* 1991; **15**: 449–54.

Murray JD, Ricketts RR. Mesenchymal hamartoma of the liver. *American Surgeon* 1998; **64**: 1097–103.

Ohtomo K, Itai Y, Hasizume K et al. CT and MR appearance of focal nodular hyperplasia of the liver in children with biliary atresia. *Clinical Radiology* 1991; **43**: 88–90.

Okeda R. Mesenchymal hamartoma of the liver: an autopsy case with serial sections and some comments on its pathogenesis. *Acta Pathologica Japan* 1976; **26**: 229–36.

Otal TM, Hendricks JB, Pharis P, Donelly WH. Mesenchymal hamartoma of the liver: DNA flow cytometric analysis of eight cases. *Cancer* 1994; **74**: 1237–42.

Pain JA, Gimson AES, Williams R, Howard ER. Focal nodular hyperplasia of the liver: results of treatment and options in management. *Gut* 1991; **32**: 524–7.

Paley MR, Mergo PJ, Torres GM, Ros PR. Characterization of focal hepatic lesions with ferumoxide-enhanced T2-weighted MR imaging. *American Journal of Roentgenology* 2000; **175**: 159–63.

Passalides A, Keramidas D, Mavrides G. Inflammatory pseudotumor of the liver in children. A case report and review of the literature. *European Journal of Pediatric Surgery* 1996; **6**: 35–7.

Petrikovsky BM, Cohen HL, Scimeca P, Bellucci E. Prenatal diagnosis of focal nodular hyperplasia of the liver. *Prenatal Diagnosis* 1994; **14**: 406–9.

Pettei MJ, Valderamma E, Levine JJ, Ilowite NT. Childhood nodular regenerative hyperplasia of the liver complicated by severe hypoxemia. *Journal of Pediatric Gastroenterology and Nutrition* 1995; **20**: 343–6.

Ramanujam TM, Ramesh JC, Goh DW et al. Malignant transformation of mesenchymal hamartoma of the liver: case report and review of the literature. *Journal of Pediatric Surgery* 1999; **34**: 1684–6.

Randolph JG, Altman RP, Arensman RM et al. Liver resection in children with hepatic neoplasms. *Annals of Surgery* 1978; **187**: 599–605.

Resnick MB, Kozakewich HP, Perez-Atayde AR. Hepatic adenoma in the pediatric age group. Clinicopathological observations and assessment of cell proliferative activity. *American Journal of Surgical Pathology* 1995; **19**: 1181–90.

Reymond D, Plaschkes J, Luthy AR *et al.* Focal nodular hyperplasia of the liver in children: review of follow-up and outcome. *Journal of Pediatric Surgery* 1995; **30**: 1590–3.

Rogers J, Mack L, Treeny P, Johnson M, Somo P. Hepatic focal nodular hyperplasia: angiography, CT, sonography, scintigraphy. *American Journal of Roentgenology* 1981; **137**: 983–90.

Rosh JR, Collins J, Groisman GM *et al.* Management of hepatic adenoma in glycogen storage disease Ia. *Journal of Pediatric Gastroenterology and Nutrition* 1995; **20**: 225–8.

Sakai M, Ikeda H, Suzuki N *et al.* Inflammatory pseudotumor of the liver: case report and review of the literature. *Journal of Pediatric Surgery* 2001; **36**: 663–6.

Sandler A, Rivlin L, Filler R *et al.* Polycythemia secondary to focal nodular hyperplasia. *Journal of Pediatric Surgery* 1997; **32**: 1386–7.

Saul SH, Titelbaum DS, Gansler ES *et al.* The fibrolamellar variant of hepatocellular carcinoma: its association with focal nodular hyperplasia. *Cancer* 1987; **60**: 3049–55.

Shuto T, Kinoshita H, Yamada C *et al.* Bilateral lobectomy excluding the caudate lobe for giant mesenchymal hamartoma of the liver. *Surgery* 1993; **113**: 215–22.

Srouji MN, Chatten J, Schulman WM, Ziegler MM, Koop CE. Mesenchymal hamartomas of the liver in infants. *Cancer* 1978; **42**: 2483–9.

Stocker JT, Ishak KG. Focal nodular hyperplasia of the liver: a study of 21 pediatric cases. *Cancer* 1981; **48**: 336–45.

Stocker JT, Ishak KG. Mesenchymal hamartoma of the liver: a report of 30 cases and a review of the literature. *Pediatric Pathology* 1983; **1**: 245–67.

Strasberg SM. Terminology of liver anatomy and liver resections: coming to grips with hepatic babel. *Journal of the American College of Surgeons* 1997; **184**: 413–34.

Stringer MD, Ramani P, Yeung CK *et al.* Abdominal inflammatory myofibroblastic tumors in children. *British Journal of Surgery* 1992; **79**: 1357–60.

Tepetes K, Selby R, Webb M *et al.* Orthotopic liver transplantation for benign hepatic neoplasms. *Archives of Surgery* 1995; **130**: 153–6.

Todani T, Tabuchi K, Watanabe Y, Tsutsumi A. True hepatic teratoma with high alpha-fetoprotein in serum. *Journal of Pediatric Surgery* 1977; **12**: 591–2.

Trenschel GM, Schubert A, Dries V, Benz-Bohm G. Nodular regenerative hyperplasia of the liver: case report of a 13-year-old girl and review of the literature. *Pediatric Radiology* 2000; **30**: 64–8.

Tsukamoto Y, Nakata H, Kimoto T *et al.* CT and angiography of peliosis hepatis. *American Journal of Roentgenology* 1984; **142**: 539–40.

Vivas Alegre S, Jorquera Plaza F, Munoz Nunez F *et al.* Multiple hepatic focal nodular hyperplasia: its presentation in childhood and atypical evolution. *Gastroenterologia y Hepatologia* 2000; **23**: 9–11.

Wang SY, Ruggles S, Vade A, Newman BM, Borge MA. Hepatic rupture caused by peliosis hepatis. *Journal of Pediatric Surgery* 2001; **36**: 1456–9.

Wanless IR, Mawdsley C, Adams R. On the pathogenesis of focal nodular hyperplasia of the liver. *Hepatology* 1985; **5**: 1194–200.

Weinberg AG, Finegold MJ. Primary hepatic tumors of childhood. *Human Pathology* 1983; **14**: 512–37.

Whelan TJ, Baugh JH, Chandor S. Focal nodular hyperplasia of the liver. *Annals of Surgery* 1973; **177**: 150–8.

Williams JG, Newman BM, Sutphen JL *et al.* Hepatobiliary cystadenoma: a rare hepatic tumor in a child. *Journal of Pediatric Surgery* 1990; **25**: 1250–2.

Yandza T, Valayer J. Benign tumors of the liver in children: analysis of a series of 20 cases. *Journal of Pediatric Surgery* 1986; **21**: 419–23.

18

Malignant tumors: hepatoblastoma and hepatocellular carcinoma

FREDERICK J RESCORLA

Hepatoblastoma (HB) and hepatocellular carcinoma (HCC) are the two most common malignant liver tumors in childhood. Surgical excision remains essential in both conditions. However, the increased use of neoadjuvant chemotherapy, new ablative methods and liver transplantation have led to a significant improvement in the management of these children.

EPIDEMIOLOGY

Liver tumors are relatively uncommon in childhood. Unfortunately, however, most of them are malignant. Liver cancer accounts for approximately 1% of childhood cancer, with approximately 79% of these cases being represented by HB (Bulterys et al., 1999), followed by HCC and then less frequently sarcoma. In children, benign lesions which may be difficult to differentiate from malignancy include vascular tumors, mesenchymal hamartoma, adenomas and focal nodular hyperplasia (see Chapter 17).

Hepatoblastoma is an embryonal tumor with a peak incidence in the first 3 years of life. Although most cases are sporadic, HB does occur with increased frequency in children with Beckwith–Wiedemann syndrome, hemihypertrophy and familial adenomatous polyposis (FAP) (Figure 18.1). The relative risk of HB in a cohort of 192 children with Beckwith–Wiedemann syndrome was 2280 (95% confidence interval, 928–11 656), and hemihypertrophy was the only clinical feature associated with an increased risk (DeBaun and Tucker, 1998). Beckwith–Wiedemann syndrome is associated with a mutation on the short arm of chromosome 11 (11p15.5). Loss of heterozygosity of one parent allele at the 11p15.5 gene locus is frequently seen in children with hepatoblastoma, suggesting the presence of a tumor suppressor gene at this site (Little et al., 1988; Montagna et al., 1994).

Hepatoblastoma has been shown to occur with increased frequency in families with a history of FAP, with an estimated rate of occurrence 1000–2000 times higher than sporadic cases from families without a history of FAP (Garber et al., 1988; Giardiello et al., 1991; Hughes and Michels, 1992). Some sporadic cases of HB have also been identified with mutation of the adenomatous polyposis coli (APC) gene (Oda et al., 1996). In addition to the close relationship between HB and FAP, there have been two pediatric cases of HCC (aged 9 and 15 years, respectively) in association with FAP and Gardner syndrome (Gruner et al., 1998). A relationship between birth weight and HB has recently been observed. Ikeda et al. (1997) reported data from the Japan Children's Cancer Registry demonstrating an association between low birth weight and HB, and this finding has also been supported by a review of patients in a recent Children's Cancer Group (CCG) study (Feusner et al., 1998).

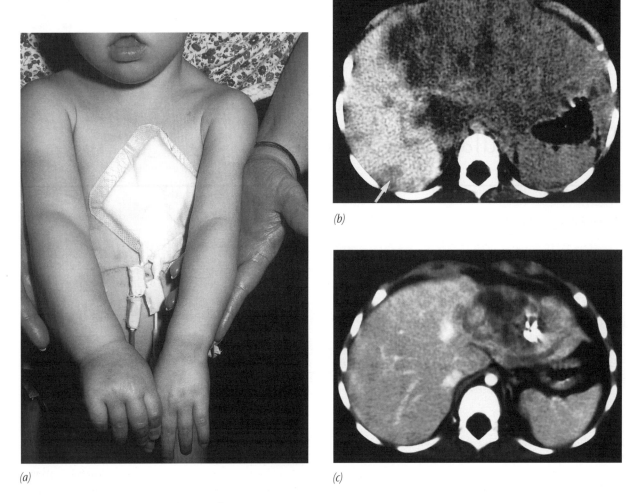

Figure 18.1 *(a) Photograph of an 18-month-old girl with Beckwith–Wiedemann syndrome with hemihypertrophy treated successfully for hepatoblastoma. (b) Initial CT demonstrates a large lesion of the entire left lobe and anterior segment of right lobe with defects in the posterior segment of the right lobe (arrow). (c) After neoadjvant chemotherapy, the tumor decreased in size to allow a left hepatic lobectomy (segments II–IV).*

Hepatocellular carcinoma can occur in children with pre-existing infectious (hepatitis B and C), metabolic (tyrosinemia, glycogen storage disease, alpha-1-anti-trypsin deficiency) or other (biliary atresia, androgen therapy, aflatoxin exposure) liver disorders. Although these disorders account for less than 10% of HCC in children in Western countries, they account for the majority of cases in parts of Asia and Africa where hepatitis B is endemic. Routine immunization with hepatitis B vaccine has decreased the incidence of childhood HCC in Taiwan (Chang *et al.*, 1997), and the effect in other countries, including the USA, remains to be seen.

CLINICAL PRESENTATION

Most children with liver tumors present with an enlarging mass or abdominal distension (Figure 18.2). Hepatoblastoma usually presents in infancy and child-

hood, with a peak incidence at around 3 years of age, whereas HCC usually presents in school-age children with a peak at around 11 years of age. In a recent CCG Pediatric Oncology Group (POG) intergroup study of 182 children with HB, 38% of these patients were less than 1 year of age at diagnosis, and only two patients were over 9 years of age (Ortega *et al.*, 2000). Both tumors occur more frequently in boys, with the recent intergroup study of HB including 62% boys. The fibrolamellar variant of HCC which usually occurs in adolescents and young adults has an equal male:female ratio (Kwee, 1989).

Serum alpha-fetoprotein (AFP) levels are elevated in nearly all children with HB and in most of those with HCC. The rate of decline during chemotherapy can indicate successful treatment, and elevations after therapy are usually indicative of recurrence. Van Tornout *et al.* (1997) noted that a two log or greater decline in the AFP level during the first four cycles of chemotherapy was strongly correlated with survival. They also noted a trend towards improved survival in HB with a high initial AFP level, whereas low levels of AFP in HB are associated with a poor outcome. Anemia and thrombocytosis are relatively common. However, most laboratory studies, including liver function tests, are usually normal. A recent report in adults (Izzo *et al.*, 1999) identified soluble interleukin-2-receptor level elevation with greater frequency than AFP elevation in patients with HCC, and found it to be a more sensitive marker of successful treatment and recurrence.

IMAGING STUDIES

Ultrasound examination is an excellent initial study for determining the characteristics of an abdominal mass (solid vs. cystic), its location, and an assessment of the status of the inferior vena cava and the hepatic and portal veins. In general, further evaluation of a liver mass will require computed tomography (CT) or magnetic resonance imaging (MRI). Calcification can frequently be identified (Figure 18.2). Both CT and MRI provide excellent delineation of the involved segments, although MRI may allow more precise assessment of the relationship between the hepatic vessels and the tumor. The accuracy of prediction of resectability is controversial. Some studies have noted excellent accuracy with MRI in predicting resectability (Boechat *et al.*, 1988), while others have noted relatively high rates of error (21%) using a combination of ultrasound with either CT or MRI (von Schweinitz *et al.*, 1994).

The use of MRI and spiral CT with reconstruction has made angiography unnecessary in nearly all cases. CT is easier to obtain and does not usually require sedation. For these reasons, MRI is rarely utilized at the author's institution. A CT scan of the chest should be obtained in order to assess the presence of metastatic disease in the lung, which is the commonest site of extrahepatic disease.

PATHOLOGY

Hepatoblastoma is an embryonal tumor classified by histology as epithelial (56% of cases) (including pure fetal, 31%; embryonal, 19%; macrotrabecular, 3%; small cell, 3%) or mixed epithelial–mesenchymal (44% of cases) (teratoid, 10%; non-teratoid, 34%) (Stocker, 1994). Completely resected pure fetal histology appears to have a survival advantage over the other histological variants. Haas *et al.* (1989), in a review of 168 cases of HB treated between 1973 and 1984, noted that children with stage I pure fetal histology had a 92% 2-year survival rate, compared with a 2-year survival rate of 57% for the other HB histological subtypes. They also noted that the absence of mitoses improved survival. Hepatoblastoma tumors are usually a solitary mass without the multicentricity and hepatic venous invasion that are commonly seen with HCC.

Hepatocellular carcinoma in childhood is similar to adult HCC. Diffuse intrahepatic dissemination is common (Figure 18.3). A small number (< 10%) of HCCs present with an associated liver disease which may prevent surgical excision. However, these children are occasionally noted with their tumor at the time of planned total hepatectomy with liver transplantation. This subgroup of incidentally detected tumors is a favorable subgroup among patients undergoing hepatic transplantation for HCC.

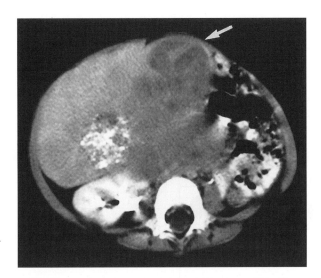

Figure 18.2   *CT scan demonstrating calcifications within a large hepatoblastoma. The protruding portion (arrow) was visible to the patient's parents as a mass.*

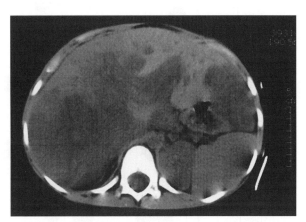

Figure 18.3   *CT scan demonstrating the appearance of a multifocal HCC in a 6-year-old boy.*

The fibrolamellar variant of HCC is usually considered to be a tumor of adolescents and young adults, with a characteristic pattern of lamellar fibrosis around neoplastic hepatocytes. Haas *et al.* (1989) noted an increased rate of complete resection but an insignificant increase in survival rate with this subtype. However, other studies have demonstrated increased rates of resectability and survival with this histological variant (Craig *et al.*, 1980; Teitelbaum *et al.*, 1985; Soreide *et al.*, 1986).

STAGING

The staging system currently being utilized by the US POG-CCG (currently merged as the Children's Oncology Group) is shown in Table 18.1. This system is dependent on the outcome of the initial operative procedure and the pathology report. In this system, the stage of the tumor is dependent on the judgement of the surgeon and oncologist. In cases in which a decision of unresectability is made based on preoperative scans, a needle or open biopsy through a limited incision is utilized initially, followed by neoadjuvant chemotherapy. In other cases, at the time of initial exploration the surgeon may lack enthusiasm for a complete resection of a large tumor. Both of these factors rely on an individual surgeon's judgement and perhaps experience, and can lead to 'stage creep', with increasing numbers of patients enrolled at stage III, some of whom might have been stage I if they had been resected at diagnosis. The argument in favor of neoadjuvant therapy is based on the good response of most HBs to chemotherapy.

Table 18.1 *Intergroup (POG-CCG) staging system*

Stage I	Complete resection, clear margins
Stage II	Gross total resection with microscopic residual or preoperative rupture
Stage III	Unresectable, or resection with gross residual or lymph-node involvement
Stage IV	Metastatic disease

The current intergroup protocol is also utilizing the pretreatment grouping developed by the International Society of Pediatric Oncology (SIOP) to evaluate the extent of disease (Figure 18.4) (MacKinlay and Pritchard, 1992; Pritchard *et al.*, 1992). According to this system the liver is divided into four sectors and the system is based on the number of free sectors. The system also accounts for vascular invasion and extrahepatic and metastatic disease.

SURGERY

The liver has excellent regenerative capabilities, and resections of up to 75–80% of the original liver mass are well tolerated. Children usually have an otherwise normal liver and are free from the limitations which underlying liver disorders place on adults who are undergoing resection. Complete initial resection of either HCC or HB provides the greatest chance of long-term survival, and this is the best treatment plan if it can be performed safely. If the procedure is considered to be unsafe or formidable, initial biopsy followed by chemotherapy is reasonable and well supported by the literature (Reynolds *et al.*, 1992; Seo *et al.*, 1998), although the postoperative

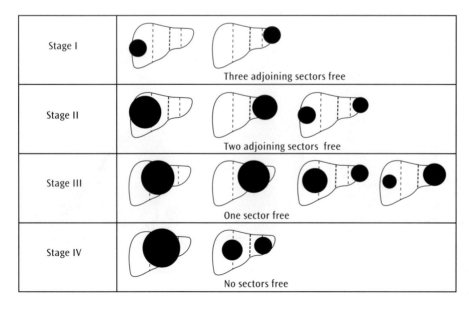

Figure 18.4 *Pretreatment grouping developed by SIOP.*

complication rate was higher in the delayed (25%) vs. initial (8%) resection in a CCG study (King *et al.*, 1991). However, Seo *et al.* (1998) claim that the delayed resection is a safer procedure. The POG study (Reynolds *et al.*, 1992) noted no major complications in patients undergoing resection at diagnosis, whereas of 26 patients undergoing post-chemotherapy resection, three patients were returned to the operating-room because of hemorrhage and three had bile duct injuries. It is most likely that the delayed resections in the CCG and POG studies were larger tumors and more difficult resections due to their size and proximity to vascular structures. As this trend has progressed, some surgeons have utilized it not only in 'unresectable' cases but also when a tumor was large enough to increase the operative morbidity (Seo *et al.*, 1998). In some reports this has included tumors which could have been resected with right or left hepatectomies. The commonest reasons for avoiding an initial resection are involvement of both right and left lobes, diffuse multifocal disease, vascular invasion and an extremely large unilobar tumor which in the surgeon's judgement may lead to excessive bleeding (Figure 18.5). King (1998) has referred to the effect of 'stage creep' as

surgeons have become less aggressive in their approach. In the recent POG-CCG intergroup study, 59 of 182 patients (32%) with HB underwent initial resection (stage I or II), compared with previous studies in which up to 66% of patients underwent initial resection (Exelby *et al.*, 1975; Ortega *et al.*, 2000).

Another area of controversy concerns the type of biopsy. The US intergroup studies have required an open biopsy with a generous (approximately 1 cm³) sample to allow biological studies. Some institutions have utilized a needle biopsy, which usually provides a diagnosis but may not allow further studies (Ehrlich *et al.*, 1997). Seo *et al.* (1998) have argued against open biopsy, and consider elevated AFP levels and radiological findings to be adequate for the diagnosis and to initiate chemotherapy. The drawback to this approach is that the tumor may be HCC, and initial aggressive surgery may be more effective than initial chemotherapy.

Although neoadjuvant chemotherapy has a definite role in unresected HB, its role in HCC carcinoma is less clear. Two recent large studies in adults have demonstrated no survival advantage for systemic chemotherapy (Rose *et al.*, 1998; Sangro *et al.*, 1998), whereas surgical

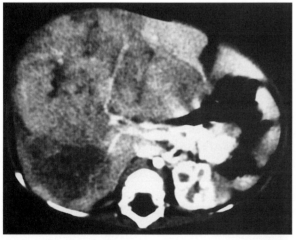

(a)

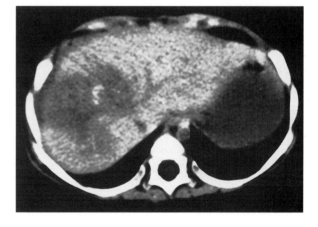

(b)

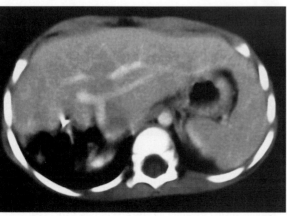

(c)

Figure 18.5 *(a) Six-month-old boy with an abdominal mass, AFP of 780 000 ng/mL and a large hepatoblastoma of the entire right lobe and medial segment left lobe. (b) After neoadjuvant therapy a significant decrease in size was observed. However, due to the central location, a right trisegmentectomy was required. (c) Postoperative CT demonstrating regenerative ability of the left lateral segment.*

resection, chemo-embolization and liver transplantation prolonged survival. In cases of HCC, the surgeon should attempt complete resection even if an extended right or left hepatectomy is required or a combination of resection and ablative therapy. If this is not possible, consideration should be given to chemo-embolization and possible transplantation.

At exploration for resection, complete mobilization of the liver is accomplished with careful examination of the entire liver for multifocal disease. A bilateral subcostal incision usually provides excellent exposure, sometimes requiring a midline extension superiorly. The utility of intraoperative ultrasound (IOUS) is particularly relevant for HCC, in which multifocal tumors are common. A recent adult series noted that IOUS identified intrahepatic disease that was not identified on a preoperative CT scan in 38% of patients (Wood et al., 2000) (Figure 18.6). This can also be useful for assessing tumor proximity to major hepatic vessels.

Various methods of describing hepatic anatomy have been utilized, leading to some confusion (see Chapter 1). The segmental anatomy system developed by Couinaud (1957) has proved to be the most useful method (Figure 18.7). This system is based on the hepatic venous anatomy, with the middle hepatic vein occupying the main portal fis-

sure dividing the liver into right and left livers or lobes. The right hepatic vein divides the right liver into an anterior and posterior portion. The left hepatic vein provides drainage of segments II and III and a portion of segment IV. The standard hepatic resections together with the segments involved are listed in Figure 18.8. Strasberg (1997) has compiled an excellent summary of the various nomenclatures of the liver, and has proposed a system based on the internal anatomy of the liver and utilized hemihepatectomy (hepatectomy in Figure 18.8) and trisectionectomy (extended hepatectomy or trisegmentectomy in Figure 18.8). The non-standardized system leads to some confusion (e.g. some surgeons may report a left lateral segmentectomy as a left lobectomy based on anatomical studies).

The surgeon must be aware of the common variations of the arterial anatomy prior to completing the hilar dissection (Michels, 1966; Suzuki et al., 1971). Although occasionally a tumor may be amenable to a wedge resection, most will be hepatectomies or extended hepatectomies. Initial dissection at the hilum allows control and ligation of the artery, bile duct and portal vein to the involved liver. This dissection is more difficult in extended hepatectomy (trisegmentectomy), in which case the structures to the remaining segments must be preserved to a portion of the liver some distance from the hilum.

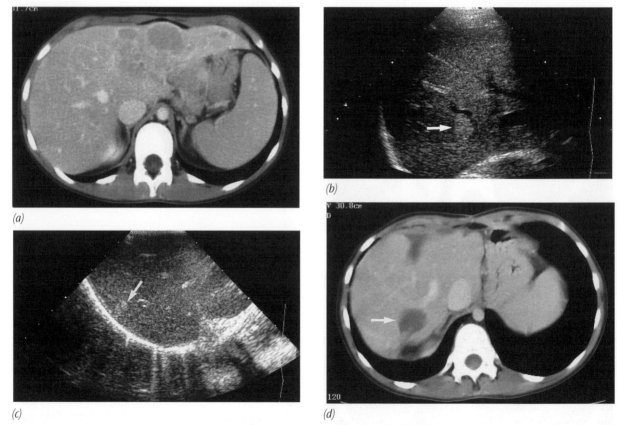

(a)

(b)

(c)

(d)

Figure 18.6 *(a) CT scan demonstrating a large hepatocellular carcinoma of the left lobe of the liver. At exploration a superficial right lobe lesion was also excised and IOUS identified a 1.5-cm lesion (arrow) lateral to the right hepatic vein (b) and a second superficial lesion (arrow) (c). Radiofrequency ablation was utilized to ablate the deep right lobe lesion, and a left trisegmentectomy was required to resect the large lesion. (d) Postoperative CT demonstrating residual defect from radiofrequency ablation (arrow) adjacent to right hepatic vein. Significant liver regeneration is also noted.*

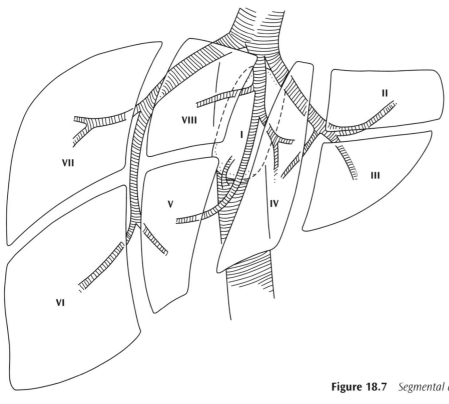

Figure 18.7 *Segmental anatomy as described by Couinaud.*

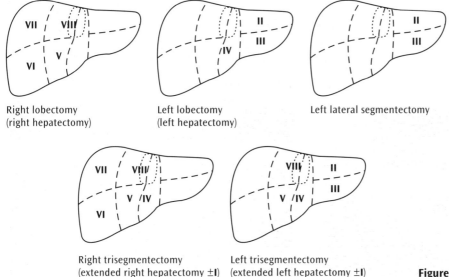

Right lobectomy
(right hepatectomy)

Left lobectomy
(left hepatectomy)

Left lateral segmentectomy

Right trisegmentectomy
(extended right hepatectomy ±I)

Left trisegmentectomy
(extended left hepatectomy ±I)

Figure 18.8 *Standard hepatic resections.*

It is useful to gain control of the inferior vena cava above and below the liver with a vessel loop prior to transecting the liver parenchyma, particularly with lobectomies and extended resections. This allows resection with the use of total vascular exclusion if necessary. In this technique the portal vein, hepatic artery and both the infrahepatic and suprahepatic vena cava are occluded. Several series have demonstrated the safety of this technique with warm ischemia times averaging 29–46 minutes (Bismuth *et al.*, 1989; Emre *et al.*, 1993). This can be tolerated for up to 60 minutes (Huguet *et al.*, 1978).

Some surgeons prefer to perform the resection without hilar ligation, and various clamps are available (Storm and Longmire, 1971; Lin, 1973) to occlude the liver parenchyma and vessels, or mattress sutures may be placed to control bleeding. In cases in which the hilar structures are not divided, selective vascular clamping may reduce blood loss during the parenchymal dissection (Malassagne *et al.*, 1998).

Various techniques are useful during the parenchymal dissection, including electrocautery, suture ligature, clips, argon-beam coagulation and ultrasonic dissectors. The Pringle maneuver (Pringle, 1908), with occlusion of the portal vein and common hepatic artery, may be useful if bleeding is encountered. The hepatic veins are usually ligated when encountered within the parenchyma, although occasionally the right hepatic vein can be controlled above the liver.

Hemorrhage remains the major intraoperative complication. This is increased with extended resections or tumors adjacent to the portal or hepatic veins. Other intraoperative complications include air embolus and bile duct or vascular injury. Postoperative complications include biliary leak, biliary obstruction, infectious problems, bleeding and bowel obstruction. Postoperative endoscopic retrograde cholangiopancreatography can identify the site of a biliary leak and can usually be therapeutic by inserting a stent to decompress the biliary tree (Figure 18.9).

The mortality for liver surgery has decreased in the past two decades. Large series in children report rare operative deaths, hemorrhage being the commonest cause (Filler *et al.*, 1991). Several recent adult studies have demonstrated low mortality in elective resections. In a series of 747 resections, Belghiti *et al.* (2000), reported a 3.9% mortality rate with elective resections, the high-risk group consisting of those patients with cirrhosis or obstructive jaundice. Melendez *et al.* (2001), in a series of 226 patients undergoing extended resection (more than four segments), reported a 6% mortality rate. They identified cholangitis, elevated creatinine levels, bilirubin levels greater than 6 mg/dL, blood loss greater than 3 L or vena caval resection as risk factors, with a mortality rate of 3% in the absence of all five risk factors.

Metastatic tumor

The commonest site of metastatic disease for both HB and HCC is the lung. A fine-cut CT scan of the lungs at the time of diagnosis may identify nodules and can be followed during initial chemotherapy. If the nodules resolve completely, continued observation after liver resection is warranted. If resolution does not occur, surgical resection should be undertaken if the lesions are amenable to resection, even if bilateral thoracotomies are necessary.

Several children have been noted with metastatic pulmonary disease after treatment for initial non-metastatic HB or HCC. Aggressive surgical excision is warranted in these cases (Figure 18.10). Black *et al.* (1991b) reported long-term survival in four out of five cases. A CCG report (Feusner *et al.*, 1993) noted long-term survival in three of six cases (one with bilateral thoracotomies), and Passmore *et al.* (1995) reported one long-term survival after repeat thoracotomies. Improved survival has been noted if the metastases develop 6 months or more after the initial tumor, respond to chemotherapy with a decrease in AFP levels, and all disease is resected.

In addition, there has been a report of one child who

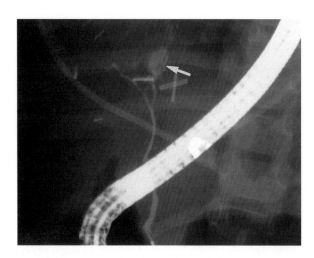

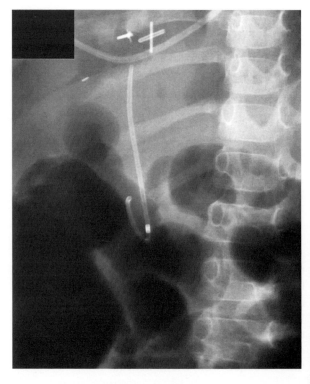

Figure 18.9 *(a) ERCP demonstrating a bile leak (arrow) after a hepatic resection. (b) Stent placement resulted in resolution of the leak within 4 days.*

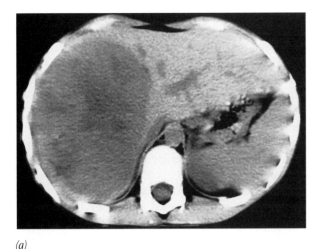

(a)

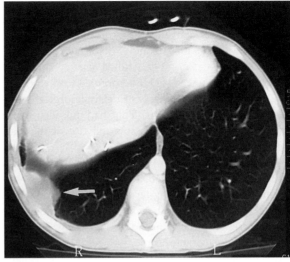

(b)

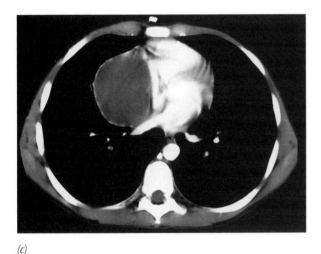

(c)

Figure 18.10 *(a) CT demonstrates a right lobe hepatoblastoma in a 6-year-old boy who was successfully treated with a right hepatic lobectomy at diagnosis. One year later he developed (b) pleural-based (arrow) and (c) mediastinal metastases which were successfully resected. He survived after further chemotherapy.*

developed pulmonary and brain metastases. The brain lesion recurred twice and was resected on all three occasions with supplemental radiation and chemotherapy. At the time of the report, the child had survived for 4.5 years after the last occurrence (Robertson *et al.*, 1997).

CHEMOTHERAPY

Significant improvements in the survival of children with HB have been noted over the past two decades, primarily as a result of effective chemotherapy. Success in the survival of children with HCC has been less striking. A survey of the Surgical Section of the Academy of Pediatrics completed in 1974 of 129 cases of HB and 98 cases of HCC reported survival rates of 35% for HB and 13% for HCC (Exelby *et al.*, 1975). Of those patients who were excised for cure, the survival rate was 60% for HB and 35% for HCC. The survival rate has improved for HB. However, the current survival rate for HCC has improved for those resected for cure but not for the entire group.

Several studies that were completed in the 1970s and 1980s demonstrated the efficacy of chemotherapy (Weinblatt *et al.*, 1982; Black *et al.*, 1991a; Filler *et al.*, 1991; Reynolds *et al.*, 1992). Andrassy *et al.* (1980) utilized preoperative Adriamycin (doxorubicin) together with other agents to achieve resection in three out of six infants. Several subsequent studies demonstrated similar results. Cisplatin was identified as an active agent in 1982 (Champion *et al.*, 1982), and several reports followed with excellent results. Quinn *et al.* (1985) reported efficacy with a combination of Adriamycin and cisplatin, with complete clearance of pulmonary metastases in one child and complete resection in two out of three initially unresectable cases. Filler *et al.* (1991) treated 15 children with HB with preoperative cisplatin and Adriamycin, and achieved complete resection with no residual tumor in 12 cases (80%). A follow-up report (Ehrlich *et al.*, 1997) from the same institution described long-term survival in 19 of 22 cases (87%), with two of the 19 patients requiring hepatic transplantation.

The CCG evaluated continuous-infusion Adriamycin with cisplatin in 46 patients with HB ($n = 32$) and HCC

($n = 14$) (King *et al.*, 1991). Delayed resections were possible in 20 out of 34 cases (59%) whose tumors were considered unresectable at diagnosis. The overall survival rate was 63% for HB and 17% for HCC. In a POG study, Reynolds *et al.* (1992) noted that 29 out of 37 patients with unresectable HB responded to chemotherapy, and 26 patients underwent delayed surgical resection. Interestingly, three patients had no identifiable tumor after neoadjuvant therapy, and two of these are long-term survivors.

The largest intergroup (POG-CCG) study (involving 242 patients) completed between 1989 and 1992 was recently reported with long-term follow-up (Ortega *et al.*, 2000). This trial treated stage I pure fetal histology with four courses of Adriamycin and then randomized all others (stage I-unfavorable histology, stages II–IV) to receive either cisplatin, vincristine and 5-fluorouracil or cisplatin and continuous-infusion Adriamycin. Of the 182 evaluable patients with HB, initial resection (stage I or II) was performed in 59 patients (32%). Survival rates are listed in Table 18.2, and were not statistically significantly different between the treatment arms, although chemotherapy toxicity was higher in the Adriamycin arm.

The German Cooperative Liver Study (HB: $n = 89$) utilized ifosfamide, cisplatin and Adriamycin for advanced HB (stages III and IV) and noted a tumor resectability rate of 89% and a survival rate of 73% (von Schweinitz *et al.*, 1995). This study noted the development of drug resistance in six of 11 patients who were treated with four or more courses. As in the other studies, complete surgical resection was essential to survival.

The approach to HB in most European countries, as in the case of Wilms' tumor, is initial chemotherapy with delayed resection (Stringer *et al.*, 1995). The International Society of Pediatric Oncology trials (SIOPEL-1) utilized primary chemotherapy with cisplatin and Adriamycin, and the current study (SIOPEL-3) randomizes standard-risk HB to cisplatin alone vs. cisplatin and Adriamycin. High-risk HB cases and all HCC cases receive carboplatin, Adriamycin and cisplatin. The results of SIOPEL-1 report a 5-year survival rate of 75% (Brown *et al.*, 2000). They utilized a pretreatment extent of disease grouping system (PRETEXT) based on the number of involved liver sections (Figure 18.4 above).

The current US intergroup Children's Oncology Group (CCG and POG) for HB was opened in March 1999, and the protocol is listed in Box 18.1. Stages II–IV are randomized to one of four arms evaluating two chemotherapy regimens, each with or without amifostine. Amifostine is a compound that was initially developed to protect against ionizing radiation. It is dephosphorylated in tissues to its active metabolite, free thiol. This protects normal tissues from the effects of radiation and chemotherapy but does not protect neoplastic tissues.

Unfortunately, the results for HCC are disappointing. The German study reported a 30% survival rate (von Schweinitz *et al.*, 1994). US studies have also reported low survival rates, with the best long-term survivors being those resected at diagnosis. There are several scattered reports with regard to children, involving the use of alternative therapy such as chemo-embolization or hepatic transplantation, which will be covered in a later section.

The major toxic side-effects of the common chemotherapeutic agents that are used to treat hepatoblastoma and HCC are listed in Table 18.3.

POSTOPERATIVE FOLLOW-UP

Postoperative follow-up in those rendered disease-free should include AFP levels, chest radiography (CXR) and abdominal CT scans. The current recommendations of the intergroup study are monthly AFP and CXR for 6 months, every 2 months for 18 months, every 3 months for an additional 2 years, and then yearly follow-up. The frequency of CT scans after completion of treatment is not specified. AFP elevation after surgical resection requires further evaluation. AFP levels can be elevated after liver resection, and the trend of the levels must be followed. Persistent elevation or an upward trend should be evaluated with a fine-cut CT scan or MRI. In addition, a careful search should be made for extrahepatic disease. Occasionally no tumor is identified, and if the AFP level is rising, consideration may be given to exploration with intraoperative ultrasound evaluation of the liver.

Table 18.2 *Survival data (%) from recent intergroup study for hepatoblastoma (Ortega et al., 2000)*

Stage	*n*	5-year event-free survival (%)	5-year survival (%)
I FH	9	100	100
I UH	43	91	98
II	7	100	100
III	83	64	69
IV	40	25	37

FH = favorable histology, UH = unfavorable histology.

Box 18.1 *Current intergroup protocol P9645 (POG-CCG) for the treatment of children with hepatoblastoma*

Stage I (favorable histology)	Surgery and observation	
Stage I (unfavorable histology)/II	Cisplatin + vincristine + 5-fluorouracil with or without amifostine	×4
Stage III/IV	Cisplatin + vincristine + 5-fluorouracil with or without amifostine	
	vs.	× 4→Surgery→ Chemotherapy × 2
	Carboplatin + cisplatin with or without amifostine	

Table 18.3 *Toxic side-effects of chemotherapeutic agents used in the treatment of hepatoblastoma and hepatocellular carcinoma*

Chemotherapeutic agent	Toxicity
Cisplatin	Renal
	Auditory
Vincristine	Neurotoxic
	Constipation
	Peripheral neuropathy
5-Fluorouracil	Diarrhea
	Pancytopenia
Adriamycin	Cardiac
	Mucositis
	Pancytopenia

Any lesion that is amenable to resection should be removed. If the lesion is unresectable due to proximity to vessels or its size, alternative therapy should be considered. For HB, consideration can be given to systemic chemotherapy with subsequent evaluation or alternative therapy as described below. HCC is usually resistant to systemic chemotherapy, and consideration should immediately be given to local therapy and infusion treatment (chemo-embolization), with consideration of transplantation if the disease can be controlled but not resected. Oue *et al.* (1998) noted postoperative elevation of AFP levels in three children with HB, and utilized two courses of aggressive chemotherapy followed by autologous bone-marrow transplant. This has not been widely used at other centers.

FURTHER THERAPY

Unfortunately, many tumors are unresectable either at presentation, after neoadjuvant chemotherapy or after resection, presenting with recurrent disease. Some of these patients may be candidates for local ablative proce-

dures, infusion therapy or hepatic transplantation. Ablative techniques include ethanol injection, microwave tumor coagulation, cryosurgical ablation and radiofrequency ablation, the latter two being the most frequently utilized procedures in the USA. These may be useful for treatment of multiple lesions or in conjunction with a resection procedure. Infusion techniques include hepatic artery infusion and chemo-embolization. Total hepatectomy with liver transplantation may be useful if the liver disease is unresectable and there is no extrahepatic disease. Alternative systemic therapy may also be considered.

Radiofrequency ablation

Radiofrequency ablation (RFA) involves the administration of high-frequency alternating current through a probe that is placed directly into the tumor, causing thermal coagulation and protein denaturation (Figure 18.6 above). This occurs when cells are heated above 45–50°C, and most RFA units have a target temperature of 90°C. The probe can be placed under ultrasound guidance at laparotomy or laparoscopy. After positioning, the probe releases curved electrode arms into the lesion to allow ablation of an area 4–5 cm in diameter. If RFA cannot be performed successfully due to heat loss from the effect of surrounding blood vessels, temporary inflow occlusion may be necessary with a Pringle maneuver (Curley *et al.*, 1999).

RFA is generally considered to be safer than cryosurgical ablation. However, it is limited by the size of the lesion (< 3–4 cm in diameter). The probes are smaller and the probe tract is cauterized during the procedure, thus limiting the risk of hemorrhage. RFA can be utilized with cryosurgery, and Bilchik *et al.* (2000) proposed that RFA could be utilized on lesions < 3 cm and cryosurgery on lesions > 3 cm in diameter. Although initial studies reported local tumor recurrence rates of 50–100% (Livraghi *et al.*, 1997; Nagata *et al.*, 1997; Solbiati *et al.*, 1997), three recent studies have reported recurrence rates in the range 1.8–18% (Curley *et al.*, 1999; Bilchik *et al.*, 2000; Wood *et al.*, 2000).

Cryosurgery

Low temperature has been used to destroy tissue since the 1800s, but it was not until 1963 that Cooper reported the use of cryosurgery to treat CNS disorders (Cooper, 1963). The mechanism of cryoablation is cell death as a result of ice crystal formation and cellular anoxia. The end result is osmotic dehydration, cell membrane destruction and cellular necrosis. The development of modern-day cryosurgery has been facilitated by the development of IOUS to allow monitoring of the iceball. This has gained popularity primarily in adults with hepatic metastases from colorectal cancer. In most cases the probe is placed at laparotomy (or laparoscopy) with ultrasound guidance after complete mobilization of the liver. Probes (3–10 mm in diameter) are selected, and after placement, liquid nitrogen is circulated within the probe, producing probe temperatures of −196°C and adjacent tissue temperature of −100°C to −160°C. The iceball is monitored by IOUS, and a 1-cm margin is utilized to ensure temperatures of −30°C to −50°C within the tumor (McCarty and Kuhn, 1998). Some surgeons place thermocouples in normal liver around the tumor and bring this area to −40°C in order to ensure complete tumor killing. A repeat cycle is often used to maximize the tumoricidal effect. Current units can treat tumors close to major vessels without a Pringle maneuver (Weber *et al.*, 1997). The probe is heated to allow removal, and the tract is packed with a hemostatic agent.

The largest reported series (involving 167 cases) that received cryosurgery for HCC is from Shanghai, China (Zhou *et al.*, 1996). This was employed as the sole therapy (46% of cases) or in combination with resection or hepatic artery ligation/infusion (54% of cases). These authors reported 1-, 3- and 5-year survival rates of 73.5%, 47.7% and 31.7%, respectively. Local recurrence

rates can vary, and may be related to lack of treatment of the entire tumor.

Complications associated with cryoablation are usually observed with treatment of larger volumes (≥ 35% of total liver volume), and they include thrombocytopenia, disseminated intravascular coagulation, renal failure, hepatic failure and adult respiratory distress syndrome. Experimental studies have demonstrated release of tumor necrosis factor-alpha and interleukin-6 after hepatic cryoablation (Seifert *et al.*, 1998), as well as increased pulmonary capillary permeability (Chapman *et al.*, 2000). Most surgeons seek to maintain relatively high urine output (fluids and mannitol) and alkalinization of the urine to protect the kidneys.

Other techniques

Percutaneous ethanol injection has been utilized for some patients, particularly those with associated parenchymal disease which may make resection a high-risk option. Usually multiple injections are required in order to achieve complete tumor necrosis. This has primarily been utilized in adults with HCC, and is currently mainly recommended for small unresectable HCC lesions and those considered to be high risk for resection. Intrahepatic tumor recurrence rates of 50–75% have been reported (Shiina *et al.*, 1993; Ebara *et al.*, 1995; Lencioni *et al.*, 1995; Livraghi *et al.*, 1995).

Microwave therapy involves the use of electrodes implanted within the tumor which emit microwaves that produce heat and coagulative necrosis (Murakami *et al.*, 1995). Adult studies have demonstrated the efficacy of this therapy, which is comparable to that of resection (Yamanaka *et al.*, 1996; Horigome *et al.*, 1999).

Intralesional injection with yttrium-90 glass microspheres has been reported to ablate entire tumors (Tian *et al.*, 1996). Injection is under ultrasound guidance, and there is some concern that intraperitoneal spill may lead to complications. Unfortunately, although these techniques have demonstrated efficacy for tumor ablation, no randomized studies exist comparing the efficacy of various techniques, and most reported series include only adults.

Chemo-embolization

Liver tumors receive nearly all of their blood supply from the hepatic artery, in contrast to the normal liver, which receives 80% of its blood supply from the portal vein. This provides the rationale for the various transarterial therapy techniques. Numerous techniques have been reported; hepatic transarterial chemo-embolization (TACE) involves embolization of the selected arterial blood supply to the tumor with a combination of gelatin sponge particles, Lipiodol and chemotherapeutic agents.

Several randomized adult studies have failed to

demonstrate improved survival rates with TACE (Pelletier *et al.*, 1990; Paye *et al.*, 1998), although non-randomized case-controlled series have demonstrated improved survival (Stefanini *et al.*, 1995). A limited number of studies have demonstrated the safety and efficacy of this technique in children. Malogolowkin *et al.* (2000) treated children with progressive, recurrent or unresectable HB (*n* = 6) and HCC (*n* = 3) with TACE, with an initial response (a 50% reduction by CT and AFP levels) in all nine cases. Two patients achieved complete resections and three achieved partial resections after several courses of TACE. Three patients (two HB cases and one HCC case) are long-term survivors, with one of the HB children surviving with a liver transplant. Oue *et al.* (1998) treated eight children with unresectable HB with TACE, and were subsequently able to achieve complete resection in all eight patients, with six surviving long term. Han *et al.* (1999) treated four children with HB with TACE, and achieved complete resection and long-term survival in all four cases. The use of iodine-131-labeled Lipiodol has been reported in adults with HCC, and appears to compare favorably with other forms of therapy (Partensky *et al.*, 2000). Although direct hepatic artery infusion with chemotherapy is rarely utilized, Yokomori *et al.* (1991) reported the case of a child who was treated for 18 months with hepatic artery infusion of several chemotherapeutic agents, with complete disappearance of the tumor.

Isolated hepatic perfusion

Isolated hepatic perfusion is a technique in which the isolated liver is infused with agents through the hepatic artery, with return of all hepatic venous blood to the perfusion circuit. Portal venous blood and infrahepatic caval venous flow are diverted through a veno–veno bypass circuit to the axillary vein. This technique allows regional treatment of the organ with high doses of agents without systemic side-effects.

Curley *et al.* (1994) treated 10 patients with unresectable HCC with an infusion of doxorubicin and noted more than 25% tumor reduction in seven cases. Of these, two showed more than 50% tumor reduction, which allowed subsequent tumor resection, and both patients were still alive with no evidence of disease at 13 and 17 months, respectively. Overall survival for responders was 13 months, compared with 2 months for non-responders. Various agents, including tumor necrosis factor (TNF), mitomycin, melphalan, cisplatin and 5-fluorouracil, have been utilized (Schwemmle *et al.*, 1987; Oldhafer *et al.*, 1998; Libutti *et al.*, 2000). Most of them utilize hyperthermia to raise the temperature of the hepatic parenchyma to 38.5–41°C. There are no reported series involving the use of this technique in children.

Liver transplantation

Some patients with unresectable liver tumors are candidates for orthotopic liver transplantation. The limited experience of reports published since 1990 is listed in Tables 18.4 and 18.5. This has been successful in unresectable or recurrent HB or HCC without extrahepatic disease, and in children with initial metastatic disease which has either responded to chemotherapy with complete resolution or has been resected.

The survival rate for the entire group of HB cases with transplant is 75%. This group included 11 patients with metastatic disease at diagnosis. The survival rate for the entire group of HCC cases was 56%. Unfortunately, the survival data for this group are affected by the inclusion of small HCCs associated with a primary liver disease for which advanced parenchymal disease leads to transplantation. The survival rate for patients with these 'incidental' tumors is very high, and the survival rate for patients

Table 18.4 *Recent results of liver transplantation for hepatoblastoma*

Author	Year	n	Metastatic at diagnosis	Survival	Follow-up
Koneru *et al.*	1991	12	0	6 (50%)	Mean 44 months
Tagge *et al.*	1992	6	0	5 (83%)	Median 1.3 years
Lockwood *et al.*	1993	1	1	1 (100%)	36 months
Otte *et al.*	1996	1	0	1 (100%)	51 months
Achilleos *et al.*	1996	2	0	2 (100%)	Mean 31 months
Ehrlich *et al.*	1997	2	1	2 (100%)	> 1 year
Bilik and Superina	1997	5	2	4 (80%)	> 2 years
Al-Qabandi *et al.*	1999	8	3	5 (63%)	Median 22 months
Perilongo and Shafford	1999	11	—	9 (82%)	Median 46 months
Reyes *et al.*	2000	12	4	10 (83%)	Mean 82 months
Total		60	—	45 (75%)	—

Table 18.5 *Recent results of liver transplantation for hepatocellular carcinoma*

Author	Year	*n*	'Incidental'	Survival	Follow-up
Tagge *et al.*	1992	9	—	4 (44%)	Median 2.3 years
Yandza *et al.*	1993	2	2	2 (100%)	> 2 years
Broughan *et al.*	1994	4	0	3 (75%)	Mean 63 months
Superina and Bilik	1996	3	2	3 (100%)	1–5 years
Otte *et al.*	1996	5	—	3 (60%)	Median 49 months
Achilleos *et al.*	1996	2	0	0	
Reyes *et al.*	2000	19	7	10	Mean 135 months
Total		44	—	25 (56%)	
Excluding incidental		33	—	14 (42%)	

presenting with HCC in a previously normal liver is therefore lower. The survival of the HCC group falls to 42% if the incidental tumors are excluded.

Reyes *et al.* (2000) performed transplants in eight HB patients with TNM stage IVA disease. Of this group, four patients had major intrahepatic venous invasion and all of them died, whereas three out of four patients without major vascular invasion survived. Of three patients with IVB (metastatic), two with major venous invasion died, whereas one patient with IVB due to contiguous extension to the diaphragm survived. In Reyes' overall group, six of the nine deaths were related to tumor recurrence, while the remaining three were non-tumor-related deaths.

The liver transplant registry report of HCC included 422 mainly adult patients (Klintmalm, 1998). The overall survival rate was 72.2% at 1 year, 63% at 2 years and 44% at 5 years. Approximately half of the deaths were due to recurrent tumor, with the liver being the most common site, followed by the lungs. Survival in this study was adversely affected by tumor size greater than 5 cm, vascular invasion and poorly differentiated tumor.

Organ availability remains a significant problem, causing a significant time interval between patient listing and actual transplant. In order to increase availability, split livers have been utilized by some centers, as well as living-related transplants. Unresolved issues include the role of preoperative systemic chemotherapy and chemoembolization, as well as the role of postoperative therapy. Tumor recurrence remains the leading cause of death in this select group, and a thorough pretransplant work-up is essential. Some centers have utilized a pretransplant laparotomy to evaluate eligibility prior to transplant.

Key references

King DR, Ortega J, Campbell J *et al.* The surgical management of children with incompletely resected hepatic cancer is facilitated by intensive chemotherapy. *Journal of Pediatric Surgery* 1991; **26**: 1074–81.

A CCG series of delayed surgical resection and a description of the associated complications.

Ortega JA, Douglass EC, Feusner JH *et al.* Randomized comparison of cisplatin/vincristine/fluorouracil and cisplatin/continuous-infusion doxorubicin for treatment of pediatric hepatoblastoma: a report from the Children's Cancer Group and the Pediatric Oncology Group. *Journal of Clinical Oncology* 2000; **18**: 2665–75.

A report of the largest randomized trial for hepatoblastoma.

Reyes JD, Carr B, Dvorchik I *et al.* Liver transplantation and chemotherapy for hepatoblastoma and hepatocellular cancer in childhood and adolescence. *Journal of Pediatrics* 2000; **136**: 795–804.

A large series of hepatic transplantations for hepatoblastoma and hepatocellular carcinoma. The article describes prognostic factors and contraindications to transplant.

Reynolds M, Douglass EC, Finegold M *et al.* Chemotherapy can convert unresectable hepatoblastoma. *Journal of Pediatric Surgery* 1992; **27**: 1080–4.

A POG report of the effect of chemotherapy on unresectable hepatoblastoma.

von Schweinitz D, Hecker H, Harms D *et al.* Complete resection before development of drug resistance is essential for survival from advanced hepatoblastoma – a report from the German Cooperative Pediatric Liver Tumor Study HB-89. *Journal of Pediatric Surgery* 1995; **30**: 845–52.

A series describing the need for surgical excision prior to development of drug resistance.

REFERENCES

Achilleos OA, Buist LJ, Kelly DA *et al*. Unresectable hepatic tumors in childhood and the role of liver transplantation. *Journal of Pediatric Surgery* 1996; **11**: 1563–7.

Al-Qabandi W, Jenkinson HC, Buckels JA *et al*. Orthotopic liver transplantation for unresectable hepatoblastoma: a single center's experience. *Journal of Pediatric Surgery* 1999; **34**: 1261–4.

Andrassy RJ, Brennan LP, Siegel MM *et al*. Preoperative chemotherapy for hepatoblastoma in children: report of six cases. *Journal of Pediatric Surgery* 1980; **15**: 517–22.

Belghiti J, Hiramatsu K, Benoist S *et al*. Seven hundred and forty-seven hepatectomies in the 1990s: an update to evaluate the actual risk of liver resection. *Journal of the American College of Surgeons* 2000; **191**: 38–46.

Bilchik AJ, Wood TF, Allegra D *et al*. Cryosurgical ablation and radiofrequency ablation for unresectable hepatic malignant neoplasms. *Archives of Surgery* 2000; **135**: 657–64.

Bilik R, Superina R. Transplantation for unresectable liver tumors in children. *Transplant Proceedings* 1997; **29**: 2834–5.

Bismuth H, Castaing D, Garden OJ. Major hepatic resection under total vascular exclusion. *Annals of Surgery* 1989; **210**: 13–19.

Black CT, Cangir A, Choroszy M *et al*. Marked response to preoperative high-dose cisplatinum in children with unresectable hepatoblastoma. *Journal of Pediatric Surgery* 1991a; **26**: 1070–3.

Black CT, Luck SR, Musemeche CA *et al*. Aggressive excision of pulmonary metastases is warranted in the management of childhood hepatic tumors. *Journal of Pediatric Surgery* 1991b; **26**: 1082–6.

Boechat MI, Kangarloo H, Ortega J *et al*. Primary liver tumors in children: comparison of CT and MRI imaging. *Radiology* 1988; **169**: 727–32.

Broughan TA, Esquivel CO, Vogt DP *et al*. Pretransplant chemotherapy in pediatric hepatocellular carcinoma. *Journal of Pediatric Surgery* 1994; **29**: 1319–22.

Brown J, Perilongo G, Shafford E *et al*. Pretreatment prognostic factors for children with hepatoblastoma – results from the International Society of Paediatric Oncology (SIOP) Study SIOPEL-1. *European Journal of Cancer* 2000; **36**: 1418–25.

Bulterys M, Goodman MT, Smith MA *et al*. Hepatic tumors. In: Reis LAG, Smith MA, Gurney JG *et al*. (eds) *Cancer incidence and survival among children and adolescents: United States SEER Program, 1975–1995*. Bethesda, MD: National Cancer Institute SEER Program, 1999: 91–7.

Champion J, Greene AA, Pratt CB. Cisplatin (DDP): An effective therapy for unresectable or recurrent hepatoblastoma. *Journal of the American Society of Clinical Oncology* 1982; **671**: 173.

Chang MH, Chen CJ, Lai MS *et al*. Universal hepatitis B vaccination in Taiwan and the incidence of hepatocellular carcinoma in children. Taiwan Childhood Hepatoma Study Group. *New England Journal of Medicine* 1997; **336**: 1855–9.

Chapman WC, Debelak JP, Blackwell TS *et al*. Hepatic cryoablation-induced acute lung injury. Pulmonary hemodynamic and permeability effects in a sheep model. *Archives of Surgery* 2000; **135**: 667–73.

Cooper IS. Cryogenic surgery. *New England Journal of Medicine* 1963; **268**: 743–9.

Couinaud CLF. *Études anatomiques et chirugicales*. Paris: Mason & Cie, 1957.

Craig JR, Peters RL, Edmondson HA *et al*. Fibrolamellar carcinoma of the liver: a tumor of adolescents and young adults with distinctive clinicopathologic features. *Cancer* 1980; **46**: 372–9.

Curley SA, Newman RA, Dougherty TM *et al*. Complete hepatic venous isolation and extracorporeal chemofiltration as treatment for human hepatocellular carcinoma: a phase I study. *Annals of Surgical Oncology* 1994; **1**: 389–99.

Curley SA, Izzo F, Delrio P *et al*. Radiofrequency ablation of unresectable primary and recurrent hepatic malignancies. *Annals of Surgery* 1999; **230**: 1–8.

DeBaun MR, Tucker MA. Risk of cancer during the first four years of life in children from the Beckwith–Weidemann Syndrome Registry. *Journal of Pediatrics* 1998; **132**: 398–400.

Ebara M, Kita K, Sugiura N *et al*. Therapeutic effect of percutaneous ethanol injection on small hepatocellular carcinoma: evaluation with CT. *Radiology* 1995; **195**: 371–7.

Ehrlich PF, Greenberg ML, Filler RM. Improved long-term survival with preoperative chemotherapy for hepatoblastoma. *Journal of Pediatric Surgery* 1997; **32**: 999–1003.

Emre S, Schwartz ME, Katz E *et al*. Liver resection under total vascular isolation: variations on a theme. *Annals of Surgery* 1993; **217**: 15–19.

Exelby PR, Filler RM, Grosfeld JL. Liver tumors in children in the particular reference to hepatoblastoma and hepatocellular carcinoma: American Academy of Pediatrics Surgical Section Survey – 1974. *Journal of Pediatric Surgery* 1975; **10**: 329–37.

Feusner J, Buckley JD, Robison L *et al*. Prematurity and hepatoblastoma: more than just an association? *Journal of Pediatrics* 1998; **133**: 585–6.

Feusner JH, Krailo MD, Haas JE *et al*. Treatment of pulmonary metastases of initial stage I hepatoblastoma in childhood. *Cancer* 1993; **71**: 859–64.

Filler RM, Ehrlich PF, Greenberg ML *et al*. Preoperative chemotherapy in hepatoblastoma. *Surgery* 1991; **110**: 591–7.

Garber JE, Li FP, Kingston JE *et al*. Hepatoblastoma and familial adenomatous polyposis. *Journal of the National Cancer Institute* 1988; **80**: 1626–8.

Giardiello FM, Offerhaus GJA, Krush AJ *et al*. Risk of

hepatoblastoma in familial adenomatous polyposis. *Journal of Pediatrics* 1991; **119**: 766–8.

Gruner BA, DeNapoli TS, Andrews W *et al*. Hepatocellular carcinoma in children associated with Gardner syndrome or familial adenomatous polyposis. *Journal of Pediatric Hematology and Oncology* 1998; **20**: 274–8.

Haas JE, Muczynski KA, Krailo M *et al*. Histopathology and prognosis in childhood hepatoblastoma and hepatocarcinoma. *Cancer* 1989; **64**: 1082–95.

Han YM, Park HH, Lee JM *et al*. Effectiveness of preoperative transarterial chemoembolization in presumed inoperable hepatoblastoma. *Journal of Vascular and Interventional Radiology* 1999; **10**: 1275–80.

Horigome H, Nomura T, Saso K *et al*. Standards for selecting percutaneous ethanol injection therapy or percutaneous microwave coagulation therapy for solitary small hepatocellular carcinoma: consideration of local recurrence. *American Journal of Gastroenterology* 1999; **94**: 1914–17.

Hughes LJ, Michels VV. Risk of hepatoblastoma in familial adenomatous polyposis. *American Journal of Medical Genetics* 1992; **43**: 1023–5.

Huguet C, Nordlinger B, Bloch P *et al*. Tolerance of the human liver to prolonged normothermic ischemia. *Archives of Surgery* 1978; **113**: 1448–51.

Ikeda H, Matsuyama S, Tanimura M. Association between hepatoblastoma and very low birth weight: a trend or a chance? *Journal of Pediatrics* 1997; **130**: 557–60.

Izzo F, Cremona F, Delrio P *et al*. Soluble interleukin-2-receptor levels in hepatocellular cancer: a more sensitive marker than alfa-fetoprotein. *Annals of Surgical Oncology* 1999; **6**: 178–85.

King DR. Liver tumors. In: O'Neill JA, Rowe MI, Grosfeld JL *et al*. (eds) *Pediatric surgery*, 5th edn. St Louis, MO: Mosby, 1998: 421–30.

King DR, Ortega J, Campbell J *et al*. The surgical management of children with incompletely resected hepatic cancer is facilitated by intensive chemotherapy. *Journal of Pediatric Surgery* 1991; **26**: 1074–81.

Klintmalm GB. Liver transplantation for hepatocellular carcinoma: a registry report of the impact of tumor characteristics on outcome. *Annals of Surgery* 1998; **228**: 479–90.

Koneru B, Flye MW, Busuttil R *et al*. Liver transplantation for hepatoblastoma. The American experience. *Annals of Surgery* 1991; **213**: 118–21.

Kwee HG. Fibrolamellar hepatocellular carcinoma. *Alpha-fetoprotein* 1989; **40**: 175–7.

Lencioni R, Bartolozzi C, Caramella D *et al*. Treatment of small hepatocellular carcinoma with percutaneous ethanol injection: analysis of prognostic factors in 105 western patients. *Cancer* 1995; **75**: 1737–46.

Libutti SK, Bartlett DL, Fraker DL *et al*. Technique and results of hyperthermic isolated hepatic perfusion with tumor necrosis factor and melphalan for the treatment of unresectable hepatic malignancies. *Journal of the American College of Surgeons* 2000; **191**: 519–30.

Lin TY. Results in 107 hepatic lobectomies with a preliminary report on the use of a clamp to reduce blood loss. *Annals of Surgery* 1973; **177**: 413–21.

Little MH, Thomson DB, Hayward NK *et al*. Loss of alleles on the short arm of chromosome 11 and a hepatoblastoma from a child with Beckwith–Weidemann syndrome. *Human Genetics* 1988; **79**: 186–9.

Livraghi T, Lazzaroni S, Meloni F *et al*. Intralesional ethanol in the treatment of unresectable liver cancer. *World Journal of Surgery* 1995; **19**: 801–6.

Livraghi T, Goldberg SN, Monti F *et al*. Saline-enhanced radiofrequency tissue ablation of liver metastases. *Radiology* 1997; **202**: 205–10.

Lockwood L, Heney D, Giles GR *et al*. Cisplatin-resistant metastatic hepatoblastoma: complete response to carboplatin, etoposide and liver transplantation. *Medical Pediatric Oncology* 1993; **21**: 517–20.

McCarty TM, Kuhn JA. Cryotherapy for liver tumors. *Oncology* 1998; **12**: 979–87.

MacKinlay GA, Pritchard J. A common language for childhood liver tumors. *Pediatric Surgery International* 1992; **7**: 325–6.

Malassagne B, Cherqui D, Alon R *et al*. Safety of selective vascular clamping for major hepatectomies. *Journal of the American College of Surgeons* 1998; **187**: 482–7.

Malogolowkin MH, Stanley P, Steele DA *et al*. Feasibility and toxicity of chemoembolization for children with liver tumors. *Journal of Clinical Oncology* 2000; **18**: 1279–84.

Melendez J, Ferri E, Zwillman M *et al*. Extended hepatic resection: a 6-year retrospective study of risk factors for perioperative mortality. *Journal of the American College of Surgeons* 2001; **192**: 47–53.

Michels NA. Newer anatomy of the liver and its variant blood supply and collateral circulation. *American Journal of Surgery* 1966; **112**: 337–47.

Montagna M, Menin C, Chieco-Bianchi L *et al*. Occasional loss of constitute heterozygosity at 11p15.5 and imprinting relaxation of the IGFII maternal allele in hepatoblastoma. *Journal of Cancer Research and Clinical Oncology* 1994; **120**: 732–6.

Murakami R, Yoshimatsu S, Yamashita Y *et al*. Treatment of hepatocellular carcinoma: value of percutaneous microwave coagulation. *American Journal of Roentgenology* 1995; **164**: 1159–64.

Nagata Y, Hiraoka M, Nishimura Y *et al*. Clinical results of radiofrequency hyperthermia for malignant liver tumors. *International Journal of Radiation Oncology, Biology, Physics* 1997; **38**: 359–65.

Oda H, Imai Y, Nakatsura Y *et al*. Somatic mutations of the APC gene in sporadic hepatoblastomas. *Cancer Research* 1996; **56**: 3320–3.

Oldhafer KJ, Lang H, Frerker M *et al*. First experience and technical aspects of isolated liver perfusion for extensive liver metastasis. *Surgery* 1998; **123**: 622–31.

Ortega JA, Douglass EC, Feusner JH *et al*. Randomized comparison of cisplatin/vincristine/fluorouracil and cisplatin/continuous-infusion doxorubicin for treatment of pediatric hepatoblastoma: a report from the Children's Cancer Group and the Pediatric Oncology Group. *Journal of Clinical Oncology* 2000; **18**: 2665–75.

Otte JB, Aronson D, Vraux H *et al.* Preoperative chemotherapy, major liver resection, and transplantation for primary malignancies in children. *Transplant Proceedings* 1996; **28**: 2393–4.

Oue T, Fukuzawa M, Kusafuka T *et al.* Transcatheter arterial chemoembolization in the treatment of hepatoblastoma. *Journal of Pediatric Surgery* 1998; **33**: 1771–5.

Partensky C, Sassolas G, Henry L *et al.* Intra-arterial iodine-131-labeled lipiodol as adjuvant therapy after curative liver resection for hepatocellular carcinoma. *Archives of Surgery* 2000; **135**: 1298–300.

Passmore SJ, Noblett HR, Wisehart JD *et al.* Prolonged survival following multiple thoracotomies for metastatic hepatoblastoma. *Medical and Pediatric Oncology* 1995; **24**: 58–60.

Paye F, Jagot P, Vilgrain V *et al.* Preoperative chemo-embolization of hepatocellular carcinoma. *Archives of Surgery* 1998; **133**: 767–72.

Pelletier G, Roche A, Ink O *et al.* A randomized trial of hepatic arterial chemoembolization in patients with unresectable hepatocellular carcinoma. *Journal of Hepatology* 1990; **11**: 181–4.

Perilongo G, Shafford EA. Liver tumors. *European Journal of Cancer* 1999; **35**: 953–9.

Pringle JH. Notes on the arrest of hepatic hemorrhage due to trauma. *Annals of Surgery* 1908; **48**: 541.

Pritchard J, Plaschkes J, Shafford EA *et al.* SIOPEL 1. The first hepatoblastoma (HB) and hepatocellular carcinoma (HCC) study. Preliminary results. *Medical and Pediatric Oncology* 1992; **20**: 389.

Quinn JJ, Altman AJ, Robinson HT *et al.* Adriamycin and cisplatin for hepatoblastoma. *Cancer* 1985; **56**: 1926–9.

Reyes JD, Carr B, Dvorchik I *et al.* Liver transplantation and chemotherapy for hepatoblastoma and hepatocellular cancer in childhood and adolescence. *Journal of Pediatrics* 2000; **136**: 795–804.

Reynolds M, Douglass EC, Finegold M *et al.* Chemotherapy can convert unresectable hepatoblastoma. *Journal of Pediatric Surgery* 1992; **27**: 1080–4.

Robertson PL, Muraszko KM, Axtell RA. Hepatoblastoma metastatic to brain: prolonged survival after multiple surgical resection of a solitary brain lesion. *Journal of Pediatric Hematology/Oncology* 1997; **19**: 168–71.

Rose AT, Rose M, Pinson CW *et al.* Hepatocellular carcinoma outcomes based on indicated treatment strategy. *American Surgeon* 1998; **64**: 1128–34.

Sangro B, Herráiz M, Martínez-González MA *et al.* Prognosis of hepatocellular carcinoma in relation to treatment: a multivariate analysis of 178 patients from a single European institution. *Surgery* 1998; **124**: 575–83.

Schwemmle K, Link KH, Rieck B. Rationale and indications for perfusion in liver tumors: current data. *World Journal of Surgery* 1987; **11**: 534–40.

Seifert JK, Finlay I, Armstrong N *et al.* Thrombocytopenia and cytokine release following hepatic cryosurgery (abstract). *Australian and New Zealand Journal of Surgery* 1998; **68**: 52.

Seo T, Ando H, Watanabe Y *et al.* Treatment of hepatoblastoma: less extensive hepatectomy after effective preoperative chemotherapy with cisplatin and Adriamycin. *Surgery* 1998; **123**: 407–14.

Shiina S, Tagawa K, Niwa Y *et al.* Percutaneous ethanol injection therapy for hepatocellular carcinoma: results in 146 patients. *American Journal of Roentgenology* 1993; **160**: 1023–8.

Solbiati L, Ierace T, Goldberg SN *et al.* Percutaneous US-guided radiofrequency tissue ablation of liver metastases: treatment and follow-up in 16 patients. *Radiology* 1997; **202**: 195–203.

Soreide O, Czerniak A, Bradpiece H *et al.* Characteristics of fibrolamellar hepatocellular carcinoma: a study of nine cases and a review of the literature. *American Journal of Surgery* 1986; **151**: 518–23.

Stefanini GF, Amorati P, Biselle M *et al.* Efficacy of transarterial targeted treatments on survival of patients with hepatocellular carcinoma: an Italian experience. *Cancer* 1995; **75**: 2427–34.

Stocker JT. Hepatoblastoma. *Seminars in Diagnostic Pathology* 1994; **11**: 136–43.

Storm FK, Longmire NP Jr. A simplified clamp for hepatic resection. *Surgery, Gynecology and Obstetrics* 1971; **133**: 103–4.

Strasberg SM. Terminology of liver anatomy and liver resection: coming to grips with hepatic babel. *Journal of the American College of Surgeons* 1997; **184**: 413–34.

Superina R, Bilik R. Results of liver transplantation in children with unresectable liver tumors. *Journal of Pediatric Surgery* 1996; **31**: 835–9.

Suzuki T, Nakayasu A, Kawabe K *et al.* Surgical significance of anatomic variations of the hepatic artery. *American Journal of Surgery* 1971; **122**: 505–12.

Tagge EP, Tagge Du, Reyes J *et al.* Resection, including transplantation, for hepatoblastoma and hepatocellular carcinoma: impact on survival. *Journal of Pediatric Surgery* 1992; **27**: 292–7.

Teitelbaum DH, Tuttle S, Carey LC *et al.* Fibrolamellar carcinoma of the liver. Review of three cases and the presentation of a characteristic set of tumor markers defining this tumor. *Annals of Surgery* 1985; **202**: 36–41.

Tian JH, Xu BX, Zhang JM *et al.* Ultrasound-guided internal radiotherapy, using yttrium-90-glass microspheres for liver malignancies. *Journal of Nuclear Medicine* 1996; **37**: 958–63.

Van Tornout JM, Buckley JD, Quinn JJ *et al.* Timing and magnitude of decline in alpha-fetoprotein levels in treated children with unresectable or metastatic hepatoblastoma are predictors of outcome: a report from the Children's Cancer Group. *Journal of Clinical Oncology* 1997; **15**: 1190–7.

von Schweinitz D, Burger D, Mildenberger H. Is laparotomy

the first step in treatment of childhood liver tumors? The experience from the German Cooperative Pediatric Liver Tumor Study HB-89. *European Journal of Pediatric Surgery* 1994; **4**: 82–6.

von Schweinitz D, Hecker H, Harms D *et al.* Complete resection before development of drug resistance is essential for survival from advanced hepatoblastoma – a report from the German Cooperative Pediatric Liver Tumor Study HB-89. *Journal of Pediatric Surgery* 1995; **30**: 845–52.

Weber SM, Lee FT Jr, Chinn DO *et al.* Perivascular and intralesional tissue necrosis after hepatic cryoablation: results in a porcine model. *Surgery* 1997; **122**: 742–7.

Weinblatt ME, Siegel SE, Siegel MM *et al.* Preoperative chemotherapy for unresectable primary hepatic malignancies in children. *Cancer* 1982; **50**: 1061–4.

Wood TF, Rose M, Chung M *et al.* Radiofrequency ablation of 231 unresectable hepatic tumors: indications, limitations and complications. *Annals of Surgical Oncology* 2000; **7**: 593–600.

Yamanaka N, Tanaka T, Oriyama T *et al.* Microwave coagulonecrotic therapy for hepatocellular carcioma. *World Journal of Surgery* 1996; **20**: 1076–81.

Yandza T, Alvarez F, Laurent J *et al.* Pediatric liver transplantation for primary hepatocellular carcinoma associated with hepatitis virus infection. *Transplant International* 1993; **6**: 95–8.

Yokomori K, Hori T, Asoh S *et al.* Complete disappearance of unresectable hepatoblastoma by continuous infusion therapy through hepatic artery. *Journal of Pediatric Surgery* 1991; **26**: 844–6.

Zhou X, Tang Z, Yu Y. Ablative approach for primary liver cancer. In: Cady B, Ravikumar T (eds) *Surgical oncology clinics of North America*. Philadelphia, PA: WB Saunders, 1996: 379–90.

Other malignant tumors

MARK D STRINGER

The spectrum of childhood liver tumors is quite different to that seen in adults (Stringer, 2000). Hepatoblastoma and hepatocellular carcinoma are by far the commonest malignant liver tumors in childhood, and both are epithelial in origin (see Chapter 18). A variety of other malignant liver tumors have been reported, but all of them are rare (Box 19.1).

Box 19.1 *Malignant tumors of the liver and bile ducts in children*

Malignant liver tumors
Hepatoblastoma
Hepatocellular carcinoma (and fibrolamellar variant)

Undifferentiated embryonal sarcoma
Angiosarcoma
Malignant epithelioid hemangioendothelioma
Rhabdomyosarcoma
Rhabdoid tumor
Liposarcoma
Fibrosarcoma

Malignant germ cell tumor
Non-Hodgkin's lymphoma

Metastases: neuroblastoma, Wilms' tumor, rhabdomyosarcoma, germ cell tumor, lymphoma, leukemia, Langerhans' cell histiocytosis, choriocarcinoma, pancreatoblastoma, carcinoid

Malignant biliary tumors
Rhabdomyosarcoma
Adenocarcinoma
Cholangiocarcinoma

PRIMARY MALIGNANT MESENCHYMAL LIVER TUMORS

Several types of malignant mesenchymal liver tumors have been described (Babin-Boilletot *et al.*, 1993).

Undifferentiated (embryonal) sarcoma

This is the third commonest malignant liver tumor in children. Also classified as malignant mesenchymal sarcoma or mesenchymoma, this tumor usually occurs in children aged between 5 and 12 years, presenting with an abdominal mass or pain. Tumors are typically large, with a transverse diameter of 10–25 cm, and have areas of necrosis, hemorrhage and cystic change. They appear predominantly solid on ultrasound (US), but often have a striking cyst-like appearance on computed tomography (CT) and magnetic resonance imaging (MRI) (Buetow *et al.*, 1997). A pseudocapsule of compressed hepatic parenchyma renders the lesion well circumscribed. Pulmonary metastases and direct tumor extension to the right side of the heart have been noted in advanced cases. The serum alpha-fetoprotein (AFP) concentration is normal.

Definitive diagnosis is usually made by laparotomy and biopsy, but there are a few reports of percutaneous fine-needle aspiration cytology yielding sufficient material for diagnosis (Pollono and Drut, 1998). Histologically, the tumor is composed of spindle- and stellate-shaped sarcomatous cells within a myxoid stroma. A consistent immunohistochemical marker is the mesenchymal filament vimentin.

Treatment is by a combination of chemotherapy and

complete resection whenever possible (Leuschner *et al.*, 1990). Biopsy followed by pre- and postoperative chemotherapy and complete resection offers the best chance of cure. Until recently, local recurrence was common and the prognosis was poor (Smithson *et al.*, 1982; Babin-Boilletot *et al.*, 1993). However, better chemotherapy regimens are beginning to improve long-term survival. Webber *et al.* (1999) reported four out of seven disease-free survivors after tumor resection and adjuvant chemotherapy. Children with unresectable disease confined to the liver should be considered for orthotopic liver transplantation (Dower *et al.*, 2000).

There have been several reports of undifferentiated sarcoma arising within a mesenchymal hamartoma in older children, and therefore the latter should be treated by complete excision (Corbally and Spitz, 1992; De Chadarevian *et al.*, 1994; Lauwers *et al.*, 1997; Ramanujam *et al.*, 1999) (see Chapter 17).

Angiosarcoma

Hepatic angiosarcomas are exceedingly rare even in pediatric hepatobiliary units (Awan *et al.*, 1996). In children, girls are more commonly affected (Selby *et al.*, 1992). Environmental carcinogens such as arsenic and vinyl chloride are potentially important etiological factors in adults, but only one such example has been reported in a child (Falk *et al.*, 1981).

The commonest presentation is with a rapidly growing liver mass in a child aged 3 to 5 years; bilobar disease and metastases occur early. Less commonly, angiosarcoma develops several years later in a child with a history of infantile hepatic hemangioendothelioma (see Chapter 15 and also Figure 19.1 and Plates 9 and 10) (Kirchner *et al.*, 1981), indicating the importance of careful follow-up

of such cases throughout childhood. Ultrasonography demonstrates an echogenic mass with increased vascularity, and CT shows a hypodense lesion with pathological arterialization on enhanced studies. Despite rapid growth suggesting a malignant liver tumor, unless there is evidence of gross venous invasion or metastatic disease, there may be no clear features on cross-sectional imaging to distinguish clearly between a benign hepatic vascular tumor and a malignant lesion (Awan *et al.*, 1996).

Histological features of malignancy include infiltration with hypercellular whorls of spindle-shaped cells with lymphatic and vascular invasion. Cells have an increased nuclear-to-cytoplasmic ratio, and they stain positive for factor-VIII-related antigen. However, histology can be misleading by indicating a benign lesion, and a high index of clinical suspicion is needed (Awan *et al.*, 1996). Adequate biopsies usually require laparotomy.

The prognosis of hepatic angiosarcoma is generally poor. A few survivors have been reported after resection and chemotherapy (Kirchner *et al.*, 1981; Gunawardena *et al.*, 1997), but radiotherapy has not achieved effective tumor control. There is one report of a child who was treated by orthotopic liver transplantation; she died 4 months later as a result of cytomegalovirus infection, but autopsy showed no evidence of residual disease (Awan *et al.*, 1996). No long-term survivors have been reported after hepatic transplantation for angiosarcoma in adults.

Rhabdomyosarcoma

Although some of these tumors arise within the liver or at the hilum, most of them are found in the extrahepatic biliary tree (Ruymann *et al.*, 1985; Horowitz *et al.*, 1987;

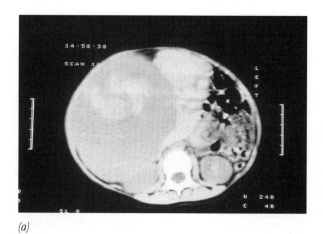

(a)

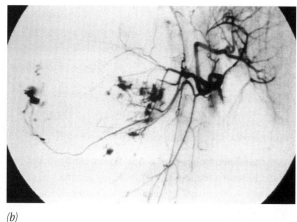

(b)

Figure 19.1 *This patient first presented at 6 months of age with a diffuse hepatic hemangioma which regressed after treatment with steroids. At 3 years of age she presented again with abdominal distension and a 20-cm-diameter mass in the left lobe, which was resected and confirmed to be a hemangioendothelioma. (a) At 4 years of age she developed a large right-sided vascular liver tumor as shown on this CT scan. (b) Arteriography demonstrated a highly abnormal tumor circulation. (Reproduced courtesy of ER Howard.)*

Mann *et al.*, 1990). These tumors are therefore discussed in more detail in Chapter 14.

Preschool children are predominantly affected, and presentation is typically with obstructive jaundice, abdominal pain, vomiting and fever. The tumor may be misdiagnosed as a choledochal cyst unless the solid content of the biliary tree is recognized on ultrasound scan or CT (Spunt *et al.*, 2000). Histologically, they are embryonal or botryoid sarcomas which are locally invasive. Approximately 20% of children have metastases at presentation (Spunt *et al.*, 2000).

Surgical excision (assisted by intraoperative cholangiography and frozen-section histology), multiagent chemotherapy and, in some cases, radiotherapy have resulted in significantly improved survival (Oelsnitz *et al.*, 1991). The Intergroup Rhabdomyosarcoma Study Group has reported their experience of 25 patients with biliary rhabdomyosarcoma treated by chemotherapy and surgery (Spunt *et al.*, 2000). They concluded first that surgical exploration is required in order to identify regional non-nodal metastases accurately, second that surgery should be used principally to determine histological diagnosis and extent of disease, and finally that, if possible, endoscopic stent placement should be used to achieve biliary drainage. The estimated 5-year survival rate was 66% overall, and was better in children without distant metastases at diagnosis.

RHABDOID TUMORS

Despite the histological resemblance to tumor cells of muscle origin implied by the term 'rhabdoid', there is no actual evidence to support such a derivation for this tumor (Scheimberg *et al.*, 1996). Indeed, malignant rhabdoid tumors may in fact have an epithelial origin. They were originally described in 1978 as a distinctive highly malignant variant of Wilms' tumor in infants (Beckwith and Palmer, 1978). Extrarenal malignant rhabdoid tumors have been described at various sites, including the central nervous system, liver, pelvis and chest. Most rhabdoid tumors occur either in infancy or in early childhood and they generally have a dismal prognosis (Gururangan *et al.*, 1993). A primary hepatic tumor with rhabdoid features was first reported by Gonzalez-Crussi *et al.* in 1982, but fewer than 20 cases had been reported up to 1998 (Kelly *et al.*, 1998). The diagnostic pathological features include the following:

- sheets of large polygonal cells with vesicular nuclei, central prominent nucleoli and abundant eosinophilic cytoplasm;
- immunohistochemical expression of vimentin and epithelial markers;
- ultrastructural demonstration of cytoplasmic inclusions composed of whorled intermediate filaments.

Primary hepatic malignant rhabdoid tumors typically present as an abdominal mass, but there are two case reports of spontaneous tumor rupture and bleeding (Kelly *et al.*, 1998; Ravindra *et al.*, in press) (Figure 19.2). Tumor rupture has also been described as the presenting feature of other malignant liver tumors, including hepatocellular carcinoma, hepatoblastoma (Stringer *et al.*, 1995) and undifferentiated sarcoma (Weinberg and Finegold, 1983).

Malignant rhabdoid liver tumors are usually associated with a normal AFP concentration, but serum lactate dehydrogenase levels may be elevated. The tumor has been associated with the secretion of parathormone-like substances causing hypercalcemia, and with vasointestinal-peptide-induced watery diarrhea (Weyman *et al.*, 1993; Jiminez-Heffernan *et al.*, 1998). There are no specific diagnostic features on imaging (Di Cori *et al.*,

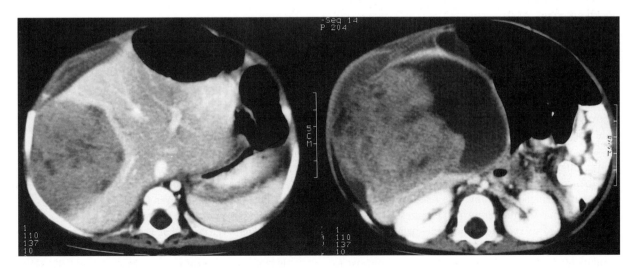

Figure 19.2 *Preoperative CT scan images of a large ruptured right lobe malignant rhabdoid liver tumor in a 13-month-old girl.*

1993). Percutaneous or open-needle biopsy has been used in diagnosis, but small samples may lead to confusion with hepatoblastoma or undifferentiated sarcoma (Scheimberg et al., 1996).

The prognosis for malignant rhabdoid tumors has been extremely poor despite surgery and chemotherapy. With one exception (Ravindra et al., in press), published survival periods have ranged from 5 days to 5 months (Scheimberg et al., 1996; Kelly et al., 1998). Gururangan et al. (1993) recommended adjuvant chemotherapy with ifosfamide either alone or in combination with carboplatin and etoposide. Our long-term survivor received ifosfamide, vincristine and actinomycin D.

Other malignant mesenchymal liver tumors in children include *liposarcoma* (Soares et al., 1989) and *leiomyosarcoma* (arising from the ligamentum teres in one case) (Weinberg and Finegold, 1983).

Key references

Awan S, Davenport M, Portmann B, Howard ER. Angiosarcoma of the liver in children. *Journal of Pediatric Surgery* 1996; **31**: 1729–32.

The largest single-center experience of angiosarcoma, consisting of four cases seen during a 20-year period at King's College Hospital, London.

Webber EM, Morrison KB, Pritchard SL, Sorensen PH. Undifferentiated embryonal sarcoma of the liver: results of clinical management in one center. *Journal of Pediatric Surgery* 1999; **34**: 1641–4.

A 15-year experience of seven children with undifferentiated embryonal sarcomas from Canada. Improved results were achieved with resection and chemotherapy.

PRIMARY MALIGNANT GERM CELL TUMORS

These tumors can arise within the liver (Hart, 1975; Mann et al., 1989, 1990) or falciform ligament (Atkinson et al., 1992). Serum AFP levels are elevated, but the protein has a different glycosylation pattern to that of liver-derived AFP (Tsuchida et al., 1997). Chemotherapy is the mainstay of treatment for extracranial nongonadal malignant germ cell tumors. Carboplatin, etoposide and bleomycin are effective and less toxic than older regimens. Surgery has a role in the treatment of well-defined tumors that can be removed without major risk.

Non-Hodgkin's lymphoma has also been described as affecting the liver as the primary site in children (Miller et al., 1983). Lymphoproliferative disease in the transplanted liver may also occur, and the imaging appearances may be similar to those seen with metastases (Pickhardt et al., 2000).

METASTATIC TUMORS

Neuroblastoma may present with massive hepatomegaly, caval compression and respiratory compromise as part of stage IV-S disease in infants (Evans et al., 1980). These infants may require surgical decompression of the abdomen with a prosthetic patch, judicious chemotherapy or even radiotherapy. The reason why infantile neuroblastoma so frequently metastasizes to the liver may be related to specific tumor-cell-surface glycoproteins preferentially adhering to extracellular matrix proteins in the liver (Kuwashima, 1997). In contrast to stage IV-S disease in infants, which generally has a good

prognosis, liver metastases in stage IV neuroblastoma are a poor prognostic factor. Surgical resection may be valuable for isolated liver metastases from Wilms' tumor.

REFERENCES

Atkinson JB, Foster CE, Lally KP, Isaacs H, Siegel SE. Primary endodermal sinus (yolk sac) tumor of the falciform ligament. *Journal of Pediatric Surgery* 1992; **27**: 105–7.

Awan S, Davenport M, Portmann B, Howard ER. Angiosarcoma of the liver in children. *Journal of Pediatric Surgery* 1996; **31**: 1729–32.

Babin-Boilletot A, Flamant F, Terrier-Lacombe MJ et al. Primitive malignant non-epithelial hepatic tumors in children. *Medical and Pediatric Oncology* 1993; **21**: 634–9.

Beckwith JB, Palmer NF. Histopathology and prognosis of Wilms' tumor: results from the first national Wilms' Tumor Study. *Cancer* 1978; **41**: 1937–48.

Buetow PC, Buck JL, Pantongrag-Brown L et al. Undifferentiated (embryonal) sarcoma of the liver: pathologic basis of imaging findings in 28 cases. *Radiology* 1997; **203**: 779–83.

Corbally MT, Spitz L. Malignant potential of mesenchymal hamartoma: an unrecognized risk. *Pediatric Surgery International* 1992; **7**: 321–2.

De Chadarevian JP, Pawel BR, Faerber EN, Weintraub WH. Undifferentiated (embryonal) sarcoma arising in conjunction with mesenchymal hamartoma of the liver. *Modern Pathology* 1994; **7**: 490–3.

Di Cori S, Oudjhane K, Neilson K. Primary malignant rhabdoid tumor of the liver. *Canadian Association of Radiologists Journal* 1993; **44**: 52–4.

Dower NA, Smith LJ, Lees G et al. Experience with aggressive therapy in three children with unresectable malignant liver tumors. *Medical and Pediatric Oncology* 2000; **34**: 132–5.

Evans AE, Chatten Y, D'Angio GJ et al. Review of 17 IVS neuroblastoma patients at the Children's Hospital of Philadelphia. *Cancer* 1980; **45**: 833–9.

Falk H, Herbert JT, Edmonds L et al. Review of four cases of childhood hepatic angiosarcoma – elevated environmental arsenic exposure in one case. *Cancer* 1981; **47**: 382–91.

Gonzalez-Crussi F, Goldschmidt RA, Hsueh W, Trujillo YP. Infantile sarcoma with intracytoplasmic filamentous inclusions. Distinctive tumor of possible histiocytic origin. *Cancer* 1982; **49**: 2365–75.

Gunawardena SW, Trautwein LM, Finegold MJ, Ogden AK. Hepatic angiosarcoma in a child: successful therapy with surgery and adjuvant chemotherapy. *Medical and Pediatric Oncology* 1997; **28**: 139–43.

Gururangan S, Bowman LC, Parham DM et al. Primitive extracranial rhabdoid tumors. Clinicopathologic features and response to ifosfamide. *Cancer* 1993; **71**: 2653–9.

Hart WR. Primary endodermal sinus (yolk sac) tumor of the liver. *Cancer* 1975; **35**: 1453–4.

Horowitz ME, Etcubanas E, Webber BL et al. Hepatic undifferentiated (embryonal) sarcoma and rhabdomyosarcoma in children. *Cancer* 1987; **59**: 396–402.

Jiminez-Heffernan JA, Lopez-Ferrer O, Burgos E, Viguer JM. Pathological case of the month. Primary hepatic malignant tumor with rhabdoid features. *Archives of Pediatrics and Adolescent Medicine* 1998; **152**: 509–10.

Kelly DM, Jones M, Humphreys S, Howard ER. Spontaneous rupture of a malignant rhabdoid tumor of the liver. *Pediatric Surgery International* 1998; **14**: 111–12.

Kirchner SG, Heller RM, Kasselberg AG et al. Infantile hepatic hemangioendothelioma with subsequent malignant degeneration. *Pediatric Radiology* 1981; **11**: 42–5.

Kuwashima N. Organ-specific adhesion of neuroblastoma cells *in vitro*: correlation with their hepatic metastasis potential. *Journal of Pediatric Surgery* 1997; **32**: 546–51.

Lauwers GY, Grant LD, Donnelly WH et al. Hepatic undifferentiated (embryonal) sarcoma arising in a mesenchymal hamartoma. *American Journal of Surgical Pathology* 1997; **21**: 1248–54.

Leuschner I, Schmidt D, Harms D. Undifferentiated sarcoma of the liver in childhood: morphology, flow cytometry and literature review. *Human Pathology* 1990; **21**: 68–76.

Mann JR, Pearson D, Barrett A et al. Results of the United Kingdom Children's Cancer Study Group's malignant germ cell tumor studies. *Cancer* 1989; **59**: 396–402.

Mann JR, Kasthuri N, Raafat F et al. Malignant hepatic tumors in children: incidence, clinical features and etiology. *Paediatric and Perinatal Epidemiology* 1990; **4**: 276–89.

Miller S, Wollner N, Meyers PA et al. Primary hepatic or hepatosplenic non-Hodgkin's lymphoma in children. *Cancer* 1983; **52**: 2285–8.

Oelsnitz G, Spaar HJ, Lieber T, Munchow B, Booss D. Embryonal rhabdomyosarcoma of the common bile duct. *European Journal of Pediatric Surgery* 1991; **1**: 161–5.

Pickhardt PJ, Siegel MJ, Hayashi RJ, Kelly M. Post-transplantation lymphoproliferative disorder in children: clinical, histopathologic and imaging features. *Radiology* 2000; **217**: 16–25.

Pollono DG, Drut R. Undifferentiated (embryonal) sarcoma of the liver: fine-needle aspiration cytology and preoperative chemotherapy as an approach to diagnosis and initial treatment. A case report. *Diagnostic Cytopathology* 1998; **19**: 102–6.

Ramanujam TM, Ramesh JC, Goh DW et al. Malignant transformation of mesenchymal hamartoma of the liver: case report and review of the literature. *Journal of Pediatric Surgery* 1999; **34**: 1684–6.

Ravindra KV, Cullinane C, Lewis IJ, Squire BR, Stringer MD. Long-term survival after spontaneous rupture of a malignant rhabdoid tumor of the liver. *Journal of Pediatric Surgery* (in press).

Ruymann FB, Raney RB, Crist WM et al. Rhabdomyosarcoma of the biliary tree in childhood. *Cancer* 1985; **56**: 575–81.

Scheimberg I, Cullinane C, Kelsey A, Malone M. Primary hepatic malignant tumor with rhabdoid features. A histological, immunocytochemical and electron microscopic study of four cases and review of literature. *American Journal of Surgical Pathology* 1996; **20**: 1394–400.

Selby DM, Stocker JT, Ishak KG. Angiosarcoma of the liver in childhood. *Pediatric Pathology* 1992; **12**: 485–98.

Smithson WA, Telander RL, Carney JA. Mesenchymoma of the liver in childhood: 5 years survival after combined-modality treatment. *Journal of Pediatric Surgery* 1982; **17**: 70–2.

Soares FA, Magnani Landell GA, Peres LC et al. Liposarcoma of hepatic hilum in childhood: report of a case and review of the literature. *Medical and Pediatric Oncology* 1989; **17**: 239–43.

Spunt SL, Lobe TE, Pappo AS et al. Aggressive surgery is unwarranted for biliary tract rhabdomyosarcoma. *Journal of Pediatric Surgery* 2000; **35**: 309–16.

Stringer MD. Liver tumors. *Seminars in Pediatric Surgery* 2000; **9**: 196–208.

Stringer MD, Hennayake S, Howard ER et al. Improved outcome for children with hepatoblastoma. *British Journal of Surgery* 1995; **82**: 386–91.

Tsuchida Y, Terada M, Honna T et al. The role of subfractionation of alpha-fetoprotein in the treatment of pediatric surgical patients. *Journal of Pediatric Surgery* 1997; **32**: 514–17.

Webber EM, Morrison KB, Pritchard SL, Sorensen PH. Undifferentiated embryonal sarcoma of the liver: results of clinical management in one center. *Journal of Pediatric Surgery* 1999; **34**: 1641–4.

Weinberg AG, Finegold MJ. Primary hepatic tumors of childhood. *Human Pathology* 1983; **14**: 512–37.

Weyman C, Dolson L, Kedar A. Secretion of vasointestinal peptide by a primary liver tumor with rhabdoid features. *Journal of Surgical Oncology* 1993; **54**: 267–70.

PART 5

Portal hypertension

20

Etiology of portal hypertension and congenital anomalies of the portal venous system

EDWARD R HOWARD

EMBRYOLOGY (SEE ALSO CHAPTER 7)

The venous system of the body is formed after a series of very complex embryological events and from two main systems. The systemic veins develop from the intra-embryonic anterior and posterior cardinal veins, whilst the portal system develops from the extra-embryonic vitelline and umbilical veins which drain from the yolk sac and placenta (Dickson, 1957; Gray and Skandalakis, 1972).

The paired vitelline veins which arise on the anterior surface of the yolk sac run in a cephalad direction to empty into the primitive sinus venosus. By the end of the fourth week of gestation, three cross-communications form between these veins (Figure 20.1). The most cranial anastomosis forms the subhepatic plexus in the region of the porta hepatis, the middle communication passes dorsal to the gut and eventually lies in a retroduodenal position, whilst the lowest communication lies distal to the origin of the common bile duct, passing ventrally.

The portal vein is fashioned into its mature S-shape by the amalgamation of the inferior section of the left vitelline vein, the middle cross communication and the superior portion of the right vein. Minor changes in this embryological formation can result in major anatomical anomalies of the portal venous system. The origin of the inferior vena cava is also very complex, and is the end-

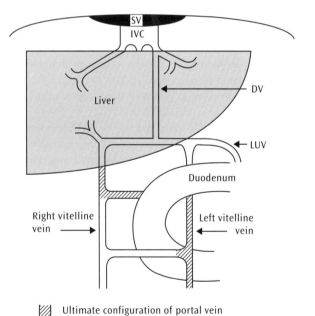

Ultimate configuration of portal vein

Figure 20.1 *Embryological development of the portal vein and relationship to the duodenum. DV, ductus venosus; IVC inferior vena cava; LUV, left umbilical vein; SV, sinus venosus. Reproduced from Joyce and Howard (1988) with the permission of the publisher.*

result of the anastomosis of several venous channels. Abnormalities in its formation may be associated with anomalies in the portal venous drainage. The common hepatic vein which gives rise to the hepatic segment of the inferior vena cava arises from the right end of the sinus venosus and the right portion of the venous plexus which joins the right and left vitelline veins in the cranial part of the liver (known as the subdiaphragmatic anastomosis).

Early in development, blood from the left umbilical vein passes through the subhepatic anastomosis and the ductus venosus to reach the retrohepatic portion of the inferior vena cava, which is known as the common hepatic vein in the embryo. The ductus venosus therefore forms a direct connection between the umbilical vein and the inferior vena cava, and provides a functional bypass through which a portion of the oxygenated umbilical blood from the placenta flows directly into the inferior vena cava (Meyer and Lind, 1966). Human fetal studies have demonstrated that the umbilical vein gives branches to the left segments of the liver, and that the opening of the ductus venosus lies opposite the junction of the umbilical vein with the left branch of the portal vein (see Chapter 2). Approximately 40–50% of umbilical blood passes through the ductus venosus, and the remainder flows through the liver sinusoids (Meyer and Lind, 1966).

Postnatal closure of the ductus venosus commences during the first day after birth but is not completed until days 15 to 20 of life. The mechanism of closure is not well understood. The wall of the ductus venosus contains only a small amount of smooth muscle and no muscular sphincter. It has been suggested that closure may be related to a decrease in portal venous pressure after cessation of umbilical vein flow (Meyer and Lind, 1966).

The portion of the vena cava below the liver is formed from extensions of both the common hepatic vein and the right subcardinal vein. The complicated origin of the inferior vena cava and its close relationship to the subdiaphragmatic anastomosis of the vitelline veins in the early embryo helps to explain the occurrence of congenital anomalies of portal venous drainage.

ANOMALIES OF PORTAL VENOUS ANATOMY

1   In the most common type of these rare anomalies, the portal vein lies in front of the duodenum, common bile duct and hepatic artery and has been described in association with biliary atresia (see Chapter 8), duodenal atresia and annular pancreas. This malformation may also be associated with malrotation of the bowel, situs inversus, polysplenia and anatomical abnormalities of the inferior vena cava, a constellation of defects that is well recognized in patients with biliary atresia (see Chapter 8).

Davenport *et al.* (1993) reported an incidence of 7.5% in 308 cases of atresia.

2   Cavernous transformation of the portal vein is the usual cause of extrahepatic portal hypertension in young children (Figure 20.2). Although some cases of portal vein obstruction are related to severe illness and umbilical catheterization in the neonatal period, many others (perhaps 60%) have no history of illness (Heaton *et al.*, 1990).

3   Duplication of the portal vein has been described. The superior and inferior mesenteric veins join to run through the transverse colon and then pass across the front of the pancreas to reach the quadrate lobe to the left of the gallbladder fossa (Marks, 1969).

4   Marks (1969) has reviewed portal venous communications with the pulmonary venous system. He described a triad which consisted of pulmonary portal venous communication, multiple intracardiac anomalies and partial situs inversus. The rarity of this abnormality is emphasized by his report of 18 patients with total anomalous pulmonary venous drainage, only three of whom had infradiaphragmatic drainage of the pulmonary veins. Only one of this group of three patients had pulmonary portal venous communications without associated cardiac defects.

5   A congenital anastomosis between the portal venous system and the inferior vena cava associated with atresia of the portal vein was first described by Abernethy in 1793. The report described the postmortem findings in a 10-month-old female who died of unknown causes. In addition to transposition of the great vessels and polysplenia, the portal vein joined the inferior vena cava at the level of the renal veins (Figure 20.3). At least 13 examples of this type of end-to-side, congenital, portosystemic anastomosis have now been recorded in females, but

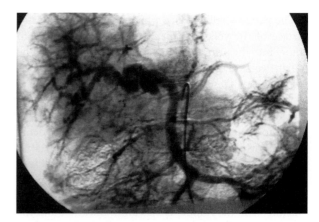

Figure 20.2 *Portal venous phase of a mesenteric angiogram in a 6-year-old girl who presented with hematemesis. The superior mesenteric vein is patent, but the portal vein is replaced by a large, tortuous collateral.*

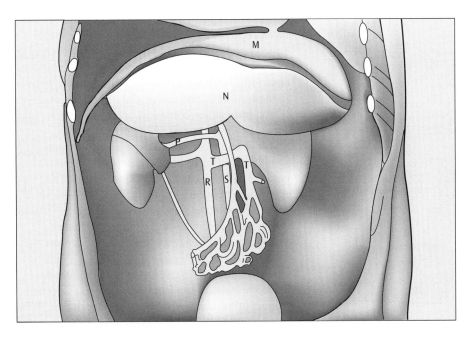

Figure 20.3 *Part of the original illustration of a congenital porto-caval shunt recorded by Abernethy in 1793. The portal vein (T) communicates directly with the inferior vena cava (R) just below the entrance of the right renal vein.*

only three cases have been recorded in boys (Kohda *et al.*, 1999). Details of the 12 female cases are shown in Table 20.1. Complications of this type of congenital shunt have included encephalopathy and a variety of liver tumors, including focal nodular hyperplasia, adenoma, hepatoblastoma and hepatoma. Howard and Davenport (1997) have suggested that a congenital end-to-side portosystemic shunt should be designated as a 'type 1' abnormality.

A second type of malformation represented by a side-to-side shunt has been described in two adult and four pediatric patients, all of whom were males. However, a 6-year-old girl has recently presented with signs of hypoxemia (Figure 20.4). Howard and

Davenport (1997) designated this as a 'type 2' abnormality, and believed it to represent a persistence of the ductus venosus. The type 2 shunt is amenable to surgical division and restoration of a normal intrahepatic flow of portal blood. This procedure was performed successfully in two children who had presented at 6 and 9 weeks of age, respectively. The extrahepatic portocaval communication in both cases was found between the right branch of the portal vein and the retrohepatic vena cava, and the livers were noted to be unusually pink due to abnormal arterialization. Temporary occlusion of the shunts was used to confirm that there was no significant rise in portal pressure before definitive shunt division. The increased intrahepatic

Table 20.1 *Congenital 'type 1' portocaval shunts: 12 reported cases of absent portal vein in female children*

Author (year)	Age	Other anomalies
Abernethy (1793)	10 months	Polysplenia, dextrocardia
Kiernan (1833)	13 years	—
Hellweg (1954)	5.5 years	Skin hemangiomata
Olling and Olsson (1974)	44 years	Encephalopathy
Marois *et al.* (1979)	4.5 years	Hepatoblastoma, VSD
Morse *et al.* (1986)	8 years	FNH, short digits, ASD
Joyce and Howard (1988)	10 years	Coarctation, hepatoma
Nakasaki *et al.* (1989)	14 years	Hepatic adenoma
Woodle *et al.* (1990)	9 years	BA, polysplenia
Matsuoka *et al.* (1992)	22 years	FNH
Morgan and Superina (1994)	14 months	BA, polysplenia, cardiac (multiple)
Morgan and Superina (1994)	1 year	BA, polysplenia, ASD

VSD, ventricular septal defect; ASD, atrial septal defect; FNH, focal nodular hyperplasia; BA, biliary atresia.

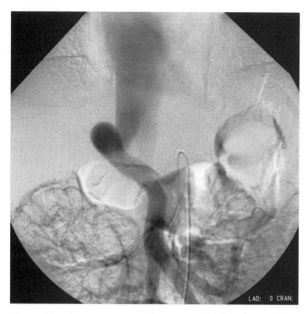

Figure 20.4 *A portovenogram in a 6-year-old girl who presented with signs of hypoxemia. The portal vein communicates with the inferior vena cava. Further imaging with ultrasound showed that this was a side-to-side shunt with a hypoplastic but patent intra-hepatic portal venous circulation. The hypoxemia was cured by surgical ligation of the shunt.*

portal flow after shunt closure was noted to cause enlargement of the livers, which also darkened in color.

The children were well at follow-up 3 and 2 years after surgery, respectively.

A familial incidence of 'type 2' shunts was reported in three young brothers who presented with encephalopathy. The symptoms and biochemical changes were successfully reversed in the two cases who underwent shunt closure (Uchino *et al.*, 1996). A second report of another family illustrated the long-term effects of these shunts in adulthood (Jacob *et al.*, 1999). Two out of three brothers, aged 36 and 43 years, respectively, showed evidence of mild encephalopathy, and one of them had renal stones. Two liver masses of focal nodular hyperplasia were detected in a third brother aged 40 years.

The complications recorded in these six male patients with side-to-side 'type 2' shunts are similar to those documented for 'type 1' shunts in Table 20.1.

Congenital portosystemic shunts may also be complicated by severe hypoxemia, known as hepatopulmonary syndrome (Kennedy *et al.*, 1977), which may be a result of the inability of the liver to metabolize vasodilator substances originating in the gut. Kamata *et al.* (2000) reported the complete disappearance of hypoxemia secondary to severe intrapulmonary shunting after surgical closure of a congenital 'type 2' shunt.

Congenital portosystemic shunts similar to those reported in humans are well recognized in several animals, including dogs, cats and cows. A progressive elevation of blood ammonia levels culminates in encephalopathy and coma. Urolithiasis is also found in these animals, and is secondary to increased rates of excretion of ammonia and urate (Rothuizen *et al.*, 1982; Hunt *et al.*, 1998).

In summary, congenital portosystemic shunts should be considered in the differential diagnosis of patients with unexplained encephalopathy. The association between shunts and liver tumors also suggests that a complete investigation of these lesions in younger patients should include a detailed assessment of the anatomy of the portal venous system. Surgical correction is possible for 'type 2' shunts, and it can reverse the signs of established hepatopulmonary syndrome and/or encephalopathy.

Liver tumors can be safely resected in patients with either type of shunt (Joyce and Howard, 1988), but severe encephalopathy or hypoxemia in 'type 1' lesions, in which the portal vein is absent, can only be relieved by liver transplantation (Orii *et al.*, 1997).

6   Portal vein drainage into the right atrium, the superior vena cava or the umbilical vein has been described by Poirier and Charpy (1903) (Figure 20.5).

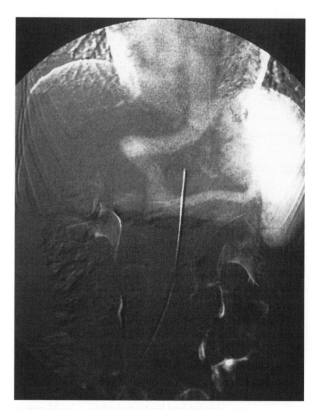

Figure 20.5 *Portovenogram in an 11-year-old boy who presented with recurrent signs of encephalopathy. The portal vein communicates directly with the heart (left atrium).*

7 Aneurysms of the portal venous system were thought to be extremely rare anomalies, but the widespread introduction of ultrasound examination has led to an increasing number of case reports (Atasoy et al., 1998; Ozbek et al., 1999).

Aneurysmal dilatation of the portal vein may be associated with portal hypertension, although the cause of this raised pressure is not clear from the published reports. Herman and Shafer (1965) reported the case of a 26-year-old woman who had been noted to have hepatosplenomegaly in childhood. Two further cases were reported by Thomas (1967), one of whom was a 13-year-old who had a sudden massive hematemesis while at school. A barium swallow examination showed esophageal varices which were treated with esophageal transection. Investigations later revealed an aneurysm of the portal vein which was saccular and thin-walled and situated approximately 3 cm away from the bifurcation of the portal vein. A side-to-side portocaval shunt was constructed using a synthetic graft. The patient did not appear to have cirrhosis, but the portal pressure was noted to be 45 cmH$_2$O before shunting.

Thomas (1967) suggested that the occurrence of portal vein aneurysms in children and the absence of obvious extrahepatic obstruction were indicative of a congenital etiology. Duodenal compression, common bile duct obstruction and acute portal hypertension from venous thrombosis are possible complications of these aneurysms, and Thomas's case (Thomas, 1967) suggests that portosystemic shunting may be a satisfactory method of management. Total excision and portal vein reconstruction would be a high-risk procedure.

PORTAL HYPERTENSION: CLASSIFICATION AND PRESENTATION

Whitington (1985) defined portal hypertension as a direct measurement of pressure in the portal system of over 11 mmHg or a splenic pulp pressure of over 16 mmHg. The etiology of portal hypertension may be simply classified as follows.

1 Cirrhotic (e.g. biliary atresia, cystic fibrosis).
2 Non-cirrhotic:
- prehepatic (e.g. portal vein thrombosis);
- intrahepatic:
  presinusoidal (e.g. portal vein sclerosis, congenital hepatic fibrosis);
  parasinusoidal (e.g. fatty liver, nodular regenerative hyperplasia);
  postsinusoidal (e.g. veno-occlusive disease);
- suprahepatic (e.g. Budd–Chiari syndrome);

- intrahepatic arteriovenous fistula:
  congenital;
  traumatic.

A clinical diagnosis of portal hypertension in children may be suspected after massive gastrointestinal hemorrhage, as esophageal varices are the commonest cause of severe hematemesis in childhood. A finding of a small liver and the absence of general signs of liver disease should lead to ultrasound examination of the portal vein for signs of portal vein obstruction. Occasionally the ultrasound scan may be misleading, as large collaterals can be misinterpreted as a normal portal vein. The demonstration of a large liver with signs of liver disease, such as jaundice, ascites and muscle wasting, should suggest intrahepatic portal hypertension.

EXTRAHEPATIC PORTAL VEIN OBSTRUCTION

Many affected patients have no obvious etiology for their portal vein obstruction, although a history of umbilical vein catheterization, abdominal sepsis, trauma or pancreatitis are all suggestive factors. More than half of the cases of cavernous transformation of the portal vein appear to be congenital in origin.

An analysis of the angiographic findings in 53 cases aged from 2 to 62 years suggested a relationship between etiology and the anatomical distribution of the portal venous occlusion (Stringer et al., 1994). The cases were classifiable into five main groups as follows.

1 Occlusion of the portal vein bifurcation and intrahepatic portal vein radicles alone (hepatoportal sclerosis). This group consisted of three children, none of whom had identifiable etiological factors.
2 Occlusion of the portal vein with or without intrahepatic branch occlusion. There were 25 patients in this group, and cavernous transformation of the portal vein was typical. Two of the patients had a history of intra-abdominal sepsis and hepatic abscess formation, and 13 cases were thought to be congenital in origin.
3 Occlusion of the portal and superior mesenteric veins. Of the 10 patients in this group, eight gave a history of umbilical vein catheterization or intra-abdominal problems. Two cases may have been congenital.
4 Total occlusion of all three segments of the portal venous system (portal, splenic and mesenteric) was observed in 15 patients (Figure 20.6). Five patients had been treated for hypercoagulable states, and three had concomitant hepatic vein occlusion. With the exception of one child, all of the remaining cases had histories of significant diseases.
5 Although not recorded in this series, occlusion of the portal and splenic veins alone is seen occasionally.

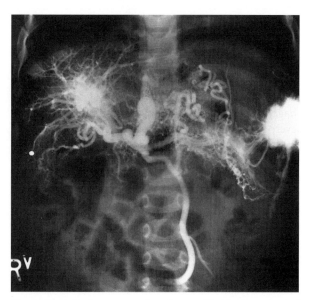

Figure 20.6 *Portovenogram in a 9-year-old girl who presented with hematemesis. There is occlusion of the portal, mesenteric and splenic regions of the portal venous system.*

In summary, these observations suggest that the splenic and superior mesenteric veins may be spared when there is a congenital anomaly of the portal venous system, and they may be useful for surgical decompression if this is indicated. However, total occlusion of the splanchnic veins may indicate an underlying hematological disorder. Occlusions of variable length may follow umbilical vein catheterization or intra-abdominal surgery and/or sepsis.

HEPATOPORTAL SCLEROSIS

There are now many reports of portal hypertension in children in which the liver architecture appears to be normal on histology, and in which the portal vein is patent. The initial reports described ascites as part of the presentation and suggested that there might be a later deterioration in liver function, and that encephalopathy and death might occur. Liver biopsies contained portal areas with increased collagen. Studies showed that the portal vein radicles were thickened and sclerotic. There was subendothelial thickening or intrahepatic branches of the portal vein, resulting in presinusoidal obstruction and increased blood flow (Nayak and Ramalingaswami, 1969). This condition is known by a variety of names, such as non-cirrhotic portal hypertension and obliterative portal venopathy, but the best known is probably hepatoportal sclerosis, suggested by Mikkelsen (1966). A 'withered-tree' appearance on angiography was described by Carson et al. (1981), who described two cases who presented with splenomegaly, portal hypertension and ascites. Liver histology was normal at first in

their cases, but periportal fibrosis appeared later. The portal vein was patent, but hepatic vein pressure suggested presinusoidal block. It is interesting that these patients presented at such a young age (20 and 21 months, respectively) with variceal bleeding.

Angiography is mandatory for diagnosis and shows a patent portal vein with a characteristic collection of large collaterals in the porta hepatis. In total, 47 out of 59 cases that were followed for over 30 years (80%) suffered variceal hemorrhage (Kingham et al., 1981). The 5-year survival rate in these cases was 90% and the actuarial survival rate was 55%. Hepatoportal sclerosis appears to be more common in India and Japan, and it has been calculated that in these countries 25–30% of portosystemic shunts are performed for this condition.

In total, 16 cases were rebiopsied after 18 years. There was no change in 11 cases, but one case showed progression to micronodular cirrhosis. It has been suggested that some of the changes recorded in these cases, particularly the deterioration in liver histology, might be due to the effects of the portosystemic shunts (Mikkelsen et al., 1965).

INTRAHEPATIC PORTAL HYPERTENSION

Intrahepatic portal hypertension may be caused by a large variety of liver diseases, such as congenital hepatic fibrosis, alpha-1-antitrypsin deficiency, biliary atresia and, in some parts of the world, schistosomiasis.

Postsinusoidal (e.g. veno-occlusive disease) and suprahepatic venous occlusion (Budd–Chiari syndrome) are occasionally seen in children. The latter is caused either by a web in the inferior vena cava above the entry of the hepatic veins, or by a thrombotic occlusion of the hepatic veins themselves (Budd-Chiari syndrome).

ARTERIOPORTAL FISTULA

Increased portal blood flow and secondary portal hypertension are very rare, but can occur in congenital arterioportal fistula (Foley et al., 1971; Heaton et al., 1995; Paley et al., 1997), hereditary hemorrhagic telangiectasia (Zentler-Munro et al., 1989) or after trauma.

An example of portal hypertension secondary to fistula formation after surgical trauma was reported by Davenport et al. (1999), who described the case of a child who presented with hematemesis from gastric varices 6 years after successful resectional surgery of a large hepatoblastoma arising in segment IV. CT scanning showed synchronous filling of the portal vein and hepatic artery in the arterial phase of the study (Figure 20.7). Hepatic angiography demonstrated a false aneurysm, retrograde filling of the portal vein and large gastric varices. The

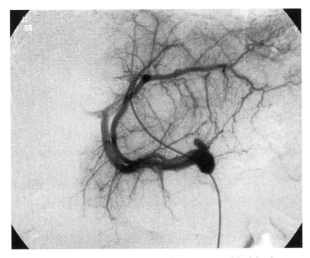

Figure 20.7 *Hepatic arteriogram in a 7-year-old girl who presented with portal hypertension and esophageal bleeding more than 6 years after resection of a hepatoblastoma. The angiogram shows rapid imaging of the intrahepatic portal venous system through an arteriovenous fistula. An aneurysmal dilatation is clearly visible at the site of the post-traumatic fistula.*

fistula was closed with selective embolization using titanium coils, and subsequent portography confirmed normal portal blood flow.

EFFECTS OF PORTAL HYPERTENSION (SEE ALSO CHAPTER 23)

Portal hypertension causes compensatory changes in venous tributaries. For example, in portal vein obstruction, hepatopetal blood flow is maintained through collateral channels in many sites, including the peritoneal attachments of the liver, the gastrohepatic omentum and the diaphragm. Intrahepatic portal hypertension, on the other hand, is associated with hepatofugal flow through the esophageal and azygos system, the periumbilical and the retroperitoneal veins.

Portal hypertension is associated with esophageal varices, the size of which is not necessarily related to the magnitude of the portal pressure. Esophageal varices are liable to bleed because of a combination of poor support within the esophageal mucosa, negative intrapleural pressure and the erosive effects of gastric juice on the esophageal epithelium. Splenomegaly is an almost invariable finding, and is associated with thrombocytopenia, leucopenia and mild anemia. A prolonged prothrombin time is an obvious feature of hepatic parenchymal disease, but a mild prolongation is also commonly seen in patients with portal vein obstruction. The reason for this is not clear. Although ascites is a common finding in advanced parenchymal disease, it may also occur after variceal hemorrhage in patients with

portal vein obstruction. In a collected series of cases of portal vein obstruction, ascites was noted in 28 out of 190 cases (14.7%), whilst 9 out of 18 cases showed an increase in prothrombin time (Clatworthy, 1974). In this series, respiratory infections preceded bleeding in 8 out of 18 cases, and the authors suggested a relationship (now accepted) between the onset of bleeding and salicylate ingestion.

Gibson *et al.* (1965) summarized the observation of the association of pyrexia and variceal bleeding when they stated that 'the association of pyrexia in bleeding (in portal hypertension) is clear, but the explanation is not'.

Encephalopathy and hepatopulmonary syndrome (hypoxemia) may be associated with portal hypertension secondary to intrahepatic disease and to congenital portosystemic fistulae in childhood (see above), but these sequelae are extremely rare in extrahepatic portal vein obstruction. However, they may be precipitated by gastrointestinal hemorrhage and absorption of blood from the gastrointestinal tract.

HEPATIC PORTAL VENOUS GAS

Gas in the intrahepatic portal vein may be associated with either primary bowel pathology (Griffiths and Gough, 1986), abdominal trauma (Ho and Hu, 1995) or iatrogenic injury (Herman and Levine, 1995). Iatrogenic causes in children include umbilical vein catheterization, barium enema examination, and colonoscopy and biopsy, particularly in the presence of inflammatory bowel disease. The mortality in this group is much lower than that in the non-iatrogenic group, and there is no reported mortality following barium enema examination.

Pathological causes are invariably associated with necrosis of the bowel mucosa and have a very poor prognosis. The commonest cause is necrotizing enterocolitis, but enterocolitis associated with intestinal aganglionosis, bowel infarction secondary to adhesive obstruction, strangulated hernias, volvulus and superior mesenteric artery occlusion have all been described. Intra-abdominal abscesses or septicemia may also cause hepatic portal venous gas.

A diagnosis of intrahepatic gas on abdominal X-ray is confirmed by the observation of tubular lucencies which branch out from the porta and run to the periphery of the liver. This appearance is caused by the centrifugal flow of venous blood. This contrasts with the appearance of gas in the biliary tree, which tends to remain within the larger ducts, close to the hilum. The presence of gas may be confirmed by ultrasound or CT examination.

The majority of affected infants are less than 3 months old. They are severely ill at presentation and deteriorate rapidly. Urgent surgical excision of necrotic bowel or drainage of pus is indicated.

The gas reaches the portal vein either directly from the bowel lumen via the damaged mucosa, or as a result of gas-forming organisms in the bowel wall or in an abscess cavity. *E. coli*, *Pseudomonas* and *Clostridium* species have been isolated from intra-abdominal pus in these patients. The gas bubbles are believed to have a direct harmful effect on the liver. Protein denaturation, activation of clotting factors, kinin release and mechanical obstruction may all play a part in causing liver injury (Griffiths and Gough, 1986).

Hepatic portal vein gas increases the morbidity and mortality of intra-abdominal disease. Persistence of the gas in the vein is associated with a poor outcome, and the mortality associated with non-iatrogenic hepatic portal venous gas is over 80%. However, effective treatment of the underlying cause results in rapid clearance of the gas from the portal vein.

Key references

Howard ER, Davenport M. Congenital extrahepatic portocaval shunts – the Abernethy malformation. *Journal of Pediatric Surgery* 1997; **32**: 271–5.

This report presents five new cases of congenital portosystemic shunts and reviews the world literature. An analysis of reported cases suggests a classification into 'type 1' and 'type 2' abnormalities. The role of surgery is also discussed.

Meyer WW, Lind J. The ductus venosus and the mechanism of its closure. *Archives of Disease in Childhood* 1966; **41**: 597–605.

This is a good introduction to the anatomical features and physiological mechanisms which govern the function of the portal venous system in the fetus and the closure of the ductus venosus around the time of birth.

Stringer MD, Heaton ND, Karani J, Olliff S, Howard ER. Patterns of portal vein occlusion and their aetiological significance. *British Journal of Surgery* 1994; **81**: 1328–31.

A well-illustrated paper describing the range of anatomical abnormalities encountered in extrahepatic portal vein occlusion. The angiographic observations are related to etiological factors.

Uchino T, Endo F, Ikeda S, Shiraki K, Sera Y. Three brothers with progressive hepatic dysfunction and severe steatosis due to patent ductus venosus. *Gastroenterology* 1996; **110**: 1964–8.

This report describes the presentation of three young brothers with complications of congenital portosystemic shunts. These included fatty infiltration of the liver, abnormal liver function tests and encephalopathy. Surgical closure of the shunts resulted in correction of the hepatic abnormalities.

Webb LJ, Sherlock S. The aetiology, presentation and natural history of extrahepatic portal venous obstruction. *Quarterly Journal of Medicine* 1979; **192**: 627–39.

This is a classic review of the natural history of 97 patients with extrahepatic portal hypertension. Etiology, age at presentation of hematemesis, morbidity and mortality are analyzed. The patients who presented in childhood were followed up into adulthood, and this provided the authors with a good overview of the problem of portal vein obstruction.

REFERENCES

Abernethy J. Account of two instances of uncommon formation in the viscera of the human body. *Philosophical Transactions of the Royal Society of London* 1793; **83**: 59–66.

Atasoy KC, Fitoz S, Akyar G, Aytac S, Erden I. Aneurysms of the portal venous system. Gray-scale and color Doppler ultrasonographic findings with CT and MRI correlation. *Clinical Imaging* 1998; **22**: 414–17.

Carson JA, Turnell WP, Barnes P, Altshuler G. Hepatoportal sclerosis in childhood: a mimic of extrahepatic portal vein obstruction. *Journal of Pediatric Surgery* 1981; **16**: 291–6.

Clatworthy HW. Extrahepatic portal hypertension. In: Child CG (ed.) *Portal hypertension*, 3rd edn. Philadelphia, PA: WB Saunders, 1974: 243–66.

Davenport M, Savage M, Mowat AP, Howard ER. Biliary atresia splenic malformation syndrome: an etiologic and prognostic subgroup. *Surgery* 1993; **113**: 662–8.

Davenport M, Redkar R, Howard ER, Karani J. Arterioportal hypertension: a rare complication of partial hepatectomy. *Pediatric Surgery International* 1999; **15**: 543–5.

Dickson AD. The development of the ductus venosus in man and the goat. *Journal of Anatomy* 1957; **91**: 358–68.

Foley WJ, Turcott JG, Hoskins PA, Brant RL, Ause RG. Intrahepatic arteriovenous fistulas between the hepatic artery and portal vein. *Annals of Surgery* 1971; **174**: 849–55.

Gibson JB, Johnston GW, Fulton TT, Rodgers HW. Extrahepatic portal venous obstruction. *British Journal of Surgery* 1965; **52**: 129.

Gray SW, Skandalakis JE. *Embryology for surgeons*. Philadelphia, PA: WB Saunders, 1972: 177.

Griffiths DM, Gough MH. Gas in the hepatic portal veins. *British Journal of Surgery* 1986; **73**: 172–6.

Heaton ND, Karani J, Howard ER. Portal vein thrombosis in myeloproliferative disease. *British Medical Journal* 1990; **300**: 945.

Heaton ND, Davenport M, Karani J, Mowatd AP, Howard ER. Congenital hepatoportal arteriovenous fistula. *Surgery* 1995; **117**: 170–4.

Hellweg G. Congenital absence of intrahepatic portal venous system simulating Eck fistula. *Archives of Pathology and Laboratory Medicine* 1954; **57**: 425–30.

Herman JB, Levine MS. Portal venous gas as a complication of ERCP and endoscopic sphincterotomy. *American Journal of Gastroenterology* 1995; **90**: 828–9.

Herman RE, Shafer WH. Aneurysm of the portal vein and portal hypertension. First reported case. *Annals of Surgery* 1965; **162**: 1101–4.

Ho MC, Hu RH. Hepatic portal vein gas following blunt colon injury. *Journal of the Formosa Medical Association* 1995; **94**: 578–80.

Howard ER, Davenport M. Congenital extrahepatic portocaval shunts – the Abernethy malformation. *Journal of Pediatric Surgery* 1997; **32**: 494–7.

Hunt GB, Bellenger CR, Borg R, Youmans KR, Tisdall PL, Malik R. Congenital interruption of the portal vein and caudal vena cava in dogs: six reports and a review of the literature. *Veterinary Surgery* 1998; **27**: 203–15.

Jacob S, Farr G, De Vun D, Takiff H, Mason A. Hepatic manifestations of familial patent ductus venosus in adults. *Gut* 1999; **45**: 442–5.

Joyce AD, Howard ER. Rare congenital anomaly of the portal vein. *British Journal of Surgery* 1988; **75**: 1038–9.

Kamata S, Kitayama Y, Usui N *et al.* Patent ductus venosus with a hypoplastic intrahepatic portal system presenting intrapulmonary shunt: a case treated with banding of the ductus venosus. *Journal of Pediatric Surgery* 2000; **35**: 655–7.

Kennedy TC, Knudson RJ. Exercise-aggravated hypoxemia and orthdeoxia in cirrhosis. *Chest* 1977; **72**: 305–9.

Kiernan F. The anatomy and physiology of the liver. *Philosophical Transactions of the Royal Society of London* 1833; **B113**: 711–70.

Kingham JGC, Levison DA, Stansfield AG, Dawson MA. Non-cirrhotic intrahepatic portal hypertension: a long-term follow-up study. *Quarterly Journal of Medicine* 1981; **199**: 259–68.

Kohda E, Saeki M, Masaki H, Ogawa K, Nirasawa M, Hiramatsu K. Congenital absence of the portal vein in a boy. *Pediatric Radiology* 1999; **29**: 235–7.

Marks C. Developmental basis of the portal venous system. *American Journal of Surgery* 1969; **117**: 671–81.

Marois D, Van Heerden JA, Carpenter HA, Sheedy PF. Congenital absence of the portal vein. *Mayo Clinic Proceedings* 1979; **54**: 55–9.

Matsuoka Y, Ohtomo K, Okubo T, Nishikawa J, Mine T. Congenital absence of the portal vein. *Gastrointestinal Radiology* 1992; **17**: 31–3.

Meyer WW, Lind J. The ductus venosus and the mechanism of its closure. *Archives of Disease in Childhood* 1966; **41**: 597–605.

Mikkelsen WP. Extrahepatic portal hypertension in children. *American Journal of Surgery* 1966; **111**: 333–40.

Mikkelsen WP, Edmondson HA, Peters RL, Redeker AG, Reynolds TB. Extra- and intrahepatic portal hypertension without cirrhosis (hepatoportal sclerosis). *Annals of Surgery* 1965; **162**: 602–20.

Morgan G, Superina R. Congenital absence of the portal vein: two cases and a proposed classification system for portosystemic vascular anomalies. *Journal of Pediatric Surgery* 1994; **29**: 1239–41.

Morse SS, Taylor KJW, Strauss EB, Ramirez E, Seashore JH. Congenital absence of the portal vein in oculovertebral dysplasia (Goldenhar syndrome). *Pediatric Radiology* 1986; **16**: 437–9.

Nakasaki H, Tanaka Y, Ohta M *et al.* Congenital absence of the portal vein. *Annals of Surgery* 1989; **210**: 190–3.

Nayak NC, Ramalingaswami V. Obliterative portal venopathy of the liver: associated with so-called idiopathic portal hypertension or tropical splenomegaly. *Archives of Pathology* 1969; **87**: 359–69.

Olling S, Olsson R. Congenital absence of the portal venous system in a 50-year-old woman. *Acta Medica Scandinavica* 1974; **155**: 527–8.

Orii T, Ohkohchi N, Kato H *et al.* Liver transplantation for severe hypoxemia caused by patent ductus venosus. *Journal of Pediatric Surgery* 1997; **32**: 1795–7.

Ozbeck SS, Killi MR, Pourbagher MA, Parildar M, Katranci N, Solak A. Portal venous system aneurysms: report of five cases. *Journal of Ultrasound Medicine* 1999; **18**: 417–22.

Paley MR, Farrant P, Kane P, Heaton ND, Howard ER, Karani JB. Developmental intrahepatic shunts of childhood: radiological features and management. *European Radiology* 1997; **7**: 1377–82.

Poirier P, Charpy A. *Anatomie humaine.* Paris: Masson & Cie, 1903.

Rothuizen J, Van den Ingh TS, Voorhout G, Van Der Luer RJT, Wouda W. Portal-systemic encephalopathy due to a congenital portocaval shunt. *Journal of Small Animal Practice* 1982; **23**: 67–81.

Stringer MD, Heaton ND, Karani J, Olliff S, Howard ER. Patterns of portal vein occlusion and their aetiological significance. *British Journal of Surgery* 1994; **81**: 1328–31.

Thomas TV. Aneurysm of the portal vein: report of two cases, one resulting in thrombosis and spontaneous rupture. *Surgery* 1967; **61**: 551–5.

Uchino T, Endo F, Ikeda S, Shiraki K, Sera Y. Three brothers with progressive hepatic dysfunction and severe steatosis due to patent ductus venosus. *Gastroenterology* 1996; **110**: 1964–8.

Whitington P. Portal hypertension in children. *Pediatric Annals* 1985; **14**: 494–9.

Woodle ES, Thistlethwaite JR, Emond JC *et al.* Successful hepatic transplantation in congenital absence of recipient portal vein. *Surgery* 1990; **107**: 475–9.

Zentler-Munro PL, Howard ER, Karani J, Williams R. Variceal haemorrhage in hereditary haemorrhagic telangiectasia. *Gut* 1989; **30**: 1293–7.

21

Pathogenesis and management of esophageal and gastric varices

MARK D STRINGER

Bleeding from esophageal varices is the commonest cause of serious gastrointestinal hemorrhage in children. This chapter focuses on portal hypertension in children, and on the pathogenesis and management of esophageal and gastric varices in particular.

DEFINITION AND PATHOPHYSIOLOGY OF PORTAL HYPERTENSION

The portal vein transports blood to the liver from the gastrointestinal tract and spleen. Intrahepatic segmental branches of the portal vein terminate in small vessels which supply the hepatic sinusoids.

Portal venous pressure is directly proportional to:

- *portal blood flow*: this is increased in cirrhotic portal hypertension due to elevated concentrations of circulating vasodilators and a decreased responsiveness to vasoconstrictors (Gupta *et al.*, 1997). The circulation is hyperdynamic as evidenced by peripheral vasodilatation, decreased systemic resistance, plasma volume expansion, increased splanchnic blood flow and a rise in the cardiac index;
- *vascular resistance*: increased resistance to portal venous blood flow may be due to portal vein obstruction, hepatic fibrosis or cirrhosis, or hepatic venous outflow obstruction. Intrahepatic disease has both fixed components (fibrosis and architectural distortion) and dynamic components (sinusoidal vascular tone under the influence of hepatic stellate cells).

A rise in portal pressure leads to splenomegaly and the development of natural portosystemic shunts:

- at the cardia via gastro-esophageal veins;
- in the anal canal via hemorrhoidal veins;
- in the falciform ligament via the umbilical vein;
- in the abdominal wall and retroperitoneum where abdominal viscera lie adjacent to systemic veins.

Variceal bleeding

Submucosal varices in the lower esophagus are particularly prone to rupture. Portal hypertension is defined by an increased hepatic venous pressure gradient (> 5 mmHg), the difference between portal venous pressure and free hepatic venous pressure. A hepatic venous pressure gradient of > 12 mmHg is necessary for the development of esophageal varices (Garcia-Tsao *et al.*, 1985) but, because of the variability in collateral pathways, some patients with pressures exceeding this value do not develop esophagogastric varices. Although the relationship is not linear, the risk of variceal bleeding is increased in larger varices and those with a higher intravariceal pressure and greater wall tension (Lebrec *et al.*, 1980; Dawson, 1983). Wall tension is inversely proportional to wall thickness. A large varix with thin walls (evidenced by 'red color signs' on endoscopy) will reach a high wall tension and risk of bleeding at much lower variceal pressures. In established cirrhosis, the risk of variceal bleeding is related to the severity of the liver disease (the Child-Pugh score).

Other effects of portal hypertension

In addition to the risk of variceal bleeding, portal hypertension may induce other harmful effects. Portal hypertensive gastropathy and enteropathy encourage malabsorption and growth retardation. This can be particularly severe in children with short bowel syndrome, where cholestatic liver disease and portal hypertension encourage bacterial translocation across the gut and have an adverse effect on intestinal adaptation (Weber, 2000). In portal vein occlusion there is a variable degree of liver atrophy and portal tract fibrosis. This may in part be related to insulin, glucagon and other hepatotrophic factors bypassing the liver and entering the systemic circulation directly through natural portosystemic shunts.

ETIOLOGY OF PORTAL HYPERTENSION

Portal hypertension in children may be due to venous obstruction at *prehepatic* (e.g. portal vein obstruction), *intrahepatic* (e.g. cirrhosis, fibrosis, nodular hyperplasia) or *posthepatic* (e.g. Budd–Chiari syndrome) sites. Occasionally, a mixed picture develops (e.g. in the child with cirrhosis complicated by secondary portal vein thrombosis). Rarely, an arterioportal venous fistula causes portal hypertension in an unobstructed system. Chronic liver disease is the commonest overall cause of portal hypertension, but portal vein obstruction is the most frequent cause of extrahepatic portal hypertension.

Prehepatic sites

PORTAL VEIN OBSTRUCTION (PVO)

PVO accounts for approximately 30% of all children presenting with bleeding esophageal varices (Howard *et al.*, 1988; Maksoud *et al.*, 1991). Many etiological factors have been implicated (Box 21.1).

Umbilical vein catheterization in the newborn, with or without infusion of irritant solutions, and umbilical sepsis are recognized precipitants (Campbell, 1971; Webb and Sherlock, 1979). There is a history of neonatal septicemia, umbilical vein catheterization or umbilical sepsis in up to 30% of patients with PVO (Yadav *et al.*, 1993; Stringer *et al.*, 1994). However, prospective ultrasound studies indicate that this is a rare complication of umbilical vein catheters used for short periods (Yadav *et al.*, 1993).

Thrombophilic states predispose to portal and/or hepatic vein thrombosis (Box 21.2) (Boughton, 1991; Brady *et al.*, 1996; Gurakan *et al.*, 1999). In the genetic conditions, homozygotes are particularly vulnerable. For the heterozygote (it is estimated that 5% of white Europeans are heterozygous for the factor V Leiden mutation) combination with other thrombotic risk factors is hazardous (Denninger *et al.*, 2000). There has long been confusion about the role of natural anticoagulant proteins (protein C, protein S and antithrombin III) in PVO. Circulating concentrations are commonly decreased *as a result* of PVO, and thus the diagnosis of inherited deficiencies is difficult (Dubuisson *et al.*, 1997; Fisher *et al.*, 2000). The minority of cases of PVO with a true inherited deficiency of one of these anticoagulant proteins tend to have very low circulating levels. They can only be identified with certainty by careful investigation of family members, although gene sequencing may be possible in the future.

Portal vein thrombosis is a rare early complication of splenectomy, occurring in up to 2% of cases, and predominantly in patients undergoing splenectomy for hematological conditions (van't Riet *et al.*, 2000). Postoperative thrombocytosis, hyperviscosity, reduced portal vein flow, and stasis of blood in the stump of the splenic vein are considered to be likely predisposing factors.

The pattern of portomesenteric venous occlusion (Figure 21.1) may provide a clue to etiology in some cases (Stringer *et al.*, 1994). In myeloproliferative disor-

---

Box 21.1 *Causes of portal vein obstruction*

General factors
Developmental anomalies
Thrombophilia
Septicemia

Local factors
Umbilical sepsis, catheterization, infusion of irritant
　　solutions
Intra-abdominal sepsis/portal pyemia
Trauma (including surgical trauma)
Structural lesions (e.g. portal vein web)
Cholangitis/choledochal cyst
Pancreatitis
Malignant disease/lymphadenopathy

Box 21.2 *Congenital and acquired causes of thrombophilia associated with portal and/or hepatic vein thrombosis*

Myeloproliferative disorders
Paroxysmal nocturnal hemoglobinuria
Protein C deficiency
Protein S deficiency
Antithrombin III deficiency
Factor V Leiden mutation
Antiphospholipid antibodies (includes lupus
　　anticoagulant and anticardiolipin)
Factor II gene mutation (prothrombin 20210A)
Carbohydrate-deficient glycoprotein syndrome

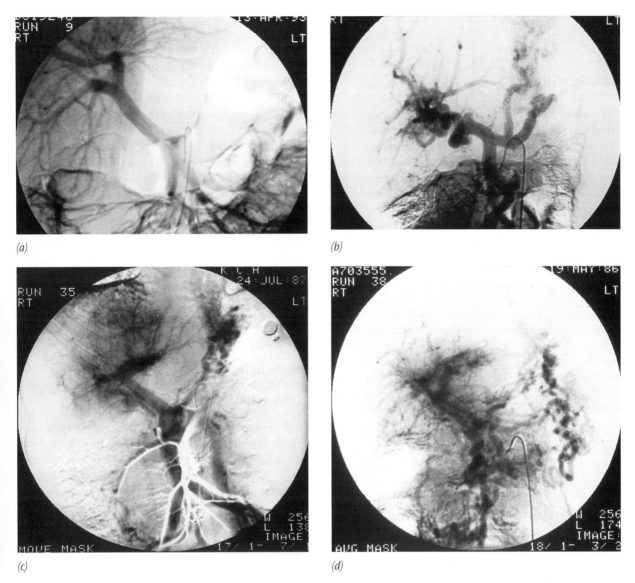

(a)

(b)

(c)

(d)

Figure 21.1 (a) Angiographic appearances of normal portal vein and intrahepatic branches following arterial injection of the superior mesenteric artery. (b) Aortoportogram demonstrating occlusion of the main portal vein with cavernomatous transformation. The origin of the portal vein at the confluence of the superior mesenteric and splenic veins is clearly visible. (c) Angiographic appearances of hepatroportal sclerosis. The superior mesenteric artery is outlined in white and the patent main portal vein is visible. The bifurcation of the portal vein and its intrahepatic radicles are replaced by multiple collateral vessels. (d) Aortoportogram demonstrating widespread venous occlusion and collateralization throughout the portal venous system.

ders and severe thrombophilia, thrombosis tends to be more extensive with frequent involvement of mesenteric, splenic, hepatic and deep veins in addition to the main portal vein. Abdominal trauma and intra-abdominal sepsis, especially if accompanied by portal pyemia, may cause PVO with or without involvement of the superior mesenteric vein. Rarely, the portal vein may be obstructed by a congenital web or externally compressed by lymphadenopathy, tumor or a choledochal cyst.

Isolated splenic vein obstruction occasionally occurs in children, and produces a picture of 'left-sided' portal hypertension with bleeding from gastro-esophageal varices but no significant portal enteropathy (Lenthall *et al.*, 1999). Unlike PVO, splenectomy may be curative in

this situation.

The majority of children with extrahepatic portal hypertension have isolated PVO and no identifiable etiological factors. The portal vein is replaced by multiple venous collaterals – the so-called portal vein cavernoma. Detailed imaging studies suggest that in some of these cases the main portal vein is actually patent but very tortuous, and its intrahepatic branches are poorly developed (Ando *et al.*, 1996). In these children PVO may be a developmental anomaly (see Chapter 20). Associations with other congenital abnormalities, such as congenital heart disease, anomalous inferior vena cava, choledochal cyst, intestinal malrotation, duodenal atresia and craniofacial dysostosis, support this hypothesis (Marks, 1974;

Odievre et al., 1977; Webb and Sherlock, 1979; Stringer et al., 1994).

Intrahepatic sites

The intrahepatic causes of portal hypertension are diverse and include several different pathological processes that lead to obstruction of portal venous flow. Some of them (hepatoportal sclerosis, schistosomiasis and veno-occlusive disease) predominantly affect the venous circulation through the liver. However, the majority (cirrhosis, fibrosis, nodular hyperplasia, malignancy, acute and chronic hepatitis) are intrinsic liver diseases which cause distortion of hepatic architecture.

CIRRHOSIS AND CONGENITAL HEPATIC FIBROSIS

Biliary atresia is the commonest cause of cirrhosis and portal hypertension in children in Western countries. Other conditions include cystic fibrosis, autoimmune hepatitis, sclerosing cholangitis, alpha-1-antitrypsin deficiency and congenital hepatic fibrosis.

HEPATOPORTAL SCLEROSIS

In a small proportion of children with portal hypertension and normal liver function the portal vein is clearly patent but there is presinusoidal venous obstruction associated with subendothelial thickening of intrahepatic portal venous radicles (Mikkelsen et al., 1965; Nayak and Ramalingaswami, 1969). Conventional liver histology is initially normal, but portal tract fibrosis is subsequently evident. The etiology of hepatoportal sclerosis is unknown. Presentation is typically with splenomegaly, ascites and variceal hemorrhage (Carson et al., 1981), and angiography confirms intrahepatic portal vein obstruction with a 'withered-tree' appearance. Most cases are not progressive and respond well to treatment of esophageal varices (see Chapter 20).

SCHISTOSOMIASIS

The eggs of this trematode are carried in the portal blood to the portal tracts, where they produce inflammatory granulomata and subsequent fibrosis leading to presinusoidal portal hypertension. In endemic areas of the world most children become infected, but the subsequent course is extremely variable.

VENO-OCCLUSIVE DISEASE

This variety of hepatic vein obstruction affects children more often than adults. Occlusion of centrilobular veins and hepatic venules causes sinusoidal congestion and hepatocyte necrosis. In South America, South Africa, India and the Middle East the condition is due to toxins found in herbal teas (Sperl et al., 1995). In the West,

veno-occlusive disease is seen after irradiation and/or cytotoxic drug-induced liver injury (Kullendorff and Bekassy, 1996). Children undergoing bone-marrow transplantation or treatment for Wilms' tumor appear to be especially at risk.

Clinical features are similar to those of acute Budd–Chiari syndrome with sudden onset of abdominal pain and distension due to hepatomegaly and ascites. If the patient survives the acute phase, cirrhosis and portal hypertension may follow. After bone-marrow transplantation, some patients with veno-occlusive disease will be asymptomatic. Others develop jaundice, painful hepatomegaly and ascites, usually within 1 month of grafting (Shulman and Hinterberg, 1992). Treatment is largely supportive. Specific therapy with thrombolytic agents such as tissue plasminogen activator, or with defibrotide, a mammalian tissue-derived polydeoxyribonucleotide with thrombolytic and antithrombotic properties, has been advocated, but no controlled data have yet been reported. Prophylactic low-dose heparin may help to prevent the condition (Attal et al., 1992).

Posthepatic sites

BUDD–CHIARI SYNDROME

The various causes of this syndrome include venous thrombosis affecting the hepatic veins or inferior vena cava (often secondary to an underlying myeloproliferative disorder, paroxysmal nocturnal hemoglobinuria or thrombophilia), an obstructing caval web, and hepatic vein injury due to trauma or tumor. The condition may also develop as a complication of orthotopic liver transplantation. The caudate lobe is frequently spared because of its independent venous drainage directly into the inferior vena cava. Caudate hypertrophy may compress the cava causing lower limb edema. Histologically, there is marked venous congestion around the central venule with hepatocyte necrosis. In chronic cases there is progression to hepatic fibrosis and cirrhosis.

CHRONIC CONSTRICTIVE PERICARDITIS

In addition to cardiac symptoms and signs, chronic constrictive pericarditis may cause liver damage similar to that seen in chronic Budd–Chiari syndrome. If it is diagnosed and treated promptly, progressive resolution of the hepatic changes can be expected.

Hepatic arterioportal venous fistula

This may occur as a consequence of blunt or penetrating liver trauma (including liver biopsy). Rarely, an arterioportal fistula is congenital, when it tends to be an isolated finding (Heaton et al., 1995; Marchand et al., 1999) but may rarely occur in association with hereditary hemorrhagic telangiectasia (Buscarini et al., 1997) or biliary atresia (see Chapters 15 and 20).

CLINICAL FEATURES OF PORTAL HYPERTENSION

In chronic liver disease, portal hypertension often firsts manifests as splenomegaly. In PVO, presentation is usually with acute gastrointestinal hemorrhage (hematemesis and/or melena) or splenomegaly. Precise diagnosis is essential because the natural history and management of the different causes of portal hypertension differ widely.

Although variceal hemorrhage may occur at any age, children with PVO typically present with bleeding at a younger mean age (5 years) than those with cirrhosis (8 years) (Howard et al., 1988). Previously, it was thought that the risk of bleeding in PVO decreased spontaneously with age, concomitant with the development of portosystemic collaterals (Webb and Sherlock, 1979; Boles et al., 1986). This concept has recently been challenged by the group from Bicêtre, France. Of a selected group of 44 children with PVO who were followed up into early adulthood, 24 cases experienced gastrointestinal bleeding after the age of 12 years (Lykavieris et al., 2000). However, the majority of these had previously bled in early childhood, but had not been treated effectively at this stage. In children with PVO who had never bled, the risk of bleeding was extremely low after the age of 15 years, and these patients tended to have small varices. Spontaneous improvement is therefore unlikely once varices have reached the critical point of bleeding, but a small proportion of children with PVO (< 10% overall) never bleed.

Upper respiratory tract infection and aspirin therapy are recognized precipitants of variceal bleeding in children. Encephalopathy may complicate the episode of bleeding in those with cirrhosis, but is rarely clinically detectable in children with PVO. Ascites usually denotes the presence of chronic liver disease, but may occur with extrahepatic portal hypertension, particularly after a major variceal bleed. An important clinical sign is the presence of dilated cutaneous veins carrying blood away from the umbilicus towards the tributaries of the vena cava (caput medusae).

Portal hypertension may cause mucosal edema, lymphatic congestion, capillary ectasia and a reduced villus/crypt ratio in the small intestine. This may lead to malabsorption, protein-losing enteropathy and failure to thrive. Impaired pancreatic exocrine function has also been described in association with extrahepatic portal hypertension (Webb et al., 1980). Growth failure is a well-recognized complication of cirrhosis, and various factors (including growth hormone resistance) have been implicated. Several studies have shown that children with PVO are also relatively growth retarded, and portal enteropathy may be the dominant cause in such cases (Sarin et al., 1992; Mehrotra et al., 1997).

The development of varices at sites other than the esophagus or stomach ('ectopic' varices) is potentially hazardous because of the risk of bleeding and other complications. Ectopic varices may occur throughout the intestine, but are more common in the duodenum, at sites of previous enteric anastomoses and around stomas. The risk of ectopic variceal hemorrhage is small, although it is significantly greater in patients with PVO compared with those with chronic liver disease (Lebrec and Benhamou, 1985; Heaton and Howard, 1993; Stringer and Howard, 1994). Anorectal varices and hemorrhoids are found in almost two-thirds of children with PVO, but in a much smaller proportion of those with chronic liver disease (Heaton et al., 1993). They represent collateral pathways between the portomesenteric and systemic venous systems. In teenagers and young adults, varices around the common bile duct may occasionally cause obstructive jaundice or a mild increase in plasma bilirubin and alkaline phosphatase (Khuroo et al., 1993).

Rarely, pulmonary hypertension may coexist with portal hypertension, either in association with cirrhosis (especially secondary to biliary atresia) or PVO, and this complication may be fatal (Boles et al., 1986, Schuijtvlot et al., 1995) (see Chapter 23).

Budd–Chiari syndrome

Most patients are young adults, but the condition may affect children (Gentil-Kocher et al., 1988). In adolescent girls, Budd–Chiari syndrome may be precipitated by the oral contraceptive pill. Clinical features include hepatomegaly, intractable ascites, portal hypertension and progressive cachexia. Jaundice is variable. Onset is more often chronic but may be acute, when abdominal pain, distension and diarrhea are predominant symptoms.

INVESTIGATION OF PORTAL HYPERTENSION

HEMATOLOGY

Hypersplenism may result in anemia and depressed white blood cell and platelet counts. In PVO, the prothrombin time is often slightly prolonged in association with a reduced factor VII concentration; plasma concentrations of both procoagulant and anticoagulant proteins are reduced, most probably as a consequence of reduced liver blood flow and/or portosystemic shunting (Fisher et al., 2000). In Budd–Chiari syndrome, an underlying myeloproliferative or thrombophilic disorder should be excluded.

BIOCHEMICAL LIVER FUNCTION

This is usually abnormal in cirrhosis but rarely deranged in PVO. In the latter, plasma albumin levels may be reduced following a variceal bleed. Severe disturbances of liver function are found in acute Budd–Chiari syndrome.

ABDOMINAL ULTRASOUND SCAN

This may show non-specific features of portal hypertension (e.g. large collateral veins and splenomegaly) as well as confirming a portal vein cavernoma and patency of the superior mesenteric and splenic veins. Doppler studies provide information about the direction, velocity and waveform characteristics of portal blood flow. In cirrhosis the maximum velocity of blood flow in the main portal trunk is inversely correlated with the severity of liver disease (Kozaiwa *et al.*, 1995). Screening for hepatic vein occlusion can be performed using duplex ultrasonography.

GASTROINTESTINAL ENDOSCOPY

Fiberoptic endoscopy enables the evaluation (and treatment) of esophageal, gastric, duodenal, colonic and anorectal varices at all ages. Various grading systems are used in the assessment of esophageal varices, and one example is shown in Box 21.3. Smaller varices are blue with a relatively thick mucosal covering, whereas large ones may have signs of recent or impending variceal hemorrhage. These stigmata include 'cherry-red spots' and 'varices on varices' (Plate 11). Variceal size may be underestimated in the presence of hypovolemia. Portal gastropathy is characterized by mucosal hyperemia with dilated submucosal veins.

COMPUTED TOMOGRAPHY AND MAGNETIC RESONANCE IMAGING

Cross-sectional imaging is particularly useful in Budd–Chiari syndrome and with focal liver lesions associated with portal hypertension (e.g. nodular regenerative hyperplasia). A variable degree of liver atrophy may be present in PVO. Magnetic resonance angiography is being increasingly used as a non-invasive alternative to conventional angiography to delineate portomesenteric venous anatomy.

ANGIOGRAPHY

This is useful for confirming the diagnosis of PVO and assessing the patency and caliber of veins throughout the portomesenteric system. Some form of angiography is essential prior to portosystemic shunt surgery liver transplantation, and in the investigation of hepatoportal sclerosis. Various angiographic techniques are described in detail in Chapter 3.

Inferior venacavography with pressure measurements is valuable in patients with Budd–Chiari syndrome in whom hepatic venography can be used to assess hepatic vein patency (Figure 21.2).

PERCUTANEOUS LIVER BIOPSY

Provided that there are no contraindications, a liver biopsy should be performed in children with portal hypertension secondary to liver disease.

TREATMENT OF PORTAL HYPERTENSION

The treatment of portal hypertension in children with intrahepatic pathology is dictated by the severity of the liver disease, and liver transplantation may be required. In contrast, patients with good liver function and bleeding varices, such as those with PVO or congenital hepatic fibrosis, can be successfully managed by treatment of their portal hypertension alone. Bleeding from esophageal varices is a life-threatening event, but mortality is largely related to the severity of any underlying liver disease.

Because of the availability of two effective therapies for the treatment of variceal bleeding, namely portosystemic shunting and endoscopic treatment, the management of

---

Box 21.3 *Assessment of esophageal varices*

Describe: location, extent, size, color, stigmata
Grading: 1 – present but small and collapsible (usually lower 5 cm)
 2 – tortuous veins filling less than one-third of esophageal lumen
 3 – tortuous veins occupying more than one-third of esophageal lumen
 4 – varices with stigmata
Stigmata: 'cherry-red spots' and 'varices on varices' (red color signs)

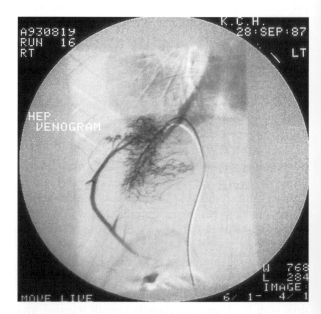

Figure 21.2 *Hepatic venogram demonstrating characteristic 'spider-web' appearance of Budd–Chiari syndrome due to hepatic vein thrombosis. There is no filling of normal hepatic veins, but a single phrenic collateral vein is outlined. (Reproduced courtesy of Dr John Karani.)*

this condition has long been controversial. There is no doubt that the results obtained with either technique in the hands of enthusiasts can be excellent. However, problems such as technical feasibility, shunt thrombosis with subsequent rebleeding, concerns about late neuropsychiatric sequelae and the recognized hazards of splenectomy in young children have limited the application of portosystemic shunt procedures (Bismuth *et al.*, 1980; Alvarez *et al.*, 1983; Pande *et al.*, 1987; Cedro *et al.*, 1993; Mitra *et al.*, 1993; Losty *et al.*, 1994; Orloff *et al.*, 1994; Prasad *et al.*, 1994; Shun *et al.*, 1997). Similarly, the availability of endoscopic expertise, problems with gastric and ectopic varices, and failures and complications of sclerotherapy have tempered enthusiasm for endoscopic sclerotherapy (Paquet, 1985; Howard *et al.*, 1988; Maksoud *et al.*, 1991). In addition to this, newer therapies have emerged in recent years (e.g. variceal banding, the mesenterico-left portal shunt, and transjugular intrahepatic portosystemic shunting), although experience with these is still limited. Dramatic advances have been made in previously experimental procedures such as liver transplantation. Consequently, the ideal treatment of variceal hemorrhage in children should be dictated by the etiology of the portal hypertension, the location of the varices and the availability of expert treatment. All therapies are complementary.

Acute variceal bleeding

Practical steps in the emergency management of bleeding esophageal varices are outlined in Box 21.4. A variety of pharmacological agents have been used to reduce portal pressure. Vasopressin (Pitressin) or its precursor, glypressin (terlipressin), may be used alone or in combination with nitrates to lower portal venous pressure. Unfortunately, these agents have side-effects related to splanchnic and systemic vasoconstriction (e.g. headache, nausea, abdominal cramps and fluid retention), which have limited their use. Somatostatin reduces splanchnic blood flow and portal pressure with minimal side-effects, but it has a short plasma half-life of less than 3 minutes. Octreotide, a long-acting analog of somatostatin, has a plasma half-life of more than 1 hour. In adults, octreotide and somatostatin perform better than vasopressin and terlipressin in the initial control of bleeding esophageal varices (Gotzsche, 2000). Although the effectiveness of octreotide has only been studied in a relatively small number of children (Siafakas *et al.*, 1998; Eroglu *et al.*, 1999), its safety and side-effect profile have encouraged its use in cases of acute variceal bleeding.

Balloon tamponade is occasionally required as a temporary measure to control active variceal bleeding. The airway should first be secured, preferably by endotracheal intubation. Only the gastric balloon is inflated, and its position should be confirmed radiographically. Bleeding can usually be controlled by moderate traction, which is obtained by taping the tube to the side of the

---

Box 21.4   *Emergency management of bleeding esophageal varices*

Resuscitation
Airway, breathing (give oxygen), circulation.
Insert two intravenous cannulae (≥ 22 G) and commence intravenous fluids.

Investigation
Full blood count, clotting, urea, creatinine, electrolytes, liver function tests ± ammonia.
Blood cultures and cross-match (at least 2 units of packed cells).
Monitor fluid balance, cardiorespiratory status and blood glucose.
Watch for encephalopathy.

Medical treatment
Transfuse packed red cells slowly, aiming for a hemoglobin concentration of *c*. 10 g/dL (avoid overtransfusion).
Give vitamin K 1 mg intravenously and correct coagulopathy with fresh frozen plasma and platelets.
Start octreotide infusion: bolus dose of 1 µg/kg intravenously (maximum 50 µg) over 5 minutes followed by infusion at 1–3 µg/kg/hour (maximum 50 µg/hour). Continue infusion until 24 hours after bleeding ceases and wean off slowly over 24 hours.
Keep nil by mouth initially.
Give gastric protection: ranitidine 1 mg/kg intravenously three times a day and sucralfate orally.
Start intravenous antibiotics if sepsis is likely.
Keep an appropriate-sized pediatric Sengstaken-type tube available to provide balloon tamponade if necessary.
Start prophylaxis against encephalopathy if there is poor liver function.

Treatment of varices
Upper gastrointestinal endoscopy within 24 hours to confirm variceal bleeding and to begin treatment by banding/sclerotherapy, if appropriate.
Note: exclude other sources of bleeding (e.g. ulcers, esophagitis, etc.).

---

face. Excessive traction can lead to esophageal ulceration or balloon displacement. The balloon is deflated after 12–24 hours, just prior to endoscopy.

Endoscopic treatment of esophageal varices

INJECTION SCLEROTHERAPY

Historical aspects
Endoscopic injection sclerotherapy was first reported in 1939 by Crafoord and Frenckner. They described the case of an 18-year-old girl who was bleeding from

esophageal varices that were controlled by serial injections of quinine via a rigid esophagoscope. By 1955, the technique had been successfully applied to children (Fearon and Sass-Kortsak, 1959). Subsequent progress was overshadowed by the development of portosystemic shunt surgery, but renewed interest was stimulated by the results obtained in adults with cirrhosis (Johnston and Rodgers, 1973; Terblanche et al., 1979). Experience with 108 children who were treated by injection sclerotherapy was reported from King's College Hospital, London, in 1988 (Howard et al., 1988), and in recent years many other large series have been published.

Technique

With modern fiberoptic endoscopes, injection sclerotherapy can be applied to all age groups, and is best performed under general anesthesia with an endotracheal tube in place. A variety of injection techniques and sclerosants have been used, and our own experience has been with 5% ethanolamine oleate (Stringer, 1998). Although good results have been obtained with paravariceal injections (Paquet, 1985), an intravariceal injection technique is preferred, and this view is supported by the results of a prospective controlled trial (Sarin et al., 1987). Between 1 and 3 mL of sclerosant are injected into each of the major variceal columns just above the gastroesophageal junction (Figure 21.3). Paravariceal injections are occasionally used to stop bleeding from a puncture site (Howard et al., 1988). During the endoscopy, care must be taken not to overdistend the stomach with air in small children. Fluids and a soft diet are allowed within a few hours. Varices are initially injected every 1–2 weeks and then at monthly intervals until sclerosis is complete. Injection is deferred for 1 week if significant esophageal mucosal ulceration is present. Patients are given oral ranitidine and sucralfate for up to 2 weeks after each injection session in an attempt to reduce post-sclerotherapy complications (Guady et al., 1989; Kumar et al., 1993). Endoscopic reviews, usually as a day-case, are conducted after 6 months and then every 6 to 18 months. Larger recurrent varices should be treated. Antibiotic prophylaxis is recommended for those with damaged/prosthetic heart valves and for the immunosuppressed (Sauerbruch et al., 1985). Patients with cystic fibrosis should receive intensive perioperative chest physiotherapy, bronchodilators and prophylactic antibiotics.

In recent years, tissue adhesives such as cyanoacrylate have been used as an alternative sclerosant in adults. This substance is transformed from liquid into solid after injection into a varix, thereby achieving hemostasis. It may be advantageous for treating gastric varices and endoscopically accessible ectopic varices, but at present reported experience is confined to adults. Post-injection embolization of cyanoacrylate is a concern, although this complication is probably rare (Roesch and Rexroth, 1998).

Efficacy

In adults with cirrhosis, endoscopic injection sclerotherapy is of proven benefit in treating acute variceal bleeding and reducing recurrent bleeding, although there is only a trend towards reduced mortality (D'Amico et al., 1995). In children who are being managed in experienced centres, endoscopic injection sclerotherapy is a highly effective treatment for esophageal varices. In a series of 108 children who presented with variceal bleeding, complete sclerosis was achieved in all 36 patients with PVO and in 84% of those with chronic liver disease (Howard et al., 1988) (Table 21.1). Of the latter, obliteration of varices was not possible in those patients with liver failure who died or were transplanted. In the subgroup of patients with biliary atresia, injection sclerotherapy proved to be effective in controlling esophageal variceal bleeding in 15 out of 16 cases (94%) (Stringer et al., 1989). However, two children in this group with insignificant esophageal varices required a portosystemic shunt for obscure small bowel bleeding. Only one child died as a direct consequence of variceal bleeding. A mean number of 5–6 injection sessions was required during a mean period of 1 year. Similar successful results have been reported by other authors using injection sclerotherapy for variceal bleeding in children (Paquet, 1985; Yachha et al., 1997).

To assess the long-term effectiveness of esophageal sclerotherapy in PVO, 32 children were followed up for a mean period of 8.7 years after complete sclerosis (Stringer and Howard, 1994). Recurrent variceal bleeding developed in 10 patients (31%), but half of these were effectively controlled by further sclerotherapy.

Table 21.1 *Results of endoscopic injection sclerotherapy (Howard* et al., *1988)*

	Extrahepatic group (n = 36)	Intrahepatic group (n = 72)
Mean age at first injection (years)	7.8 (0.7–16.0)	8.4 (0.6–17.2)
Successful obliteration	100%	84%
Mean number of injections to obliteration	5.4 (3–13)	6.2 (2–15)
Mean time to obliteration (years)	0.7 (0.1–2.7)	0.9 (0.1–5.0)
Mean volume of sclerosant per injection session (mL)	9	9

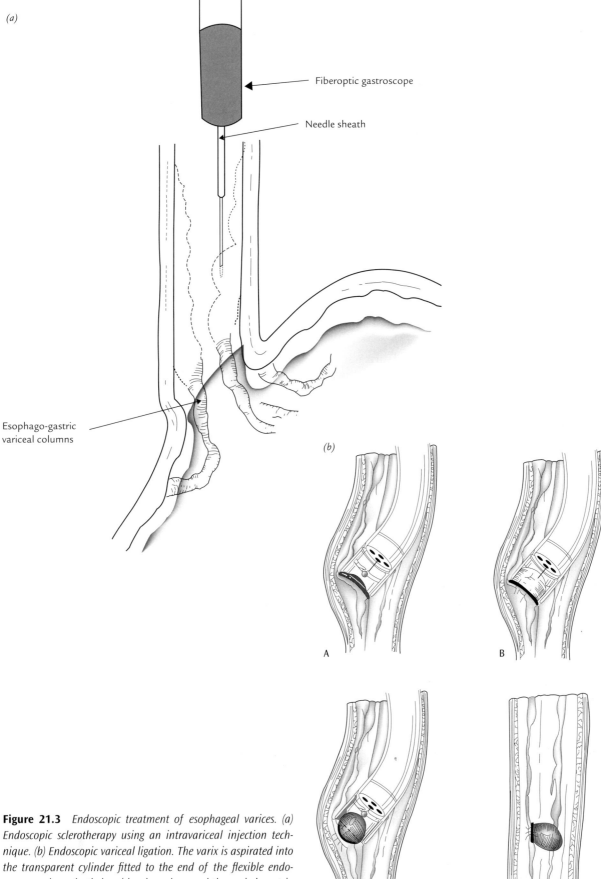

(a)

Fiberoptic gastroscope

Needle sheath

Esophago-gastric
variceal columns

(b)

A

B

C

D

Figure 21.3 *Endoscopic treatment of esophageal varices. (a) Endoscopic sclerotherapy using an intravariceal injection technique. (b) Endoscopic variceal ligation. The varix is aspirated into the transparent cylinder fitted to the end of the flexible endoscope, and an elastic band is released around the varix by a trip wire passing through the biopsy channel.*

Gastric variceal bleeding that was not amenable to sclerotherapy necessitated portosystemic shunt surgery in four cases (13%). Two patients required a splenectomy for symptomatic hypersplenism, and three children required a variety of local treatments for bleeding anorectal varices (Heaton *et al.*, 1992). Endoscopic injection sclerotherapy alone proved safe and effective in the long-term control of variceal bleeding from portal hypertension in more than 80% of children with PVO. Others have reported similar favorable long-term outcomes (Hassall *et al.*, 1989; Paquet and Lazar, 1994).

In children with cirrhosis, the long-term outcome is jeopardized not only by the complications of portal hypertension but also by deteriorating liver function. Primary treatment of bleeding esophageal varices is effective in controlling hemorrhage and, unlike portosystemic shunting, it does not reduce portal perfusion or carry the risk of encephalopathy, and it does not add to the technical difficulties of liver transplantation.

Pathological effects of sclerotherapy

Injection of sclerosant into the esophageal varix results in venous thrombosis, localized chemical esophagitis and mucosal ulceration (Evans *et al.*, 1982). The esophageal mucosa heals leaving residual mucosal tags (Plates 12 and 13) and the esophageal wall becomes more rigid. This may lead to esophageal dysmotility, gastro-esophageal reflux and stricture formation. Distant effects from the passage of sclerosant into systemic veins or tributaries of the portal venous system may also occur, but these are uncommon (Stringer and Howard, 1994).

Complications

Retrosternal discomfort and transient fever are common after injection sclerotherapy and usually resolve within 48 hours. Chemical phlebitis and/or transient bacteremia may be responsible for the fever (Sauerbruch *et al.*, 1985), and children with significant pyrexia ($> 38°C$) should be treated with intravenous antibiotics pending the results of blood cultures.

Injection sclerotherapy has been associated with numerous complications (Box 21.5). Most of these have been described in the vast numbers of adults with cirrhosis treated by sclerotherapy. Serious complications of the technique in children are rare. However, more significant complications of sclerotherapy in children include esophageal stricture in 16% of cases (responding to simple dilatation), recurrent esophageal varices, and bleeding before complete variceal obliteration in 40% of cases (Howard *et al.*, 1988). The latter is usually due to a non-thrombosed varix or an injection ulcer. Most sclerotherapy ulcers are asymptomatic and an inevitable temporary consequence of the sclerosant (Reilly *et al.*, 1984; Sarin *et al.*, 1986). They more often follow frequent or large-volume injections, but may also be related to the depth of injection. In recent years, local complication

---

Box 21.5 *Reported complications of endoscopic injection sclerotherapy for esophageal varices (Stringer, 1998)*

Esophageal ulceration and stricture
Esophageal perforation and mediastinitis
Variceal hemorrhage (uncontrolled or recurrent varices)
Esophageal dysmotility and gastro-esophageal reflux

Broncho-esophageal fistula
Pleural effusion/chylothorax/empyema
Thoracic duct perforation
Respiratory distress syndrome
Pulmonary collapse/consolidation/embolism
Pericardial effusion/tamponade/pericarditis

Portal vein thrombosis

Paraplegia
Cerebral abscess
Digital gangrene
Bacteremia/septicemia
Transient coagulopathy/disseminated intravascular coagulation
Anaphylaxis
Acute renal failure

---

rates have been significantly lower in the author's practice (without any reduction in efficacy), probably as a result of injecting smaller volumes of sclerosant.

Bleeding after variceal obliteration may be due to recurrent varices or to other pathology, such as peptic ulceration. The impact of esophageal variceal sclerotherapy on gastric varices is variable. Gastric varices have been observed to develop (Mathur *et al.*, 1990), disappear (Sarin *et al.*, 1988) or persist unchanged during esophageal variceal sclerotherapy. Contrast studies indicate that the disappearance of gastric varices is due to retrograde flow of sclerosant from esophageal to gastric varices (Grobe *et al.*, 1984). The low incidence of bleeding from gastric varices after obliteration of esophageal varices in children is reassuring.

Some children develop esophageal dysmotility and gastro-esophageal reflux which may cause intermittent dysphagia and heartburn (Greenholz *et al.*, 1988). Systemic dissemination of the injected sclerosant leading to distant complications has been reported, but it appears to be rare in children (Stringer, 1998). The potential long-term risk of neoplasia from childhood sclerotherapy remains a concern but, despite the global application of this technique in patients with variceal bleeding, there are only a few isolated reports of this potential association in adults (Kokudo *et al.*, 1990). Moreover, recognized risk factors for esophageal cancer have coexisted in these cases, and a study using brush cytology failed to support an association (Dina *et al.*, 1992). Nevertheless, the long-term morbidity of sclerotherapy must remain under review.

VARICEAL LIGATION (BANDING)

Introduced by Stiegmann and Goff in 1988, this technique involves the endoscopic application of an elastic band to a variceal column. The strangulated varix subsequently thromboses and sloughs (Figure 21.3 above). The ligating device is attached to the end of the endoscope, which must be introduced gently, and an overtube is not used in children. Treatment begins with ligation of the most distal variceal column in the esophagus just above the gastro-esophageal junction. Usually up to three bands are applied at each session, one on each of the major variceal columns. Multi-band devices allow the application of several bands without the need for reloading. Treatments are performed initially at 1- to 2-weekly intervals, extending to monthly intervals once the larger varices have been treated.

In adults, endoscopic variceal ligation is of comparable efficacy to injection sclerotherapy in controlling active variceal bleeding, but it appears to achieve more rapid eradication, with fewer treatment sessions and lower complication rates. Esophageal ulcers caused by banding are more superficial and resolve more quickly than sclerotherapy-induced ulcers (Marks et al., 1993; Young et al., 1993). The incidence of esophageal stricture and systemic side-effects is lower (Binmoeller and Soehendra, 1996). As a result, endoscopic variceal ligation is now regarded as the optimum method for treating active variceal bleeding and preventing re-bleeding from esophageal varices in adults. The synchronous use of band ligation and sclerotherapy has not been shown to be superior to band ligation alone, but a metachronous approach using sclerotherapy to treat recurrent varices after band ligation has been shown to be beneficial (Binmoeller and Borsatto, 2000).

Several small studies of endoscopic variceal ligation have been reported in children, confirming both its safety and its efficacy (Cano et al., 1995; Fox et al., 1995; Price et al., 1996; Reinoso et al., 1997; Sasaki et al., 1998; McKiernan and Davison, 1999). The largest of these reported on 22 children who were treated during a 9-year period (Price et al., 1996). Variceal eradication was achieved after a mean of four sessions. Complications included bleeding between sessions (n = 6), cervical esophageal perforation (n = 1) and recurrent varices (n = 1). In another series which included 11 patients with biliary atresia and esophageal varices, 73% were improved after one to seven sessions of variceal ligation (Sasaki et al., 1998). At present, equipment limitations make the technique difficult to use in small children (< 2 years of age), but technical modifications or endoscopic clipping devices may overcome these obstacles. Long-term follow-up data on larger cohorts of patients are required to determine whether variceal recurrence rates in children are comparable to those after sclerotherapy.

Gastric varices

Many gastric varices are fundal and directly contiguous with lower esophageal varices (gastro-esophageal varices) (Plate 14). These are usually observed at endoscopy for bleeding esophageal varices, and are frequently eradicated during the treatment of esophageal varices by injection sclerotherapy (Stringer, 1998). However, 5–10% of patients will develop significant gastric varices after eradication of esophageal varices. Bleeding from gastric varices may respond to injection sclerotherapy, but this is much less likely if the gastric varices are not contiguous with esophageal varices (isolated gastric varices) (Sarin, 1997). Alternative sclerosants, such as bovine thrombin and cyanoacrylate, have been used successfully in adults with gastric varices (Binmoeller and Soehendra, 1996; Binmoeller and Borsatto, 2000) but have not been formally evaluated in children. Band ligation of gastric varices is associated with a high re-bleeding rate. If sclerotherapy is ineffective or inappropriate, then portosystemic shunting or under-running of the bleeding varix, with or without a local devascularization procedure, may be necessary (Heaton and Howard, 1993).

It is important to exclude isolated splenic vein obstruction as a cause of gastric varices, since this condition may be treated effectively by splenectomy.

Ectopic varices

Bleeding from suspected ectopic varices is best investigated by endoscopy and angiography (see Chapter 23). Although local resection may be effective in the short term, recurrence is common and portosystemic shunting (see Chapter 22) or liver transplantation, depending on the presence and severity of any underlying liver disease, is usually required for persistent bleeding. Bleeding from anorectal varices is uncommon and can usually be controlled by local measures such as injection sclerotherapy or banding, but occasionally portosystemic shunting is necessary (Heaton et al., 1992).

Primary prophylaxis of variceal bleeding

BETA-BLOCKERS

Propranolol reduces portal pressure by causing splanchnic vasoconstriction and reducing cardiac output. Several randomized controlled trials have demonstrated its efficacy in preventing both the first variceal bleed and re-bleeding in adults with cirrhosis (Hayes et al., 1990; Binmoeller and Borsatto, 2000). If there are no contraindications to beta-blockade (e.g. asthma), treatment is aimed at reducing the resting pulse rate by 25%. Uncontrolled studies in children suggest a possible benefit with minimal side-effects (Shashidhar et al., 1999). Children with PVO and those with cirrhosis and large varices may particularly benefit from primary prophylaxis with beta-blockers.

ENDOSCOPIC THERAPY

The value of primary prophylactic injection sclerotherapy is controversial. A small proportion of patients with PVO never bleed (Lykavieris *et al.*, 2000). The single prospective randomized controlled trial in children (predominantly with intrahepatic disease) showed no survival advantage for prophylactic sclerotherapy during a median follow-up period of 4.5 years, and suggested that prophylactic treatment of esophageal varices may actually encourage the development of portal gastropathy and gastric varices which are less amenable to treatment (Goncalves *et al.*, 2000). Results from the many trials performed in adults with cirrhosis have been conflicting, and routine primary prophylaxis in children cannot be recommended on the basis of these data. The availability of local resources is probably a more important factor influencing prophylactic therapy in the individual child.

The safety and efficacy of band ligation have stimulated renewed interest in primary endoscopic prophylaxis of variceal bleeding. Although randomized trials in adults have shown a benefit for band ligation compared with no active treatment (Lay *et al.*, 1997), any advantage of this intervention over beta-blocker therapy has not been established (Binmoeller and Borsatto, 2000). Moreover, variceal recurrence after band ligation may eliminate any theoretical advantage.

Transjugular intrahepatic portosystemic shunt (TIPS)

This intervention involves the percutaneous transjugular insertion of an expandable metallic stent between a hepatic and portal vein under radiological guidance. Under fluoroscopic guidance, a guidewire is passed into a hepatic vein. A needle is then advanced over the guidewire into the hepatic vein and thence to the portal vein. A balloon catheter is then used to dilate the intrahepatic tract and the stent is deployed (Heyman and LaBerge, 1999) (Figure 21.4).

The indications for TIPS in children include uncontrolled acute variceal bleeding, and also control of recurrent variceal bleeding in patients who are awaiting liver transplantation (a 'bridge to transplantation') (Schweizer *et al.*, 1995; Heyman and LaBerge, 1999). Selected patients with Budd–Chiari syndrome (Figure 21.4) or intractable ascites may also benefit. Portal vein occlusion, intrahepatic malignancy, bacterial sepsis, hepatic arterial insufficiency and uncorrected coagulopathy are contraindications.

In adults, effective portal decompression is achieved with low procedural complication rates, but there are medium- and long-term risks of stent occlusion and hepatic encephalopathy (Jalan *et al.*, 2000). The incidence of shunt occlusion, which is usually secondary to pseudointimal hyperplasia, increases with time. This complication may lead to portomesenteric venous thrombosis. Regular shunt surveillance and prophylactic dilatation or the use of coated stents may reduce the risk of stent thrombosis. These and other complications, and the technical demands of the procedure in smaller patients, have limited its role in children (Heyman and LaBerge, 1999). Nevertheless, TIPS has been successfully performed in children as young as 3 years of age and as small as 13 kg in weight. The long-term patency rates in children are not yet known.

TIPS is also discussed in Chapters 22 and 23 in the context of surgical management of portal hypertension in children.

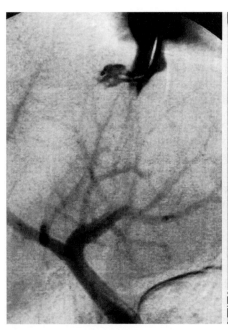 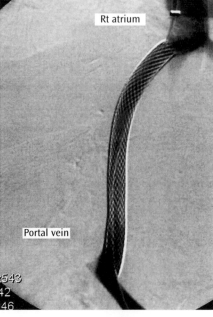

Figure 21.4 *Transjugular intrahepatic portosystemic shunt (TIPS) in a patient with Budd–Chiari syndrome due to hepatic vein occlusion. Images have been taken before and after stent deployment between the stump of the hepatic vein above and the portal vein below. (Reproduced courtesy of Dr David Kessel, Leeds.)*

Surgery for portal hypertension

A variety of surgical treatments may be required for the management of portal hypertension in children, and these are discussed in detail in Chapter 22.

Endoscopic therapy offers effective primary treatment of bleeding esophageal varices in the majority of children with reasonable liver function. Nevertheless, surgical intervention is indicated for the following:

- uncontrolled bleeding from esophageal varices (not responding to at least two sessions of banding or sclerotherapy);
- bleeding gastric or ectopic varices (not controlled endoscopically);
- massive splenomegaly causing symptoms or severe hypersplenism;
- lack of access to expert endoscopic therapy;
- symptomatic biliary obstruction from choledochal varices;
- variceal bleeding complicating severe chronic liver disease;
- selected patients with Budd–Chiari syndrome.

Portosystemic shunt surgery should be regarded as a complementary therapy to endoscopic treatment. Portomesenteric venous anatomy does not permit successful shunt surgery in every child, and shunt thrombosis has been recorded with all types of shunts, especially in small children (Bismuth et al., 1980; Mitra et al., 1993; Orloff et al., 1994; Prasad et al., 1994). Endoscopic treatment may be the only possible approach to bleeding esophageal varices in such patients. The recent introduction of the mesenterico-left portal (Rex) shunt is certain to broaden the indications once more for shunt surgery as the *primary* treatment for children with PVO (de Ville de Goyet et al., 1998, 1999; Bambini et al., 2000). This shunt, which was first developed as a portal vein bypass in patients with portal vein thrombosis complicating liver transplantation, utilizes an interposition graft between the superior mesenteric vein and the intrahepatic portion of the left portal vein which is identified in the Rex recessus adjacent to the falciform ligament. By restoring hepatic portal blood flow and correcting portal hypertension, the technique is more physiological and obviates the potential disadvantages of portosystemic shunts.

Both endoscopic therapy and surgical portosystemic shunting may be effective in children with variceal bleeding complicating cystic fibrosis, provided that they have reasonably satisfactory liver and lung function (Stringer et al., 1993; Debray et al., 1999). Although choledochal varices rarely cause symptomatic bile duct obstruction in children, experience in adults indicates that portosystemic shunting rather than a direct approach to the biliary tract is the optimum treatment in most cases (Chaudhary et al., 1998).

Splenectomy may be necessary for massive splenomegaly causing severe hypersplenism or abdominal pain, and may be combined with a portosystemic shunt. Splenic embolization is an alternative, but the effects may be temporary and the procedure may be associated with significant morbidity (Brandt et al., 1989).

Liver transplantation is the treatment of choice for children with variceal bleeding complicating end-stage chronic liver disease. Survival after transplantation is not compromised by previous portosystemic shunt for surgery, although operative morbidity may be higher if the porta hepatis has been disturbed by the shunt procedures (Mazzaferro et al., 1990).

In the absence of a surgically treatable cause such as a caval web, many patients with Budd–Chiari syndrome can be successfully managed by medical therapy aimed at controlling ascites and preventing progressive hepatic vein thrombosis. Portal decompression by portosystemic shunting, rather than endoscopic therapy, is often required in patients with variceal bleeding. Mesocaval shunting is usually performed unless there is significant caval compression by caudate lobe hypertrophy in which case TIPS or mesoatrial shunting has to be considered (Slakey et al., 2001). Liver transplantation is required for patients with acute liver failure or advanced cirrhosis. Recurrence of Budd–Chiari syndrome in the liver graft is a recognized hazard, and patients with an underlying thrombophilia usually require lifelong anticoagulation (Halff et al., 1990).

Treatment of an arterioportal fistula is directed at the fistula rather than the varices. Selective angiography and arterial embolization is the treatment of choice for an acquired arterioportal fistula. Arterial embolization, hepatic artery ligation and hepatic resection are the usual options for a congenital fistula, but transplantation is occasionally necessary (Marchand et al., 1999; Stringer et al., 1999).

CONCLUSIONS

The management of children with bleeding esophageal varices demands the use of a variety of complementary techniques, each of which may be limited by its applicability, efficacy and complications. Endoscopic sclerotherapy is highly effective and has an established track record. Banding techniques may prove even more effective, with fewer complications, but greater experience is needed in children. Bleeding from gastric fundal varices may respond to injection with newer sclerosants. Portosystemic shunting has a definite place in the treatment of bleeding esophageal varices that are unresponsive to endoscopic therapy, and for bleeding from gastrointestinal varices. Liver transplantation is the procedure of choice for patients with complications of portal hypertension associated with end-stage liver disease. The role of novel therapies such as TIPS and the Rex shunt has yet to be precisely determined, but the latter in particular offers the exciting prospect of cure in selected children with PVO.

Key references

de Ville de Goyet J, Alberti D, Clapuyt P et al. Direct bypassing of extrahepatic portal venous obstruction in children: a new technique for combined hepatic portal revascularization and treatment of extrahepatic portal hypertension. *Journal of Pediatric Surgery* 1998; **33**: 597–601.

This article contains a detailed description of this novel portal bypass procedure applicable to selected patients with extrahepatic portal hypertension. Technical variations and results in seven children are reported.

Goncalves ME, Cardoso SR, Maksoud JG. Prophylactic sclerotherapy in children with esophageal varices: long-term results of a controlled prospective randomized trial. *Journal of Pediatric Surgery* 2000; **35**: 401–5.

The only prospective randomized study to examine the role of prophylactic injection sclerotherapy in children. The study population consisted of 100 consecutive children with cirrhotic and non-cirrhotic portal hypertension from Brazil. Prophylactic sclerotherapy was safe and reduced the incidence of bleeding from esophageal varices, but it increased the risk of bleeding from gastric varices and portal gastropathy. The overall survival rate (83%) was not improved by prophylactic sclerotherapy during a median follow-up period of 4.5 years.

Heyman MB, LaBerge JM. Role of transjugular intrahepatic portosystemic shunt in the treatment of portal hypertension in pediatric patients. *Journal of Pediatric Gastroenterology and Nutrition* 1999; **29:** 240–9.

A useful review article on TIPS therapy in children.

Howard ER, Stringer MD, Mowat AP. Assessment of injection sclerotherapy in the management of 152 children with oesophageal varices. *British Journal of Surgery* 1988; **75**: 404–8.

Experience of endoscopic injection sclerotherapy is described in a consecutive series of 108 children presenting with bleeding esophageal varices at King's College Hospital, London. This paper details the safety and efficacy of this technique in a broad spectrum of patients. The complications of sclerotherapy may have decreased since this publication.

Price MR, Sartorelli KH, Karrer FM et al. Management of esophageal varices in children by endoscopic variceal ligation. *Journal of Pediatric Surgery* 1996; **31**: 1056–9.

An early report of experience with endoscopic variceal ligation in children from the Pediatric Liver Center in Denver, Colorado.

REFERENCES

Alvarez F, Bernard O, Brunelle F, Hadchouel P, Odievre M, Algille D. Portal obstruction in children. II. Results of surgical portosystemic shunts. *Journal of Pediatrics* 1983; **103**: 703–7.

Ando H, Kaneko K, Ito F, Seo T, Watanabe H, Ito T. Anatomy and etiology of extrahepatic portal vein obstruction in children leading to bleeding esophageal varices. *Journal of the American College of Surgeons* 1996; **183**: 543–7.

Attal M, Huguet F, Rubie H et al. Prevention of hepatic veno-occlusive disease after bone marrow transplantation by continuous infusion of low-dose heparin: a prospective randomized trial. *Blood* 1992; **79**: 2834–40.

Bambini DA, Superina R, Almond PS, Whitington PF, Alonso E. Experience with the Rex shunt (mesenterico-left portal bypass) in children with extrahepatic portal hypertension. *Journal of Pediatric Surgery* 2000; **35**: 13–19.

Binmoeller KF, Soehendra PS. Treatment of esophagogastric varices. *Endoscopy* 1996; **28**: 44–53.

Binmoeller KF, Borsatto R. Variceal bleeding and portal hypertension. *Endoscopy* 2000; **32**: 189–99.

Bismuth H, Franco D, Alagille D. Portal diversion for portal hypertension in children. *Annals of Surgery* 1980; **192**: 18–24.

Boles ET, Wise WE, Birken G. Extrahepatic portal hypertension in children: long-term evaluation. *American Journal of Surgery* 1986; **151**: 734–9.

Boughton BJ. Hepatic and portal vein thrombosis. *British Medical Journal* 1991; **302**: 192–3.

Brady L, Magilavy D, Black DD. Portal vein thrombosis associated with antiphospholipid antibodies in a child. *Journal of Pediatric Gastroenterology and Nutrition* 1996; **23**: 473.

Brandt CT, Rothbarth LJ, Kumpe DA et al. Splenic embolization in children: long-term efficacy. *Journal of Pediatric Surgery* 1989; **24**: 642–5.

Buscarini E, Buscarini L, Danesino C et al. Hepatic vascular malformations in hereditary hemorrhagic telangiectasia: Doppler sonographic screening in a large family. *Journal of Hepatology* 1997; **26**: 111–18.

Campbell RE. Roentgenologic features of umbilical vascular catheterization in the newborn. *American Journal of Roentgenology* 1971; **112**: 68–76.

Cano I, Urruzuno P, Medina E et al. Treatment of esophageal varices by endoscopic ligation in children. *European Journal of Pediatric Surgery* 1995; **5**: 299–302.

Carson JA, Tunell WP, Barnes P, Altshuler G. Hepatoportal sclerosis in childhood: a mimic of extrahepatic portal vein obstruction. *Journal of Pediatric Surgery* 1981; **16**: 291–6.

Cedro A, Kaminski W, Bokszczanin L, Ismall H. Surgical treatment of portal hypertension in children: experience with portosystemic shunts. *Surgery in Childhood International* 1993; **1**: 42–6.

Chaudhary A, Dhar P, Sarin SK *et al.* Bile duct obstruction due to portal biliopathy in extrahepatic portal hypertension: surgical management. *British Journal of Surgery* 1998; **85**: 326–9.

Crafoord C, Frenckner P. New surgical treatment of varicose veins of the oesophagus. *Acta Otolaryngologica* 1939; **27**: 422–9.

D'Amico G, Pagliaro L, Bosch J. The treatment of portal hypertension: a meta-analytic review. *Hepatology* 1995; **22**: 332–54.

Dawson JL. Oesophageal varices: curiosities. *British Medical Journal* 1983; **286**: 826.

Debray D, Lykavieris P, Gauthier F *et al.* Outcome of cystic fibrosis-associated liver cirrhosis: management of portal hypertension. *Journal of Hepatology* 1999; **31**: 77–83.

Denninger MH, Chait Y, Casadevall N *et al.* Cause of portal or hepatic venous thrombosis in adults: the role of multiple concurrent factors. *Hepatology* 2000; **31**: 587–91.

de Ville de Goyet J, Alberti D, Clapuyt P *et al.* Direct bypassing of extrahepatic portal venous obstruction in children: a new technique for combined hepatic portal revascularization and treatment of extrahepatic portal hypertension. *Journal of Pediatric Surgery* 1998; **33**: 597–601.

de Ville de Goyet J, Alberti D, Falchetti D *et al.* Treatment of extrahepatic portal hypertension in children by mesenteric-to-left portal vein bypass: a new physiological procedure. *European Journal of Surgery* 1999; **165**: 777–81.

Dina R, Cassisa A, Baroncini D, D'Imperio N. Role of esophageal brushing cytology in monitoring patients treated with sclerotherapy for esophageal varices. *Acta Cytologica* 1992; **36**: 477–9.

Dubuisson C, Boyer-Neumann C, Wolf M, Meyer D, Bernard O. Protein C, protein S and antithrombin III in children with portal vein obstruction. *Journal of Hepatology* 1997; **27**: 132–5.

Eroglu Y, Emerick KM, Whitington PF, Alonso EM. Octreotide is effective in controlling gastrointestinal bleeding in children. *Journal of Pediatric Gastroenterology and Nutrition* 1999; **29**: 512.

Evans D, Jones D, Cleary B, Smith P. Oesophageal varices treated by sclerotherapy: a histopathological study. *Gut* 1982; **23**: 615–20.

Fearon B, Sass-Kortsak A. The management of esophageal varices in children by injection of sclerosing agents. *Annals of Otology, Rhinology and Laryngology* 1959; **68**: 906–15.

Fisher NC, Wilde JT, Roper J, Elias E. Deficiency of natural anticoagulant protein C, S and antithrombin in portal vein thrombosis: a secondary phenomenon? *Gut* 2000; **46**: 534–9.

Fox VL, Carr-Locke DL, Connors PJ, Leichtner AM. Endoscopic ligation of esophageal varices in children. *Journal of Pediatric Gastroenterology and Nutrition* 1995; **20**: 202–8.

Garcia-Tsao G, Groszmann RJ, Fisher RL *et al.* Portal pressure, presence of gastrovarices and variceal bleeding. *Hepatology* 1985; **5**: 419–24.

Gentil-Kocher S, Bernard O, Brunelle F *et al.* Budd–Chiari syndrome in children: report of 22 cases. *Journal of Pediatrics* 1988; **113**: 30–8.

Goncalves ME, Cardoso SR, Maksoud JG. Prophylactic sclerotherapy in children with esophageal varices: long-term results of a controlled prospective randomized trial. *Journal of Pediatric Surgery* 2000; **35**: 401–5.

Gotzsche PC. Somatostatin or octreotide for acute bleeding oesophageal varices (Cochrane Review). In: *The Cochrane Library. Issue 2*. Oxford: Update Software, 2000.

Greenholz SK, Hall RJ, Sonheimer JM, Lilly JR, Hernandez-Cano AM. Manometric and pH consequences of esophageal endosclerosis in children. *Journal of Pediatric Surgery* 1988; **23**: 38–41.

Grobe JL, Kozarek RA, Sanowski RA, Le Grand J, Kovac A. Venography during endoscopic injection sclerotherapy of oesophageal varices. *Gastrointestinal Endoscopy* 1984; **30**: 6–8.

Guady H, Rosman A, Korssen M. Prevention of stricture formation after endoscopic sclerotherapy of esophageal varices. *Gastrointestinal Endoscopy* 1989; **35**: 377–80.

Gupta TK, Chen L, Groszmann RJ. Pathophysiology of portal hypertension. *Clinical Liver Disease* 1997; **1**: 1–12.

Gurakan F, Gurgey A, Bakkaloglu A, Kocak N. Homozygous factor V Leiden mutation in a child with Budd–Chiari syndrome. *Journal of Pediatric Gastroenterology and Nutrition* 1999; **28**: 516–17.

Halff G, Todo S, Tzakis AG, Gordon RD, Starzl TE. Liver transplantation for the Budd–Chiari syndrome. *Annals of Surgery* 1990; **211**: 43–9.

Hassall E, Berquist WE, Ament ME, Vargas J, Dorney S. Sclerotherapy for extrahepatic portal hypertension in childhood. *Journal of Pediatrics* 1989; **115**: 69–74.

Hayes PC, Davis JM, Lewis JA, Bouchier IA. Meta-analysis of the value of propranolol in the prevention of variceal haemorrhage. *Lancet* 1990; **336**: 153–6.

Heaton ND, Howard ER. Complications and limitations of injection sclerotherapy in portal hypertension. *Gut* 1993; **34**: 7–10.

Heaton ND, Davenport M, Howard ER. Symptomatic haemorrhoids and anorectal varices in children with portal hypertension. *Journal of Pediatric Surgery* 1992; **27**: 833–5.

Heaton ND, Davenport M, Howard ER. Incidence of haemorrhoids and anorectal varices in children with portal hypertension. *British Journal of Surgery* 1993; **80**: 616–18.

Heaton ND, Davenport M, Karani J, Mowat AP, Howard ER. Congenital hepatoportal arteriovenous fistula. *Surgery* 1995; **117**: 170–4.

Heyman MB, LaBerge JM. Role of transjugular intrahepatic portosystemic shunt in the treatment of portal hypertension in pediatric patients. *Journal of Pediatric Gastroenterology and Nutrition* 1999; **29**: 240–9.

Howard ER, Stringer MD, Mowat AP. Assessment of injection sclerotherapy in the management of 152 children with oesophageal varices. *British Journal of Surgery* 1988; **75**: 404–8.

Jalan R, Lui HF, Redhead DN, Hayes PC. TIPSS 10 years on. *Gut* 2000; **46**: 578–81.

Johnston GW, Rodgers HW. A review of 15 years' experience in the use of sclerotherapy in the control of acute haemorrhage from oesophageal varices. *British Journal of Surgery* 1973; **60**: 797–800.

Khuroo MS, Yattoo GN, Zargar SA *et al.* Biliary abnormalities associated with extrahepatic portal venous obstruction. *Hepatology* 1993; **17**: 807–13.

Kokudo N, Sanio K, Umekita N, Harihara Y, Tada Y, Idezuki Y. Squamous-cell carcinoma after endoscopic injection sclerotherapy for esophageal varices. *American Journal of Gastroenterology* 1990; **85**: 861–4.

Kozaiwa K, Tajiri H, Yoshimura N *et al.* Utility of duplex Doppler ultrasound in evaluating portal hypertension in children. *Journal of Pediatric Gastroenterology and Nutrition* 1995; **21**: 215–19.

Kullendorff CM, Bekassy AN. Hepatic veno-occlusive disease in Wilms' tumor. *European Journal of Pediatric Surgery* 1996; **6**: 338–40.

Kumar A, Mehta SR, Joshi V, Kasthuri AS, Narayanan VA. Ranitidine for the prevention of complications following endoscopic sclerotherapy for esophageal varices. *Journal of the Association of Physicians of India* 1993; **41**: 584–9.

Lay CS, Tsai YT, Teg CY *et al.* Endoscopic variceal ligation in prophylaxis of first variceal bleeding in cirrhotic patients with high-risk esophageal varices. *Hepatology* 1997; **25**: 1346–50.

Lebrec D, Benhamou JP. Ectopic varices in portal hypertension. *Clinical Gastroenterology* 1985; **14**: 105–21.

Lebrec D, DeFleury P, Rueff B *et al.* Portal hypertension, size of esophageal varices, and risk of gastrointestinal bleeding in alcoholic cirrhosis. *Gastroenterology* 1980; **79**: 1139–44.

Lenthall R, Kane PA, Heaton ND, Karani JB. Segmental portal hypertension due to splenic vein obstruction: imaging findings and diagnostic pitfalls in four cases. *Clinical Radiology* 1999; **54**: 540–4.

Losty PD, Lynch MJ, Guiney EJ. Long-term outcome after surgery for extrahepatic portal vein thrombosis. *Archives of Disease in Childhood* 1994; **71**: 437–40.

Lykavieris P, Gauthier F, Hadchouel P, Duche M, Bernard O. Risk of gastrointestinal bleeding during adolescence and early adulthood in children with portal vein obstruction. *Journal of Pediatrics* 2000; **136**: 805–8.

McKiernan PJ, Davison SM. A prospective study of endoscopic oesophageal variceal ligation using a multi-band ligator. *Journal of Pediatric Gastroenterology and Nutrition* 1999; **28**: 583.

Maksoud JG, Goncalves ME, Porta G, Miura I, Velhote MC. The endoscopic and surgical management of portal hypertension in children: analysis of 123 cases. *Journal of Pediatric Surgery* 1991; **26**: 178–81.

Marchand V, Uflacker R, Baker SS, Baker RD. Congenital hepatic arterioportal fistula in a 3-year-old child. *Journal of Pediatric Gastroenterology and Nutrition* 1999; **28**: 435–41.

Marks C. Surgical implications of portal venous system malformation. *Annals of the Royal College of Surgeons of England* 1974; **55**: 299–306.

Marks RD, Arnold MD, Baron TH. Gross and microscopic findings in the human esophagus after esophageal variceal band ligation: a postmortem analysis. *American Journal of Gastroenterology* 1993; **88**: 272–4.

Mathur SK, Dalvi AN, Someshwar V, Supe AN, Ramakantan R. Endoscopic and radiological appraisal of gastric varices. *British Journal of Surgery* 1990; **77**: 432–5.

Mazzaferro V, Todo S, Tzakis AG, Stieber AC, Makowka L, Starzl TE. Liver transplantation in patients with previous portasystemic shunts. *American Journal of Surgery* 1990; **160**: 111–16.

Mehrotra RN, Bhatia V, Dabadghao P, Yachha SK. Extrahepatic portal vein obstruction in children: anthropometry, growth hormone, and insulin-like growth factor I. *Journal of Pediatric Gastroenterology and Nutrition* 1997; **25**: 520–3.

Mikkelsen WP, Edmondson HA, Peters RL, Redeker AG, Reynolds TB. Extra- and intrahepatic portal hypertension without cirrhosis (hepatoportal sclerosis). *Annals of Surgery* 1965; **162**: 602–20.

Mitra SK, Rao KLN, Narasimhan KL *et al.* Side-to-side lienorenal shunt without splenectomy in non-cirrhotic portal hypertension in children. *Journal of Pediatric Surgery* 1993; **28**: 398–402.

Nayak NC, Ramalingaswami V. Obliterative portal venopathy of the liver: associated with so-called idiopathic portal hypertension or tropical splenomegaly. *Archives of Pathology* 1969; **87**: 359–69.

Odievre M, Pige G, Alagille D. Congenital abnormalities associated with extrahepatic portal hypertension. *Archives of Disease in Childhood* 1977; **52**: 383–5.

Orloff MJ, Orloff MS, Rambotti M. Treatment of bleeding oesophagogastric varices due to extrahepatic portal hypertension: results of portal-systemic shunts during 35 years. *Journal of Pediatric Surgery* 1994; **29**: 142–54.

Pande GK, Reddy VM, Kar P *et al.* Operations for portal hypertension due to extrahepatic obstruction: results and 10-year follow-up. *British Medical Journal* 1987; **295**: 1115–17.

Paquet KJ. Ten years' experience with paravariceal injection sclerotherapy of esophageal varices in children. *Journal of Pediatric Surgery* 1985; **20**: 109–12.

Paquet KJ, Lazar A. Current therapeutic strategy in bleeding esophageal varices in babies and children and long-term results of endoscopic paravariceal sclerotherapy over 20 years. *European Journal of Pediatric Surgery* 1994; **4**: 165–72.

Prasad AS, Gupta S, Kohli V, Pande GK, Sahni P, Nundy S. Proximal splenorenal shunts for extrahepatic portal venous obstruction in children. *Annals of Surgery* 1994; **219**: 193–6.

Price MR, Sartorelli KH, Karrer FM *et al*. Management of esophageal varices in children by endoscopic variceal ligation. *Journal of Pediatric Surgery* 1996; **31**: 1056–9.

Reilly JJ, Schade RR, Van Rhiel DS. Esophageal function after injection sclerotherapy: pathogenesis of esophageal stricture. *American Journal of Surgery* 1984; **147**: 85–8.

Reinoso MA, Sharp HL, Rank J. Endoscopic variceal ligation in pediatric patients with portal hypertension secondary to liver cirrhosis. *Gastrointestinal Endoscopy* 1997; **46**: 244–6.

Roesch W, Rexroth G. Pulmonary, cerebral and coronary emboli during bucrylate injection of bleeding fundic varices. *Endoscopy* 1998; **30**: S89–90.

Sarin SK. Long-term follow-up of gastric variceal sclerotherapy: an 11-year experience. *Gastrointestinal Endoscopy* 1997; **46**: 8–14.

Sarin SK, Nanda R, Vij JC, Anand BS. Esophageal ulceration after endoscopic sclerotherapy – an accompaniment or a complication? *Endoscopy* 1986; **18**: 44–5.

Sarin SK, Nanda R, Sachdev G, Chari S, Anand BS, Broor SI. Intravariceal versus paravariceal sclerotherapy: a prospective, controlled, randomised trial. *Gut* 1987; **28**: 657–62.

Sarin SK, Sachdev G, Nanda R, Misra SP, Broor SL. Endoscopic sclerotherapy in the treatment of gastric varices. *British Journal of Surgery* 1988; **75**: 747–50.

Sarin SK, Bansal A, Sasan S, Nigam A. Portal vein obstruction in children leads to growth retardation. *Hepatology* 1992; **15**: 229–33.

Sasaki T, Hasegawa T, Nakajima K *et al*. Endoscopic variceal ligation in the management of gastroesophageal varices in postoperative biliary atresia. *Journal of Pediatric Surgery* 1998; **33**: 1628–32.

Sauerbruch T, Holl J, Ruckdeschel G. Bacteraemia associated with endoscopic sclerotherapy of oesophageal varices. *Endoscopy* 1985; **17**: 170–2.

Schuijtvlot ET, Bax NMA, Houwen RHJ, Hruda J. Unexpected lethal pulmonary hypertension in a 5-year-old girl successfully treated for biliary atresia. *Journal of Pediatric Surgery* 1995; **4**: 589–90.

Schweizer P, Brambs HJ, Schweizer M, Astfalk W. TIPS: a new therapy for esophageal variceal bleeding caused by EHBA. *European Journal of Pediatric Surgery* 1995; **5**: 211–15.

Shashidhar H, Langhans NA, Grand RJ. Propranolol in prevention of portal hypertensive haemorrhage in children: a pilot study. *Journal of Pediatric Gastroenterology and Nutrition* 1999; **29**: 12–17.

Shulman HM, Hinterberg W. Hepatic veno-occlusive disease – liver toxicity syndrome after bone marrow transplantation. *Bone Marrow Transplantation* 1992; **10**: 197–214.

Shun A, Delaney DP, Martin HC *et al*. Portosystemic shunting for paediatric portal hypertension. *Journal of Pediatric Surgery* 1997; **32**: 489–93.

Siafakas C, Fox VL, Nurko S. Use of octreotide for the treatment of severe gastrointestinal bleeding in children. *Journal of Pediatric Gastroenterology and Nutrition* 1998; **26**: 356–9.

Slakey DP, Klein AS, Venbrux AC, Cameron JL. Budd–Chiari syndrome: current management options. *Annals of Surgery* 2001; **233**: 522–7.

Sperl W, Stuppner H, Gassner I, Judmaier W, Dietze O, Vogel W. Reversible hepatic veno-occlusive disease in an infant after consumption of pyrrolizidine-containing herbal tea. *European Journal of Pediatrics* 1995; **154**: 112–16.

Stiegmann GV, Goff JS. Endoscopic oesophageal varix ligation. Preliminary clinical experience. *Gastrointestinal Endoscopy* 1988; **34**: 113–17.

Stringer MD. Injection sclerotherapy of esophageal varices. In: Stringer MD, Oldham KT, Mouriquand PDE, Howard ER (eds) *Pediatric surgery and urology: long-term outcomes*. Philadelphia, PA: WB Saunders Co., 1998: 430–8.

Stringer MD, Howard ER. Long-term outcome after injection sclerotherapy for oesophageal varices in children with extrahepatic portal hypertension. *Gut* 1994; **35**: 257–9.

Stringer MD, Howard ER, Mowat AP. Endoscopic sclerotherapy in the management of esophageal varices in 61 children with biliary atresia. *Journal of Pediatric Surgery* 1989; **24**: 438–42.

Stringer MD, Price JF, Mowat AP, Howard ER. Liver cirrhosis in cystic fibrosis. *Archives of Disease in Childhood* 1993; **69**: 407.

Stringer MD, Heaton ND, Karani J, Olliff S, Howard ER. Patterns of portal vein occlusion and their aetiological significance. *British Journal of Surgery* 1994; **81**: 1328–31.

Stringer MD, McClean P, Heaton ND, Karani J, Mieli-Vergani G. Congenital hepatic arterioportal fistula. *Journal of Pediatric Gastroenterology and Nutrition* 1999; **29**: 487–8.

Terblanche J, Northover JM, Bornman P *et al*. A prospective evaluation of injection sclerotherapy in the treatment of acute bleeding from esophageal varices. *Surgery* 1979; **85**: 239–45.

van't Riet M, Burger JW, van Muiswinkel JM *et al*. Diagnosis and treatment of portal vein thrombosis following splenectomy. *British Journal of Surgery* 2000; **87**: 1229–33.

Webb LJ, Sherlock S. The aetiology, presentation and natural history of extra-hepatic portal venous obstruction. *Quarterly Journal of Medicine* 1979; **192**: 627–39.

Webb L, Smith-Laing G, Lake-Bakaar G, McKavanagh S, Sherlock S. Pancreatic hypofunction in extrahepatic portal venous obstruction. *Gut* 1980; **21**: 227–31.

Weber TR. Adverse effects of liver disease and portal hypertension on intestinal adaptation in short bowel syndrome (SBS). Paper presented at the British Association of Paediatric Surgeons XLVII Annual International Congress, Sorrento, Italy, July 2000.

Yachha SK, Sharma BC, Kumar M, Khanduri A. Endoscopic sclerotherapy for esophageal varices in children with extrahepatic portal venous obstruction: a follow-up study. *Journal of Pediatric Gastroenterology and Nutrition* 1997; **24**: 49–52.

Yadav S, Dutta AK, Sarin SK. Do umbilical vein catheterization and sepsis lead to portal vein thrombosis? A prospective, clinical, and sonographic evaluation. *Journal of Pediatric Gastroenterology and Nutrition* 1993; **17**: 392–6.

Young MF, Sanowski RA, Rasche R. Comparison and characterization of ulcerations induced by endoscopic ligation of esophageal varices versus endoscopic sclerotherapy. *Gastrintestinal Endoscopy* 1993; **39**: 119–22.

22

Surgery for portal hypertension

FREDERIC GAUTHIER

INTRODUCTION

The common aim of surgical and alternative treatments of portal hypertension (PH) is the prevention of the life-threatening risk of bleeding from gastrointestinal varices. In the first edition of this book the chapter on the surgical treatment of PH focused on technical aspects and the results of portosystemic shunt surgery in the various types of PH. The difference in results between cirrhotic and non-cirrhotic patients, the adverse effects of shunts, and the indications for shunting were emphasized (Valayer, 1991).

During the past 10 years the framework of treatment of PH has changed because of the simultaneous development of pediatric liver transplantation (LT), new surgical techniques for the treatment of portal vein thrombosis, and radiological techniques. The new surgical techniques were initially designed for the treatment complications of LT.

The treatment of PH patients should be planned according to the cause. The portal hypertension itself is the main target of treatment in a patient with normal liver function, as in most cases of portal vein thrombosis. On the other hand, in a patient who is a candidate for LT the treatment of PH should be viewed as a temporary measure, and a technique should be chosen which will both preserve liver function and avoid adding surgical difficulties to the transplant procedure.

This chapter starts with a description of the surgical techniques and radiological procedures available for portal system decompression. The following section gives a brief overview of the technical problems related to PH in liver transplantation. The last section suggests guidelines for a strategy for the management of portal hypertensive patients, and treatment options which are based on the various etiologies.

SURGICAL TECHNIQUES AND RADIOLOGICAL PROCEDURES

Shunt surgery

PRINCIPLE

The principle of portosystemic shunt surgery is to restore normal pressure within the portal system by constructing a low-resistance channel between a vessel of the portal system and a systemic vein related to the caval system. This shunt may consist either of a direct end-to-side or side-to-side anastomosis between both vessels, or of an H-shunt using autologous vein interposed between the two vessels. The latter technique is described as the favored procedure, and it has been used with increasing frequency in our hospital during the last 22 years (Valayer et al., 1985; Gauthier et al., 1989).

PREOPERATIVE VASCULAR INVESTIGATIONS FOR SHUNT SURGERY

The anatomical arrangement of the portal venous system should be thoroughly evaluated prior to surgery. In cases without portal vein obstruction, patency of portal, mesenteric and splenic veins may be demonstrated with minimally invasive imaging techniques such as Doppler ultrasound, spiral CT scan or MR angiography. Useful information on the length and diameter of both superior mesenteric and splenic veins may also be obtained on the venous phases of successive superior mesenteric and splenic angiograms, and this may be particularly useful in patients with portal vein thrombosis. Normal anatomy and patency of the inferior vena cava (IVC) and left renal vein are usually easily assessed by non-invasive techniques.

A special note must be made of any anomalies in the distribution or location of the left renal vein when a splenorenal shunt is planned. The extent of obstruction in hepatic veins in Budd–Chiari patients should always be investigated by cavography, and sometimes by transhepatic venography, to assess the patency of the IVC and to measure the cavo-atrial blood pressure gradient. Ultrasound is very helpful for assessment of the internal jugular veins which are to be used for interposition grafts, especially in children who have previously undergone surgical insertion of central venous lines.

Both in cases of portal vein obstruction and in cases of intrahepatic PH the pressure gradient between the portal venous system and the IVC is usually high enough to ensure a satisfactory flow through the shunt, and preoperative hemodynamic studies are not necessary. On the other hand, a staged study of caval pressures remains mandatory in Budd–Chiari cases.

TECHNIQUE OF MESOJUGULAR–CAVAL (MJC) H-SHUNT

This shunt has been the most commonly performed technique in our practice, as it is in many other centers in the world. The right internal jugular vein is chosen as the graft as often as possible, in order to avoid the risk of injury of the thoracic duct during retrieval of a left jugular vein.

The child is placed in a supine position, with the head turned to the left. A pillow is placed posteriorly under the shoulders and the upper part of the abdomen to aid both abdominal and cervical exposures. A transverse abdominal incision transects both rectus muscles and extends to the costal margin on the right side.

The first step of the operation is the exposure of the superior mesenteric vein (SMV) through the root of the mesentery. Dissection should be performed with careful ligation of all lymphatic channels in order to prevent the occurrence of postoperative chylous ascites. The right aspect of the SMV is exposed from the right superior colic vein to the ileocolic vein, and is carefully unbedded from the fibrous tissue at the inferior border of the pancreas. It is sometimes necessary to divide small pancreatic tributaries of the SMV to free its right aspect, but dissection of its posterior aspect should be extremely careful and limited in order to avoid injury to the short and fragile posterior pancreatic veins. As a general rule, encircling of the vein is not necessary to allow safe clamping.

The IVC is next exposed from the third part of the duodenum to the right iliac artery through the retroperitoneal tissue, which is usually thickened and hypervascular. The duodenum should be well mobilized on each side so that it will not cause kinking of the venous graft. The root of the mesentery is then tunneled from the IVC to the right side of the SMV, crossing the duodenum, to allow the most direct route for the graft. The lateral approach of the IVC with retraction of the right colon to the midline (Cardenas and Bussutil, 1982) is not recommended because of the increased risks of bleeding and injury to the right ureter.

The cervical approach is the third step of the operation. It is performed through a longitudinal incision, which allows safe dissection and retrieval of the whole length of the internal jugular vein from above the thyrofacial branch to a point as far behind the clavicle as possible.

Portal and caval pressures are recorded before construction of the shunt. The distal end of the graft is sutured to the anterior aspect of the IVC after removal of a small elliptic patch of the caval wall, with a double running 6/0 absorbable suture. The IVC is unclamped whilst the graft is occluded with a small clamp, and the free end of the graft is brought to the SMV through the mesenteric tunnel. The position and length of the graft should be carefully adjusted when it is filled with blood in order to avoid excessive shortening, kinking or torsion of the graft. The proximal end of the internal jugular vein is then sutured to a simple incision on the lateral aspect of the SMV. Small (6/0 or 7/0) absorbable running or interrupted sutures are used for this anastomosis, and the posterior row is performed from the inside of the lumen.

The abdomen is closed without drainage and a suction tube is placed in the neck. The average operating time is 3–4 hours, and minimal blood loss does not usually require replacement. No anticoagulant therapy is prescribed.

VARIANTS OF H-SHUNTS

The mesojugular–caval shunt is the most popular H-shunt, but other types of H-shunts may be constructed when necessary, depending on the anatomy of the portal vessels.

Splenosystemic H-shunts

A splenorenal H-shunt may be a good alternative when the SMV is narrow, or in patients with dense mesenteric adhesions due to previous bowel surgery. The splenic vein (SV) can usually be exposed through the root of the mesocolon, without division of the omentum and mobilization of the stomach, using the inferior mesenteric vein as a guide for dissection. Dissection of the SV from its pancreatic bed should be sufficient to allow safe lateral clamping or double-cross clamping. The distance between the SV and the left renal vein is usually so short that it is possible to restrict the retrieval of the jugular vein from below the level of the thyrofacial vein. In a few patients the SV forms large loops and it is possible to construct a side-to-side, X-shaped, splenorenal anastomosis. A disadvantage of the splenorenal H-shunt is the frequent need for division of large chyliferous lymphatic ducts on the anterior aspect of the left renal vein, which results in a risk of prolonged chylous ascites. The construction of a splenocaval H-shunt, requiring a minimal retroperitoneal dissection, avoids this complication (Yandza et al., 1998).

Makeshift H-shunts

In some cases of extensive thrombosis of the portal venous system, both the SMV and the SV are unsuitable for a shunt, and a 'makeshift' H-shunt between a jejunal or a pancreaticoduodenal vein (or any large vein of the portal system) and the IVC or left renal vein may be a satisfactory solution.

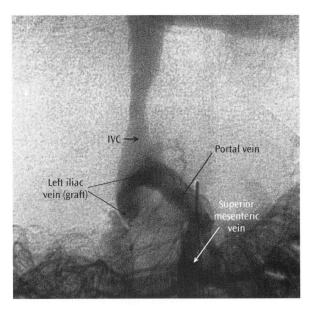

Figure 22.1 *'Discardable' H-shunt between the right branch of the portal vein and the inferior vena cava (IVC) in a patient with sclerosing cholangitis. Note the preserved large size of the trunk of the portal vein.*

H-TYPE SHUNTS IN CHILDREN WHO ARE POTENTIAL CANDIDATES FOR TRANSPLANTATION

H-type shunts have been performed in our hospital in children with intrahepatic PH (e.g. in 25 patients after successful Kasai operation for biliary atresia) who were not considered as candidates for LT in the short term. Our experience with 10 cases of LT after shunt surgery confirmed that H-shunts do not jeopardize the feasibility of LT and are usually easy to disconnect. In three cases of cirrhosis with satisfactory anatomy, 'temporary' H-shunts were constructed between the trunk or the right branch of the portal vein and the suprarenal IVC (Figure 22.1). This type of shunt offers an advantage for LT in that there is preservation of a wide portal trunk.

CHOOSING A VENOUS GRAFT

The left iliac vein may be used as a free graft, provided that the distance between the portal vessel and the caval vessel is not too great (e.g. in cases of splenorenal or portocaval H-shunts). The esthetic advantage of this choice, rather than the use of an internal jugular vein, is obvious, but the possible consequences in adulthood of the loss of an iliac venous axis have not been evaluated to date. It is not usually advisable to use a vein smaller than the iliac or the internal jugular vein, since a large-diameter graft helps to avoid thrombosis.

OTHER TYPES OF INTRA-ABDOMINAL SHUNTS

Pioneering shunts

The superior mesenteric–iliocaval shunt, which has been extensively used in the past (Auvert et al., 1973), was abandoned because of the better results of the H-shunt and also because of the risk or late venous complications related to interruption of both iliac axes (Boles et al., 1986). The central splenorenal shunt with associated splenectomy, still advocated recently (Prasad et al., 1994), is no longer justified in our view because of the well-known risk of overwhelming sepsis associated with splenectomy, especially in younger children.

Selective shunts

The distal selective splenorenal shunt was designed to protect cirrhotic patients from encephalopathy induced by deprivation of hepatopetal portal blood flow after complete portosystemic diversion (Warren et al., 1974). The splenic vein is approached in the same manner as for the construction of a splenorenal H-shunt, but this is a delicate and time-consuming procedure. An extensive dissection of the vein from its pancreatic bed is necessary to obtain an adequate length of the vessel, in order to avoid any kinking after anastomosis. The renal vein is dissected through retroperitoneal lymphatic tissue. After division of the SV with suture ligation of its medial end, the distal segment is apposed to the renal vein with a vascular clamp, taking care to avoid any twist of the anastomosis. The portal–azygous disconnection recommended by Warren et al. (1974) is achieved by ligation of the coronary vein and the major tributaries in the area. An alternative technique to the original Warren operation is the construction of a short interposition splenorenal shunt, followed by ligation or interruption by vascular clips of the SV distal to the H-shunt, and also of the coronary vein. These selective shunts have been advocated during the past 10 years, especially in children suffering from severe thrombocytopenia secondary to PH (Evans *et al.*, 1995; Shilyansky *et al.*, 1999).

ABDOMINOTHORACIC SHUNTS

The poor pressure gradient between the portal system and the IVC in some cases of Budd–Chiari syndrome represents an absolute contraindication to any intra-abdominal shunt. In such cases only an abdominothoracic shunt will provide satisfactory portal decompression. A mesoatrial shunt from the SMV to the right atrium may be performed through an abdominal approach followed by a transdiaphragmatic anastomosis to the atrium (Soyer *et al.*, 1993). The use of a prosthetic graft, usually a ringed polytetrafluorethylene graft, is necessary because of the long gap between the SMV and the atrium. In young children the interposition of a jugular free graft between the SMV and the lower end of the prosthesis has been advocated to allow growth (Gentil-Kocher *et al.*, 1988). More recently, meso-innominate shunts between the SMV and the left innominate vein via a retrosternal route have been described.

INTRA- AND POSTOPERATIVE ASSESSMENT OF SHUNT PATENCY

Intraoperative assessment

The best way to check the patency of a shunt during surgery is to measure the portal pressures successively whilst occluding and opening the shunt. A quick drop of at least one-third in the pressure at shunt opening indicates a satisfactory result.

Postoperative assessment

Postoperative assessment of patency may be achieved by means of abdominal Doppler ultrasound. If the shunt cannot be directly visualized because of the presence of intestinal gas, indirect signs of changes in portal flow can be observed, such as decreasing thickness of the lesser omentum and an increasing diameter of the inferior vena cava. MR imaging or CT scan may also be helpful. In our experience the disappearance or significant shrinking of esophageal varices is demonstrated in 50% of cases 6 months after surgery. An angiographic study should be performed only in cases where doubt persists for 6 to 12 months after surgery. A patent shunt is associated with complete diversion of portal blood from the liver into the vena cava on the venous phase of mesenteric or splenic arteriography.

OVERALL RESULTS OF SHUNT SURGERY

A survey of the world literature on shunt surgery, conducted in the mid-1990s, demonstrated that a patency rate ranging from 87% to 98% could be expected after shunt surgery performed by skilled pediatric surgical teams who had experience of more than 100 cases each. In our experience the success rates were higher in older children, with shunt patency rates of 80% and 89% before and after 5 years of age, respectively. However, the difference was not statistically significant (Valayer and Branchereau, 1998).

In cases of portal vein obstruction, the expected patency rate depends on the general pattern of the portal system. Preoperative angiograms were reviewed in our hospital and assigned to either a confluent (Figure 22.2a) or a scattered (Figure 22.2b) pattern in a cohort of 76 consecutive patients who received an H-shunt for portal vein obstruction. In total, 59 of 62 patients with the confluent pattern had patent shunts, compared with 7 of 14 patients with the scattered pattern ($P < 0.001$).

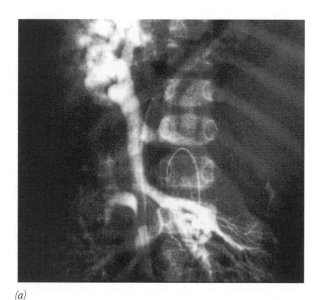

(a)

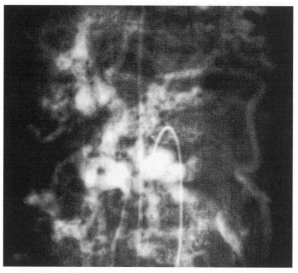

(b)

Figure 22.2 *Patterns of extrahepatic portal venous system. (a) 'Confluent' pattern. (b) 'Scattered' pattern.*

MANAGEMENT OF FAILED SHUNTS

Failure of a shunt and recurrent PH may result from postoperative thrombosis, which may require the construction of a second shunt. Percutaneous iliocavography sometimes allows retrograde catheterization of the shunt and successful balloon dilatation of an anastomotic stricture. This technique was found to be successful in a patient with Budd–Chiari syndrome who suffered from thrombosis of a mesocaval shunt soon after surgery. The patency of the shunt was re-established 6 years later by endoluminal dilatation. Refractory ascites disappeared within 2 weeks. We now recommend that the margins of the caval or renal end of the shunt should be marked with small titanium clips in order to facilitate any future endoluminal procedure.

LONG-TERM BENEFITS OF SHUNT SURGERY

Long-term patency

In a series of 190 patients, 135 children were reviewed less than 5 years and 55 children were reviewed more than 5 years after shunt surgery (Valayer and Branchereau, 1998). Shunt patency was achieved in 165 out of 190 cases (87%), including 10 cases that had undergone a second surgical procedure. From an analysis of the 55 patients who were reviewed more than 5 years after operation, it appeared that confirmation of the patency of a shunt during the year following operation was a good indication of future patency. This was confirmed by subsequent clinical and ultrasonographic examinations.

Clearance of gastrointestinal varices

A total of 147 patients have undergone at least one fiberoptic esophagoscopy approximately 6 months after operation. Complete disappearance or a marked improvement of varices was observed in 71 (48%) and 60 (41%) cases, respectively. The varices remained unchanged in the other 16 patients (11%) (Valayer and Branchereau, 1998).

Correction of hypersplenism

It often takes several months before there is complete reversal of hypersplenism – that is, it does not occur rapidly after surgery. Patency of the shunt should be followed by an obvious rise in the platelet count, but normal levels are not usually achieved for several weeks or months. Complete disappearance of splenomegaly was observed in only 119 out of 147 patients (81%) with a patent shunt.

Acceleration of growth

A striking acceleration of the growth curve has been reported in 16 out of 25 children who underwent successful shunt surgery for portal vein obstruction in a previous study from Bicêtre Hospital (Alvarez et al., 1983).

Correction of biliary anomalies associated with portal vein obstruction (PVO)

Biliary tract abnormalities associated with PVO include bile duct dilatation caused by the compressive effect of periductal collateral veins, ischemic damage and cholelithiasis. Reversal of PH after successful shunt surgery usually, but not always, results in regression of the signs of biliary obstruction (Khuroo et al., 1993; Chaudhary et al., 1998; Dhiman et al., 1999).

ADVERSE EFFECTS OF SHUNT SURGERY

Postoperative mortality and morbidity

Deaths following shunt surgery are now rare, but associated complications include encephalopathy, cardiopulmonary problems and rare changes in liver histology.

Portosystemic encephalopathy (PSE)

PSE detected either clinically or by electroencephalographic abnormalities is a well-recognized complication of shunt surgery in patients with cirrhosis. At least one episode of PSE occurred in nine out of 37 cirrhotic patients (24%) who underwent shunt surgery in our hospital (Bernard et al., 1985).

Some controversy arose among surgeons after Vorhees et al. (1973) suggested that non-cirrhotic children who were subjected to shunt surgery could also develop postoperative PSE. However, this has not been borne out in more recent studies of 251 children, which reported no patients suffering from late neuropsychiatric sequelae (Alagille et al., 1986; Boles et al., 1986; Mohapatra et al., 1992; Prasad et al., 1994). Thus the risk of PSE after shunt surgery for PVO can be regarded as negligible.

Cardiovascular complications

Pulmonary arteriovenous shunting (PAVS) and pulmonary artery hypertension (PAHT) are two rare but severe complications of PH. They may occur in patients with cirrhosis and in those who have undergone surgical portosystemic shunt surgery.

PAVS (hepatopulmonary syndrome) is caused by a progressive dilatation of pulmonary capillaries resulting in chronic hypoxemia with finger clubbing, cyanosis and dyspnea. PAVS may be demonstrated by technetium Technetium-99m-labeled microaggregated albumin pulmonary scanning and/or an increased alveolo-arterial oxygen gradient. The mechanism of PAVS is not clearly understood. It can occur at any age in children with PH, but the risk is highest and occurs earlier in children with biliary atresia and associated polysplenia syndrome. In the majority of cases with liver disease, PAVS may be reversed after liver transplantation (Barbe et al., 1995; Uemoto et al., 1996). A single case of postoperative PAVS occurred in our series of 190 patients who underwent shunt surgery. That patient had received a splenorenal shunt for extrahepatic portal vein obstruction, and the PAVS responded completely to aspirin administration.

The anatomical basis of PAHT is a plexiform pulmonary arteriopathy, which may be associated with fibrinous thrombi. The etiology in cases of PH with natural or surgical shunts remains unclear, but is likely to involve the shunting of vasoactive agents from the splanchnic circulation to the pulmonary vascular bed, thus escaping metabolism in the liver. Clinical manifestations such as exertional dyspnea, chest pain or syncope reflect an advanced stage of the disease, and several cases of sudden death in unsuspected cases of PAHT have been reported (Moscoso *et al.*, 1991; Tokiwa *et al.*, 1993). We have experienced only one case of PAHT followed by death, which occurred several years after a shunt operation for congenital hepatic fibrosis (Valayer and Branchereau, 1998).

Liver tumors and tumor-like lesions

A promoting effect of portocaval anastomosis in the development of hyperplastic nodules or, as a cofactor, in hepatocarcinogenesis has been reported in experimental studies in rats (Weinbren and Washington, 1976; Préat *et al.*, 1984). Cases of focal nodular hyperplasia (Guariso *et al.*, 1998) and hepatoblastoma occurring during childhood, and associated with a congenital absence of the portal vein and congenital portocaval fistula, have also been reported (Barton and Keller, 1989; Howard and Davenport, 1997). However, no case of a malignant liver tumor developing in a previously normal liver has yet been reported after a portosystemic shunt performed during childhood.

Transjugular intrahepatic portosystemic shunt

Transjugular intrahepatic portosystemic shunt (TIPS) is a variant shunt procedure which was developed by radiologists as an alternative to surgery for the treatment of complications of portal hypertension in adults. The TIPS procedure has been used less frequently in children.

PRINCIPLE

The principle of TIPS is to make an intrahepatic conduit between a main branch of the portal vein and one of the main hepatic veins, usually the right one (Figure 22.3). A TIPS resembles a portosystemic surgical shunt in that it offers portal blood an outlet with a low resistance. However, it differs from surgical shunts in three respects. First, a TIPS, when feasible, avoids the need for a laparotomy and its complications. Second, the diameter of the intrahepatic channel and then the degree of portal blood diversion may be adjusted. Third, the passage of the portal blood through at least one hepatic vein is preserved.

TECHNICAL ASPECTS

The radiological technique used to perform TIPS placement in adults is well established (La Berge *et al.*, 1993).

The first step of the procedure is the introduction of a long, curved needle from the right internal jugular vein into the hepatic vein. The needle is then advanced through the liver parenchyma into a branch of the portal vein (Figure 22.3a). The resultant intrahepatic channel is catheterized and dilated (Figure 22.3b), and an expandable metallic stent is deployed across this channel as a support (Figure 22.3c). According to the extent of portal venous decompression assessed by intraoperative portal venography, the stent can be dilated with a larger balloon and residual varices may be embolized.

Technical modifications had to be introduced in order to facilitate placement of TIPS in children (Heyman *et al.*, 1997). As with most prolonged radiological percutaneous pediatric procedures, general anesthesia is required to provide adequate sedation and analgesia. Because of the smaller size of children, shorter needles and stents were designed.

Routine assessment of TIPS patency during follow-up is performed with repeat clinical examination and Doppler ultrasound. In patients with recurrent symptoms of PH, and/or with evidence of shunt dysfunction on ultrasound examination, transjugular portal venography allows accurate diagnosis of shunt obstruction and attempts at restoration of patency by balloon dilation and placement of a new stent if necessary.

RESULTS OF TIPS

There have been encouraging results in five reports of treatment of PH by TIPS in a total of 27 children, with an overall success rate of 92% (Table 22.1).

Bypass surgery: the Rex shunt

PRINCIPLE

The principle of bypass surgery – the so-called 'Rex shunt' – is to offer patients with prehepatic portal obstruction both portal decompression and liver reperfusion while constructing a conduit between the extrahepatic portal system and the left branch of the portal vein (Figure 22.4). This technique was developed for the treatment of portal vein thrombosis after liver transplantation, and was then applied to selected cases of idiopathic or iatrogenic portal vein obstruction with cavernous transformation.

PREOPERATIVE INVESTIGATIONS FOR BYPASS SURGERY

Two criteria must be fulfilled before any attempt at bypass surgery. The first is the presence of a large extrahepatic vessel suitable for interposition anastomosis. The second and most important criterion is the presence of sufficiently large and well-communicating intrahepatic

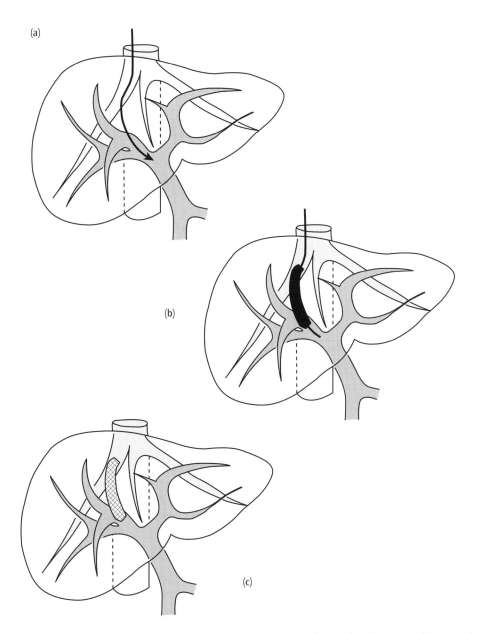

Figure 22.3 *Principle of a transjugular intrahepatic portosystemic shunt (TIPS). (a) Creation of a channel between the right hepatic vein and the right portal branch. (b) Balloon dilatation of the channel. (c) Insertion of a metallic stent in the channel.*

Table 22.1 *Results of TIPS in children from five series*

Author (Year)	Number of patients	Age range	Success rate	Shunt duration
Berger *et al.* (1994)	2	10 and 11 years	2/2	1 year
Johnson *et al.* (1996)	3	6–11 years	3/3	Not known
Cao *et al.* (1997)	1	10 months	Yes	Not known
Heyman *et al.* (1997)	9	5–15 years	7/9	1–800 days
Hackworth *et al.* (1998)	12	2.5–16 years	12/12 (1 redone)	10 patent at LT (median = 53 days) 2 patent at 1 year

LT, liver transplantation.

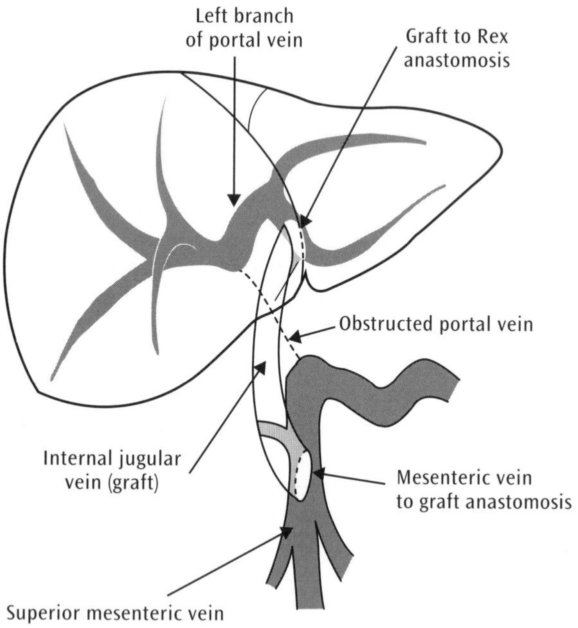

Figure 22.4 *Principle of bypass surgery. This diagram represents a mesentric-to-Rex shunt with interposition of an internal jugular venous graft.*

portal branches, so that resistance to blood flow will be low. An angiographic study is usually necessary to assess the extrahepatic portal system. Assessment of intrahepatic portal vessels may be more difficult. In cases of portal vein thrombosis following LT, Doppler ultrasound readily demonstrates the patency of portal branches within the liver parenchyma, especially when the thrombotic occlusion is recent. In cases of idiopathic or iatrogenic portal vein obstruction, the patency of the left portal branch in the umbilical fissure is more difficult to prove and must be studied carefully with Doppler ultrasound. Preliminary surgical experience suggests that a portal branch of diameter 5 mm, associated with a good flow, correlates with a reasonable likelihood of successful surgery. Preoperative transhepatic portography may be helpful for obtaining more complete preoperative information.

OPERATIVE TECHNIQUE

The abdominal approach must be large enough to give good exposure of both the hepatic umbilical fissure and the extrahepatic portal vessels. The first step in the operation is needle puncture of the Rex recess in order to obtain a measurement of intrahepatic portal blood pressure and to perform portography through the same catheter. Provided that there is a normal intrahepatic portal pressure, a satisfactory pattern of intrahepatic

portal vein branches and an observable retrograde flow, then a bypass procedure may be performed. The distal part of the left portal vein runs within the umbilical fissure up to the point where the left branch of the hepatic artery and the left bile duct cross the vein. Transection of a parenchymal bridge and removal of a small amount of liver parenchyma on each side of the umbilical fissure are usually necessary in order to facilitate exposure of the vessels. Special care must be taken to avoid any injury to the bile ducts during this dissection. Segmental portal pedicles supplying segment III and the anterior part of segment IV are gently encircled and the extrahepatic portal vein is exposed. Most authors have described anastomosis of the superior mesenteric vein to the left portal vein, but a large splenic vein was used satisfactorily in three of our cases of idiopathic portal vein thrombosis (Figure 22.5).

The distance between the extrahepatic portal vessel and the left portal vein is measured after normal positioning of the liver and removal of cushions from behind the patient, to avoid any kinking of the venous conduit. A long jugular graft is retrieved from the neck using the same technique as that described for H-shunts.

After cross-clamping of the left portal vein and occlusion of segmental collaterals, a triangular end-to-side anastomosis is performed between the proximal end of the jugular graft and the left portal vein with 7/0 absorbable running sutures. The left portal vein and the portal collaterals are unclamped while the graft is filled with heparinized saline and its distal extremity is occluded with a small clamp. The liver is returned to its definitive position and the length of the filled graft is carefully adjusted. The distal extremity of the conduit is

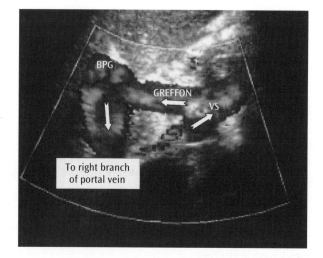

Figure 22.5 *Doppler ultrasonographic appearance of a successful splenic-to-Rex shunt. VS, splenic vein; GREFFON, jugular venous graft; BPG, left branch of the portal vein. White arrows indicate the direction of the venous flow.*

sutured to the mesenteric or to the splenic vein with an absorbable running suture. Since there is usually a very slow flow in intrahepatic portal veins, and therefore a high risk of thrombosis, it is most important to flush the venous conduit repeatedly.

Bypass surgery may not be possible in some cases of idiopathic portal vein obstruction, because of either an unfavorable intrahepatic portal venous pattern or extensive thrombosis of the extrahepatic portal vessels. Furthermore, in cases of portal vein thrombosis following a liver transplantation with a partial graft, difficulties may arise because of the large distance between the mesenteric vein and a left portal branch located far on the right side. In such cases, the use of an allogenic preserved venous graft or a prosthetic graft may be considered.

RESULTS OF BYPASS SURGERY

De Ville de Goyet et al. (1996) first reported encouraging preliminary results in a series of seven cases of portal vein thrombosis after LT, and more recently in 11 selected cases of idiopathic portal vein thrombosis (de Ville de Goyet et al., 1999). An American team reported on another short series of five cases (Bambini et al., 2000). Immediate patency of the shunt was achieved in all reported cases, with relief of PH-related symptoms. Two late stenoses occurred in each of the series, and these were treated successfully by either redoing the shunt or dilating with percutaneous endoluminal angioplasty.

We now have experience of 10 cases, including two portal thromboses after LT. Seven patients are free of PH symptoms with a patent bypass, two patients required a second portosystemic shunt after unsuccessful attempts to refashion the bypass, and one child was treated by endoscopic sclerotherapy (unpublished data).

The initial results suggest that bypass surgery is a promising technique, but its evaluation needs careful and prolonged follow-up. It is still too early to regard it as a 'routine' procedure.

Surgical alternatives to vascular procedures

SURGICAL LIGATION OF VARICES

Transthoracic variceal ligation was one of the first techniques to be introduced for the local treatment of esophageal varices, but late re-bleeding was a frequent occurrence in both adults and children (Martelli et al., 1982). Endoscopic sclerotherapy has now been accepted as a safer and more efficient technique (see Chapter 21).

PORTO-AZYGOS DISCONNECTION

The Sugiura operation has been used to treat portal hypertension in children (Sugiura and Futagawa, 1973). The principle of the procedure is an extensive devascularization of the stomach and the abdominal esophagus to interrupt blood flow to the esophageal varices. Additional steps in the operation include truncal vagotomy, pyloroplasty and esophageal transection and anastomosis. The last step may be performed with an EEA stapler inserted into the esophagus via a gastrotomy (Van Kemmel, 1976). An additional fundoplication has been recommended as a preventive measure against postoperative reflux (Sapenna et al., 1983). A splenectomy was recommended by Sugiura and Futagawa (1973) to allow better access to the cardiogastric region and to treat hypersplenism. We have reservations about the use of the Sugiura procedure in children, particularly in relation to the problems of infection after splenectomy, the risk of iatrogenic complications due to dissection of the esophagus and the performance of a pyloroplasty.

Techniques that include resection of the distal thoracic esophagus and the fundus of the stomach with colon interposition are technically difficult and prone to iatrogenic complications. Sclerotherapy will achieve a similar interruption of varicose venous channels within the esophagus and is a much less aggressive technique.

Satisfactory long-term results of the Sugiura procedure and other 'non-shunt' operations in children have been reported in two short series of 15 patients by Belloli et al. (1992) and Uchiyama et al. (1994).

OTHER NON-SHUNT OPERATIONS

Total splenectomy has no effect on the long-term prognosis of PH and should not be advised.

Partial splenectomies with or without transposition of the spleen, and with or without gastro-esophageal devascularization, have been proposed (Kheradpir, 1990; El-Banna et al., 1991; Louis and Chazalette, 1993).

SURGICAL PROBLEMS RELATED TO pH IN LIVER TRANSPLANTATION

Liver transplantation is now accepted as the routine treatment of end-stage liver diseases, and more than 50% of the children undergoing LT have previously undergone portoenterostomy for biliary atresia. This previous surgery often causes additional difficulties with regard to the transplant procedure.

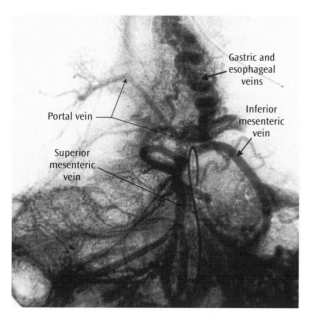

Figure 22.6 *Venous phase of a superior mesenteric angiogram of a child with biliary atresia waiting for liver transplantation. Note the very narrow portal vein compared to the mesenteric veins.*

Bleeding from adhesion-related varices

Difficulties may be encountered at the start of the total hepatectomy in the recipient who has suffered with severe portal hypertension after a previous laparotomy.

Early access to the hepatic artery, the portal vein and many of the collateral veins in the liver hilum may not be possible in portoenterostomy patients because of the previous anastomosis of jejunum to the liver hilum. The preliminary division of vascular adhesions surrounding the liver may therefore result in profuse bleeding from the liver surface before it is possible to occlude the hepatic artery and portal vein. Prophylactic administration of aprotinin and transfusion of fresh frozen plasma and platelets may improve blood coagulation, and the use of an argon-beam coagulator may be helpful.

Construction of portal vein anastomosis

The portal vein may be extremely narrow in liver transplant recipients, especially in patients with biliary atresia (Figure 22.6), either because of the severity of cirrhosis or because of the previous construction of a surgical shunt. In some of these patients the construction of a portal vein wide enough to ensure a satisfactory blood flow may be very difficult. The difficulties may be compounded by a discrepancy in the diameters of the vessels of an adult donor and those of a very young recipient, and/or by the short length of the portal vein of a left lobe taken from a living donor. Techniques that are available to minimize the risk of portal vein thrombosis in these patients include end-to-side anastomosis between the conflu-

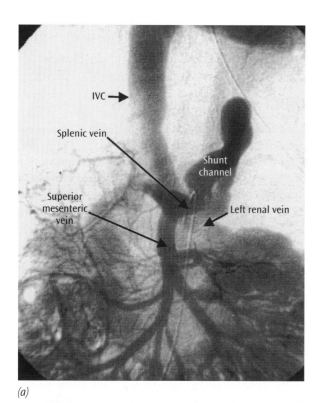

(a)

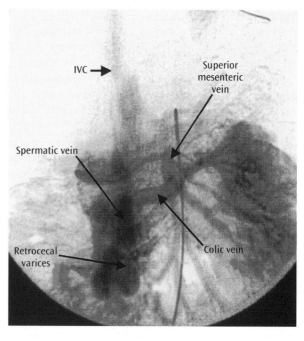

(b)

Figure 22.7 *Two examples of large spontaneous portosystemic shunts in children awaiting liver transplantation. (a) A classical splenorenal shunt. (b) A rare type of shunt through the right spermatic vein.*

ence of the origin of the superior mesenteric vein and the portal vein in the recipient with the portal vein of the donor organ. The interposition of a venous graft from the same donor, or of an autologous graft from the recipient, may be helpful in the case of a very short portal vein on the graft side of the anastomosis. Complete thrombosis of the portal vein, with development of a portal cavernoma in the recipient, is not an absolute contraindication to LT. However, angiographic studies must demonstrate that at least the mesenteric vein, or the distal part of the splenic vein, is suitable for an anastomosis to the portal vessel of the graft.

Spontaneous portosystemic shunts

Spontaneous portosystemic shunts may develop in patients with severe PH, either as multiple small-size veins or as a single wide vascular channel. Ligation of these large shunts at the time of unclamping may help to prevent postoperative portal vein thrombosis. Shunts develop most frequently between the splenic vein and the left renal vein (Figure 22.7a), but a search should be made for shunts at other sites. We have noted significant shunts communicating between cecal varices and the IVC via the right spermatic vein and the right ovarian vein (Figure 22.7b) in one boy and one girl, respectively. The presence of a significant shunt should be suspected in all patients with reversed portal flow, especially when the left renal vein or the IVC appears to be enlarged on US, CT scan or MR imaging. In such cases, splenic and/or mesenteric angiography should be performed to demonstrate the shunt prior to surgery.

GUIDELINES FOR A STRATEGY FOR MANAGEMENT OF PORTAL HYPERTENSION

General considerations

Satisfactory results with regard to the management of PH have been reported for a wide range of non-surgical and surgical approaches to the problem. Some of these treatment options (e.g. the choice between surgery and sclerotherapy as first-line treatment, or between portosystemic shunt procedures and transection surgery) depend to some extent on local availability of particular techniques. Nevertheless, a few clear rules based on the etiology of the PH and on tests of liver function have emerged since liver transplantation became more widely available for patients with end-stage liver disease.

Portal vein obstruction

Patients suffering from idiopathic or traumatic portal vein obstruction usually have normal liver function, and PVO may therefore be regarded more as a vascular problem than as a liver disease. The life-threatening risk of bleeding from gastrointestinal varices or from portal hypertensive gastropathy has been well established in these patients (Bernard et al., 1985), and a recent retrospective study suggests that this risk does not decrease with age. The risk may be greater than 50% during adolescence and early adulthood, depending on the severity of the varices at the beginning of puberty (Lykavieris et al., 2000). Splenomegaly and secondary hypersplenism with a low platelet count and repeated gastrointestinal hemorrhage are well known signs of PVO. Hilar and intrahepatic varices developing close to bile ducts can cause ductal compression and dilatation. Although this portal biliopathy can result in symptomatic biliary obstruction with jaundice in rare cases (Chaudhary et al., 1998; Dhiman et al., 1999), it has only been an asymptomatic observation made during ultrasonographic examination of some of our cases.

Pulmonary arteriovenous shunting or pulmonary hypertension in the absence of previous portosystemic shunt surgery are unusual complications in these patients (Tokiwa et al., 1993; Barbé et al., 1995). The most frequent indication for surgery in PVO patients is still therefore the prevention of gastrointestinal bleeding. We recommend that patients should be considered for surgical treatment soon after a first bleeding episode, but the question of prophylactic surgery remains unanswered. However, it should be noted that a definite risk of portosystemic encephalopathy has not been confirmed in recent short- and long-term studies of patients who underwent shunt surgery for PVO (Alagille et al., 1986; Mitra et al., 1993; Prasad et al., 1994; Valayer and Branchereau, 1998).

Cases of idiopathic PVO with large mesenteric or distal splenic veins should be considered for a bypass operation ('Rex operation'). This should now be the first choice of an experienced surgeon, provided that the intrahepatic portal branches are patent and large enough to achieve a satisfactory left portal branch–jugular vein anastomosis. When operative findings show that the bypass operation is not possible, then a portosystemic shunt should be performed. Preoperative Doppler ultrasonographic studies have shown that approximately two-thirds of PVO patients might be suitable for bypass surgery (de Ville de Goyet et al., 1999). Bypass surgery (the Rex operation) provides both relief of portal hypertension and the restoration of a normal physiological liver circulation, and again it raises the possibility of prophylactic surgery in selected cases. However, more experience of the procedure is necessary before this can be recommended as a routine approach to the treatment of PVO.

Percutaneous angioplasty has been widely and successfully used to treat portal venous stenoses after LT (Funaki et al., 2000). It is interesting to speculate that it might be useful as a minimally invasive alternative to bypass surgery in a few cases of PVO. No such cases have been reported to date.

Children with idiopathic PVO who have a poor intrahepatic portal network but a favorable extrahepatic portal pattern remain, in our view, good candidates for shunt surgery. Surgical treatment offers a one-stage treatment with a high probability of a normal life with relief from the complications of portal hypertension and a very low risk of long-term complications (Valayer and Branchereau, 1998). Transection surgery or endoscopic sclerotherapy represents a more conservative approach, with portosystemic shunt surgery being reserved as a second-line treatment (Maksoud and Goncalves, 1994).

Intrahepatic branches of the portal vein usually remain patent in cases of portal vein thrombosis or symptomatic portal stenosis complicating liver transplantation. The portal vein obstruction is therefore suitable for either endoluminal dilatation procedures or bypass surgery, and an attempt at dilatation of the portal vein should be the first-line treatment, with bypass surgery reserved as a second option in the event of failure. A recent report suggests that shunt surgery in liver transplant recipients might cause an increased risk of portosystemic encephalopathy, and should therefore be avoided wherever possible (Tissières et al., 2000).

Intrahepatic portal hypertension

The treatment for children with intrahepatic portal hypertension should be chosen according to the cause of the disease. Patients with hepatoportal sclerosis, and the majority of those with congenital hepatic fibrosis, are likely to maintain normal liver function for life, and PH appears to be the major complication of their disease. They can be subjected to any of the surgical procedures except bypass surgery, as the risks of portosystemic encephalopathy (Bernard et al., 1985) or cardiovascular complications (Valayer and Branchereau, 1998) in the absence of cirrhosis are very low. However, most patients with intrahepatic PH have liver cirrhosis.

Biliary atresia is the predominant cause of ongoing fibrosis/cirrhosis in the pediatric population, followed by progressive familial intrahepatic cholestasis, ductular paucity, alpha-1-antitrypsin deficiency, cystic fibrosis and rare biliary or metabolic disorders. The diagnosis of the disease has usually been made before signs of PH appear, and the risk of gastrointestinal bleeding has been shown to be lower and later than in children with PVO or congenital hepatic fibrosis

(Bernard et al., 1985).

The risk of portosystemic encephalopathy following surgical portosystemic shunts in cirrhotic children has been well established for many years (Bernard et al., 1985), so only cirrhotic patients classified as Child-Pugh class A should be considered for a surgical shunt procedure. Pulmonary arteriovenous shunting and, to a lesser extent, pulmonary hypertension are more likely to occur in these cirrhotic patients (Nakatani et al., 1988; Moscoso et al., 1991). A higher and earlier risk of pulmonary shunting has been identified in children with biliary atresia and polysplenia syndrome compared with those who have biliary atresia without polysplenia or those who have other types of cirrhosis (Barbé et al., 1995). The presence of either of these cardiovascular complications is an absolute contraindication to any type of surgical portosystemic shunt, which could worsen the pulmonary disease. Liver transplantation should be considered for these cases (Uemoto et al., 1996; Losay et al., 1998).

Shunt surgery for intrahepatic PH should only be considered if the patient has normal liver function and no cardiovascular complications. TIPS should probably be avoided until there is further experience of the long-term results of the technique. Non-shunt surgical procedures can increase the difficulty of any future LT and should be avoided, as they may increase the collateral portal venous circulation and stimulate the formation of intra-abdominal adhesions. Alternative non-surgical treatments with propranolol and sclerotherapy are preferred.

Budd–Chiari syndrome

The major complications of Budd–Chiari syndrome are intractable ascites and progressive destruction of liver, rather than gastrointestinal bleeding (Bernard et al., 1985). The surgical technique used for decompression of the portal venous system depends on the cause of the syndrome. Budd–Chiari syndrome due to an obstructive abnormality of either the IVC (e.g. a caval diaphragm) or the termination of the hepatic veins may be cured by surgical correction of the obstruction or by percutaneous angioplasty. Unfortunately, most cases of Budd–Chiari syndrome are unsuitable for such direct procedures, as they are the result of an extensive thrombosis of all three main hepatic veins. Destruction of the hepatic parenchyma can be arrested in these cases by reducing intrasinusoidal blood pressure with portosystemic shunts. The type of shunt is selected on the basis of measurements of the porto–caval–atrial pressure gradients, and these data provide the rationale for the construction of either an intra-abdominal (mesenterico-caval) or an abdominothoracic (mesenterico-atrial) shunt.

Key references

Barbé T, Losay J, Grimon G *et al.* Pulmonary arteriovenous shunting in children with liver disease. *Journal of Pediatrics* 1995; **126**: 571–9.

Losay J, Piot D, Bougaran *et al.* Early liver transplantation is crucial in children with liver disease and pulmonary artery hypertension. *Journal of Hepatology* 1998; **28**: 337–42.
Two relevant studies of cardiovascular complications in children with liver disease and portal hypertension, with emphasis on the need for early liver transplantation.

de Ville de Goyet J, Alberti D, Falchetti D *et al.* Treatment of extrahepatic portal hypertension in children by mesenteric-to-left portal vein bypass: a new physiological procedure. *European Journal of Surgery* 1999; **165**: 777–81.

A critical study of the preliminary promising results obtained with a new and more physiological surgical approach to the treatment of extrahepatic portal hypertension in children.

Hackworth CA, Leef JA, Rosenblum JD *et al.* Transjugular intrahepatic portosystemic shunt creation in children: initial clinical experience. *Radiology* 1998; **206**: 109–14.

The most recent information to date on technical problems and the results of TIPS in children.

Valayer J, Brancereau S. Portal hypertension: portosystemic shunts. In: Stringer MD *et al.* (eds) *Pediatric surgery and urology: long-term outcomes.* London: WB Saunders, 1998: 439–46.

An overview of short- and long-term results of shunt surgery for portal hypertension in childhood during the last 30 years. There is special emphasis on the overall good results and on the limitations of the procedures in patients with either poor venous patterns and/or impairment of liver function.

REFERENCES

Alagille D, Carlier AC, Chiva M, Ziade R, Ziade M, Moy F. Long-term neuropsychological outcome in children undergoing portal–systemic shunts for portal vein obstruction without liver disease. *Journal of Pediatric Gastroenterology and Nutrition* 1986; **5**: 861–6.

Alvarez F, Bernard O, Brunelle F, Hadchouel P, Odièvre M, Alagille D. Portal obstruction in children. II. Results of portosystemic shunts. *Journal of Pediatrics* 1983; **103**: 703–7.

Auvert J, Farge D, Weisgerber G. Traitement de l'hypertension portale de l'enfant par implantation de l'axe cavo-iliaque retourné dans la veine mésentérique inférieure. *Annales de Chirurgie Thoracique et Cardio-Vasculaire* 1973; **12**: 165–73.

Bambini DA, Superina R, Almond PS, Whitington PF, Alonso E. Experience with the Rex shunt (mesenterico–left portal bypass) in children with extrahepatic portal hypertension. *Journal of Pediatric Surgery* 2000; **35**: 13–18.

Barbé T, Losay J, Grimon G *et al.* Pulmonary arteriovenous shunting in children with liver disease. *Journal of Pediatrics* 1995; **126**: 571–9.

Barton JW III, Keller MS. Liver transplantation for hepatoblastoma in a child with congenital absence of the portal vein. *Pediatric Radiology* 1989; **20**: 113–14.

Belloli G, Campobasso P, Musi L. Sugiura procedure in the surgical treatment of bleeding esophageal varices in children: long-term results. *Journal of Pediatric Surgery* 1992; **27**: 1422–6.

Berger H, Bugnon F. Goffette P *et al.* Percutaneous transjugular intrahepatic stent shunt for treatment of intractable varicose bleeding in paediatric patients. *European Journal of Pediatrics* 1994; **153**: 721–5.

Bernard O, Alvarez F, Brunelle F, Hadchouel P, Alagille D. Portal hypertension in children. *Clinics in Gastroenterology* 1985; **14**: 33–54.

Boles ET, Wise WE, Birken G. Extrahepatic portal hypertension in children: long-term evaluation. *American Journal of Surgery* 1986; **151**: 734–9.

Cao S, Monge H, Semba *et al.* Emergency transjugular intrahepatic portosystemic shunt (TIPS) in an infant: a case report. *Journal of Pediatric Surgery* 1997; **32**: 125–7.

Cardenas A, Bussutil RW. A comparative analysis of the mesocaval H-graft versus the distal splenorenal shunt. *Current Surgery* 1982; **39**: 151–7.

Chaudhary A, Dhar P, Sarin SK *et al.* Bile duct obstruction due to portal biliopathy in extrahepatic portal obstruction: surgical management. *British Journal of Surgery* 1998; **85**: 326–9.

de Ville de Goyet J, Gibbs P, Clapuyt P *et al.* Original extrahilar approach for hepatic portal revascularization and relief of extrahepatic portal hypertension related to late portal vein thrombosis after pediatric liver transplantation. Long-term results. *Transplantation* 1996; **62**: 71–5.

de Ville de Goyet J, Alberti D, Falchetti D *et al.* Treatment of extrahepatic portal hypertension in children by mesenteric-to-left portal vein bypass: a new physiological procedure. *European Journal of Surgery* 1999; **165**: 777–81.

Dhiman RK, Puri P, Chawla Y *et al.* Biliary changes in extrahepatic portal venous obstruction: compression by collaterals or ischemia? *Gastrointestinal Endoscopy* 1999; **50**: 646–52.

El-Banna I, Fathy M, Baza O, Gaber A, el-Sheikh M. Segmental splenectomy and extrapyramidal splenic transposition with gastroesophageal devascularization in treatment of esophageal varices. A new technique. *International Surgery* 1991; **76**: 6–11.

Evans S, Stovroff M, Heiss K, Ricketts R. Selective distal splenorenal shunts for intractable variceal bleeding in pediatric portal hypertension. *Journal of Pediatric Surgery* 1995; **30**: 1115–18.

Funaki B, Rosenblum JD, Leef JA et al. Percutaneous treatment of portal venous stenosis in children and adolescents with segmental hepatic transplants: long-term results. Radiology 2000; 215: 247–51.

Gauthier F, de Dreuzy O, Valayer J, Montupet P. H-type shunt with an autologous venous graft for treatment of portal hypertension in children. Journal of Pediatric Surgery 1989; 24: 1041–3.

Gentil-Kocher S, Bernard O, Brunelle F et al. Budd–Chiari syndrome in children. Journal of Pediatrics 1988; 113: 30–8.

Guariso G, Fiorio S, Altavilla G et al. Congenital absence of the portal vein associated with focal nodular hyperplasia of the liver and cystic dysplasia of the kidney. European Journal of Pediatrics 1998; 157: 287–90.

Hackworth CA, Leef JA, Rosenblum JD, Whitington PF, Millis JM, Alonso EM. Transjugular intrahepatic portosystemic shunt creation in children: initial clinical experience. Radiology 1998; 206: 109–14.

Heyman MB, LaBerge JM, Somberg KA et al. Transjugular portosystemic shunts (TIPS) in children. Journal of Pediatrics 1997; 131: 914–19.

Howard ER, Davenport M. Congenital extrahepatic portocaval shunts – the Abernethy malformation. Journal of Pediatric Surgery 1997; 32: 494–7.

Johnson SP, Leyendecker JR, Joseph FB et al. Transjugular portosystemic shunts in pediatric patients awaiting liver transplantation. Transplantation 1996; 27: 1178–81.

Kheradpir MH. Partial splenectomy and partial splenic attachment for the treatment of portal hypertension. Zeitschrift für Kinderchirurgie 1990; 45: 98–9.

Khuroo MS, Yattoo GN, Zargar SA. Biliary abnormalities associated with extrahepatic portal venous obstruction. Hepatology 1993; 17: 807–13.

La Berge JM, Ring EJ, Gordon RL, Lake JR, Doherty MM, Somberg KA. Creation of transjugular intrahepatic portosystemic shunts with the Wallstent endoprosthesis: results in 100 patients. Radiology 1993; 187: 413–20.

Losay J, Piot D, Bougaran J. et al. Early liver transplantation is crucial in children with liver disease and pulmonary artery hypertension. Journal of Hepatology 1998; 28: 337–42.

Louis D, Chazalette JP. Cystic fibrosis and portal hypertension: interest of partial splenectomy. European Journal of Pediatric Surgery 1993; 3: 22–4.

Lykavieris P, Gauthier F, Hadchouel P, Duché M, Bernard O. Risk of gastrointestinal bleeding during adolescence and early adulthood in children with portal vein obstruction. Journal of Pediatrics 2000; 136: 805–8.

Maksoud JG, Goncalves ME. Treatment of portal hypertension in children. World Journal of Surgery 1994; 18: 251–8.

Martelli H, Carlier JC, Descos B, Alagille D, Valayer J. Traitment chirurgical de l'hypertension portale: etude retrospective de 157 cas. Chirurgie Pediatrique 1982; 23: 171–8.

Mitra SK, Rao KL, Narasimhan KL et al. Side-to-side lienorenal shunt without splenectomy in non-cirrhotic portal hypertension in children. Journal of Pediatric Surgery 1993; 28: 398–402.

Mohapatra MK, Mohapatra AK, Acharya SK, Sahni P, Nundy S. Encephalopathy in patients with extrahepatic obstruction after lienorenal shunts. British Journal of Surgery 1992; 79: 1103–5.

Moscoso G, Mieli-Vergani G, Mowat AP, Portmann B. Sudden death caused by unsuspected pulmonary arterial hypertension, 10 years after surgery for biliary atresia. Journal of Pediatric Gastroenterology and Nutrition 1991; 12: 388–93.

Nakatani Y, Ogawa N, Sasaki Y, Yamada R, Misugi K. Pulmonary hypertension associated with portal hypertension in childhood. Case report of a 6-year-old child and review of literature. Acta Pathologica Japan 1988; 38: 897–907.

Prasad AS, Gupta S, Kohli V, Pande GK, Sahni P, Nundy S. Proximal splenorenal shunts for extrahepatic portal venous obstruction in children. Annals of Surgery 1994; 219: 193–6.

Préat V, Pector JC, Taper H, Lans M, de Gerlache J, Roberfrold M. Promoting effect of portocaval anastomosis in rat hepatocarcinogenesis. Carcinogenesis 1984; 5: 1151–4.

Sapenna RA, Weber JL, Shandling B. A modified Sugiura operation for bleeding varices in children. Journal of Pediatric Surgery 1983; 18: 794–7.

Shilyansky J, Roberts EA, Superina RA. Distal splenorenal shunt for the treatment of severe thrombocytopenia from portal hypertension in children. Journal of Gastrointestinal Surgery 1999; 3: 167–72.

Soyer P, Debrouker F, Zeitoun G, Caudron C, Hay JM, Levesque M. Mesoinnominate shunt for the treatment of Budd–Chiari syndrome; evaluation with multimodality imaging. European Journal of Radiology 1993; 16: 131–7.

Sugiura M, Futagawa S. A new technique for treating esophageal varices. Journal of Thoracic and Cardiovascular Surgery 1973; 66: 677–85.

Tissières P, Pariente D, Chardot C, Gauthier F, Devictor D, Debray D. Postshunt encephalopathy in liver-transplanted children with portal vein thrombosis. Transplantation 2000; 70: 1536–9.

Tokiwa K, Ikai N, Nakamura K, Shiraishi I, Hayashi S, Onouchi Z. Pulmonary hypertension as a fatal complication of extrahepatic portal hypertension. European Journal of Pediatric Surgery 1993; 3: 373–5.

Uchiyama M, Iwafuchi M, Ohsawa Y et al. Long-term results after non-shunt operations for esophageal varices in children. Journal of Pediatric Surgery 1994; 29: 1429–33.

Uemoto S, Inomata Y, Tanaka K et al. Living related liver transplantation in children with hypoxemia related to intrapulmonary shunting. Transplant International 1996; 9 (Supplement 1): S157–9.

Valayer J. Portosystemic shunt surgery. In: Howard ER (ed.) Surgery of liver disease in children. Oxford: Butterworth-Heinemann, 1991: 171–80.

Valayer J, Branchereau S. Portal hypertension: portosystemic shunts. In: Stringer MD, Oldham KT, Mouriquand PDE, Howard ER (eds) *Pediatric surgery and urology: long-term outcomes*. London: WB Saunders, 1998: 439–46.

Valayer J, Hay JM, Gauthier F, Broto J. Shunt surgery for treatment of portal hypertension in children. *World Journal of Surgery* 1985; **9**: 258–68.

Van Kemmel M. Resection anastomose de l'oesophage suscardial pour rupture de varices oesophagiennes. Bilan d'une technique nouvelle. *Nouvelle Presse Medicale* 1976; **5**: 1123–4.

Vorhees AB, Chaitman E, Schneider S, Nicholson JF, Kornfeld DS, Price JB. Portasystemic encephalopathy in the non-cirrhotic patient. *Archives of Surgery* 1973; **107**: 659–62.

Warren D, Salam AA, Hutson D, Zeppa R. Selective distal spleno-renal shunt. *Archives of Surgery* 1974; **108**: 306–14.

Weinbren K, Washington SLA. Hyperplastic nodules after portal anastomosis in rats. *Nature* 1976; **264**: 440–2.

Yandza T, Mayer S, Dubois J, Blanchard H. Splenocaval shunt in children using internal jugular vein graft: a case report. *European Journal of Pediatric Surgery* 1998; **8**: 58–60.

23

Complications of portal hypertension and their management

KATHLEEN B SCHWARZ

The various etiologies of portal hypertension in children and the management of esophageal and gastric varices have been described in Chapters 20 and 21. This chapter begins with a brief overview of the pathophysiology of portal hypertension. Since there are few data for children, the relevant information is largely derived from studies of experimental animals and of human adults. The complications of portal hypertension are reviewed, including gastrointestinal bleeding, hypersplenism, ascites, hepatorenal syndrome and hepatopulmonary syndrome. Medical and surgical management strategies are outlined for each complication, and the indications for and timing of liver transplantation relative to these complications are considered. Finally, areas for future research to advance knowledge with regard to pathophysiology, natural history, and management of the infant, child and adolescent with portal hypertension are suggested.

PATHOPHYSIOLOGY

In the normal liver, the portal vein supplies about 70% of the liver blood flow and 40–70% of the oxygen consumed (Lautt and Greenway, 1987; Ballet, 1990). The nutrient-rich, low-pressure, less well-oxygenated portal blood mixes with the high-pressure, well-oxygenated hepatic arterial blood in the hepatic sinusoids. The pressure gradient between the hepatic veins and the portal vein is the main determinant of the movement of portal blood across the liver. Hepatic venous pressure usually reflects central venous filling pressure. Portal venous pressure is determined by the product of the vascular resistance to flow and the portal venous inflow. Ordinarily, the difference between the portal venous pressure and hepatic venous pressure is 5 mmHg or less. In portal hypertension there is both increased resistance to flow and increased portal venous blood flow.

In portal hypertension, portal venous pressure is somewhat higher than wedged hepatic vein pressure, indicating a presinusoidal component, most probably due to inflammatory activity or fibrotic changes in the portal triads (Pomier-Layragues et al., 1985). The space of Disse may contain deposits of collagen which also contribute to the resistance (Orrego et al., 1981). In addition to these structural changes, vasoactive mediators may play a role in portal hypertension. Contractile cells known as myofibroblasts are present in perivenous and perisinusoidal areas of cirrhotic but not normal livers, and infusion of vasodilators into the cirrhotic liver decreases portal pressure, perhaps by effects on these contractile cells. In contrast, vasodilators do not affect portal venous pressure in the normal liver (Housset et al., 1993). Plasma endothelin levels are increased in patients with cirrhosis (Sanyal et al., 1994; Moller et al., 1995), and endothelin causes myofibroblasts to contract (Rockey et al., 1993).

In portal hypertension, portal venous blood flow is markedly increased secondary to blood flowing through portosystemic collaterals (Vorobioff et al., 1984). In contrast, portal venous perfusion of the liver is diminished.

The role of the increased portal venous blood flow in maintaining elevated portal pressure is less important than is increased resistance to flow (Wright and Boyer, 1990). The major circulatory change accompanying portal hypertension is hyperdynamic circulation, which is characterized by peripheral vasodilatation, reduced peripheral vascular resistance and increased plasma volume. Patients with portal hypertension thus have an increased cardiac output and heart rate.

Two major theories have been proposed to explain the systemic vascular changes which occur in portal hypertension. The first is the peripheral vasodilatation theory, which is a refinement of the classic underfill hypothesis (Schrier et al., 1998). According to this theory, arterial vasodilatation, primarily in the splanchnic circulation, results from the effects of a factor or factors associated with cirrhosis. Vasodilatation then leads to decreased effective circulating volume, and sodium retention occurs in order to compensate for this decreased volume. Vasodilatation may result from diminished responsiveness of gut vascular endothelium to endogenous vasoconstrictors (Finberg et al., 1981). Endogenous vasodilators which accumulate in cirrhotics, including glucagon, nitric oxide and prostacyclin, may play a role in vasodilatation (Benoit et al., 1986; Bomzon and Blendis, 1994).

Alternatively, the overflow theory proposes that there is a primary stimulus (hepatorenal reflex) to sodium retention which is directly related to portal hypertension (Groszmann, 1994). According to this theory, sodium retention is primary and results in increased total blood volume, leading to increased cardiac output.

DIAGNOSIS

Portal hypertension is defined in terms of the difference between portal venous pressure and hepatic venous pressure. Although direct pressure measurements are the standard for experimental animal models of portal hypertension, and can be performed intraoperatively in humans, in clinical practice the diagnosis is usually deduced by the presence of splenomegaly and cytopenia. Imaging techniques to diagnose portal hypertension include B-mode ultrasound and duplex Doppler ultrasound, in which the maximal velocity of blood flow in the main portal trunk is decreased in patients with portal hypertension (Kozaiwa et al., 1995). However, ultrasound may be problematic because of the presence of abdominal gas and anatomical variations and, in particular, it may fail to diagnose cavernous transformation of the portal vein, a common cause of extrahepatic portal hypertension, in which occlusion of the portal vein is associated with small periportal collaterals. Glassman et al. (1993) have shown that magnetic resonance imaging can be very useful for establishing this diagnosis in

patients with splenomegaly in whom Doppler ultrasound has failed to identify a normal portal vein (Figure 23.1). A more direct way of diagnosing portal hypertension is to determine the difference between free and wedged hepatic venous pressure (an approximate measure of portal vein pressure). A difference greater than 5 mmHg is diagnostic of portal hypertension.

COMPLICATIONS OF PORTAL HYPERTENSION

Gastrointestinal bleeding

ESOPHAGEAL AND GASTRIC VARICES

Variceal hemorrhage is the most serious complication of portal hypertension, accounting for about one-third of deaths in adult cirrhotic patients (Wright and Boyer, 1990). The mechanisms that explain why esophageal varices bleed have not been fully delineated for either adults or children. According to the 'corrosion' hypothesis, gastric acid refluxing into the lower part of the esophagus subsequently eroded into submucosal varices. However, there is no evidence for increased gastroesophageal reflux in patients with portal hypertension who have bled from esophageal varices (Eckardt and Grace, 1979). Recently, more credence has been given to the 'explosion' theory, in which rupture is postulated to occur when esophageal wall tension reaches a critical level (Lebrec et al., 1980). The distal esophagus is the most common site of bleeding. In adults, several factors are thought to predict risk of bleeding, including the size

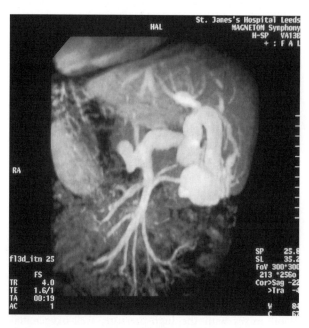

Figure 23.1 *Magnetic resonance angiogram demonstrating portal vein obstruction with marked cavernous transformation in a child with situs inversus. (Reproduced courtesy of MD Stringer.)*

of the varices, intravariceal pressure, the severity of liver disease according to Child's classification, red wale marks and cherry-red spots on the varices.

Approximately 20% of adults with esophageal varices develop gastric varices (Sarin *et al.*, 1992b). Gastroesophageal varices which extend into the fundus of the stomach and intragastric varices in the antrum or body of the stomach are particularly prone to bleeding. Gastric varices usually occur in patients who also have esophageal varices. Isolated gastric varices should raise the suspicion of splenic vein thrombosis, but they are most often a manifestation of portal hypertension. Varices associated with isolated splenic vein thrombosis originate from the short gastric and epiploic veins (Sarin and Kumar, 1989). Portal hypertension often leads to portal hypertensive gastropathy, secondary to increased gastric mucosal blood flow. Previous sclerotherapy of esophageal varices increases the risk of gastropathy in adults (McCormack *et al.*, 1985), but may not necessarily do so in children. Mild portal hypertensive gastropathy is characterized by a mosaic vascular pattern, and carries a 35% risk of bleeding (Hyams and Treem, 1993). Severe gastropathy, which is characterized by cherry-red spots and granular mucosa, carries a 90% risk of bleeding (McCormack *et al.*, 1985). In adults, the factors that have been shown to increase the risk of re-bleeding are bleeding from gastric rather than esophageal varices, thrombocytopenia, encephalopathy, large varices, and active bleeding at the time of endoscopy (de Franchis and Primignani, 1992).

ECTOPIC VARICES

Ectopic varices are defined as varices arising in sites other than the esophagus and stomach. They may occur in isolation or in association with varices at other sites. They may develop spontaneously (Figure 23.2) or as a

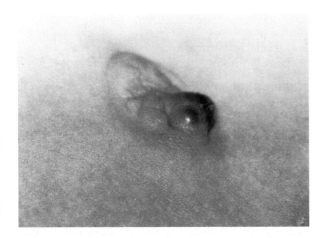

Figure 23.2 *An umbilical varix in a child with cirrhosis and portal hypertension. Variceal bleeding from this site was successfully controlled by local injection sclerotherapy. (Reproduced courtesy of ER Howard.)*

result of surgery and subsequent adhesion formation. They may also follow injection sclerotherapy and obliteration of esophageal varices. Ectopic varices are an uncommon cause of gastrointestinal bleeding, with a reported incidence of hemorrhage in cirrhotic portal hypertension of 1–5% (Stephan and Miething, 1968; Kinkhabwala *et al.*, 1977; Lebrec and Benhamou, 1985).

Ectopic varices may arise at several sites.

Duodenal varices

Duodenal varices account for one-third of bleeding episodes from ectopic varices (Lebrec and Benhamou, 1985). Most reported cases have been in adults (Khoqeer *et al.*, 1987). Duodenal varices in children may be associated with extrahepatic portal hypertension, and there is a history of previous surgery in almost half of the cases. The patients present with gastrointestinal bleeding, and can be diagnosed by upper gastrointestinal endoscopy and angiography. Treatment by injection sclerotherapy may be successful, but surgical excision or ligation is usually required. Duodenal varices may develop either via adhesion collaterals after previous surgery, or from collaterals between the portal vein and the superior mesenteric vein.

Jejunal and ileal varices

These constitute about one-third of all bleeding ectopic varices, and the majority of affected patients have a history of previous abdominal or pelvic surgery (Lebrec and Benhamou, 1985). Venous collaterals develop via adhesions between the gastrointestinal tract and the abdominal wall. Patients present with bleeding from large submucosal veins within the small bowel (Figure 23.3). Surgical excision of the affected segment of bowel may provide long-term relief, but recurrent bleeding can occur after further adhesion formation.

Colonic varices

It is well known that adults with cirrhosis can develop large hemorrhoids, colorectal varices and generalized hypervascularity of the colon (Hosking *et al.*, 1989). Kozarek *et al.* (1991) reported finding multiple vascular ectasias of the colon in a series of adult cirrhotics who had previously undergone a course of sclerotherapy for esophageal varices. Some of the patients required heater probe therapy for actively oozing lesions, or sclerotherapy for bleeding midrectal varices. Fortunately, bleeding from colonic varices is a rare clinical problem in children, accounting for about a quarter of reported cases of ectopic variceal bleeding (Lebrec and Benhamou, 1985). Around 40–50% of large bowel varices are localized to the rectum and sigmoid colon (Rabinowitz *et al.*, 1990), and approximately one-fifth of the patients have had previous surgical operations which may have predisposed them to the development of varices (Lebrec and Benhamou, 1985). The varices are recognized by their appearance at colonoscopy. The mortality rate following

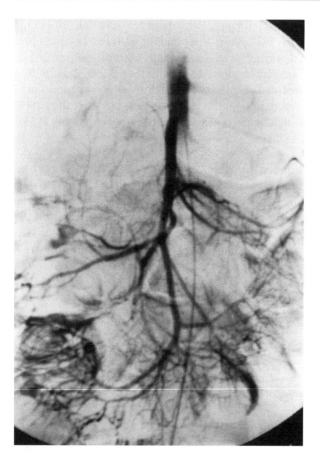

Figure 23.3 *A mesenteric angiogram in a child with portal hypertension and intestinal bleeding demonstrating ectopic small bowel varices in the right lower quadrant of the abdomen. (Reproduced courtesy of ER Howard.)*

partial or total colectomy in adult patients with cirrhosis is more than 60% (Lebrec and Benhamou, 1985).

Rectal varices and hemorrhoids

Anorectal varices represent collateral formation between the superior rectal vein which drains the submucosa of the lower rectum and upper part of the anal canal and the systemic venous drainage at the anus. In a prospective study of 100 cirrhotic adult patients, Hosking *et al.* (1989) found anorectal varices in 44% and hemorrhoids in 63% of cases. They further subdivided hemorrhoids into the external hemorrhoidal plexus and hemorrhoids within the anal canal, identified by the appearance of purple vascular mucosal cushions. These could be differentiated from varices, which were most commonly found in the anal canal, extending distally on to the anal margin and proximal into the rectum. They found no direct relationship between the presence and severity of the portal hypertension and hemorrhoids. This finding may have been expected, as hemorrhoids have previously been shown to have no direct communication with the portal vein (Thomson, 1975).

Heaton *et al.* (1993) noted a significant incidence of hemorrhoids (33%), anorectal varices (35%) and

external anal varices (15%) in children with portal hypertension. In addition, there was a small group of patients who had inflammatory changes in the rectal mucosa, which appeared erythematous, granular or friable.

Stomal varices

The formation of portosystemic collaterals at small or large bowel stomas is frequent and serious (Plate 15). In children, stomas are sometimes used to assess bile excretion after portoenterostomy for biliary atresia. Bleeding can only be controlled by intraperitoneal closure of the stoma (Smith *et al.*, 1988), but a late complication of this may be adhesion-related varices.

Other sites of varices

Spontaneous rupture of intraperitoneal varices has not been reported in children and is rare in adults. The typical presentation is one of sudden onset of acute abdominal pain, hypotension and increasing abdominal girth. The diagnosis can be made by paracentesis and laparotomy. Early surgical treatment by direct suture ligation is the treatment of choice (Fox *et al.*, 1982). Gallbladder varices as seen on duplex sonogram have been reported in children with portal hypertension. These are mainly of significance because they tend to bleed during biliary surgery (Rathi *et al.*, 1996). Rarely, choledochal varices are a cause of obstructive jaundice (see Chapter 21).

Adhesion-related varices

These patients present with melena but not hematemesis. All have a history of previous surgery, and varices occur along adhesions between the abdominal wall and the intestines, particularly the small bowel (Bloor and Orr, 1961; Fry *et al.*, 1988). The varices tend to be localized to the site of adhesions. Investigations with labeled red blood cells or selective visceral angiography have been recommended for this problem (Moncure *et al.*, 1976). Localized resection of the affected segment has been advised (Moncure *et al.*, 1976), but adhesion-related varices are likely to recur, and in children they are best treated by portosystemic shunting.

Hypersplenism

Hypersplenism is a syndome characterized by congestive splenomegaly accompanied by pancytopenia. As noted above, the thrombocytopenia that accompanies hypersplenism is a risk factor for variceal re-bleeding. Adult patients with extrahepatic portal hypertension exhibit abnormalities of cell-mediated immunity, including anergy to delayed hypersensitivity skin testing and reduced T-lymphocyte concentration and mitogen responsiveness (Webb *et al.*, 1980). Symptomatic hypersplenism or massive splenic enlargement accompanied by left-sided abdominal pain or discomfort can be responsible for long-term problems in a small proportion of patients with extrahepatic portal hypertension successfully treated by endoscopic sclerotherapy (Stringer and Howard, 1994).

Ascites

Ascites refers to the presence of fluid within the peritoneal cavity. Portal hypertension frequently results in ascites, a complication that is thought to be secondary to rising sinusoidal pressure and subsequent loss of the permeability barrier in the space of Disse. With the loss of this barrier, Starling forces cannot limit the entry of protein and fluid into the interstitial space. Large increases in lymph formation result from small increases in sinusoidal pressure. The capacity of the lymphatic system is overwhelmed, and ascites results (Wright and Boyer, 1990). From a clinical perspective, ascites becomes particularly problematic in infants with portal hypertension, since ascitic fluid together with the enlarged liver and spleen may limit diaphragmatic excursion and lead to respiratory embarrassment. Ascitic fluid can easily become infected, leading to the development of spontaneous bacterial peritonitis (Larcher et al., 1985).

Hepatorenal syndrome

Hepatorenal syndrome occurs in patients with chronic liver disease and portal hypertension. Portal hypertension has profound effects on renal hemodynamics. Although renal blood flow and glomerular filtration rate (GFR) may actually increase in the early stages of portal hypertension (Wong et al., 1993), as portal hypertension increases, renal blood flow and GFR decrease (Anderson et al., 1976). There is intense vasoconstriction of the renal circulation, and blood flow is redistributed away from cortical and juxtamedullary nephrons. Avid renal sodium retention results in a urinary sodium concentration of less than 10 mmol/L, and there is dilutional hyponatremia. The condition must be distinguished from prerenal failure due to hypovolemia and other causes. In adults, the condition carries a poor prognosis (Gines and Arroyo, 1999).

Hepatopulmonary syndrome

This syndrome is characterized by arterial hypoxemia in the absence of cardiorespiratory disease. Pulmonary vasodilatation is thought to result in a ventilation perfusion (V/Q) mismatch, leading to a low V/Q ratio and arterial hypoxemia. Intrapulmonary shunting contributes to the clinical picture. More severe cases manifest clubbing, cyanosis and dyspnea. Cyanotic congenital heart disease must be excluded. Barbe et al. (1995) showed that macroaggregated albumin is useful for demonstrating right-to-left shunting in children

with cirrhosis, and they also noted regression of shunting post transplant. Children with cirrhosis secondary to biliary atresia appear to be at greatest risk of this complication.

Pulmonary arterial hypertension

This complication of portal hypertension can occur at any age in children with portal hypertension secondary to either portal vein obstruction or cirrhosis, although the pathogenetic mechanisms may be different in these two conditions (Silver et al., 1992). Shunting of vasoactive agents from the splanchnic circulation to the pulmonary vascular bed and increased pulmonary blood flow may contribute in both conditions, whereas in portal vein obstruction a pulmonary arteriopathy has been described which may in turn be a consequence of portosystemic shunting. Pulmonary arterial hypertension can develop before or after portosystemic shunt surgery (Valayer and Branchereau, 1998). Clinical presentation is usually with exertional dyspnea and fatigue, progressing to right heart failure and death. The interval between the onset of portal hypertension and pulmonary symptoms is extremely variable, ranging from a few months to many years.

Other respiratory complications of chronic liver disease and portal hypertension include pleural effusions, respiratory compromise from organomegaly and ascites, and primary pathology such as cystic fibrosis.

Encephalopathy

As portal hypertension progresses, spontaneous splenorenal shunts may develop. In extrahepatic portal hypertension, these shunts may be beneficial in that they may decrease portal pressure. On the other hand, in intrahepatic portal hypertension secondary to cirrhosis, these spontaneous shunts may aggravate hepatic encephalopathy, since portal blood is diverted from the first-pass detoxification of the liver, including the hepatic urea cycle. Cerebral blood flow is increased in the early stages of portal hypertension. However, as liver disease progresses, cerebral blood flow and cerebral metabolic rate decrease (Posner and Plum, 1960). In contrast, in hepatic coma a hyperdynamic cerebral circulation may play a role in intracranial hypertension (Rockey et al., 1992).

Growth failure and malnutrition

Growth failure is a significant problem complicating portal hypertension. In addition, chronic liver disease is associated with growth hormone resistance. Sarin et al. (1992a) noted that children with extrahepatic portal vein obstruction had stunted growth (height for age < 90% of normal). Holt *et al.* (1999) reported that children with liver disease and portal hypertension have a poor IGF-1 response to exogenous growth hormone, an effect which could be partially overcome by supraphysiological administration of growth hormone. Ksiazyk *et al.* (1996) reported that children with portal hypertension are susceptible to malnutrition and have an elevated resting energy expenditure compared with healthy controls.

Splenic artery aneurysms are more common in patients with portal hypertension than in those without portal hypertension (Kobori *et al.*, 1997). The risk of rupture of these aneurysms is about 10%, with mortality rates in the range 10–75% (Fukunaga *et al.*, 1990).

MANAGEMENT OF COMPLICATIONS

Gastrointestinal bleeding

The major life-threatening complication of portal hypertension is gastrointestinal bleeding, and there is a growing literature with regard to the various medical and surgical methods of managing this problem in children (see Chapters 21 and 22). This section will review some of the published experience of medical management, partial splenic embolization and transjugular intrahepatic portosystemic shunt (TIPS). Finally, the various types of surgical management of gastrointestinal bleeding in children secondary to portal hypertension will be reviewed in relation to complications of portal hypertension. The ultimate therapy for intractable bleeding secondary to liver-disease related portal hypertension is, of course, liver transplantation.

Shashidhar *et al.* (1999) reported an uncontrolled pilot study of the use of propranolol for the prevention of portal hypertensive hemorrhage in children. Their results suggested that the drug was well tolerated and that administration of propranolol in doses of no less than 1 mg/kg/day to reduce resting heart rate by 25% was effective in preventing variceal bleeding. However, a prospective controlled trial is needed before firm conclusions can be drawn.

Prophylactic endoscopic sclerotherapy in children with esophageal varices from either cirrhotic or non-cirrhotic portal hypertension has been examined in a randomized controlled trial (Goncalves *et al.*, 2000). Sclerotherapy eliminated esophageal varices in 94% of treated patients, but 24% of these experienced intercurrent upper gastrointestinal bleeding. In contrast, 48% of the untreated controls experienced bleeding. The sclerotherapy group bled primarily from the stomach and had higher rates of congestive gastropathy (16%), whereas the control group bled from the esophagus and had lower rates of congestive gastropathy (6%). The

mortality rate was 18% in the sclerotherapy group, which was not significantly different from that of the controls (16%). Yachha *et al.* (1996) performed variceal obliteration by endoscopic sclerotherapy in children with extrahepatic portal venous obstruction, and noted that portal hypertensive gastropathy was more extensive following sclerotherapy. Sokal *et al.* (1992) found that emergency sclerotherapy for acute gastrointestinal bleeding effectively controlled bleeding in all but one of 19 children with end-stage liver disease who were awaiting transplantation. Complications of esophageal variceal sclerotherapy in children include esophageal stricture, esophageal ulceration, dysphagia and odynophagia, pleural effusion, fever, sepsis, pneumonia and spinal cord paralysis (Howard *et al.*, 1988; Sarin *et al.*, 1988; Hassall *et al.*, 1989; Thapa and Mehta, 1990; Hill and Bowie, 1991; Maksoud *et al.*, 1991) (see Chapter 21).

In 1986, Stiegmann *et al.* reported on a new technique for obliteration of esophageal varices, namely endoscopic ligation (see Chapter 21). In adults, the technique has been shown to be as effective as sclerotherapy, and to be associated with dramatically fewer complications (Stiegmann *et al.*, 1992). Fox *et al.* (1995) reported the successful application of this technique to seven children aged from 2.4 to 14.5 years. These patients required a mean of four treatment sessions for elimination of varices, and transient mild dysphagia occurred in all patients. However, 75% of the patients experienced recurrence of varices. Nijhawan *et al.* (1995) and Price *et al.* (1996) reported similar successful application of the technique, but complications in the latter report included bleeding between sessions, cervical esophageal perforation and transient fever. Ohnuma *et al.* (1997) used a clipping device to perform endoscopic variceal ligation in children with portal hypertension, with successful ligation in 414 of 417 clipping procedures.

If endoscopic variceal sclerotherapy or variceal ligation is unsuccessful, or if there is intractable bleeding from gastric or ectopic varices, then consideration of a percutaneous TIPS shunt is warranted. The procedure has the benefit of being totally intrahepatic, thereby interfering minimally with any subsequent liver transplant procedure. It has become an effective 'bridge to transplant', helping to avoid both emergency portosystemic shunt and emergency liver transplantation in the face of uncontrolled variceal bleeding. It is also preferred to portosystemic shunt procedures, which may complicate the outcome of liver transplantation because of adhesions in the porta hepatis (Turrian *et al.*, 1991). There are at least three reports of the use of this procedure in children (Berger *et al.*, 1994; Heyman *et al.*, 1997; Hackworth *et al.*, 1998). A total of 23 children have received a TIPS, their ages ranging from 2 to 17 years and weight ranging from 13.9 to 80.9 kg. The initial procedures were successful in 20 out of 23 children; three patients required repeat procedures. TIPS resulted in cessation of bleeding and reduction of ascites. Five children experienced shunt stenosis, four children had patent shunts 1 year post procedure, and the remainder were either transplanted, underwent surgical shunts or died of underlying liver disease.

In the era of liver transplantation, the role of surgical portosystemic shunting for gastrointestinal bleeding secondary to portal hypertension associated with chronic liver disease requires reappraisal. Although most such patients appropriately undergo liver transplantation to manage this problem, there are exceptions. Debray et al. (1999) reported that 86% of children with cystic-fibrosis-associated liver cirrhosis developed esophageal varices, and that 50% of these children experienced variceal bleeding for which sclerotherapy was largely ineffective. Elective surgical portosystemic shunting was successfully performed in 9 out of 11 patients, allowing postoperative survival for up to 15 years. Reyes et al. (1999) have emphasized that portosystemic shunting can occasionally be used to avoid retransplantation or multivisceral transplantation. These authors have devised a technique for distal spleno-adrenal shunting which utilizes the enlarged left adrenal vein, thereby minimizing tension on the vascular anastomosis (Mazariegos and Reyes, 1998).

In extrahepatic portal hypertension, portosystemic shunting can be extremely valuable for the treatment of complications such as uncontrolled esophageal bleeding or hemorrhage from ectopic varices (see Chapters 21 and 22). Treatment of uncomplicated extrahepatic portal hypertension by a novel shunt designed to restore hepatopetal portal blood flow has also been described in recent years. Bambini et al. (2000) have utilized a mesenterico–left portal bypass (Rex shunt) in such cases. Gastrointestinal bleeding did not recur, the ascites resolved, spleen size decreased and the mean platelet count and white blood cell count increased. The shunt has the notable potential advantage of restoring liver portal perfusion after years of diversion of portal blood away from the liver (de Ville de Goyet et al., 1998).

The treatment of bleeding anorectal varices has included injection sclerotherapy, banding, cryosurgery, under-running of varices, embolization and portosystemic shunting (Weinshel et al., 1986; Hosking and Johnson, 1988). Injection sclerotherapy is usually satisfactory for treating true hemorrhoids, but direct suture or banding is probably the most effective treatment for bleeding anorectal varices (Heaton et al., 1993).

If hypersplenism is thought to contribute significantly to thrombocytopenia and gastrointestinal bleeding, then in the past splenectomy would have been performed. However, that procedure has major drawbacks. It may jeopardize a portosystemic shunt procedure, increase the difficulty of liver transplantation because of adhesions, and be associated with a significant postoperative morbidity (Cooper and Williamson, 1984). In addition, individuals have a 1–2% lifetime risk of overwhelming infection (Dickerma, 1979). Israel et al. (1993) reported their experience with successful partial splenic embolization in children with hypersplenism. Antibiotic administration before and after the procedure, as well as effective pain control, were important components of the procedure, which resulted in a reduction of splenic volume to 25% of the original size and a dramatic increase in platelets and leukocyte counts. Symptomatic hypersplenism may also be treated by portosystemic shunting.

Ascites is typically managed by gentle diuresis with spironolactone and a low-salt diet. Large-volume paracentesis is avoided unless there is respiratory embarrassment. Spontaneous bacterial peritonitis should be treated with appropriate antibiotic therapy and albumin infusions. Although hepatorenal syndrome is a feared complication of liver failure in adults, who may be salvaged by liver transplantation, there is little knowledge of the incidence and natural history of this condition in children with end-stage liver disease. Hepatopulmonary syndrome, once thought to be a contraindication to liver transplantation, will definitely reverse postoperatively, although these patients are more at risk of surgical complications after liver transplantation (Egawa et al., 1999). Severe intrapulmonary shunting is now a recognized indication for liver transplantation, even in the presence of cirrhosis and good liver function (Lange and Stoller, 1995). Early liver transplantation is crucial in children with liver disease and pulmonary hypertension (Losay et al., 1998). Encephalopathy is typically managed with lactulose, neomycin and restriction of dietary protein. The report of Stewart et al. (1991), which demonstrated that neuropsychological outcome after pediatric liver transplantation is abnormal, and that liver transplant patients had significantly lower scores on non-verbal intelligence tests, lower levels of academic achievement, and lower z-scores for age in all areas of visual and motor function, suggests that subtle subclinical hepatic encephalopathy may be present in many children with portal hypertension, particularly intrahepatic portal hypertension, prior to transplant. Systematic assessment of pretransplant neuropsychological function might suggest ways of improving the outcome after transplant.

There is still much to be learned about the natural history of portal hypertension in children, risk factors for variceal bleeding and re-bleeding, and the impact of portal hypertension on immune function. These topics have assumed much greater importance in the era of liver transplantation, where detailed knowledge of these complications can be translated into better timing of liver transplantation and avoidance of the complications of portal hypertension which may jeopardize the success of the procedure.

The sections on ectopic varices and pulmonary arterial hypertension were written jointly by ERH and MDS.

Key references

Lebrec D, Benhamou J-P. Ectopic varices in portal hypertension. *Clinics in Gastroenterology* 1985; **14**: 105–21.

An excellent account of the problem of ectopic varices in portal hypertension from an internationally renowned unit in France which has contributed many definitive publications, both clinical and experimental, on the subject of portal hypertension during the past two decades.

Stringer MD, Howard ER. Long-term outcome after injection sclerotherapy for oesophageal varices in children with extrahepatic portal hypertension. *Gut* 1994; **35**: 257–9.

A rare long-term outcome study in children with extrahepatic portal hypertension. A consecutive series of 36 children with bleeding esophageal varices were successfully treated by endoscopic injection sclerotherapy and followed up for a mean period of 9 years. Approximately 20% of patients subsequently required surgery for complications of portal hypertension; four underwent portosystemic shunt surgery for bleeding gastric varices, and two required splenectomy for painful splenomegaly/hypersplenism.

REFERENCES

Anderson RJ, Cronin RE, McDonald KM, Schrier RW. Mechanisms of portal hypertension-induced alterations in renal hemodynamics, renal water excretion, and renin secretion. *Journal of Clinical Investigation* 1976; **58**: 964–70.

Ballet F. Hepatic circulation: potential for therapeutic intervention. *Pharmacology and Therapeutics* 1990; **47**: 281–328.

Bambini DA, Superina R, Almond PS *et al.* Experience with the Rex shunt (mesenterico–left portal bypass) in children with extrahepatic portal hypertension. *Journal of Pediatric Surgery* 2000; **35**: 13–19.

Barbe T, Losay J, Grimon G *et al.* Pulmonary arteriovenous shunting in children with liver disease. *Journal of Pediatrics* 1995; **126**: 571–9.

Benoit JN, Zimmermann B, Preman AJ *et al.* Role of glucagon in splanchnic hyperemia of chronic portal hypertension. *American Journal of Physiology* 1986; **251**: G674–7.

Berger H, Bugnon F, Goffette P *et al.* Percutaneous transjugular intrahepatic stent shunt for treatment of intractable varicose bleeding in paediatric patients. *European Journal of Pediatrics* 1994; **153**: 721–5.

Bloor K, Orr W. A case of haemorrhage from varices in the small intestine due to portal hypertension. *British Journal of Surgery* 1961; **48**: 423–4.

Bomzon A, Blendis LM. The nitric oxide hypothesis and the hyperdynamic circulation in cirrhosis. *Hepatology* 1994; **20**: 1343–50.

Cooper MJ, Williamson RCN. Splenectomy: indications, hazards and alternatives. *British Journal of Surgery* 1984; **71**: 173–80.

Debray D, Lykavieris P, Gauthier F *et al.* Outcome of cystic fibrosis-associated liver cirrhosis: management of portal hypertension. *Journal of Hepatology* 1999; **31**: 77–83.

de Franchis R, Primignani M. Why do varices bleed? *Gastroenterology Clinics of North America* 1992; **21**: 85–101.

de Ville de Goyet J, Alberti D, Clapuyt P *et al.* Direct bypassing of extrahepatic portal venous obstruction in children: a new technique for combined hepatic portal revascularization and treatment of extrahepatic portal hypertension. *Journal of Pediatric Surgery* 1998; **33**: 597–601.

Dickerma G. Splenectomy and sepsis: a warning. *Pediatrics* 1979; **63**: 938–41.

Eckardt VF, Grace ND. Gastroesophageal reflux and bleeding esophageal varices. *Gastroenterology* 1979; **76**: 39–42.

Egawa H, Kasahara M, Inomata Y *et al.* Long-term outcome of living related liver transplantation for patients with intrapulmonary shunting and strategy for complications. *Transplantation* 1999; **67**: 712–17.

Finberg JP, Syrop HA, Better OS. Blunted pressor response to angiotensin and sympathomimetic amines in bile-duct ligated dogs. *Clinical Science* 1981; **61**: 535–9.

Fox L, Crane SA, Bidari C, Jones A. Intra-abdominal hemorrhage from ruptured varices. *Archives of Surgery* 1982; **117**: 953–6.

Fox VL, Carr-Locke DL, Connors P, Leichtner M. Endoscopic ligation of esophageal varices in children. *Journal of Pediatric Gastroenterology and Nutrition* 1995; **20**: 202–8.

Fry RD, Fischer KC, Susma N, Shatz BA, Hulbert B. Adhesions-related variceal hemorrhage following sclerosis of esophageal varices. *Archives of Surgery* 1988; **123**: 94–5.

Fukunaga Y, Usui N, Hirohashi K *et al.* Clinical courses and treatment of splenic artery aneurysms – report of three cases and review of literature in Japan. *Osaka City Medical Journal* 1990; **36**: 161–73.

Gines P, Arroyo V. Hepatorenal syndrome. *Journal of the American Society of Nephrology* 1999; **10**: 1833–9.

Glassman MS, Klein SA, Spivak W. Evaluation of cavernous transformation of the portal vein by magnetic resonance imaging. *Clinical Pediatrics* 1993; **32**: 77–80.

Goncalves ME, Cardoso SR, Maksoud JG. Prophylactic sclerotherapy in children with esophageal varices: long-term results of a controlled prospective randomized trial. *Journal of Pediatric Surgery* 2000; **35**: 401–5.

Groszmann RJ. Hyperdynamic circulation of liver disease 40 years later: pathophysiology and clinical consequences. *Hepatology* 1994; **20**: 1359–63.

Hackworth CA, Leef JA, Rosenblum JD, Whitington PF, Millis JM, Alonso EM. Transjugular intrahepatic portosystemic shunt creation in children: initial clinical experience. *Radiology* 1998; **206**: 109–14.

Hassall E, Berquist WE, Ament ME, Vargas J, Dorney S. Sclerotherapy for extrahepatic portal hypertension in childhood. *Journal of Pediatrics* 1989; **115**: 69–74.

Heaton ND, Davenport M, Howard ER. Incidence of haemorrhoids and anorectal varices in children with portal hypertension. *British Journal of Surgery* 1993; **80**: 616–18.

Heyman MB, LaBerge JM, Somberg KA et al. Transjugular intrahepatic portosystemic shunts (TIPS) in children. *Journal of Pediatrics* 1997; **131**: 914–19.

Hill ID, Bowie MD. Endoscopic sclerotherapy for control of bleeding varices in children. *American Journal of Gastroenterology* 1991; **86**: 472–6.

Holt RI, Jones JS, Baker AJ, Buchanan CR, Miell JP. The effect of short stature, portal hypertension and cholestasis on growth hormone resistance in children with liver disease. *Journal of Clinical Endocrinology and Metabolism* 1999; **84**: 3277–82.

Hosking SW, Johnson AG. Bleeding anorectal varices – a misunderstood condition. *Surgery* 1988; **104**: 70–3.

Hosking SW, Smart HL, Johnson AG, Triger DR. Anorectal varices, haemorrhoids, and portal hypertension. *Lancet* 1989; **i**: 349–52.

Housset C, Rockey DC, Bissell DM. Endothelin receptors in rat liver: lipocytes as a contractile target for endothelin-1. *Proceedings of the National Academy of Sciences of the USA* 1993; **90**: 9266–70.

Howard ER, Stringer MD, Mowat AP. Assessment of injection sclerotherapy in the management of 152 children with oesophageal varices. *British Journal of Surgery* 1988; **75**: 404–8.

Hyams JS, Treem WR. Portal hypertensive gastropathy in children. *Journal of Pediatric Gastroenterology and Nutritious* 1993; **17**: 13–18.

Israel DM, Hassall E, Culham JAG, Phillips RR. Partial splenic embolization in children with hypersplenism. *Journal of Pediatrics* 1993; **124**: 95–100.

Khoqueer F, Morrow C, Jordan P. Duodenal varices as a case of massive upper gastrointestinal bleeding. *Surgery* 1987; **102**: 548–52.

Kinkhabwala M, Mousavi A, Iyer S, Adamsons R. Bleeding ileal varicosity demonstrated by transhepatic portography. *American Journal of Radiography* 1977; **129**: 514–16.

Kobori L, van der Kolk MJ, de Jong KP et al. Splenic artery aneurysms in liver transplant patients. *Journal of Hepatology* 1997; **27**: 890–3.

Kozaiwa K, Tajiri H, Yoshimura N et al. Utility of duplex Doppler ultrasound in evaluating portal hypertension in children. *Journal of Pediatric Gastroenterology and Nutrition* 1995; **21**: 215–19.

Kozarek RA, Botoman VA, Bredfeldt JE et al. Portal colopathy: prospective study of colonoscopy in patients with portal hypertension. *Gastroenterology* 1991; **101**: 1192–7.

Ksiazyk J, Lyszkowska M, Kierkus J. Energy metabolism in portal hypertension in children. *Nutrition* 1996; **12**: 469–74.

Lange PA, Stoller JK. The hepatopulmonary syndrome. *Annals of Internal Medicine* 1995; **122**: 521–9.

Larcher VF, Manolaki N, Vegnente A, Vergani D, Mowat AP. Spontaneous bacterial peritonitis in children with chronic liver disease: clinical features and etiological factors. *Journal of Pediatrics* 1985; **106**: 907–10.

Lautt W, Greenway C. Conceptual review of the hepatic vascular bed. *Hepatology* 1987; **7**: 952–63.

Lebrec D, Benhamou J-P. Ectopic varices in portal hypertension. *Clinics in Gastroenterology* 1985; **14**: 105–21.

Lebrec D, De Fleury P, Rueff B, Nahum H, Benhamou J. Portal hypertension, size of esophageal varices, and risk of gastrointestinal bleeding in alcoholic cirrhosis. *Gastroenterology* 1980; **79**: 1139–44.

Losay J, Piot D, Bougaran J et al. Early liver transplantation is crucial in children with liver disease and pulmonary artery hypertension. *Journal of Hepatology* 1998; **28**: 337–42.

McCormack TT, Sims J, Eyre-Brook I et al. Gastric lesions in portal hypertension: inflammatory gastritis or congestive gastropathy? *Gut* 1985; **26**: 1226–32.

Maksoud JG, Goncalves ME, Porta G, Miura I, Velhote MC. The endoscopic and surgical management of portal hypertension in children: analysis of 123 cases. *Journal of Pediatric Surgery* 1991; **26**: 178–81.

Mazariegos GV, Reyes J. A technique for distal splenoadrenal shunting in pediatric portal hypertension. *Journal of the American College of Surgeons* 1998; **187**: 634–6.

Moller S, Gulberg V, Henriksen JH et al. Endothelin-1 and endothelin-3 in cirrhosis: relations to systemic and splanchnic haemodynamics. *Journal of Hepatology* 1995; **23**: 135–44.

Moncure AC, Waltman AC, Vandersalm T et al. Gastrointestinal hemorrhage from adhesion-related mesenteric varices. *Annals of Surgery* 1976; **183**: 24–9.

Nijhawan S, Patni T, Sharma U, Rai RR, Miglani N. Endoscopic variceal ligation in children. *Journal of Pediatric Surgery* 1995; **30**: 1455–6.

Ohnuma N, Takahashi H, Tanabe M, Yoshida H, Iwai J, Muramatsu T. Endoscopic variceal ligation using a clipping apparatus in children with portal hypertension. *Endoscopy* 1997; **29**: 86–90.

Orrego H, Blendis LM, Crossley IR et al. Correlation of intrahepatic pressure with collagen in Disse space and hepatometaly in humans and the rat. *Gastroenterology* 1981; **80**: 546–56.

Pomier-Layragues G, Kusielewicz D, Willems B et al. Presinusoidal portal hypertension in non-alcoholic cirrhosis. *Hepatology* 1985; **5**: 415–18.

Posner JB, Plum F. The toxic effects of carbon dioxide and acetazolamide in hepatic encephalopathy. *Journal of Clinical Investigation* 1960; **39**: 1246–58.

Price MR, Sartorelli KH, Karrer FM, Narkewicz MR, Sokol RJ, Lilly JR. Management of esophageal varices in children by endoscopic variceal ligation. *Journal of Pediatric Surgery* 1996; **31**: 1056–9.

Rathi PM, Soni A, Nanivadekar SA *et al.* Gallbladder varices: diagnosis in children with portal hypertension on duplex sonography. *Journal of Clinical Gastroenterology* 1996; **23**: 228–31.

Reyes J, Mazariegos GV, Bueno J, Cerda J, Towbin RB, Kocoshis S. The role of portosystemic shunting in children in the transplant era. *Journal of Pediatric Surgery* 1999; **34**: 117–23.

Rockey DC, Housset CN, Friedman SL. Contractility of hepatic lipocytes: implications for the pathogenesis of portal hypertension. *Hepatology* 1992; **16**: 316A.

Rockey DC, Housset CN, Friedman SL. Activation-dependent contractility of rat hepatic lipocytes in culture and *in vivo*. *Journal of Clinical Investigation* 1993; **92**: 1795–804.

Sanyal AJ, Gehr T, Freedman AM *et al.* Increased splanchnic endothelin-1 plays a role in the pathogenesis of ascites. *Hepatology* 1994; **20**: 67.

Sarin SK, Kumar A. Gastric varices: profile, classification and management. *American Journal of Gastroenterology* 1989; **84**: 1244–9.

Sarin S, Misra S, Singal A, Thorat V, Broor S. Endoscopic sclerotherapy for varices in children. *Journal of Pediatric Gastroenterology and Nutrition* 1988; **7**: 662–6.

Sarin SK, Bansal A, Sasan S, Nigam A. Portal-vein obstruction in children leads to growth retardation. *Hepatology* 1992a; **15**: 229–33.

Sarin SK, Lahoti D, Saxena SP, Murthy NS, Makwana UK. Prevalence, classification and natural history of gastric varices: a long-term follow-up study in 568 portal hypertension patients. *Hepatology* 1992b; **16**: 1343–9.

Schrier RW, Arroyo V, Bernardi M *et al.* Peripheral arterial vasodilation hypothesis: a proposal for the initiation of renal sodium and water retention in cirrhosis. *Hepatology* 1998; **8**: 1151–7.

Shashidhar H, Langhans N, Grand RJ. Propranolol in the prevention of portal hypertensive hemorrhage in children: a pilot study. *Journal of Pediatric Gastroenterology and Nutrition* 1999; **29**: 12–17.

Silver MM, Bohn D, Shawn DH *et al.* Association of pulmonary hypertension with congenital portal hypertension in a child. *Journal of Pediatrics* 1992; **120**: 321–9.

Smith S, Weiner ES, Starzl TE, Rowe MI. Stoma-related variceal bleeding: an under-recognized complication of biliary atresia. *Journal of Pediatric Surgery* 1988; **23**: 243–5.

Sokal EM, Van Hoorebeeck N, Van Obbergh L, Otte JB, Buts JP. Upper gastrointestinal tract bleeding in cirrhotic children candidates for liver transplantation. *European Journal of Pediatrics* 1992; **151**: 326–8.

Stiegmann GV, Cambre T, Sen JH. A new endoscopic elastic band ligating device. *Gastrointestinal Endoscopy* 1986; **32**: 230–3.

Stiegmann GV, Goff JS, Michaletz-Onedy PA *et al.* Endoscopic sclerotherapy as compared with endoscopic ligation for bleeding esophageal varices. *New England Journal of Medicine* 1992; **326**: 1527–32.

Stephan C, Miething R. Rontgendiagnostik varicoser duodenal-veranderungen by portaler hypertension. *Der Radiology* 1968; **3**: 90–5.

Stewart SM, Hiltebeitel C, Nici J, Waller DA, Uauy R, Andrews WS. Neuropsychological outcome of pediatric liver transplantation. *Pediatrics* 1991; **87**: 367–76.

Stringer MD, Howard ER. Long-term outcome after injection sclerotherapy for oesophageal varices in children with extrahepatic portal hypertension. *Gut* 1994; **35**: 257–9.

Thapa BR, Mehta S. Endoscopic sclerotherapy of esophageal varices in infants and children. *Journal of Pediatric Gastroenterology and Nutrition* 1990; **10**: 430–4.

Thomson WHF. The nature of haemorrhoids. *British Journal of Surgery* 1975; **62**: 542–52.

Turrian VS, Mora NP, Cofer JB, Soloman H, Morris CA, Ganna TA. Retrospective evaluation of liver transplantation for cirrhosis: a comparative study of 100 patients with or without portosystemic shunt. *Transplantation Proceedings* 1991; **23**: 1570–1.

Valayer J, Branchereau S. Portal hypertension: portosystemic shunts. In: Stringer MD, Oldham KT, Mouriquand PDE, Howard ER (eds) *Pediatric surgery and urology: long-term outcomes*. Philadelphia, PA: WB Saunders Co., 1998: 438–46.

Vorobioff J, Bredfeldt JE, Groszmann RJ. Increased blood flow through the portal system in cirrhotic rats. *Gastroenterology* 1984; **87**: 1120–6.

Webb LJ, Ross M, Markham RL, Webster AD, Thomas HC, Sherlock S. Immune function in patients with extrahepatic portal venous obstruction and the effect of splenectomy. *Gastroenterology* 1980; **79**: 99–103.

Weinshel E, Chen W, Falkenstein DB, Kessler R, Raicht RF. Haemorrhoids or rectal varices: defining the cause of massive rectal haemorrhage in patients with portal hypertension. *Gastroenterology* 1986; **90**: 744–7.

Wong F, Massie D, Colman J, Dudley F. Glomerular hyperfiltration in patients with well-compensated alcoholic cirrhosis. *Gastroenterology* 1993; **104**: 884–9.

Wright TI, Boyer TD. Diagnosis and management of cirrhotic ascites. In: Zakim D, Boyer TD (eds) *Hepatology*, 2nd edn. Philadelphia, PA: WB Saunders Co., 1990: 616–34.

Yachha SK, Ghoshal UC, Gupta R, Sharma BC, Ayyagari A. Portal hypertensive gastropathy in children with extrahepatic portal venous obstruction: role of variceal obliteration by endoscopic sclerotherapy and *Helicobacter pylori* infection. *Journal of Pediatric Gastroenterology and Nutrition* 1996; **23**: 20–3.

Liver infection and trauma

Liver abscesses

VT JOSEPH

HEPATIC ABSCESSES

Hepatic abscess is an uncommon condition in childhood that nevertheless needs prompt diagnosis and treatment, as it is still associated with significant morbidity and mortality. Although the condition has been recognized since ancient times, the first detailed study was only published in 1938 (Ochsner et al., 1983). Liver abscesses are generally pyogenic or amebic. Other causative agents, such as candidiasis, actinomycosis, tuberculosis and echinococcal disease (see Chapter 25), are rare.

PYOGENIC LIVER ABSCESS

Pyogenic liver abscess in children is a serious, life-threatening disease. Indeed, earlier studies consisted only of autopsy cases, indicating the high mortality associated with this condition (Dehner and Kissane, 1969).

Incidence

The incidence of pyogenic liver abscess varies in different population groups, and is probably influenced by the frequency of occurrence of various etiological conditions. In children it ranges from 3 to 25 per 100 000 hospital admissions (Arya et al., 1982; Chusid, 1987; Pineiro-Carrero and Andres, 1989). In some areas, such as South India, unusually high rates of 78.9 per 100 000 hospital admissions have been recorded (Kumar et al., 1998). The rise in incidence is due to better diagnosis with the use of modern imaging techniques, and the

increased survival rate of children with immunodeficient states, who have a special predilection towards hepatic abscesses.

Age and sex

Pyogenic liver abscess may occur in any age group, from neonatal cases to children and adolescents. There has been a shift towards the older age groups in recent years, with 50% of cases occurring in children over 6 years of age since 1977, compared with 66% in children under 5 years prior to 1977. The sex distribution shows a slightly increased male:female ratio in patients who do not have chronic granulomatous disease. In a review of 109 patients, 67% were boys and 33% were girls (Pineiro-Carrero and Andres, 1989). However, as would be expected, in patients with chronic granulomatous disease there is an overwhelming male preponderance (5:1).

Liver abscess in the neonate

Hepatic abscess in the neonatal period is a rare condition, and is usually secondary to sepsis (Moss and Pysher, 1981; Altman and Stolar, 1985). A particular feature of the disease in this age group is that it is unusual to see opportunistic or parasitic infections. Infection most commonly occurs in premature infants following umbilical vein cannulation (Brans et al., 1984), or secondary to surgery for necrotizing enterocolitis (Doerr et al., 1994).

BACTERIOLOGY

A wide variety of Gram-positive and Gram-negative bacteria have been isolated from the pus in the liver.

Staphylococcus aureus accounts for one-third of the infections, with *Klebsiella*, *Pseudomonas* and *Escherichia coli* being present in the others.

CLINICAL FEATURES

There are no specific signs to establish the diagnosis in the neonate. Abdominal distension, hepatomegaly, abnormal gas patterns in the right upper quadrant and elevation of the right hemidiaphragm with pleural effusion are some of the findings (Vade *et al.*, 1998). In 30% of cases the hepatic lesion is solitary and may be evident on the scans. However, in 70% of patients the abscesses are small and multiple, being scattered diffusely throughout the whole liver (Figure 24.1).

TREATMENT

In the majority of cases surgical drainage is not possible, and treatment consists of intensive antibiotic therapy with supportive measures (Kays, 1992). Laparotomy is sometimes necessary to establish the diagnosis and obtain pus for bacteriological studies. Solitary abscesses have been successfully treated with antibiotics combined with aspiration or percutaneous catheter drainage (Vade *et al.*, 1998).

Liver abscess in older children

Pyogenic liver abscess may occur in previously normal patients (Moore 1994; Moore *et al.*, 1994) but is generally more common in immunocompromised children (Chusid, 1987; Pineiro-Carrero and Andres, 1989). These abscesses are usually cryptogenic, and they may show evidence of opportunistic infection.

ETIOLOGY

Pyogenic liver abscess is usually associated with infection from the bile ducts, portal vein or hepatic artery. It may also develop following spread from adjacent areas, or be introduced as a result of penetrating trauma (Pitt and Zuidema, 1975).

BILIARY TRACT DISEASE

Cholelithiasis and cholecystitis have been increasingly documented in children. In neonates, cholelithiasis is most commonly associated with total parenteral nutrition, but is also seen after ileal resection (Akierman *et al.*, 1984). In older children, hemoglobinopathies, dehydration associated with debilitating illnesses, inflammatory bowel disease and choledochal cyst may be underlying causes (Nanni, 1983) (Figure 24.2). Although hemolytic disorders are common in childhood, they seldom give rise to gallbladder disease (Sears *et al.*, 1973). In infants, congenital deformities of the ducts predispose to the disorder (Arnspiger *et al.*, 1960).

Oriental cholangiohepatitis or recurrent pyogenic cholangitis is a clinical syndrome that is especially prevalent in South-East Asia and the Far East, with 3% of all cases occurring in children (Figure 24.3). It is characterized by repeated infections of the bile ducts by pyogenic organisms, with fibrosis of the duct wall, strictures and formation of pigment stones composed of calcium bilirubinate (Saing *et al.*, 1988). The presence of

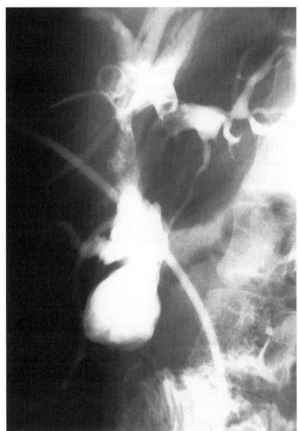

Figure 24.2 *Choledochal cyst – ascending cholangitis with liver abscess.*

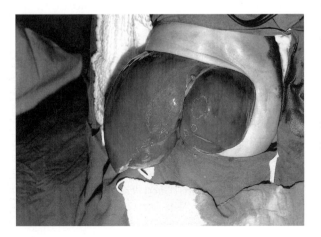

Figure 24.1 *Neonate with massive hepatomegaly due to multiple liver abscesses.*

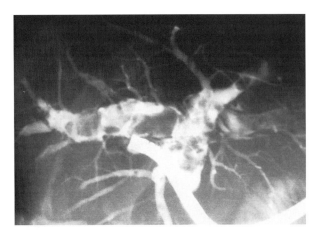

Figure 24.3 *Oriental cholangiohepatis – bile ducts choked with stones and sludge.*

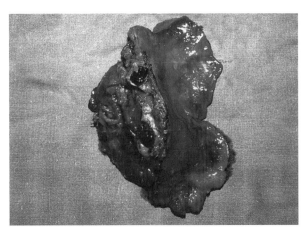

Figure 24.5 *Resected left lobe showing stones and pus in the bile ducts.*

obstruction and infection of the biliary tract, especially in the intrahepatic ducts, often gives rise to the development of pyogenic liver abscesses (Figures 24.4 and 24.5). They are usually multiple, small, purulent collections, and they may contain biliary mud or sludge and pigment stones.

In Third World countries, parasitic infections such as ascariasis are common in childhood (see Chapter 12). The peak incidence in African children was noted to occur at 4–8 years of age, and 28% of cases developed biliary lesions (Cremin and Fisher, 1976). The finding of *Ascaris* in the abscess cavity clearly indicates a direct etiological role, probably related to parenchymal necrosis (Javid *et al.*, 1999). Patients with biliary atresia sometimes develop intrahepatic bilomas after hepatic portoenterostomy, which may form abscesses following ascending infection (Tam *et al.*, 1983; Khuroo and Zargar, 1985) (Figure 24.6).

PORTAL PYEMIA

Although Schatten *et al.* (1955) demonstrated that bacteria could be isolated during routine sampling of portal venous blood in up to 32% of patients, the liver is essentially a sterile organ, presumably because of the excellent phagocytic function of its reticuloendothelial system. There is evidence to suggest that ischemia may play an important role in facilitating suppurative infection in the

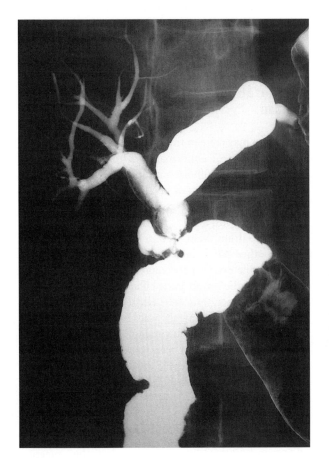

Figure 24.4 *Stricture of left hepatic duct with stones and abscess in the left lobe of the liver.*

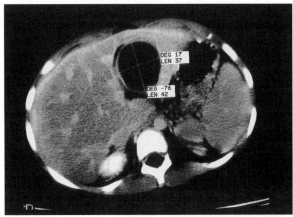

Figure 24.6 *Biliary atresia patient with large biloma and multiple bouts of infection.*

liver. When infection does occur via the portal vein, it is usually secondary to an infective lesion in the gastrointestinal tract. Acute appendicitis has a significantly reduced role, accounting for only 7.9% of cases in a series of 397 cases (Sorenson *et al.*, 1983). Other diseases of the digestive system, such as regional enteritis and foreign body perforation of the gut, have also been reported to give rise to infection of the liver (Altemeier *et al.*, 1970; Lowry and Rollins, 1993).

TRAUMA

In cases of blunt and penetrating trauma liver abscesses may develop as a result of infection in the intrahepatic hematomas (Figure 24.7). In blunt injuries the superior segments of the right lobe are most frequently involved, with formation of subcapsular and intraparenchymal hematomas (Vock *et al.*, 1986). In the case of penetrating wounds the organisms are carried from the external surface into the traumatized liver tissue, and thus initiate the infective process (Figure 24.8). Infection of intrahepatic hematomas may also occur along drains which may have been placed in the perihepatic space during laparotomy for abdominal injuries (Taguchi *et al.*, 1988).

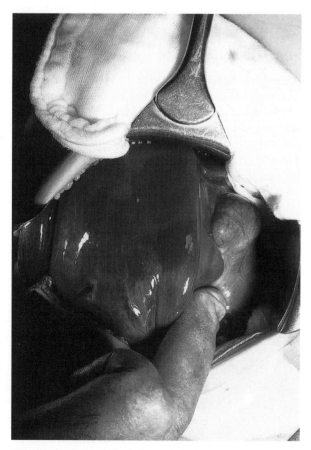

Figure 24.7 *Intrahepatic hematoma following blunt trauma which subsequently needed drainage due to infection.*

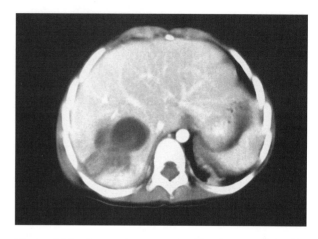

Figure 24.8 *Penetrating trauma with abscess within liver parenchyma.*

SEPSIS

A focus of infection elsewhere in the body may give rise to bacterial infection of the liver through dissemination of the organisms via the systemic circulation. Liver abscesses have occurred in patients with pneumonia, bacterial endocarditis, otitis media and osteomyelitis. However in 15% of patients, no source of preceding disease can be identified to account for the hepatic lesion. This cryptogenic group excludes cases of septicemia in which microabscesses may be demonstrated in other organs in addition to the liver.

Hepatic abscess with pre-existing liver disease

An abscess may arise in the liver in association with pre-existing disease or abnormality of that organ. Cysts of the liver may be solitary, multiple, exist in association with polycystic disease, or be a manifestation of Caroli's disease. Simple solitary cysts may remain asymptomatic, and infection with abscess formation may in fact follow attempts to drain them (Tetz *et al.*, 1973) (Figure 24.9). On the other hand, infection may occur without any demonstrable extrahepatic cause. In Caroli's disease the cysts arise in the intrahepatic biliary ducts. Infection can result in a tremendous increase in the size of the cysts, and over a period of time the walls become thick and calcified (Figure 24.10). Surprisingly, the other normal areas of the biliary tract seem to be unaffected by this infective process. In endemic areas, infected echinococcal cyst as a cause of pyogenic liver abscess must always be considered.

PATHOGENESIS AND GROSS FEATURES

Ultrasound and CT scans show that the infection spreads to the liver from the primary focus (perforated appendicitis) as a septic thrombus in the portal vein

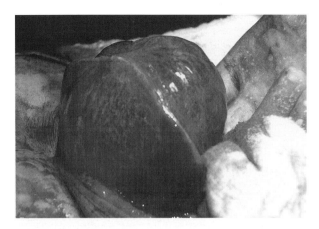

Figure 24.9 *Large solitary cyst of the liver. Infection in such cysts may result in hepatic abscess.*

(Chan *et al.*, 1988). The hepatic lesion evolves from an initial solid inflammatory focus to a well-defined fluid-filled cavity over a period of time. Antibiotic treatment at the stage of a 'hepatitis'-type lesion may result in resolution without abscess formation. The right lobe is involved in 73% of cases, presumably due to its greater size and the larger volume of blood flow. Multiple abscesses are usually associated with biliary tract disease.

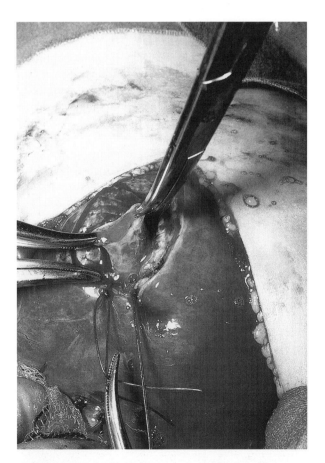

Figure 24.10 *Caroli's disease involving right lobe. Cysts became infected, with large amounts of pus and thick, calcified wall.*

At laparotomy, pyogenic liver abscess appears as a pale-yellowish circumscribed nodule. The cavity may be loculated, giving it a honeycomb-like appearance. The wall may be thin and indistinct, but in longstanding cases it becomes very thick and even calcified, reaching very large dimensions without rupture (Sorenson *et al.*, 1983).

BACTERIOLOGY

Staphylococcus aureus and *E. coli* are the commonest organisms (Frey *et al.*, 1989; Pineiro-Carrero and Andres, 1989; Rustgi and Richter, 1989). Anaerobic organisms should be strongly suspected in cases where gas is present in the cavity and the aspirate is found to be sterile (Table 24.1) (Sabbaj *et al.*, 1972; Perera *et al.*, 1980). *Haemophilus influenzae* has recently been recognized as a causative agent, especially in unvaccinated young children (Hartwig *et al.*, 1999).

CLINICAL FEATURES

Pyogenic liver abscess most commonly presents as a febrile illness with right upper quadrant pain (Table 24.2). The duration of symptoms ranges from 1 to 90 days, but is usually less than 3 weeks. In a review of 397 cases, constitutional symptoms were predominant, with a clinical picture of a flu-like illness associated with malaise and weakness (Sorenson *et al.*, 1983). Other symptoms include weight loss, cough with dyspnea, right shoulder pain and abdominal distension. Physical examination reveals a febrile, lethargic, ill-looking child. Jaundice is present in about 25% of cases, and the liver is tender and enlarged in 70% of patients. In more severe cases, signs of right-sided pleural effusion may be present.

Patients who develop liver abscess following cholangiohepatitis usually have an acute clinical course with fever, chills and rigors, right upper quadrant pain and jaundice. The liver is enlarged and tender. Often a distended gallbladder may be palpated. Cryptogenic liver abscess in infants may present initially as a non-specific febrile illness, and rapidly progress to a fulminating sepsis with marked abdominal distension due to hepatomegaly.

Table 24.1 *Common pathogens in pyogenic liver abscess*

	Gram-negative pathogens	Gram-positive pathogens
Aerobes	*E. coli* *Klebsiella*	*Staphylococcus aureus* *Streptococcus pyogenes* *Streptococcus milleri*
Anaerobes	*Bacteroides* *Fusobacterium*	*Peptostreptococcus*

Table 24.2 *Findings in pyogenic liver abscess*

Finding	Frequency (%)
Sex (male/female)	67/33
Age > 5 years	55
Abdominal pain	90
Fever	80
Anemia	90
Hepatomegaly	73
Raised ESR	100
Leukocytosis	70
Multiple abscesses	50
Right lobe involvement	70

ESR, erythrocyte sedimentation rate.

LABORATORY FINDINGS

The most consistent abnormal finding in pyogenic liver abscess is an elevated erythrocyte sedimentation rate, which is present in almost all patients in the range 32–122 mm/hour, with a mean value of 77 mm/hour. Anemia is seen in 90% of cases, leukocytosis in 70%, and abnormalities in the liver function tests, including raised serum alkaline phosphatase and transaminase levels with significant hypoalbuminemia, in up to 50% of patients.

DIAGNOSIS

The diagnosis of pyogenic liver abscess must be suspected in any child who presents with fever, abdominal pain and hepatomegaly (Karrar and Abdullah, 1985). Confirmation of the diagnosis ultimately depends on the aspiration of pus from the abscess cavity. A number of conditions, such as cysts, arteriovenous malformations, intrahepatic hematomas and tumors with necrosis, can be confused with abscess (Northover *et al.*, 1982; Vock *et al.*, 1986).

DIAGNOSTIC INVESTIGATIONS

The ready availability of ultrasound and its diagnostic accuracy have made it the investigation of choice for pre-operative and intraoperative localization of hepatic abscess (Glen *et al.*, 1984; Salama *et al.*, 1988). Plain chest X-rays may show elevated right hemidiaphragm, pleural effusion or gas/fluid level, but fluoroscopy is not useful (Clark and Towbin, 1983). Other investigations, such as cholangiography and radionuclide scans, have very limited applications (Tetz *et al.*, 1973; Rubinson *et al.*, 1980; Laurin and Kaude, 1984; Denison and Wallerstedt, 1989).

Computed tomography currently provides the best method of detecting pyogenic liver abscess (Halvorsen *et al.*, 1984). The CT appearances of liver abscess are variable, and include gas within a fluid collection in 19% of cases, a single, low-density area in 38% of cases, and a single cavity appearing as a heterogeneous, lower-density area compared with its surroundings in 34% of cases (Figures 24.11, 24.12, 24.13 and 24.14).

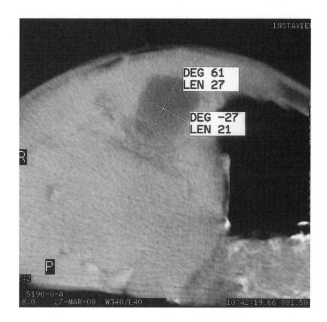

Figure 24.11 *CT scan showing typical solitary liver abscess.*

COMPLICATIONS

The commonest complication associated with pyogenic liver abscess is septicemia, which is associated with a significantly higher mortality (Altemeier *et al.*, 1970). Another complication that may be encountered is rupture, especially in left-sided abscesses (Moore, 1994; Moore *et al.*, 1994). This may occur into the subphrenic space, into the right pleural cavity with empyema, or into the peritoneal cavity, resulting in generalized peritonitis. Other problems associated with liver abscess include obstruction of the intrahepatic biliary ducts and recurrence of the lesion.

Pyogenic liver abscess may sometimes give rise to unusual and dramatic complications, such as hemobilia presenting as life-threatening upper gastrointestinal hemorrhage (Larsen and Raffensperger, 1979; Khalil *et*

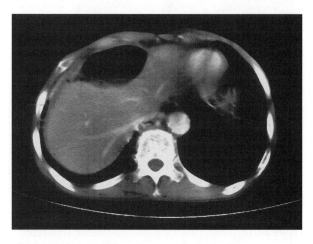

Figure 24.12 *Gas filling abscess cavity in the liver.*

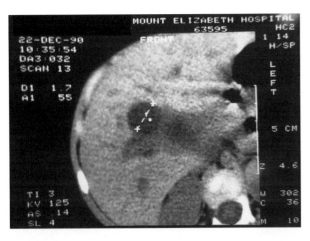

Figure 24.13 *Heterogeneous appearance of abscess cavity on CT. Note the presence of smaller abscesses.*

al., 1991). Selective arterial embolization has replaced open surgery as the treatment of choice.

Septic endophthalmitis has been reported in 7.8% of patients with liver abscess, and the organism involved is *Klebsiella* (Chiu *et al.*, 1988).

TREATMENT

The principles of management of pyogenic liver abscess are as follows:

1 Establish the diagnosis, location and number of abscesses.

2 Start treatment with broad-spectrum antibiotics (Loh *et al.*, 1987; Moore, 1994; Moore *et al.*, 1994; Kumar *et al.*, 1998).

3 Drain the abscess if there is no response clinically and on imaging.

Antibiotics are generally given for an extended period of 6 to 8 weeks, but this may not always be necessary (Bowers *et al.*, 1990). The underlying disease must also be treated at the same time to prevent recurrence (Crass, 1983).

PERCUTANEOUS DRAINAGE

Needle aspiration has been successfully used to drain abscesses which showed a poor response to conservative therapy (McFadzean *et al.*, 1953; Vachon *et al.*, 1986). Lavage is not used unless the material is very viscous (Taguchi *et al.*, 1988).

Percutaneous catheter drainage has now become the procedure of choice for the drainage of uncomplicated abscesses including those which are multilocular (Greenwood *et al.*, 1982; Clark and Towbin, 1983; Skibber *et al.*, 1986). Many types of catheter have been used, and they are passed into the abscess cavity under ultrasound or CT guidance. Drainage is continued until there is scan evidence of resolution (Liu *et al.*, 1990).

OPEN SURGICAL DRAINAGE

This approach is useful in cases where the primary source of infection needs to be surgically treated at the same time. The transperitoneal route is used, and biopsy of the wall with adjacent liver is performed in order to exclude amebic infection and multiple microscopic abscesses (Pitt and Zuidema, 1975). Multiple lesions associated with septicemia are not amenable to surgical drainage (Altemeier *et al.*, 1970).

RESULTS

The mortality rate of pyogenic liver abscess has steadily declined from 36% prior to 1977 to almost zero at the present time (Moore *et al.*, 1994). However, the presence of associated disease, multiple abscesses, mixed organisms and complications can result in significant morbidity (Northover *et al.*, 1982; Bergamini *et al.*, 1987).

AMEBIC LIVER ABSCESS

Amebic liver abscess has been recognized as a distinct entity since the nineteenth century. It is found in about 10% of patients who have amebic infestation of the intestinal tract. The disease is uncommon in children, with less than 5% of abscesses occurring in the pediatric population.

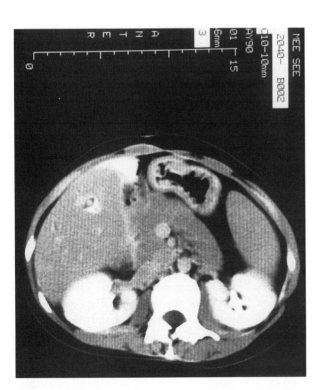

Figure 24.14 *Dense peripheral enhancement surrounding abscess cavity in liver.*

INCIDENCE AND EPIDEMIOLOGY

Amebiasis is endemic in the tropical and subtropical regions of Asia, Africa and Latin America, and is typically associated with poor sanitary conditions. Amebic liver abscess is the commonest extraintestinal site of invasive amebiasis, and mainly affects infants and young children (McCarty *et al.*, 1973; Das *et al.*, 1976; Merten and Kerkes, 1984).

In contrast to the striking male preponderance in adult cases, there is little difference in the sex distribution of amebic abscess in children (Scragg, 1975).

PATHOLOGY

Amebic liver abscess results from invasion of the liver by trophozoites from the bowel through the radicals of the portal vein. In the liver, thrombosis of the portal vessels occurs, leading to infarction and areas of focal necrosis which are further aggravated by the cytolytic activity of the parasite. These changes can be visualized sonographically (Hayden *et al.*, 1984). Multiple abscesses occur more frequently in children, being present in 54% of cases. A solitary abscess in the right lobe occurs in 37% of cases, while single left lobe abscesses are found in only 9% of cases.

CLINICAL FEATURES

Amebic liver abscess presents as a fairly acute illness in childhood, with a clinical picture of a high, swinging fever, tender hepatomegaly and abdominal distension (Figure 24.15). The patient is anemic, but jaundice is not usually present. A previous history of diarrhea with blood in the stools may be obtained in 50% of cases. The combination of fever with a tender, enlarged liver in a child living in an endemic area is sufficient to warrant a clinical diagnosis of this condition (Table 24.3).

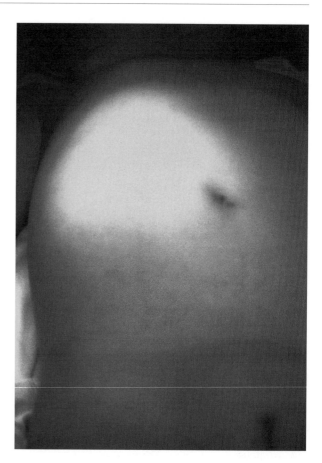

Figure 24.15 *Marked abdominal distension with pointing of the abscess.*

UNUSUAL PRESENTATIONS

Many patients with this condition may present only with prolonged fever without any apparent cause. Left lobe abscesses may give rise to an epigastric mass, and abscesses which are centrally situated may obstruct the bile ducts, causing severe jaundice. Paralytic ileus with toxemia mimicking typhoid fever and abdominal findings mimicking perforated appendicitis may lead to an erroneous diagnosis (Harrison *et al.*, 1979).

DIAGNOSIS

In endemic areas, the clinical picture alone is often sufficient to make the diagnosis, and the response to drug therapy can provide useful confirmatory evidence. Laboratory investigations show a raised erythrocyte sedimentation rate, anemia and leukocytosis. The liver function tests do not show any marked deviations. A raised serum bilirubin level is noted in less than 10% of cases.

Isolation of cysts or trophozoites of *Entamoeba histolytica* in the stool can only be achieved in 35% of patients. Serological tests that detect the presence of antibodies to amebic antigen are positive in more than 90% of cases, but do not differentiate between recent and previous infection.

Table 24.3 *Findings in amebic liver abscess*

Finding	Frequency (%)
Sex (male/female)	54/46
Age < 3 years	70
Fever	100
Abdominal distension	90
Diarrhea	50
Anemia	90
Hepatomegaly	90
Jaundice	10
Leukocytosis	80
E. histolytica positive in pus	60
Multiple abscesses	55
Solitary abscess, right lobe	35
Solitary abscess, left lobe	10

IMAGING

A plain X-ray of the chest will show abnormalities in 50% of patients with amebic liver abscess, including an elevated right hemidiaphragm, right pleural effusion, right lower lobe infiltration and hepatomegaly (Figure 24.16). Radionuclide scans, ultrasound CT and magnetic resonance imaging (MRI) have all been successfully used to identify amebic liver abscess (Figure 24.17). Ultrasound provides the best imaging modality, and the characteristic features of a peripheral halo with central liquefaction are well recognized (Ralls *et al.*, 1982; Moore *et al.*, 1994). MRI can detect early lesions at the stage of granulomatous amebic hepatitis which show up as low-intensity areas surrounded by a double-layered wall (Giovagnoni *et al.*, 1993).

ASPIRATION

Diagnostic needle aspiration of liver abscesses has been used in several centers to establish the presence of an amebic liver abscess. The fluid has been described as having a yellowish color. Gram staining shows no organisms, and culture of the pus is sterile. Amebae can be recovered from the pus in 56–60% of cases.

COMPLICATIONS

The incidence of complications in amebic liver abscess has decreased considerably as a result of earlier diagnosis and effective therapy. However, 17% of patients still present with this clinical problem, and the mortality rate

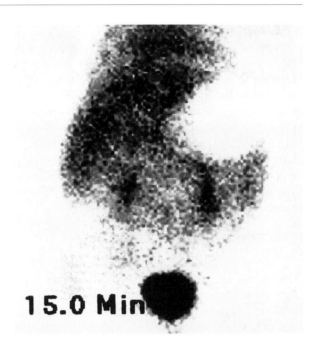

Figure 24.17 *Technetium scan showing filling defect corresponding to abscess cavity.*

is significantly higher in this group. The commonest complication is rupture into the pleural cavity and lung, which occurs in 6% of cases. The clinical features include dyspnea, tachypnea, crepitations at the lung base and evidence of pleural effusion. Rupture into the peritoneal cavity presents as generalized or localized peritonitis with subphrenic and intra-abdominal abscesses. Extension into adjacent viscera such as the stomach and duodenum can give rise to hematemesis. In some patients, abdominal pain, distension and ileus may be present without peritonitis – a condition that is referred to as 'pre-rupture'. Clinical indicators that can be used to predict rupture include a diameter greater than 5–10 cm, progressive increase in size and left lobe location (Baijal *et al.*, 1995).

The most serious complication is extension into the pericardial cavity from left lobe abscesses, resulting in signs of cardiac tamponade or congestive cardiac failure. Other less common complications include hemobilia and hepatic failure associated with thrombosis of the portal vein.

TREATMENT

The management of amebic liver abscess is based on two fundamental principles, namely medical therapy and drainage.

MEDICAL MANAGEMENT

Uncomplicated cases of amebic liver abscess, especially when situated deep within the liver, can be managed by drug therapy alone (Nazir and Moazam, 1993;

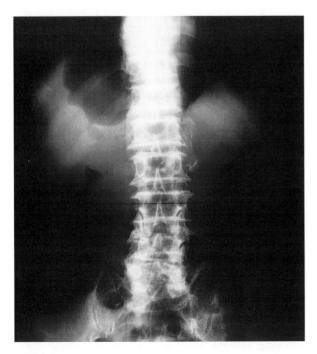

Figure 24.16 *Gas-containing subdiaphragmatic collection following rupture.*

Porras-Ramirez *et al.*, 1995). The drug of choice is metronidazole, which is effective against both tissue and intestinal parasites. The recommended dose schedule is 35–50 mg/kg in three doses daily for 10 days. As a result of the availability of an intravenous form of the drug, it can be used even in situations where the patient is unable to tolerate oral ingestion. The vast majority of patients will show a rapid improvement with defervescence within 72 hours (Barnes *et al.*, 1987). Percutaneous needle aspiration is indicated if symptoms persist or if the abscess is large and rupture imminent, and it has given excellent results (Adams and MacLeod, 1977; Gupta, 1984).

PERCUTANEOUS CATHETER DRAINAGE

The use of ultrasound-guided, percutaneously placed catheters for amebic liver abscess is occasionally indicated, especially in non-endemic areas, in order to differentiate pyogenic from amebic abscess, and also in cases of failure to respond to drug treatment, imminent rupture and left lobe abscess (VanSonnenberg *et al.*, 1985; Singh and Kashyap, 1989). The use of laparoscopic techniques may facilitate catheter placement in difficult cases (e.g. when the abscess is adherent to the diaphragm) (Salky and Finkel, 1985).

SURGICAL DRAINAGE

Although open surgical drainage has been advocated as the primary treatment, this approach is generally restricted to the treatment of complications (Balasegaram, 1981; Basile *et al.*, 1983). Drainage should be performed using catheters placed within the abscess cavity. Needle aspiration and drains placed in the perihepatic space are not effective (Grewal, 1984).

TREATMENT OF SPECIFIC COMPLICATIONS

Extension of amebic abscess into the pleural cavity is best treated with tube thoracostomy drainage. Pericardial extension requires urgent decompression using needle aspiration or percutaneous catheter drainage of the hepatic abscess (Adams and MacLeod, 1977; Takhtani *et al.*, 1995). The latter technique is successful because there is free communication between the pericardial space and the cavity in the liver. Rupture or leakage into the abdominal cavity is best treated by laparotomy. The liver abscess and associated active colitis must also be appropriately treated, in addition to its extension (Harrison *et al.*, 1979).

RESULTS

The mortality rates for amebic liver abscess have declined to very low levels, ranging from 0% to 11% since the introduction of accurate methods of diagnosis and the use of specific drug therapy. The disease has a more fulminating course in infants and in cases where complications have occurred (Jessee *et al.*, 1985).

CONCLUSION

Although hepatic amebiasis is no longer associated with high death rates, it is still a cause of considerable morbidity among the millions of individuals in Third World countries where it is endemic. Transmission by person-to-person contact correlates with overcrowding in slum areas. It is only by implementing public health measures that the enormous social and economic burden of this disease can be alleviated.

Key references

Adams EB, MacLeod IN. Invasive amebiasis. II. Amebic liver abscess and its complications. *Medicine* 1977; **56**: 325–34.

This report is one of the most comprehensive reviews in the published literature on amebic liver abscess. It is based on the large clinical experience of the authors in an endemic area, and it describes in detail all aspects of this condition.

Altman RP, Stolar CJH. Pediatric hepatobiliary disease. *Surgical Clinics of North America* 1985; **65**: 1245–67.

This paper discusses hepatobiliary disease in children and includes a useful section on neonatal liver abcess.

Clark RA, Towbin R. Abscess drainage with CT and ultrasound guidance. *Radiologic Clinics of North America* 1983; **21**: 445–59.

This paper discusses the technical aspects of interventional radiology in the drainage of liver abscesses and provides much helpful practical advice.

Pineiro-Carrero VM, Andres JM. Morbidity and mortality in children with pyogenic liver abscess. *American Journal of Diseases in Children* 1989; **143**: 1424–7.

This reference discusses the epidemiological features of pyogenic liver abscess in children.

REFERENCES

Adams EB, MacLeod IN. Invasive amebiasis. II. Amebic liver abscess and its complications. *Medicine* 1977; **56**: 325–34.

Akierman A, Elliott PD, Gall DG. Association of cholelithiasis with total parenteral nutrition and fasting in a preterm infant. *Canadian Medical Association Journal* 1984; **131**: 122–3.

Altemeier WA, Schowengerdt CG, Whiteley DH. Abscesses of the liver: surgical consideration. *Archives of Surgery* 1970; **101**: 258–66.

Altman RP, Stolar CJH. Pediatric hepatobiliary disease. *Surgical Clinics of North America* 1985; **65**: 1245–67.

Arnspiger LA, Martin JG, Krempin HO. Acute non-calculous cholecystitis in children. *American Journal of Surgery* 1960; **100**: 103–6.

Arya LS, Ghani R, Abdali S, Singh M. Pyogenic liver abscess in children. *Clinical Pediatrics* 1982; **2**: 89–93.

Baijal SS, Agarwal DK, Roy S, Choudhuri G. Complex ruptured amebic liver abscesses: the role of percutaneous catheter drainage. *European Journal of Radiology* 1995; **20**: 65–7.

Balasegaram M. Management of hepatic abscess. *Current Problems in Surgery* 1981; **18**: 282–340.

Barnes PF, De Cock KM, Reynolds TN, Ralls PW. A comparison of amebic and pyogenic abscess of the liver. Medicine 1987; **66**: 472–83.

Basile JA, Klein SR, Worthen NJ, Wilson SE, Hiatt JR. Amebic liver abscess: the surgeon's role in management. *American Journal of Surgery* 1983; **146**: 67–71.

Bergamini TM, Larson GM, Malangoni MA, Richardson JD. Liver abscess: review of a 12-year experience. *American Surgeon* 1987; **53**: 596–9.

Bowers ED, Robinson DJ, Doberneck RC. Pyogenic liver abscess. *World Journal of Surgery* 1990; **14**: 128–32.

Brans YW, Ceballos R, Cassady G. Umbilical catheters and hepatic abscesses. *Pediatrics* 53: 264–6.

Chan SC, Chan FL, Chau EM, Mok FP. Portal thrombosis complicating appendicitis: ultrasound detection and hepatic computed tomography lobar attenuation alteration. *Journal of Computed Tomography* 1988; **12**: 208–10.

Chiu CT, Lin DY, Liaw YF. Metastatic septic endophthalmitis in pyogenic liver abscess. *Journal of Clinical Gastroenterology* 1988; **10**: 524–7.

Chusid MJ. Pyogenic hepatic abscess in infancy and childhood. *Pediatrics* 1987; **62**: 554–9.

Clark RA, Towbin R. Abscess drainage with CT and ultrasound guidance. *Radiologic Clinics of North America* 1983; **21**: 445–59.

Crass JR. Liver abscess as a complication of regional enteritis: interventional considerations. *American Journal of Gastroenterology* 1983; **78**: 747–9.

Cremin BJ, Fisher RM. Biliary ascariasis in children. *American Journal of Roentgenology* 1976; **126**: 352–7.

Das BN, Mitra SK, Walia BNS, Mahajan RC, Pathak IC. Amoebic liver abscess in children: a report of five cases. *Indian Pediatrics* 13: 113–17.

Dehner LP, Kissane JM. Pyogenic hepatic abscesses in infancy and childhood. *Journal of Pediatrics* 1969; **74**: 763–73.

Denison H, Wallerstedt S. Diagnosis of pyogenic liver abscess via liver scanning with indium-111 labelled granulocytes. *Scandinavian Journal of Infectious Diseases* 1989; **21**: 345–8.

Doerr CA, Demmler GJ, Garcia-Prats JA, Brandt ML. Solitary pyogenic liver abscess in neonates: report of three cases and review of the literature. *Pediatric Infectious Disease Journal* 1994; **13**: 64–9.

Frey CF, Zhu Y, Suzuki M, Isaji S. Liver abscesses. *Surgical Clinics of North America* 1989; **69**: 259–71.

Glovagnoni A, Gabrielli O, Coppa GV, Paci E, Catassi C, Giorgi P. MRI appearances in amoebic granulomatous hepatitis: a case report. *Pediatric Radiology* 1993; **23**: 536–7.

Glen PM, Noseworthy J, Babcock DS. Use of intraoperative ultrasonography to localise a hepatic abscess. *Archives of Surgery* 1984; **119**: 347–8.

Greenwood LH, Collins TL, Yrizarry JM. Percutaneous management of multiple liver abscesses. *American Journal of Roentgenology* 1982; **139**: 390–2.

Grewal RS. Amebic liver abscess. *International Surgery* 1984; **69**: 137–9.

Gupta RK. Amebic liver abscesses: a report of 100 cases. *International Surgery* 1984; **69**: 261–4.

Halvorsen RA, Korobkin M, Foster WL, Silverman PM, Thompson WM. The variable CT appearance of hepatic abscesses. *American Journal of Roentgenology* 1984; **141**: 941–6.

Harrison HR, Crowe CP, Fulginiti VA. Amebic liver abscess in children: clinical and epidemiologic features. *Pediatrics* 1979; **64**: 923–8.

Hartwig NG, Sinaasappel M, Robben SGF, de Groot R. Liver abscess caused by *Haemophilus influenzae* b in an infant. *Pediatric Infectious Disease Journal* 1995; **14**: 3.

Hayden CK Jr, Toups M, Swischuk LE, Amparo EG. Sonographic features of hepatic amebiasis in childhood. *Journal of Canadian Association of Radiology* 1984; **35**: 282–99.

Javid G, Wani NA, Gulzar GM et al. *Ascaris*-induced liver abscess. *World Journal of Surgery* 1999; **23**: 1191–4.

Jessee WF, Ryan JM, Fitzgerald JF, Grosfeld JL. Amebic liver abscess in childhood. *Clinical Pediatrics* 1985; **14**: 134–45.

Karrar ZA, Abdullah MA. Pyogenic liver abscess in children: a report of three patients and review of the literature. *Annals of Tropical Pediatrics* 1985; **5**: 97–101.

Kays DW. Pediatric liver cysts and abscesses. *Seminars in Pediatric Surgery* 1992; **1**: 107–14.

Khali A, Chadha V, Mandapati R et al. Hemobilia in a child with liver abscess. *Journal of Pediatric Gastroenterology and Nutrition* 1991; **12**: 136–8.

Khuroo MS, Zargar SA. Biliary ascariasis. *Gastroenterology* 1985; **88**: 418–23.

Kumar A, Srinivasan S, Sharma AK. Pyogenic liver abscess in children – South Indian experiences. *Journal of Pediatric Surgery* 1998; **33**: 417–21.

Larsen LR, Raffensperger J. Liver abscess. *Journal of Pediatric Surgery* 1979; **14**: 329–31.

Laurin S, Kaude JV. Diagnosis of liver–spleen abscesses in children – with emphasis on ultrasound for the initial and follow-up examinations. *Pediatric Radiology* 1984; **14**: 198–204.

Liu KW, Fitzgerald RJ, Blake NS. An alternative approach to pyogenic hepatic abscess in childhood. *Journal of Paediatric Child Health* 1990; **26**: 92–4.

Loh R, Wallace G, Thong VH. Successful non-surgical management of pyogenic liver abscess. *Scandinavian Journal of Infectious Diseases* 1987; **19**: 137–40.

Lowry P, Rollins NK. Pyogenic liver abscess complicating ingestion of sharp objects. *Pediatric Infectious Disease Journal* 1993; **12**: 4.

McCarty E, Pathmanand C, Sunakron P, Scherz RG. Amebic liver abscess in childhood. *American Journal of Diseases in Children* 1973; **126**: 67–70.

McFadzean JS, Chang KPS, Wong CC. Solitary pyogenic abscess of the liver treated by closed aspiration and antibiotics: a report of 14 consecutive cases with recovery. *British Journal of Surgery* 1953; **41**: 141–52.

Merten DF, Kerkes DR. Amebic liver abscess in children: the role of diagnostic imaging. *American Journal of Roentgenology* 1984; **143**: 1325–9.

Moore SW. Left-sided liver abscess in childhood. *South African Journal of Surgery* 1994; **32**: 4.

Moore SW, Millar JW, Cywes S. Conservative initial treatment for liver abscesses in children. *British Journal of Surgery* 1994; **81**: 872–4.

Moss TJ, Pysher TJ. Hepatic abscess in neonates. *American Journal of Diseases of Children* 1981; **135**: 726–8.

Nanni G. Acute acalculous cholecystitis in childhood. *Postgraduate Medicine* 1983; **74**: 269–74.

Nazir Z, Moazam F. Amebic liver abscess in children. *Pediatric Infectious Disease Journal* 1993; **12**: 929–32.

Northover JMA, Jones BJM, Dawson JL, Williams R. Difficulties in the diagnosis and management of pyogenic liver abscess. *British Journal of Surgery* 1982; **69**: 48–51.

Ochsner A, Debakey M, Murray S. Pyogenic abscess of the liver. *American Journal of Surgery* 1983; **40**: 292–319.

Perera MR, Kirk A, Noone P. Presentation, diagnosis and management of liver abscess. *Lancet* 1980; **2**: 629–32.

Pineiro-Carrero VM, Andres JM. Morbidity and mortality in children with pyogenic liver abscess. *American Journal of Diseases in Children* 1989; **143**: 1424–7.

Pitt HA, Zuidema GD. Factors influencing mortality in the treatment of pyogenic hepatic abscess. *Surgery, Gynecology and Obstetrics* 1975; **140**: 228–34.

Porras-Ramirez G, Hernandez-Herrera MH, Porras-Hernandez JD. Amebic liver abscess in children. *Journal of Pediatric Surgery* 1995; **30**: 662–4.

Ralls PW, Colletti PM, Quinn MF, Halls J. Sonographic findings in hepatic amebic abscess. *Radiology* 1982; **145**: 123–6.

Rubinson HA, Isikoff MB, Hill MC. Diagnostic imaging of hepatic abscesses: a retrospective analysis. *American Journal of Roentgenology* 1980; **135**: 735–40.

Rustgi AK, Richter JM. Pyogenic and amebic liver abscess. *Medical Clinics of North America* 1989; **13**: 847–58.

Sabbaj J, Sutter VL, Finegold SM. Anaerobic pyogenic liver abscess. *Annals of Internal Medicine* 1972; **77**: 629–38.

Saing H, Tam PKH, Choi TK, Wong J. Childhood recurrent pyogenic cholangitis. *Journal of Pediatric Surgery* 1988; **23**: 424–9.

Salama HM, Abdel-Wahab MF, Farid Z. Hepatobiliary disorders presenting as fever of unknown origin in Cairo, Egypt: the role of diagnostic ultrasonography. *Journal of Tropical Medicine and Hygiene* 1988; **91**: 147–9.

Salky B, Finkel S. Laparoscopic drainage of amebic liver abscess. *Gastrointestinal Endoscopy* 1985; **31**: 30–2.

Schatten WE, Desprez JD, Holden WD. A bacteriologic study of portal-vein blood in man. *AMA Archives of Surgery* 1955; **71**: 404–9.

Scragg JN. Hepatic amoebiasis in childhood. *Tropical Doctor* 1975; **5**: 132–4.

Sears HF, Golden GT, Horsley JS III. Cholecystitis in childhood and adolescence. *Archives of Surgery* 1973; **105**: 651–3.

Singh JP, Kashyap A. A comparative evaluation of percutaneous catheter drainage of resistant amebic liver abscesses. *American Journal of Surgery* 1989; **158**: 58–62.

Skibber JM, Lotze MT, Garra B, Fauci A. Successful management of hepatic abscesses by percutaneous catheter drainage in chronic granulomatous disease. *Surgery* 1986; **99**: 626–9.

Sorenson MR, Baekgaard N, Kirkegaard P. Pyogenic liver abscess. *Acta Chirurgica Scandinavica* 1983; **149**: 437–9.

Taguchi T, Ikeda K, Yakabe S, Kimura S. Percutaneous drainage for post-traumatic hepatic abscess in children under ultrasound imaging. *Pediatric Radiology* 1988; **18**: 85–7.

Takhtani D, Kalagara S, Trehan MS, Chawla Y, Suri S. Intrapericardial rupture of amebic liver abscess managed with percutaneous drainage of liver abscess alone. *American Journal of Gastroenterology* 1996; **91**: 7.

Tam PKH, Saing H, Lau JTK. Three successfully treated cases of nonamoebic liver abscess. *Archives of Disease in Childhood* 1983; **58**: 828–9.

Tetz EM, Reeves CD, Longerbeam JK. Treatment of liver abscesses. *American Journal of Surgery* 1973; **126**: 263–70.

Vachon L, Diament MJ, Stanley P. Percutaneous drainage of hepatic abscesses in children. *Journal of Pediatric Surgery* 1986; **21**: 366–8.

Vade A, Sajous C, Anderson B, Challapalli M. Neonatal hepatic abscess. *Computerized Medical Imaging and Graphics* 1998; **22**: 357–9.

VanSonnenberg E, Mueller PR, Schiffman HR *et al.* Intrahepatic amebic abscesses: Indications for and results of percutaneous catheter drainage. *Radiology* 1985; **156**: 631–5.

Vock P, Kehrer B, Tschaeppeler H. Blunt liver trauma in children: the role of computed tomography in diagnosis and treatment. *Journal of Pediatric Surgery* 1986; **21**: 413–18.

25

Hydatid disease

SN CENK BÜYÜKÜNAL

INTRODUCTION

Hydatid disease is a slow and silent infestation which can be caused by two closely related species of cestode, namely *Echinococcus granulosus* and *Echinococcus multilocularis*. The most common form, unilocular hydatid cyst, is caused by *E. granulosus*.

E. multilocularis is extremely rare in children, and differs biologically and morphologically from the other species, causing multilocular cysts of the liver (Braun and Seifert, 1941; Unat, 1966; Taspinar *et al.*, 1980).

The incidence of this infestation is particularly high in sheep grazing areas in the Mediterranean and Balkan countries, Turkey, the Middle East, Australia, New Zealand, South America, and North and South Africa (Unat, 1966; Monroe, 1985; Senyüz *et al.*, 1988; Schwartz, 1994). The following discussion refers primarily to *E. granulosus*.

LIFE CYCLE

Life cycle of *E. granulosus* and related pathology (FIGURE 25.1)

The parasite *Echinococcus granulosus* is a small worm, measuring 5–6 mm in length, that consists of a scolex (a head-like segment), a neck, and usually three or four seg-

ments. The scolex is the first segment and the smallest one. In the vertical part of the scolex there is a retractable area which is called the rostellum, on which a double row of hooklets with extremely sharp tips is located. Four suckers, located circumferentially, are found behind these hooklets. The second segment is immature and the third is a mature segment containing the sex organs. The gravid terminal segment is the largest segment of all, and it contains 400–800 ova (Dagher, 1983).

The life cycle of the adult worm is closely linked to an intermediate host and a definitive host. The worm is found in the small intestine of a definitive host (e.g. dog, wolf, jackal). The ova are ingested by an intermediate host (e.g. sheep, cattle, human adults and children) (Unat, 1966; Dagher, 1983).

Life cycle in a definitive host

Adult parasites develop within 4 weeks of the ova reaching the intestine of the definitive host (commonly the dog). The adult parasites develop hooklets with which they become attached to the intestinal mucosa, and nutrition is obtained via the developing suckers. The terminal segment of the worm, containing ova, becomes separated and thousands of eggs spread into the feces of the host. Grass and vegetables are then contaminated by these eggs, which are swallowed by sheep, cattle or humans (Hiçsönmez, 1982; Senyüz *et al.*, 1983; Rizalar *et al.*, 1994).

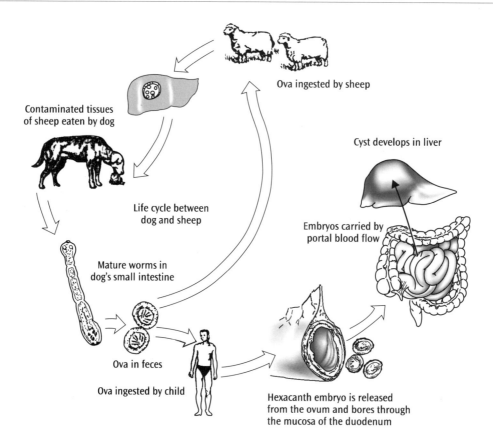

Figure 25.1 *Life cycle of* Echinococcus granulosus.

Life cycle in intermediate host

After ingestion, many of the ova are destroyed by gastric juice. However, some escape from this acidic environment and reach the duodenum, where alkaline digestive juice and the tryptic activity of pancreatic enzymes help to dissolve the rigid membrane of the ovum, releasing the embryo into the duodenal cavity. By means of its sharp spicules, the embryo penetrates the duodenal mucosa and is carried by the bloodstream until it is filtered out in small capillaries within the liver. Although the liver is the site most frequently affected by these embryos, some may reach the lung. Small larvae may also escape from the liver and the lungs and gain access to the heart and general circulation.

The surviving embryos in the liver reach a length of 40 μm before changing into small cysts, known as acephalocysts, which develop and differentiate into mature hydatids. The normal liver tissue around the cyst develops a zone of connective tissue called the *pericyst* or *ectocyst*. This layer consists of fibroblasts, epithelial cells, giant cells and eosinophils, and as the cyst grows, a thick fibrous connective tissue cyst wall is formed which is intimately related to the parenchyma of affected organs such as the liver, spleen and kidney. This thick pericyst layer is not easily separated from the surrounding parenchyma. Attempts to dissect the fibrous tissue away from the parenchyma may cause severe bleeding and tissue damage, and should therefore be avoided.

An *endocyst* lies on the inner surface of the pericyst, and it is possible to separate the two layers (Figure 25.2). The endocyst itself consists of an outer thicker layer and an inner laminated layer, called the *germinal layer*, which is approximately 15 μm in thickness. The outer layer protects the cyst and enhances nutrition by permeation. The inner layer has a granular surface and is responsible for the formation of hydatid fluid and the growth of small capsules and scolices.

The clear fluid within the cyst is highly antigenic and can cause anaphylactic reactions in the host.

The diameter of the cysts within the liver reaches 2 mm by the end of the third month after infestation. Cysts that are located centrally grow more slowly than those on the periphery of the liver, where there is less resistance to spherical growth. There is also a close relationship between the growth rate of the cyst and the age

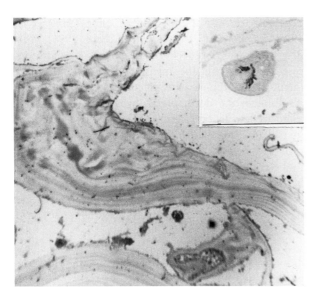

Figure 25.2 *Part of a hydatid cyst removed from a 13-year-old girl. The membrane is composed of fibrillary eosinophilic material (×80). Inset (top right): a small daughter cyst composed of laminated acellular material in which echinococcal hooklets are seen (×200). (Reproduced courtesy of J Stamatakis.)*

of the host. The cysts appear to grow faster in childhood, and scolices reach the size of an adult worm's head. Both the scolices and the small capsules are shed into the bottom of the cystic cavity to form *hydatid sand*.

As the cyst grows, the germinal layer produces increasing numbers of daughter cysts which float in the hydatid cyst fluid. Like the mother cyst, each daughter cyst has a germinal layer and produces both scolices and daughter cysts of its own. Hydatid fluid which contains scolices is highly infectious, and spillage of this fluid during an open or laparoscopic operation, or during any invasive diagnostic procedure, may result in the development of new secondary cysts on the peritoneal surface (Braun and Seifert, 1941; Unat, 1966; Dagher, 1983; Monroe, 1985; Schwartz, 1994).

The life cycle is completed when, for example, a dog eats sheep offal containing viable scolices which then develop into mature worms within the dog's small intestine. Humans are 'incidental' intermediate hosts following ingestion of ova as a result of contact with an infected dog or contaminated environment.

PATHOLOGY

Hydatid cysts are most commonly found within the liver, where the growth process tends to be rather slow. In adults growth may continue for 15 years or more,

although in children very large cysts may appear within a much shorter period of time, and extremely large cysts have been observed in children as young as 3 to 5 years of age (Senyüz *et al.*, 1983). Almost all cysts in children are univesicular, and daughter cysts are commonly absent. The right lobe of the liver is affected more commonly than the left (85% vs. 15% of cases).

Hydatid cysts in the liver can be classified into two major groups, namely uncomplicated and complicated. The intact uncomplicated cysts themselves are usually asymptomatic, although clinical signs may result from pressure or displacement of surrounding organs. For example, a large cyst may induce pressure over the extrahepatic biliary system and cause obstructive jaundice. Furthermore, a cyst in the subdiaphragmatic surface may induce right shoulder pain.

Major complications of hydatid cysts include the following:

- rupture into the peritoneal cavity and allergic or severe anaphylactic reactions (Placer *et al.*, 1988). Large hepatic cysts are at risk from minor blunt abdominal trauma, and may rupture into the peritoneal cavity (Büyükünal *et al.*, 1988);
- jaundice caused by external pressure on the extrahepatic bile ducts (Ceyhan and Büyükpamukçu, 1985);
- infection within the biliary system with transient jaundice, fever, pain from cholangitis and allergic reactions (Marti-Bonmati *et al.*, 1988);
- frank rupture into the major extrahepatic bile ducts causing severe obstructive jaundice (Paksoy *et al.*, 1998);
- rupture into the pleural space and biliopleural or biliobronchial fistulas (Taspinar *et al.*, 1978);
- bacterial infection within the cyst.

Infection within cysts is not uncommon. A cyst may become infected from the biliary tract or, less commonly, through the bloodstream. These infections lead to suppuration or even degeneration of the cyst, and death of the parasite. Calcification is observed in many of these degenerate cysts, and in our practice a 'calcified hydatid cyst' is identical to a 'dead cyst' (Unat, 1966; Dagher, 1983; Monroe, 1985; Senyüz *et al.*, 1999).

CLINICAL FINDINGS

In our experience, hydatid cyst can be diagnosed from as early as 3 to 5 years of age (Senyüz *et al.*, 1983; Zorludemir *et al.*, 1987). Children with simple or uncomplicated cysts are usually asymptomatic, but the cysts are frequently detected on routine abdominal ultrasonography (US) that is performed for some other rea-

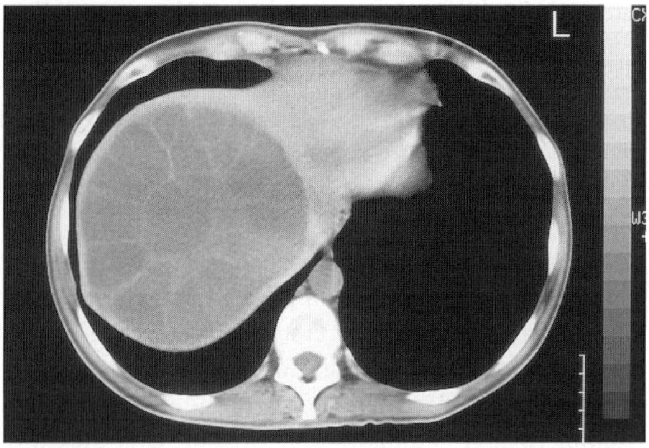

Figure 25.3 *CT scan of a young adult female who had experienced right-sided abdominal pain from the age of 10 years. The cyst in the right lobe of the liver shows septa associated with daughter cysts ('cartwheel sign').*

son. In endemic areas, all symptomatic and asymptomatic cystic masses should be suspected of being hydatid and should be included in the initial differential diagnosis. We are very suspicious of hydatid disease in all children who present with cystic masses in the abdominal and thoracic cavities.

The diagnostic value of specific tests for hydatid disease is still far from satisfactory. The following tests are performed;

- Casoni skin test;
- indirect hemagglutination tests;
- enzyme-linked immunosorbent assay (ELISA).

The most reliable results have been obtained with the ELISA and hemagglutination tests (Yalin *et al.*, 1989a; Baveja *et al.*, 1997; Senyüz *et al.*, 1999). The reliability of the Casoni test is generally less than 50%. It should be noted that cross-reactivity with antigens from other helminth infections reduces the sensitivity of these tests (El Mufti, 1989).

Ultrasonography and CT are now the most commonly performed diagnostic tests for hydatid disease of the liver, and Yalin *et al.* (1989a) reported that CT was more reliable than US in the evaluation of residual disease after surgical treatment (Figure 25.3). However, US is a simple and useful diagnostic test in pediatric patients, and it can image daughter cysts and hydatid sand in most cases.

MEDICAL TREATMENT

The medical treatment of hydatid disease with the antiscolicides mebendazole and albendazole has been the subject of several clinical trials, but these have mainly

been restricted to adult patients (Tsimoyiannis *et al.*, 1995; Vagianos *et al.*, 1995; Aktan and Yalin, 1996). These drugs are especially effective in the larval stage of the disease. By rupturing the microtubules of the germinal membrane of the parasite, glucose uptake is decreased, resulting in the death of the hydatid cysts. However, there are few data concerning the effects of these drugs in pediatric patients, and controversy continues with regard to the dose and duration of treatment in relation to the age of the patient and the size, location and number of cysts. Side-effects caused by the drugs include hepatotoxicity, and frequent liver function tests should be performed during treatment (Morris and Smith, 1987).

A randomized controlled trial of the efficacy of albendazole in adult patients with hydatid disease of the liver has been reported by Gil-Grande *et al.* (1993). In this study the best results were obtained in a group of patients who were treated with 10 mg/kg daily of albendazole prescribed for 3 months. The non-viability rate of the protoscolices and daughter cysts was 94%, and successful treatment was associated with disintegration of the cyst membrane. Echographic changes were observed in 68% of the cysts treated for 3 months, and at the end of this period only one of the 20 cysts was believed to be viable.

Messaritakis *et al.* (1991) reported their experience with pulmonary and liver hydatid disease in the pediatric age group. The authors concluded that success rates were higher in cases with cysts less than 5 cm in diameter. This study showed that 30% of liver hydatid cysts disappeared and did not relapse later.

Since 1995, Senyüz, in Istanbul, has treated pediatric patients with hydatid disease with 1 month of preoperative albendazole. Complete remission has been observed in five patients with cysts smaller than 5 cm in diameter. During the last 3 years, larger cysts have been treated with longer courses of albendazole. Unpublished data on cysts as large as 18 cm in diameter suggest that successful treatment can be achieved with albendazole alone (Senyüz, personal communication, May 2000), using a dose of 10 mg/kg/daily for a period of 3 weeks. Blood analysis and liver tests were performed monthly with a repeat US every 3 months. The total treatment period in these children was 6 months, and calcification, disintegration or shrinkage of the germinal membrane were the positive US findings indicative of successful treatment (Figures 25.4 and 25.5).

As noted above, reversible toxicity has been reported with long-term albendazole treatment, and therapeutic treatment should therefore be monitored carefully with liver function tests. Percutaneous drainage of liver hydatid disease has been recommended during the last decade. Tan *et al.* (1998) reported on the results obtained in 36 adult patients with hydatid disease of the liver. In selected cases with small cysts, the

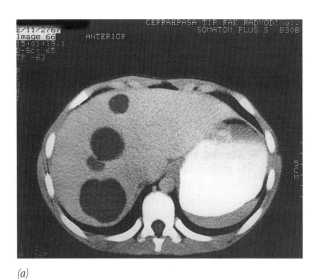

(a)

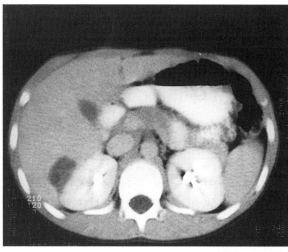

(b)

Figure 25.4 (a) CT of a 9-year-old boy with multiple hydatid cysts, the largest of which is 4 × 4 cm in diameter. (b) The same patient 6 months after mebendazole treatment. Significant shrinkage of the cyst has occurred.

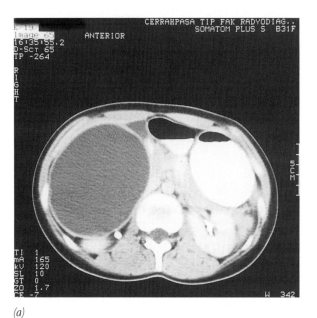

(a)

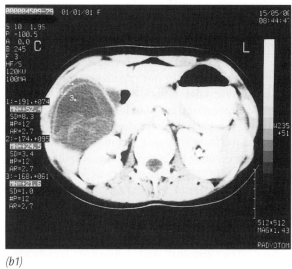

(b1)

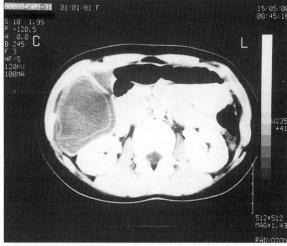

(b2)

Figure 25.5 (a) CT of a teenage girl. A 15 × 13 cm single cyst is present in the right lobe of the liver. (b) CT of the same patient after 6 months of albendazole treatment. Disintegration and shrinkage of the germinal membrane can be seen.

percutaneous drainage technique was reported to be more successful than surgery in terms of complication rate, duration of hospitalization and recurrence rate. However, this was a pilot study involving only a small number of pediatric patients, and there are no data on long-term follow-up.

SURGICAL TREATMENT

Endoscopic treatment of hydatid cysts has been reported (Akkiz et al., 1996), but as yet there are no significant data for the pediatric age group.

The conventional surgical technique can be summarized as follows:

- evacuation of the cyst contents without any spillage;
- closure of minor biliary channels;
- preservation of as much of the liver parenchyma as possible.

In the past, scolicidal agents such as formaldehyde, hypertonic saline, povidone iodine, hypertonic dextrose, hydrogen peroxide, 3% saline or 0.9% saline solution were used (Hiçsönmez, 1982; Zorludemir et al., 1987; Ergüney et al., 1994). In our experience, formaldehyde and hypertonic saline solution may be associated with serious complications, and should be avoided (Senyüz et al., 1999). Preoperative prophylactic albendazole treatment and meticulous surgical technique should be successful in preventing the complications of spillage of cyst fluid. The use of colored agents such as povidone iodine may mask evidence of bile leakage from small biliary channels into the cystic cavity, and is therefore best avoided. The cyst is decompressed with a large cannula and opened between stay sutures in order to prevent spillage. The germinal and laminated membranes, together with all scolices and daughter cysts, are then removed using a combination of suction and blunt dissection.

Various surgical techniques have been recommended for closing the residual cavity after evacuation of the cyst material, including the following:

- free peritoneal drainage;
- partial cystectomy plus capitonnage (closing with mass sutures);
- partial cystectomy and omentoplasty;
- partial cystectomy and marsupialization, or tube drainage (Yalin et al., 1989b; Rizalar et al., 1994; Senyüz et al., 1999).

In endemic areas, many experienced surgeons recommend capitonnage of the remaining cyst without any drainage procedure (Akinoglu et al., 1985; Senyüz et al., 1999). Papadimitrioau and Mandrekas (1970) empha-

sized the usefulness of filling the remaining cavity with a pedunculated mass of omental tissue (omentoplasty), and several authors have reported successful results using this technique (Xynos et al., 1991; Aktan et al., 1993).

In our experience of more than 100 pediatric cases of hepatic hydatid disease, partial cystectomy plus capitonnage has been the simplest and most effective method of treatment. The use of partial cystectomy and free peritoneal drainage has been reserved for cysts located on the convex subdiaphragmatic surface of the liver. We have not found it necessary to use omentoplasty in children, and indeed the omentum is often very rudimentary in the pediatric age group.

Indications for surgery

We suggest that surgical treatment should be reserved for the following cases:

- those with simple cysts over 5 cm in diameter;
- those with cysts that have complications such as intraperitoneal perforation, or fistula formation involving adjacent abdominal organs, the pleural space, the bronchial tree, etc.

Children with cysts smaller than 5 cm in diameter, multiple cysts and involvement of adjacent organs should initially be treated with albendazole or mebendazole.

Surgery of complicated hydatid cysts

BILIARY FISTULA

Small biliary channels should be looked for on the inner surface of the cyst wall, using magnifying spectacles. Any leaking biliary channels must be closed with non-absorbable sutures. Internal or external drainage techniques should be considered for large biliary fistulas. Subdiaphragmatic cysts with biliobronchial fistulas require treatment using combination of abdominal and thoracic approaches. Bronchial communications are closed with non-absorbable sutures.

The closure of persistent postoperative biliary fistulas may be hastened by sphincteroplasty and bile duct intubation (stenting).

PERFORATED HYDATID CYSTS

Cyst perforation should be treated urgently. Due to the high risk of anaphylactic shock, high doses of steroids should be prescibed during the preoperative period. Treatment with albendazole or mebendazole is advised in this group of patients.

Experience of the Cerrahpasa Group in Istanbul

During the period 1978–97, 100 pediatric patients with hydatid disease were treated (Senyüz et al., 1999; Senyüz, personal communication, May 2000). The male.female ratio was 57:43 and the average age was 9.14 years. The liver was the only organ involved in 46 patients, but both liver and lung were affected in 15 patients. In 61 cases with liver involvement, a total of 121 liver cysts were found.

Non-specific abdominal pain in association with a mass was the most frequent clinical symptom and sign at presentation, and ELISA and hemagglutination tests were the most useful diagnostic tests.

Partial cystectomy and capitonnage was the treatment of choice in 45 of the 61 cases. Cystectomy and omentoplasty were used in five patients, whilst five were treated by cystectomy alone and one by marsupialization alone.

Two patients were treated with albendazole alone (10 mg/kg/day for 6 months). The first of these had multiple liver cysts, and the second patient had multiple liver, pulmonary and thoracic wall cysts. In the remaining three patients, a 4-week period of medical treatment was combined with surgical treatment.

Serious postoperative complications were detected in only four children. These were subdiaphragmatic abscess formation ($n = 1$), wound infection ($n = 1$), bowel obstruction ($n = 1$) and biliary leakage ($n = 1$). Only two recurrent cysts were observed.

Two patients with multiple hepatic cysts (one with five and the other with seven cysts) died during the postoperative period. We believe that formaldehyde and hypertonic saline solutions, which were used as scolicidal agents during the surgical intervention, may have been responsible for these deaths. Since these fatalities we have not used any intraoperative scolicidal agents apart from isotonic saline solution.

SUMMARY

Hydatid disease of the liver is still a major problem in some areas of the world. From a public health viewpoint, the breaking of the life cycle between sheep and dogs is the key measure in the prevention of the disease. Six-monthly deworming of dogs, strict disposal of sheep offal and general hygiene in the home all play a part in disease control. Meat from sheep and cattle should also be inspected thoroughly before sale.

Medical treatment of hydatid disease of the liver is now effective in many pediatric cases, although surgery is required for large and complicated cysts. Public health education is the key to reducing the incidence of this disease in endemic areas.

Key references

Hiçsönmez A. Hydatid cyst in childhood. *Progress in Pediatric Surgery* 1982; **15**: 87–94.

This paper provides useful information about the problem of hydatidosis in Turkey and Middle Eastern countries. Details of the role of surgical treatment modalities in pediatric hydatid disease are given.

Messaritakis J, Psychou P, Nicolaidou P et al. High mebendazole doses in pulmonary and hepatic hydatid disease. *Archives of Disease in Childhood* 1991; **66**: 532–3.

Striking and successful long-term results of mebendazole treatment in up to 30% of a group of pediatric patients with hydatid disease of the liver are reported. The success rate in cases of pulmonary hydatid disease was even higher.

Paksoy M, Karahasanoglu T, Carkman S et al. Rupture of hydatid disease of the liver into the biliary tracts. *Digestive Surgery* 1998; **15**: 25–9.

This paper presents clinical experience of one of the major complications of hydatid disease of the liver. Clinical pictures, treatment modalities and the outcomes of this complication are discussed.

Senyüz OF, Celayir AC, Kliç N et al. Hydatid disease of the liver in childhood. *Pediatric Surgery International* 1999; **15**: 217–20.

A clinical study involving a large group of pediatric patients. This is an informative study of medical and surgical treatment modalities.

REFERENCES

Akinoglu A, Bilgin I, Erkoçak EU. Surgical management of hydatid disease of the liver. *Canadian Journal of Surgery* 1985; **28**: 171–4.

Akkiz H, Akinoglu A, Çolakoglu S, Demiryürek H, Yagmur O. Endoscopic management of biliary hydatid disease. *Canadian Journal of Surgery* 1996; **39**: 287–92.

Aktan AO, Yalin R. Preoperative albendazole treatment for liver hydatid disease decreses the viability of the cyst. *European Journal of Gastroenterology and Hepatology* 1996; **8**: 877–9.

Aktan AO, Yalin R, Yegen C, Okbay N. Surgical treatment of hepatic hydatid cysts. *Acta Chirurgica Belgique* 1993; **93**: 151–3.

Baveja UK, Basak S, Thusoo TK. Immunodiagnosis of human hydatid disease. *Journal of Communicable Disease* 1997; **29**: 313–19.

Braun M, Seifert O (eds) *Insanin hayvani parazitleri*. Istanbul: Maarif Matbaasi, 1941 (translated from German).

Büyükünal SNC, Senyüz OF, Erdogan E et al. Importance of underlying anomalies in paediatric trauma. In:

Proceedings of the Thirteenth Annual International Meeting of the Greek Associations of Paediatric Surgeons, 1988: 12.

Ceyhan M, Büyükpamukçu N. Obstructive jaundice due to hydatid cyst in a rare location. *Turkish Journal of Pediatrics* 1985; **27**: 177–80.

Dagher FJ. Echinococcal liver disease. In: Shackelford RT, Zuidema GD (eds) *Surgery of the alimentary tract. Volume IV*, 2nd edn. Philadelphia, PA: WB Saunders Co., 1983: 498–512.

El Mufti M. *Surgical management of hydatid disease: immunological aspects*. Oxford: Butterworth-Heinemann, 1989.

Ergüney S, Önes S, Özcan M. *L'effet scolocide du peroxyde d'hydrogene et du cetrimide dans la chirurgie du kiste hydatique*. Paper presented at XVIII Semaine Medicale Balkanique, Istanbul, 30 August–4 September 1994.

Gil-Grande LA, Rodriguez-Caabeiro F, Prieto JG *et al*. Randomized controlled trial of efficacy of albendazole in intra-abdominal hydatid disease. *Lancet* 1993; **342**: 1269–72.

Hiçsönmez A. Hydatid cyst in childhood. *Progress in Pediatric Surgery* 1982; **15**: 87–94.

Marti-Bonmati L, Menor F, Ballesta A. Hydatid cyst of the liver: rupture into the biliary tree. *American Journal of Radiology* 1988; **150**: 1051–3.

Messaritakis J, Psychou P., Nicolaidou P *et al*. High mebendazole doses in pulmonary and hepatic hydatid disease. *Archives of Disease in Childhood* 1991; **66**: 532–3.

Monroe LS. Gastrointestinal parasites. In: Berk JE, Haubrich WS, Kalser MH, Roth JLA, Schaffner F (eds) *Bockus gastroenterology. Volume VII*, 4th edn. Philadelphia, PA: WB Saunders Co., 1985: 4312–14.

Morris DL, Smith PG. Albendazole in hydatid disease – hepatocellular toxicity. *Transactions of the Royal Society of Tropical Medicine and Hygiene* 1987; **87**: 343–4.

Paksoy M, Karahasanoglu T, Carkman S *et al*. Rupture of hydatid disease of the liver into the biliary tract. *Digestive Surgery* 1998; **15**: 25–9.

Papadimitrioau J, Mandrekas A. The surgical treatment of hydatid disease of the liver. *British Journal of Surgery* 1970; **57**: 431–3.

Placer C, Martin R, Sanchez E, Soleto E. Rupture of abdominal hydatid cysts. *British Journal of Surgery* 1988; **75**: 157.

Rizalar R, Günayd M, Gürses N, Aritürk E, Bernay F, Gürses N. Hydatid cyst of childhood. *Ondokuz Mays Ü. T p Fakültesi Dergisi* 1994; **11**: 197–204.

Schwartz SI. Liver. In: Schwartz SI, Shires GT, Spencer FC (eds) *Principles of surgery. Volume II*, 6th edn. New York: McGraw Hill, 1994; 1319–66.

Senyüz OF, Büyükünal SNC, Yeker D, Danismend N, Söylet Y. Hydatid disease in children. In: *Proceedings of the Twenty-First Turkish National Meeting of Paediatrics*, 1983: 537–42.

Senyüz OF, Erdogan E, Büyükünal SNC *et al*. Benign and malignant lesions of the liver. In: *Proceedings of the Twenty-Seventh Turkish National Meeting of Paediatrics*, 1988: 27–9.

Senyüz OF, Celayir AC, Kiliç N *et al*. Hydatid disease of the liver in childhood. *Pediatric Surgery International* 1999; **15**: 217–20.

Tan A, Yakut M, Kaymakçioglu N, Özerhan IH, Cetiner S, Akdeniz A. The results of surgical treatment and percutaneous drainage of hepatic hydatid disease. *International Surgery* 1998; **83**: 314–16.

Taspinar AH, Büyükünal SNC, Güoney E. A biliobronchial fistula due to hydatid disease of the liver. In: *Proceedings of the Second Turkish National Meeting of Hepatology with International Participation*, 1978: 234–6.

Taspinar AH, Koç AE, Önes S, Akçal T, Büyükünal SNC. L'echinococcose alvoilaire du foi en Turquie. *Archives de l'Union Medicale Balkanique* 1980; **2–3**: 359–61.

Tsimoyiannis EC, Siakas P, Mautesidou KI, Karayianni M, Kontoyiannis DS, Gossios KJ. Perioperative benzimidazole therapy in human hydatid liver disease. *International Surgery* 1995; **80**: 131–3.

Unat EK (ed.) *Tropikal hastaliklar ve parazitoloji. Volume I*. Istanbul: Nurettin Uycan Matbaasi, 1966.

Vagianos CE, Karavias DD, Kakkos SK, Vagenas CA, Androukkakis JA. Conservative surgery in the treatment of hepatic hydatidosis. *European Journal of Surgery* 1995; **161**: 415–20.

Xynos E, Pechlivanides G, Tzortzinis A, Papageorgiou A, Vassilakis JS. Hydatid disease of the liver. Diagnosis and surgical treatment. *HPB Surgery* 1991; **4**: 59–66.

Yalin R, Aktan AÖ, Açikgözoglu S. Computed tomography and sonography of hydatid cyst of the liver after surgical management. *Journal of Medical Imaging* 1989a; **3**: 301–5.

Yalin R, Oguz M, Yildirir C, Dülger M. Surgical treatment of hepatic hydatid cysts. *Medical Principles and Practice* 1989b; **1**: 154–9.

Zorludemir Ü, Okuyan H, Yücesan S, Olcay I. Analysis of 64 patients with hydatid disease. A retrospective study. *Pediatrik Cerrahi Dergisi* 1987; **3**: 113–17.

26

Liver and biliary trauma

PAUL M COLOMBANI

Liver and biliary tract injuries in the pediatric patient have been diagnosed with increasing frequency with the advent of sophisticated technologies for assessing patients with blunt abdominal trauma. Since the liver is the largest abdominal organ in the pediatric patient, it is not surprising that it is now one of the commonest injuries found by CT scanning and other methods. Fortunately, in the pediatric patient the majority of injuries to the liver can be managed non-operatively, and injuries to the biliary tract, although managed operatively, remain quite rare. In general, the management of liver and biliary tract injuries has undergone considerable development over the last 50 years. This chapter outlines the current diagnosis and management of liver and biliary tract injuries in children.

HISTORICAL PERSPECTIVE

Liver injuries have been described since classical times, beginning with the legend of Prometheus. His punishment by the Gods for giving humans the gift of fire was to be chained to a stone in the Caucasus mountains and have an eagle dine each day on a part of his liver until he was saved by Hercules (Hamilton, 1969). From classical times to the twentieth century, anecdotal descriptions of liver injuries were described, and most of them were managed non-operatively. Not surprisingly, these reported injuries were usually fatal (Edler, 1887; Beck, 1902).

During the twentieth century, operative repairs were routinely performed and various operative maneuvers, such as the Pringle maneuver, hepatic artery ligation and other vascular isolation methods, were described (Pringle, 1908; Lucas and Ledgerwood, 1976; Flint and Polk, 1979). Early in the twentieth century, the operative packing of complex liver injuries was used, but the result was a very high infection rate and accompanying mortality. As a result, this approach was abandoned in favor of more aggressive surgical repairs (Madding, 1942; Beebe and DeBakey, 1952).

Despite this aggressive surgical management, a subset of patients with high-grade complex liver and vascular injuries continued to suffer a high operative mortality during attempted resection and repair (Bass et al., 1984; Beal, 1990). These results led to the resurgence of judicious packing for patients with complex injuries. Packing allowed more complete resuscitation of these patients and a better chance of survival (Feliciano et al., 1981, 1986).

During the last 25 years, non-operative management of liver injuries has been the mainstay of therapy for the pediatric patient, and more than 90% of patients are managed in this way. However, successful non-operative management requires continuous clinical monitoring and pediatric ICU capability (Cheatham et al., 1980; Karp et al., 1983; Giacomantonio et al., 1984; Cywes et al., 1985).

In the pediatric age group, biliary tract injuries have always been rare and have usually been associated with iatrogenic or penetrating injuries. In most series, biliary tract injuries usually represent less than 1% of trauma cases. The management of biliary tract injuries has also advanced from attempts to repair damaged bile ducts directly to meticulous reconstruction of the biliary tract with intestinal bypass (Roux-en-Y choledocho- or hepaticojejunostomy). This evolution of definitive repair with intestinal bypass has yielded excellent long-term patency and low complication rates (Burt and Nelson, 1981; Posner and Moore, 1985; Bade et al., 1989).

LIVER INJURIES

Etiology

The majority of injuries to the liver in the pediatric age group are blunt, and less than 10% of injuries are secondary to penetrating trauma. The commonest etiologies include passenger motor vehicle accidents, pedestrian motor vehicle accidents, bicycle injuries and child abuse (O'Neill et al., 1973; Oldham et al., 1986; McGarvey and Indeck, 1991). The mechanism of injury that is common to all of these etiologies is high-speed deceleration and energy transfer to the abdomen and lower right chest (Lau et al., 1987). Liver injuries due to iatrogenic causes, such as massive fluid resuscitation or traumatic delivery in the neonate, external cardiac massage, intraoperative damage during neonatal surgery or laceration from percutaneous liver biopsy, are fortunately rare events (Mason-Brown, 1957).

Attempts to quantify the severity of injury in order to assess outcomes have focused on the type of injury (laceration vs. hematoma), or the extent of injury including vascular disruption, or the method of classification (surgical vs. radiographic description). Liver injuries can be graded at operation using severity criteria established by the American Association for the Surgery of Trauma (Moore et al., 1989). Liver injuries are graded from 1 to 6, ranging from minor injuries (small subcapsular hematoma or minimal lacerations) to major vascular injuries and hepatic avulsion. Table 26.1 provides a detailed description of this grading system. Grading of liver injuries is useful when comparing results obtained from different institutions. Variations in management, complications and outcomes with different grades of injury can be analyzed and the best treatment methods identified.

For the pediatric patient, who is generally managed non-operatively, other grading systems using non-invasive imaging techniques have been developed. The most recent grading system utilizes CT to grade liver injuries ranging from minor lacerations to complex injuries (Moore et al., 1995). Table 26.2 details the CT grading system for pediatric liver injuries.

Table 26.1 *Liver Injury Scale (intraoperative)*

Grade		Description
I	Hematoma	Subcapsular, non-expanding, < 10 cm^2 in surface area
	Laceration	Capsular tear, non-bleeding, < 1 cm in depth
II	Hematoma	Subcapsular, non-expanding, 10–50% surface area
		Intraparenchymal, non-expanding, < 10 cm in diameter
	Laceration	Capsular tear, bleeding, 1–3 cm in depth, < 10 cm in length
III	Hematoma	Subcapsular, > 50% surface area/expanding/ruptured with active bleeding
		Intraparenchymal hematoma, > 10 cm/expanding
	Laceration	> 3 cm in depth
IV	Hematoma	Ruptured intraparenchymal: bleeding
	Laceration	Parenchymal disruption, 25–75% hepatic lobe
		1–3 Couinaud's segment, single lobe
V	Laceration	Parenchymal disruption > 75% lobe, > three segments
	Vascular	Intrahepatic venous injuries
VI	Vascular	Hepatic avulsion

Table 26.2 *CT grading of liver injuries*

Grade	CT description
I	Subcapsular hematoma
II	Contusion or laceration, 1–3 cm in depth
III	Laceration > 3 cm in depth, intraparenchymal hematoma
IV	Hepatic transection; extensive lacerations, stellate dome, posterior right lobe injury

Diagnosis

As with any trauma patient, attention to airway, breathing and circulation is the priority during the initial assessment of the injured child. During this primary survey and the resuscitation period, hemodynamic stability is determined and continuously monitored. Patients with tachycardia, hypotension, decreased capillary refill and cool extremities should be assessed for blood loss. In the multiply injured patient with head, thoraco-abdominal and extremity trauma, a careful frequent assessment of vital signs is required, as a sudden change in vital signs may indicate ongoing bleeding. It is also important to remember that the pediatric patient has considerable cardiorespiratory reserve, and can experience considerable blood loss with minimal objective evidence of shock. It is important to avoid hypothermia in the pediatric patient, and this may be achieved by the use of warmed fluids, heating blankets, and covering the patient's head. In addition, the stomach of hypothermic patients can be lavaged with warm nasogastric fluid. During an operation, intra-abdominal irrigation with warm saline may help to prevent further hypothermia.

Following the initial assessment of vital signs and neurological status, a thorough head-to-toe examination of the patient should be performed (secondary survey). This may reveal external evidence of injury to the right side of the chest or upper abdomen, with soft tissue bruising, hematoma, abrasions or tire marks. Abdominal distension and firmness may also be found on abdominal examination with intra-abdominal blood loss and hematoma. It is important to note that the commonest cause of abdominal distension and pain in the injured child is acute gastric dilatation caused by crying. It can be promptly treated with a nasogastric tube. Penetrating injuries to the right side of the abdomen and the right lower chest below the nipple, with or without exit wounds on the abdomen or back, might also indicate a liver injury.

A number of adjunctive tests are currently in use to assess pediatric patients. Historically, diagnostic peritoneal lavage was performed on patients who showed evidence of blood loss in the abdomen (Root et al., 1965; Olsen et al., 1972; Bivins et al., 1976). A positive peritoneal tap would indicate immediate surgical exploration. With the widespread use of non-operative management of liver and spleen injuries for the pediatric age group, this procedure is now out of date. Diagnostic peritoneal lavage may still be utilized in patients who are unstable and who are being taken immediately to the operating-room for neurological or orthopedic injuries. Warm saline or Ringer's lactate solution (15 mL/kg body weight) is instilled directly into the abdominal cavity and drained back. A positive peritoneal lavage with more than 100 000 red blood cells/mm³ or bile-stained debris would warrant abdominal exploration. Box 26.1 outlines the criteria for a positive peritoneal lavage.

For pediatric patients who are managed non-operatively, the immediate availability of other diagnostic testing is required. Abdominal CT scanning has been used with success to diagnose liver, spleen and other injuries in the abdomen of pediatric patients (Karp et al., 1981; Lino et al., 1981). CT scanning can give the examiner an exact depiction of the location and severity of the liver injury, as well as an idea of how much blood loss has occurred and evidence of active bleeding (Goldstein et al., 1985; Trunkey and Federele, 1986).

Ultrasound scanning in the emergency resuscitation area to assess patients rapidly for potential abdominal injury has also been successfully used in the adult population (Bode et al., 1993; Jehle et al., 1993). Focused abdominal sonography for trauma (FAST) utilizes bedside real-time ultrasound examination to screen for abdominal injury in the trauma admissions area. Four areas of the abdomen are scanned for free fluid and solid organ injury. It is unclear whether FAST will be an effective diagnostic tool for the pediatric patient. One recent study demonstrated a high false-negative rate using FAST in pediatric patients with blunt abdominal trauma, compared with CT scanning (Mutabagani et al., 1999).

Laparoscopy has also been used as an adjunct to the assessment of patients for potential intra-abdominal injuries (Ivatury et al., 1993; Rossi et al., 1993; Gandhi and Stringel, 1997). Certainly laparoscopy may have a role in the assessment of patients for possible intestinal injuries with perforation following low-velocity penetrating injuries. However, for the average liver trauma patient with minor injury secondary to blunt trauma, diagnostic laparoscopy has no role.

MANAGEMENT OF LIVER INJURIES

General measures

Patients who are clinically unstable in the admissions area require immediate fluid resuscitation. One or two 20 mL/kg body weight boluses of Ringer's lactate solution may be given and the patient's clinical response assessed. Persistent tachycardia and hypotension, an altered sensorium and low urine output warrant the administration of blood products. A blood bank that is capable of immediately providing packed red blood cells, plasma and platelets is an absolute requirement. Patients who remain unstable despite fluid and blood administration are taken to the operating-room for exploration. Patients who are stable or who stabilize with fluid resuscitation may then be taken for CT scanning for assessment.

Following initial assessment and diagnosis by CT scanning, most patients with liver injuries are hemodynamically stable and will be observed in a hospital setting (Hepp, 1985; Pearl et al., 1989; Coburn et al., 1995). A number of supportive measures are required for safe monitoring. The pediatric trauma team must be in-house to monitor patients frequently for clinical deterioration. Patients should have one or two large-bore intravenous lines in the upper extremities (above the diaphragm) in preparation for the potential need for

---

Box 26.1 *Criteria for positive peritoneal lavage*

1 Gross blood
2 More than 100 000 red blood cells/mm³
3 More than 500 white blood cells/mm³
4 Presence of bile, bacteria and amylase

rapid fluid or blood administration. The patient should be continuously monitored (cardiopulmonary and/or oxygen saturation). He or she is initially placed on bowel rest with nothing by mouth and a nasogastric tube on suction. A Foley catheter is placed to monitor urine output continuously for most patients. Serial hematocrits or hemoglobin concentrations should be measured every 4 hours for the first 24 hours. In the second 24 hours after admission, basic metabolic and liver chemistry panels are drawn, in addition to hematocrit or hemoglobin. Short-acting narcotics may be used for pain relief, particularly in the multiply injured patient.

Management of blunt injuries

As mentioned above, non-operative management of blunt hepatic injuries is the mainstay of therapy for the pediatric age group. Patients who are hemodynamically stable with no evidence of peritoneal irritation may be managed in the ICU or ward setting, depending on the grade of liver injury diagnosed by CT scan. Patients who are stable with CT grade I and II injuries may be safely monitored in a hospital ward (Figure 26.1). Stable patients with more extensive CT grade III and IV injuries should be monitored in an ICU setting (Figures 26.2 and 26.3). Recently, a multicenter study of resource utilization showed that grade III injuries can also be managed on the pediatric ward (Miller *et al.*, 1998). The actual specific grade of liver injury is not quite as important as the presence of hemodynamic stability and the trend in the patients' vital signs and their hemoglobin level following injury. In patients who have neurological or other multiple injuries, non-operative management of liver injuries may still be possible, but will require more careful monitoring in the ICU setting. Using this approach, more than 90% of liver injuries may be managed non-operatively (Stylianos, 2000). Patients with evidence of ongoing blood loss with a falling hematocrit/hemoglobin level and the need for blood administration will need a reassessment of a non-operative management schema. Blood loss of more than 40 mL/kg body weight is often used as an indicator for operative intervention. This may be by angiography to embolize bleeding vessels, or by surgical exploration. Patients with evidence of ongoing blood loss who are hemodynamically stable are candidates for angiographic localization and embolization of active bleeding sites (Figure 26.4). Patients who deteriorate rapidly and are hemodynamically unstable should undergo prompt surgical exploration. Figure 26.5 shows an algorithm for the management of the pediatric patient with suspected liver injury.

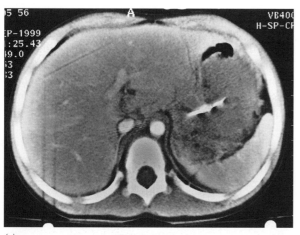

(a)

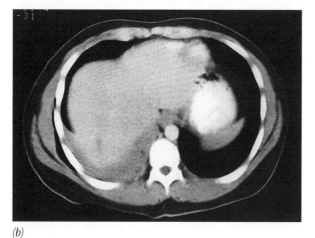

(b)

Figure 26.1 *(a) CT scan radiographically demonstrating a grade I liver injury following blunt abdominal injury. Contusion to the posterior medial right lobe with minimal hematoma. (b) CT scan radiographically demonstrating a grade II liver injury. The patient suffered a stab wound to the posterior chest/flank area. Tract of stab wound in the posterior right lobe of the liver with surrounding hematoma.*

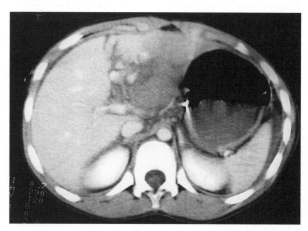

Figure 26.2 *Abdominal CT demonstrating evidence of extensive grade IV injury to the left lobe of the liver with deep lacerations. Active extravasation of intravenous contrast as well as evidence of decreased perfusion to the left lateral segment of the liver.*

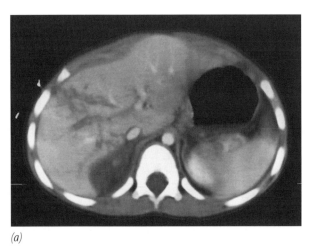

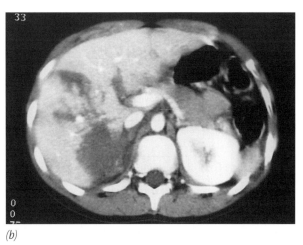

(a)   (b)

Figure 26.3 *(a) CT scan radiographically demonstrating a grade III liver injury. CT scan demonstrates deep lacerations involving the medial left lobe and the medial area of the right lobe of the liver. (b) CT scan radiographically demonstrating a grade IV liver injury. CT scan demonstrates extensive lacerations and intraparenchymal hematoma involving the right lobe and medial left lobe of the liver, with extravasation of contrast.*

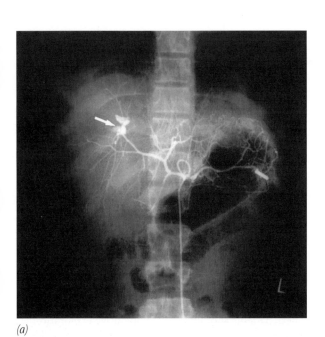

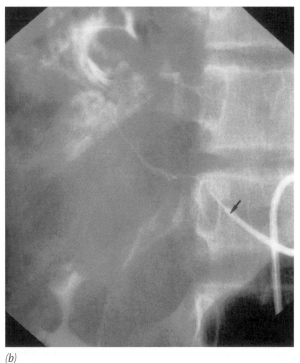

(a)   (b)

Figure 26.4 *(a) Celiac axis arteriogram demonstrating extravasation of contrast into the liver parenchyma in a patient who developed continuing blood loss following blunt injury. Arteriogram demonstrates site of active intraparenchymal bleeding. (b) Embolization of blood vessels feeding bleeding sites was successful in stopping blood loss and avoiding the need for surgical exploration. (Reproduced courtesy of ER Howard.)*

Penetrating injuries

Penetrating injuries may be divided into low-velocity (e.g. stab wounds, foreign bodies) and high-velocity (e.g. gunshot) injuries. Patients with absent peritoneal signs after low-velocity injuries may be safely managed non-operatively. If there is evidence of peritoneal signs or ongoing blood loss occurs, the patient should be explored. Exploration may begin with diagnostic laparoscopy in some centers. High-velocity penetrating gunshot wounds to the abdomen in children should be explored if the peritoneal cavity has been entered or traversed. There is a higher incidence of organ injury in children secondary to this type of penetrating injury. Persistent hemorrhage after percutaneous needle liver biopsy can be managed by urgent angiography and embolization, or by surgical exploration.

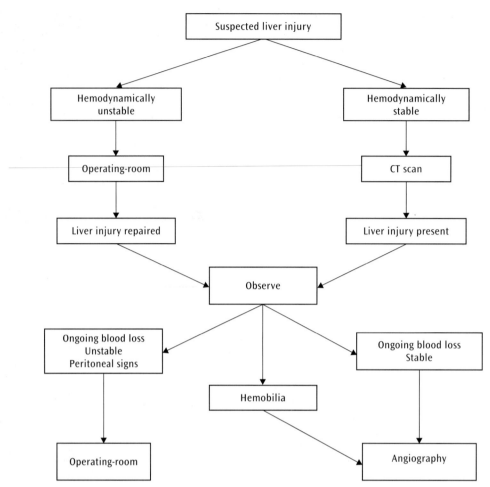

Figure 26.5 *Algorithm for the management of pediatric liver injuries.*

Liver rupture in the neonate

Fortunately, liver rupture in the neonate is a rare occurrence. A traumatic vaginal delivery may injure the neonatal liver, with intra-abdominal hemorrhage. Massive fluid resuscitation in the preterm infant with acute right heart overload may lead to passive congestion and enlargement of the liver. Capsular rupture and intra-abdominal bleeding may then occur. These patients should be managed expectantly as for blunt traumatic injury in older patients. Operative intervention is required for ongoing bleeding. Operative packing is the initial management of choice to allow for complete resuscitation. Similarly, intraoperative liver capsule rupture during neonatal surgery is best managed by judicious packing to stop ongoing blood loss. Packs may be removed after 48 hours.

OPERATIVE APPROACH

Patients who have sustained penetrating or blunt injuries with hemodynamic instability and evidence of ongoing blood loss or peritoneal signs are candidates for operative intervention. Hemodynamic instability in the emergency area with evidence of major liver injury requires early operative intervention. Early signs of peritonism might indicate intestinal perforation, and the late appearance of peritoneal signs might indicate a bile leak. These patients should undergo operative exploration.

Numerous repair techniques have been developed during the last century for the management of hepatic injuries. A successful operative approach requires an intimate knowledge of the perihepatic anatomy for rapid and safe exposure and vascular control. Detailed knowledge of the segmental anatomy of the liver is also essential (Couinaud, 1957; Bismuth, 1982; Buechter *et al.*, 1990). Patients who require operation should have a laparotomy through a midline incision. Rapid evacuation of the hematoma and manual compression of the liver with or without a Pringle maneuver are then performed. If the patient continues to bleed actively despite these measures, particularly in the presence of hypothermia and coagulopathy, then packing of the right upper quadrant and perihepatic area is recommended. In this situation, patients with bleeding that is controlled by packing may be brought back to the ICU for continued resuscitation, correction of coagulopathy and rewarming (Krige *et al.*, 1992). Packs may be left in place for 48–72 hours, and the patient is then taken back to the operating-room for re-exploration and definitive repair of the injury (Svoboda *et al.*, 1982; Baracco-Gandolfo *et al.*, 1986; Cue *et al.*, 1990).

Patients who are stable with bleeding controlled by compression and minimal packing should undergo a more detailed assessment of the extent of their injuries. Depending on the depth and extent of injury, repair may involve simple debridement with ligation of vascular or biliary duct structures which are actively bleeding or leaking bile. For more extensive injuries, patients may undergo a non-anatomical resection or debridement of devitalized injured liver tissue or formal lobar resection (Pachter *et al.*, 1981). Occasionally, complex injuries may require selective hepatic artery ligation (Mays *et al.*, 1979). Some centers have proposed the use of fibrin glue or vicryl mesh to bolster and repair extensive lacerations within the liver.

Patients with retrohepatic major vascular injuries have been managed by a variety of techniques, including atrial–caval shunting, retrohepatic caval balloon shunting, and more recently vascular isolation and direct repair without the use of intraoperative shunting (Yellin *et al.*, 1971; Pilcher *et al.*, 1977; Coln *et al.*, 1980; Rovito, 1987). Finally, patients may undergo transplant for extensive avulsion and irreversible injury to the entire liver (Esquivel *et al.*, 1987; Ringe *et al.*, 1991).

COMPLICATIONS

For the non-operatively managed patient, complications of management are in fact quite rare. Delayed or continued bleeding occurs in a very small number of patients, but the majority (> 90%) are successfully managed non-operatively without exploration. Occasionally, a patient may develop gastrointestinal bleeding suggestive of hemobilia (Figure 26.6). An arteriovenous fistula may also rarely occur within the liver following traumatic injury (Figure 26.7). Intra-abdominal infection, intra-hepatic abscess and bile leaks into the peritoneal cavity may occur, but are also quite rare in these patients. For the operatively managed patient, postoperative hematoma with or without infection, hemobilia and bile leaks may all occur. Most patients are drained following repair in order to control a bile leak if it occurs.

Patients who develop these complications can often be managed non-operatively. Those with evidence of slow ongoing blood loss, but who are hemodynamically stable, may benefit from angiography and selective embolization (Hendren *et al.*, 1971; Wagner *et al.*, 1985) (Figure 26.4 above). Patients with hemobilia or arteriovenous fistulas may also require selective embolization of the offending arterial branch within the liver

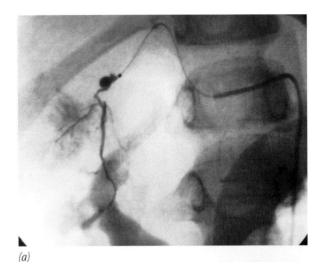

(a)

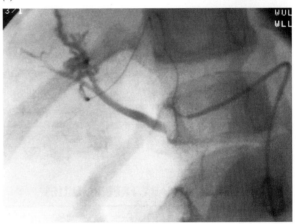

(b)

Figure 26.6 *Hemobilia. The patient developed gastrointestinal bleeding 3 weeks after suffering blunt abdominal trauma. (a) Distal selective right hepatic arteriogram demonstrating false aneurysm and extravasation of contrast. (b) Contrast beginning to fill right hepatic bile duct.*

(Heimbach *et al.*, 1978; Franklin *et al.*, 1980; Tanaka *et al.*, 1991). Percutaneous drainage of perihepatic or intra-hepatic abscesses or biliary collections may avoid operative drainage (Gerzof *et al.*, 1981, 1985).

OUTCOMES

More than 90% of children with a liver injury are managed non-operatively, and the mortality rate in these patients is less than 10%. Most of the patients who require surgery come to the emergency room *in extremis* with severe hypotension, evidence of obvious abdominal bleeding and hemodynamic instability. The survival rate in these patients is less than 50%. In the multiply injured patient, outcome is also related to the pattern of concomitant injuries, with serious head injury being a major determinant of survival.

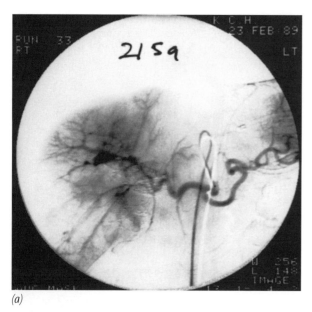

(a)

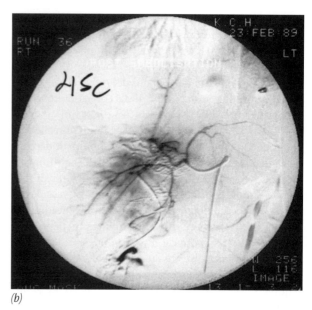

(b)

Figure 26.7 (a) Selective celiac axis injection showing pathological arterioportal shunting at an area of liver disruption following penetrating injury. (b) Venous phase of the superior mesenteric artery injection, showing shunting between the portal vein and the middle hepatic vein at the same site. (c) Selective arterial embolization of the site of arterial disruption was used to ablate the shunts. (Reproduced courtesy of ER Howard.)

EXTRAHEPATIC BILIARY TREE INJURIES

Etiology

In the pediatric patient, intrahepatic biliary tract injuries are extremely rare, representing less than 1% of injuries. The commonest etiology is penetrating trauma. Biliary tract injuries also occur in association with injuries to the liver and other organs in the upper abdomen, such as the duodenum and pancreas (Busuttil *et al.*, 1980; Kitahama *et al.*, 1982; Burgess and Fulton, 1992). Iatrogenic biliary tract injury during the course of routine or laparoscopic cholecystectomy or endoscopic retrograde cholangiopancreatography may also occur (Hepp, 1985; Pitt *et al.*, 1989).

Diagnosis

Since most biliary tract injuries are secondary to penetrating trauma, these injuries are most often encountered during surgical exploration. A careful assessment should be made of all potential organs injured and the extent of the biliary injury.

Given the infrequency of extrahepatic biliary injury secondary to blunt trauma, the diagnosis of these injuries is usually delayed. The diagnosis may not be made until the actual onset of peritoneal irritation or signs of a fluid collection in the upper abdomen or biliary obstruction secondary to a stricture at the injury site (Figure 26.8). In the patient who has sustained an iatrogenic injury, the diagnosis should be entertained in the presence of a fluid collection in the upper abdomen with or without peritoneal signs in the context of recent upper abdominal surgery. Evidence of liver enzyme elevation, bacteremia or sepsis may also be present.

A number of adjunctive studies are available to diagnose biliary tract injuries. These include abdominal CT scanning to assess fluid collections and technetium-99m-hydroxyimidoacetic acid (HIDA) scanning to look for extravasation of tracer from the biliary tree (Sty *et al.*,

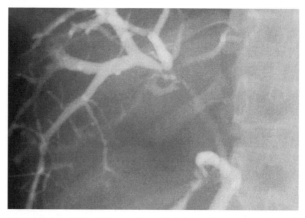

Figure 26.8 Hilar biliary stricture involving the common hepatic duct and first-order intrahepatic ducts 3 months after blunt trauma. (Reproduced courtesy of ER Howard.)

1982). In addition, endoscopic retrograde cholangio-pancreatography or percutaneous transhepatic cholangiography may be used with success to diagnose biliary tract or pancreatic duct injuries (see Chapter 35).

Classification

As for liver injuries, the American Association for the Surgery of Trauma has also classified extrahepatic biliary tract injuries according to a grading system (Burgess and Fulton, 1992). Box 26.2 outlines the grading system.

Box 26.2 *Extrahepatic biliary tract injury score*

Grade

1   Contusion of gallbladder/portal triad
2   Laceration/perforation/partial avulsion of gallbladder
3   Complete gallbladder avulsion; cystic duct injury
4   Any injuries to right or left hepatic ducts; common hepatic duct injury ≤ 50% transection
5   > 50% transection of common hepatic or bile duct; intraduodenal or intrapancreatic common bile duct injury

Adapted from Moore EE, Shackford SR, Pachter HL *et al.* Organ injury scaling: spleen, liver and kidney. *Journal of Trauma* 1989; **29**: 1664–6.

Management

The clinical setting for biliary tract injuries is usually the patient with an intra-abdominal penetrating injury. Patients with high-velocity injuries are explored, since there is a high incidence of injuries that require surgical correction. Patients with stab wounds that are being managed expectantly may require exploration if peritoneal signs develop. At operation, the upper abdomen and porta hepatis are assessed. Extrahepatic biliary tract injuries will usually be found if there is evidence of bile staining and hematoma in the porta hepatis. An assessment of the gallbladder and extrahepatic bile ducts should be made. Hematoma or bile staining in the region of the porta hepatis mandate that a Kocher maneuver be performed to mobilize the duodenum and head of the pancreas for a complete assessment. If the gallbladder is found to be injured, it should be removed rather than repaired. A clean laceration of the common bile duct or common hepatic duct with minimal blast injury can be repaired using a simple repair with T-tube stenting and

drainage. This may be the case with stab wounds. However, patients who have more complex injuries, with segmental loss of more than 50% of the wall of the bile duct, circumferential injuries or transections, should undergo a formal biliary–enteric anastomosis. A number of different methods for reconstructing the biliary tract have been described. The method which has the lowest rate of long-term complications is a Roux-en-Y choledochojejunostomy.

Complications

Patients who require extrahepatic biliary tract repairs may develop a number of complications. A bile leak into the abdomen may occur following repair which would yield a biliary collection or fistula. In the absence of downstream stricture or obstruction, simple drainage should allow healing of the biliary leak. Endoscopic retrograde cholangiopancreatography and temporary stenting of the bile duct may encourage resolution by facilitating internal bile drainage. More commonly, a stricture may develop during the postoperative period. This is more likely to occur with a primary repair, even with the use of T-tube stenting. Stricture formation is rare when a careful Roux-en-Y choledocho jejunostomy is performed using healthy proximal bile duct tissue.

Outcomes

When extrahepatic biliary tract injuries are managed by primary repair or reconstruction using a biliary–enteric anastamosis, these injuries should be treated successfully with minimal long-term morbidity and mortality (Millar and Bass, 1998).

SUMMARY

In summary, liver and biliary tract injuries represent an important group of injuries in the pediatric age group following blunt or penetrating trauma. In some series, more than 50% of the abdominal injuries identified are liver injuries. The mechanism of injury, physical findings and a high index of suspicion of hepatobiliary injury should prompt diagnostic studies to identify specific injuries. Most liver injuries are identified promptly and successfully managed non-operatively. However, operative or angiographic intervention is necessary in a minority of patients. Biliary tract injuries are often diagnosed at the time of exploration for penetrating trauma and repaired primarily. Overall morbidity and mortality rates are low when a standard treatment algorithm is followed.

Key references

Bismuth H. Surgical anatomy and anatomical surgery of the liver. *World Journal of Surgery* 1982; **6**: 3–9.

This article outlines the internal anatomy of the liver and is essential reading for all liver surgeons.

Feliciano DV, Mattox KL, Birch JM. Packing for control of hepatic hemorrhage: 58 consecutive patients. *Journal of Trauma* 1986; **26**: 738–43.

This paper resurrects the use of intraoperative packing of the bleeding damaged liver to stabilize the patient.

Karp MP, Cooney DR, Pros GA *et al.* The non-operative management of pediatric hepatic trauma. *Journal of Pediatric Surgery* 1983; **18**: 512–18.

This article documents the use of non-operative management for pediatric blunt liver injuries. It applies the techniques and guidelines used for managing splenic injury.

REFERENCES

Bade PG, Thomson SR, Hirschberg A *et al.* Surgical options in traumatic injury to the extrahepatic biliary system. *British Journal of Surgery* 1989; **76**: 256–8.

Baracco-Gandolfo V, Vidarte O, Baracco-Miller V *et al.* Prolonged closed liver packing in severe hepatic trauma: experience with 36 patients. *Journal of Trauma* 1986; **26**: 754–6.

Bass BL, Eichelberger MR, Schisgall R *et al.* Hazards of non-operative therapy of hepatic injury in children. *Journal of Trauma* 1984; **24**: 978–82.

Beal SL. Fatal hepatic hemorrhage: an unresolved problem in the management of complex liver injuries. *Journal of Trauma* 1990; **30**: 163–9.

Beck C. Surgery of the liver. *Journal of the American Medical Association* 1902; **38**: 1063–70.

Beebe GW, DeBakey ME (eds) *Battle casualties.* Springfield, IL: Charles C Thomas, 1952.

Bismuth H. Surgical anatomy and anatomical surgery of the liver. *World Journal of Surgery* 1982; **6**: 3–9.

Bivins BA, Jona JZ, Belin RP. Diagnostic peritoneal lavage in pediatric trauma. *Journal of Trauma* 1976; **16**: 739–42.

Bode PJ, Niezen RA, Van-Vugt AB *et al.* Abdominal ultrasound as a reliable indicator for conclusive laparotomy in blunt abdominal trauma. *Journal of Trauma* 1993; **34**: 27–31.

Buechter KJ, Zeppa R, Gomez G. The use of segmental anatomy for an operative classification of liver injuries. *Annals of Surgery* 1990; **211**: 669–73.

Burgess P, Fulton RL. Gallbladder and extrahepatic biliary duct injury following abdominal trauma. *Injury* 1992; **23**: 413–14.

Burt TB, Nelson JA. Extrahepatic biliary duct trauma – spectrum of injuries. *Western Journal of Medicine* 1981; **134**: 283–9.

Busuttil RW, Kitahama A, Cerise E *et al.* Management of blunt and penetrating injuries to the porta hepatis. *Annals of Surgery* 1980; **191**: 641–8.

Cheatham JE, Smith IE, Tunnell WP *et al.* Non-operative management of subcapsular hematomas of the liver. *American Journal of Surgery* 1980; **140**: 852–7.

Coburn MC, Pfeifer J, DeLuca FG. Nonoperative management of splenic and hepatic trauma in the multiply injured pediatric and adolesceut patient. *Archives of Surgery* 1995; **130**: 332–8.

Coln D, Crighton J, Schorn L. Successful management of hepatic vein injury from blunt trauma in children. *American Journal of Surgery* 1980; **140**: 858–64.

Couinaud C. *Le foie. Etudes anatomiques et chirurgicales.* Paris: Masson, 1957.

Cue JI, Cryer HG, Miller FB *et al.* Packing and planned re-exploration for hepatic and retroperitoneal hemorrhage: critical refinements of a useful technique. *Journal of Trauma* 1990; **30**: 1011–13.

Cywes S, Rode H, Millar AJW. Blunt liver trauma in children: nonoperative management. *Journal of Pediatric Surgery* 1985; **20**: 14–18.

Edler L. Die traumatischen Verletzungen der parenchymatosen Unterleibsorgane. *Archiv der Klinische Chirurgie* 1887; **34**: 343, 573, 738.

Esquivel CO, Bernardos A, Makowka L *et al.* Liver replacement after massive hepatic trauma. *Journal of Trauma* 1987; **27**: 800–2.

Feliciano DV, Mattox KL, Jordan GL Jr. Intra-abdominal packing for control of hepatic hemorrhage: a reappraisal. *Journal of Trauma* 1981; **21**: 285–90.

Feliciano DV, Mattox KL, Birch JM. Packing for control of hepatic hemorrhage: 58 consecutive patients. *Journal of Trauma* 1986; **26**: 738–43.

Flint LM Jr, Polk HC Jr. Selective hepatic artery ligation: limitation and failures. *Journal of Trauma* 1979; **19**: 319–23.

Franklin RH, Bloom WI, Schottstal RO. Angiographic embolization as a definite treatment for hemobilia. *Journal of Trauma* 1980; **20**: 702–5.

Gandhi RR, Stringel G. Laparoscopy in pediatric abdominal trauma. *Journal of the Society for Laparoendoscopic Surgery* 1997; **1**: 349–51.

Gerzof SG, Coggins AH, Johnson WC *et al.* Percutaneous catheter drainage in abdominal abscesses. *New England Journal of Medicine* 1981; **305**: 653–7.

Gerzof SG, Johnson WC, Robbin AH. Intrahepatic pyogenic abscesses: treatment by percutaneous drainage. *American Journal of Surgery* 1985; **149**: 487–94.

Giacomantonio M, Filler RM, Rich RH. Blunt hepatic trauma in children: experience with operative and nonoperative management. *Journal of Pediatric Surgery* 1984; **54**: 443–5.

Goldstein AS, Sclafani SJA, Kupferstein NH *et al.* The diagnostic superiority of computerized tomography. *Journal of Trauma* 1985; **25**: 938–46.

Hamilton E. How the world and mankind were created. In: *Mythology: timeless tales of gods and heroes*. New York: The New American Library, Inc., 1969: 70–3.

Heimbach OM, Ferguson GS, Harley JD. Treatment of traumatic hemobilia with angiographic embolization. *Journal of Trauma* 1978; **18**: 221–4.

Hendren WH, Warshaw AL, Fleischli DJ *et al.* Traumatic haemobilia: non-operative management with healing documented by serial angiography. *Annals of Surgery* 1971; **174**: 991–3.

Hepp J. Hepaticojejunostomy using the left biliary trunk for iatrogenic biliary lesions: the French connection. *World Journal of Surgery* 1985; **9**: 507–11.

Ivatury RR, Simon RJ, Stahl WM. A critical evaluation of laparoscopy in penetrating abdominal trauma. *Journal of Trauma* 1993; **34**: 822–7.

Jehle D, Guarino J, Karamanoukian H. Emergency department ultrasound in the evaluation of blunt abdominal trauma. *American Journal of Emergency Medicine* 1993; **11**: 342–6.

Karp MP, Cooney DR, Berger PE *et al.* The role of computed tomography in the evaluation of blunt abdominal trauma in children. *Journal of Pediatric Surgery* 1981; **16**: 316–23.

Karp MP, Cooney DR, Pros GA *et al.* The non-operative management of pediatric hepatic trauma. *Journal of Pediatric Surgery* 1983; **18**: 512–18.

Kitahama A, Elliott LF, Overby JL. The extrahepatic biliary tract injury. *Annals of Surgery* 1982; **196**: 536–40.

Krige JE, Bornman PC, Terblanche J. Therapeutic perihepatic packing in complex liver trauma. *British Journal of Surgery* 1992; **79**: 43–6.

Lau IV, Horsch JD, Viano DG *et al.* Biomechanics of liver injury by steering wheel loading. *Journal of Trauma* 1987; **27**: 225–35.

Lino S, Sawada T, Kusonoki T. Computed tomography in neonatal subcapsular hemorrhage of the liver. *Journal of Computed-Assisted Tomography* 1981; **5**: 416–17.

Lucas CE, Ledgerwood AM. Prospective evaluation of hemostatic techniques for liver injuries. *Journal of Trauma* 1976; **16**: 442–51.

McGarvey N, Indeck M. Epidemiology of liver trauma. *Trauma Quarterly* 1991; **7**: 22–6.

Madding GF, Lawrence KB, Kennedy DA. Forward surgery of the severely injured. *Second Auxiliary Surgical Group* 1942; **1**: 307–10.

Mason-Brown HH. Hepatic haemorrhage in the newborn. *Archives of Disease in Childhood* 1957; **32**: 480–3.

Mays ET, Conti S, Fallah Zadkh H *et al.* Hepatic artery ligation. *Surgery* 1979; **86**: 536–43.

Millar AJW, Bass D. Liver and biliary trauma. In: Stringer MD, Oldham KT, Mouriquand PDE, Howard ER (eds) *Pediatric surgery and urology: long-term outcomes*. Philadelphia, PA: WB Saunders Co., 1998: 465–74.

Miller K, Kou D, Sivit C *et al.* Pediatric hepatic trauma: does clinical course support intensive-care-unit stay? *Journal of Pediatric Surgery* 1998; **33**: 1459–62.

Moore EE, Shackford SR, Pachter HL *et al.* Organ injury scaling: spleen, liver and kidney. *Journal of Trauma* 1989; **29**: 1664–6.

Moore EE, Cogbill TH, Jurkovich GJ *et al.* Organ injury scaling: spleen, liver. *Journal of Trauma* 1995; **38**: 323–4.

Mutabagani KH, Coley BD, Zumberge N *et al.* Preliminary experience with focused abdominal sonography for trauma (FAST) in children: is it useful? *Journal of Pediatric Surgery* 1999; **34**: 48–52.

O'Neill JA, Meacham WF, Griffin PP *et al.* Patterns of injury in the battered child syndrome. *Journal of Trauma* 1973; **13**: 332–9.

Oldham KT, Guice KS, Ryckman F *et al.* Blunt liver injury in childhood: evolution of therapy and current perspective. *Surgery* 1986; **100**: 542–9.

Olsen WR, Redman HC, Hildreth DH. Quantitative peritoneal lavage in blunt abdominal trauma. *Archives of Surgery* 1972; **104**: 536–43.

Pachter LH, Spencer FC, Hofstetler SR *et al.* Experience with the finger fracture technique to achieve intrahepatic hemostasis in 75 patients with severe injuries of the liver. *Annals of Surgery* 1981; **197**: 771–8.

Pearl RH, Wesson DE, Spence LJ *et al.* Splenic injury: a five-year update with improved results and changing criteria for conservative management. *Journal of Pediatric Surgery* 1989; **24**: 428–31.

Pilcher DB, Harman PK, Moore EE. Retrohepatic vena cava balloon shunt introduced via the sapheno-femoral junction. *Journal of Trauma* 1977; **17**: 837–41.

Pitt HA, Kaufman SL, Coleman J *et al.* Benign postoperative biliary strictures: operate or dilate? *Annals of Surgery* 1989; **210**: 417–25.

Posner MC, Moore EE. Extrahepatic biliary tract injury: operative management plans. *Journal of Trauma* 1985; **25**: 833–7.

Pringle JH. Notes on the arrest of hepatic hemorrhage due to trauma. *Annals of Surgery* 1908; **48**: 541–4.

Ringe B, Pichlmayr R, Ziegler H *et al.* Management of severe hepatic trauma by two-stage total hepatectomy and subsequent liver transplantation. *Surgery* 1991; **109**: 792–5.

Root HD, Hauser CW, McKinley CR *et al.* Diagnostic peritoneal lavage. *Surgery* 1965; **57**: 633–7.

Rossi P, Mullins D, Thal E. Role of laparoscopy in the evaluation of abdominal trauma. *American Journal of Surgery* 1993; **166**: 707–10.

Rovito PF. Atrial caval shunting in blunt hepatic vascular injury. *Annals of Surgery* 1987; **205**: 318–21.

Sty JR, Starshak RJ, Hubbard AM. Radionuclide hepatobiliary imaging in the detection of traumatic biliary tract disease in children. *Pediatric Radiology* 1982; **12**: 115–18.

Stylianos S. Evidence-based guidelines for resource utilization in children with isolated spleen or liver injury. The APSA Trauma Committee. *Journal of Pediatric Surgery* 2000; **35**: 164–7.

Svoboda JA, Peter ET, Dan CU *et al.* Severe liver trauma in the face of coagulopathy – a case for temporary packing and early re-exploration. *American Journal of Surgery* 1982; **144**: 717–21.

Tanaka H, Iwai A, Sugimoto H. Intrahepatic arterioportal fistula after blunt hepatic trauma: case reports. *Journal of Trauma* 1991; **31**: 143–6.

Trunkey D, Federele MP. Computed tomography in perspective. *Journal of Trauma* 1986; **26**: 660–1.

Wagner WH, Lundell CJ, Donovan AJ. Percutaneous angiographic embolization for hepatic arterial hemorrhage. *Archives of Surgery* 1985; **120**: 1241–9.

Yellin AE, Chaffee CB, Donovan AJ. Vascular isolation in treatment of juxtahepatic venous injuries. *Archives of Surgery* 1971; **102**: 566–73.

PART 7

Liver transplantation

27

Indications, timing and preoperative preparation

MAX R LANGHAM Jr

INTRODUCTION

Replacement of human livers has become the standard therapy for a wide variety of disease in children. Dramatic improvements in and standardization of technique (Kramer *et al.*, 1994) and medication (Borel *et al.*, 1976; Ochiai *et al.*, 1987) have transformed liver transplantation into a useful tool that is applicable to a variety of clinical problems. Orthotopic liver transplantation (OLT) may be used to provide adequate hepatic synthetic function, relieve portal hypertension and correct selected genetic disorders, and for liver replacement after aggressive resection of certain benign or malignant tumors of the liver.

Once restricted to a few centers in the USA and Europe, liver transplantation is now available in most developed countries worldwide. Of 80 221 OLTs performed worldwide and reported by 1999 to the Worldwide Transplant Center Directory (Cecka and Terasaki, 1999), 44 053 operations had been performed in the USA and, with a few exceptions, the rest were performed in Established Market Economies or Formerly Socialist Economies of Europe (World Health Organization designations).

Murray and Lopez (1996) estimate that these countries contain approximately 20% of the world's population, but together bear less than 12% of the global disease burden. Their combined gross domestic products represent the majority of the world's economic resources, and provide the means with which to extend costly treatment to patients who survive long term only with continued provision of expensive medications and ongoing medical care. The age weighting that they use to calculate the disability-adjusted life year dramatically limits the weight assigned to children under 5 years of age. However, it is clear that even if diseases which burden infants and young children were equally weighted, liver disease would lag far behind other causes of childhood death. It is noteworthy that the six most significant contributors to the total disease burden worldwide in 1990 included alcohol abuse, and that this particular burden was heaviest in men in developed countries (Murray and Lopez, 1996). Thus in precisely those areas where pediatric liver transplantation is a fiscal and technical possibility, adult substance abuse creates intense competition for a limited organ supply.

Children in all areas of the world suffer liver dysfunction that is caused by a different set of diseases to those which affect adults. Childhood diseases that lead to liver transplantation in the state of Florida, USA, are listed in Tables 27.1 and 27.2. However, it is important to make a distinction between diagnosis and indications for transplantation. This distinction is obvious if one considers the impact of the disease on an individual. The goal in managing childhood disease should be the attainment of adulthood and the prospects of a good quality of life. Transplantation is simply a tool that is used to achieve this goal.

To my knowledge, no research has been conducted to examine population-based variations in childhood liver disease, or the extent to which the accepted indications

Table 27.1 *Diseases leading to liver transplantation in Florida: data from the State of Florida Pediatric Liver Transplant Program, University of Florida, University of Miami, and Children's Medical Services, Department of Health – diagnoses leading to first isolated liver transplant*

Diagnosis	n^*	Percentage†
Alpha-1-antitrypsin deficiency	14	4.8
Acute hepatic necrosis (various etiologies)	26	8.9
Autoimmune hepatitis	8	2.7
Alagille's syndrome and variants	14	4.8
Arteriovenous malformation	1	0.3
Biliary atresia	119	40.8
Biliary cirrhosis	2	0.7
Budd–Chiari syndrome	2	0.7
Cirrhosis/fibrosis	2	0.7
Cryptogenic (chronic liver failure)	6	2.1
Cystic fibrosis	9	3.0
Drug toxicity	1	0.3
Histiocytosis	2	0.7
Metabolic diseases	13	4.4
Viral hepatitis	8	2.7
Neonatal hepatitis	7	2.4
Primary liver tumor	7	2.4
Sickle-cell disease	1	0.3
Total parenteral nutrition-related cholestasis	1	0.3
Retransplantation	49	15

* Total n = 292.
† Rounding prevents addition giving a total of 100%.

Table 27.2 *Diagnoses leading to retransplantation*

Diagnosis	n^*	Percentage of total transplants (N = 292)
Abscess	1	0.3
Acute rejection (incompatible blood type)	2	0.7
Arterial stenosis/aneurysm	2	0.7
Chronic rejection	7	2.4
Hepatic arterial thrombosis	12	4.1
Primary non-function	17	5.5
Portal vein thrombosis	6	2.1
Recurrent disease	2	0.7

* Total n = 49.

for pediatric liver transplantation vary among different regions of the world and within countries. Likewise, no data have been collected on variations in timing and preoperative preparation for the operation. Certainly some variation is expected due to patient factors, societal norms and medical resources available to the physicians who care for these children. The applicability of specific recommendations for a treatment as complex and expensive as replacement of the human liver must therefore be viewed in the context of the individual patient and his or her local environment. The one overriding principle for application of liver transplantation is that the benefits to the patient in terms of quality and duration of life should be expected to outweigh the considerable risks and cost of a procedure whose current acceptance has been due to the absence of effective alternative therapies for many of the problems that lead to substantial morbidity and mortality in children with acute and chronic liver disease. In my opinion, the complexity of any evaluation of a child's need for liver transplantation may be best managed by answering the following questions.

1 Is liver transplantation the best treatment for the specific problems of this child and his or her family?
2 Do any contraindications exist?
3 What educational and financial resources do the family need to care for the child before and after transplantation?
4 How urgent is transplantation (i.e. how likely is the child to die during the preoperative waiting period)?
5 What medical interventions might improve the child's condition before transplantation?

This standard will work well in those centers that have mature transplant programs and where demonstration of success after liver transplantation is no longer itself a goal.

SPECIFIC PROBLEMS THAT ARE TREATED WITH LIVER TRANSPLANTATION

Specific problems that are directly treatable with liver transplantation include failing hepatic synthetic function, portal hypertension, genetic mutations which lead to the absence of key enzyme functions located in the liver or which cause hepatic disease, and the freedom to resect aggressively certain benign or malignant tumors of the liver which cannot be resected with preservation of adequate native hepatocyte mass. Frequently, more than one of these problems will exist in an individual patient. Biliary atresia and hepatitis C are both diseases that usually cause severe portal hypertension and significant abnormalities in hepatic synthetic function. Liver transplantation is a robust therapy that can frequently solve multiple related problems simultaneously. In such circumstances, it represents the logical treatment.

Replacement of failing hepatic synthetic function is the commonest reason for consideration of transplantation. Replacement of failed hepatic synthetic function is the indication for transplantation in virtually all patients with acute liver failure, and is a significant factor in the majority of patients with chronic liver disease.

Acute hepatic failure due to a variety of conditions is relatively easy to recognize. In these children, the usual dilemma is whether the acute condition might resolve without the need to resort to liver transplantation. Chronic hepatic failure is more difficult to recognize. Long-term disability due to failure to grow and develop normally is common. Failure of children to exhibit 'catch-up growth' has led to modulation of immunosuppression and a perception that liver transplantation *per se* has unacceptably high morbidity. Although incomplete correction of abnormal hepatic synthetic function is common after transplantation, delay in providing complete restoration of this function by timely transplantation is an under-appreciated contributor to chronic illness in children with liver disease. The best assessment of the adequacy of liver function is a careful assessment of growth and development, and this is particularly important during the first few years of life (McDiarmid *et al.*, 1998).

Portal hypertension is the next commonest complication of liver disease leading to consideration of liver transplantation. It may represent the most pressing problem in children with biliary atresia, hepatitis C, cystic fibrosis, Budd–Chiari syndrome and congenital hepatic fibrosis. Bleeding from esophageal or gastric varices should prompt at least a consideration of liver transplantation (Iwatsuki *et al.*, 1988; Wood *et al.*, 1990; Henderson, 1992). Long-term management depends primarily on the presence or absence of hepatic parenchymal disease. Those patients with cirrhosis, severe hepatic fibrosis or hepatitis are potential candidates for transplantation. Endoscopic sclerotherapy and banding of varices are useful first-line management tools in patients with acute bleeding (Terblanche *et al.*, 1979, 1989; Stiegmann *et al.*, 1992; Karrer *et al.*, 1994). Portosystemic shunts are a good option in two distinct settings. In the patient who will require transplantation and who cannot be managed safely using endoscopy, transjugular intrahepatic portosystemic shunt (TIPS) offers a relatively safe and very effective method of acutely lowering portal pressures, thereby decreasing bleeding from varices. TIPS has a number of advantages over traditional operative shunts, but has a much higher failure rate during intermediate-length follow-up, and its long-term patency has not been studied in children (Heyman and LaBorge, 1999). Surveillance with ultrasound or angiography and repeated dilatations improve the outcome of this procedure, and are an essential part of management if TIPS is chosen (Grace, 1997). Portal vein thrombosis is the most vexing complication of TIPS for the transplant surgeon, closely followed by placement that is either too low, making control of the portal vein problematic (Clavien *et al.*, 1998), or too high, making control of the suprahepatic vena cava difficult (Wilson *et al.*, 1995).

Traditional surgical shunts have a better long-term patency rate and are effective in treatment of portal hypertension, but are associated with a much higher procedure-related mortality and make transplantation rather more difficult (Esquivel *et al.*, 1987; Brems *et al.*, 1989; Lagnas *et al.*, 1992). Mesocaval or splenorenal shunts are excellent long-term treatments for patients with presinusoidal portal hypertension (cavernous transformation of the portal vein) (see Chapter 22), and in a few patients with postsinusoidal obstruction (Budd–Chiari syndrome) (Mitchell *et al.*, 1982). In the author's opinion, it is imperative to have a liver biopsy when considering these procedures, since significant parenchymal abnormalities greatly reduce the likelihood of long-term success.

SPECIFIC DISEASES THAT ARE TREATED WITH LIVER TRANSPLANTATION

Biliary atresia (See Chapters 8 and 9)

> Congenital atresia of the bile ducts is the darkest chapter in pediatric surgery. The etiology is unknown . . . In the light of our present knowledge, unless bile can be shunted to the gastrointestinal tract, early death is inevitable.
>
> (Willis Potts, 1959)

Biliary atresia is a disorder of infancy that is characterized by progressive hepatic fibrosis, bile ductular proliferation, and scarring of the major bile ducts (both intra- and extrahepatic). Electron microscopy reveals hepatocellular cholestasis, marked loss of bile canalicular microvilli, bile duct cell degeneration, and periductal inflammatory fibrosis (Park *et al.*, 1996). The etiology of this disease is still unknown. In this respect, therefore, we are no better off than Willis Potts. Two significant treatments have changed the outlook for children with the disorder, namely the Kasai portoenterostomy and liver transplantation, primarily pioneered by Starzl (Starzl *et al.*, 1982). The frequent failure of the first treatment has led to an explosion in the use of the second one. In every country and every series, biliary atresia is the commonest childhood disorder leading to liver transplantation.

Biliary atresia presents clinically with an apparently well infant with direct hyperbilirubinemia and a large, firm liver. Indeed, the apparent health of the baby often contributes to a delay in the diagnosis. The natural history of the disorder has been outlined by Potts (1959) and Ladd and Gross (1941), who found that 5% and 20%, respectively, of cases were operable (defined as having a patent hepatic duct or common bile duct). In the 80–95% of cases that were not so fortunate, the average age at subsequent death was 5 months.

Population-based estimates of the incidence of biliary atresia range from 5.12 in 100 000 live births to 29.4 in 100 000 (Yoon *et al.*, 1997; Chardot *et al.*, 1999a; McKiernan *et al.*, 2000) with conflicting data on seasonal variability (Ayas *et al.*, 1996). White patients were found to have a lower incidence than those of other races in the

USA, but these differences were not controlled for socioeconomic status. No population-based evidence points to heredity as a factor in the disease. Indirect evidence from twins supports the concept that biliary atresia is acquired, not inherited (Poovorawan et al., 1996). The long-term survival rate for biliary atresia has been so poor that few affected children have survived to have offspring. Future studies of subsequent generations could help to determine whether a spontaneous mutation contributes to the pathogenesis of biliary atresia.

Although clinical recognition of biliary atresia may be delayed, its origins are probably prenatal (see Chapter 8). Certainly it is associated with a higher than normal incidence of associated congenital anomalies, including splenic malformations, malrotation, Meckel's diverticulum, jejunal atresia and vascular anomalies (Tanano et al., 1999). Choledochal cysts are commonly related to biliary atresia (Cheng et al., 2000). The results of transplantation in patients with associated anomalies have been good (Varela-Fascinetto et al., 1998), and the presence of serious associated anomalies is not per se a contraindication to living-related liver transplantation (Maggard et al., 1999), even if the child has situs inversus (Mattei et al., 1998).

An infectious etiology of biliary atresia has not been convincingly demonstrated. Human papillomavirus types 6 and 18 have been found in pathological specimens from patients with biliary atresia by amplified polymerase chain reaction, but not in controls (Drut et al., 1998). These viruses are so common in most populations that this may be a chance observation. Cytomegalovirus (CMV) has also been implicated (Fischler et al., 1998), but other authors have not been able to confirm this association (Jevon and Dimmick, 1999). Reovirus-3 IgM levels have been more prevalent in babies with a variety of cholestatic liver disorders, including biliary atresia (Richardson et al., 1994). Reovirus (Tyler et al., 1998) and retrovirus-like DNA (Mason et al., 1998) has also been found in specimens from affected patients. There is no evidence that rotavirus is involved (Bobo et al., 1997).

Over the past few years, a description of the molecular events associated with biliary atresia has started to emerge. Stem cells that are capable of differentiating into hematopoietic precursors of liver have been identified (Peterson et al., 1999). The putative hepatic progenitors include oval cells in rodents (which stain with OV-6) (Crosby et al., 1998) and small epithelial cells (hepatoblasts). Cells with similar ultrastructural characteristics are seen in biliary atresia (Xiao et al., 1999), but not in normal babies. OV-6 expression is increased with biliary atresia (Crosby et al., 1998). There may be phenotypic switching in biliary atresia between hepatocytes and epithelial cells (Cocjin et al., 1996), which would account for some of the ductal proliferation that is commonly seen. Proliferating cell nuclear antigen is increased in hepatocytes in biliary atresia (Hossain et al., 1995), but

stem-cell factor/c-kit ligand–receptor system is not (Baumann et al., 1999). Bile duct proliferation as determined by anticytokeratin 7 staining (Kinugasa et al., 1999) and the Ki67 index is increased, but apoptosis as determined by the TUNEL method is also increased (Funaki et al., 1998).

The inflammatory process in biliary atresia is also receiving attention. Increased expression of intracellular adhesion molecule 1 on ductal epithelial cells (Dillon et al., 1994, 1997; Broome et al., 1997) is found in biliary atresia. CD68 and CD14 (macrophage markers) are also increased (Tracy et al., 1996; Kobayashi et al., 1997). It is agreed that there is abnormal expression of major histocompatibility complex (MHC) by biliary epithelium in the condition, although there are conflicting reports about MHC 1 and MHC 2 expression (Broome et al., 1997; Dillon et al., 1997; Kobayashi et al., 1997). Not surprisingly, TGF-β 1 and PDGF-α are expressed (Malizia et al., 1995; Lamireau et al., 1999), as are procollagen and collagen I and IV. Increased levels of both the protein- and mRNA-encoding metalloproteinases 1 and 2 are found in biliary atresia (Benyon et al., 1996). Superoxide dismutase is increased in biliary atresia, Alagille's syndrome and portal vein thrombosis (Broide et al., 2000). Plasma endothelin (Kobayashi et al., 1998a) and CD26 levels are also elevated (Perner et al., 1999). Finally, it is possible to detect collagen type IV (Kobayashi et al., 1998b), laminin (Shirahase et al., 1995) and connective tissue growth factor in the serum of infants who are severely affected by biliary atresia. Many of these changes are not specific for this disease, but have been found in other forms of end-stage liver disease. An improved understanding of their role in the mechanism of the disease might lead to novel treatment strategies which may improve the health of patients while they are awaiting transplantation, or even remove the need for transplantation.

A Kasai portoenterostomy performed well in a young baby results in relief of jaundice in between one- and two-thirds of patients (see Chapters 8 and 9) (Karrer et al., 1990; Ohi and Nio, 1998). No other effective therapy is known. While the benefits of a Kasai procedure in those children who clear their jaundice clearly justify its use in all babies with a diagnosis of biliary atresia, revision of a Kasai procedure that has been well performed is controversial. It may be of benefit to those children who have cleared their jaundice and have a sudden recurrence of acholic stools (Ibraham et al., 1991; Altman et al., 1997).

Chardot et al. (1999b) found that the overall 10-year survival rate of babies with biliary atresia in France, a country with a modern medical system and mature pediatric liver transplant programs, was 68%. McKiernan et al. (2000) examined the outcomes of babies treated in the UK and Ireland over a 24-month period. Babies who were cared for in centers that saw more than five cases per year had a 5-year overall survival rate of 91.2%, compared with 75% for those who were treated in hospitals seeing fewer cases. The 5-year survival rates without transplantation were 61.3% and 13.7%, respectively. Survival without transplantation after a Kasai procedure shows a steady decline, and currently more than 80% of children with biliary atresia will eventually need a liver transplant.

Biliary hypoplasia and Alagille's syndrome

Cholestatic disorders other than biliary atresia are less common but nevertheless important causes of childhood liver disease. According to current concepts, affected children are categorized as syndromic (Alagille's syndrome) or non-syndromic. Alagille et al. (1987) described a genetic syndrome transmitted as an autosomal-dominant trait whose phenotype includes chronic cholestasis, posterior embryotoxon, butterfly-like vertebral arch defects and peripheral pulmonary artery stenosis. The disorder is caused by a single defect in the Jagged1 gene (Li et al., 1997; Oda et al., 1997). The usual symptoms that lead to evaluation for liver transplant include intense itching and (less frequently) complications of portal hypertension. The levels of serum bile acids, triglycerides and cholesterol are elevated. Growth velocity and ultimate height are usually decreased. Emerick et al. (1999) have reviewed 92 children with the disorder, of whom 19 children were transplanted. Transplantation resulted in relief of icterus, pruritis and portal hypertension.

Non-syndromic paucity has an identical morphological appearance on liver biopsy, but is not associated with the other components of Alagille's syndrome. The prognosis is worse, with at least 50% of cases developing cirrhosis, and portal hypertension and dying in the first years of life (Ohi and Nio, 1998). Transplantation appears to be curative in this disorder. No other surgical therapy has been shown to be of lasting benefit, although in non-cirrhotic patients bypass of the distal ileum may result in lower levels of serum bile salts and less itching (see Chapter 12).

Fulminant hepatic failure

Fulminant hepatic failure is defined as the presence of acute liver failure with superimposed hepatic encephalopathy within 8 weeks of the onset of illness (Trey and Davidson, 1970). There is some evidence that fulminant liver failure is increasing as an indication for liver transplantation in the USA (Belle et al., 1995). Drug toxicity, including acetaminophen overdose, toxicity related to antibiotics used to treat tuberculosis, idiosyncratic responses to neuroleptic medications or chemotherapeutic drugs (Zimmerman, 1978; Lee et al., 1989) and viral hepatitis, especially hepatitis B (Bernuau et al., 1986), are well-defined causes of fulminant hepatic failure. However, in children in the USA these cases are the exception, and in most cases the etiology is unclear. Two distinct populations have presented to our center. The commonest is the onset of jaundice and liver failure in previously healthy children with no previous drug exposure and negative serological markers for known viruses causing hepatitis. The second population is that of newborns presenting with liver failure at the time of birth. These infants undoubtedly have prenatal liver disease, but they benefit from the mother's intact hepatic function and the placenta's ability to exchange most nutrients and toxins. Shortly after delivery, these babies exhibit profound life-threatening liver failure, but are otherwise intact.

Independent of the etiology, fulminant liver failure represents a challenging problem for the entire health care team. Under considerable time pressure, a diagnosis must be made, supportive treatment initiated, a transplant planned, a donor identified, and the procedure completed before irreversible neurological damage or cardiovascular collapse occurs. The King's College criteria were developed using both children and adults (O'Grady et al., 1989). Indications for transplantation in non-acetaminophen-induced acute liver failure are as follows:

the presence of three of the following:
   age < 10 years
   etiology of non-A, non-B hepatitis or drug-induced fulminant liver failure
   bilirubin > 300 μmol/L
   jaundice to encephalopathy time > 7 days
   prothrombin time > 50 seconds

OR

prothrombin time > 100 seconds.

Most children who develop encephalopathy from fulminant liver failure are under 10 years of age, have non-A, non-B hepatitis or idiosyncratic drug reactions and are coagulopathic, thus fulfilling the criteria for transplantation based on these criteria. Survival rates without transplantation in this group are quite low. Immediate evaluation and expeditious liver transplantation represent the child's best hope. Specific supportive measures are described below.

Non-function of a transplanted organ

Hepatic failure after liver transplantation is now the second commonest indication for liver transplantation in children (Table 27.1 above). Graft failure commonly occurs early after a previous transplant because of 'primary' non-function of the graft or thrombosis of the hepatic artery or portal vein. Less commonly, chronic rejection or recurrent disease will lead to graft loss months to years after a successful liver transplant (Langham et al., 2001).

University of Wisconsin's preservation solution (Kalayoglu et al., 1988) has dramatically improved graft function after prolonged cold ischemia. However, the shortage of suitable organs for transplantation has simultaneously increased the desirability of using 'marginal' donors (Mirza et al., 1994). Advanced donor age (Hoofnagle et al., 1996) significantly increases the likelihood of graft failure. The role of hepatic steatosis in the graft in contributing to non-function is less clear, but the data suggest that this and other 'soft' reasons why surgeons reject livers as unsuitable indeed correlate with graft outcome (Yamada et al., 2000). A major advantage of living-related donation is the lower incidence of graft loss due to both technical problems and primary non-function, which is quite rare in this setting (Reding et al., 1999). Techniques such as graft reduction and ex-vivo division of the liver into two usable organs have been associated with increased non-function (Dunn et al., 1997). Grafts prepared using in-situ split techniques (Rogiers et al., 1996; Goss et al., 1997) appear to be superior to those which are prepared ex vivo (Reyes et al., 2000). Thus the current practice in the USA balances donor mortality on the waiting-list with risk of non-function associated with suboptimal donors, the added morbidity associated with creating segmental grafts, or the ethical dilemmas presented by living donation. The data from our study show that 44% of retransplants in Florida have been due to primary non-function of the first graft (Langham et al., 2001).

Hepatic artery thrombosis and portal vein thrombosis are presumably technical complications. In most series they occur in 5–10% of pediatric transplants. Surveillance with Doppler ultrasound (Gilabert et al., 1996; Cook and Crofton, 1997) is used to aid prompt recognition of these problems. Portal vein thrombosis, if not corrected before hepatic necrosis occurs, usually requires retransplantation or else results in the patient's death. Hepatic artery thrombosis may be relatively well tolerated with long-term survival which is often complicated by a cholangiopathy (Stringer et al., 2001). Prompt revascularization is the best treatment. Hyperbaric oxygen therapy has been recommended, but its benefits are unproven (Mazariegos et al., 1999). Various risk factors have been associated with increased risk of vascular thrombosis, including auxiliary transplants (van Hoek et al., 1999), donor and recipient age (Cacciarelli et al., 1997; Praghakaran et al., 1999) and use of segmental grafts (Sieders et al., 1999 (see Chapter 3)). Use of a high-power operating microscope, especially in segmental grafts from living donors, has been advocated as a method of reducing these complications (Tanaka et al., 1994; Sieders et al., 1999). Evidence of massive hepatic necrosis is an indication for emergent retransplantation in this population.

Recurrent disease is predominantly a problem in children with viral hepatitis (Davison et al., 1998) or autoimmune hepatitis (Birnbaum et al., 1997). Treatment of viral hepatitis after transplantation with interferon (Nour et al., 1995) or prostaglandin E (Flowers et al., 1994) has been reported, but its benefit is unproven. Chronic rejection is a surprisingly rare cause of late graft loss. In 292 transplants performed in the state of Florida, chronic rejection leading to retransplantation has occurred only seven times (2.4% of cases, unpublished data). Non-compliance with complex drug regimens which have significant undesirable side-effects is responsible for most such problems. The low incidence in our state may in part be due to a multidisciplinary statewide program aimed at focused case management and pre- and post-transplant education for patients and their families. Retransplantation for chronic rejection can be successful, but is associated with a higher complication rate and lower rates of patient and graft survival (Nicolette et al., 1998).

Viral hepatitis

Although it is common in some parts of the world, acute fulminant liver failure associated with hepatitis B is very uncommon in the USA. Early aggressive recurrence of hepatitis B has diminished enthusiasm for transplanting patients with actively replicating virus. Hepatitis C, a common cause of liver failure in adults, is uncommon as an etiology of liver failure in children.

Malignancy

Liver tumors are uncommon in children, representing approximately 1.1% of all childhood malignancies. Benign lesions represent 25% of the total, and include mesenchymal hamartomas, hemangioendotheliomas, adenomas and true hemangiomas. Of the malignant tumors, hepatoblastoma is the most common cell type in the USA, representing 43% of the total, with hepatocellular carcinomas and sarcomas accounting for 23% and 6%, respectively (Finegold, 1994) (see Chapters 18 and 19). Liver transplantation is an important option for unresectable malignant tumors localized to the liver (see Chapter 18). In early reports there were no long-term survivors (Starzl et al., 1976). Subsequent reports held more promise, and transplantation has been advocated for children with hepatoblastomas whose disease is localized to the liver (Superina and Bilik, 1996; Douglass, 1997). This enthusiasm must be tempered somewhat, particularly in those children with stage 4 hepatoblastomas, since recurrence is almost universal (R Superina, personal communication, 1999).

It is important to recognize the potential for benign liver tumors to cause the death of a child. Of 60 children who were treated for hepatic tumors at our institution, 21 patients had benign disease, four of whom died from complications of the tumors or from their treatment. With survival rates after liver transplantation approaching 90%, those children with unresectable or untreatable benign tumors are likely to benefit from liver replacement. We have transplanted eight children with isolated primary liver tumors at our institution (three with benign disease, three with hepatoblastoma and two with hepatocellular carcinoma). There have been two deaths from recurrent disease, 2 and 4 years after initial transplantation.

Based on the literature and our limited personal experience, transplantation for highly selected children with isolated liver tumors does appear to be warranted. Multi-institutional trials through organizations such as the Children's Oncology Group would be the ideal way to determine the true efficacy of this approach and to define the best adjunctive chemotherapy strategy. In the absence of such data, we have adopted a general strategy of treatment consisting of four courses of appropriate chemotherapy followed by transplantation and early post-transplant consolidation therapy using two further courses of chemotherapy.

Correction of selected genetic disorders

Spontaneous and inherited genetic mutations leading to liver disease have historically been the second commonest indication for liver transplantation in children. However, data from the state of Florida (Tables 27.1 and 27.2) suggest that this is no longer true. Both acute fulminant hepatic failure and retransplantation after a failed first transplant are now more common indications for

transplantation. Nevertheless, metabolic disorders are a significant source of morbidity and mortality in children. This can best be minimized by early diagnosis and appropriate treatment, which may include liver transplantation. The complexity of the biology involved may lead physicians to delay diagnosis until irreversible and unnecessary harm has been done to the child (Box 27.1).

CYSTIC FIBROSIS

The commonest genetic disorder in the USA, which can cause chronic liver disease, is cystic fibrosis. This disorder occurs in approximately 1 in 3000 white live births and 1 in 17 000 black infants in the USA (Fitzsimmoms, 1993). Liver disease associated with cystic fibrosis is characterized by severe portal fibrosis, bile duct proliferation, a mononuclear periportal infiltrate and portal hypertension. The etiology of the fibrosis is unclear, but it is probably related to abnormal chloride transport leading to bile inspissation. Abnormalities of the cystic fibrosis transmembrane conductance regulator in gallbladder epithelium have been reported (Dray-Charier et al., 1999). Hepatic synthetic function as measured by coagulation studies, serum ammonia and transferrin is usually well preserved. The commonest event precipitating referral to a liver transplant center is variceal bleeding. Successful management with portosystemic shunts has been described (Shun et al., 1997), but the potential for subsequent hepatic decompensation prompts caution in applying such therapy in this patient population. We have used TIPS in two patients with severe variceal bleeding as a successful bridge to liver transplantation.

Box 27.1 *Summary recommendations for liver transplantation in patients with metabolic disorders*

Alpha-1-Antitrypsin deficiency	< 5% homozygous Pi type ZZ
Caution: arteriovenous shunts may complicate transplant and post-transplant course	
Crigler-Najjar type 1	OLT indicated before age of 6 years
Homozygous familial hypercholesterolemia	Indicated for coronary artery disease despite other treatment; 50% reduction in plasma low-density lipoprotein expected
Methylmalonic acidemia	No recommendation
Neonatal hemochromatosis	OLT indicated for infants who do not respond to 3–4 months of antioxidant and chelating therapy
Primary hyperoxaluria I	Pre-emptive OLT indicated before development of renal failure
Tyrosinemia type 1	OLT indicated if no response to NTBC
Urea cycle disorders	Pre-emptive OLT may be indicated
Wilson's disease	OLT indicated for fulminant liver failure or failure of medical therapy
Glycogen storage disease types I, III, IV	OLT indicated for liver failure or malignancy and for classic progressive hepatic form of type IV
Maple syrup urine disease	OLT not indicated
Propionic acidemia	OLT indicated for patients with severe recurrent metabolic decompensation
Mitochondrial respiratory chain disorders	OLT only indicated for patients with isolated hepatic disorders

OLT, orthotopic liver transplantation.

Relatively little has been written about liver transplantation for cystic fibrosis, although several authors list this disorder as a diagnosis leading to liver replacement (Revell *et al.*, 1993; Pratschke *et al.*, 1998). At the University of Florida we have performed seven liver transplants for cystic fibrosis. One of these patients required retransplantation due to chronic rejection, and subsequently died from pneumocystis pneumonia. The other patients are alive, although one experienced terminal pulmonary dysfunction 8 years after liver transplantation. Pulmonary function in the remaining patients is still surprisingly good.

A difficult dilemma arises when a patient presents with both poor lung function and advanced liver disease. Successful simultaneous lung/liver transplantation has been reported (Zimmerman *et al.*, 1999). The hemodynamic difficulties that are commonly encountered early after lung transplantation make sequential transplantation more appealing, and our center has performed lung transplants in two patients with advanced liver disease without simultaneous liver transplantation. Both have survived the procedure and have not experienced rapid progression of their liver disease. As survival increases worldwide, more patients with cystic fibrosis can be expected to develop complications of liver disease (Fogarty *et al.*, 2000).

SICKLE-CELL ANEMIA

Sickle-cell anemia is another common genetic anomaly that may be associated with liver disease. The etiology of the liver disorder in this condition is probably linked to iron overload. We have transplanted two patients with sickle-cell disease. One had a post-transplant lung infarction and stroke, despite an aggressive pretransplant transfusion protocol. He survived for several years with a reasonable quality of life, but eventually succumbed to complications of sickle-cell anemia. We do not believe that liver transplantation for sickle-related liver disease has yet been established as beneficial.

Other genetic problems that are treatable by liver transplantation are much less common. The pathophysiology of many of these disorders centers on abnormal function of the mitochondria (Treem and Sokol, 1998). This may be primary or secondary (Box 27.2). Diagnosis is difficult, but patients with elevated blood lactate levels and characteristic liver pathology should be evaluated further. The following discussion of these problems is incomplete and focuses mainly on those disorders for which liver transplantation has been considered to be therapeutic. The extrahepatic effects of most of these disorders are not corrected by liver transplantation. The decision as to whether to use orthotopic liver transplantation as a treatment therefore rests on a judgement of the impact of the disorder on the patient's quality of life.

WILSON'S DISEASE

Wilson's disease is an autosomal-recessive disorder characterized by a defect in biliary copper excretion. The

---

> **Box 27.2** *Mitochondrial disorders that cause liver disease*
>
> *Primary mitochondrial disorders*
> Respiratory chain defects
> Defects of oxidative phosphorylation
> Fatty acid oxidation
> Urea cycle defects
> Electron transport protein deficiency
> Pearson's disease
> Alper's disease
> Mitochondrial neurogastrointestinal
>   encephalomyelopathy syndrome
> Navajo neuropathy
>
> *Secondary mitochondrial disorders*
> Wilson's disease
> Neonatal hemochromatosis
> Heritable hemochromatosis
> Drug-induced hepatic injury

---

disease-associated gene (ATP7B) encodes a copper-transporting P-type ATPase – the Wilson's disease protein – which has been localized to both the trans-Golgi network and the mitochondria (Lutsenko and Cooper, 1998). The presentation can be variable, with fulminant or chronic liver disease, neurodegenerative disease and hemolysis being the commonest symptoms. Some patients who remain entirely asymptomatic are discovered through genetic linkage studies (Gow *et al.*, 2000). Hepatic toxicity may be mediated via a CD95-dependent pathway (Strand *et al.*, 1998). Wide variations in symptoms and age at presentation necessitate consideration of this diagnosis in any patient with liver disease of obscure origin. In most cases, diagnosis is clinical, with Kayser–Fleischer rings and low ceruloplasmin levels constituting the most standard diagnostic findings. Cauza *et al.* (1997) found that serum ceruloplasmin levels have a low positive predictive value (5.9%), and concluded that this is not a useful screening test in a population with liver disease. Tissue copper levels are more specific, but genetic testing will probably supplant most of these tests.

There appears to be some correlation between the specific genetic mutation and the severity of liver disease at diagnosis (Okada *et al.*, 2000). Liver transplantation may normalize copper metabolism in some patients (Chen *et al.*, 1996), although this is not certain (Diaz *et al.*, 1995). Excellent results have been reported after liver transplantation (Rela *et al.*, 1995; Chen *et al.*, 1996; Pratschke *et al.*, 1998) in some centers. The potential for major neurotoxicity and an increased cardiovascular risk (Tallgren *et al.*, 1996) exist with late-stage disease, and these represent relative contraindications to transplantation.

HEMOCHROMATOSIS

Neonatal hemochromatosis is characterized by severe hepatic fibrosis or cirrhosis which begins *in utero* and results in death in the first days or weeks of life (Rodriguez-Velasco *et al.*, 1999). It is distinct from hereditary hemochromatosis, a disorder that is caused by mutation of the HFE (Fiel *et al.*, 1999) gene, which encodes a protein with structural homology with MHC class 1 (Parkkila *et al.*, 1997). The etiology of neonatal hemochromatosis has not been characterized, and it remains a difficult dilemma. The diagnosis can be made by minor salivary gland biopsy. Initial treatment recommendations now include antioxidant chelation cocktails including desferrioxamine, vitamin E, *N*-acetylcysteine, selenium and prostaglandin E1. Survival with no specific therapy has been reported (Muller-Berghaus *et al.*, 1997), but most children die even with aggressive medical therapy and transplantation (Sigurdsson *et al.*, 1998). Nevertheless, successful outcome has been reported after transplantation. Progressive hemosiderosis and death after orthotopic liver transplantation was described in one case (Egawa *et al.*, 1996).

Hereditary hemochromatosis rarely causes liver failure in children. Iron overload is common in older patients with liver disease. Brandhagen *et al.* (2000) reported that nearly 10% of 456 adult transplant recipients had quantified hepatic iron stores in the liver high enough to warrant a diagnosis of hemosiderosis. Of these, only four cases (1%) were C282Y homozygotes. Increased iron stores substantially increased the likelihood of death within 5 years of transplant due to a higher rate of lethal infections, cardiac complications and recurrent tumors (Farrell *et al.*, 1994). The development of primary liver cancer is quite common in this condition, and may represent an indication for early transplantation. In total, 13 of 37 patients reported by Kowdley *et al.* (1995) had either a hepatocellular carcinoma or a cholangiocarcinoma in their explants. Survival rates were significantly lower than in patients who were transplanted for other indications.

MITOCHONDRIAL RESPIRATORY CHAIN DISORDERS

Much rarer than Wilson's disease or hemochromatosis are mitochondrial respiratory chain disorders, which are also frequently associated with neurodegenerative symptoms (Sokal *et al.*, 1999). Tyrolean infantile cirrhosis may be a related disorder (Wijmenga *et al.*, 1998). Babies with these disorders usually present early in life with severe liver disease. Few patients have been transplanted, but it is clear that extrahepatic manifestations may progress and cause a patient's death even after successful transplantation (Sokal *et al.*, 1999). Simple diagnostic tests for these disorders are not readily available. Assay of respiratory chain enzyme activity in affected organs is necessary for definitive diagnosis, and must be performed on tissue frozen at $-80°C$.

TYROSINEMIA

Tyrosinemia type I is an autosomal-recessive deficiency of fumarylacetoacetase, the last enzyme in the tyrosine catabolic pathway. Lack of the enzyme results in the formation of maleylacetoacetate and fumarylacetoacetate, which cause both liver and kidney injury. Mohan *et al.* (1999) reported on 17 patients, most of whom presented with hepatomegaly, coagulopathy and failure to thrive. All of them had elevated transaminase and alpha-fetoprotein values. Variable clinical presentations can include progressive liver damage and failure, a high risk of developing hepatocellular carcinoma, renal tubular dysfunction with hypophosphatemic rickets, hypertrophic cardiomyopathy, porphyria-like symptoms, and neurological crises. Classic treatment includes dietary restriction of protein with selective supplements of amino acids. Treatment with 2-(2-nitro-4-trifluoromethyl benzoyl)-1,3-cyclohexanedione (NTBC) therapy inhibits the second step of tyrosine metabolism, thereby preventing the formation of maleylacetoacetate and fumarylacetoacetate and the resultant symptoms. NTBC therapy does not allow normalization of diet and may not prevent the onset of hepatic malignancy (Dionisi-Vici *et al.*, 1997), which was present at transplantation in 10% of the collected cases reported by Mohan *et al.* (1999). Hypertrophic cardiomyopathy appears to regress after transplantation, but renal dysfunction may persist.

ALPHA-1-ANTITRYPSIN DEFICIENCY

Alpha-1-antitrypsin deficiency is a common inborn error of metabolism that is most commonly recognized in patients who are homozygous for the PiZZ gene. Most patients with this genotype develop chronic obstructive lung disease in adulthood, but some children develop cholestasis as neonates and may have progressive cirrhosis during childhood. Heterozygotes for the PiZZ gene may be at increased risk of liver failure in adulthood (Grazuadei *et al.*, 1998).

Lung disease is uncommon in children with liver disease due to alpha-1-antitrypsin deficiency. There is a single report of increased risk of splenic artery aneurysms in patients with alpha-1-antitrypsin deficiency who are undergoing liver transplantation (Gaglio *et al.*, 2000). The major comorbidity that merits consideration is renal failure, which occurs at an increased rate in children with alpha-1-antitrypsin deficiency (Németh, 1999). Our experience concurs with that of Németh in that this can usually be handled conservatively without renal transplantation. A profound leukocytosis (WBC $> 70\,000$/mL) has occurred post transplant in two of our patients with alpha-1-antitrypsin deficiency, although this did not appear to cause any specific problems. The etiology of this interesting phenomenon is unclear.

There is an interesting and impressive difference in the rate of transplantation for alpha-1-antitrypsin deficiency between the USA and two recent large reports from Europe. United Network for Organ Sharing data report 255 recipients of liver transplants for alpha-1-antitrypsin deficiency, compared with 40 recipients for Wilson's disease (ratio 6.4:1), by comparison with European reports which document 17 recipients with alpha-1-antitrypsin deficiency vs. 30 recipients who had Wilson's disease (ratio 1:1.8) (Rela et al., 1995; Pratschke et al., 1998). Whether this represents a difference in the prevalence of these genetic defects or a difference in transplant practices is unclear. However, what is clear is that progression of liver disease in alpha-1-antitrypsin deficiency is often quite slow, with excellent long-term survival for most affected patients (Németh and Strandvick, 1982; Németh and Möller, 1987). However, children with the disease can decompensate quite rapidly, which leads most transplant centers in the USA to list these children early so that they may start to accrue waiting time. It is possible that the urinary excretion pattern of bile acids may predict the prognosis (Németh and Strandvik, 1984) while human leukocyte antigen phenotype, birth weight, duration and grade of cholestasis and viral infections do not. We have not routinely monitored urinary bile acid levels in children who are awaiting liver transplant.

ORNITHINE DECARBOXYLASE DEFICIENCY AND OTHER UREA CYCLE DEFECTS

The urea cycle plays a critical role in hepatic metabolism. Components of the cycle include arginase, which is conserved genetically across the primary biological kingdoms, suggesting that it is a primordial enzyme which was possibly present in the universal common ancestor and useful as a phylogenetic marker (Ouzounis and Kyrpides, 1994). Abnormalities in the pathway are frequently fatal and often present as acute hepatic failure. Thus a basic familiarity is important for the liver transplant physician and surgeon. The principal disorders are ornithine transcarbamylase (OTC) deficiency, carbamoyl phosphate synthase (CPS) deficiency, citrullinemia and arginosuccinic aciduria.

CPS is the first committed step in the cycle (Lawson et al., 1996). CPS-deficient patients usually die during the immediate postnatal period as a result of severe hyperammonemic coma (Saudubray et al., 1999b). Rare patients with residual enzyme activity may do well. To my knowledge, successful liver transplantation has not been reported.

Citrullinemia is caused by argininosuccinic synthetase deficiency, and is also usually fatal in infancy. Some patients with partial enzyme activity will present later and may have good neurological function. At least one patient has been transplanted at the age of 5 years with a good long-term outcome. He has high plasma citrulline levels due to a renal argininosuccinic synthetase deficiency.

Argininosuccinic aciduria is caused by argininosuccinic lyase deficiency. The series of Saudubray et al.

(1999a) suggests that although a higher proportion of these patients survive infancy (9 out of 15 cases), all of them have some developmental sequelae.

OTC deficiency is the commonest of these disorders. It is transmitted as a sex-linked trait with the clinical phenotype affecting both males and heterozygous females, and a spectrum of severity ranging from neonatal death to asymptomatic survival into adulthood (Tuchman et al., 1998). Good long-term survival and neurological outcome have been reported after liver transplantation (Saudubray et al., 1999a, b). Late-onset disease is still associated with a high mortality rate and a high rate of devastating neurological impairment in both sexes. Low plasma citrulline levels may persist due to persistent intestinal OTC defects (Saudubray et al., 1999a, b).

GLYCOGEN STORAGE DISEASES

Glycogen storage disease (GSD) types I, III and IV can be associated with the development of hepatic failure and hepatocellular carcinoma. Glycogen storage diseases are inherited disorders in which the concentration and/or structure of glycogen in body tissues is abnormal. Not surprisingly, liver and muscle are the most commonly affected tissues. Type I (glucose-6-phosphatase deficiency), type III (debrancher deficiency) and type IV (brancher deficiency) cause the most severe liver disorders. Clinical manifestations of these disorders are summarized from Matern et al. (1999) and are outlined in Table 27.3. These authors reviewed the results of 25 patients with GSDs treated with liver transplantation. Diagnoses included seven patients with GSD Ia, two with GSD Ib, three with GSD III and 13 patients with GSD IV. Liver transplantation corrected the presenting symptoms in all patients with GSD Ia and Ib, but did not reverse the neutropenia in GSD Ib, which does respond to granulocyte colony-stimulating factor (Donadieu et al., 1993). Ages at transplantation for GSD types Ia and Ib ranged from 7.6 to 27.5 years (mean 19.2 years) (Matern et al., 1999). All three patients with GSD III were transplanted as adults. The mean age of the 13 patients who were transplanted for GSD IV was 3.2 years (range 0.9–12 years). Two children died perioperatively, and one died from heart failure 9 months post transplant. No progressive cardiomyopathy or neuromuscular symptoms occurred in 10 long-term survivors. There is no direct evidence that liver transplantation alters neuromuscular symptoms, but cardiac amylopectin levels decreased in one patient following liver transplantation (Selby et al., 1993; Starzl et al., 1993).

Current treatment recommendations for GSD, based on type, are as follows.

- *Type Ia and Ib*: nocturnal nasogastric infusion of glucose or orally administered uncooked cornstarch (Greene et al., 1976; Chen et al., 1988); liver transplantation for adenoma or small hepatocellular carcinoma.

Table 27.3 *Clinical manifestations of glycogen storage disease (GSD)*

Disorder	Enzyme defect	Presenting symptoms	Predictable outcome
GSD type Ia (von Gierke disease)	Deficiency of glucose-6-phosphatase	Growth retardation, hepatomegaly, hypoglycemia, lactic acidemia, hyperuricemia, hyperlipidemia	Gout, short stature, osteoporosis, renal failure, pulmonary hypertension, hepatic adenomas
GSD type Ib	Defect in transport of glucose-6-phosphate	Type Ia symptoms plus neutropenia, neutrophil dysfunction, bacterial infections, oral and gastrointestinal ulcerations	Gout, short stature, osteoporosis, renal failure, pulmonary hypertension, hepatic adenomas
GSD type IIIb (liver involvement only)	Deficiency of glycogen debranching enzyme	Hepatomegaly, hypoglycemia, hyperlipidemia, growth retardation	Usually improves with age, cirrhosis and hepatocellular carcinoma possible
GSD type IV	Deficiency of branching enzyme	Presents in first year of life with hepatosplenomegaly and failure to thrive	Cirrhosis, with portal hypertension, variceal bleeding, hypotonia, muscle wasting, cardiomyopathy

- *Type III*: high-protein diet; if hypoglycemia is present, increase carbohydrates and add nocturnal feeds or cornstarch (Matern *et al.*, 1999); transplantation for small hepatocellular carcinoma or cirrhosis with liver failure.
- *Type IV*: liver transplantation for progressive liver failure with portal hypertension in those patients without debilitating neuromuscular or cardiac disease.

GALACTOSEMIA AND FRUCTOSEMIA

In general, these disorders of carbohydrate metabolism do not require liver transplantation. Although both can cause severe liver disease, this is usually reversed after withdrawal of the offending carbohydrate. Strict dietary control must be observed in both instances. Hepatocellular carcinoma may arise in adolescence, and represents a late indication for transplantation (Otto *et al.*, 1989).

CRIGLER–NAJJAR'S SYNDROME TYPE 1

Unconjugated hyperbilirubinemia that persists after the first few weeks of life (Crigler-Najjar syndrome) (Crigler and Najjar, 1952) can be due to complete deficiency of the enzyme bilirubin-UPD-glucuronosyltransferase (type 1), or a partial deficiency (type 2). Type 2 is treated with phenobarbital. Type 1, which is clinically determined by resistance to treatment with phenobarbital, is treated with exchange transfusions shortly after birth and phototherapy (Gorodischer *et al.*, 1970; Karon *et al.*, 1970). Liver transplantation is curative for these patients (Kaufmann *et al.*, 1986). Success with auxiliary transplantation has been reported (Whitington *et al.*, 1993),

but complication rates are higher than with liver replacement. Jansen (1999) collected 57 patients from a multicenter survey and found that 26% of them had developed some form of brain damage. In total, 37% of the transplanted patients already had brain damage at the time of transplantation.

Burdelski and Ullrich (1999) have summarized the findings of a symposium on liver transplantation for metabolic diseases. Their recommendations are presented in Box 27.1.

CONTRAINDICATIONS TO LIVER TRANSPLANTATION IN CHILDREN

There are relatively few absolute contraindications to liver transplantation. Chief among them are concurrent medical problems that preclude successful transplantation. Significant cardiac, renal, pulmonary and neurological dysfunction may be tolerated and improve dramatically after transplantation if it is related to the underlying cause of liver failure. On the other hand, if liver failure is secondary to ischemia caused by an uncorrectable cardiac anomaly, or fixed pulmonary dysfunction, or severe renal failure exists, consideration of a multi-organ transplant is the only context within which orthotopic liver transplantation may be rationally discussed. Successful management of these problems is a real challenge, and should not be underestimated.

Extrahepatic malignancy and actively replicating viral diseases, including HIV (Gordon *et al.*, 1998), hepatitis B, Epstein–Barr virus and several respiratory viruses, often blossom after a transplant recipient has been immunosuppressed, and may lead to rapid post-transplant death.

Active bacterial and fungal infections are less problematic, but none the less must be regarded as very real risks. Anatomical abnormalities may make the procedure difficult. Portal vein thrombosis, large portosystemic shunts (both natural and man-made) and abnormalities of venous return to the heart must be defined preoperatively. In experienced hands, most of these problems can be overcome (Shaw et al., 1985). Arterial anomalies are less important if the surgeon is experienced, but may be crucial in certain graft/patient combinations, particularly with living donors. Finally, social issues that preclude follow-up or compliance with immunosuppressive regimens are frequent causes of post-transplant mortality, and represent relative contraindications.

TIMING OF LIVER TRANSPLANTATION IN CHILDREN

The one overriding principle for application of liver transplantation is that the benefits to the patient in terms of quality and duration of life should be expected to outweigh the considerable risks and cost of the procedure. As the results of liver transplantation have improved, patient referral has occurred earlier in the disease process. This has further improved transplant results and decreased the costs of the procedure. This success has revolutionized the practice of hepatology, and over the past 10 years the number of liver transplants has increased dramatically, putting increasing pressure on a limited donor pool, and resulting in longer waiting periods for cadaveric donors. United Network for Organ Sharing data (current data can be found at http://www.unos.org) show that from 1995 the number of deaths on the waiting-list in the USA began to climb rapidly. By far the highest rate of death on the waiting-list is in children under 1 year of age. In 1990, the overall rate for all ages was 462 deaths per 1000 years at risk on the waiting-list. By 1998, this rate had decreased to 167 per 1000 years at risk. This improvement, despite the increasing pressure of larger waiting-lists, reflects the maturation of liver transplantation as a therapy.

Our ability to predict the course of liver disease is fair at best, but depends absolutely on making a diagnosis and establishing as accurate an estimate as possible of the severity of the disease. This is the most important activity during preparation for a possible transplant procedure. Those disorders that have unpredictable clinical courses present the greatest challenge. Without question liver disease affects infants much more profoundly than older children. We are therefore increasingly aggressive in listing and transplanting children in this age group.

Prognostic models for risk of death in transplantation have been mainly derived from adult data, especially for patients with primary sclerosing cholangitis (Kim et al., 2000) and primary biliary cirrhosis (Grambsch et al.,

1989). No such prognostic model has been developed for biliary atresia or other disorders leading to liver transplantation in children. Thus the timing of transplantation must be based on the clinical judgement of experienced clinicians.

Living donation of segmental grafts still represents only a small fraction of all transplants performed in the USA and Europe, although it is the rule in Japan. One major advantage of living donation is the ability to schedule the transplant electively when the time appears to be most propitious for the patient. Ethical issues surrounding informed consent and avoidance of coercion have been addressed (Singer et al., 1989), but will increase as greater pressure is placed on families and transplant teams by the current shortage of appropriate cadaveric organs.

PRINCIPLES OF PREOPERATIVE ASSESSMENT AND PREPARATION

A thorough preoperative assessment before liver transplantation is a crucial component of care necessary for obtaining a good long-term outcome. When done properly, the assessment educates the transplant team about the child's medical condition and family structure, with its strengths and weaknesses. It also provides the family with an opportunity to learn about their child's medical condition and to begin the process of learning about post-transplant care. Both functions are necessary in order to facilitate the transplant process and ensure a good outcome. At its core, the evaluation needs to answer the five questions listed in the introduction to this chapter.

Box 27.3 shows the standard evaluation for a potential recipient in the Pediatric Liver Transplant Program at the University of Florida and Shands Hospital. A multidisciplinary team of surgeons, anesthesiologists, pediatricians, nurses, social workers and psychologists, all with special expertise and interest in transplantation, assesses each potential patient. A treatment-planning meeting is then held, and each potential issue is discussed prior to any decision being made about offering transplantation. In children with acute hepatic failure, unscheduled urgent meetings are held as needed.

If donation from a living relative or loved one is being considered, an equally careful evaluation of the donor must be performed. If the surgeon is inexperienced in this procedure, we would recommend transfer of the patient to a surgeon and center with appropriate training and experience, since the procedure represents a real risk to the donor. Certain institutions manage this risk by caring for the donor and the recipient in separate facilities (Revillon et al., 1999), while others prefer to provide simultaneous care for the donor and the recipient in a single institution. In all cases it is essential to have

Box 27.3 *Standard evaluation for a potential pediatric recipient*

Diagnosis:

Admission Weight: Height:

Medications:

Allergies:

Laboratory tests:	
Complete blood count with differential	
Basic metabolic panel; sodium, potassium, chloride, CO_2, blood urea nitrogen, creatinine, glucose, calcium	
Hepatic function panel: total protein, albumin, total and direct bilirubin, AST, ALT, alkaline phosphatase	
Prothrombin time with international normalized ratio, APTT, fibrinogen	
Urinalysis	
HIV antibody	
Pre-albumin	
Chronic hepatitis profile: Hep B: Surface Ag (HBsAg); Hep B: Surf Ab; Hep C: Ab	
Lipase	
CMV IgG	
Rapid plasma reagin	
Alpha-fetoprotein	
Tissue typing and lymphocytic antibody screen (PRA)	
ABO typing and antibody screen	
Other:	
Chest X-ray (posterior-anterior and lateral)	
Doppler ultrasound: pre liver transplant (assess portal vein patency, color flow)	
Consults:	
Pediatric surgery	
Anesthesiology	
Clinical psychology	
Social work	
Dietitian	
□ Cardiology consult if indicated	
□ Physiotherapy consult (gross motor and developmental skills) if indicated	
□ Occupational therapy consult (developmental, feeding and activities of daily living (ADL) skills)	
□ Speech therapy consult (language skills and swallowing) if indicated	
Additional orders:	
□ Alpha-1-antitrypsin if not previously done	
□ Antimurine antibody for transplant only if given OKT3	
□ Ceruloplasmin if > 5 years of age	
□ Ammonia if albumin < 3.0 g/dL and PT > 13.5 seconds	
□ 24-hour urine for creatinine clearance if serum creatinine > 2 mg/dL	
□ Urine culture and sensitivity if indicated	
□ Arterial blood gas if indicated	
□ Pulmonary functions if arterial blood gases abnormal	
□ Sinus X-rays if history of infection or cystic fibrosis	
□ ECG, 12-lead if indicated	

personnel who are capable of providing uncompromised care for both the donor and the recipient.

As transplants have increasingly become a 'standard of care' for many childhood liver diseases, pediatric patients are not excluded by psychosocial criteria. Like treatment for childhood tumors or diabetes, liver transplantation has matured as a therapy to the point where the question for families and physicians has increasingly become what resources and programs will need to be used to manage the child's long-term care successfully. If a transplant is indicated, the extended health care team must then, in a coordinated fashion, identify what resources are needed and develop a plan to help families who will require intensive psychosocial support services. At the University of Florida, our social workers stratify families into three simple categories to help us to determine the level of support that will be necessary for successful transplantation (Box 27.4). Level 1 requires the most intervention, while level-3 families are usually self-sufficient.

There are occasional families whose resources are so depleted that even the minimum requirements are not present. In such situations, foster care may be necessary or transplant may have to be withheld. If a family has several of the characteristics listed in Box 27.5, we feel that their child is at high risk for potentially avoidable morbidity and mortality after liver transplant. Child protective services should be involved as early as possible when considering children from such homes for transplantation.

Box 27.4 *Stratification used at University of Florida to help plan family support*

Level 1 (meets all minimal concrete needs)
- Adequate housing, indoor plumbing, not overly crowded, heat or air conditioning based on diagnosis, free from potential toxins, access to telephone, same address for over one year.
- US citizen, or legally in country, or sponsorship with adequate ongoing medical coverage and emotional support.
- Health insurance eligibility or Social Security Income eligibility.
- Minimal family support. Identifiable relative to assume care of child.
- Desire to have transplantation for their child or, in the older teenager, the patient him- or herself desires transplant.
- Has had intermittent employment or child support.
- No significant psychiatric history.
- No current history of substance abuse.

Level 2
- Meets all of the level 1 criteria.
- Understands the process of transplantation and the expected outcomes, and has the capability to obtain resources above the minimal criteria listed under Level 1.
- Has maintained employment for a period of more than one year.
- Maintains meaningful stable relationships with family members and friends. Can provide childcare for other children, maintain household while hospitalized, and has adequate organizational and processing skills.
- Derives some support from organized religious or social structures.
- Maintains working transportation, and can provide transport for the child and family to and from hospital.
- Understands and acknowledges the complexity of transplant process and management, and works to obtain knowledge and provide stability for the patient.
- No language barriers (i.e. reading, language).
- Health care coverage.

Level 3
- Meets all of the level 1 and 2 criteria.
- Has strong interpersonal bonds and highly functional relationships both at work and at home.
- Has family support available and present.
- No history of major psychological problems. Presents as well adjusted, appropriately concerned, and demonstrates age-appropriate parenting skills to meet patient's needs.
- History of using coping skills and demonstrating problem solving.
- Flexibility to change lifestyle. Willing to obtain education and make life changes to accommodate patient's new health care needs.
- No history of drug or alcohol abuse.
- Has excellent organizational skills and is willing to become knowledgeable about medications.
- Knowledgeable and able to state risks and benefits of transplant and to identify additional areas of self-learning.

In several situations it may be appropriate to respect a family's wish not to transplant their child. Medically complex cases in which liver transplantation is heroic and not the standard of care, or where treatment would be an unusually difficult burden on the family, are examples of such situations. Older teenage patients who are judged to be free of depression and mentally competent, but who do not desire a transplant, are unusual but particularly difficult patients for health care teams that are committed to caring for children with end-stage liver disease.

Medical issues that should be addressed in all patients who are considered for transplant include nutrition and immunizations. Intervening in these areas before transplantation can have a major impact in reducing the morbidity and mortality of the procedure.

Nutrition is a frequent problem in children with end-stage liver disease (see Chapter 5). After a careful nutritional assessment, a specific feeding plan is provided for patients who are judged to be nutritionally deficient. This may include the use of special diets containing predigested formulas and branch-chain amino acids. In patients with poor appetites or oral aversions, alternate routes of administration for these unpalatable diets should be considered. We prefer the use of nasoduodenal tubes to surgical gastrostomies, because of the propensity of patients with portal hypertension to develop variceal communications between the stomach and the abdominal wall. This frequently leads to massive bleeding that requires blood transfusions and emergency operations. We have not experienced problems with bleeding from esophageal varices while using nasoduodenal tubes. Parenteral nutrition should be avoided if possible because of the increased risks of sepsis and further hepatic decompensation.

Immunizations are an important part of pre- and post-transplant care. Education of primary care providers and families about the risks associated with certain vaccines in immunosuppressed patients is crucial to patient safety. Immunizations should be given before transplantation in immunocompetent patients according to the recommendations of local health authorities. In the USA these recommendations are codified in the Report of the Committee on Infectious Diseases (American Academy of Pediatrics, 2000). Table 27.4 is a compilation of these recommendations that we have adopted for immunizations in our pediatric transplant programs. We consider that OPV (live oral polio virus vaccine – Sabin) should not be used, since it results in active viral replication for 6–8 weeks, precluding transplant during that time. Instead, IPV (inactivated poliovirus vaccine) should be used both for potential patients and for all household contacts. In other countries where different live vaccines may be available, we would recommend extreme caution in their application, and suggest substitution of noninfectious alternatives where possible. After transplantation, approved immunizations may be resumed when the patient is more than 6 months post transplant and the prednisone dose is less than 0.5 mg/kg/day. Postimmunization titers should be drawn 30 days after the vaccine is administered for those children on steroids at > 0.2 mg/kg/day to ensure effectiveness. Vaccinations that are received less than 2 weeks prior to transplant should be repeated after transplant. Multiple vaccines can be given in one visit.

Several cautions with regard to specific vaccines are important. No MMR (measles, mumps, rubella) vaccines should be given post transplant. MMR can be given as early as 6 months of age, and should be given before transplantation, with a booster after 12 months if the child has not been transplanted in the interim. MMR may be given to household contacts after transplantation. Primary caregivers or parents should contact the transplant center about any measles exposure in post-transplant patients. Severely immunocompromised patients may require passive immunity even if they were vaccinated pre transplant. If a non-vaccinated transplanted patient is exposed to measles, they should receive measles immune globulin 0.5 mL/kg (maximum dose 15 mL) intramuscularly (IM) within 6 days of exposure.

Varivax should not be given after transplant. Pretransplant Varivax can be given as early as 6 months of age. We recommend vaccinating household contacts prior to transplant or when the patient is hospitalized for the transplant. Varivax may be given to household contacts 6 months after transplant, when immunosuppression doses are lower, although there is still a risk of exposure. It would therefore seem wise to contact the transplant center before administering this vaccination. Any household member who develops a rash after receiving this vaccination needs to be isolated from the patient. If a transplant recipient has a significant exposure to varicella, varicella zoster immune globulin (VZIG) 125 U (1 vial)/10 kg IM should be given within 72 hours of exposure. The maximum dose is 625 U (5 vials). If VZIG is not available, intravenous immune globulin, 400 mg/kg IV, may be substituted. The transplant center should be notified of the date on which both of these vaccinations are administered. We

Table 27.4 *Immunization protocol for pediatric liver transplant program, Shands Hospital at the University of Florida*

Immunization(s)	Pre transplant	Post transplant	Household
HBV (hepatitis B vaccine)	Yes Birth, 1–2 months, 6–18 months Start in any non-immunized patient who is HBsAg negative	Yes	Yes
MMR (measles, mumps, rubella)	Yes Age ≥ 6 months, booster at 12–15 months, if given before age 1 year; if given at 12–15 months, booster at 11–12 years, unless two doses are given after first birthday	**No**	Yes
Havrix (hepatitis A vaccine) *or*	Yes Age 2–18 years, can administer in two doses (initial, 6–12 months later) or three doses (initial, 1 month, 6–12 months). If > 18 years, administer in two doses (initial, 6–12 months later)	Yes	Yes
Vaqta (hepatitis A vaccine)	Yes Age 2–18 years, two doses (initial, 6–18 months later). Age > 18 years, two doses (initial, 6–12 months later)	Yes	Yes
DTaP (diphtheria, tetanus, acellular pertussis)	Yes 2 months, 4 months, 6 months, 15 months, booster at 4–6 years; use Td for patients ≥ 7 years	Yes	Yes
Td (tetanus, diphtheria)	Yes 14–16 years, and every 10 years thereafter	Yes	Yes
OPV (live oral polio virus vaccine – Sabin)	**No**	**No**	**No**
IPV (inactivated poliovirus vaccine, injection)	Yes 2 months, 4 months, 6–18 months, booster at 4–6 years	Yes	Yes
HbOC = HIBTITER; PRPT = ActHIB, OmniHIB; Tetramune = HbOC-DTP (*Haemophilus influenzae* b conjugate vaccines) *or*	Yes 2 months, 4 months, 6 months, booster at 12–15 months	Yes	Yes
PRP-OMP = PedvaxHIB (*Haemophilus influenzae* b conjugate vaccine)	Yes 2 months, 4 months, booster at 12–15 months	Yes	Yes
Varivax (Varicella vaccine)	Yes Age > 6 months, booster at 1 year if given before age 1 year; if age > 13 months, booster 1–2 months later	**No**	Yes
Influenza virus vaccine	Yes Age ≥ 6 months, booster 1 month after initial dose if age ≤ 9 months, then yearly (split virus vaccine if ≤ 12 months)	Yes	Yes
Pneumococcal vaccine	Yes After the age of 2 years	Yes If not done pre-treatment: age ≤ 10 years, revaccinate every 3–5 years; age > 10 years, revaccinate every 6 years	Yes

recommend that no transplantation takes place for 30 days after the patient receives MMR or Varivax vaccines.

Several other general precautions pertain to transplant patients. Hepatitis vaccines pose little risk but may not be effective. Post-immunization testing for both hepatitis B antibodies (HBsAB) and hepatitis A antibodies (HAV IGG) should be performed 1–2 months after the series is completed. HBsAB should be repeated yearly in order to determine the timing of booster doses. Either of two hepatitis A vaccines may be used, but the products should not be interchanged in an individual. Acellular pertussis vaccines are recommended. Pneumococcal vaccines are safe, but they may not work well if the patient is transplanted within 2 weeks of the vaccine administration. Immunization guidelines change continually as new information and vaccines become available. The Committee on Infectious Diseases of the American Academy of Pediatrics maintains up-to-date recommendations and is a valuable resource when caring for transplant recipients.

Meaningful exploration of the current state of the art in critical care related to liver failure is beyond the scope of this chapter. The care of those patients with acute fulminant liver failure or rapid worsening of chronic liver disease is taxing and complex, and often fails to stabilize patients for more than a few days. This area represents one of the principal challenges with regard to future work. Alternate therapy has also received little attention, but this situation will undoubtedly change rapidly with the anticipated advent of effective gene therapy. Finally, nuances of the cultural and political systems within which we live have a major impact on the provision of liver transplant services worldwide. In the USA, funding is often the deciding issue with regard to access to health care. Over the next decade our society will have to address issues of funding necessary to sustain these patients through a productive life. With appropriate preoperative preparation and careful postoperative care, a child undergoing liver transplantation for a variety of diseases can expect to grow to adulthood, succeed in academic or business ventures, and have children of his or her own. These pioneers represent the first generation of people to live as functional chimeras. Undoubtedly there will be much that they can teach us as they grow and mature, and clearly we have much left to learn about how best to provide for their needs.

Acknowledgment

I would like to thank Cheryl McGinnis ARNP and Jean Osbrach MSW for providing information relating to patient assessment and preoperative preparation at the University of Florida, and Dawn Maillart for her help in preparing the manuscript.

Key references

Burdelski M, Ullrich K. Liver transplantation in metabolic disorders: summary of the general discussion. *European Journal of Pediatrics* 1999; **158 (Supplement 2)**: S95–6.

This reference summarizes the recommendations of a recent consensus conference on liver transplantation for metabolic disorders. The entire supplement contains the most current and comprehensive review of this subject.

Cecka JM, Terasaki PI. *Clinical Transplants* 1999. Los Angeles, CA: UCLA Immunogenetics Center, 1999.

Published yearly, *Clinical Transplants* provides the best summary data on the status of liver (as well as other solid organ) transplantation. These data are especially useful for assessing current transplant outcomes.

Chardot C, Carton M, Spire-Bendelac N. Prognosis of biliary atresia in the era of liver transplantation: French national study from 1986 to 1996. *Hepatology* 1999; **30**: 606–11.

This study sets a standard for population-based outcomes research focused on children with the commonest disorder leading to transplantation.

Murray CSL, Lopez AD. *Global burden of disease: a comprehensive assessment of mortality and disability from diseases, injuries and risk factors in 1990 and projected to 2020.* Cambridge, MA: Harvard University Press, 1996.

This is a highly readable survey that provides a clear picture of which diseases cause the greatest burden to mankind. Improvements in assessment of the burden of childhood disease are clearly needed, but this book provides the reader who is interested in pediatric liver diseases with a valuable perspective.

Singer PA, Siegler M, Lantos J *et al.* Ethics of liver transplantation with living donors. *New England Journal of Medicine* 1989; **321**: 620–1.

This article has become a classic reference for living-related transplantation, and it deserves periodic rereading as living donor transplants become increasingly common.

REFERENCES

Alagille D, Odievre M, Dommergues JP. Hepatic ductular hypoplasia associated with characteristic facies, vertebral malformations, retarded physical, mental and sexual development, and cardiac murmur. *Journal of Pediatrics* 1987; **110**: 195–200.

Altman RP, Lilly JR, Greenfeld J. A multivariable risk factor analysis of the portoenterostomy (Kasai) procedure for biliary atresia: twenty-five years of experience from two centers. *Annals of Surgery* 1997; **226**: 348–53.

American Academy of Pediatrics. Immunizations in special clinical circumstances. In: Pickering LK (ed.) *Red Book: Report of the Committee on Infectious Diseases*, 25th edn. Elk Grove Village, IL: American Academy of Pediatrics, 2000.

Ayas MF, Hillemeier AC, Olson AD. Lack of evidence for seasonal variation in extrahepatic biliary atresia during infancy. *Journal of Clinical Gastroenterology* 1996; **22**: 292–4.

Baumann U, Crosby HA, Ramani P. Expression of the stem cell factor receptor c-kit in normal and diseased pediatric liver: identification of a human hepatic progenitor cell? *Hepatology* 1999; **30**: 112–17.

Belle S, Beringer K, Detre K. An update on liver transplantation in the United States: recipient characteristics and outcome. *Clinical Transplants* 1995; 19–33.

Benyon RC, Iredale JP, Goddard S. Expression of tissue inhibitor of metalloproteinases 1 and 2 is increased in fibrotic human liver. *Gastroenterology* 1996; **110**: 821–31.

Bernuau J, Rueff B, Benhamou JP. Fulminant and subfulminant liver failure: definitions and causes. *Seminars in Liver Disease* 1986; **6**: 97–106.

Birnbaum A, Benkov K, Pittman N. Recurrence of autoimmune hepatitis in children after liver transplantation. *Journal of Pediatric Gastroenterology and Nutrition* 1997; **25**: 20–5.

Bobo L, Ojeh C, Chiu D. Lack of evidence for rotavirus by polymerase chain reaction/enzyme immunoassay of hepatobiliary samples from children with biliary atresia. *Pediatric Research* 1997; **11**: 229–34.

Borel J, Feurer C, Gubler HC *et al*. Biologic effects of cyclosporine A: a new antilymphocytic agent. *Agents and Actions* 1976; **6**: 468–75.

Brandhagen DJ, Alvarez W, Therneau TM. Iron overload in cirrhosis-HFE genotypes and outcome after liver transplantation. *Hepatology* 2000; **31**: 456–60.

Brems JJ, Hiat JR, Klein AS *et al*. Effect of prior portosystemic shunt on subsequent liver transplantation. *Annals of Surgery* 1989; **209**: 51–6.

Broide E, Klinowski E, Koukoulis G. Superoxide dismutase activity in children with chronic liver disease. *Journal of Hepatology* 2000; **32**: 188–92.

Broome U, Nemeth A, Hultcrantz R. Different expression of HLA-DR and ICAM-1 in livers from patients with biliary atresia and Byler's disease. *Journal of Hepatology* 1997; **26**: 857–62.

Cacciarelli TV, Esquivel CO, Moore DH. Factors affecting survival after orthotopic liver transplantation in infants. *Transplantation* 1997; **64**: 242–8.

Cauza E, Maier-Dobersberger T, Polli C *et al*. Screening for Wilson's disease in patients with liver diseases by serum ceruloplasmin. *Journal of Hepatology* 1997; **27**: 358–62.

Cecka JM, Terasaki PI. *Clinical transplants 1999*. Los Angeles, CA: UCLA Immunogenetics Center, 1999.

Chardot C, Carton M, Spire-Bendelac N. Epidemiology of biliary atresia in France: a national study 1986–1996. *Journal of Hepatology* 1999a; **31**: 1006–13.

Chardot C, Carton M, Spire-Bendelac N *et al*. Prognosis of biliary atresia in the era of liver transplantation: French national study from 1986 to 1996. *Hepatology* 1999b; **30**: 606–11.

Chen CL, Chen YS, Chiang YC. Paediatric liver transplantation: a 10-year experience in Taiwan. *Journal of Gastroenterology and Hepatology* 1996; **11**: S1–3.

Chen Y-T, Coleman RA, Scheinman JI. Renal disease in type I glycogen storage disease. *New England Journal of Medicine* 1988; **318**: 7–11.

Cheng MT, Chang MH, Hsu HY. Choledochal cyst in infancy: a follow-up study. *Chung Hua Min Kuo Hsiao Erh Ko I Hsueh Hui Tsa Chih* 2000; **41**: 13–17.

Clavien PA, Selzner M, Tuttle-Newhall JM *et al*. Liver transplantation complicated by misplaced TIPS in the portal vein. *Annals of Surgery* 1998; **227**: 440–5.

Cocjin J, Rosenthal P, Buslon V. Bile ductule formation in fetal, neonatal and infant livers compared with extrahepatic biliary atresia. *Hepatology* 1996; **24**: 568–74.

Cook GJ, Crofton ME. Hepatic artery thrombosis and infarction: evolution of the ultrasound appearances in liver transplant recipients. *British Journal of Radiology* 1997; **70**: 248–51.

Crigler JF, Najjar VA. Congenital familial nonhemolytic jaundice with kernicterus. *Pediatrics* 1952; **10**: 169–79.

Crosby HA, Hubscher SG, Joplin RE. Immunolocalization of OV-6, a putative progenitor cell marker in human fetal and diseased pediatric liver. *Hepatology* 1998; **28**: 980–5.

Davison SM, Skidmore SJ, Collingham KE *et al*. Chronic hepatitis in children after liver transplantation: role of hepatitis C virus and hepatitis G virus infections. *Journal of Hepatology* 1998; **28**: 764–70.

Diaz J, Acosta F, Canizares F *et al*. Does orthotopic liver transplantation normalize copper metabolism in patients with Wilson's disease? *Transplantation Proceedings* 1995; **27**: 2306.

Dillon P, Belchis D, Tracy TF Jr. Increased expression of intercellular adhesion molecules in biliary atresia. *American Journal of Pathology* 1994; **145**: 263–7.

Dillon PW, Belchis D, Minnick KE. Differential expression of the major histocompatibility antigens and ICAM-1 on bile duct epithelial cells in biliary atresia. *Tohoku Journal of Experimental Medicine* 1997; **181**: 33–40.

Dionisi-Vici C, Boglino C, Marcellini M. Tyrosinaemia type I with early metastatic hepatocellular carcinoma: combined treatment with NTBC, chemotherapy and surgical mass removal (abstract). *Journal of Inherited Metabolic Disease* 1997; **20 (Supplement 1)**: 3.

Donadieu J, Bader-Meunier B, Bertrand EA. Recombinant human G-CSF (lenograstim) for infectious complications in glycogen storage disease type Ib – report of 7 cases. *Revue Francaise de Hematologie* 1993; **35**: 529–34.

Douglass E. Hepatic malignancies in children and adolescents (hepatoblastoma, hepatocellular carcinoma and embryonal sarcoma). *Cancer Treatment and Research* 1997; **92**: 201–12.

Dray-Charier N, Paul A, Scoazec JY. Expression of delta F508 cystic fibrosis transmembrane conductance regulator protein and related chloride transport properties in the gallbladder epithelium from cystic fibrosis patients. *Hepatology* 1999; **29**: 1624–34.

Drut R, Drut RM, Gomez MA *et al.* Presence of human papillomavirus in extrahepatic biliary atresia. *Journal of Pediatric Gastroenterology and Nutrition* 1998; **27**: 530–5.

Dunn SP, Haynes JH, Nicolette LA. Split liver transplantation benefits the recipient of the 'leftover liver'. *Journal of Pediatric Surgery* 1997; **32**: 252–4.

Egawa H, Berquist W, Garcia-Kennedy R. Rapid development of hepatocellular siderosis after liver transplantation for neonatal hemochromatosis. *Transplantation* 1996; **62**: 1511–13.

Emerick KM, Rand EB, Goldmuntz E *et al.* Features of Alagille syndrome in 92 patients: frequency and relation of prognosis. *Hepatology* 1999; **29**: 822–9.

Esquivel CO, Klintmalm G, Iwatsuki S *et al.* Liver transplantation in patients with patent splenorenal shunts. *Surgery* 1987; **101**: 430–2.

Farrell FJ, Nguyen M, Woodley S. Outcome of liver transplantation in patients with hemochromatosis. *Hepatology* 1994; **20**: 404–10.

Fiel MI, Schiano TD, Bodenheimer HC. Hereditary hemochromatosis in liver transplantation. *Liver Transplant Surgery* 1999; **5**: 50–6.

Finegold MJ. Tumors of the liver. *Seminars in Liver Disease* 1994; **14**: 270–81.

Fischler B, Ehrnst A, Forsgren M. The viral association of neonatal cholestasis in Sweden: a possible link between cytomegalovirus infection and extrahepatic biliary atresia. *American Journal of Pathology* 1998; **153**: 527–35.

Fitzsimmons SC. The changing epidemiology of cystic fibrosis. *Journal of Pediatrics* 1993; **122**: 1–9.

Flowers M, Sherker A, Sinclair SB *et al.* Prostaglandin E in the treatment of recurrent hepatitis B infection after orthotopic liver transplantation. *Transplantation* 1994; **58**: 183–92.

Fogarty A, Hubbard R, Britton J. International comparison of median age at death from cystic fibrosis. *Chest* 2000; **117**: 1656–60.

Funaki N, Sasano H, Shizawa S. Apoptosis and cell proliferation in biliary atresia. *Journal of Pathology* 1998; **186**: 429–33.

Gaglio PJ, Regenstein F, Slakey D. Alpha-1-antitrypsin deficiency and splenic artery aneurysm rupture: an association? *American Journal of Gastroenterology* 2000; **95**: 1531–4.

Gilabert R, Bargallo X, Forns X *et al.* Value of duplex-Doppler ultrasound findings in liver transplant recipients with poor graft function. *Transplantation* 1996; **61**: 832–5.

Gordon FH, Mistry PK, Sabin CA *et al.* Outcome of orthotopic liver transplantation in patients with haemophilia. *Gut* 1998; **42**: 744–9.

Gorodischer R, Levy G, Krasner J *et al.* Congenital non-obstructive, non-hemolytic jaundice: effect of phototherapy. *New England Journal of Medicine* 1970; **282**: 375–7.

Goss JA, Yersiz H, Shackleton CR *et al. In-situ* splitting of the cadaveric liver for transplantation. *Transplantation* 1997; **64**: 871–7.

Gow PJ, Smallwood RA, Angus PW. Diagnosis of Wilson's disease: an experience over three decades. *Gut* 2000; **46**: 415–19.

Grace ND. TIPS: the long and the short of it. *Gastroenterology* 1997; **112**: 1040–3.

Grambsch PM, Dickson ER, Kaplan M *et al.* Extramural cross-validation of the Mayo primary biliary cirrhosis survival model establishes its generalizability. *Hepatology* 1989; **10**: 846–50.

Grazuadei IW, Joseph JJ, Wiesner RH. Increased risk of chronic liver failure in adults with heterozygous alpha-1-antitrypsin deficiency. *Hepatology* 1998; **28**: 1058–63.

Greene HL, Slonim AE, O'Neill JA *et al.* Continuous nocturnal intragastric feeding for management of type I glycogen storage disease. *New England Journal of Medicine* 1976; **294**: 423–5.

Henderson JM. Liver transplantation for portal hypertension. *Gastroenterology Clinics of North America* 1992; **21**: 197–213.

Heyman MB, LaBorge JM. Role of transjugular intrahepatic portosystemic shunt in the treatment of portal hypertension in pediatric patients. *Journal of Pediatric Gastroeuterology and Nutrition* 1999; **29**: 240–9.

Hoofnagle JH, Lombardero M, Zetterman RK. Donor age and outcome of liver transplantation. *Hepatology* 1996; **24**: 89–96.

Hossain M, Murahashi O, Ando H. Immunohistochemical study of proliferating cell nuclear antigen in hepatocytes of biliary atresia: a parameter to predict clinical outcome. *Journal of Pediatric Surgery* 1995; **30**: 1297–301.

Ibraham M, Ohi R, Chiba T, Nio M. *Indications and results of reoperation for biliary atresia.* Tokyo: Icon Associates, 1991.

Iwatsuki S, Starzl TE, Todo S *et al.* Liver transplantation in the treatment of bleeding esophageal varices. *Surgery* 1988; **104**: 697–705.

Jansen PLM. Diagnosis and management of Crigler–Najjar syndrome. *European Journal of Pediatrics* 1999; **158 (Supplement 2)**: S89–94.

Jevon GP, Dimmick JE. Biliary atresia and cytomegalovirus infection: a DNA study. *Pediatric Developmental Pathology* 1999; **2**: 11–14.

Kalayoglu M, Sollinger HW, D'Alessandro AM. Successful extended preservation of the liver for clinical transplantation. *Lancet* 1988; **1**: 617–20.

Karon M, Imach D, Schwarz A. Effective phototherapy in congenital, non-obstructive, non-hemolytic jaundice. *New England Journal of Medicine* 1970; **282**: 377–81.

Karrer FM, Lilly JR, Stewart BA, Hall RJ. Biliary atresia registry, 1976 to 1989. *Journal of Pediatric Surgery* 1990; **25**: 1076–80.

Karrer FM, Holland RM, Allshouse MJ, Lilly JR. Portal vein thrombosis: treatment of variceal hemorrhage by endoscopic variceal ligation. *Journal of Pediatric Surgery* 1994; **29**: 1149–51.

Kaufmann SS, Wood RP, Shaw JBW *et al.* Orthotopic liver transplantation for type 1 Crigler–Najjar syndrome. *Hepatology* 1986; **6**: 1259–62.

Kim WR, Therneau TM, Wiesner RH *et al.* A revised natural history model for primary sclerosing cholangitis. *Mayo Clinic Proceedings* 2000; **75**: 688–94.

Kinugasa Y, Nakashima Y, Matsuo S. Bile ductular proliferation as a prognostic factor in biliary atresia: an immunohistochemical assessment. *Journal of Pediatric Surgery* 1999; **34**: 1715–20.

Kobayashi H, Puri P, O'Briain DS. Hepatic over-expression of MHC class II antigens and macrophage-associated antigens (CD68) in patients with biliary atresia of poor prognosis. *Journal of Pediatric Surgery* 1997; **32**: 590–3.

Kobayashi H, Miyano T, Horikoshi K. Clinical significance of plasma endothelin levels in patients with biliary atresia. *Pediatric Surgery International* 1998a; **13**: 491–3.

Kobayashi H, Miyano T, Horikoshi K. Prognostic value of serum procollagen III peptide and type IV collagen in patients with biliary atresia. *Journal of Pediatric Surgery* 1998b; **33**: 112–14.

Kowdley KV, Hassanein T, Kaur S. Primary liver cancer and survival in patients undergoing liver transplantation for hemochromatosis. *Liver Transplant Surgery* 1995; **1**: 237–41.

Kramer B, Broolsch CE, Henne-Bruns D (eds). *Atlas of liver, pancreas and kidney transplantation*. New York: Thieme Medical Publishers, Inc., 1994.

Ladd WE, Gross RE (eds). *Abdominal surgery of infancy and childhood*. Philadelphia, PA: WB Saunders, 1941.

Lagnas AN, Marujo WC, Stratta RJ *et al.* Influence of a prior portosystemic shunt on outcome after liver transplantation. *American Journal of Gastroenterology* 1992; **87**: 714–18.

Lamireau T, LeBail B, Boussarie L. Expression of collagens type I and IV, osteonectin and transforming growth factor beta-a (TGF-beta-1) in biliary atresia, and paucity of intrahepatic bile ducts during infancy. *Journal of Hepatology* 1999; **31**: 248–55.

Langham MR, Tzakis AG, Gonzalez-Peralta R *et al.* Graft survival in pediatric liver transplantation. *Journal of Pediatric Surgery* 2001; **36**: 1205–9.

Lawson F, Charlebois R, Dillon J. Phylogenetic analysis of carbamoylphosphate synthetase genes: complex evolutionary history includes an internal duplication within a gene which can root the tree of life. *Molecular Biology and Evolution* 1996; **13**: 970–7.

Lee MG, Hanchard B, Williams NP. Drug-induced acute liver disease. *Postgraduate Medical Journal* 1989; **65**: 367–70.

Li L, Krantz ID, Deng Y *et al.* Alagille syndrome is caused by mutations in human Jagged1, which encodes a ligand for Notch1. *Nature Genetics* 1997; **16**: 243–51.

Lutsenko S, Cooper MJ. Localization of the Wilson's disease protein product to mitochondria. *Proceedings of the National Academy of Sciences of the USA* 1998; **95**: 6004–9.

McDiarmid SV, Millis MJ, Olthoff KM *et al.* Indications for pediatric liver transplantation. *Pediatric Transplantation* 1998; **2**: 106–16.

McKiernan PJ, Baker AJ, Kelly DA. The frequency and outcome of biliary atresia in the UK and Ireland. *Lancet* 2000; **355**: 25–9.

Maggard MA, Goss JA, Swenson KL. Liver transplantation in polysplenia syndrome: use of a living-related donor. *Transplantation* 1999; **68**: 1206–9.

Malizia G, Brunt EM, Peters MG. Growth factor and procollagen type I gene expression in human liver disease. *Gastroenterology* 1995; **108**: 145–56.

Mason AL, Xu L, Guo L. Detection of retroviral antibodies in primary biliary cirrhosis and other idiopathic biliary disorders. *Lancet* 1998; **351**: 1620–4.

Matern D, Starzl TE, Arnaout W. Liver transplantation for glycogen storage disease types I, III and IV. *European Journal of Pediatrics* 1999; **158 (Supplement 2)**: S43–8.

Mattei P, Wise B, Schwarz K. Orthotopic liver transplantation in patients with biliary atresia and situs inversus. *Pediatric Surgery International* 1998; **14**: 104–10.

Mazariegos GV, O'Toole K, Mieles LA *et al.* Hyperbaric oxygen therapy for hepatic artery thrombosis after liver transplantation in children. *Liver Transplant Surgery* 1999; **5**: 429–36.

Mirza DF, Gunson BK, Da Silva RF *et al.* Policies in Europe on 'marginal quality' donor livers. *Lancet* 1994; **344**: 1480–3.

Mitchell MC, Boitnott JK, Kaufman S *et al.* Budd–Chiari syndrome: etiology, diagnosis and management. *Medicine* 1982; **61**: 199–205.

Mohan N, McKiernan PJ, Preece MA. Indications and outcome of liver transplantation in tyrosinaemia type I. *European Journal of Pediatrics* 1999; **158 (Supplement 2)**: S49–54.

Muller-Berghaus J, Knisely AS, Zaum R *et al.* Neonatal haemachromatosis: report of a patient with favorable outcome. *European Journal of Pediatrics* 1997; **156**: 296–8.

Murray CSL, Lopez AD. *Global burden of disease: a comprehensive assessment of mortality and disability from diseases, injuries and risk factors in 1990 and projected to 2020*. Cambridge, MA: Harvard University Press, 1996.

Németh A. Liver transplantation in α-1-antitrypsin deficiency. *European Journal of Pediatrics* 1999; **158 (Supplement 2)**: S85–8.

Németh A, Möller E. HLA in juvenile liver disease with α-1-antitrypsin deficiency. *Acta Paediatrica Scandinavica* 1987; **76**: 603–7.

Németh A, Strandvick B. Natural history of children with α-1-antitrypsin deficiency and neonatal cholestasis. *Acta Paediatrica Scandinavica* 1982; **71**: 993–9.

Németh A, Strandvick B. Urinary excretion of tetrahydroxylated bile acids in children with α-1-antitrypsin deficiency and neonatal cholestasis. *Scandinavian Journal of Clinical and Laboratory Investigation* 1984; **44**: 387–92.

Nicolette LA, Reichard KW, Falkenstein K. Results of transplantation for acute and chronic hepatic allograft rejection. *Journal of Pediatric Surgery* 1998; **33**: 909–12.

Nour B, Tzakis AG, Van Thiel DH. The use of interferon for the treatment of viral hepatitis in pediatric liver transplant recipients. *Journal of the Oklahoma State Medical Association* 1995; **88**: 109–13.

Ochiai T, Nakajima K, Nagata M *et al.* Studies of the induction and maintenance of long-term graft acceptance by treatment with FK 506 in heterotopic cardiac allotransplantation in rats. *Transplantation* 1987; **44**: 734–8.

Oda T, Elkahloun AG, Pike BL *et al.* Mutations in the human Jagged1 gene are responsible for Alagille syndrome. *Nature Genetics* 1997; **16**: 235–43.

O'Grady JG, Alexander GJ, Hayllar KM. Early indicators of prognosis in fulminant hepatic failure. *Gastroenterology* 1989; **97**: 439–45.

Ohi R, Nio M. *The jaundiced infant: biliary atresia and other obstructions in pediatric surgery*, 5th edn. St Louis, MO: Mosby 1998.

Okada A, Morise T, Takeda Y. A new variant deletion of a copper-transporting P-type ATPase gene found in patients with Wilson's disease presenting with fulminant hepatic failure. *Journal of Gastroenterology* 2000; **35**: 278–83.

Otto G, Herfarth C, Senninger N *et al.* Hepatic transplantation in galactosemia. *Transplantation* 1989; **47**: 902–3.

Ouzounis CA, Kyrpides NC. On the evolution of arginases and related enzymes. *Journal of Molecular Evolution* 1994; **39**: 101–4.

Park WH, Kim SP, Park KK *et al.* Electron microscopic study of the liver with biliary atresia and neonatal hepatitis. *Journal of Pediatric Surgery* 1996; **31**: 367–74.

Parkkila S, Waheed A, Britton RS. Association of the transferrin receptor in human placenta with HFE, the protein defective in hereditary hemochromatosis. *Proceedings of the National Academy of Sciences of the USA* 1997; **94**: 13198–202.

Perner F, Gyuris T, Rakoczy G. Dipeptidyl peptidase activity of CD26 in serum and urine as a marker of cholestasis: experimental and clinical evidence. *Journal of Laboratory and Clinical Medicine* 1999; **134**: 56–67.

Peterson BE, Bower WC, Patrene KD *et al.* Bone marrow as a potential source of hepatic oval cells. *Science* 1999; **284**: 1168–70.

Poovorawan Y, Chongsrisawat V, Tanunytthawongse C. Extrahepatic biliary atresia in twins: zygosity determination by short tandem repeat loci. *Journal of the Medical Association of Thailand* 1996; **79** (**Supplement 1**): S119–24.

Potts WJ. *The surgeon and the child*. Philadelphia, PA: WB Saunders, 1959.

Praghakaran K, Wise B, Chen A. Rational management of post-transplant lymphoproliferative disorder in pediatric recipients. *Journal of Pediatric Surgery* 1999; **34**: 112–15.

Pratschke J, Steinmuller T, Bechstein WO *et al.* Orthotopic liver transplantation for hepatic associated metabolic disorders. *Clinical Transplants* 1998; **12**: 228–32.

Reding R, de Ville de Goyet J, Delbeke I. Pediatric liver transplantation with cadaveric or living related donors: comparative results in 90 elective recipients of primary grafts. *Journal of Pediatrics* 1999; **134**: 280–6.

Rela M, Muiesan P, Heaton ND *et al.* Orthotopic liver transplantation for hepatic-based metabolic disorders. *Transplant International* 1995; **8**: 41–4.

Revell SP, Noble-Jamieson G, Roberton NRC *et al.* Liver transplantation in cystic fibrosis. *Journal of the Royal Society of Medicine* 1993; **86**: 111–12.

Revillon Y, Michel JL, Lacaille F *et al.* Living-related liver transplantation in children: the 'Parisian' strategy to safely increase organ availability. *Journal of Pediatric Surgery* 1999; **34**: 851–3.

Reyes J, Gerber D, Mazariegos GV. Split-liver transplantation: a comparison of *ex-vivo* and *in-situ* techniques. *Journal of Pediatric Surgery* 2000; **35**: 283–90.

Richardson SC, Bishop RF, Smith AL. Reovirus serotype 3 infection in infants with extrahepatic biliary atresia or neonatal hepatitis. *Journal of Gastroenterology and Hepatology* 1994; **9**: 264–8.

Rodriguez-Velasco A, Garcia GR, Tejeda-Vega S. Neonatal hemochromatosis. Report of three autopsy cases. *Revista de Investigacion Clinica* 1999; **51**: 81–7.

Rogiers X, Malago M, Gawad K. *In-situ* splitting of cadaveric livers. The ultimate expansion of a limited donor pool. *Annals of Surgery* 1996; **224**: 331–9.

Saudubray JM, Touati G, Delonlay P *et al.* Liver transplantation in propionic acidaemia. *European Journal of Pediatrics* 1999a; **158** (**Supplement 2**): S65–9.

Saudubray JM, Touati G, Delonlay P *et al.* Liver transplantation in urea cycle disorders. *European Journal of Pediatrics* 1999b; **158** (**Supplement 2**): S55–9.

Selby R, Starzl TE, Yunis E *et al.* Liver transplantation for type I and type IV glycogen storage disease. *European Journal of Pediatrics* 1993; **152** (**Supplement 1**): S71–6.

Shaw JBW, Iwatsuki S, Bron K *et al.* Portal vein grafts in hepatic transplantation. *Surgery, Gynecology and Obstetrics* 1985; **161**: 66–8.

Shirahase I, Ooshima A, Tanaka K *et al.* The slow progression of hepatic fibrosis in intrahepatic cholestasis as compared with extrahepatic biliary atresia. *European Journal of Pediatric Surgery* 1995; **5**: 77–81.

Shun A, Delaney DP, Martin HC *et al.* Portosystemic shunting for paediatric portal hypertension. *Journal of Pediatric Surgery* 1997; **32**: 489–93.

Sieders E, Peeters PM, TenVergert EM *et al.* Analysis of survival and morbidity after pediatric liver transplantation with full-size and technical-variant grafts. *Transplantation* 1999; **68**: 540–5.

Sigurdsson L, Reyes J, Kocoshis SA *et al.* Neonatal hemochromatosis: outcomes of pharmacologic and surgical therapies. *Journal of Pediatric Gastroenterology and Nutrition* 1998; **26**: 85–90.

Singer PA, Siegler M, Lantos J *et al.* Ethics of liver transplantation with living donors. *New England Journal of Medicine* 1989; **321**: 620–1.

Sokal EM, Sokol RJ, Cormier V *et al.* Liver transplantation in mitochondrial respiratory chain disorders. *European Journal of Pediatrics* 1999; **158 (Supplement 2)**: S81–4.

Starzl TE, Porter KA, Putnam CW *et al.* Orthotopic liver transplantation in ninety-three patients. *Surgery, Gynecology and Obstetrics* 1976; **142**: 487–505.

Starzl TE, Iwatsuki S, Van Thiel DH *et al.* Evolution of liver transplantation. *Hepatology* 1982; **2**: 614–36.

Starzl TE, Demetris AJ, Trucco M *et al.* Chimerism after liver transplantation for type IV glycogen storage disease and type I Gaucher's disease. *New England Journal of Medicine* 1993; **328**: 745–9.

Stiegmann GV, Goff JS, Michaletz-Onody PA *et al.* Endoscopic sclerotherapy as compared with endoscopic variceal ligation for bleeding esophageal varices. *New England Journal of Medicine* 1992; **326**: 1527–32.

Strand S, Hofmann WJ, Grambihler A *et al.* Hepatic failure and liver cell damage in acute Wilson's disease involve CD95 (APO-1/Fas) mediated apoptosis. *Nature Medicine* 1998; **4**: 588–93.

Stringer MD, Marshall MM, Muiesan P *et al.* Survival and outcome after hepatic artery thrombosis complicating pediatric liver transplantation. *Journal of Pediatric Surgery* 2001; **36**: 888–91.

Superina R, Bilik R. Results of liver transplantation in children with unresectable liver tumors. *Journal of Pediatric Surgery* 1996; **31**: 835–9.

Tallgren M, Hockerstedt K, Makinen J *et al.* Cardiac evaluation of liver transplant recipients: QT dispersion in electrocardiogram. *Clinical Transplants* 1996; **10**: 408–13.

Tanaka K, Uemoto S, Tokunaga Y *et al.* Living related liver transplantation in children. *American Journal of Surgery* 1994; **168**: 41–8.

Tanano H, Hasegawa T, Kawahara H *et al.* Biliary atresia associated with congenital structural anomalies. *Journal of Pediatric Surgery* 1999; **34**: 1687–90.

Terblanche J, Northover JM, Bornman P *et al.* A prospective controlled trial of sclerotherapy in long-term management of patients after esophageal variceal bleeding. *Surgery, Gynecology and Obstetrics* 1979; **148**: 323–33.

Terblanche J, Burroughs AK, Hobbs KE. Controversies in the management of bleeding esophageal varices. *New England Journal of Medicine* 1989; **320**: 1469–75.

Tracy TF Jr, Dillon PW, Fox EK *et al.* The inflammatory response in pediatric biliary disease; macrophage phenotype and distribution. *Journal of Pediatric Surgery* 1996; **31**: 121–5.

Treem WR, Sokol JR. Disorders of the mitochondria. *Seminars in Liver Disease* 1998; **18**: 237–53.

Trey C, Davidson CS. *The management of fulminant hepatic failure.* New York: Grune & Stratton 1970.

Tuchman M, Morizono H, Rajagopal BS *et al.* The biochemical and molecular spectrum of ornithine transcarbamylase deficiency. *Journal of Inherited Metabolic Disease* 1998; **21 (Supplement 1)**: 40–58.

Tyler KL, Sokol RJ, Oberhaus SM *et al.* Detection of reovirus RNA in hepatobiliary tissues from patients with extrahepatic biliary atresia and choledochal cysts. *Hepatology* 1998; **27**: 1475–82.

van Hoek B, de Boer J, Boudjema K *et al.* Auxiliary versus orthotopic liver transplantation for acute liver failure. EURALT Study Group. European Auxiliary Liver Transplant Registry. *Journal of Hepatology* 1999; **30**: 699–705.

Varela-Fascinetto G, Castaldo P, Fox IJ *et al.* Biliary atresia–polysplenia syndrome: surgical and clinical relevance in liver transplantation. *Annals of Surgery* 1998; **227**: 583–9.

Whitington PF, Emond JC, Heffron T *et al.* Orthotopic auxiliary liver transplantation for Crigler–Najjar syndrome type 1. *Lancet* 1993; **342**: 779–80.

Wijmenga C, Muller T, Murli IS *et al.* Endemic Tyrolean infantile cirrhosis is not an allelic variant of Wilson's disease. *European Journal of Human Genetics* 1998; **6**: 624–8.

Wilson MW, Gordon RL, Laborge JM *et al.* Liver transplantation complicated by malpositioned transjugular intrahepatic portosystemic shunts. *Journal of Vascular and Interventional Radiology* 1995; **6**: 695–9.

Wood RP, Shaw BW, Rikkers LF. Liver transplantation for variceal hemorrhage. *Surgical Clinics of North America* 1990; **70**: 449–61.

Xiao JC, Ruck P, Kaiserling E. Small epithelial cells in extrahepatic biliary atresia: electron microscope and immunoelectron microscopic findings suggest a close relationship to liver progenitor cells. *Histopathology* 1999; **35**: 454–60.

Yamada S, Iida T, Tabata T *et al.* Alcoholic fatty liver differentially induces a neutrophil-chemokine and hepatic non-ischemia-reperfusion in rat. *Hepatology* 2000; **32**: 278–88.

Yoon PW, Bresee JS, Olney RS *et al.* Epidemiology of biliary atresia: a population-based study. *Pediatrics* 1997; **99**: 376–82.

Zimmerman AA, Howard TK, Huddleston CB *et al.* Combined lung and liver transplantation in a girl with cystic fibrosis. *Canadian Journal of Anaesthesia* 1999; **46**: 571–5.

Zimmerman HJ. *Hepatotoxicity: the adverse effects of drugs and other chemicals on the liver.* New York: Appleton-Century-Crofts, 1978.

28

Operative strategies and techniques

RICCARDO A SUPERINA

INTRODUCTION

Liver transplantation in children has undergone a radical evolution from its first description by Starzl et al. (1968), when it varied little from the operation as it was performed in adults. The necessities imposed by the ever-increasing demand for more organs and the relatively high mortality on waiting-lists for children led to innovative techniques and strategies to increase organ availability for children.

The first human orthotopic liver transplant was performed by Starzl in a 3-year-old with biliary atresia in 1963, and he reported the first long-term survivor, a 1-year-old girl with a hepatoma (Starzl et al., 1968). Over the next 20 years, the scarcity of size-matched donor organs in children stimulated the development of three innovative techniques, namely reduced-size (Bismuth and Houssin, 1984), living-related (Strong et al., 1990) and split-liver transplantation (Pichlmayr et al., 1988; Riuge et al., 1990). These surgical innovations led to shorter waiting times and fewer deaths on the waiting-list. Improved postoperative survival was a result of children undergoing transplantation in a more timely fashion, and improved results led to a greater acceptance of the procedure among both the medical community and the public at large. The improved efficacy of immunosuppressive medication and advances in anesthesia and critical care medicine have also contributed to the improvement in long-term survival, which is now routinely in the range 80–90% at 1 year post transplant (McDiarmid, 1996a; Kelly, 1998a, b; Otte et al., 1998; Reyes and Mazariegos, 1999).

As progress has been made in obtaining organs for children and increasing survival after transplantation, the long-term problems of reintegration into normal childhood have become a focus of increasing interest for those who care for children after liver transplantation. The treatment of chronic viral diseases, the monitoring, prevention and treatment of lymphoproliferative disease, and the focus on growth and nutrition have become issues with a uniquely pediatric perspective, which children, their parents and their caregivers have taken the lead in developing.

Statistics

A total of 1541 children (aged < 18 years) were listed for liver transplantation in the USA in 1998, and 573 were transplanted (US Department of Health and Human Services, 1998). This constituted 13% of all liver transplants performed in that year. In total 7.5% of the children who were listed died while on the waiting-list.

According to data from the United States Bureau of Vital Statistics, 55% of children with liver disease die before the age of 2 years, and a second mortality peak occurs after the age of 10 years. In contrast, the pediatric donor population consists of predominantly preschool and school-age children.

LIVER DISEASE IN CHILDREN

Liver disease in infancy interferes with the critical period of growth and development in the early years of life, and adds to the urgency of transplantation so that losses can be regained. The decision to list for transplant must be made in the context of maximizing whatever potential for growth and development still exists without a transplant, balanced by the knowledge that as nutrition and metabolic reserves suffer, the likelihood of a successful outcome also decreases.

The commoner indications for liver transplantation in children are listed in Figure 28.1 (see also Chapter 27).

Cholestatic diseases

BILIARY ATRESIA

The commonest indication for liver transplantation in children is biliary atresia (Superina, 1992; Miyano et al., 1993; Otte et al., 1994), a progressive fibro-inflammatory destruction of the extrahepatic biliary tree, which develops in approximately 1 in 15 000 newborns (Figure 28.1). The etiology of the disorder remains unknown, but as many as 10% of affected children will have

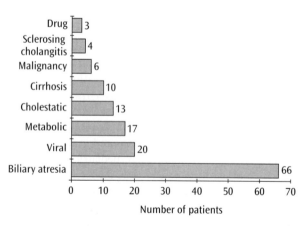

Figure 28.1 *Biliary atresia accounted for almost half of 137 patients coming to liver transplant over a 10-year period at the Hospital for Sick Children in Toronto. Viral hepatitis presented as acute or subacute fulminant disease in 20 patients and included syncytial giant-cell hepatitis. It was the second commonest reason for transplantation, followed by a variety of metabolic diseases including tyrosinemia, alpha-1-antitrypsin deficiency, glycogen storage disease and mitochondrial depletion syndromes. Cholestatic diseases included Alagille's syndrome and progressive familial intrahepatic cholestasis. Malignant diseases included hepatoblastoma and hepatocellular carcinoma.*

associated developmental abnormalities such as polysplenia, malrotation and intra-abdominal vascular anomalies. Some infants will benefit from the Kasai procedure, but the majority will have progressive biliary cirrhosis despite surgical intervention (Azarow et al., 1997; Ryckman et al., 1998; Chardot et al., 1999; Okazaki et al., 1999). A minority of infants with biliary atresia should be considered for primary transplantation if the likelihood of successful portoenterostomy is remote, whether due to lateness of the diagnosis or other poor prognostic factors (Sandler et al., 1997). A previous Kasai procedure adds to the difficulty of a subsequent transplant, but the benefits of delaying the transplant until the child is older are substantial.

OTHER CHOLESTATIC DISEASES

Other cholestatic diseases for which there is no effective surgical therapy include Alagille's syndrome (Alagille, 1985), progressive familial intrahepatic cholestasis (Whitington and Whitington, 1988; Rebhandl et al., 2000), and primary sclerosing cholangitis. The course of these diseases is variable. Some children may present with minimal and stable disease which does not progress to decompensated cirrhosis. Transplantation becomes an option as the complications of the liver disease become more apparent. These include growth retardation, bleeding from portal hypertension, ascites and bacterial peritonitis, and encephalopathy.

METABOLIC LIVER DISEASE

Metabolic liver diseases that result in cirrhosis, such as alpha-1-antitrypsin deficiency (Nemeth, 1999), (tyrosinemia Superina et al., 1989; Mieles et al., 1990; Freese et al., 1991), glycogen storage diseases (Malatack et al., 1983; Matern et al., 1999), neonatal hemochromatosis (Vohra et al., 2000) and Wilson's disease (DuBois et al., 1971; Sokol et al., 1985; Schilsky et al., 1994) are also common indications for liver transplantation in children. In addition, a new form of zinc storage disease has recently been described in children (Phillips et al., 1996).

INBORN ERRORS OF METABOLISM

Inborn errors of metabolism without cirrhosis, such as Crigler–Najjar syndrome or ornithine transcarbamylase deficiency, as well as others (Pett and Mowat, 1987; Whitington et al., 1993; Batshaw, 1994; Sokal et al., 1995; Odaib et al., 1998; Whitington et al., 1998; Saudubray et al., 1999), are also uncommon but important indications.

CHRONIC HEPATITIS

Cirrhosis due to chronic viral diseases is uncommon in children, but may include survivors of neonatal hepatitis, cytomegalovirus (CMV) hepatitis and other forms of unknown viral infections (Phillips et al., 1991; Langnas et al., 1995; Verboon-Maciolek et al., 1997; Cuffari et al., 1998; Egawa et al., 1998a; Sokal et al., 1998; Bernuau et al., 1999; Munoz et al., 1999; Ben-Ari et al., 2000; Hanna et al., 2000).

MALIGNANCY

Children with unresectable liver tumors represent a small but significant proportion of patients who undergo transplantation. Hepatoblastoma is the commonest childhood liver tumor, but transplantation for hepatocellular carcinoma and sarcomas has been reported (Koneru et al., 1991; Superina and Bilik, 1996; Bilik and Superina, 1997; Al-Qabandi et al., 1999; Reyes et al., 2000a). Care must be taken to exclude patients with extrahepatic malignant disease.

Acute liver disease

Patients with fulminant failure represent a significant proportion of those children who require transplantation (Phillips et al., 1991; Goss et al., 1998; Nicolette et al., 1998). Jaundice, coagulopathy and encephalopathy following a short prodrome of a flu-like illness are hallmarks of acute liver failure in children. Most have markedly raised liver enzyme levels and an associated hyperbilirubinemia, although the latter may not be very prominent (Alonso et al., 1995).

Children with acute liver failure must be assessed, diagnosed and treated rapidly. These patients may remain relatively stable for days or weeks with increasing jaundice and persistent coagulopathy, or they may deteriorate rapidly within hours of presentation, with progressive neurological, cardiovascular and renal dysfunction which complicates the care of the patient pre- and intraoperatively and increases the post-transplant morbidity and mortality.

These patients may recover spontaneously from liver failure, and therefore the decision to transplant must not be taken prematurely. The King's College criteria are useful as guidelines for listing for transplantation (O'Grady et al., 1989; Pauwels et al., 1993; Williams and Wendon, 1994). The commonest cause of fulminant failure in children is viral hepatitis (A, B and non A-G) (Langnas et al., 1995; Verboon-Maciolek et al., 1997; Cuffari et al., 1998; Egawa et al., 1998a; Sokal et al., 1998; Bernuau et al., 1999). Giant-cell hepatitis has been identified as an entity with a particularly poor prognosis (Phillips et al., 1991) once it progresses to cause jaundice and an uncorrectable coagulopathy, even in the absence of overt encephalopathy.

Metabolic diseases may also present with fulminant failure. These include neonatal hemochromatosis and Wilson's disease, among others.

Liver failure in association with neurological disturbances that are not due to encephalopathy may be secondary to mitochondrial respiratory chain disorders (Goncalves et al., 1995; Morris et al., 1998; Odaib et al., 1998; Berk and Stump, 1999; Sokal et al., 1999). Unless the mitochondriopathy is confined to the liver, transplantation should be avoided, since continued neurological deterioration may be expected even if the liver is successfully replaced.

TIMING OF TRANSPLANTATION

Patients with chronic liver disease are not actively listed for transplant unless they are judged to have less than 6 to 12 months' life expectancy. Predicting life expectancy is dependent on the form of liver disease. For example, biliary atresia has a very predictable progression. Patients who do not have successful biliary drainage following the Kasai procedure invariably reach end-stage liver disease with hepatic insufficiency by 2 years of age (Grosfeld et al., 1989; Otte et al., 1994). It is best to proceed with transplantation when they begin to exhibit linear growth failure and the first complications of portal hypertension. Patients with familial cholestatic syndromes, which ultimately lead to cirrhosis, may have a less predictable course (Rebhandl et al., 2000). Growth failure is characteristic of these syndromes even when liver function is preserved. Signs of advancing portal hypertension and liver synthetic failure are the earliest indications for transplant in this group. Children with metabolic defects, which are corrected by transplantation, are approached with a different strategy. In this setting, the goal should be to perform the transplant before the patient develops significant complications from the metabolic defect. The child with fulminant hepatic failure should undergo transplant as soon as a suitable organ is available, since fewer than 25% of these patients will survive without transplantation (Anand et al., 1997).

The preoperative evaluation of a child who is awaiting liver transplantation includes establishing the etiology, predicting the timing of the need for transplant, and identifying anatomical abnormalities or other organ system impairment which would complicate the surgical procedure. Children with cirrhosis should show signs of hepatic insufficiency, such as growth failure or coagulopathy, or have significant complications of portal hypertension, such as ascites or variceal bleeding before liver transplant is performed. A child who has not developed these complications may enjoy many years of good quality of life before they require transplantation.

RADIOLOGICAL AND LABORATORY TESTS IN PREPARATION FOR TRANSPLANTATION

Laboratory data

A complete blood count, electrolytes, blood urea nitrogen, serum cholesterol and bile salts, liver function tests, prothrombin and partial thromboplastin times, and alpha-fetoprotein are necessary. Viral serology is obtained (antibodies against CMV, Epstein–Barr virus, measles, varicella and HIV), and a hepatitis screen (antibodies against hepatitis C and A and measurement of hepatitis B surface antigen and antibody to surface antigen) is also performed.

CONFIRMATION OF DIAGNOSIS

The majority of children at our institution undergo a percutaneous liver biopsy using the 15-gauge Menghini needle. In patients with significant coagulation defects, a transjugular liver biopsy may be safely performed by the interventional radiology service, or alternatively, particularly in babies, through an open operative approach to ensure hemostasis. A liver biopsy in the setting of fulminant liver disease may not only aid the diagnosis, but also indicate the prognosis and likelihood of recovery without a transplant (Sokol et al., 1985; Gallinger et al., 1989).

Radiological investigations

The single most useful test before a possible liver transplant is an abdominal ultrasound with Doppler examination of intra-abdominal vessels. The patency and cross-sectional diameter of the portal vein are useful for assessing the possible need for portal reconstruction using vein grafts.

The presence of a preduodenal portal vein may sometimes be detected by ultrasound. Other relevant potential anomalies include azygos continuation of the inferior vena cava, congenital absence of the portal vein, anomalous drainage of the hepatic veins directly into the atrium, and situs inversus abdominis (Morgan and Superina, 1994a). Vascular anomalies and splenic malformations, such as polysplenia, are common in children with biliary atresia and must always be suspected and anticipated (Karrer et al., 1991; Davenport et al., 1993). Mesenteric angiography or more recently magnetic resonance angiography may be requested if important information cannot be obtained using ultrasound.

CT scanning may be useful for detecting previously unsuspected anomalies of other intra-abdominal organs. In children with hepatic malignancy, it is important to monitor for the presence of metastatic disease at frequent intervals.

In patients with fulminant failure, MR or CT imaging of the brain is necessary in order to rule out catastrophic intracranial bleeding as a cause of sudden changes in neurological status. Catastrophic intracranial events may preclude transplantation, as they make acceptable neurological recovery impossible.

Tissue matching

In general, blood group compatibility is desirable between donor and recipient. However, blood group incompatibility does not preclude successful transplantation (Gordon et al., 1986). In children with urgent indications for transplantation, blood-group-incompatible transplants have been successfully performed, and protocols have been proposed to decrease the likelihood of catastrophic rejection. Closer tissue typing and cytotoxic antibody cross-matching have not been consistently demonstrated to have any effect on short- or long-term outcome in liver transplantation, and they are not used when matching donors to recipients (Markus et al., 1988; Wall, 1988).

Miscellaneous considerations

Malnutrition is a very common condition in children who are referred for liver transplantation (Pierro et al., 1989; Kelly, 1998; van Mourik et al., 2000). Nutrition is optimized by the provision of adequate calories and fat-soluble vitamin supplements in order to correct deficiencies. In babies, formulae with medium- chain-triglyceride supplementation are substituted for regular formulae, and may be supplemented with carbohydrates to increase caloric density (see Chapter 5).

Regular childhood immunizations, including hepatitis B, measles, mumps, Haemophilus influenzae, polio and varicella, are completed whenever possible. Complications of liver disease, such as coagulopathy, pruritus, cholestasis, ascites and encephalopathy, are managed medically.

In the setting of acute liver failure, intracranial pressure monitoring has not been universally accepted as a useful management tool in children, and it is not without risk. Most pediatric centers manage raised intracranial pressure by using clinical criteria without the aid of intracranial pressure monitors.

PREOPERATIVE CONSIDERATIONS

Adequate intravenous access is perhaps the most important requirement for proceeding with the operation (Chapin et al., 1989).

In general, a triple-lumen central line is placed in the subclavian vein to serve as a central venous pressure monitoring line and for the administration of medications. Another large-bore line is required in the internal jugular vein for rapid volume replacement. In babies, a surgically placed tunneled line is often desirable as a secure access route which can be kept long after the operation is over as a site from which to draw blood on the ward and even as an outpatient.

A peripheral intravenous line as well as an arterial line completes the vascular access requirements preoperatively.

In children who weigh more than 10 kg, a cell saver should be available for autotransfusion of suctioned blood whenever possible. In smaller children this device can still be used, but we have found that the volume of blood which is recycled does not justify the expense involved.

A rapid-infusion device for the administration of blood and blood products is a valuable adjunct in the event that blood loss is brisk and requires replacement more rapidly than can be achieved with conventional intravenous administration sets.

Other surgical equipment includes the argon-beam coagulator, as well as a conventional cautery unit. In our experience, the argon-beam cautery unit is a valuable device for stopping or reducing small vessel bleeding from raw peritoneal surfaces, the retroperitoneum and the liver itself.

Hypothermia is a frequent complication during a liver transplant, and temperature control may be difficult in very small children. Low body temperature can lead to cardiovascular instability, troublesome bleeding due to coagulation factor dysfunction and, in extreme cases, cardiac arrest. Equipment designed to direct the flow of warm air along the body of an infant underneath the surgical drapes is an essential accessory for helping to maintain acceptable body temperature in these very young patients.

Other surgical equipment

Self-retaining adjustable retractors are essential for providing adequate exposure of the surgical site for the many hours that may be necessary to complete a liver transplant operation.

Surgical loupes that provide 2.5 to 4.5 times magnification are indispensable aids in the transplantation of infants and small children. With the advent of microsurgical techniques for sewing the hepatic artery in some settings, access to an operating microscope and microsurgical instruments and equipment is essential.

Vascular clamps and forceps which are reserved for liver transplantation operations alone are the best way to ensure that these instruments do not malfunction at critical moments. A variety of vascular clamps, forceps and scissors suitable for use in small infants are necessary, which enable the surgeon to clamp, cut and sew fragile vessels in as precise and atraumatic a manner as possible.

Finally, a device for measuring the quality and quantity of blood flow through the hepatic artery and portal vein has in our experience been found to be an invaluable adjunct in pediatric transplantation. Flow probes of different sizes are used to measure the quantity of blood flow after reperfusion and at the end of the operation (Rasmussen et al., 1997). Doppler probes can also be used to indicate the presence but not the quantity of flow by placing them directly on the liver surface and listening for venous and arterial signals.

TRANSPLANT OPERATION

The most commonly used incision is the transverse incision in the upper abdomen that extends from the right subcostal margin to the left one. In older children, a midline vertical incision to the xiphisternum is often necessary to provide adequate exposure of the subphrenic areas, including the suprahepatic vena cava.

As much of the operation as possible is performed with cautery in order to minimize bleeding.

Hepatectomy

The hepatectomy is the first phase of the transplant operation. Patients with extensive previous right upper quadrant surgery may present a significant challenge when dissecting the liver and preparing it for removal. Since patients with biliary atresia and failed previous Kasai procedures are the commonest pediatric candidates for liver transplantation, extensive adhesions between bowel and liver and between bowel and abdominal wall are very commonly encountered. Every effort must be made to keep bleeding to a minimum by means of meticulous surgical technique, ligation of even small vessels and extensive use of cautery. The combination of portal hypertension and coagulation defects from liver disease can lead to steady bleeding, which over the course of a lengthy operation can result in a surprising amount of blood loss unless efforts are made to minimize bleeding from the start (Sandler et al., 1997).

The liver is mobilized by first dividing the round and falciform ligaments, the left triangular ligament and adhesions between the anterior edge of the liver and the transverse colon if there has been previous surgery. Incision of the lesser omentum and division of any aberrant left hepatic artery opens up the left approach to the hilum of the liver.

At this point, the right lobe can be mobilized by dividing the adhesions to the right parietal peritoneum, and mobilizing the hepatic flexure of the colon from the Roux loop (if there is one) and away from the liver.

Dissection of the hilum and proper identification of the hilar structures are essential for the later anastomosis of the new liver to the recipient portal vein and hepatic artery.

In children who have undergone previous biliary enteric procedures for biliary atresia, the safest way to dissect the bowel away from the vascular structures underneath is to incise the anterior bowel wall first. The posterior wall of the bowel can then be gently separated from the underlying structures, staying very close to the liver. Division of the posterior bowel wall allows the surgeon to reflect the loop of bowel away from the liver, thus exposing the tissue which contains the arterial and portal venous supply.

If the child has an intact biliary tree, the common

hepatic duct is identified, encircled and divided proximal to the cystic duct insertion.

The hepatic arteries are traced to beyond their segmental divisions and divided. This will allow the surgeon maximum flexibility in reconstructing the arterial supply later. It is not uncommon in children with biliary atresia to encounter a left hepatic artery that originates directly from the aorta and runs through the lesser omentum. Aberrant right hepatic arteries are also not uncommon. All vessels should be carefully preserved for the maximum length possible.

The portal vein is usually the most posterior structure. In children with biliary atresia, a small percentage of cases will have preduodenal portal veins that are encountered in a more anterior position.

The portal vein in babies with biliary atresia may be hypoplastic and narrow (Shaw et al., 1985; Tzakis et al., 1989a). The vein must be dissected distal to its bifurcation so that a branch patch may later be fashioned for the anastomosis. The vein is then traced proximally. It may often be necessary to find a portion of portal vein of a wider caliber near the spleno-mesenteric vein confluence or near the location of the coronary vein.

The lower infrahepatic vena cava is encircled, and the suprahepatic vena cava and hepatic veins must then be approached. The native vena cava is simply mobilized posteriorly and separated from the adrenal vein. The dissection must be taken cephalad so that a venous clamp may be placed around the upper cava.

The piggyback technique must be used when the donor liver is transplanted without its own vena cava, as in living-donor transplants (Strong et al., 1988). The native liver must then be dissected off the vena cava by dividing and oversewing the individual minor, accessory and major hepatic veins. It is faster and safer to dissect the liver sharply off the vena cava after the upper and lower caval clamps have been applied and the portal vein ligated, rather than attempting to individually isolate and ligate all of the retrohepatic veins with blood still flowing through the liver and the inferior vena cava.

After the native liver has been removed, the individual orifices of the retrohepatic venous branches can be clearly seen and oversewn with monofilament sutures. The right, middle and left hepatic veins may then be oversewn or left open, depending on the technique and location chosen for the hepatic venous anastomosis.

After the liver has been removed, every effort must be made to dry the field from ongoing blood loss. This will allow both for a more stable recipient during the critical implantation phase, and for better visibility of the vascular anastomoses for the surgeon and assistants.

Implantation

VENOUS DRAINAGE

Implantation of a whole liver starts with the sewing of the donor upper vena cava to the recipient cava. The recipient hepatic veins are opened to form a venous confluence, allowing for construction of a very wide venous anastomosis. The donor cava above the liver must be trimmed back to excise any pericardium or atrium if the donor heart was not procured. The two lateral corners of the anastomosis are then aligned with two double-armed monofilament absorbable sutures with as fine a gauge as possible. From the operator's side, the suture on the left corner is then used to complete the posterior venous wall in a continuous fashion, turning around the right corner. The anterior wall is then completed in a similar manner.

The infrahepatic vena cava anastomosis is performed with a running monofilament absorbable suture. During completion of the anterior wall anastomosis, the liver is flushed through the portal vein with lactated Ringer's solution in order to evacuate the solution that was used to preserve the organ.

Some authors have advocated the routine use of the piggyback technique in which the recipient vena cava is preserved and the hepatic veins of the donor liver are anastomosed to the recipient veins or to a large venotomy on the recipient vena cava (Tzakis et al., 1989b).

The portal vein anastomosis must be performed with great care. Sutures must be precise and placed close together in order not to constrict veins that are already small. The knot of the anastomosis must be tied away from the venous wall in order to allow for expansion of the circumference of the anastomosis after restitution of blood flow (Starzl et al., 1984). For babies, 7–0 absorbable monofilament suture is used, and in older children 6–0 is used.

Usually the venous clamps can be removed at this stage, restoring blood flow to the liver. All bleeding points at the anastomoses are suture ligated, and the liver is quickly inspected for adequate perfusion.

Bleeding may be exacerbated after venous reperfusion. Heparin that is still present in the graft may reach the circulation. In addition, dermatan sulphates and other heparin-like molecules appear after reperfusion (Mitchell et al., 1995), with the result that the partial thromboplastin time may rise significantly. Unless the bleeding is severe and unrelenting, support with volume and fresh frozen plasma is adequate for control. Fibrinolysis may play a significant role in the persistence of bleeding, and may require antifibrinolytic therapy for control (Kang et al., 1987, 1989).

ARTERIAL ANASTOMOSIS

The artery can be sewn using a variety of techniques. For whole-liver transplants, the anastomosis is most reliably performed by joining the celiac axis of the donor with a Carrel patch to the branching point of the recipient proper hepatic and gastroduodenal arteries using a continuous non-absorbable monofilament suture. However, some prefer the bifurcation of the proper hepatic artery of the recipient as an anastomotic site (Busuttil *et al.*, 1987).

In small babies, some have advocated the routine use of arterial conduits to the supraceliac or infrarenal aorta because of the small caliber of the native hepatic artery and the higher incidence of arterial thrombosis (Stevens *et al.*, 1992; Bilik *et al.*, 1995).

Preparation of the infrarenal aorta can be accomplished relatively quickly, although bleeding from retroperitoneal venous collaterals may be troublesome. An iliac artery, usually procured from the cadaveric donor, can be sewn to the recipient artery first, followed by anastomosis between the distal end of the conduit and the donor hepatic artery. Alternatively, if the entire abdominal aorta or thoracic aorta is procured in continuity with the donor liver, an aortic conduit to the infrarenal aorta of the recipient can be constructed. This method of reconstruction has been associated with a higher incidence of arterial thrombosis (personal experience of the author) and should only be used as a last resort.

BILIARY ANASTOMOSIS

A bile duct anastomosis to a Roux loop of bowel is the preferred method of biliary reconstruction in most children. The anastomosis is performed with interrupted absorbable sutures, and the loop may be positioned either in front of or behind the colon.

For small bile ducts, it is preferable to use an internal stent fashioned from a size 5 or 3.5 feeding tube which spans the anastomosis and prevents anterior wall sutures from catching the back wall. The stent may be secured to the bowel with a fine catgut suture that will dissolve rapidly and allow the stent to pass spontaneously. For larger bile ducts, no stent is necessary.

Duct-to-duct anastomoses are less commonly performed in pediatric transplantation, because of the small caliber of the ducts in infants and small children. If the size of the ducts permits a direct ductal anastomosis, internal stents or T-tubes may be used to stent the ducts, but have been associated with complications after removal (Shuhart *et al.*, 1998; Johnston *et al.*, 2000). No stents are necessary for these wider anastomoses (Randall *et al.*, 1996).

After the completion of the bile duct, the field is inspected for adequate hemostasis and the abdomen is closed.

Drains may be placed on both left and right sides. They serve to evacuate blood and fluid from the abdominal cavity, and alert the surgeon to the presence of a bile leak before it may otherwise be noted. Drains are not completely sensitive to either bleeding or a bile leak, and are usually only indicators of what may be happening in the abdomen. The drains should be removed after the second or third day, but the drain below the biliary anastomosis is usually left in for 7 days.

SPECIAL PEDIATRIC TECHNIQUES

Reduced-size transplantation

Reduced-size transplantation was first described in 1984 by Bismuth and Houssin. This technique allows for transplantation of a portion of a liver from an adult or older child cadaveric donor into an infant or smaller child. Segments 2 and 3 or 2, 3 and 4 are separated from the right side of the liver in continuity with the main portal vein, celiac axis and common hepatic duct. The vascular and ductal branches to the right side, and segment 4 if indicated, are ligated, and the liver is divided in the interlobar plane or along the falciform ligament. The right side of the liver is then discarded. In general, the size differential between the donor and recipient dictates how much of the liver should be transplanted. For donors who weigh less than four times the weight of the recipient, the entire left lobe can be transplanted. For donors who weigh more than four times the weight of the recipient, transplanting more than segments 2 and 3 is inadvisable, since this may delay or prevent primary abdominal wall closure. For discrepancies larger than weight ratios of 10 and above, even transplanting only segments 2 and 3 may be impossible. This is particularly true of newborn recipients with acute disease and very small abdominal cavities.

Reduced-size transplants have been used less commonly as the demand for livers for adult recipients has increased, leading to techniques which allow for transplantation of both lobes whenever possible.

Split-liver transplantation

The remnant of liver following segment 2 and 3 resection from a cadaveric liver or from a living donor is essentially identical, and is illustrated in Figure 28.2.

Dividing the liver for use in two recipients is an attractive hypothesis (Pichlmayr *et al.*, 1988) for dealing with the shortage of organs, but not every liver can be split (Strasberg *et al.*, 1999), and there may be circumstances in which it would be inadvisable to split a liver. Splitting livers also makes greater technical demands on both recipient teams than either would face without having to split the liver. Splitting may increase the risk of complications in the recipient to whom the liver was originally allocated, and it increases the logistical complexity associated with the coordination of two transplants instead of one, particularly if both sides of the split liver are used by the same program.

Split-liver transplantation is most commonly performed between an adult who receives the right lobe and segment 4, and a child who is small enough to receive segments 2 and 3. Full-lobe splits are possible but are less commonly performed (de Ville de Goyet, 1995; Otte *et al.*, 1998).

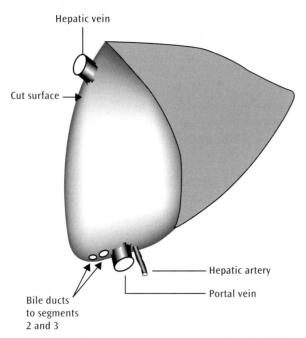

Figure 28.2 *The cut surface of segments 2 and 3 after division of the liver in the living-donor operation and split-liver operation. Segmental bile ducts may require separate anastomoses of ducts draining segments 2 and 3.*

ANATOMICAL CONSIDERATIONS WHEN DIVIDING A LIVER FOR TWO RECIPIENTS

The relationship between the middle and left hepatic veins is very important in determining the feasibility and ease with which segments 2 and 3 can be used separately from the rest of the liver. The middle hepatic vein usually joins with the left one at or near the junction of the veins with the vena cava. The junction between the two hepatic veins can usually be visualized above the liver by dissecting back the substance of the liver from the connective tissue which contains the vena cava. If the junction of the two veins is deeply intrahepatic, or if the middle vein is small and the left hepatic vein cannot be separated from the middle vein without significantly compromising flow within the latter, it may be inadvisable to proceed with the split. Interfering with the flow of the middle hepatic vein may cause engorgement of segment 4 as well as segments 5 and 8 in the right lobe, and result in severe bleeding from the cut surface of the lobe. In unusual circumstances where the middle vein is the principal drainage route of the anterior segments of the right lobe, the results of the transplant in the recipient for whom the liver was originally intended may be jeopardized if flow within the middle hepatic vein is compromised.

The liver may be split *in situ* or *ex situ* (Rogiers *et al.*, 1995; Goss *et al.*, 1997; Busuttil and Goss, 1999; Reyes *et al.*, 2000b). We prefer the *ex-situ* technique, as this alternative reduces operative time in the donor and avoids delaying other procurement teams. Only ideal donors are usually selected for liver splitting. We prefer donors under the age

of 40 years with normal or near-normal enzymes, who are on minimal vasopressor support. The macrovesicular fat content of the liver must be less than 10%. Using strict donor criteria for splitting, we have split approximately 20% of transplantable livers. This figure is similar to that reported by other centers (Azoulay *et al.*, 1996).

The preparation of the liver starts on the back table in the usual fashion. All vessels are inspected. The hepatic venous anatomy is determined first by looking down the suprahepatic vena cava and visualizing the junction of the middle and left hepatic veins. These are separated first and the middle vein is repaired, or the split attempt is abandoned if this cannot be done safely.

The dissection then proceeds to the right of the round ligament, dividing all portal vein branches to segment 4. In this fissure, the artery to segment 4 is encountered and carefully preserved. The artery is traced back to the main left hepatic and the branch to segments 2 and 3 is divided. This branch varies greatly in length, and its origin from the left hepatic artery must be located precisely in order to gain the maximum length possible for later reconstruction in the pediatric recipient. By carefully preserving the arterial supply to segment 4, its viability is ensured and the likelihood of biliary leaks in the recipient of the right liver is greatly reduced.

Once the artery and hepatic vein to the segment 2 and 3 block have been dissected out, then the left portal vein is transected just distal to the bifurcation, and the parenchyma of the liver is divided just to the right of the Rex fissure. All vascular and biliary structures encountered within the liver are meticulously ligated. Crossover branches between the middle hepatic vein on the right and the left hepatic vein are identified and suture-ligated. Biliary anatomy can vary greatly. We have encountered large anomalous ducts in the liver bridge between segments 3 and 4. The bile ducts are encountered at the liver plate just posterior to the portal vein, and form a network within the connective tissue which envelops the ducts at the liver plate. The bile duct to segment 4 may be encountered here and may join with the ducts from segments 2 and 3 to the left of the falciform ligament. It may have to be ligated in the right part of the split liver. Usually one or two ducts from the left side are encountered here, but we have seen as many as three.

The tissue posterior to the portal vein is divided with a scalpel to enable transected ducts to be seen as clearly as possible and identified for later anastomosis.

The portion of the liver that is ready for a transplant is identical to that which is procured from a living donor, and the recipient procedure is identical.

Recipient procedure for living-donor and split-liver transplants

There are a number of important technical differences between transplants that are performed using livers originating from split operations (Broelsch *et al.*, 1990; Langnas *et al.*, 1992; Rogiers *et al.*, 1995; Azoulay *et al.*, 1996; Malago *et al.*, 1997; Otte *et al.*, 1998) and living donors (Strong *et al.*, 1990; Broelsch *et al.*, 1991, 1993) on the one hand and whole-organ and reduced-size transplants on the other. Living-donor and split-liver transplants demand a higher level of expertise in order to obtain acceptable results, and should only be attempted after the surgeon has gained a reasonable amount of experience with whole-organ and reduced-size transplants. A number of techniques must be mastered in order to achieve acceptable success rates.

The liver is always piggybacked on to the recipient cava with a split or living donor transplant. A number of methods have been described for hepatic venous reconstruction, all in an attempt to reduce the incidence of venous outflow obstruction (Tanaka *et al.*, 1993; Yamaguchi *et al.*, 1993). In general, two principles should guide the hepatic venous reconstruction. The first is that the venous orifice on the recipient should match the donor hepatic vein in size. Too small an orifice on the recipient will not provide for adequate flow. On the other hand, too large an opening may result in stretching of the donor vein, and the orifice will resemble a slit that will be susceptible to twisting and obstruction with even small alterations in the orientation of the transplanted liver. The second principle is that the reconstructed hepatic vein should be kept as short as possible. This will reduce the likelihood of twisting with subsequent obstruction to flow. Thus there should be no attempt to procure a long segment of hepatic vein from the donor, since the anastomosis should be performed almost flush with the parenchymal edge.

The recipient hepatic veins should all be available for use in the hepatic venous reconstruction. Our preferred method is to open the orifices of the middle and left recipient hepatic veins, and to oversew the right vein. The confluence of the middle and left veins can then be extended in a caudal direction along the vena cava if necessary in order to match the donor vein in diameter. The orientation of the anastomosis will then be in a predominantly longitudinal direction, with a slight left-to-right orientation going down from the diaphragm. The upper and lower corners of the venotomy on the recipient will then be aligned with the corners of the left hepatic vein, allowing the segment to rotate slightly in a counterclockwise manner on the axis of the recipient cava. This will rotate the hilum of the liver medially and enable an easier anastomosis between the artery and portal vein.

The portal vein anastomosis must also be oriented in the proper manner in order to prevent twisting or kinking. The cut surface of the liver must be allowed to fall posteriorly to mimic its final position in the recipient at completion of the operation. Thus the donor portal vein also falls posteriorly, allowing the surgeon to judge the orientation of the vein properly, as well as its length, so that the recipient vein can then be prepared appropri-

ately. The bifurcation of the recipient vein should always be preserved so that it is available if necessary. The full length of the vein will be necessary in many circumstances in order to bridge the distance to the donor vein stump. Furthermore, large size discrepancies are not uncommon between the recipient and donor veins, and the branch patch of the recipient vein bifurcation is very helpful in dealing with the size differential that is often seen. A number of other techniques have been described for either lengthening or widening the recipient portal vein (Harihara *et al.*, 1999; Marwan *et al.*, 1999).

The arterial anastomosis in living-donor and split-liver transplants requires high magnification with either surgical loupes or an operating microscope (Tanaka *et al.*, 1993; Inomoto *et al.*, 1996; Shackleton *et al.*, 1997). Experience in microvascular surgery is essential before tackling these small vessels under sometimes difficult conditions. Appropriate equipment is essential, and includes microvascular forceps and needle holders, microvascular suction mats to remove blood and fluid from the operative field, and a microscope which can focus from a relatively high position into a narrow field and provide good depth of field. The hepatic artery on split and living-donor livers is often very short, measuring 3 to 4 cm in length, and just a few millimeters in diameter. All of our anastomoses of arteries from segment 2–3 grafts are performed with an operating microscope at 7-power magnification. The sutures are interrupted 9–0 non-absorbable nylon sutures. Often only 8 to 10 sutures are necessary to complete the anastomosis. Precise placement of sutures, only possible at this magnification, has resulted in very low rates of arterial thromboses in these very small vessels.

Arterial anomalies in the liver are commonplace. Accessory left hepatic arteries are encountered in over 25% of donors. When a dual arterial supply to the left lobe or to segments 2 and 3 is present in a living-donor or split-liver transplant, the surgeon must decide whether to anastomose both donor arteries or just the dominant one (Inomoto *et al.*, 1996) (Figure 28.3).

When procuring the graft from the donor, both arterial branches must be carefully preserved to allow for a possible reconstruction for each of them. The accessory vessel may be harvested with a portion of the left gastric artery to allow for a technically larger-diameter anastomosis.

In the recipient, whenever possible the hepatic artery must be divided distal to its bifurcation to allow for the possibility of two anastomoses. If accessory vessels are present in the recipient, these are also dissected and divided as close to the liver as possible, and may also serve as locations for second arterial anastomoses.

The surgeon must choose which artery in the donor is the dominant one, and proceed with the reconstruction of that vessel. If, after arterial reperfusion, brisk retrograde bleeding occurs from the smaller of the two donor arteries, the smaller artery may be safely tied off. This is

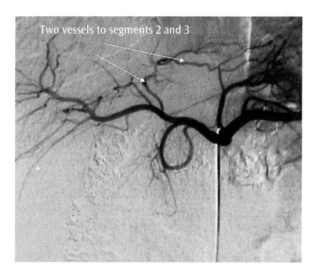

Figure 28.3 *An arteriogram demonstrating a dual arterial supply to segments 2 and 3, one from an aberrant left hepatic artery and one from the left hepatic artery. There is a separate artery to segment 4 from the left hepatic artery. In the recipient, either artery or both may be anastomosed to recipient arteries depending on the degree of intrahepatic communication between the terminal branches of the two hepatic arteries. It is usually only necessary to anastomose the larger of the two donor vessels.*

done with the proof that there is a rich intragraft network between the two arteries which allows the entire graft to enjoy excellent perfusion through only one vessel. On the other hand, if there is poor retrograde bleeding from the secondary artery, one should proceed with the second anastomosis. In the latter case, segments 2 and 3 may each have a relatively independent arterial supply.

Bile duct branching patterns often mimic the arterial supply. If arterial anomalies are present, one must be very attentive to the possibility of unusual biliary drainage patterns. Bile duct branching is highly variable, and may be difficult to sort out completely even when the liver is on the back table.

More than one bile duct may be encountered as the liver parenchyma is transected at or near the falciform ligament (Figure 28.2). Great care must be taken either *in situ* or *ex situ* to identify correctly any significant bile ducts running in the hilar plate posterior to the portal vein. On rare occasions, large bile ducts to segment 3 have been encountered in the liver bridge between segments 3 and 4. Inadvertent ligation of segmental ducts may result in significant biliary complications. If all transected bile ducts are not correctly identified and anastomosed, troublesome bile leaks are certain to occur, which will require reoperation and anastomosis to the bowel.

In our experience, approximately 50% of transplants that are performed with segments obtained from living donors or cadaveric split operations will require more than one biliary anastomosis. The anastomoses are performed with interrupted 6–0 monofilament absorbable suture. For the very small ducts, it is preferable to use internal stents to prevent inadvertent inclusion of the back wall while placing the front wall sutures. The internal stent may be secured to the front bowel wall with a fine catgut suture which will allow for passage of the stent as the suture dissolves. An internal stent may also allow for freer bile flow in the immediate postoperative period, when edema may cause almost complete obstruction of these small ducts.

At the conclusion of the operation, one must decide whether abdominal closure is possible without causing excessive compression of the liver and adversely affecting ventilatory parameters. Oversize grafts, particularly in small babies, and bowel wall edema may not permit abdominal wall closure without deleterious consequences for graft and kidney perfusion and pulmonary gas exchange. We have adopted a very liberal policy of approximating only skin, and delaying abdominal wall closure until most of the perioperative edema has resolved. This may take a few days. In more extreme cases, a marlex-reinforced piece of silastic is used to allow temporary abdominal wall closure (de Ville de Goyet *et al.*, 1998). The silastic is sewn to the fascial edges circumferentially as with omphalocele or gastroschisis closures. This permits a more gradual reapproximation of the fascial edges, with ultimate closure within the first or second postoperative week.

Drains are placed along the cut edge of the liver and above and below the biliary anastomosis. These allow for fluid evacuation which may cause an undesirable rise in intra-abdominal pressure, and they also facilitate the early detection of biliary leaks.

POSTOPERATIVE MANAGEMENT

Antithrombosis prophylaxis

Low-dose heparin (10 units/kg/hour) is started in the postoperative period for the prevention of arterial thrombosis. Aspirin is started orally in patients who weigh less than 15 kg, as soon as the patient can eat or tolerate medications down the nasogastric tube, at which time the heparin is stopped. There have been no clinical trials to assess the value of prophylactic heparin in the prevention of arterial thrombosis, but most pediatric programs implement some regimen to prevent clotting of the artery (Mazzaferro *et al.*, 1989; Stahl *et al.*, 1990; Vazquez *et al.*, 1991; Hashikura *et al.*, 1995).

Fresh frozen plasma

It has been demonstrated that the post-transplant period is characterized by a hypercoagulable state, in which the rate of return to normal concentrations of coagulation factors is not equal (Stahl et al., 1990; Leaker et al., 1995). Factors that promote clot lysis are relatively deficient. This state may lead to an increased rate of small vessel thrombosis. Correction of this hypercoagulable state in vitro may be effected by the addition of fresh frozen plasma. We therefore replace all drain losses with fresh frozen plasma even when the prothrombin time is near normal in all children under 10 kg in weight, who are most at risk for arterial thrombosis.

Doppler ultrasound

Doppler examination of the vessels is routinely undertaken on the first and second postoperative days. Absence of flow within either the artery or the portal vein warrants an early return to the operating-room for revision and attempts to restore flow. Angiography is rarely necessary to confirm ultrasound findings, and may only cause further delay in taking the appropriate steps.

Antibiotics

Cefotaxime and ampicillin are started before the operation and are continued for 48 hours after it. Changes in the choice of antibiotics are made based on whether there has been pretransplant sepsis with a known organism whose sensitivities are established, or on the basis of septic complications after the transplant with resistant organisms.

Routine antifungal prophylaxis is advocated by some programs (Viviani et al., 1992; Reents et al., 1993), while others have identified predictors of fungal sepsis which may warrant the implementation of antifungal therapy even in the absence of positive cultures (Gladdy et al., 1999; Singhal et al., 2000).

Antiviral prophylaxis

Routine ganciclovir is started in all babies under 1 year of age, or in older patients if the donor is serologically positive for CMV. Prophylaxis is continued for 2 to 4 weeks at a dose of 5 mg/kg/day in the absence of abnormal renal function. The cost-effectiveness of anti-CMV prophylaxis and its importance in the prevention of serious disease have been the subject of numerous studies (Greig et al., 1989a; King et al., 1990, 1997; Gane et al., 1997; Gavalda et al., 1997; Green et al., 1997; Seu et al., 1997).

Immunosuppression

Induction immunosuppression in children is based primarily on calcineurin inhibitors (see Chapter 29). Our immunosuppressive regimen is currently cyclosporine based, with the addition of azathioprine and methylprednisolone intravenously. Tacrolimus may be chosen as the primary immunosuppressant if there is a history of graft loss from rejection, cyclosporine neurotoxicity or other undesirable side-effects of cyclosporine, such as hirsutism. Children who are older than 10 years are started directly on the microemulsion formulation of oral cyclosporine by a nasogastric tube until oral intake is commenced (Superina et al., 1994; Alvarez et al., 1998). Cyclosporine trough levels of between 250 and 400 ng/mL are maintained by daily monitoring until a steady state is achieved. Due to the high metabolic rate of small children, the relatively short gastrointestinal tract of babies and the relatively high frequency of return to the operating-room within the first few days after transplantation, the immunosuppressive management of children after liver transplants requires close vigilance and dose adjustment (Whitington et al., 1990).

The popularity of induction immunosuppression with polyclonal (Greig et al., 1989b) or monoclonal antibodies (Cosimi et al., 1990; McDiarmid et al., 1991) directed against the immune cells which initiate and propagate the rejection response has waxed and waned. Antibodies against human T-lymphocytes are raised in a variety of animals, including the mouse, horse and rabbit. The specificity of these antibodies has improved over time, so that platelets and B-lymphocytes which may share epitopes with T-cells have been spared in the more recent generation of anti-T-cell antibodies. Many of these antibodies are themselves immunogenic to the human recipient because of species-specific differences in parts of the immunoglobulin molecule, and they therefore elicit a response in the host which may limit more than one application of the antibody (Schroeder et al., 1989). Humanized hybrid antibodies may circumvent some of the antispecies response.

Antibody-based induction therapy has not been shown to improve graft or patient survival over calcineurin-inhibitor-based immunosuppression (Neuhaus et al., 2000), and may result in a more frequent rate of viral infections and lymphoproliferative disorders. Furthermore, the development of anti-idiotypic and anti-isotypic antibodies has limited the repeated use of anti-T-cell regimens. Because of their profound immunosuppressive properties, it has been suggested that extensive use of anti-T-cell antibodies may increase the incidence of post-transplant lymphoproliferative disease (PTLD) (Morgan and Superina, 1994b; Newell et al., 1996).

A new class of antibody for induction immunosuppression has recently become available that has improved specificity for immunologically activated cells, and which is directed primarily against the interleukin-2 receptor (Kovarik et al., 1998; Berard et al., 1999; Onrust and Wiseman, 1999). Further studies in children still need to be undertaken in order to understand the long-term benefits and risks of this type of therapy.

COMPLICATIONS

Complications after liver transplantation may be numerous (see Chapter 30), and only some of the more important ones will be discussed here.

Bleeding

Patients who undergo reduction procedures are at increased risk of bleeding compared with the recipients of whole organs (Bilik *et al.*, 1992). Persistent bleeding often occurs from small arterial branches near the hilum of the liver, or from the cut surface. Bleeding is rarely rapid, but it may be persistent. Mild to moderate bleeding is managed by blood transfusion and administration of fresh frozen plasma. Temporary cessation or reduction of the heparin dose may be necessary. If bleeding persists, or causes unacceptable intra-abdominal distension with compromised renal and pulmonary function, a return to the operating-room is necessary. Evacuation of blood clot and inspection of all of the vascular anastomoses and the hilar area will often identify a small arterial bleeding point. Bleeding from a venous site (either hepatic or portal) is rarely the cause of persistent postoperative bleeding.

Vascular thrombosis

ARTERIAL THROMBOSIS

Arterial thrombosis may cause devastating damage to the liver, or it may be silent. It may occur early or late (Tan *et al.*, 1988; Superina *et al.*, 1989; Bilik *et al.*, 1992a). However, in most cases, even if it does not result in early graft loss, biliary tract damage is a very frequent consequence (Bilik *et al.*, 1995; Valente *et al.*, 1996). Bile leaks can occur from the biliary–enteric anastomosis, or intrahepatic bile collections can cause sepsis which may be difficult to treat. Early biliary complications resulting from an arterial thrombosis are usually an indication for retransplantation.

Arterial thrombosis may also result in late bile duct strictures which may present many months after the transplant. If the strictures are numerous and present throughout the liver, retransplantation may be the only solution. A single stricture may be amenable to surgical correction (Schlitt *et al.*, 1999) or transhepatic balloon dilatation and stenting (Zajko *et al.*, 1995; Rieber *et al.*, 1996).

In the past, arterial thrombosis was treated expectantly (Bilik *et al.*, 1992a, 1995). Attempts to correct or reverse the thrombosis in children were not generally successful (Yanaga *et al.*, 1990), although attempts to restore arterial flow in adult transplants met with encouraging results (Langnas *et al.*, 1991). Treatment

included prolonged antibiotic therapy to treat septic infarcts and infected bile collections, ursodeoxycholic acid to delay or prevent biliary cirrhosis due to imperfect biliary drainage, and retransplantation when necessary (Bilik *et al.*, 1995).

More recently we have adopted an aggressive approach to the problem of arterial thrombosis, with early attempts at revision of the anastomosis and restitution of arterial flow to the liver (Ferrario *et al.*, 2000). If the thrombosis is detected early on, before the liver has sustained permanent damage, this approach has yielded excellent results with long-term patency of most of the thrombosed vessels.

If the postoperative Doppler ultrasound examination does not demonstrate good arterial flow, the patient is returned to the operating-room. Angiography is rarely necessary on a routine basis, but is reserved for cases where the results of the ultrasound examination are equivocal.

Once the thrombosis has been confirmed, the anastomosis is undone and the distal and proximal arteries are thrombectomized. A small embolectomy catheter is passed up into the liver to remove all particulate clot in the macroscopic vessels. Thrombolytic agents such as urokinase or tissue plasminogen activator are then injected into the donor artery and allowed to remain undisturbed for 15 minutes. The donor artery is then flushed with saline containing heparin, and the arterial anastomosis is redone using an operating microscope. Arterial flow is usually restored, and the patient is then placed on full anticoagulation therapy with intravenous heparin.

In a recent series of patients who had suffered from arterial thrombosis during the immediate postoperative period, all but one anastomosis was restored to excellent flow. The overall resultant rate of arterial thrombosis was in the range 1–2%.

PORTAL VEIN THROMBOSIS

Portal vein thrombosis is uncommon and almost always occurs secondary to a mechanical problem such as kinking, twisting or compression. The increasing frequency of technically more complicated transplants has contributed to more portal venous occlusions. Aligning the donor and recipient portal veins correctly and eliminating excess length will reduce the possibility of significant twisting or kinking. Doppler ultrasound examination of the portal vein is a very rapid method of determining the presence of portal venous flow, and re-exploration must be done quickly.

In children with small portal veins, thrombectomy of the vein through a small venotomy is rarely sufficient to re-establish permanent flow (Bilik *et al.*, 1992a). The anastomosis must be taken down, and both sides of the anastomosis need to be examined for thrombi. All clot must be removed. The surgeon must seek to correct whatever caused the thrombosis in the first place. If the veins are too long, shortening each side may correct kinking. Reorienting the vein ends so that they are properly aligned, and redoing the anastomosis with as little constriction as possible, will almost always result in restored patency of the venous circulation.

Hypoplasia of the portal vein is a frequent finding in babies with biliary atresia after the Kasai procedure (Hernandez-Cano et al., 1987) or in those with a pre-duodenal portal vein. Congenital absence of the portal vein can also occur (Morgan and Superina, 1994a). In these situations, reconstruction of the portal vein is always an option by using an iliac vein graft from a cadaveric donor (Shaw et al., 1985). A vein graft may be anastomosed to the confluence of the splenic and superior mesenteric veins during the anhepatic phase. The distal end of the graft is then joined to the donor portal vein. The resultant larger vein allows a considerably increased blood flow to the liver compared with that which would have been possible through the original hypoplastic vein. A vein graft also enables the anastomosis to be performed with less tension between the ends of the veins, particularly when using a split-liver graft in which only the left branch of the portal vein is available.

In situations when a cadaveric graft is not available (e.g. with living donors), an anastomosis between the bifurcation of the recipient vein using a branch patch and the left donor vein is usually acceptable in terms of length and resultant flow. On one occasion we used the internal jugular vein of the recipient as a vein graft when the recipient native portal vein could not support acceptable flow and had thrombosed.

Late portal vein thrombosis will result in progressive splenic enlargement and bleeding from upper gastrointestinal varices. The diagnosis can be made by Doppler ultrasound examination and angiography. Partial venous occlusion or stenosis may be successfully managed by placement of a transanastomotic indwelling stent after the stenosis has been dilated with a balloon introduced through the liver (Funaki et al., 2000).

In cases where a portal vein thrombosis results in complete occlusion of the vein, it may be possible to restore portal flow to the liver by means of a so-called Rex shunt. A shunt between the superior mesenteric vein proximal to the occlusion and the intrahepatic portion of the left portal vein is fashioned using an autologous jugular vein graft (de Ville de Goyet et al., 1996). It has been shown that this technique can result in the resolution of the symptoms of portal hypertension and avoid the need for retransplantation. This technique has also been successfully applied in a patient after a living-donor transplant in whom the portal vein was completely obstructed (Bambini et al., 2000).

HEPATIC VENOUS OUTFLOW OBSTRUCTION

Venous outflow occlusion is the most devastating thrombotic complication after liver transplantation, and fortunately it is also the least common (Settmacher et al., 2000). Hepatic vein occlusion may be observed immediately after reperfusion. Graft failure will rapidly ensue if the problem is not corrected.

A number of techniques have been described for preventing outflow obstruction in reduced-size transplantation (Emond et al., 1993; Someda et al., 1995; Inomata et al., 1997; Kubota et al., 2000; Sieders et al., 2000). The problem is more likely to occur in piggybacked livers (Stieber et al., 1997; Sze et al., 1999). Twisting of the graft on the venous pedicle must be prevented by performing an anastomosis that is correctly oriented and generous in diameter. The diameter of the venotomy on the recipient cava must not be much larger than the hepatic venous orifice on the donor liver (Kubota et al., 2000), since this will result in stretching of the donor vein orifice with a resultant slit for the blood to flow through. If the donor vein orifice is stretched into a slit, it will also be more susceptible to complete occlusion by only minor twisting movements.

Correction of a venous outflow occlusion must be done rapidly with temporary occlusion of portal and arterial inflow. The liver will thus be subjected to a period of warm ischemia which, if kept to a minimum, will not result in graft loss. Correction of the problem will involve obtaining control of the upper and lower vena cava, opening the anastomosis, inspecting it for errant sutures which may have compromised the lumen, and either enlarging or reducing the size of the anastomosis.

If the problem cannot be corrected, the patient will require immediate retransplantation.

Late outflow obstruction may also cause progressive graft dysfunction (Dousset et al., 1997). Transjugular venous stenting may be used as a means of salvaging the liver (Sze et al., 1999).

Biliary complications

Biliary complications have been referred to as the Achilles heel of liver transplantation (Krom et al., 1985; Yanaga and Sugimachi, 1992; Webb et al., 1998; Davidson et al., 1999). An incidence of bile leakage of 19% from the cut parenchymal surface and 5% from the biliary anastomosis has been found after routine re-exploration on the seventh postoperative day (Renz et al., 1997). However, routine re-exploration is not commonly undertaken, and most bile leaks are detected from bile in the abdominal drains, or are found at re-exploration for signs and symptoms of intra-abdominal sepsis. Significant complications include anastomotic leaks, leaks from the cut surface in segmental or lobar transplantation, or anastomotic obstruction. Biliary complications occur in 15–30% of patients, and in approximately equal frequency in whole-liver and in reduced-size and living-donor transplants (Letourneau *et al.*, 1989; Heffron *et al.*, 1992; Lallier *et al.*, 1993; Peclet *et al.*, 1994; Egawa *et al.*, 1998b; Otte *et al.*, 1999).

Bile leaks are often related to arterial thrombosis, with ischemia of the distal duct at the anastomosis. A leak which occurs in association with arterial thrombosis is not usually amenable to surgical correction, and retransplantation is usually necessary (Schindel *et al.*, 2000a).

All bile leaks in asymptomatic patients which do not resolve spontaneously after a few days (Johnston *et al.*, 2000) should lead to Doppler examination of the artery and surgical correction. Leaks may be secondary to aberrant ducts that were not detected at the time of the transplant, particularly in the setting of split or living-related transplants. Major missed ducts require a second enteric anastomosis, whereas small ducts can safely be oversewn.

All patients who suffer from an arterial thrombosis (Valente *et al.*, 1996) with no immediate serious consequences may present with late biliary strictures, which may be localized or diffuse. Anastomotic strictures may be dilated and stented with good long-term patency. Diffuse biliary damage may lead to recurrent cholangitis and the need for retransplantation.

Primary graft non-function

Primary non-function constitutes one of the most serious complications of liver transplantation. The reported incidence of primary non-function is generally in the range 5–10% (Bilik *et al.*, 1992a; Vazquez *et al.*, 1995).

Graft dysfunction may occur immediately after reperfusion, as indicated by vasomotor instability and the requirements for ionotropic support, renal dysfunction and progressive pulmonary dysfunction.

More commonly, primary graft non-function is characterized by sustained and severe coagulopathy as manifested by a prolonged prothrombin time (> 30 seconds) and low levels of factors V and VII, accompanied by very high transaminase levels (Bilik *et al.*, 1992b). Later manifestations include hypoglycemia, encephalopathy and metabolic acidosis. In our experience the most sensitive and specific early indicator of the need for retransplantation is endogenous factor VII production. If, by 48 hours after transplantation, the factor VII level is below 10% of normal, retransplantation will be necessary. The measurement of liver metabolism of lignocaine has been used to predict early graft survival, as it converts the parent drug to its metabolite monoethylglycinexylidide (MEGX) (Potter *et al.*, 1993; Freys *et al.*, 1997).

Donor characteristics associated with graft non-function are age > 30 years, elevated serum bilirubin levels, hospital stay longer than 3 days, cold ischemia time longer than 6 hours, and fatty infiltration of the graft (Greig *et al.*, 1990; Urena *et al.*, 1999). Donor age has been the subject of significant debate, particularly in the context of an interest in extending the age range of acceptable donors into the older age range. Most reviews favor the use of organs from older donors and show that the risk of poor post-transplant function is minimal if careful selection criteria are maintained (Emre *et al.*, 1996; Oh *et al.*, 2000).

Urgent retransplantation is necessary in cases of primary graft non-function. In cases of serious hemodynamic instability and acidosis, removal of the graft while waiting for a new liver may help to temporarily improve the cardiovascular stability of the recipient and will allow also a longer waiting period in order to find a new organ (Oldhafer *et al.*, 1999).

Delayed graft non-function has also been reported, with apparent early satisfactory graft function, which then deteriorates during the end of the first month after transplantation. It may be related to immunological factors (Ogura *et al.*, 1994).

If poor graft function is suspected or anticipated, early use of intravenous prostaglandin E1 may improve liver function, stop reperfusion injury and reduce the need for retransplantation (Greig *et al.*, 1989a, c; Neumann *et al.*, 2000).

During the operation, good graft function may be anticipated if bile production is observed after restoration of blood flow, if bicarbonate production increases, if the intraoperative calcium requirements decrease, and if serum potassium levels fall spontaneously.

Pancreatitis

Pancreatitis occurs uncommonly after liver transplantation in the absence of specific viral infections, but has serious consequences when it does occur (Bilik *et al.*, 1992a; Tissieres *et al.*, 1998; Verran *et al.*, 2000). Pancreatitis after liver transplantation has been associated with increased mortality, arterial thrombosis and hemorrhagic complications. Treatment consists of supportive measures, control of sepsis, debridement of necrotic pancreatic tissue and elimination of all possible contributing medications, including corticosteroids.

Intestinal perforations

Intestinal perforations should always be suspected in patients with prolonged ileus or the clinical symptoms suggestive of ongoing intra-abdominal sepsis (Bilik *et al.*, 1992a; Yamanaka *et al.*, 1994; Beierle *et al.*, 1998; Vilca Melendez *et al.*, 1998). Perforations may occur at anastomotic suture lines, or in a delayed fashion from inadvertent cautery burns. Spontaneous perforations in apparently normal bowel have also been described. Timely repair is obviously the treatment of choice. Patients who have undergone surgery prior to the liver transplant have a higher likelihood of post-transplant perforations (Yamanaka *et al.*, 1994; Sandler *et al.*, 1997; Beierle *et al.*, 1998).

Perforations due to ulcers, bowel lymphoproliferative

disorders or viral enteritides are rare in children, but should always be kept in mind.

Delayed perforations may occur as a result of intestinal involvement with lymphoproliferative disease (Liu *et al.*, 1998).

Miscellaneous complications

Prolonged ascites, splenic infarction and infected intra-abdominal collections may occur after transplantation. Although the majority of these complications may be treated medically or with interventional radiological techniques, occasional operative intervention may be necessary.

Thoracic complications

Pleural effusions are the commonest thoracic complication following liver transplantation (Mack *et al.*, 2000a). Although most effusions are sterile, some may be infected. Tube thoracostomy is usually adequate for the diagnosis and treatment of most pleural effusions. Sometimes a pleural effusion is an indicator of a serious subphrenic process such as an infected collection or graft rejection.

Diaphragmatic paralysis with paradoxical motion of the diaphragm may be an indication for operative intervention (Bilik *et al.*, 1992a). Clamp injury of the phrenic nerve as it innervates the diaphragm may cause prolonged diaphragmatic paresis. The commonest manifestation of this disorder is failure of the patient to tolerate extubation. Since the work of breathing is increased by a wide variety of factors in children after liver transplantation, the need for operative intervention must be weighed carefully against the risks of a thoracotomy.

Real-time ultrasound examination of the diaphragm while the child breathes spontaneously is the best way to diagnose paradoxical motion of the diaphragm. In the appropriate setting, diaphragmatic plication through the chest may greatly hasten the respiratory recovery of an affected child.

Bronchoalveolar lavage and open lung biopsies may be necessary to diagnose pulmonary infections from bacterial, viral or fungal infections (Winthrop *et al.*, 1990).

MEDICAL COMPLICATIONS

Hypertension

Hypertension is a very common occurrence after liver transplantation (Textor *et al.*, 1995). Cyclosporine and corticosteroids are believed to play an etiological role, but the pathogenesis is not fully understood (Reding, 2000). The use of antihypertensive agents may be necessary to bring the blood pressure under control.

Infection

BACTERIAL INFECTION

Bacterial infections are common after liver transplantation, and they are one of the more frequent causes of severe morbidity and mortality (Green *et al.*, 1991; Saint-Vil *et al.*, 1991; Uemoto *et al.*, 1994; Alonso and Ryckman, 1998). Sources of bacterial infections are numerous and include the biliary tract, intravascular catheters and the respiratory tract (George *et al.*, 1992). Bacterial infections range in severity from those that are easily treatable, such as catheter-related sepsis or urinary tract infections, to the very serious ones, such as cholangitis or arterial thrombosis and septic hepatic infarcts.

The commonest pathogens include Gram-negative bacilli, enterococci and staphylococci. Antibiotic sensitivities may be predicted by the location of the sepsis and local bacterial susceptibility patterns. Venous catheter infections with Gram-positive cocci should always be treated with methicillin or vancomycin. Cholangitis and other forms of biliary tract sepsis should always be treated with antibiotics that are active against enterococci and *Enterobacter* species.

VIRAL INFECTION

Historically, viral infections have been a major source of morbidity and mortality following liver transplantation. Cytomegalovirus, Epstein–Barr virus, herpes simplex, varicella, adenovirus and respiratory syncytial virus are all potential pathogens.

CMV can cause a wide variety of symptoms after liver transplantation, including fever and malaise, pneumonia, gastrointestinal bleeding, pancreatitis and numerous other serious disorders. The diagnosis of CMV after liver transplantation has improved with technological advances in early detection of CMV antigens after primary infections (Kalicinski *et al.*, 1996; Evans *et al.*, 1998). With the advent of ganciclovir, CMV infections became more easily treatable and preventable (King *et al.*, 1990, 1997; Gane *et al.*, 1997; Green *et al.*, 1997; Seu *et al.*, 1997; Das, 2000). CMV prophylaxis is instituted in CMV-positive recipients and CMV-negative patients transplanted with CMV-positive grafts with ganciclovir, immunoglobulin or both.

Herpes simplex and varicella viruses should be watched for, and should be treated with acyclovir at the first sign of infection. Herpes simplex infections may be superficial and localized, as with herpes stomatitis, or systemic and invasive, as with esophagitis and hepatitis. Varicella infections may present as chickenpox or shingles and should respond to prompt institution of acyclovir.

Serial monitoring of EBV using the polymerase chain reaction is recommended to facilitate early detection of EBV infection (Rogers et al., 1997; Green et al., 1998; Rogers et al., 1998; Kogan et al., 1999), and thus to decrease the risk of PTLD by decreasing the dose of immunosuppression and administering ganciclovir (McDiarmid et al., 1998) (see Chapter 30).

Adenovirus infections may cause significant respiratory problems after transplantation, as well as severe hepatic dysfunction and hepatitis with graft necrosis (Cames et al., 1992; Michaels et al., 1992). Treatment is supportive, and includes withdrawal of immunosuppression. Ribavirin has been used, although with no proven benefit, for severe adenoviral infections (Shetty et al., 2000).

Unfortunately, few other effective antiviral agents are available for the treatment of other pathogens after transplantation. If the diagnosis of a viral infection following transplantation is made, care must be supportive and coupled with a reduction in immunosuppressive therapy.

FUNGAL INFECTION

Infections with *Candida* species may be difficult to diagnose (Gladdy et al., 1999). Blood cultures may not turn positive even in the presence of invasive abdominal or pulmonary candidiasis. Multiple positive cultures in locations which are not defined as invasive infections may indicate a more serious problem or the potential for serious infection. Treatment with amphotericin may be started after multiple superficial cultures turn positive, such as urine, endotracheal aspirates and wound cultures, even in the absence of proven invasive disease.

Bile leakage, hepatic artery thrombosis, preoperative steroid use, transfusion requirement and the duration of intubation have been identified as independent risk factors for invasive *Candida* infection (Gladdy et al., 1999). Treatment consists of intravenous amphotericin for 14 to 21 days. The use of routine antifungal prophylaxis has not been demonstrated to improve patient survival, and has been associated with drug-related complications (Winston et al., 1999).

Rejection

Acute rejection is T-cell-mediated and complicates 30–70% of orthotopic liver transplants (Sokal et al., 1990; Colombani et al., 1996; Alvarez et al., 2000). Clinical manifestations of acute rejection include fever, hyperbilirubinemia, raised transaminases, raised alkaline phosphatase, increased prothrombin time and decreased production of bile, which becomes lighter and thinner. The diagnosis is confirmed by liver biopsy. About 50–75% of acute rejection episodes are controlled by pulse methylprednisolone therapy consisting of

10 mg/kg/day for 3 days. Conversion from cyclosporine to tacrolimus (Jara et al., 1998; Reggiani et al., 1998; Klein, 1999) or treatment with anti-CD3 monoclonal antibody (Cosimi et al., 1987; Esquivel et al., 1987; Goldstein et al., 1987; Woodle et al., 1991) for steroid-resistant rejection can reverse acute rejection in 90% of cases. Recently, mycophenolate mofetil has been demonstrated to be effective in treating steroid-resistant rejection and as an alternative drug in patients with cyclosporine and tacrolimus toxicity (McDiarmid, 1996b).

Cyclosporine- and tacrolimus-based immunosuppressive regimens are both widely used. Comparative trials of the two medications in pediatric liver transplantation indicate equivalent results, with a subtle difference in the spectrum of the drug-related side-effects (McDiarmid et al., 1995; Alberti et al., 1996; Cacciarelli et al., 1996; Mirza et al., 1997). Importantly, it has been suggested that post-transplant lymphoproliferative disorders are more common after primary immunotherapy with tacrolimus (Younes et al., 2000).

Chronic rejection is a serious cause of graft loss in children (Achilleos et al., 1999). It is diagnosed on the basis of deteriorating liver function tests, which are often characterized by increasing bilirubin, deteriorating synthetic function and a biopsy that exhibits the characteristic features of chronic rejection, namely bile duct destruction with a paucity of bile ducts relative to the number of visible portal triads. Foam-cell arteritis may also be seen, but is more commonly seen in medium-size arteries. Clinical features associated with the development of chronic rejection are the number and severity of acute rejection episodes and donor age over 40 years (Blakolmer et al., 2000).

Chronic rejection may be reversible, but not if bile duct loss is severe or if there are significant amounts of fibrosis on biopsy (Blakolmer et al., 1999).

Intervention involving alternative drug therapy with tacrolimus or, more recently, mycophenolate mofetil has been shown to reverse the changes of chronic rejection if the intervention occurs before the onset of severe cholestatic changes (Sher et al., 1997; Kato et al., 1999).

Humorally mediated rejection is less common, and is more difficult to confirm and treat.

Raised liver enzymes accompanied by centrilobular necrosis in the absence of vascular problems may indicate humorally mediated rejection (Sebagh et al., 1999). Treatment may consist of plasmapheresis and implementation of tacrolimus therapy.

Immunosuppression-related problems

Significant toxic side-effects are associated with the use of cyclosporine, tacrolimus and OKT3, and they have been well documented (see Chapter 29).

Among the most serious problems are renal toxicity, which is usually reversible up to a point. Long-term use of both cyclosporine and tacrolimus has been associated with permanent impairment of renal function (Iwatsuki *et al.*, 1985; McDiarmid, 1996c). Young children may be relatively more resistant to the nephrotoxic side-effects of these medications than older children and young adults (Bilik *et al.*, 1993a).

Severe neurotoxicity may be seen with both cyclosporine and tacrolimus, and may include seizures and tremors. Specific side-effects of tacrolimus include gastrointestinal symptoms, cardiotoxicity and hyperglycemia, all of which may be improved by conversion of the patient to cyclosporine (Emre *et al.*, 2000).

Anti-CD3 therapy may produce a serious first-dose effect characterized by fever, pulmonary edema and anaphylaxis in extreme cases (Thistlethwaite *et al.*, 1988; Ryckman *et al.*, 1994). Patients require premedication with corticosteroids, antihistamines and antipyretics before the first dose. Undulating fever, photophobia and aseptic meningitis may further complicate the course of therapy.

One of the most serious complications of immunosuppressive therapy is the development of PTLD. The reported incidence of PTLD is 22% in patients receiving tacrolimus and 4% in those who are not receiving tacrolimus (McDiarmid *et al.*, 1995). It is thought that the incidence of PTLD is an indication of the cumulative effect of immunosuppressive therapy (Morgan and Superina, 1994b). Most PTLD is a result of B-cell transformation by Epstein–Barr virus, with the resultant polyclonal activation of B-cells in the host. PTLD can then evolve into monoclonal disease and frank immunoblastic lymphoma (Rogers *et al.*, 1998).

Monitoring of Epstein–Barr virus activity in transplant recipients is a fertile area of research, and it is hoped that PTLD can be prevented by earlier detection of viral proliferation and infection of B-lymphocytes (Rogers *et al.*, 1997; Egawa *et al.*, 1998c; Green *et al.*, 1998; Kogan *et al.*, 1999). Restoration of host immunity remains the best weapon for fighting this very troublesome problem.

Treatment of PTLD consists of the reduction or elimination of all immunosuppressive medications (Dror *et al.*, 1999). Ganciclovir or acyclovir coupled with immunoglobulin therapy has been implemented, but there is little or no proof that it affects the course of the disease.

RESULTS OF TRANSPLANTATION

Most pediatric liver transplant centers now routinely report 1-year patient survival rates of over 80% after transplantation. Most of the variability is dependent on the state of the recipient and the underlying diagnosis at the time of the transplant, rather than on the type of graft (Figure 28.4) (see Chapter 31).

Living-donor transplantation (LDT)

At its outset, LDT was reserved for patients who were in a stable condition and in whom a good result could be

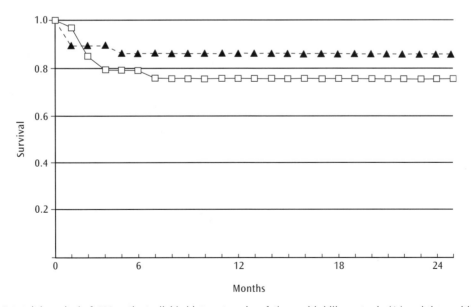

Figure 28.4 *Actuarial survival of 100 patients divided into categories of those with biliary atresia (▲) and those with other diseases (□) including fulminant hepatic failure and metabolic diseases. The metabolic disease group included four children with mitochondrial disorders who presented with liver disease and varying degrees of neurological impairment. All four children died of progressive neurological deterioration between 2 weeks and 4 years after the transplant. One of the four patients had been thought to have valproate toxicity, but was later found to have a mitochondrial respiratory chain disorder. The valproate had been taken for severe and intractable seizures. The survival rate for children with biliary atresia was 85% at 1 and 2 years post transplant, whereas in all others it was 77%.*

expected (Broelsch et al., 1991). This approach was used in order to obtain the best possible patient survival given the sacrifice and risks taken by the donor (Singer et al., 1989).

As the rate of success with LDT increased and the risks to the donors remained minimal, the living-donor operation was extended to include patients with less stable conditions (Emre et al., 1999; Fischer et al., 1999; Vemoto et al., 2000), those whose chances of survival were not excellent (Tokunaga et al., 1993), and even those who had relative contraindications for transplantation (Casas et al., 1999). Predictably, the survival data changed and mirrored the conditions which preceded the transplant. Success rates still remain excellent in stable patients, who represent by far the largest cohort of patients who are transplanted with organs from living donors (Heffron, 1993; Whitington et al., 1994; Colombani et al., 1996; Inomoto et al., 1996; Otte et al., 1999).

However, recent reports from various centers have shown that acceptable results can be expected in patients who are waiting in intensive-care settings, those who are waiting for second organs, and in children with multisystem organ failure (Mack et al., 2000b).

At the present time LDT constitutes only a very small percentage of the overall transplant activity in the USA, representing less than 5% of the entire liver transplant output (US Department of Health and Human Services, 1998, 1999). At some large pediatric centers up to one-third of the total transplant activity takes place with living donors (Otte et al., 1998). Emergency transplants with living donors have been performed for primary non-function of the first graft, arterial thrombosis, fulminant liver failure and patients with decompensated cirrhosis and multisystem organ failure (Mack et al., 2000b).

Living-donor transplant survival rates are 84% at 1 year after the transplant (Inomata et al., 1999; Otte et al., 1999; Revillon et al., 1999; Rogiers et al., 1999; Colombani et al., 2000). However, if such transplants are performed under urgent indications in the setting of multisystem organ failure, survival rates drop to 60% (Casas et al., 1999; Emre et al., 1999; Mack et al., 2000b; Uemoto et al., 2000). This represents an improvement in the survival of these very sick children compared with rates which have been reported in the past, and it may be due to improved timing of the transplant with a readily available living donor.

Split-liver transplantation

In the first report of the European Split Liver Registry, results obtained for the recipients of split livers were shown to be as good as those for patients who received whole organs (de Ville de Goyet, 1995). As more centers develop the expertise to successfully transplant two patients with one organ (Rela et al., 1998), it may be expected that the number of complications following

transplantation will increase to accommodate the rise of the learning curve (Broelsch et al., 1990).

At our center, approximately 20% of pediatric transplants are performed with segments from livers assigned to adult recipients. At the present time survival rates are excellent, since patients are chosen carefully to maximize the potential for success. Of 14 patients who were transplanted with split-liver grafts, 12 patients are alive and well. Two patients died, one from pancreatitis and one from overwhelming CMV pneumonia following retransplantation after primary non-function of the split graft.

Overall survival rates are comparable to those obtained for whole and reduced-size transplantation in stable recipients.

In a recent review of one of the largest pediatric liver transplant programs in Europe, 6% of children received a split liver and 13% received an organ from a living donor, with equally good results (Reding et al., 1999). This review extends over a lengthy period, and one must assume that all busy pediatric programs have increased the proportion of transplants that employ these innovative techniques. Although routine splitting of livers would quickly remove the waiting-list for children awaiting liver transplants, consensus with regard to the risks to the adult recipient and the type of donor who would make a good split-liver candidate has yet to be reached (Superina et al., 1999).

Risk factors for success

Survival has been shown in the past to be due to recipient factors and not to the type of transplant. Important factors include pretransplant status, type of disease, recipient age and number of liver transplants.

PRETRANSPLANT STATUS

Recipient status has been shown to affect survival significantly, regardless of the type of transplant (Bilik et al., 1993b; Cacciarelli et al., 1999).

Reduced-size grafting has been reported by others to yield survival rates that are lower than those obtained with whole organs (Cacciarelli et al., 1999), although this is not the universal experience. Patients who are waiting at home fare better than those in intensive-care units or those with renal failure or fulminant hepatic failure.

TYPE OF DISEASE

Patients with stable cholestatic liver disease have been reported to have better survival rates than patients with rapidly progressive liver disease and those whose organs other than the liver are also failing (Pitre et al., 1996).

Patients with malignancies have historically had very poor survival rates (Koneru et al., 1991), but with improved patient selection, success in this area has increased. Children with malignant liver disease that is unresectable by conventional criteria have been reported to have poorer survival rates than those with benign disease. Patients with unresectable hepatoblastoma and hepatocellular carcinoma have been reported to have 1-year tumor-free survival rates in the range 60–90% (Superina and Bilik, 1996; Bilik and Superina, 1997; Al-Qabandi et al., 1999).

Patients with mitochondriopathies may have a particularly poor prognosis, and should be carefully screened for neurological abnormalities which may cause death despite successful liver grafting (Morris et al., 1998; Sokal et al., 1999; Delarue et al., 2000).

AGE

Babies under 3 months of age have been reported to have lower survival rates than older children (Bonatti et al., 1997; Woodle et al., 1998) (see Chapter 31).

The lack of suitable organ donors for small babies is largely responsible for the reported lower survival rates. Because of the severe size constraints in small babies, even reduction procedures and living-donor transplants may not result in donor organs that are small enough. Moreover, disease states which cause liver failure in newborn babies often cause rapid liver deterioration, resulting in malnutrition, failure of growth and early death.

If a suitable organ can be found, the results should not be that different to those obtained in older children, although the technical challenges of transplanting small infants are not inconsiderable. Single segmental transplantation (Srinivasan et al., 1999) and hepatocyte transplantation may offer more hope for babies under 3 months of age.

NUMBER OF LIVER TRANSPLANTS

Acute retransplantation after primary non-function and arterial thrombosis has been reported to have variable success (Achilleos et al., 1999). If transplantation can take place before the onset of serious infection or the advent of deterioration of other organ systems, the likelihood of a successful outcome is reasonable (Schindel et al., 2000b). The decision to retransplant must be made early on in order to maximize the likelihood of a successful outcome.

Late retransplantation has also been associated with a poorer prognosis (Newell et al., 1998). Late graft failure is usually due to chronic rejection or progressive biliary cirrhosis resulting from bile duct complications. Malnutrition and the effects of chronic immunosuppression may weaken the resistance of the host. The likelihood of success decreases with increasing number of retransplants (Pitre et al., 1997), although the results are still acceptable (Schindel et al., 2000b). Decisions to retransplant must be taken carefully, with consideration of the reasons for previous graft failure and the likelihood that these can be avoided if the decision is taken to transplant again.

CHRONIC IMMUNOSUPPRESSION AND GROWTH

The issues which determine the delicate balance between graft and host immune defenses have yet to be elucidated. Liver transplants are less frequently lost to chronic rejection compared with other organ transplants, such as those of kidney and heart. For this reason, liver transplant patients are more likely than others to tolerate a planned, deliberate reduction in immunosuppression. Protocols have been suggested to wean patients off all immunosuppression (Superina et al., 1993), but no reliable predictor of success has been found. It remains a trial-and-error field.

It has been well demonstrated that patients with chronic advanced liver disease suffer from malnutrition and growth retardation (Pierro et al., 1989). Successful transplantation can reverse malnutrition and result in catch-up growth (van Mourik et al., 2000).

Growth after transplantation is directly related to the total cumulative dose of corticosteroids, and reduction of steroids with a view to eliminating them altogether can result in excellent linear growth (Superina et al., 1998).

Reduction of all immunosuppressants is not a reliable science, but it can be undertaken safely in an algorithmic way. Breakthrough rejection can usually be easily reversed (Superina et al., 1998).

Lack of serious clinical rejection and an absence of pathological rejection on biopsies may serve as criteria for proceeding with a planned protocol for elimination of immunosuppressants. This must be done carefully, since subclinical chronic rejection may cause late graft loss. Although the dangers of chronic immunosuppression are considerable, graft loss due to insidious chronic rejection with the resultant need for retransplantation is a devastating complication. Any regimen which reduces immunosuppression must be undertaken with strict surveillance criteria for the detection of occult rejection. The long-term effects of a reduction in immune suppression must still be determined.

Efforts must be directed at detecting the immunological markers which can serve as more reliable biological indicators of operational tolerance (Devlin et al., 1998; Wong et al., 1998; Riordan and Williams, 1999).

There are many examples of patients who were taken off immunosuppression for treatment of serious viral disease or PTLD and who have remained well and were never restarted on their medications (Mazariegos et al., 1997). There are also those patients who decided to take themselves off immune suppression and who have fortunately remained well. However, there are as many (if not more) who were taken off immune suppression, either for medical indications or because of non-compliance, who suffered from serious rebound rejection which required aggressive therapy to save the graft.

For the present, a reduction of corticosteroids in order to maximize growth should remain a priority for pediatric transplant programs. The elimination of all immune suppression from most patients in a controlled way is an area which still requires much work.

SUMMARY

The challenges involved in transplanting children with liver disease are considerable. Much progress has been made in the areas of organ availability for children, advanced techniques for splitting organs, operative strategies and the management of post-transplant complications. Areas such as xenotransplantation and the achievement of tolerance remain long-term goals which may yet do much to improve the likelihood of survival of children who are waiting for liver transplants. As the mortality rate on waiting-lists has decreased for children and postoperative survival rates continue to improve, the focus has started to shift towards the task of returning a child who has had a liver transplant to as normal a life as possible.

Long-term strategies to improve growth, reduce immunosuppression and detect potentially serious infections and rejections at an earlier stage remain the challenges for the future.

Key references

Broelsch CE, Whitington PF, Emond JC *et al*. Liver transplantation in children from living related donors. Surgical techniques and results. *Annals of Surgery* 1991; **214**: 428–37.

Early pioneering experience with left lateral segment living-donor liver transplantation in children from Chicago.

Emond JC, Heffron TG, Whitington PF, Broelsch CE. Reconstruction of the hepatic vein in reduced-size hepatic transplantation. *Surgery, Gynecology and Obstetrics* 1993; **176**: 11–17.

An evaluation of different techniques of hepatic vein anastomosis in the implantation of reduced/split livers, which demonstrates the superiority of the triangulation technique for preventing venous outflow obstruction.

O'Grady JG, Alexander GJ, Hayllar KM, Williams R. Early indicators of prognosis in fulminant hepatic failure. *Gastroenterology* 1989; **97**: 439–45.

The King's College Hospital criteria were developed in order to determine which patients with acute liver failure should be listed for urgent transplantation. Although these criteria have been challenged and modified, they continue to provide useful and practical guidance.

Tanaka K, Uemoto S, Tokunaga Y *et al*. Surgical techniques and innovations in living related liver transplantation. *Annals of Surgery* 1993; **217**: 82–91.

Initial experience from Japan with living-donor liver transplantation in children. The technical surgical innovations of the Kyoto group have not only fostered the continuing development of living-related liver transplantation, but have also had a significant positive impact on the whole process of reduced/split cadaveric liver transplantation.

REFERENCES

Achilleos OA, Mirza DF, Talbot D *et al*. Outcome of liver retransplantation in children. *Liver Transplant Surgery* 1999; **5**: 401–6.

Alagille D. Management of paucity of interlobular bile ducts. *Journal of Hepatology* 1985; **1**: 561–5.

Alberti D, Wallemacq P, Falchetti D *et al*. Microemulsion formulation of cyclosporine in pediatric liver transplantation. *Transplantation* 1996; **61**: 512–14.

Alonso MH, Ryckman FC. Current concepts in pediatric liver transplant. *Seminars in Liver Disease* 1998; **18**: 295–307.

Alonso EM, Sokol RJ, Hart J *et al*. Fulminant hepatitis associated with centrilobular hepatic necrosis in young children. *Journal of Pediatrics* 1995; **127**: 888–94.

Al-Qabandi W, Jenkinson HC, Buckels JA *et al*. Orthotopic liver transplantation for unresectable hepatoblastoma: a single center's experience. *Journal of Pediatric Surgery* 1999; **34**: 1261–4.

Alvarez F, Atkison P, Grant D *et al*. NOF-11: a one-year randomized double-blind comparison of Neoral versus Sandimmune in pediatric liver transplantation. *Transplantation Proceedings* 1998; **30**: 1961.

Alvarez F, Atkison PR, Grant DR *et al*. NOF-11: a one-year pediatric randomized double-blind comparison of neoral versus sandimmune in orthotopic liver transplantation. *Transplantation* 2000; **69**: 87–92.

Anand AC, Nightingale P, Neuberger JM. Early indicators of prognosis in fulminant hepatic failure: an assessment of the King's criteria. *Journal of Hepatology* 1997; **26**: 62–8.

Azarow KS, Phillips MJ, Sandler AD, Hagerstrand I, Superina RA. Biliary atresia: should all patients undergo a portoenterostomy? *Journal of Pediatric Surgery* 1997; **32**: 168–72.

Azoulay D, Astarcioglu I, Bismuth H *et al*. Split-liver transplantation. The Paul Brousse policy. *Annals of Surgery* 1996; **224**: 737–46.

Bambini DA, Superina R, Almond PS *et al*. Experience with the Rex shunt (mesenterico-left portal bypass) in children with extrahepatic portal hypertension. *Journal of Pediatric Surgery* 2000; **35**: 13–18.

Batshaw ML. Inborn errors of urea synthesis. *Annals of Neurology* 1994; **35**: 133–41.

Beierle EA, Nicolette LA, Billmire DF *et al.* Gastrointestinal perforation after pediatric orthotopic liver transplantation. *Journal of Pediatric Surgery* 1998; **33**: 240–2.

Ben-Ari Z, Samuel D, Zemel R *et al.* Fulminant non-A-G viral hepatitis leading to liver transplantation. *Archives of Internal Medicine* 2000; **160**: 388–92.

Berard JL, Velez RL, Freeman RB, Tsunoda SM. A review of interleukin-2 receptor antagonists in solid organ transplantation. *Pharmacotherapy* 1999; **19**: 1127–37.

Berk PD, Stump D. Acute hepatic failure and defective fatty acid transport: clinical proof of a physiologic hypothesis. *Hepatology* 1999; **29**: 1607–9.

Bernuau J, Durand F, Valla D. Parvovirus B19 infection and fulminant hepatitis. *Lancet* 1999; **353**: 754–5.

Bilik R, Superina R. Transplantation for unresectable liver tumors in children. *Transplantation Proceedings* 1997; **29**: 2834–5.

Bilik R, Yellen M, Superina RA. Surgical complications in children after liver transplantation. *Journal of Pediatric Surgery* 1992a; **27**: 1371–5.

Bilik R, Superina RA, Poon AO. Coagulation plasma factor levels are early indicators of graft non-function following liver transplantation in children. *Journal of Pediatric Surgery* 1992b; **27**: 302–6.

Bilik R, Superina RA, Hu X. Long-term effect of cyclosporine on renal function in children after liver transplantation. *Transplantation Proceedings* 1993a; **25**: 2578–9.

Bilik R, Greig P, Langer B, Superina RA. Survival after reduced-size liver transplantation is dependent on pretransplant status. *Journal of Pediatric Surgery* 1993b; **28**: 1307–11.

Bilik R, Superina RA, Phillips J, Edwards V. Prevention of biliary cirrhosis following hepatic arterial thrombosis after liver transplantation in children by using ursodeoxycholic acid. *Journal of Pediatric Surgery* 1995; **30**: 49–52.

Bismuth H, Houssin D. Reduced-sized orthotopic liver graft in hepatic transplantation in children. *Surgery* 1984; **95**: 367–70.

Blakolmer K, Seaberg EC, Batts K *et al.* Analysis of the reversibility of chronic liver allograft rejection implications for a staging schema. *American Journal of Surgical Pathology* 1999; **23**: 1328–39.

Blakolmer K, Jain A, Ruppert K *et al.* Chronic liver allograft rejection in a population treated primarily with tacrolimus as baseline immunosuppression: long-term follow-up and evaluation of features for histopathological staging. *Transplantation* 2000; **69**: 2330–6.

Bonatti H, Muiesan P, Connelly S *et al.* Hepatic transplantation in children under 3 months of age: a single centre's experience. *Journal of Pediatric Surgery* 1997; **32**: 486–8.

Broelsch CE, Lloyd DM. Living related donors for liver transplants. *Advances in Surgery* 1993; **26**: 209–31.

Broelsch CE, Emond JC, Whitington PF *et al.* Application of reduced-size liver transplants as split grafts, auxiliary orthotopic grafts and living related segmental transplants. *Annals of Surgery* 1990; **212**: 368–75.

Broelsch CE, Whitington PF, Emond JC *et al.* Liver transplantation in children from living related donors. Surgical techniques and results. *Annals of Surgery* 1991; **214**: 428–37.

Busuttil RW, Goss JA. Split liver transplantation. *Annals of Surgery* 1999; **229**: 313–21.

Busuttil RW, Colonna JO, Hiatt JR *et al.* The first 100 liver transplants at UCLA. *Annals of Surgery* 1987; **206**: 387–402.

Cacciarelli TV, Esquivel CO, Cox KL *et al.* Oral tacrolimus (FK506) induction therapy in pediatric orthotopic liver transplantation. *Transplantation* 1996; **61**: 1188–92.

Cacciarelli TV, Dvorchik I, Mazariegos GV *et al.* An analysis of pretransplantation variables associated with long-term allograft outcome in pediatric liver transplant recipients receiving primary tacrolimus (FK506) therapy. *Transplantation* 1999; **68**: 650–5.

Cames B, Rahier J, Bustomboy G *et al.* Acute adenovirus hepatitis in liver transplant recipients. *Journal of Pediatrics* 1992; **120**: 33–7.

Casas A, Falkenstein K, Gallagher M, Dunn SP. Living donor liver transplantation in critically ill children. *Pediatric Transplantation* 1999; **3**: 104–8.

Chapin JW, Newland MC, Hurlbert BJ. Anesthesia for liver transplantation. *Seminars in Liver Disease* 1989; **9**: 195–201.

Chardot C, Carton M, Spire-Bendelac N *et al.* Prognosis of biliary atresia in the era of liver transplantation: French national study from 1986 to 1996. *Hepatology* 1999; **30**: 606–11.

Colombani PM, Cigarroa FG, Schwarz K *et al.* Liver transplantation in infants younger than 1 year of age. *Annals of Surgery* 1996; **223**: 658–62.

Colombani PM, Lau H, Prabhakaran K *et al.* Cumulative experience with pediatric living related liver transplantation. *Journal of Pediatric Surgery* 2000; **35**: 9–12.

Cosimi AB, Cho SI, Delmonico FL *et al.* A randomized clinical trial comparing OKT3 and steroids for treatment of hepatic allograft rejection. *Transplantation Proceedings* 1987; **19**: 2431–3.

Cosimi AB, Jenkins RL, Rohrer RJ *et al.* A randomized clinical trial of prophylactic OKT3 monoclonal antibody in liver allograft recipients. *Archives of Surgery* 1990; **125**: 781–4.

Cuffari C, Brochu P, Russo P, Alvarez F. A case of non-A, non-B, non-C hepatitis that relapsed into fulminant hepatic failure. *Hepatogastroenterology* 1998; **45**: 2348–51.

Das A. Cost-effectiveness of different strategies of cytomegalovirus prophylaxis in orthotopic liver transplant recipients. *Hepatology* 2000; **31**: 311–17.

Davenport M, Savage M, Mowat AP, Howard ER. Biliary atresia splenic malformation syndrome: an etiologic and prognostic subgroup. *Surgery* 1993; **113**: 662–8.

Davidson BR, Rai R, Kurzawinski TR *et al.* Prospective randomized trial of end-to-end versus side-to-side biliary reconstruction after orthotopic liver transplantation. *British Journal of Surgery* 1999; **86**: 447–52.

Delarue A, Paut O, Guys JM et al. Inappropriate liver transplantation in a child with Alpers–Huttenlocher syndrome misdiagnosed as valproate-induced acute liver failure. Pediatric Transplantation 2000; 4: 67–71.

de Ville de Goyet J. Split liver transplantation in Europe – 1988 to 1993. Transplantation 1995; 59: 1371–6.

de Ville de Goyet J, Gibbs P, Clapuyt P et al. Original extrahilar approach for hepatic portal revascularization and relief of extrahepatic portal hypertension related to later portal vein thrombosis after pediatric liver transplantation. Long-term results. Transplantation 1996; 62: 71–5.

de Ville de Goyet J, Struye de Swieland Y, Reding R et al. Delayed primary closure of the abdominal wall after cadaveric and living related donor liver graft transplantation in children: a safe and useful technique. Transplant International 1998; 11: 117–22.

Devlin J, Doherty D, Thomson L et al. Defining the outcome of immunosuppression withdrawal after liver transplantation. Hepatology 1998; 27: 926–33.

Dousset B, Legmann P, Soubrane O et al. Protein-losing enteropathy secondary to hepatic venous outflow obstruction after liver transplantation. Journal of Hepatology 1997; 27: 206–10.

Dror Y, Greenberg M, Taylor G et al. Lymphoproliferative disorders after organ transplantation in children. Transplantation 1999; 67: 990–8.

DuBois RS, Rodgerson DO, Martineau F et al. Orthotopic liver transplantation for Wilson's disease. Lancet 1971; 1: 505–8.

Egawa H, Inomata Y, Nakayama S et al. Fulminant hepatic failure secondary to herpes simplex virus infection in a neonate: a case report of successful treatment with liver transplantation and perioperative acyclovir. Liver Transplant Surgery 1998a; 4: 513–15.

Egawa H, Uemoto S, Inomata Y et al. Biliary complications in pediatric living related liver transplantation. Surgery 1998b; 124: 901–10.

Egawa H, Ohishi T, Arai T et al. Application of in situ hybridization technique for quantitative assessment of ongoing symptomatic Epstein–Barr virus infection after living-related liver transplantation. Clinical Transplantation 1998c; 12: 116–22.

Emond JC, Heffron TG, Whitington PF, Broelsch CE. Reconstruction of the hepatic vein in reduced-size hepatic transplantation. Surgery, Gynecology and Obstetrics 1993; 176: 11–17.

Emre S, Schwartz ME, Altaca G et al. Safe use of hepatic allografts from donors older than 70 years. Transplantation 1996; 62: 62–5.

Emre S, Genyk Y, Schluger LK et al. Treatment of tacrolimus-related adverse effects by conversion to cyclosporine in liver transplant recipients. Transplant International 2000; 13: 73–8.

Emre S, Schwartz ME, Shneider B et al. Living related liver transplantation for acute liver failure in children. Liver Transplant Surgery 1999; 5: 161–5.

Esquivel CO, Fung JJ, Markus B et al. OKT3 in the reversal of acute hepatic allograft rejection. Transplantation Proceedings 1987; 19: 2443–6.

Evans PC, Soin A, Wreghitt TG, Alexander GJ. Qualitative and semiquantitative polymerase chain reaction testing for cytomegalovirus DNA in serum allows prediction of CMV-related disease in liver transplant recipients. Journal of Clinical Pathology 1998; 51: 914–21.

Ferrario M et al. Early re-arterialization of thrombosed hepatic arteries in pediatric liver transplants. International Liver Transplant Society, Buenos Aires, Argentina, 2000.

Fischer L, Sterneck M, Rogiers X. Liver transplantation for acute liver failure. European Journal of Gastroenterology and Hepatology 1999; 11: 985–90.

Freese DK, Tuchman M, Schwarzenberg SJ et al. Early liver transplantation is indicated for tyrosinemia type I. Journal of Pediatric Gastroenterology and Nutrition 1991; 13: 10–15.

Freys G, Pottecher T, Calon B et al. Early assessment of transplanted liver function: lignocaine clearance test (MEGX). European Journal of Anaesthesiology 1997; 14: 397–405.

Funaki B, Rosenblum JD, Leef JA et al. Percutaneous treatment of portal venous stenosis in children and adolescents with segmental hepatic transplants: long-term results. Radiology 2000; 215: 147–51.

Gallinger S, Greig PD, Levy G et al. Liver transplantation for acute and subacute fulminant hepatic failure. Transplantation Proceedings 1989; 21: 2435–8.

Gane E, Saliba F, Valdecasas GJ et al. Randomised trial of efficacy and safety of oral ganciclovir in the prevention of cytomegalovirus disease in liver-transplant recipients. The Oral Ganciclovir International Transplantation Study Group. Lancet 1997; 350: 1729–33.

Gavalda J, deOtero J, Murio E et al. Two grams daily of oral acyclovir reduces the incidence of cytomegalovirus disease in CMV-seropositive liver transplant recipients. Transplant International 1997; 10: 462–5.

George DL, Arnow PM, Fox A et al. Patterns of infection after pediatric liver transplantation. American Journal of Diseases in Children 1992; 146: 924–9.

Gladdy RA, Richardson SE, Davies HD, Superina RA. Candida infection in pediatric liver transplant recipients. Liver Transplant Surgery 1999; 5: 16–24.

Goldstein G, Kremer AB, Barnes L, Hirsch L. OKT3 monoclonal antibody reversal of renal and hepatic rejection in pediatric patients. Journal of Pediatrics 1987; 111: 1046–50.

Goncalves I, Hermans D, Chretien D et al. Mitochondrial respiratory chain defect: a new etiology for neonatal cholestasis and early liver insufficiency. Journal of Hepatology 1995; 23: 290–4.

Gordon RD, Iwatsuki S, Esquivel CO et al. Liver transplantation across ABO blood groups. Surgery 1986; 100: 342–8.

Goss JA, Yersiz H, Shackleton CR et al. In situ splitting of the cadaveric liver for transplantation. Transplantation 1997; 64: 871–7.

Goss JA, Shackleton CR, Maggard M et al. Liver transplantation for fulminant hepatic failure in the pediatric patient. *Archives of Surgery* 1998; **133**: 839–46.

Green M, Tzakis A, Reyes J *et al.* Infectious complications of pediatric liver transplantation under FK 506. *Transplantation Proceedings* 1991; **23**: 3038–9.

Green M, Kaufmann M, Wilson J, Reyes J. Comparison of intravenous ganciclovir followed by oral acyclovir with intravenous ganciclovir alone for prevention of cytomegalovirus and Epstein–Barr virus disease after liver transplantation in children. *Clinical Infectious Diseases* 1997; **25**: 1344–9.

Green M, Cacciarelli TV, Mazariegos GV *et al.* Serial measurement of Epstein–Barr viral load in peripheral blood in pediatric liver transplant recipients during treatment for post-transplant lymphoproliferative disease. *Transplantation* 1998; **66**: 1641–4.

Greig PD, Woolf GM, Sinclair SB *et al.* Treatment of primary liver graft nonfunction with prostaglandin E1. *Transplantation* 1989a; **48**: 447–53.

Greig PD, Levy G, Superina RA *et al.* Antilymphoblast globulin (ALG) as initial prophylaxis against rejection following liver transplantation. *Transplantation Proceedings* 1989b; **21**: 2244–6.

Greig PD, Woolf GM, Abecassis M *et al.* Prostaglandin E1 for primary non-function following liver transplantation. *Transplantation Proceedings* 1989c; **21**: 3360–1.

Greig PD, Forster J, Superina RA *et al.* Donor-specific factors predict graft function following liver transplantation. *Transplantation Proceedings* 1990; **22**: 2072–3.

Grosfeld JL, Fitzgerald JF, Predaina R *et al.* The efficacy of hepatoportoenterostomy in biliary atresia. *Surgery* 1989; **106**: 692–700.

Hanna JN, Warnock TH, Shepherd RW, Selvey LA. Fulminant hepatitis A in indigenous children in north Queensland. *Medical Journal of Australia* 2000; **172**: 19–21.

Harihara Y, Makuuchi M, Kawarasaki H *et al.* Portal venoplasty for recipients in living-related liver transplantation. *Transplantation* 1999; **68**: 1199–200.

Hashikura Y, Kawasaki S, Okumura N *et al.* Prevention of hepatic artery thrombosis in pediatric liver transplantation. *Transplantation* 1995; **60**: 1109–12.

Heffron TG. Living-related pediatric liver transplantation. *Seminars in Pediatric Surgery* 1993; **2**: 248–53.

Heffron TG, Emond JC, Whitington PF *et al.* Biliary complications in pediatric liver transplantation. A comparison of reduced-size and whole grafts. *Transplantation* 1992; **53**: 391–5.

Hernandez-Cano AM, Geis JR, Rumack CH *et al.* Portal vein dynamics in biliary atresia. *Journal of Pediatric Surgery* 1987; **22**: 519–21.

Inomata Y, Tanaka K, Egawa H *et al.* Application of a tissue expander for stabilizing graft position in living-related liver transplantation. *Clinical Transplantation* 1997; **11**: 56–9.

Inomata Y, Tanaka K, Uemoto S *et al.* Living donor liver transplantation: an 8-year experience with 379 consecutive cases. *Transplantation Proceedings* 1999; **31**: 381.

Inomoto T, Nishizawa F, Sasaki H *et al.* Experiences of 120 microsurgical reconstructions of hepatic artery in living related liver transplantation. *Surgery* 1996; **119**: 20–6.

Iwatsuki S, Esquivel CO, Klintmalm GB *et al.* Nephrotoxicity of cyclosporine in liver transplantation. *Transplantation Proceedings* 1985; **17** (**Supplement 1**): 191–5.

Jara P, Robledo MJ, Frauca E *et al.* Tacrolimus for steroid-resistant liver rejection in children. *Transplant International* 1998; **11** (**Supplement 1**): S275–7.

Johnston TD, Gates R, Reddy KS *et al.* Non-operative management of bile leaks following liver transplantation. *Clinical Transplantation* 2000; **14**: 365–9.

Kalicinski P, Kaminski A, Prokurat A *et al.* Diagnosis and monitoring of cytomegalovirus infection after liver transplantation in children. *Annals of Transplantation* 1996; **1**: 13–14.

Kang Y, Lewis JH, Navalgund A *et al.* Epsilon-aminocaproic acid for treatment of fibrinolysis during liver transplantation. *Anesthesiology* 1987; **66**: 766–73.

Kang Y, Borland LM, Picone J, Martin LK. Intraoperative coagulation changes in children undergoing liver transplantation. *Anesthesiology* 1989; **71**: 44–7.

Karrer FM, Hall RJ, Lilly JR. Biliary atresia and the polysplenia syndrome. *Journal of Pediatric Surgery* 1991; **26**: 524–7.

Kato T, Ruiz P, DeFaria W *et al.* Mycophenolate mofetil rescue therapy in patients with chronic hepatic allograft rejection. *Transplantation Proceedings* 1999; **31**: 396.

Kelly DA. Pediatric liver transplantation. *Current Opinion in Pediatrics* 1998a; **10**: 493–8.

Kelly DA. Current results and evolving indications for liver transplantation in children. *Journal of Pediatric Gastroenterology and Nutrition* 1998b; **27**: 214–21.

King SM, Petric M, Superina R *et al.* Cytomegalovirus infections in pediatric liver transplantation. *American Journal of Diseases in Children* 1990; **144**: 1307–10.

King SM, Superina R, Andrews W *et al.* Randomized comparison of ganciclovir plus intravenous immune globulin (IVIG) with IVIG alone for prevention of primary cytomegalovirus disease in children receiving liver transplants. *Clinical Infectious Diseases* 1997; **25**: 1173–9.

Klein A. Tacrolimus rescue in liver transplant patients with refractory rejection or intolerance or malabsorption of cyclosporine. The US Multicenter FK506 Liver Study Group. *Liver Transplant Surgery* 1999; **5**: 502–8.

Kogan DL, Burroughs M, Emre S *et al.* Prospective longitudinal analysis of quantitative Epstein–Barr virus polymerase chain reaction in pediatric liver transplant recipients. *Transplantation* 1999; **67**: 1068–70.

Koneru B, Flye MW, Busuttil RW *et al.* Liver transplantation for hepatoblastoma. The American experience. *Annals of Surgery* 1991; **213**: 118–21.

Kovarik J, Breidenbach T, Gerbeau C *et al.* Disposition and immunodynamics of basiliximab in liver allograft recipients. *Clinical Pharmacology and Therapeutics* 1998; **64**: 66–72.

Krom RA, Kingma LM, Haagsma EB et al. Choledocho-choledochostomy, a relatively safe procedure in orthotopic liver transplantation. Surgery 1985; 97: 552–6.

Kubota K, Makuuchi M, Takayama T et al. Successful hepatic vein reconstruction in 42 consecutive living related liver transplantations. Surgery 2000; 128: 48–53.

Lallier M, St Vil D, Luks FI et al. Biliary tract complications in pediatric orthotopic liver transplantation. Journal of Pediatric Surgery 1993; 28: 1102–5.

Langnas AN, Marujo W, Stratta RJ et al. Hepatic allograft rescue following arterial thrombosis. Role of urgent revascularization. Transplantation 1991; 51: 86–90.

Langnas AN, Marujo WC, Inagaki M et al. The results of reduced-size liver transplantation, including split livers, in patients with end-stage liver disease. Transplantation 1992; 53: 387–91.

Langnas AN, Markin RS, Cattral MS, Naides SJ. Parvovirus B19 as a possible causative agent of fulminant liver failure and associated aplastic anemia. Hepatology 1995; 22: 1661–5.

Leaker MT, Brooker LA, Mitchell LG et al. Fibrin clot lysis by tissue plasminogen activator (tPA) is impaired in plasma from pediatric patients undergoing orthotopic liver transplantation. Transplantation 1995; 60: 144–7.

Letourneau JG, Hunter DW, Ascher NL et al. Biliary complications after liver transplantation in children. Radiology 1989; 170: 1095–9.

Liu PP, Chen CL, Eng HL et al. Lymphoproliferative disorder after liver transplantation. Journal of the Formosan Medical Association 1998; 97: 59–62.

McDiarmid SV. Risk factors and outcomes after pediatric liver transplantation. Liver Transplant Surgery 1996a; 2 (Supplement 1): 44–56.

McDiarmid SV. Mycophenolate mofetil in liver transplantation. Clinical Transplantation 1996b; 10: 140–5.

McDiarmid SV. Renal function in pediatric liver transplant patients. Kidney International 1996c; 53 (Supplement 1): S77–84.

McDiarmid SV, Millis MJ, Terasaki PI et al. OKT3 prophylaxis in liver transplantation. Digestive Diseases and Sciences 1991; 36: 1418–26.

McDiarmid SV, Busuttil RW, Ascher NL et al. FK506 (tacrolimus) compared with cyclosporine for primary immunosuppression after pediatric liver transplantation. Results from the US Multicenter Trial. Transplantation 1995; 59: 530–6.

McDiarmid SV, Jordan S, Lee GS et al. Prevention and pre-emptive therapy of posttransplant lymphoproliferative disease in pediatric liver recipients. Transplantation 1998; 66: 1604–11.

Mack CL, Millis JM, Whitington PF, Alonso EM. Pulmonary complications following liver transplantation in pediatric patients. Pediatric Transplantation 2000a; 4: 39–44.

Mack C et al. Urgent living-donor liver transplantation in children with fulminant hepatic failure or acute decompensated cirrhosis. International Liver Transplant Society, Buenos Aires, Argentina, 2000b.

Malago M, Rogiers X, Broelsch CE. Liver splitting and living donor techniques. British Medical Bulletin 1997; 53: 860–7.

Malatack JJ, Finegold DN, Iwatsuki S et al. Liver transplantation for type I glycogen storage disease. Lancet 1983; 1: 1073–5.

Markus BH, Duquesnoy RJ, Gordon RD et al. Histocompatibility and liver transplant outcome. Does HLA exert a dualistic effect? Transplantation 1988; 46: 372–7.

Marwan IK, Fawzy AT, Egawa H et al. Innovative techniques for and results of portal vein reconstruction in living-related liver transplantation. Surgery 1999; 125: 265–70.

Matern D, Starzl TE, Arnaout W et al. Liver transplantation for glycogen storage disease types I, III and IV. European Journal of Pediatrics 1999; 158 (Supplement 2): S43–8.

Mazariegos GV, Reyes J, Marino IR et al. Weaning of immunosuppression in liver transplant recipients. Transplantation 1997; 63: 243–9.

Mazzaferro V, Esquivel CO, Makowka L et al. Hepatic artery thrombosis after pediatric liver transplantation – a medical or surgical event? Transplantation 1989; 47: 971–7.

Michaels MG, Green M, Wald ER, Starzl TE. Adenovirus infection in pediatric liver transplant recipients. Journal of Infectious Diseases 1992; 165: 170–4.

Mieles LA, Esquivel CO, van Thiel DH et al. Liver transplantation for tyrosinemia. A review of 10 cases from the University of Pittsburgh. Digestive Diseases and Sciences 1990; 35: 153–7.

Mirza DF, Gunson BK, Soonawalla Z et al. Reduced acute rejection after liver transplantation with Neoral-based triple immunosuppression. Lancet 1997; 349: 701–2.

Mitchell L, Superina R, Delorme M et al. Circulating dermatan sulfate and heparin sulfate/heparin proteoglycans in children undergoing liver transplantation. Thrombosis and Haemostasis 1995; 74: 859–63.

Miyano T, Fujimoto T, Ohya T, Shimomura H. Current concept of the treatment of biliary atresia. World Journal of Surgery 1993; 17: 332–6.

Morgan G, Superina R. Congenital absence of the portal vein: two cases and a proposed classification system for portosystemic vascular anomalies. Journal of Pediatric Surgery 1994a; 29: 1239–41.

Morgan G, Superina RA. Lymphoproliferative disease after pediatric liver transplantation. Journal of Pediatric Surgery 1994b; 29: 1192–6.

Morris AA, Taanman JW, Blake J et al. Liver failure associated with mitochondrial DNA depletion. Journal of Hepatology 1998; 28: 556–63.

Munoz SJ, Alter HJ, Nakatsuji Y et al. The significance of hepatitis G virus in serum of patients with sporadic fulminant and subfulminant hepatitis of unknown etiology. Blood 1999; 94: 1460–4.

Nemeth A. Liver transplantation in alpha(1)-antitrypsin deficiency. European Journal of Pediatrics 1999: 158 (Supplement 2): S85–8.

Neuhaus P, Klupp J, Langrehr JM et al. Quadruple tacrolimus-based induction therapy including azathioprine and

ALG does not significantly improve outcome after liver transplantation when compared with standard induction with tacrolimus and steroids: results of a prospective, randomized trial. *Transplantation* 2000; **69**: 2343–53.

Neumann UP, Kaisers U, Langrehr JM *et al.* Administration of prostacyclin after liver transplantation: a placebo-controlled randomized trial. *Clinical Transplantation* 2000; **14**: 70–4.

Newell KA, Alonso EM, Whitington PF *et al.* Post-transplant lymphoproliferative disease in pediatric liver transplantation. Interplay between primary Epstein–Barr virus infection and immunosuppression. *Transplantation* 1996; **62**: 370–5.

Newell KA, Millis JM, Bruce DS *et al.* An analysis of hepatic retransplantation in children. *Transplantation* 1998; **65**: 1172–8.

Nicolette L, Billmire D, Faulkenstein K *et al.* Transplantation for acute hepatic failure in children. *Journal of Pediatric Surgery* 1998; **33**: 998–1002.

Odaib AA, Shneider BL, Bennet MJ *et al.* A defect in the transport of long-chain fatty acids associated with acute liver failure. *New England Journal of Medicine* 1998; **339**: 1752–7.

O'Grady JG, Alexander GJ, Hayllar KM, Williams R. Early indicators of prognosis in fulminant hepatic failure. *Gastroenterology* 1989; **97**: 439–45.

Ogura K, Terasaki PI, Koyama H *et al.* High one-month liver graft failure rates in flow cytometry crossmatch-positive recipients. *Clinical Transplantation* 1994; **8**: 111–15.

Oh CK, Sanfey HA, Pelletier SJ *et al.* Implication of advanced donor age on the outcome of liver transplantation. *Clinical Transplantation* 2000; **14**: 386–90.

Okazaki T, Kobayashi H, Yamataka A *et al.* Long-term postsurgical outcome of biliary atresia. *Journal of Pediatric Surgery* 1999; **34**: 312–15.

Oldhafer KJ, Bornscheuer A, Fruhauf NR *et al.* Rescue hepatectomy for initial graft non-function after liver transplantation. *Transplantation* 1999; **67**: 1024–8.

Onrust SV, Wiseman LR. Basiliximab. *Drugs* 1999; **57**: 207–13.

Otte JB, de Ville de Goyet J, Reding R *et al.* Sequential treatment of biliary atresia with Kasai portoenterostomy and liver transplantation: a review. *Hepatology* 1994; **20**: 41–8S.

Otte JB, de Ville de Goyet J, Reding R *et al.* Pediatric liver transplantation: from the full-size liver graft to reduced, split and living related liver transplantation. *Pediatric Surgery International* 1998; **13**: 308–18.

Otte JB, Reding R, de Ville de Goyet J *et al.* Experience with living related liver transplantation in 63 children. *Acta Gastroenterologica Belgica* 1999; **62**: 355–62.

Pauwels A, Mostefarkara N, Dumonte J *et al.* Emergency liver transplantation for acute liver failure. Evaluation of London and Clichy criteria. *Journal of Hepatology* 1993; **17**: 124–7.

Peclet MH, Rykman FC, Pedersoen SH *et al.* The spectrum of bile duct complications in pediatric liver transplantation. *Journal of Pediatric Surgery* 1994; **29**: 214–19.

Pett S, Mowat AP. Crigler–Najjar syndrome types I and II. Clinical experience – King's College Hospital 1972–1978. Phenobarbitone, phototherapy and liver transplantation. *Molecular Aspects of Medicine* 1987; **9**: 473–82.

Phillips MJ, Blender LM, Poucell S *et al.* Syncytial giant-cell hepatitis. Sporadic hepatitis with distinctive pathological features, a severe clinical course, and paramyxoviral features. *New England Journal of Medicine* 1991; **324**: 455–60.

Phillips MJ, Ackerley CA, Superina RA *et al.* Excess zinc associated with severe progressive cholestasis in Cree and Ojibwa–Cree children. *Lancet* 1996; **347**: 866–8.

Pichlmayr R, Ringe B, Gubernati SG *et al.* Transplantation of a donor liver to two recipients (splitting transplantation – a new method in the further development of segmental liver transplantation. *Langenbecks Archiv für Chirurgie* 1988; **373**: 127–30.

Pierro A, Koletzko B, Carnielli V *et al.* Resting energy expenditure is increased in infants and children with extrahepatic biliary atresia. *Journal of Pediatric Surgery* 1989; **24**: 534–8.

Pitre J, Soubrane O, Dousset B *et al.* How valid is emergency liver transplantation for acute liver necrosis in patients with multiple-organ failure? *Liver Transplant Surgery* 1996; **2**: 1–7.

Pitre J, Soubrane O, Dousset B *et al.* Rationale and technical constraints of a tertiary liver transplantation. *Liver Transplant Surgery* 1997; **3**: 624–7.

Potter JM, Wright M, Lynch SV *et al.* Lignocaine metabolism and liver function testing in primary graft failure following orthotopic liver transplantation. *Medical Journal of Australia* 1993; **158**: 125–6.

Randall HB, Wachs ME, Somberg KA *et al.* The use of the T-tube after orthotopic liver transplantation. *Transplantation* 1996; **61**: 258–61.

Rasmussen A, Hjortrup A, Kirkegaard P. Intraoperative measurement of graft blood flow – a necessity in liver transplantation. *Transplant International* 1997; **10**: 74–7.

Rebhandl W, Felberbauer FX, Huber WD *et al.* Progressive familial intrahepatic cholestasis (Byler disease): current genetics and therapy. *Klinische Pädiatrie* 2000; **212**: 64–70.

Reding R. Steroid withdrawal in liver transplantation: benefits, risks, and unanswered questions. *Transplantation* 2000; **70**: 405–10.

Reding R, Genari F, Janssen M *et al.* The pediatric liver transplant program at the Université Catholique de Louvain, Cliniques Saint-Luc, Brussels: overall results in 444 children (1984–1997). *Acta Gastroenterologica Belgica* 1999; **62**: 285–9.

Reents S, Goodwin SD, Singh V. Antifungal prophylaxis in immunocompromised hosts. *Annals of Pharmacotherapy* 1993; **27**: 53–60.

Reggiani P, Gridelli B, Colledan M *et al.* Rescue FK506 early conversion for refractory rejection after pediatric liver transplantation: experience in 20 children. *Transplant International* 1998; **11** (**Supplement 1**): S272–4.

Rela M, Vougas V, Muiesan P *et al.* Split liver transplantation: King's College Hospital experience. *Annals of Surgery* 1998; **227**: 282–8.

Renz JF, Rosenthal P, Roberts JP *et al.* Planned exploration of pediatric liver transplant recipients reduces post-transplant morbidity and lowers length of hospitalization. *Archives of Surgery* 1997; **132**: 950–5.

Revillon Y, Michel JL, Lacaille F *et al.* Living-related liver transplantation in children: the 'Parisian' strategy to safely increase organ availability. *Journal of Pediatric Surgery* 1999; **34**: 851–3.

Reyes J, Mazariegos GV. Pediatric transplantation. *Surgical Clinics of North America* 1999; **79**: 163–89.

Reyes JD, Carr B, Dvorchik I *et al.* Liver transplantation and chemotherapy for hepatoblastoma and hepatocellular cancer in childhood and adolescence. *Journal of Pediatrics* 2000a; **136**: 795–804.

Reyes J, Gerber D, Mazariegos GV *et al.* Split-liver transplantation: a comparison of *ex vivo* and *in situ* techniques. *Journal of Pediatric Surgery* 2000b; **35**: 283–9.

Rieber A, Brambs HJ, Lauchart W. The radiological management of biliary complications following liver transplantation. *Cardiovascular and Interventional Radiology* 1996; **19**: 242–7.

Ringe B, Burdelski M, Rodeck B, Pichlmayr R. Experience with partial liver transplantation in Hannover. *Clinical Transplants* 1990; **135**: 135–44.

Riordan SM, Williams R. Tolerance after liver transplantation: does it exist and can immunosuppression be withdrawn? *Journal of Hepatology* 1999; **31**: 1106–19.

Rogers BB, Conlin C, Timmons CF *et al.* Epstein-Barr virus PCR correlated with viral histology and serology in pediatric liver transplant patients. *Pediatric Pathology and Laboratory Medicine* 1997; **17**: 391–400.

Rogers BB, Sommerauer J, Quan A *et al.* Epstein–Barr virus polymerase chain reaction and serology in pediatric post-transplant lymphoproliferative disorder: three-year experience. *Pediatric Developmental Pathology* 1998; **1**: 480–6.

Rogiers X, Malago M, Habib N *et al. In situ* splitting of the liver in the heart-beating cadaveric organ donor for transplantation in two recipients. *Transplantation* 1995; **59**: 1081–3.

Rogiers X, Broering DC, Mueller L, Burdelski M. Living-donor liver transplantation in children. *Langenbecks Archiv für Chirurgie* 1999; **384**: 528–35.

Ryckman FC, Schroeder TJ, Pedersen SH *et al.* Induction therapy with OKT3 in pediatric liver-transplant recipients. *Transplantation Science* 1994; **4** (**Supplement 1**): S20–5.

Ryckman FC, Alonso MH, Bucuvalas JC, Balistreri WF. Biliary atresia – surgical management and treatment options as they relate to outcome. *Liver Transplant Surgery* 1998: **4** (**Supplement 1**): S24–33.

Saint-Vil D, Luks FI, Lebel P *et al.* Infectious complications of pediatric liver transplantation. *Journal of Pediatric Surgery* 1991; **26**: 908–13.

Sandler AD, Azarow KS, Superina RA. The impact of a previous Kasai procedure on liver transplantation for biliary atresia. *Journal of Pediatric Surgery* 1997; **32**: 416–19.

Saudubray JM, Touati G, Delonlay P *et al.* Liver transplantation in urea cycle disorders. *European Journal of Pediatrics* 1999; **158** (**Supplement 2**): S55–9.

Schilsky ML, Scheinberg IH, Sternlieb I. Liver transplantation for Wilson's disease: indications and outcome. *Hepatology* 1994; **19**: 583–7.

Schindel D, Dunn S, Casas A *et al.* Characterization and treatment of biliary anastomotic stricture after segmental liver transplantation. *Journal of Pediatric Surgery* 2000a; **35**: 940–2.

Schindel DT, Dunn SP, Casas AT *et al.* Pediatric recipients of three or more hepatic allografts: results and technical challenges. *Journal of Pediatric Surgery* 2000b; **35**: 297–300.

Schlitt HJ, Meier PN, Nashan B *et al.* Reconstructive surgery for ischemic-type lesions at the bile duct bifurcation after liver transplantation. *Annals of Surgery* 1999; **229**: 137–45.

Schroeder TJ, First MR, Hurtubise PE *et al.* Immunologic monitoring with Orthoclone OKT3 therapy. *Journal of Heart Transplantation* 1989; **8**: 371–80.

Sebagh M, Debette M, Samuel D *et al.* 'Silent' presentation of veno-occlusive disease after liver transplantation as part of the process of cellular rejection with endothelial predilection. *Hepatology* 1999; **30**: 1144–50.

Settmacher U, Nussler NC, Glanemann M *et al.* Venous complications after orthotopic liver transplantation. *Clinical Transplantation* 2000; **14**: 235–41.

Seu P, Winston DJ, Holt CD *et al.* Long-term ganciclovir prophylaxis for successful prevention of primary cytomegalovirus (CMV) disease in CMV-seronegative liver transplant recipients with CMV-seropositive donors. *Transplantation* 1997; **64**: 1614–17.

Shackleton CR, Goss JA, Swenson K *et al.* The impact of microsurgical hepatic arterial reconstruction on the outcome of liver transplantation for congenital biliary atresia. *American Journal of Surgery* 1997; **173**: 431–5.

Shaw BW, Iwatsuki S, Bron K, Starzl TE. Portal vein grafts in hepatic transplantation. *Surgery, Gynecology and Obstetrics* 1985; **161**: 66–8.

Sher LS, Cosenza CA, Michel J *et al.* Efficacy of tacrolimus as rescue therapy for chronic rejection in orthotopic liver transplantation: a report of the US Multicenter Liver Study Group. *Transplantation* 1997; **64**: 258–63.

Shetty AK, Gans HA, So S *et al.* Intravenous ribavirin therapy for adenovirus pneumonia. *Pediatric Pulmonology* 2000; **29**: 69–73.

Shuhart MC, Kowdley KV, McVicar JP *et al.* Predictors of bile leaks after T-tube removal in orthotopic liver transplant recipients. *Liver Transplant Surgery* 1998; **4**: 62–70.

Sieders E, Peeters PM, Ten Vergert EM *et al.* Early vascular complications after pediatric liver transplantation. *Liver Transplant* 2000; **6**: 326–32.

Singer PA, Siegler M, Whitington PF et al. Ethics of liver transplantation with living donors. New England Journal of Medicine 1989; 321: 620–2.

Singhal S, Ellis RW, Jones SG et al. Targeted prophylaxis with amphotericin B lipid complex in liver transplantation. Liver Transplant 2000; 6: 588–95.

Sokal EM, Veyckemans F, de Ville de Goyet J et al. Liver transplantation in children less than 1 year of age. Journal of Pediatrics 1990; 117: 205–10.

Sokal EM, Silva ES, Hermans D et al. Orthotopic liver transplantation for Crigler–Najjar type I disease in six children. Transplantation 1995; 60: 1095–8.

Sokal EM, Melchior M, Cornu C et al. Acute parvovirus B19 infection associated with fulminant hepatitis of favourable prognosis in young children. Lancet 1998; 352: 1739–41.

Sokal EM, Sokol R, Cormier V et al. Liver transplantation in mitochondrial respiratory chain disorders. European Journal of Pediatrics 1999; 158 (Supplement 2): S81–4.

Sokol RJ, Francis PD, Gold SH et al. Orthotopic liver transplantation for acute fulminant Wilson's disease. Journal of Pediatrics 1985; 107: 549–52.

Someda H, Moriyasu F, Fujimoto M et al. Vascular complications in living-related liver transplantation detected with intraoperative and postoperative Doppler US. Journal of Hepatology 1995; 22: 623–32.

Srinivasan P, Vilca Melendez H, Muiesan P et al. Liver transplantation with monosegments. Surgery 1999; 126: 10–12.

Stahl RL, Duncan A, Hooks MA et al. A hypercoagulable state follows orthotopic liver transplantation. Hepatology 1990; 12: 553–8.

Starzl TE, Groth CG, Brettschneider L et al. Extended survival in three cases of orthotopic homotransplantation of the human liver. Surgery 1968; 63: 549–63.

Starzl TE, Iwatsuki S, Shaw B. A growth factor in fine vascular anastomoses. Surgery, Gynecology and Obstetrics 1984; 159: 164–5.

Stevens LH, Emond JC, Piper JB et al. Hepatic artery thrombosis in infants. A comparison of whole livers reduced-size grafts, and grafts from living-related donors. Transplantation 1992; 53: 396–9.

Stieber AC, Gordon RD, Bassi N. A simple solution to a technical complication in 'piggyback' liver transplantation. Transplantation 1997; 64: 654–5.

Strasberg SM, Lowell JA, Howard TK. Reducing the shortage of donor livers: what would it take to reliably split livers for transplantation into two adult recipients? Liver Transplant Surgery 1999; 5: 437–50.

Strong R, Ong TH, Pillay P et al. A new method of segmental orthotopic liver transplantation in children. Surgery 1988; 104: 104–7.

Strong RW, Lynch SV, Ong TH et al. Successful liver transplantation from a living donor to her son. New England Journal of Medicine 1990; 322: 1505–7.

Superina RA. Liver transplantation in children: an update. Surgery Annual 1992; 1: 195–226.

Superina R, Bilik R. Results of liver transplantation in children with unresectable liver tumors. Journal of Pediatric Surgery 1996; 31: 835–9.

Superina RA, Pearl RH, Roberts EA et al. Liver transplantation in children: the initial Toronto experience. Journal of Pediatric Surgery 1989; 24: 1013–19.

Superina R, Acal L, Bilik R, Zaki A. Growth in children after liver transplantation on cyclosporine alone or in combination with low-dose azathioprine. Transplantation Proceedings 1993; 25: 2580.

Superina RA, Strong DK, Acal LE, DeLuca E. Relative bioavailability of Sandimmune and Sandimmune Neoral in pediatric liver recipients. Transplantation Proceedings 1994; 26: 2979–80.

Superina RA, Zangari A, Acal L et al. Growth in children following liver transplantation. Pediatric Transplantation 1998; 2: 70–5.

Superina RA, Harrison C, Alonso EM, Whitington PF. Ethical issues in pediatric liver transplantation. Transplantation Proceedings 1999; 31: 1342–4.

Sze DY, Semba CP, Razavi MK, et al. Endovascular treatment of hepatic venous outflow obstruction after piggyback technique liver transplantation. Transplantation 1999; 68: 446–9.

Tan KC, Yandza T, de Hemptinne B et al. Hepatic artery thrombosis in pediatric liver transplantation. Journal of Pediatric Surgery 1988; 23: 927–30.

Tanaka K, Uemoto S, Tokunaga Y et al. Surgical techniques and innovations in living related liver transplantation. Annals of Surgery 1993; 217: 82–91.

Textor SC, Canzanello VJ, Taler SJ et al. Hypertension after liver transplantation. Liver Transplant Surgery 1995; 1: 20–8.

Thistlethwaite JR, Stuart JK, Mayer JT et al. Complications and monitoring of OKT3 therapy. American Journal of Kidney Diseases 1988; 11: 112–19.

Tissieres P, Simon L, Debray D et al. Acute pancreatitis after orthotopic liver transplantation in children: incidence, contributing factors and outcome. Journal of Pediatric Gastroenterology and Nutrition 1998; 26: 315–20.

Tokunaga Y, Tanaka K, Fujita S et al. Living related liver transplantation across ABO blood groups with FK506 and OKT3. Transplant International 1993; 6: 313–18.

Tzakis A, Todo S, Stieber A, Starzl TE. Venous jump grafts for liver transplantation in patients with portal vein thrombosis. Transplantation 1989a; 48: 530–1.

Tzakis A, Todo S, Starzl TE. Orthotopic liver transplantation with preservation of the inferior vena cava. Annals of Surgery 1989b; 210: 649–52.

Uemoto S, Tanaka K, Fujita S et al. Infectious complications in living related liver transplantation. Journal of Pediatric Surgery 1994; 29: 514–17.

Uemoto S, Inomata Y, Sakurai T et al. Living donor liver transplantation for fulminant hepatic failure. Transplantation 2000; 70: 152–7.

Urena MA, Moreno Gonzalez E, Romero CJ et al. An approach to the rational use of steatotic donor livers in liver transplantation. *Hepatogastroenterology* 1999; **46**: 1164–73.

US Department of Health and Human Services. *UNOS annual report*. Richmond, VA: United Network for Organ Sharing.

US Department of Health and Human Services. *UNOS ninth annual report of the US Scientific Registry of Transplant Recipients and the Organ Procurement and Transplantation Network*. Richmond, VA: United Network for Organ Sharing, 1999.

Valente JF, Alonso MH, Weber FL, Hanto DW. Late hepatic artery thrombosis in liver allograft recipients is associated with intrahepatic biliary necrosis. *Transplantation* 1996; **61**: 61–5.

van Mourik ID, Beath SV, Brook GA *et al.* Long-term nutritional and neurodevelopmental outcome of liver transplantation in infants aged less than 12 months. *Journal of Pediatric Gastroenterology and Nutrition* 2000; **30**: 269–75.

Vazquez J, Santamaria ML, Gamez M *et al.* Hepatic artery thrombosis in the pediatric liver transplant. *Cirugia Pediatrica* 1991; **4**: 185–9.

Vazquez J, Santamaria ML, Murcia J *et al.* Our first 100 consecutive pediatric liver transplants. *European Journal of Pediatric Surgery* 1995; **5**: 67–71.

Verboon-Maciolek MA, Swanink CM, Krediet TG *et al.* Severe neonatal echovirus 20 infection characterized by hepatic failure. *Pediatric Infectious Disease Journal* 1997; **16**: 524–7.

Verran DJ, Gurkan A, Chui AK *et al.* Pancreatitis in adult orthotopic liver allograft recipients: risk factors and outcome. *Liver Transplant* 2000; **6**: 362–6.

Vilca Melendez H, Vougas V, Muiesan P *et al.* Bowel perforation after paediatric orthotopic liver transplantation. *Transplant International* 1998; **11**: 301–4.

Viviani MA, Tortorano AM, Malaspina C *et al.* Surveillance and treatment of liver transplant recipients for candidiasis and aspergillosis. *European Journal of Epidemiology* 1992; **8**: 433–6.

Vohra P, Haller C, Emre S *et al.* Neonatal hemochromatosis: the importance of early recognition of liver failure. *Journal of Pediatrics* 2000; **136**: 537–41.

Wall WJ. Liver transplantation: current concepts. *Canadian Medical Association Journal* 1988; **139**: 21–8.

Webb M, Puig R, Khan F *et al.* Intraoperative donor cholangiography. *Liver Transplant Surgery* 1998; **4**: 297–9.

Whitington PF, Whitington GL. Partial external diversion of bile for the treatment of intractable pruritus associated with intrahepatic cholestasis. *Gastroenterology* 1988; **95**: 130–6.

Whitington PF, Emond JC, Whitington SH *et al.* Small-bowel length and the dose of cyclosporine in children after liver transplantation. *New England Journal of Medicine* 1990; **322**: 733–8.

Whitington PF, Emond JC, Heffron T, Thistlethwaite JR. Orthotopic auxiliary liver transplantation for Crigler–Najjar syndrome type 1. *Lancet* 1993; **342**: 779–80.

Whitington PF, Alonso EM, Piper JB. Pediatric liver transplantation. *Seminars in Liver Disease* 1994; **14**: 303–17.

Whitington PF, Alonso EM, Boyle JT *et al.* Liver transplantation for the treatment of urea cycle disorders. *Journal of Inherited Metabolic Disease* 1998; **1**: 112–18.

Williams R, Wendon J. Indications for orthotopic liver transplantation in fulminant liver failure. *Hepatology* 1994; **20**: S5–10.

Winston DJ, Pakrasi A, Busuttil RW. Prophylactic fluconazole in liver transplant recipients. A randomized, double-blind, placebo-controlled trial. *Annals of Internal Medicine* 1999; **131**: 729–37.

Winthrop AL, Waddell T, Superina RA. The diagnosis of pneumonia in the immunocompromised child: use of bronchoalveolar lavage. *Journal of Pediatric Surgery* 1990; **25**: 878–80.

Wong T, Nouri-Aria KT, Devlin J *et al.* Tolerance and latent cellular rejection in long-term liver transplant recipients. *Hepatology* 1998; **28**: 443–9.

Woodle ES, Thistlethwaite JR, Emond JC *et al.* OKT3 therapy for hepatic allograft rejection. Differential response in adults and children. *Transplantation* 1991; **51**: 1207–12.

Woodle ES, Millis JM, So SK *et al.* Liver transplantation in the first three months of life. *Transplantation* 1998; **66**: 606–9.

Yamaguchi T, Yamaoka Y, Mori K *et al.* Hepatic vein reconstruction of the graft in partial liver transplantation from living donor: surgical procedures relating to their anatomic variations. *Surgery* 1993; **114**: 976–83.

Yamanaka J, Lynch SV, Ong TH *et al.* Post-transplant gastrointestinal perforation in pediatric liver transplantation. *Journal of Pediatric Surgery* 1994; **29**: 635–8.

Yanaga K, Sugimachi K. Biliary tract reconstruction in liver transplantation. *Surgery Today* 1992; **22**: 493–500.

Yanaga K, Lebeau G, Marsh JN *et al.* Hepatic artery reconstruction for hepatic artery thrombosis after orthotopic liver transplantation. *Archives of Surgery* 1990; **125**: 628–31.

Younes BS, McDiarmid SV, Martin MG *et al.* The effect of immunosuppression on post-transplant lymphoproliferative disease in pediatric liver transplant patients. *Transplantation* 2000; **70**: 94–9.

Zajko AB, Sheng R, Zetti GM *et al.* Transhepatic balloon dilation of biliary strictures in liver transplant patients: a 10-year experience. *Journal of Vascular and Interventional Radiology* 1995; **6**: 79–83.

Clinical immunosuppression

PAUL M COLOMBANI

Advances in clinical immunosuppression for the pediatric liver transplant recipient have made a significant contribution to the overall success of liver transplantation. These advances over the last two decades have paralleled technical advances in the operative procedure as well as advances in post-transplant critical and ongoing care. This section describes the current state of clinical immunosuppression for pediatric liver transplant recipients.

HISTORICAL PERSPECTIVE

Clinical immunosuppression has been required for any transplant procedure other than transplantation between identical twins. In the 1940s, Medawar and colleagues outlined the process of transplant rejection and defined the ability to induce transplant tolerance in neonatal animals (Gibson and Medawar, 1943; Medawar, 1944). By the 1950s, technical advances allowed for clinical renal transplantation in identical twins (Merrill et al., 1956; Starzl and Butz, 1962). During the 1960s and 1970s, renal transplantation came into its own as an acceptable practice for the treatment of end-stage renal disease and much of the success could be attributed to advances in immunosuppression (Dempster, 1953; Merrill et al., 1960).

The first non-identical twin transplants with disparate human lymphocyte antigen (HLA) types required mea-

sures to prevent rejection. The last 50 years have seen a progressive improvement in clinical immunosuppression, first in renal transplantation and then in other solid organ transplants (Murray et al. 1968; Brent, 1997). These advances are summarized in Table 29.1 First, irradiation of the graft to kill invading lymphocytes proved successful (Hamburger et al., 1962). Following that, high-dose corticosteroids were utilized with success to treat and prevent rejection, but at the high cost of infectious complications. During the 1960s, 6-mercaptopurine and its more palatable oral analog azathioprine began to be used in combination with corticosteroids (Calne, 1960). By the 1970s, antithymocyte preparations were developed to provide rather more specific immunosuppression (Levey and Medawar, 1966). The first compound, namely antilymphocyte serum, was utilized to eliminate circulating T- and B-cells (Najarian et al., 1969). Following this, an antithymocyte globulin was clinically available to specifically eliminate circulating T-cells (Kohler and Milstein, 1975). Both of these polyclonal antibodies caused considerable systemic side-effects in transplant recipients.

From the 1980s to the present day, clinical liver transplantation has been acceptable practice for end-stage liver disease. One of the principal reasons for the success of clinical liver transplantation was the introduction of the more specific anti-T-cell agent, cyclosporine (Borel et al., 1976). With Food and Drug Administration (FDA) approval of cyclosporine in 1984, clinical liver transplantation became a widely accepted practice (Starzl et al.,

Table 29.1 *Historical advances in clinical immunosuppression*

1950s	X-irradiation
1960s	High-dose corticosteroids
	Azathioprine
1970s	Antilymphocyte serum (polyclonal)
	Antithymocyte globulin (polyclonal)
1980s	Cyclosporine
	Anti-CD3 antibody (monoclonal)
1990s	Tacrolimus
	Anti-IL2 receptor antibody (monoclonal)
	Mycophenolate mofetil
	Rapamycin

1981). During the 1980s, monoclonal antibodies were developed to provide anti-T-cell effects, the principal agent being the anti-CD3 monoclonal antibody (Cosimi *et al.*, 1981). Survival rates in patients during this period increased from 25% to more than 80% with the introduction of cyclosporine into a multiple-drug immunosuppressive regimen (Starzl *et al.*, 1989).

During the 1990s, further refinements of T-cell inhibition were made with the introduction of tacrolimus and rapamycin (Armitage *et al.*, 1991; Fung *et al.*, 1991; Stepkowski *et al.*, 1991; Klintmalm, 1994; Groth *et al.*, 1999). These two agents further refined specific anti-T-cell effects and provided further improvements in graft and patient survival. In addition to these agents, the 1990s also brought another generation of 'humanized' antibody therapies which have provided more specific immunosuppression with markedly reduced toxicities (Woodle *et al.*, 1999). These more specific monoclonal antibodies are hybrid human/mouse monoclonal antibodies which provide fewer allergic responses and toxicities. These new agents include the anti-IL-2-receptor monoclonal antibodies which are in current clinical use (Nashan *et al.*, 1999; Benjaminovitz *et al.*, 2000).

In summary, over the last four decades there has been significant progress in providing more specific immunosuppression to prevent graft rejection. Many of these newer and more specific agents are used sequentially or in combination. Over the past two decades these advances have made clinical liver transplantation as well as pediatric liver transplantation an extremely successful endeavor in cases of end-stage liver disease.

OVERVIEW OF TRANSPLANT IMMUNOLOGY

As mentioned in the previous section, clinical transplantation beyond identical twins was a significant barrier to success. This was primarily related to the HLA complex, which is also known as the major histocompatibility complex (MHC). The genes that encode for the HLA complex are found on chromosome 6. These MHC antigens are divided into specific families, and each individual has a specific and unique MHC identity. In order to transplant across MHC barriers, the recipient's immune system must be inhibited to prevent allograft rejection (Terasaki, 1990).

The principal cells involved in allograft rejection are the T-lymphocytes and, to a lesser extent, preformed or generated antibody synthesized by B-lymphocytes. In addition, natural killer cells, monocytes and other accessory cells play a non-specific role in the overall immune response (Cooper *et al.*, 1966; Gatti *et al.*, 1968).

MHC non-identity and thus graft rejection is discriminated by the specific immune system of T- and B-cells. Within populations of T-cells there is also a class restriction whereby certain subpopulations of T-helper or killer cells are restricted to identifying only class I of the MHC (HLA A, B and C loci). Other populations of T-cells are restricted to identifying only the class II MHC (HLA) (D and DR loci) (Amos and Bach, 1968). Not only are cells restricted in their identity pattern, but they may also be restricted in their ability to process and identify antigen. Cell presentation of antigen by accessory cells, such as the monocyte–macrophage lineage, that have processed foreign antigen is known as the indirect method of stimulating and sensitizing T- and B-cells. This process is probably the main method by which the human organism is sensitized and responds to foreign infectious antigens. In addition, T- and B-cells have the capability within class restrictions to directly identify MHC antigens on foreign cells. This direct sensitization by circulating immune-competent T- and B-cells may play a major role in the patient's immune response to vascularized solid organ grafts.

Further specificity and target homing is provided by adhesion molecules ICAM-1 and LFA-2. The ICAM-1 site is found on sensitizing transplanted tissue, while the LFA-1 or CD2 locus is found on the recipient's sensitized responding T- and B-cells. In addition to MHC antigens, these adhesion molecules help to provide specific binding and sensitization of the responding cell populations (Dragun *et al.*, 1998; Abraham *et al.*, 1999; Berlin-Rufenach *et al.*, 1999).

At the subcellular level, T-lymphocyte activation undergoes a sequential cascade beginning at the cell membrane and creating calcium-dependent and calcium-independent cytoplasmic events leading to nuclear activation, *de-novo* gene expression and eventual synthesis of proteins required for cell proliferation and clonal expansion of cell populations. The calcium-dependent pathway is well documented and is considered to operate via the T-cell receptor (CD3) where a calcium flux activates protein kinase C and other calcium-dependent proteins, such as calmodulin, and the calcium-dependent phosphatases, such as calcineurin (Kissinger *et al.*, 1995; Batiuk *et al.*, 1997). In addition, an accessory pathway exists through the CD28 membrane receptor which is calcium-independent and may directly activate protein kinases (Li *et al.*, 1999).

The activation of cellular protein kinases leads to the activation of nuclear factors which migrate to the nucleus to activate certain genes (Frantz *et al.*, 1994; Sugimoto *et al.*, 1997). These factors include NFA-T, NFA-κβ and AF-1. These nuclear binding proteins serve to deform the chromosome, and expose and activate the genes involved in the T-cell activation. This T-cell activation leads to the synthesis of new proteins such as lymphokines, and cell receptors specific for activated T-cells and those proteins necessary for the initiation of cell division.

Numerous proteins are involved but the principal T-cell lymphokine is interleukin-2 and the principal T-cell-activation receptor is the IL-2 receptor. The generation of IL-2 by helper T-cells and the IL-2 receptor expression on cytotoxic T-cells and B-cells allow for the clonal expansion of responsive sensitized MHC-specific T- and B-cells (Wicker *et al.*, 1990; Hultsch *et al.*, 1991; Werlen *et al.*, 1998).

CLINICALLY RELEVANT IMMUNOSUPPRESSIVE AGENTS

A variety of antimetabolites, bacterially or fungally derived antibiotics and alkylating agents that have been used for cancer chemotherapy have been utilized to provide clinical immunosuppression. However, this discussion is limited to those agents that have been or are in current clinical use.

Box 29.1 *Classification of clinically useful immunosuppressive drugs*

Non-specific agents
Corticosteroids
Antimetabolites
  Azathioprine
  Mycophenolate mofetil

Specific agents
Calcineurin inhibitors
  Cyclosporine
  Tacrolimus
Unknown T- and B-cell targets
  Rapamycin
Antilymphocyte preparations
  Polyclonal antibodies
    Antilymphocyte globulin (ALG)
    Antithymocyte globulin (ATG)
    Thymoglobulin
Monoclonal antibodies
  Anti-CD3 antibodies
  Anti-IL-2 receptor antibodies

Immunosuppressive drugs may be classified by a variety of methods. A common method divides them into specific and non-specific agents. The non-specific agents include anti-inflammatory drugs such as corticosteroids, antiproliferative agents such as azathioprine (6-mercaptopurine), and new antiproliferative agents such as mycophenolate mofetil.

Agents that provide more specific immunosuppres-

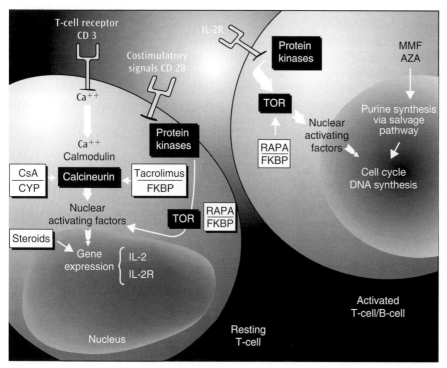

Figure 29.1 *Graphic depiction of the naive T-cell (left) and activated T- or B-cell (right). The common cellular pathways of activation and the sites of action of clinically relevant immunosuppressive agents are depicted. CsA, cyclosporine; CYP, cyclophilin; FKBP, FK binding protein; RAPA, rapamycin; AZA, azathioprine; MMF, mycophenolate; TOR, target of rapamycin; IL-2, interleukin-2; IL-2R, interleukin-2 receptor.*

sion can be divided into the calcineurin (or other cytoplasmic enzyme)-inhibiting agents (e.g. cyclosporine, FK506 (tacrolimus) and rapamycin), agents that block antigen recognition (e.g. many of the monoclonal antibodies) and agents that are specifically cytotoxic to T-cells or that remove them from the circulation. This last group includes mechanical methods such as graft irradiation, ultraviolet-light photophoresis, thoracic duct drainage, total lymphoid radiation and thymectomy. Box 29.1 summarizes this classification of clinically useful immunosuppressive drugs. In general, this drug classification is arbitrary and there may be considerable overlap between categories for some of these drugs (e.g. corticosteroids). These agents have specific mechanisms of action that sometimes overlap. Figure 29.1 depicts the cellular sites of action of a number of these clinically used and investigational agents. The following descriptions of these agents also delineate potential toxicities, common routes of administration and dosages.

Corticosteroids

The corticosteroids methylprednisolone and prednisone have been the mainstay of clinical immunosuppression since the 1950s. Corticosteroids have potent anti-inflammatory membrane stabilization effects. They provide general inhibition of anabolic activities and gene activation (Stellato et al., 1999; McNally et al., 2000). There may also be a direct cytotoxic effect on lymphocytes with higher doses. Steroids are used both for induction therapy and for the treatment of rejection. Pediatric patients are usually pulsed with higher doses of steroids (10 mg/kg/day), with the dosage tapering over time. The maintenance therapy dose is usually in the range 0.1–0.3 mg/kg/day. These relatively low maintenance doses of steroids are achieved because of the availability of other immunosuppressive agents for use in combination with corticosteroids. The clinical use of long-term high-dose steroids was associated with significant morbidity and mortality secondary to opportunistic infections. In addition to these infection risks, the acute toxicity effects of steroids include potent sodium and water retention with secondary hypertension. Chronic use of low-dose steroids may lead to decreased bone mineralization with osteoporosis, growth retardation, effects on gastric acidity and gastritis. As a result, a number of centers attempt alternate-day low-dose steroids or complete steroid withdrawal.

Azathioprine (Imuran)

Azathioprine and its metabolic end-product 6-mercaptopurine are purine analogs which competitively bind to and inhibit the enzyme phosphoribosyl pyrophosphate amidotransferase, thereby preventing purine biosynthesis in all mammalian cells. This effectively blocks DNA synthesis and cell division. Azathioprine and 6-mercaptopurine may both be incorporated into RNA and DNA strands, blocking transcription (Hitchings and Elion, 1954; Murray et al., 1964). Azathioprine may be the most commonly used agent in clinical organ transplantation. It is well absorbed orally, but can also be given intravenously. Dosing of azathioprine is usually 1–2 mg/kg in a single daily dose. The major toxicity seen with azathioprine is bone-marrow suppression. All precursors in the bone marrow may be affected, with neutropenia, anemia and thrombocytopenia being seen. Most commonly, neutropenia develops first in patients. Early in the course of azathioprine administration, white blood cell counts should be followed and dose adjustments made for patients whose white blood cell counts fall below 5000/mm³. Late toxicity of azathioprine is occasionally seen and includes red-cell aplasia, hepatitis and pancreatitis.

Mycophenolate mofetil (Cellcept)

Mycophenolate mofetil is an antimetabolite that was approved for clinical use in 1995. It competitively inhibits inositol monophosphate dehydrogenase, which is a critical enzyme in the purine salvage pathway. The use of mycophenolate mofetil exploits the fact that the purine salvage pathway is absolutely critical for purine biosynthesis in lymphocytes. Other mammalian cells are able to synthesize purines *de novo*, and thus are not affected by mycophenolate mofetil. DNA synthesis and cell division of T- and B- lymphocytes are markedly inhibited by mycophenolate (Cohn et al., 1999). Like azathioprine, mycophenolate is well absorbed orally, and the usual dose for adults is 1–2 g/day divided into two doses every 12 hours. In the pediatric population, little is known about adequate dosing and pharmacokinetics. Children are given a 600 mg/m² dose orally every 12 hours in divided doses for clinical immunosuppressive regimens. The principal toxicities of mycophenolate are gastrointestinal, including anorexia, nausea, vomiting, crampy abdominal pain and diarrhea. With high doses, bone-marrow suppression with anemia and neutropenia may develop (Chardot et al., 2001).

Cyclosporine

Cyclosporine is an intracellular fungal metabolite whose immunosuppressive activity was first identified in 1976. It was quickly brought to clinical use in the 1980s. Cyclosporine is a cyclic peptide consisting of 11 amino acids. The native compound is extremely hydrophobic and easily partitions into lipid membranes. Cyclosporine appears to impart specific immunosuppression by inhibiting T-lymphocyte activation events (Emmel et al., 1989; Ivery, 1999). This inhibition of early activation events results in a failure of helper T-cells to synthesize and release IL-2, a potent cytokine and inducer of cytotoxic T-cell activity. It appears that the site of action of cyclosporine is along the calcium-dependent activation pathway via the T-cell receptor, and it involves calcineurin, a calcium–calmodulin-dependent phosphatase, a cyclosporine-binding protein (cyclophilin) and the cyclosporine molecule. This cytoplasmic inhibition mechanisms prevents nuclear activation and the expression of early genes of cell activation, including the genes for IL-2 and IL-2 receptor. Cyclosporine may be administered intravenously or orally. It is poorly absorbed from the gastrointestinal tract and must be dissolved in oil. After absorption, cyclosporine is metabolized by the cytochrome P-450 system, resulting in an extensive number of both clinically active and inactive metabolites. Drugs that are similarly metabolized by or that alter the activity of cytochrome P-450 also alter the pharmacokinetics and levels of cyclosporine. The usual dose for solid organ transplantation patients is 10 mg/kg/day, administered orally and divided every 12 hours, or 5 mg/kg/day administered intravenously in three divided doses (every 8 hours) or as a continuous infusion. Trough levels of cyclosporine are monitored on a daily basis. Trough levels in the range 150–250 ng/mL are commonly acceptable levels for clinical organ transplantation, depending on the assay method used. Neoral, a micro-emulsion preparation of cyclosporine, may offer improved oral absorption and simpler dosing. Pharmacokinetic analysis demonstrates an improved area under the curve. Better oral absorption may provide improved immunosuppression, but may also increase toxicity. Intravenous administration may be necessary during the early post-transplant period.

Cyclosporine may be administered intravenously at 2 mg/kg/dose every 8 hours or by continuous infusion to achieve serum levels in the range 150–250 ng/mL. Toxic side-effects of cyclosporine include neurological symptoms (tremor, seizures), hypertension, hirsutism, hypercholesterolemia, hepatotoxicity and nephrotoxicity. All of these toxic side-effects are dose related, and many of them are alleviated by dose reduction.

Tacrolimus (Prograf)

Tacrolimus is a macrolide antibiotic derived from *Streptomyces tsukabiensis*. It has been shown to have potent immunosuppressive activity, apparently 100-fold more potent than that of cyclosporine. Like cyclosporine, tacrolimus inhibits early T-cell activation events. It also appears to affect the calcium–calmodulin–calcineurin axis, but has its own unique binding peptide (FK binding protein) to form a molecular complex with these compounds in the cytoplasm (Liu *et al.*, 1991). For all practical purposes, both cyclosporine and tacrolimus have the same mechanism of action, although there are subtle differences in the spectra of activity. Tacrolimus may be administered intravenously or given orally. It is rapidly absorbed from the gastrointestinal tract with good pharmacokinetic activity. Given this easy absorption, even with postopera-

tive ileus, most transplant centers rarely use intravenous tacrolimus. The adult oral dosage is 0.10 mg/kg/day divided every 12 hours, and pediatric patients are administered tacrolimus orally beginning at 0.15 mg/kg/day divided every 12 hours. Occasionally a patient requires intravenous administration. This is given either by continuous infusion or by intermittent doses of 0.05 mg/kg/day divided every 12 hours. Trough levels of tacrolimus are followed daily until they are stable. Individual pediatric patients can have widely disparate serum trough levels on standard dosing and, as a result, levels are required for optimal management. Trough levels in the range 5–10 ng/mL are initial targets, but higher levels should be obtained during rejection treatment and lower levels tolerated in stable patients. Tacrolimus is also metabolized by the cytochrome P-450 system in the liver, and dose adjustments should be made in patients with significant liver insufficiency. Patients may require a single daily dose or doses held for high trough levels or early liver dysfunction. As with cyclosporine, significant dose adjustments of tacrolimus may be necessary when it is used with other drugs that affect cytochrome P-450 activity. The principal toxicities of tacrolimus are neurological (tremor, seizures, nervousness, sleeplessness and nightmares), hypertension, gastric upset with nausea, vomiting, and diarrhea, hyperglycemia, hyperkalemia and nephrotoxicity. As with cyclosporine, most of these toxic side-effects are dose-related and they usually respond to dose adjustment. Guidelines for the use of tacrolimus in pediatric recipients have been published (Esquivel *et al.*, 1996).

Rapamycin

Rapamycin is a macrolide antibiotic similar to tacrolimus but derived from a different fungal species. Although it binds to FK binding protein, rapamycin probably does not significantly affect the calcium–calmodulin–calcineurin axis. It most probably affects a downstream activation event, and as a result is a potent inhibitor of late activation events. More specifically, rapamycin may have effects on a novel pathway that is critical for T-cell function independent of the T-cell-receptor activation cascade, and may inhibit calcium-independent cell activation events. The target of rapamycin is also required for B-cell antibody production and proliferation, which are thus inhibited by this drug (Abraham and Wiederrecht, 1964; Nave *et al.*, 1999; Peterson *et al.*, 1999).

Currently, rapamycin is being utilized in pediatric liver recipients as salvage therapy for patients with chronic or steroid-resistant rejection, and as substitute therapy for patients with complications of cyclosporine or tacrolimus treatment. There has been little experience with the use of rapamycin alone or in combination regimens for primary liver recipients.

Dosing in pediatric patients is not well documented. Patients receive 1 mg/m²/day as a single daily dose. A loading dose of three times the maintenance dose is given initially. Rapamycin levels are followed and doses adjusted to maintain trough levels in the range 5–10 ng/mL.

Adverse reactions that require dose adjustment include thrombocytopenia, hyperlipidemia, hypokalemia, hypertension, gastrointestinal distress and anemia.

Anti-CD3 (OKT3) monoclonal antibody

The OKT3 monoclonal antibody is a murine antibody raised against the human T-cell receptor (CD3) on human T-lymphocytes (McDiarmid et al., 1992; Bonnefoy-Berard and Revillard, 1996). This antibody binds directly to the T-cell receptor on the T-lymphocyte. After binding, cross-linking of receptors with complement deposition and direct cytotoxicity may occur. Alternatively, capping and internalization of the receptor after antibody binding may also serve to inhibit the activity of the affected T-lymphocyte. This is a non-specific action on all T-lymphocytes, because the T-cell receptor is present on all mature T-lymphocytes. The usual dose of OKT3 is 2.5 mg/day intravenously for patients under 20 kg body weight, and 5 mg/kg/day intravenously for patients weighing more than 20 kg. The white blood counts of patients are monitored, and circulating CD3 cells assessed in the blood. The percentage of CD3 lymphocytes in the blood should be less than 2–3% in order to achieve the therapeutic goal. Patients may require higher doses of OKT3 in order to achieve an adequate drop in circulating CD3 lymphocytes. Dose escalation to 7.5 mg or even 10 mg daily may occasionally be necessary. Patients who have had previous exposure to the OKT3 antibody may express antimurine antibodies, which block OKT3 activity directly. In this situation, higher intravenous doses of OKT3 may be necessary in order to overcome these inhibitory antibodies or other agents used. The principal toxicity of OKT3 is directly related to the intravenous administration of foreign protein. Fever, myalgia, stiff neck and headache are all seen, particularly during the first few days of administration. With the rapid lysis of T-cells after the initial doses of OKT3, a cytokine release syndrome may also develop, with secondary reactive pulmonary edema and respiratory distress. Patients may occasionally have a meningitis-like syndrome that requires cessation of treatment. Before OKT3 administration, patients are given corticosteroids, diphenhydramine and acetaminophen. They should also be assessed for fluid overload. Patients who are hypervolemic with potential for impending or early pulmonary edema should undergo diuresis or dialysis before receiving the first dose of OKT3, in order to prevent reactive pulmonary edema during cytokine release. Fluid restriction, dialysis, anti-inflammatories, antipyretics and antihistamines all serve to minimize patient symptoms.

Antithymocyte globulin (ATGAM)

Antithymocyte globulin is a polyclonal antibody, derived from horse sera, that is specific for human T-lymphocytes (Steininger et al., 1991). This agent is given intravenously in order to bring about rapid destruction of T-lymphocytes. The dosage is 15 mg/kg/day given as a single intravenous dose. Significant side-effects are related to the administration of a foreign protein, and patients are pretreated and treated in a similar way to those who are receiving OKT3.

Thymoglobulin

Like antithymocyte globulin, thymoglobulin is a polyclonal antibody. It is derived from rabbit sera. The agent is given intravenously, and the dose is 1.5 mg/kg/day given as a single dose (Gaber et al., 1998). Like OKT3 and ATGAM, thymoglobulin has significant systemic side-effects which must be alleviated during treatment.

Other monoclonal antibodies

ANTI-IL-2 RECEPTOR

Two anti-interleukin-2 receptors (CD25) antibodies are clinically available, namely basiliximab and daclizumab. Basiliximab is a mouse–human chimeric antibody, and daclizumab is fully humanized. The interleukin-2 receptor is found only on activated T-lymphocytes. Thus these agents inhibit only activated T-lymphocytes and have no effect on resting inactive T-cells (i.e. those cells that are not sensitized and responding to the allograft). Both agents have been used as part of induction protocols in renal transplant recipients to significantly decrease rejection episodes. The agents are now being utilized in liver transplant recipients. Basiliximab has been given to adults as a 20 mg/kg/day dose intravenously, while daclizumab is given intravenously at a dose of 1 mg/kg/day. Unlike anti-CD3 and the polyclonal antithymocyte globulins, these agents have minimal systemic or local infusion site side-effects. They may also be used repetitively, given little or no immunogenicity. They have been shown to be effective only at induction to decrease first rejection episodes. There have been no studies demonstrating efficacy in the treatment of established rejection.

TREATMENT STRATEGIES

Overview

All of the agents described above can be used alone or in combination to provide an adequate strategy to maintain a graft in the transplant recipient, with the goal of reduced rejection or toxicity. The general trend in therapy with the availability of more specific agents has been to minimize general non-specific agents and use combination therapies involving more specific agents. As further refined and more specific agents become available, therapies will be tailored to individual patient requirements (Kahan, 1992). Treatment strategies for clinical immunosuppression may be divided into three groups, namely induction, maintenance and treatment of rejection. Drug combination strategies and drug withdrawal plans also play an important role in immunosuppressive regimens for children in order to minimize acute toxicity and late effects (Kahan *et al.*, 1991).

Induction therapy

Induction therapy may be thought of as the immunosuppression that is administered to the patient at the time of implantation of the graft and for the first few weeks after transplantation. Induction therapy may simply involve the initiation of maintenance immunosuppressive therapy with a high-dose steroid pulse and taper after the implantation of the transplanted organ. More commonly it consists of the administration of an antithymocyte preparation (antilymphocyte globulin, OKT3 monoclonal or anti-IL-2-receptor antibodies) to provide potent T-cell inhibition or elimination of the sensitized T-lymphocyte at the initiation of the transplant procedure and engraftment. Box 29.2 outlines the pediatric induction protocol for clinical liver transplantation immunosuppression at Johns Hopkins Hospital. The advantage of induction therapy is that it provides potent and specific T-cell immunosuppression before sensitization of the recipient to the engrafted allo-antigens. Induction therapy is not universally practised in pediatric transplant recipients because of the potential complications that may attend the use of such potent immunosuppression. The incidence of opportunistic infections (viral, fungal and protozoal) and secondary malignancies (post-transplant lymphoproliferative disease) appears to be higher in patients who have received treatment with ATGAM or OKT3 monoclonal antibody. However, short courses of induction may not place the recipient at increased risk for these complications. In addition, as clinical experience with antithymocyte preparations increases, dose reductions will most probably be made. These reductions may serve to increase safety while at the same time preserving efficacy. More recently, the use of the specific anti-IL-2-receptor antibodies has been shown not to increase complications. In addition to these induction agents, the drugs planned for maintenance therapy are started as early as is clinically feasible.

Maintenance therapy

After induction therapy, whether this involves high-dose steroids and a taper or an antithymocyte preparation, maintenance therapy involves maintaining the program of conventional immunosuppression in order to prevent graft rejection. Conventional maintenance therapy has evolved over the years and now includes multiple immunosuppressive agents that are given in non-toxic doses. Historically, corticosteroids and azathioprine were used to maintain grafts after induction therapy. Cyclosporine was then added to the armamentarium for maintenance therapy. This triple-drug therapy using cyclosporine, azathioprine and prednisone is the commonest regimen for many transplant recipients. Triple-drug therapy permits lower doses of cyclosporine and azathioprine to be given, as well as allowing the use of low-dose steroids or every-other-day steroid therapy.

Since 1995, mycophenolate mofetil has been available for substitution for azathioprine in clinical immunosuppressive protocols. In stable liver transplant patients,

---

Box 29.2 *Immunosuppression protocols for pediatric liver transplant recipients at Johns Hopkins Hospital*

Induction

1 *Daclizumab (Zenapax)*: 1 mg/kg/dose given IV intraoperatively and on days 7, 14, 28 and 42.
2 *Corticosteroids*: 10 mg/kg/dose given intraoperatively and every day for 2 days, then decrease dose to 2 mg/kg/day every 2 days until 1 mg/kg/day.
3 *Mycophenolate mofetil (Cellcept)*: 600 mg/m^2/dose every 12 hours orally.
4 *Tacrolimus (Prograf)*: 0.15 mg/kg/dose every 12 hours orally to obtain trough levels of approximately 10 ng/mL (may need to withhold tacrolimus dosing at induction of significant liver or kidney dysfunction).

Maintenance

1 *Corticosteroids*: Gradual taper to 0.2–0.3 mg/kg/day oral prednisone by 3 months and every-other-day dosing by 6 months. The goal is corticosteroid withdrawal by 12 months.
2 *Tacrolimus*: Maintain trough levels at 5–7 ng/mL.
3 *Mycophenolate mofetil*: 600 mg/m^2/day for 6–12 months; may continue for problem rejection or to decrease dosing of other drug.

Rejection

1 Initial rejection episode.
 Corticosteroids: Methylprednisolone 10 mg/kg IV every day for 3 days, then taper to 2 mg/kg/day every until other day achieve 1 mg/kg/day and hold (may convert to oral prednisone during taper).
2 Persistent steroid-resistant rejection.
 OKT3 monoclonal antibody: 2.5–5.0 mg/day IV for 10–14 days (use 2.5 mg if the patient weighs < 20 kg and 5.0 mg if weight is > 20 kg).
 ATGAM polyclonal antibody: 15 mg/kg/day IV for 10–14 days.

cyclosporine may be discontinued and the recipient maintained on azathioprine or mycophenolate and every-other-day steroids. Alternatively, patients have been maintained on cyclosporine monotherapy with complete withdrawal of azathioprine/mycophenolate and steroids.

With the clinical introduction of tacrolimus, this potent agent rapidly gained popularity in maintenance therapy for liver transplant recipients. Tacrolimus-based therapy usually includes very-low-dose prednisone, but may also utilize azathioprine or mycophenolate. The potent activity of tacrolimus allows more rapid steroid withdrawal, and many patients can be maintained off steroids altogether with the use of tacrolimus. Box 29.2 also outlines the Johns Hopkins Hospital pediatric liver transplantation protocol for maintenance immunosuppression with tacrolimus.

Anti-rejection strategy

A number of strategies are available for the patient who undergoes an acute rejection episode. For typical patients, alteration in clinical graft function prompts a liver biopsy and pathological evaluation of the graft for rejection. The first-line treatment for rejection is a high-dose corticosteroid pulse (10 mg/kg/day for 2 to 3 days) and taper using methylprednisolone. Patients who fail to respond adequately to a steroid pulse may undergo a second steroid pulse or be placed on an antithymocyte preparation. Both OKT3 monoclonal antibody and antithymocyte polyclonal antibody preparations are available, and provide a potent treatment for rejection. More than 90% of patients will respond to corticosteroid pulse or antithymocyte preparations.

With the availability of tacrolimus, mycophenolate and rapamycin, a number of pediatric and adult patients have been treated for steroid- and cyclosporine-resistant rejection without the need for repeated steroid pulses and antithymocyte preparations. Conversion from one immunosuppressive drug combination to another may successfully treat acute rejection. In general, a combination of these approaches is adequate for the treatment of an acute rejection episode in most patients.

For the patient with chronic rejection, newer agents may be on the horizon to slow down or reverse the rejection process. In the liver transplant recipient whose organ has significant regenerative abilities, the use of high-dose tacrolimus appears to have some effect in reversing chronic rejection, if the patient is seen early in its course. With potent inhibitory action on B-lymphocytes, mycophenolate mofetil may play a future role in the treatment of chronic rejection. Similarly, rapamycin – which has a broader effect on T- and B-cell function – may help to decrease the incidence of chronic rejection and retransplantation.

Drug combinations

With the availability of a growing number of therapeutic agents which may prevent or treat rejection, the trend in clinical immunosuppression has been towards the use of multiple agents either sequentially (induction) or simultaneously (combination therapy). From a pharmacological viewpoint, combination therapy may allow for dose reduction, which may alter harmful drug toxicities or interactions with other medications. In addition, the combination use of agents that affect different points along the same cellular pathway of immune activation may lead to a more potent immunosuppression. Agents that affect different pathways often produce additive immunosuppressive effects.

These theoretical advantages have spurred the trend towards the use of combination therapies. Most centers have adopted some form of induction therapy using monoclonal or polyclonal antibodies followed by multidrug maintenance immunosuppression, and most of them use cyclosporine or tacrolimus (calcineurin inhibitors) in combination with an antimetabolite (azathioprine or mycophenolate) and corticosteroids (Cao et al., 1999; Renz et al., 1999; Colombani et al., 2000). The recent clinical availability of rapamycin may lead to drug regimens which eliminate the need for a calcineurin inhibitor. Box 29.2 summarizes the immunosuppressive protocol that is used at the Johns Hopkins Hospital for pediatric liver transplant recipients.

Immunosuppressive drug withdrawal

The alternative to multiple low-dose drug combinations is the use of more potent single immunosuppressive agents to allow the gradual withdrawal of other agents. This procedure is a common practice, and will continue to be used as more potent agents are developed. At present, multiple drugs are used early in the transplant patient's postoperative course. These combination drugs allow for a significant rejection-free stabilization period, as well as possible accommodation of the patient's immune system to the new organ. Over time, stable patients may have some of their immunosuppressive drugs withdrawn. In the pediatric age group, steroid withdrawal has been used clinically with success (Mckee et al., 1997). Both cyclosporine- and tacrolimus-based therapies allow for every-other-day steroids and potential steroid withdrawal. A certain percentage of patients who have steroids completely withdrawn will experience a late rejection episode, but these are usually well treated with reinstitution of pulse-and-taper steroids. Patients may subsequently undergo successful steroid withdrawal if cyclosporine and tacrolimus are maintained at higher serum levels.

Patients have also had their azathioprine and steroid treatment withdrawn, to be maintained on cyclosporine or tacrolimus alone as the sole immunosuppressive agent

(Mckee *et al.*, 1997; Varela-Fascinetto *et al.*, 1997). This cyclosporine or tacrolimus monotherapy requires slightly higher dosing with cyclosporine or tacrolimus. Although monotherapy avoids the use of steroids or long-term azathioprine, it may lead to long-term hypertension and nephrotoxicity related to the use of these drugs at higher levels. A recent trend in adult patients has been to switch to rapamycin therapy in order to avoid the nephrotoxic side-effects of cyclosporine or tacrolimus.

GENERAL COMPLICATIONS OF IMMUNOSUPPRESSION

Clinical immunosuppressive strategies involve striking a balance between freedom from rejection episodes and freedom from the toxicity and complications of immunosuppression. In simple terms, the more potent the immunosuppressive regimen, the fewer the number of rejection episodes, but the greater the likelihood of opportunistic infection, late malignancy and drug toxicity. Box 29.3 summarizes the general complications of immunosuppression.

The specific toxicities of the immunosuppressive drugs are described in the sections pertaining to each drug. In general, the goal of multidrug therapy is to decrease the toxicities of the drugs used. In addition, the more severe the toxicities that are seen with higher doses of these agents, the greater the likelihood of poor patient compliance with drug regimens, or more general difficulties with patients.

Opportunistic infections are problematic in patients who are undergoing significant chronic clinical immunosuppression. As the potency of the agents and the number of drugs used increase, so does the likelihood of opportunistic infections. These infections are particularly problematic for the pediatric recipient (Saint-Vil *et al.*, 1991). In general, the pediatric patient has not been exposed to a wide variety of bacterial, fungal or viral agents prior to transplantation. As a result, they have not had time or opportunity to develop specific immunity to many of these infectious agents, and consequently they are at risk for significant opportunistic infection, particularly from parasitic and viral pathogens. In the early post-transplant period, both bacterial and fungal infections have higher frequencies than in the adult population. Aggressive surveillance and vigilance for enteric pathogens and fungi are important. In addition, these patients are at risk for development of *Pneumocystis carinii* pneumonia. It is recommended that patients who are undergoing induction immunosuppression or rejection treatment with monoclonal or polyclonal antibodies receive antifungal and *Pneumocystis* prophylaxis with trimethoprim-sulfamethoxazole.

Viral infections are also problematic for the pediatric

Box 29.3 *Complications of immunosuppression*

Infection
Bacterial, fungal (*Staphylococcus* species, *Candida* species)
Protozoons (*Pneumocystis carinii*, toxoplasmosis)
Viral (cytomegalovirus, Epstein–Barr virus, herpes virus, varicella zoster virus, adenovirus)

Secondary malignancy
Post-transplant lymphoproliferative disorder (PTLD)
Kaposi's sarcoma
Other lymphoma/leukemia
Other primary cancers (skin, colon, breast, lung)

Toxicities
Corticosteroids: osteoporosis, avascular necrosis of femur, cataracts, gastritis
Azathioprine: neutropenia, red-cell aplasia, pancreatitis, hepatitis
Cyclosporine: hypertension, nephrotoxicity, hirsutism, hypercholesterolemia, neurotoxicity
Tacrolimus: hypertension, nephrotoxicity, neurotoxicity, hyperkalemia, insulin-dependent hyperglycemia
Rapamycin: hypertension, hyperlipidemia, thrombocytopenia, neutropenia
Mycophenolate: gastrointestinal upset, neutropenia

---

recipient. The typical pediatric organ transplant recipient is usually seronegative for cytomegalovirus (CMV) and other herpes viruses, such as herpes simplex virus type 1 (HSV-1), varicella zoster virus (VZV) and Epstein–Barr virus (EBV). All four of these viral pathogens can wreak havoc on the pediatric transplant recipient. Pediatric patients who receive a CMV-seropositive donor organ should undergo CMV prophylaxis with a specific anti-CMV immunoglobulin, intravenous ganciclovir, or both. Fortunately, the clinical prophylactic use of immunoglobulins and ganciclovir has markedly decreased the incidence of life-threatening CMV infections in pediatric organ transplant recipients (Hibberd and Rubin, 1991). Similarly, patients who are undergoing induction therapy or being treated for rejection with antithymocyte preparations should receive acyclovir prophylaxis for HSV-1 and VZV. Both of these herpes viruses can either produce a primary infection in naive recipients or reactivate infection in seropositive individuals. Treatment with intravenous acyclovir for HSV-1 and VZV is required for initial primary infections. EBV infection is also problematic with regard to the management of the post-transplantation organ recipient. Although 80% of the adult population are seropositive for EBV, few children are seropositive. EBV infection causes the mononucleosis syndrome, and EBV directly targets and transfects B-lymphocytes. The infected B-lymphocyte is 'transformed' in these patients into a state of continuous cell division, like a lymphoma or leukemia cell. In the immunologically normal patient in whom mononucleosis develops, there is a secondary effector T-cell response that eliminates these clones of immortalized B-cells. In the immunosuppressed patient, the EBV-transformed B-lymphocyte may continue to grow unchecked because the T-cell arm of the immune system is compromised by the drugs. The EBV-negative transplant recipient who receives either an EBV-positive donor organ or acquires EBV from the community may contract a significant EBV infection. The first phase is a mononucleosis syndrome, characterized by typical features of mononucleosis, including fever, chills, hepatosplenomegaly and lymphadenopathy. At this stage, the patient should be treated with acyclovir or ganciclovir, and immunosuppression tapered if possible. The patient may go on to manifest a polyclonal lymphoproliferative disorder secondary to the EBV transformation of B-lymphocytes and their unchecked proliferation. At this point, immunosuppression should be further reduced or discontinued. Finally, a monoclonal lymphoproliferative syndrome may develop in these patients, which is essentially a B-cell leukemia or lymphoma. With the development of an overt monoclonal lymphoproliferative syndrome, immunosuppression must be withdrawn. If the patient does not respond, he or she should receive chemotherapy to treat the lymphoma or leukemia (Hanto *et al.*, 1985; Kuo *et al.*, 1995). With active drug withdrawal, there is always a risk of loss of the organ due to rejection. Liver transplant recipients may need to be retransplanted if they go on to develop chronic rejection.

In addition to post-transplantation lymphoproliferative disease, other malignancies may develop in patients, as discussed below.

LATE EFFECTS OF IMMUNOSUPPRESSION

The long-term survival of liver transplant recipients requires lifelong treatment with immunosuppressive drugs. Despite the use of multiple agents in smaller doses, significant toxicities (both specifically and non-specifically related to the immunosuppression) occur. The primary long-term effects of corticosteroids include growth inhibition, Cushing's syndrome, osteoporosis, avascular femoral head necrosis, cataracts, glaucoma, cardiovascular disease and gastritis–peptic ulcer disease. The long-term effects of azathioprine include hepatitis, pancreatitis and red-cell aplasia. The long-term effects of cyclosporine include hypercholesterolemia, arteriosclerosis, hypertension and nephrotoxicity. The long-term effects of tacrolimus may include hypertension and nephrotoxicity, but it is too early to determine what other side-effects may develop over time.

The most serious long-term effects of immunosuppression are the late malignancies that may be seen in these patients. Kaposi's sarcoma may develop, as well as the post-transplantation lymphoproliferative diseases that are specific to chronically immunosuppressed patients. In addition, patients are at higher risk for the common malignancies that are seen in non-immunosuppressed patients. The commonest cancer seen in immunosuppressed patients is skin cancer, which mimics its frequency in the general population. Slightly higher incidences of Hodgkin's disease, non-Hodgkin's lymphoma, and breast, colon, lung, uterine and ovarian cancer have been seen in transplant recipients. For this reason, patients should undergo yearly cancer surveillance, including chest radiography, Pap smear and pelvic examination for women, and a general physical examination to look for new skin lesions (Penn, 1991).

In summary, significant progress has been made in developing effective immunosuppressive protocols in children undergoing liver transplantation. These protocols rely on combination therapy using multiple drugs at low dosage to prevent rejection, treat established rejection episodes and minimize the short-term toxicities and long-term complications of therapy.

Key references

Amos DB, Bach FH. Phenotypic expressions of the major histocompatibility locus in man (HLA): leukocyte antigens and mixed leukocyte culture reactivity. *Journal of Experimental Medicine* 1968; **128**: 623–37.

This is the classic paper describing the HLA locus and its critical role in alloreactivity and transplantation.

Esquivel CO, So SK, McDiarmid SV *et al.* Suggested guidelines for the use of tacrolimus in pediatric liver transplant patients. *Transplantation* 1996; **61**: 847–8.

This paper provides a useful guide to the safe use of tacrolimus. The paper summarizes the peculiarities of the pharmacokinetics and pharmacology of tacrolimus and strategies for avoiding over- and under-immunosuppression.

Klintmalm G. US Multicenter FK506 Liver Study Group: a comparison of tacrolimus (FK506) and cyclosporine for immunosuppression in liver transplantation. *New England Journal of Medicine* 1994; **331**: 1110–15.

This randomized clinical trial demonstrated the equivalence of immunosuppression and the comparative morbidity and mortality in liver transplant recipients of cyclosporine and tacrolimus.

Starzl TE, Klintmalm GBG, Porter KA, Iwatsuki S, Schroter GPJ. Liver transplantation with use of cyclosporin A and prednisone. *New England Journal of Medicine* 1981; **305**: 266–9.

This paper summarizes the successful use of cyclosporine and steroids for clinical liver transplant recipients.

REFERENCES

Abraham RT, Wiederrecht GJ. Immunopharmacology of rapamycin. *Annual Review of Immunology* 1996; **14**: 483–510.

Abraham C, Griffith J, Miller J. The dependence of leukocyte function-associated antigen-1/ICAM-1 interactions in T-cell activation cannot be overcome by expression of high-density TCR ligand. *Journal of Immunology* 1999; **162**: 4399–405.

Amos DB, Bach FH. Phenotypic expressions of the major histocompatibility locus in man (HLA): leukocyte antigens and mixed leukocyte culture reactivity. *Journal of Experimental Medicine* 1968; **128**: 623–37.

Armitage JM, Kormos RL, Griffith BP *et al.* The clinical trial of FK506 as primary and rescue immunosuppression in cardiac transplantation. *Transplantation Proceedings* 1991; **23**: 1149–52.

Batiuk TD, Kung L, Halloran PF. Evidence that calcineurin is rate-limiting for primary human lymphocyte activation. *Journal of Clinical Investigation* 1997; **100**: 1894–901.

Benjaminovitz A, Itescu S, Lietz K *et al.* Prevention of rejection in cardiac transplantation by blockade of the interleukin-2 receptor with a monoclonal antibody. *New England Journal of Medicine* 2000; **342**: 613–19.

Berlin-Rufenach C, Otto F, Mathies M *et al.* Lymphocyte migration in lymphocyte function-associated antigen (LFA)-1-deficient mice. *Journal of Experimental Medicine* 1999; **189**: 1467–78.

Bonnefoy-Berard N, Revillard JP. Mechanisms of immunosuppression induced by antithymocyte globulins and OKT3. *Journal of Heart and Lung Transplantation* 1996; **15**: 435–42.

Borel JF, Feurer C, Gubler HU, Stahelin H. Biological effects of cyclosporine A: a new antilymphocyte agent. *Agents and Actions* 1976; **6**: 468–75.

Brent L (ed.) *A history of transplantation immunology.* San Diego, CA: Academic Press, 1997.

Calne RY. The rejection of renal homografts: inhibition in dogs by 6-mercaptopurine. *Lancet* 1960; **1**: 417–18.

Cao S, Cox KL, Berquist W *et al.* Long-term outcomes in pediatric liver recipients: comparison between cyclosporin A and tacrolimus. *Pediatric Transplant* 1999; **3**: 22–6.

Chardot C, Nicoluzzi JE, Janssen M *et al.* Use of mycophenolate mofetil as rescue therapy after pediatric liver transplantation. *Transplantation* 2001; **71**: 224–9.

Cohn RG, Mirkovich A, Dunlap B *et al.* Mycophenolic acid increases apoptosis, lysosomes and lipid droplets in human lymphoid and monocytic cell lines. *Transplantation* 1999; **68**: 411–18.

Colombani PM, Lau H, Prabhakaran K *et al.* Cumulative experience with pediatric living related liver transplantation. *Journal of Pediatric Surgery* 2000; **35**: 9–12.

Cooper MD, Raymond DA, Peterson RDA *et al.* The functions of the thymus system and bursa system in the chicken. *Journal of Experimental Medicine* 1966; **123**: 75–102.

Cosimi AB, Colvin RB, Burton RC *et al.* Use of monoclonal antibodies to T-cell subsets for immunological monitoring and treatment in recipients of renal allografts. *New England Journal of Medicine* 1981; **305**: 308–14.

Dempster WJ. Kidney homotransplantation. *British Journal of Surgery* 1953; **40**: 447–65.

Dragun D, Lukitsch I, Tullius SG *et al.* Inhibition of intercellular adhesion molecule-1 with antisense deoxynucleotides prolongs renal isograft survival in the rat. *Kidney International* 1998; **54**: 2113–22.

Emmel EA, Verweij CL, Durand DB *et al.* Cyclosporine A specifically inhibits function of nuclear proteins involved in T-cell activation. *Science* 1989; **246**: 1617–20.

Esquivel CO, So SK, McDiarmid SV *et al.* Suggested guidelines for the use of tacrolimus in pediatric liver transplant patients. *Transplantation* 1996; **61**: 847–8.

Frantz B, Nordby EC, Bren G *et al.* Calcineurin acts in synergy with PMA to inactivate IkB/MAD3, an inhibitor of NF-κB. *EMBO Journal* 1994; **13**: 861–70.

Fung JJ, Todo S, Jain A *et al.* Conversion of liver allograft recipients from cyclosporine to FK506-based immunosuppression: benefits and pitfalls. *Transplant Proceedings* 1991; **23**: 14–21.

Gaber AO, First MR, Tesi RJ *et al.* Results of the double-blind, randomized, multicenter phase III clinical trial of thymoglobulin versus ATGAM in the treatment of acute graft rejection episodes after renal transplantation. *Transplantation* 1998; **66**: 29–37.

Gatti RA, Meuwissen HJ, Allen HD, Hong R, Good RA. Immunological reconstitution of sex-linked lymphopenic immunological deficiency. *Lancet* 1968; **2**: 1366–9.

Gibson T, Medawar PB. The fate of skin homografts in man. *Journal of Anatomy* 1943; **77**: 299–310.

Groth C, Backman L, Moralcs JM *et al.* For the Sirolimus Renal Transplant Study Group. Sirolimus (rapamycin)-based therapy in human renal transplantation: similar efficacy and different toxicity compared with cyclosporine. *Transplantation* 1999; **67**: 1036–42.

Hamburger J, Vaysse J, Crosnier J, Auvert J, Lalanne CL, Hopper J Jr. Renal homotransplantation in man after radiation of the recipient. *American Journal of Medicine* 1962; **32**: 854–71.

Hanto DW, Firizzera G, Gajl-Pezalska KJ *et al.* Epstein–Barr virus immunodeficiency and B-cell lymphoproliferation. *Transplantation* 1985; **39**: 461–72.

Hibberd PL, Rubin RH. Prevention of cytomegalovirus infection in the pediatric renal transplant recipient. *Pediatric Nephrology* 1991; **5**: 112–17.

Hitchings GH, Elion GB. The chemistry and biochemistry of purine analogs. *Annals of the New York Academy of Sciences* 1954; **60**: 195–9.

Hultsch T, Albers MW, Schreiber SL, Hohman RJ. Immunophilin ligands demonstrate common features of signal transduction leading to exocytosis or transcription. *Proceedings of the National Academy of Sciences of the USA* 1991; **88**: 6229–33.

Ivery M. A proposed molecular model for the interaction of CN with the CsA-CyPA complex. *Bioorganic and Medicinal Chemistry* 1999; **7**: 1389–402.

Kahan BD. Immunosuppressive therapy. *Current Opinion in Immunology* 1992; **4**: 553–60.

Kahan BD, Gibbons S, Tejpal N *et al.* Synergistic effect of the rapamycin–cyclosporin combination: median effect analysis of *in vitro* immune performances by human T-lymphocytes in PHA, CD3 and MLR proliferative and cytotoxic assay. *Transplant Proceedings* 1991; **23**: 1090–91.

Kissinger CR, Parge HE, Knighton DR *et al.* Crystal structure of human calcineurin and the human FKBP12-FK506–calcineurin complex. *Nature* 1995; **378**: 641–4.

Klintmalm G. US Multicenter FK506 Liver Study Group: a comparison of tacrolimus (FK506) and cyclosporine for immunosuppression in liver transplantation. *New England Journal of Medicine* 1994; **331**: 1110–15.

Kohler G, Milstein C. Continuous culture of fused cells secreting antibody of predefined specificity. *Nature* 1975; **256**: 495–7.

Kuo PC, Dafoc DC, Alfrey EJ *et al.* Post-transplant lymphoproliferative disorders and Epstein–Barr virus prophylaxis. *Transplantation* 1995; **59**: 135–8.

Levey RH, Medawar PB. Nature and mode of action of antilymphocytic antiserum. *Proceedings of the National Academy of Sciences of the USA* 1966; **56**: 1130–7.

Li Y, Li XC, Zheng XX *et al.* Blocking both signal 1 and signal 2 of T-cell activation prevents apoptosis of alloreactive T-cells and induction of peripheral allograft tolerance. *National Medicine* 1999; **5**: 1298–302.

Liu J, Farmer JD Jr, Lane WS *et al.* Calcineurin is a common target of cyclophilin–cyclosporin A and FKBP-FK506 complexes. *Cell* 1991; **66**: 807–15.

McDiarmid SV, Busittil RN, Terasaki P *et al.* OKT3 treatment of steroid-resistant rejection in pediatric liver transplant recipients. *Journal of Pediatric Gastroenterology and Nutrition* 1992; **14**: 86–92.

Mckee M, Mattei P, Schwarz K, Wise B, Colombani P. Steroid withdrawal in tacrolimus (FK506)-treated pediatric liver transplant recipients. *Journal of Pediatric Surgery* 1997; **32**: 973–5.

McNally JG, Muller WG, Walker D *et al.* The glucocorticoid receptor: rapid exchange with regulatory sites in living cells. *Science* 2000; **287**: 1262–5.

Medawar PB. The behavior and fate of skin autografts and skin homografts in rabbits. *Journal of Anatomy* 1944; **78**: 176–99.

Merrill JP, Murray JE, Harrison JH, Guild WR. Successful homotransplantation of the human kidney between identical twins. *Journal of the American Medical Association* 1956; **160**: 277–82.

Merrill JP, Murray JE, Harrison JH, Friedman EA, Dealy JB Jr Dammin GJ. Successful homotransplantation of the kidney between non-identical twins. *New England Journal of Medicine* 1960; **262**: 1251–63.

Murray JE, Sheil AGR, Moseley R, Knoght PR, McGavice JD, Dammin GJ. Analysis of the mechanism of immunosuppressive drugs in renal homotransplantation. *Annals of Surgery* 1964; **160**: 449–73.

Murray JE, Merrill JP, Harrison JH, Wilson RE, Dammin GJ. Prolonged survival of human-kidney homografts by immunosuppressive drug therapy. *New England Journal of Medicine* 1968; **268**: 1315–23.

Najarian JS, Simmons RL, Gewurz H, Moberg A, Merkel F, Moore GA. Antiserum to cultured human lymphoblasts: preparation, purification and immunosuppressive properties in man. *Annals of Surgery* 1969; **170**: 617–32.

Nashan B, Light S, Hardie IR *et al.* for the Daclizumab Double Therapy Study Group. Reduction of acute renal allograft rejection by daclizumab. *Transplantation* 1999; **67**: 110–15.

Nave BT, Ouwens DM, Withers DJ *et al.* Mammalian target of rapamycin as a direct target for protein kinase B: identification of a convergence point for opposing effects of insulin and amino-acid deficiency on protein translation. *Biochemistry Journal* 1999; **344**: 427–31.

Penn I. The changing pattern of post-transplant malignancies. *Transplant Proceedings* 1991; **23**: 1101–13.

Peterson RT, Desai BN, Hardwick JS, Schreiber SL. Protein phosphatase 2A interacts with the 70-kDa S6 kinase and is activated by inhibition of FKBP12-rapamycin-associated protein. *Proceedings of the National Academy of Sciences of the USA* 1999; **96**: 4438–42.

Renz JF, Lightdale J, Mudge C *et al.* Mycophenolate mofetil, microemulsion cyclosporine, and prednisone as primary immunosuppression for pediatric liver transplant recipients. *Liver Transplant Surgery* 1999; **5**: 136–43.

Saint-Vil D, Luks FI, Lebel P *et al.* Infectious complications of pediatric liver transplantation. *Journal of Pediatric Surgery* 1991; **26**: 908–13.

Starzl TE, Butz GW Jr. Surgical physiology of the transplantation of tissues and organs. *Surgical Clinics of North America* 1962; **42**: 55–67.

Starzl TE, Klintmalm GBG, Porter KA, Iwatsuki S, Schroter GPJ. Liver transplantation with use of cyclosporin A and prednisone. *New England Journal of Medicine* 1981; **305**: 266–9.

Starzl TE, Demetris AJ, Van Thiel DH. Medical progress: liver transplantation. *New England Journal of Medicine* 1989; **321**: 1014–22.

Steininger R, Muhlbacher F, Hamilton G *et al.* Comparison of CYA, OKT3 and ATG immunoprophylaxis in human liver transplantation. *Transplantation Proceedings* 1991; **23**: 2269–71.

Stellato C, Matsukura S, Fal A *et al.* Differential regulation of epithelial-derived C-C chemokine expression by IL-4 and the glucocorticoid budesonide. *Journal of Immunology* 1999; **163**: 5624–32.

Stepkowski SM, Chen H, Daloze P *et al.* Rapamycin, a potent immunosuppressive drug for vascularized heart, kidney and small bowel transplantation in the rat. *Transplantation* 1991; **51**: 22–6.

Sugimoto T, Stewart S, Guan KL. The calcium/calmodulin-dependent protein phosphatase calcineurin is the major Elk-1 phosphatase. *Journal of Biological Chemistry* 1997; **272**: 29415–18.

Terasaki PI (ed.) *History of HLA: ten recollections*. Los Angeles, CA: UCLA Tissue Typing Laboratory, 1990.

Varela-Fascinetto G, Treaey SJ, Vacanti JP. Approaching operational tolerance in long-term pediatric liver transplant recipients receiving minimal immunosuppression. *Transplantation Proceedings* 1997; **29**: 449–51.

Werlen G, Jacinto E, Xia Y, Karin M. Calcineurin preferentially synergizes with PKC-theta to activate JNK and IL-2 promoter in T-lymphocytes. *EMBO Journal* 1998; **17**: 3101–11.

Wicker LS, Boltz RC, Matt V. Suppression of B-cell activation by cyclosporine-A, FK506. *European Journal of Immunology* 1990; **20**: 2277–83.

Woodle ES, Xu D, Zivin RA *et al.* Phase 1 trial of a humanized Fe receptor nonbinding OKT3 antibody, huOKT3gamma 1 (Ala Ala) in the treatment of acute renal graft rejection. *Transplantation* 1999; **68**: 608–16.

30

Complications and their management

MARK D STRINGER

INTRODUCTION

This chapter focuses on the complications of orthotopic liver transplantation (OLT) in children and their treatment. Progress in all aspects of liver transplantation has helped to minimize these problems, so that many children are now discharged home within a few weeks of their operation. Many factors have a significant impact on eventual outcome, including patient selection (e.g. underlying diagnosis, urgency of the transplant, comorbidity) preoperative preparation, donor availability and selection, organ preservation and preparation, operative techniques, choice of immunosuppressive regimen, and the child's psychosocial background. Many of these aspects are discussed in detail in related chapters in this section (see Chapters 27 to 29).

If early graft function is good, early postoperative recovery is more likely to be straightforward. In contrast, significant graft dysfunction may rapidly result in a hemodynamically unstable patient with severe metabolic disturbance progressing to multi-organ failure. Good early graft function is manifested by the following:

- hemodynamic stability;
- early bile production;
- progressive improvement in base excess and arterial pH;
- falling serum lactate and international normalized ratio (INR);
- normal blood glucose;

Box 30.1 *An overview of postoperative complications after liver transplantation*

Primary non-function and poor early graft function
Hemorrhage (intra-abdominal, gastrointestinal)
Vascular complications:
    Hepatic artery thrombosis/stenosis/pseudoaneurysm
    Portal vein thrombosis/stenosis
    Venous outflow obstruction
Biliary complications: leaks and strictures
Bowel perforation/obstruction
Wound complications
Mismatch problems (size, ABO, cytomegalovirus, gender)
Respiratory complications
Renal failure
Acute/chronic rejection
Graft disease (transmission, recurrence, *de novo*, graft-vs.-host disease)
Complications of immunosuppressive therapy:
    Infection: bacterial, fungal, viral, etc.
    Drug toxicity/side-effects: hypertension, nephropathy, hyperlipidemia, diabetes mellitus, etc.
    Post-transplant lymphoproliferative disease
    Other malignancies
    Non-compliance
Nutritional complications
Neurological complications
Psychosocial problems

Donor complications after living-related liver transplantation

- serum aspartate transaminase (AST) levels of
  < 2000 IU/L on the first postoperative day, and halv-
  ing daily from 48 hours onward.

Anticipation of potential postoperative complications
is fundamental to their prevention and prompt treatment. For example, maintaining the hemoglobin concentration at 9–10 g/dL and the hematocrit below 35%
reduces the risk of hepatic artery thrombosis. Daily postoperative Doppler ultrasound examination of the
hepatic vasculature in the immediate postoperative
period can detect major vascular complications at a stage
when timely surgical intervention can salvage the graft.
Meticulous hygiene in the management of catheters and
intravenous lines may avoid life-threatening sepsis.

> **Box 30.2** *Potential factors contributing to primary non-function or poor early graft function*
>
> Donor-related factors:
>   Prolonged hypoxia or hypotension
>   Severe biochemical disturbance (e.g. plasma Na^+
>   > 155 mmol/L)
>   Prolonged intensive-care stay ($\geq$ 5 days)
>   Severe fatty liver
> Problems with organ retrieval or preservation
> Prolonged cold (> 16 hours) or warm (> 1 hour) ischemia
>   of the graft
> Profound reperfusion hypotension
> ABO incompatibility and other immunological factors

POST-TRANSPLANT COMPLICATIONS

There are numerous complications, both medical and
surgical, associated with solid organ transplantation
(Box 30.1). Although these will be discussed separately,
many of them are closely interrelated. The incidence of
surgical complications has declined steadily in recent
years in parallel with technical improvements, but reoperative surgery is none the less required in up to 50% of
children after cadaveric or living-related liver transplantation (Yandza *et al.*, 1992; Revillon *et al.*, 1999; Sieders
et al., 1999). Vascular, biliary and hemorrhagic complications account for most of these cases.

Primary non-function

Primary non-function (PNF) of the transplanted liver,
characterized by absent metabolic and synthetic activity, is uncommon and affects between 4% and 7% of
pediatric recipients (Achilleos *et al.*, 1999; Sieders *et
al.*, 1999; Migliazza *et al.*, 2000). A variety of factors
may contribute to PNF or poor early graft function.
These include adverse conditions in the donor prior to
organ retrieval, problems with organ procurement or
preservation, and complications following implantation (Box 30.2) (Ploeg *et al.*, 1993; Zamboni *et al.*,
2001). Recipient factors are less important (Ploeg *et
al.*, 1993).

Signs of poor graft function include hemodynamic
instability requiring inotrope support, persistent or
increasing acidosis, and bleeding due to persistent coagulopathy. A postoperative INR of > 4 and first-day AST
levels of > 2000 IU/L indicate severe graft dysfunction,
but even grafts with AST levels of > 5000 IU/L may
recover and be associated with good long-term graft
function (Muiesan and Heaton, 1998). The arterial
ketone body ratio has been used to predict graft recovery
in children. The liver is the only organ that is capable of
producing ketone bodies from acetyl-CoA derived from

fatty acid oxidation. Poor early graft function is reflected
by a ratio of < 0.7, whilst a value of > 1.0 within 40 hours
of reperfusion is associated with a good outcome.
However, the specificity of this test is less than 80%, limiting its value in clinical practice (Kitabayashi *et al.*,
1998). The only treatment for primary non-function is
urgent retransplantation, and 1-year survival rates in this
group of patients are less than 50%.

Hemorrhage

Postoperative intra-abdominal bleeding occurs in
approximately 5–10% of patients. Risk factors include
poor graft function, renal failure, high intraoperative
blood loss, and technical variant grafts (reduced or split
livers). Correction of coagulopathy or a low platelet
count will often secure hemostasis. Persistent bleeding
from the cut surface of a reduced or split liver graft may
be due to venous outflow obstruction. Occasionally,
parenchymal injury of the liver allograft is a cause of
bleeding in adults (Soliman *et al.*, 2000), but this is rarely
encountered in children, in whom smaller, non-steatotic
grafts are used. Major intra-abdominal hemorrhage
requires prompt re-exploration once acidosis, coagulopathy and hypothermia have been corrected. In many
cases no specific bleeding point is identified after evacuation of blood clots, but the release of any abdominal
tamponade helps to avoid additional complications such
as renal and respiratory failure. Excessive blood loss has
been identified as a factor that adversely affects graft and
patient survival.

Gastrointestinal bleeding may occur from a variety
of sources after orthotopic liver transplantation,
including the enteric anastomosis (after Roux-en-Y
loop construction), gastroduodenal ulceration, infective enteritis and hemobilia. Ulcers from recent
esophageal injection sclerotherapy may bleed or perfo-
rate (Vickers *et al.*, 1989).

Vascular complications

HEPATIC ARTERY THROMBOSIS

In the denervated transplanted liver there are initially no collateral arterial pathways, and the normally reciprocal blood flow between the portal vein and the hepatic artery is lost. After clamping the hepatic artery, compensatory flow in the portal vein is inadequate to restore normal blood flow to the graft (Payen *et al.*, 1990). The transplanted liver is therefore uniquely dependent on hepatic arterial inflow, particularly in the early postoperative period. Hepatic artery thrombosis (HAT) is a major cause of graft loss and mortality after pediatric liver transplantation. The incidence of this complication is between 7% and 17% in large cadaveric programs (Tan *et al.*, 1988; Lopez Santamaria *et al.*, 1996; Rela *et al.*, 1996; Shackleton *et al.*, 1997; Mazariegos *et al.*, 1999; Migliazza *et al.*, 2000; Sieders *et al.*, 2000a). HAT is less frequent after living-related liver transplantation (Inomoto *et al.*, 1996), which may be due to the use of microvascular anastomotic techniques, immunological factors and short cold ischemic times. In recent years, the introduction of similar microsurgical techniques into cadaveric transplantation has reduced the incidence of HAT (Goss *et al.*, 1998). In small children (< 5 years) the incidence of HAT in reduced or split grafts is significantly less than that in whole grafts (Stevens *et al.*, 1992; Rela *et al.*, 1996). A whole graft with recipient hepatic arterial inflow is a particularly high-risk situation in a small child, and such grafts are often better supplied by an arterial conduit from the aorta. There is an unacceptably high incidence of HAT in grafts from donors under 3 months of age (Yokoyama *et al.*, 1992).

A large number of potential risk factors for HAT have been identified, and these are summarized in Box 30.3. The clinical presentation of HAT encompasses a spectrum of manifestations, ranging from graft necrosis with acute liver failure to asymptomatic thrombosis with minimally disturbed liver function. In between these extremes, HAT may be associated with septicemia, biliary leakage or stricture, cholangitis, liver abscess, or an insidious onset with fever and graft dysfunction.

Color Doppler sonography is particularly valuable for the detection of hepatic arterial complications after orthotopic liver transplantation (Gaetano *et al.*, 2000). The complete absence of an arterial signal at the porta hepatis and within the liver suggests HAT. A *tardus parvus* waveform (prolonged systolic acceleration time and low flow velocity) at the porta hepatis or in the intrahepatic arteries indicates significant impairment of hepatic arterial perfusion, usually as a result of either arterial stenosis (when it may be accompanied by turbulent distal flow in the main arterial trunk) or thrombosis. This requires further investigation by angiography (Figure 30.1). False-negative results from Doppler sonography may occur in children in cases where collat-

---

Box 30.3 *Risk factors for the development of hepatic artery thrombosis after OLT*

Surgical

Small vessel size (especially recipients < 3 years or < 15 kg or donors < 3 months)

Technical failure (excess length or angulation, faulty suture technique, intimal dissection during graft preparation or implantation)

Multiple donor hepatic arteries

Multiple transplants

Arterial anastomosis to a previous aortic conduit?

Medical

Thrombophilia

Overzealous correction of intraoperative coagulopathy

Elevated hematocrit (PCV > 35%)

Severe acute rejection with increased hepatic arterial resistance (decreases diastolic blood flow)

Prolonged cold ischemia

Cytomegalovirus mismatch (D+/R–)

ABO-incompatible graft

Tan et al., *1988; Tisone* et al., *1988; Yanaga* et al., *1989; Stevens* et al., *1992; Yokoyama* et al., *1992; Rela* et al., *1996; Shackleton* et al., *1997; Mazariegos* et al., *1999; Migliazza, 2000; Oh* et al., *2001; Pastacaldi* et al., *2001*

---

eralization has restored the intrahepatic arterial waveform, and angiography should be performed if there is strong clinical suspicion of hepatic arterial insufficiency, even in the presence of an apparently normal Doppler examination (Hall *et al.*, 1990).

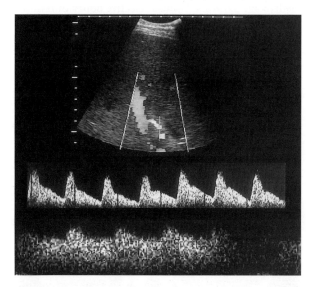

Figure 30.1 *Doppler ultrasound scan of the hepatic artery after liver transplantation. The artery is localized using color Doppler and the arterial waveform is recorded. The upper horizontal trace shows a normal arterial waveform, whilst the lower trace demonstrates a* tardus parvus *waveform suggestive of hepatic artery stenosis (see Figure 30.3).*

The speed of onset and timing of HAT are two of the factors that are likely to be paramount in determining the extent of graft necrosis (and ultimately graft survival). Collateral arterialization may develop as early as 3 weeks after OLT, and may be sufficient to sustain the graft after HAT (Hall *et al.*, 1990; Stringer *et al.*, 2001). Treatment options after HAT include early revascularization, urgent retransplantation or, in some cases, a conservative approach. If HAT is detected within the first few days after OLT, early revascularization before the onset of extensive necrosis may salvage the graft (Langnas *et al.*, 1991; Stevens *et al.*, 1992; Garcia-Gallont *et al.*, 1999). If this is inappropriate or unsuccessful, urgent retransplantation is usually necessary. Retransplantation for HAT is associated with a patient survival rate of 50–70% (Stevens *et al.*, 1992; Stringer *et al.*, 2001). In some centers, hyperbaric oxygen has been used to provide a bridge to retransplantation (Mazariegos *et al.*, 1999). Conservative management is possible in patients without evidence of irreversible liver failure, extensive graft necrosis and/or uncontrolled sepsis. This is more likely in patients who have received reduced or split livers than in those with whole grafts, which may reflect the earlier development of substantial bridging collateral vessels in grafts with a cut surface. Critical to successful conservative management is expert radiological assessment and intervention, particularly in managing biliary strictures and intrahepatic abscesses. Computed tomographic scanning is a useful adjunctive investigation when defining the presence and extent of graft necrosis (Figure 30.2). In the King's College Hospital series of pediatric liver transplants, there were 31 (7.8%) confirmed instances of HAT in 29 children of median age 3.8 years. Using a selective policy of retransplantation, revascularization and conservative treatment, 83% of children survived HAT complicating OLT,

and approximately 40% survived without retransplantation (Stringer *et al.*, 2001).

There is no consensus about the role of heparin or aspirin in the prevention of HAT after OLT (Salt *et al.*, 1992; Wolf *et al.*, 1997; Sieders *et al.*, 2000a). Most pediatric centers use one or both of these agents prophylactically.

HEPATIC ARTERY STENOSIS

Hepatic artery stenosis after OLT is uncommon, usually occurs at the site of anastomosis, and may cause graft dysfunction or be associated with biliary complications. The cause may be technical, immunological or a result of intimal hyperplasia, when it usually presents as a late complication after OLT. Hepatic artery stenosis may be suspected from Doppler studies, but angiography is required to confirm the diagnosis and quantify the degree of narrowing (Figure 30.3). Hemodynamically significant stenoses that occur more than 2 weeks after OLT can be effectively treated by percutaneous transluminal angioplasty (Mondragon *et al.*, 1994).

PSEUDOANEURYSM

A pseudoaneurysm affecting the arterial inflow to the graft is a rare but potentially devastating complication after OLT (Bonham *et al.*, 1999). It may develop after conventional hepatic arterial reconstruction or affect an aortic conduit. Although rare, this complication has been reported more often in association with supraceliac conduits (Marcucci *et al.*, 1999; Verzaro *et al.*, 2001). The

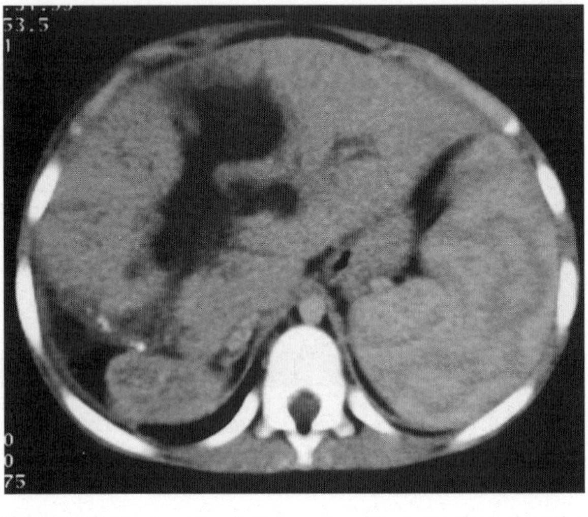

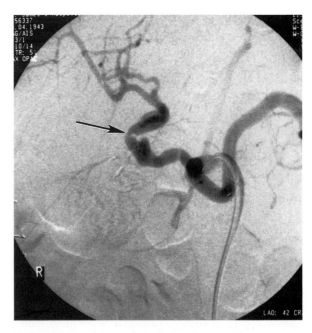

Figure 30.3 *Anastomotic stenosis of the hepatic artery 5 days after transplantation of a whole graft in a teenager. The anastomosis was revised surgically with a successful outcome. An intraoperative liver biopsy demonstrated severe acute cellular rejection which may have exacerbated the stenosis.*

Figure 30.2 *A computed tomographic scan demonstrating extensive graft necrosis after hepatic artery thrombosis. This patient was successfully retransplanted.*

predominant cause is intra-abdominal bacterial infection or fungal sepsis (mycotic aneurysms), but technical failure and anatomical defects account for some cases. Pseudoaneurysm formation may be asymptomatic, cause mild abdominal discomfort and fever, or result in catastrophic bleeding. Angiography is used to define the aneurysm (Figure 30.4). Prompt treatment with antimicrobial therapy and either ligation or (preferably) excision and revascularization of the graft is necessary in order to avoid fatal rupture; retransplantation may be the only solution in some cases.

PORTAL VEIN THROMBOSIS/STENOSIS

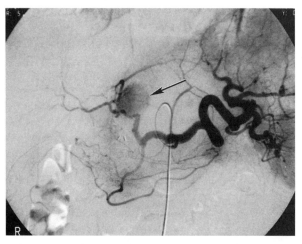

Figure 30.4 *A pseudoaneurysm of the hepatic artery in an adult following liver transplantation. There was no evidence of fungal infection. The aneurysm was excised and the graft was revascularized via an aortic conduit.*

The incidence of portal vein thrombosis (PVT) after pediatric OLT is very variable, ranging from 1% to 10% (Millis *et al.*, 1996; Cacciarelli *et al.*, 1997; Chardot *et al.*, 1997; Goss *et al.*, 1998; Sieders *et al.*, 2000a). Recognized factors predisposing to this complication are summarized in Box 30.4. Children who are transplanted for biliary atresia are particularly at risk because their main portal vein tends to be narrow. Chardot *et al.* (1997) reported 16 PVTs and three portal vein stenoses during a median follow-up period of 50 months in 96 children with biliary atresia undergoing 115 transplants, representing a portal vein complication rate of 16.5%. Almost all of the episodes of PVT occurred within 2 weeks of transplantation.

The presenting features of PVT occurring soon after transplantation include a prolonged prothrombin time, a rise in AST and, in severe cases, a persistent metabolic acidosis. Doppler ultrasound is both sensitive and specific in diagnosis. Urgent re-exploration, thrombectomy and revision of the portal vein anastomosis will often rescue the graft, but retransplantation is usually necessary if this is unsuccessful (Bilik *et al.*, 1992; Hamada *et al.*, 1995; Millis *et al.*, 1996; Chardot *et al.*, 1997; Sieders

---

> **Box 30.4** *Risk factors for the development of portal vein thrombosis after OLT*
>
> Narrow-caliber portal vein (< 4 mm) (e.g. biliary atresia with cirrhosis)
> Infants and small children
> Split-liver grafts
> Large-for-size grafts (graft-to-body weight ratio > 3%)
> Hypercoagulability
> Technical (e.g. anastomotic stenosis, kinking, torsion, excess tension, cryopreserved venous conduits)
> Concomitant splenectomy
> Composite interposition grafts
> Preoperative portal vein thrombosis
> Portosystemic shunts: e.g. unligated large spontaneous shunts
> High intra-abdominal pressure
>
> *Payen* et al., *1990; Chardot* et al., *1997; Kiuchi* et al., *1999; Lyass* et al., *2000*

et al., 2000a). Aspirin may have a protective role in PVT (Chardot *et al.*, 1997).

In recent years, late portal vein complications have been increasingly reported after cadaveric and living-related liver transplantation in children (Lee *et al.*, 1996; Millis *et al.*, 1996; Funaki *et al.*, 1997). The problem is recognized by the onset of portal hypertension with variceal hemorrhage and/or increasing splenomegaly. The underlying cause of portal vein thrombosis or, more frequently, stenosis in these cases may be technical or related to growth and remodeling of the segmental graft, or it may be secondary to other factors, such as rejection or biliary tract infection (Figure 30.5). The risks of both early and late portal vein thrombosis and stenosis may be

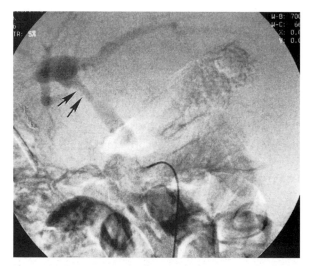

Figure 30.5 *Late portal vein stenosis in a 3-year-old girl following a left lateral segment liver transplant in infancy. She developed increasing splenomegaly and variceal bleeding and was managed with a Rex shunt.*

higher after living related transplantation than for reduced or split cadaveric grafts (Millis *et al.*, 1996). Possibly the short length of donor left portal vein is a contributory factor in such cases. Use of cadaveric cryopreserved donor iliac or femoral vein contributes further to the risk of late thrombosis. The problem of late portal vein stenosis may be largely avoidable in children with biliary atresia and a narrow portal vein undergoing transplantation with a reduced size cadaveric graft. In such cases the donor left portal vein can either be anastromosed to the recipient's superior mesenteric/splenic vein confluence (Shaw *et al.*, 1985) or a segment of donor iliac vein can be interposed between the two.

Although portal vein complications contribute to post-transplant morbidity, overall 5-year graft and patient survival rates are not markedly decreased (Chardot *et al.*, 1997). Many children with late-onset portal vein obstruction develop a venous collateral circulation and remain well in the short term. For those with symptomatic portal hypertension, treatment options include interventional radiology (balloon dilatation or stenting of the portal vein), direct revisional surgery, portosystemic shunting or conventional management of the consequences of portal hypertension (e.g. banding of esophageal varices). In one series from France, percutaneous transhepatic portal vein recanalization and endoluminal angioplasty were successful in 6 out of 10 transplanted children with PVT (Tissieres *et al.*, 2000). Similar success rates have been reported following percutaneous transhepatic portal venoplasty for portal vein stenosis, although most of these patients require intravascular stenting rather than angioplasty alone (Funaki *et al.*, 1997). Post-shunt encephalopathy has now been reported in two children with PVT complicating OLT. In one child, fatal encephalopathy developed 2.5 years after a mesocaval shunt, and in the other encephalopathy was noted 6 months after OLT in association with a large spontaneous splenorenal shunt (Tissieres *et al.*, 2000). A further option is the Rex mesenterico–left portal venous bypass, which is an attractive alternative as it restores hepatopetal portal blood flow (see Chapters 21 and 22) (de Ville de Goyet *et al.*, 1998a).

Nodular regenerative hyperplasia in the graft, which may occur as a complication of azathioprine treatment, is a further cause of late portal hypertension in adults (Gane *et al.*, 1994). In the majority of cases the disorder improves on withdrawal of the drug, but a small group of patients develop progressive graft failure.

VENOUS OUTFLOW OBSTRUCTION

This is a relatively rare event after OLT, and is usually due to technical problems. In most units, the frequency of this complication is less than 5% with segmental liver grafts, and even less with whole grafts. An incidence of 4% has been reported after living-related liver transplantation (Egawa *et al.*, 1997a). Venous outflow obstruction

occurs as a consequence of suprahepatic caval anastomotic stenosis or thrombosis, or compression or torsion of hepatic vein(s). Graft remodeling with hepatic vein distortion may contribute to late-onset cases. Venous outflow complications are associated with significant morbidity and mortality (Mazariegos *et al.*, 2000).

Presentation is usually with acute Budd–Chiari syndrome (i.e. a combination of abdominal pain, ascites, hepatomegaly, pericardial and pleural effusions, lower trunk and leg edema, signs of portal hypertension, coagulopathy and renal impairment). Doppler ultrasound and cavography with pressure measurements confirm the diagnosis (Figure 30.6). An underlying prothrombotic

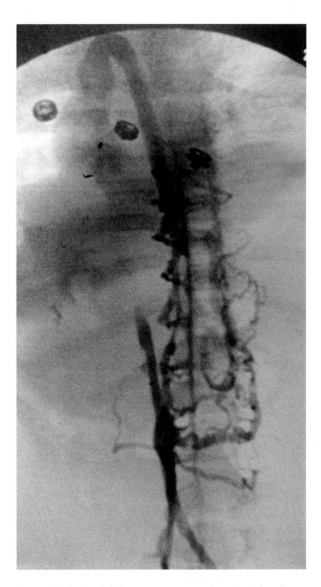

Figure 30.6 *An inferior vena cavogram demonstrating thrombotic caval occlusion after segmental liver transplantation in a 2-year-old boy. Note the collateral veins draining to the azygos system. Thrombus was identified within the retrohepatic cava and left hepatic vein. Treatment was by interventional radiological techniques and anticoagulation, which led to a resolution of the acute Budd–Chiari syndrome.*

state should be considered if a technical cause is not apparent. Various therapeutic alternatives are available, including interventional radiology, surgery (which may involve retransplantation) and thrombolysis and/or anti-coagulation. Early hepatic vein thrombosis due to torsion of a segmental graft may be salvaged by urgent thrombectomy and fixation of the liver (Sieders *et al.*, 2000a). Percutaneous balloon dilatation or stenting may lead to a dramatic resolution of the venous obstruction, sufficient to precipitate acute cardiac failure. After stenting, long-term patency is a cause for concern (Mazariegos *et al.*, 2000). Late-onset cases are best managed initially by balloon angioplasty (Egawa *et al.*, 1997b).

In segmental liver transplantation, venous outflow obstruction is largely preventable by technical modifications – using a short segment of hepatic vein, a triangular anastomosis, and securing the falciform ligament of the graft to the anterior abdominal wall (Emond *et al.*, 1993b).

Biliary complications

Biliary drainage in children undergoing liver transplantation is usually achieved with a Roux-en-Y hepatico-jejunostomy, although a duct-to-duct anastomosis is sometimes used in older children who are receiving a whole graft (see Chapter 28). Biliary complications are relatively frequent, with an average incidence of approximately 10% (range 5–30%) and a small but significant mortality (Heffron *et al.*, 1992; Lallier *et al.*, 1993; Chaib *et al.*, 1994; Bhatnagar *et al.*, 1995; Chardot *et al.*, 1997; Goss *et al.*, 1998; Reichert *et al.*, 1998; Sieders *et al.*, 1999). The risk of biliary complications with whole grafts, reduced or split livers, and after living-related liver transplantation, appears to be similar (Heffron *et al.*, 1992; Lallier *et al.*, 1993; Egawa *et al.*, 1998). Hepatic artery thrombosis has been reported to be responsible for up to 25% of all biliary complications (Peclet *et al.*, 1994), and should be specifically excluded in all cases.

Bile leaks occur early in the postoperative period, and may arise from the biliary anastomosis, the cut surface of a technical variant graft, or an unrecognized or abnormal segmental duct. The patient is usually febrile with mild graft dysfunction, and may go on to develop biliary peritonitis. Cut-surface leaks often settle with drainage alone, whereas more complex leaks may require ultrasound-guided percutaneous drainage with or without endoscopic or percutaneous cholangiography and stenting. Surgical reconstruction can be avoided in the majority of cases.

Most biliary strictures occur within 1 year of transplantation and present with cholangitis or obstructive jaundice. Gamma-glutamyl transferase is the most sensitive biochemical marker of bile duct obstruction. Ultrasonography will usually reveal dilated bile ducts proximal to the biliary stricture, which in early cases will respond to balloon dilatation with or without temporary stenting (Figure 30.7). Anastomotic biliary strictures presenting 6 months or more after OLT tend to recur after dilatation, and almost invariably require surgical revision. Non-anastomotic biliary strictures are less common and usually present late. Multiple intrahepatic strictures are associated with hepatic artery thrombosis, prolonged cold ischemia or ABO-incompatible transplants. Intraductal stones and bile plugs may form within the damaged ducts and cause recurrent cholangitis. Treatment with ursodeoxycholic acid, antibiotics and percutaneous stricture dilatation may be helpful, but the majority of these cases require retransplantation.

Bowel perforation/obstruction

These complications develop in approximately 5–10% of patients, but the incidence is higher in children with biliary atresia who have undergone a previous portoenterostomy (Shaked *et al.*, 1993; Chardot *et al.*, 1997; Goss *et al.*, 1998; Vilca-Melendez *et al.*, 1998). Perforations occur in the small bowel and Roux loop more commonly

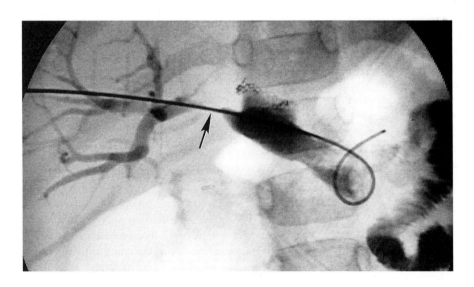

Figure 30.7 *A post-transplant stricture at the biliary–enteric anastomosis successfully treated by percutaneous balloon dilatation. Hepatic artery stenosis/ thrombosis must always be excluded in such cases.*

than in the large bowel. Roux loop perforations accounted for 62% of all cases in the UCLA series (Shaked *et al.*, 1993), but only 23% in the King's College series (Vilca-Melendez *et al.*, 1998). Duodenal perforations are particularly hazardous. Factors which predispose to bowel perforation include previous upper abdominal surgery (including retransplantation), cytomegalovirus (CMV) infection, and malnutrition. There is less agreement about the role of corticosteroid therapy and a prolonged portal venous cross-clamp time (Soubrane *et al.*, 1995). Lymphoproliferative disease is an additional cause of late perforation.

Intestinal perforation usually manifests in the second week after OLT, and the clinical features, which may be partially masked by immunosuppression, include fever, leukocytosis, abdominal distension and tenderness. Contaminated abdominal drain fluid and/or free air on a plain abdominal radiograph are generally diagnostic. Ultrasound and computed tomography are useful investigations in those presenting with features of sepsis and few abdominal signs.

Most perforations are adequately treated by local excision and repair of healthy vascular tissues, but intestinal resection or an enterostomy is occasionally required. Most patients suffer no long-term sequelae, but there is a high incidence of reperforation of the bowel, either at the same or a distant site, and this is associated with a significant mortality (Shaked *et al.*, 1993). Fungal sepsis is particularly hazardous and should be treated aggressively. The mortality from intestinal perforation may be reduced by adopting a low threshold for surgical re-exploration in patients with suspicious clinical signs.

Mechanical bowel obstruction is rarely encountered, and may be due to factors that are avoidable (e.g. Roux loop obstruction or internal hernias associated with mesenteric defects) or unavoidable (e.g. intra-abdominal adhesions).

Wound complications

Wound infections after OLT in children are uncommon despite immunosuppressive therapy. Incisional hernias and dehiscence are essentially technical failures, but primary fascial closure is not always possible with large-for-size grafts. In the presence of large-volume ascites, wound problems can be minimized by the placement of large-caliber drains. Post-transplant ascitic losses tend to resolve rapidly unless there is evidence of hepatic or portal venous obstruction, poor graft function or chylous ascites. Albumin, immunoglobulins and clotting factors may need to be replaced if losses are persistent.

Mismatch problems

A variety of different mismatch issues can lead to complications after OLT. Minor size discrepancies are not important, as the volume of the transplanted liver tends to converge towards the normal standard liver volume with time, regardless of whether the initial graft was small or large (Kawasaki *et al.*, 1992). However, major size mismatch may lead to complications. Reduced or split-liver grafts (technical variant grafts) have largely overcome the commonest difficulty, namely that of transplanting too large a graft into infants and small children. Thus an infant can accept a left lateral segment from a donor weighing 10 to 15 times more than his or her own body weight. An even greater increase in this ratio is possible after non-anatomical reduction of a left lateral segment, or by using a monosegmental graft (e.g. segment 3) (Srinivasan *et al.*, 1999). The donor:recipient weight ratio for a left lobe graft is about 3:1. Despite this flexibility, there are occasions when a graft is too large for the recipient and attempted closure of the abdominal wall incurs risks of partial liver necrosis, vascular insufficiency or thrombosis (Payen *et al.*, 1990), wound dehiscence and respiratory compromise. In such cases, either skin closure alone or repair with prosthetic material, with or without delayed primary closure 1 to 2 weeks later, is advisable (de Ville de Goyet *et al.*, 1998b).

Small-for-size grafts pose a different set of problems. In healthy adults, the liver accounts for 2–3% of the total body weight, but this proportion is higher in children. Experience with living-donor liver transplantation has shown that the minimum safe graft:recipient weight ratio is 0.8%. For cadaveric transplantation, where the graft is less optimal, this should be at least 1%. A left lateral segment graft (Couinaud segments 2 and 3) generally weighs 200–300 g and is therefore suitable for a child weighing < 30 kg. A left lobe graft (Couinaud segments 2, 3 and 4) weighs approximately 300–500 g and can therefore be transplanted into recipients weighing up to 50 kg. Small-for-size grafts from living-related donors (< 1.0%) tend to be associated with delayed resolution of pretransplant cholestasis, a higher prothrombin time, higher AST levels in the early post-transplant period, and more frequent hemorrhagic complications (Kiuchi *et al.*, 1999). Graft survival rates are reduced.

Most liver transplants are either ABO-identical or ABO-compatible (e.g. group O donor and group A or B recipient). The latter are associated with a small risk of ABO alloantibody-mediated hemolysis towards the end of the first postoperative week (Angstadt *et al.*, 1987). This is usually self-limiting provided that the patient is supported with donor-type blood transfusions; plasmapheresis is rarely required. Several centers have described the outcome of children with ABO-incompatible transplants. Lo *et al.* (1994) reported their experience of emergency liver transplantation with ABO-incompatible allografts. One-year graft and patient survival rates were less than 50%, and were particularly poor in patients who were not of blood group O. They noted a significantly higher incidence of rejection (including antibody-mediated hyperacute rejection), hepatic artery thrombosis and biliary stricture in such cases. They concluded that the use of an ABO-incompatible graft is only justified in patients of blood group O in an emergency when no other donor is available. Others have reported apparently satisfactory results after ABO-incompatible transplants in infants of blood group O who lack ABO alloantibodies at the time of transplant (Yandza *et al.*, 1994).

Gender mismatch and CMV mismatch are both considered in subsequent sections of this chapter.

Respiratory complications

Right-sided pleural effusions, basal pulmonary atelectasis and an elevated right hemidiaphragm are common respiratory complications after OLT, and these usually resolve without specific intervention. Perioperative chest physiotherapy and adequate analgesia are useful both prophylactically and therapeutically. Rarely, small children develop a right-sided diaphragmatic paralysis secondary to phrenic nerve injury either from vascular clamping of the suprahepatic vena cava or from local diathermy (Smyrniotis *et al.*, 1998). This causes an inability to wean from the ventilator in association with right-sided pulmonary atelectasis/infection. Paradoxical diaphragmatic movement is seen with fluoroscopy or real-time ultrasound. This complication can be successfully treated by diaphragmatic plication.

Renal failure

Minor degrees of renal impairment are common after OLT in children, but the incidence of renal dysfunction before and after transplantation is lower than that observed in adults. Assessment of renal function in children can be problematic. Plasma creatinine levels and creatinine clearance may not accurately reflect renal function in children with chronic liver disease. Renal impairment may be present despite a normal serum creatinine level because the loss of muscle mass associated with chronic liver disease leads to decreased creatinine production. In addition, serum bilirubin levels higher than 200–500 µmol/L can interfere with the laboratory measurement of serum creatinine, resulting in an artificially low estimation of creatinine levels. Intrinsic glomerular abnormalities commonly occur in association with liver cirrhosis, regardless of the etiology of the liver disease.

Renal failure after OLT has many potential causes, including pre-existing nephropathy (e.g. alpha-1-antitrypsin deficiency, Alagille's syndrome), prolonged caval cross-clamping time, intraoperative hypotension, intra-abdominal bleeding, drug toxicity (e.g. calcineurin inhibitors, aminoglycosides, amphotericin, ganciclovir), sepsis, poor graft function, and the hepatorenal syndrome. Temporary renal support may be required using hemofiltration or dialysis. In the Chicago series, the incidence of acute renal failure requiring dialysis after pediatric OLT was 6%, but the mortality rate was 85% (Bartosh *et al.*, 1997).

Acute/chronic rejection

Acute cellular rejection affects 40–70% of children within 1 month of transplantation, and typically responds to pulsed corticosteroid therapy. Later-onset acute cellular rejection may be precipitated by a reduction in immunosuppression due to gastrointestinal malabsorption, biliary obstruction, non-compliance or inadequate dosing. Late acute rejection can be more difficult to reverse and may evolve into chronic rejection. The etiology and pathogenesis of chronic rejection after OLT remain unclear. Several risk factors have been identified, including pediatric recipients, retransplantation for chronic rejection (Cho *et al.*, 1997), CMV infection, late (after 1 month) steroid-resistant acute rejection, and recipients who are non-indigenous to the donor population. The relevance of HLA mismatch is uncertain. Approximately 5–10% of children will develop chronic rejection after transplantation, but the incidence has been declining during the last decade due to more effective immunosuppression. The use of tacrolimus as either primary or rescue therapy has been associated with a lower incidence (McDiarmid *et al.*, 1993; Reyes *et al.*, 2000).

Chronic rejection can occur as early as 1 month post transplant, and most cases present within the first year after OLT. However, it can occur many years later, particularly as a consequence of late acute rejection secondary to poor drug compliance. Presentation is with jaundice and pruritus, and liver function tests reveal marked cholestasis with only mild to moderate elevation of serum transaminases. Hepatic synthetic function is usually relatively well preserved. Histological appearances are those of a cellular infiltrate of lymphocytes, macrophages and plasma cells within the portal tracts. There is loss of intrahepatic bile ducts (ductopenia), an obliterative arteriopathy with foam cells, and evidence of perivenular cell dropout (Figure 30.8). Retransplantation is the only realistic option if rescue therapy with tacrolimus or mycophenolate mofetil (Chardot *et al.*, 2001) is unsuccessful.

Graft disease

A diverse spectrum of pathological conditions may affect the transplanted liver. Vascular, biliary and infective complications are discussed elsewhere in this chapter, but there are numerous examples of specific graft diseases which deserve comment (Box 30.5).

The risk of malignancy transmitted via the liver allograft is extremely small with current donor criteria (Kauffman *et al.*, 2000). Infection is a greater hazard, and viral transmission is inevitable if adult livers are trans-

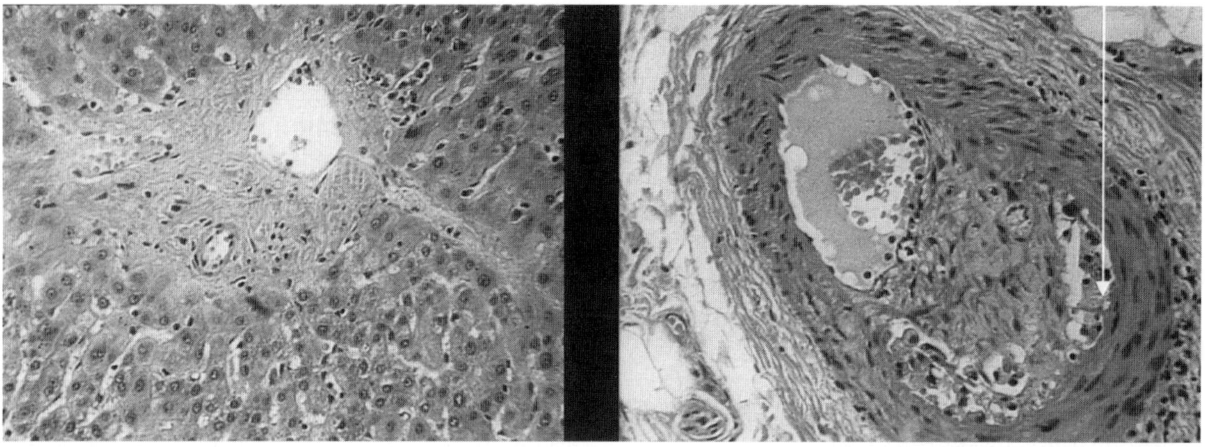

Figure 30.8 *Typical histological features of chronic rejection. In the high-power view of the portal tract (left), the bile duct has disappeared, and there is a chronic inflammatory cell infiltrate. The intrahepatic artery (right) shows obliterative changes with foam cells (arrow). (Reproduced courtesy of Dr J Wyatt.)*

Box 30.5 *Examples of specific graft disease after pediatric liver transplantation*

Disease transmission: infection, malignancy, Gilbert's disease, thrombophilia

Recurrent disease in the transplanted liver:
 Viral hepatitis B and C
 Malignancy
 Autoimmune hepatitis
 Langerhan's cell histiocytosis
 Giant-cell hepatitis (with autoimmune hemolytic anemia)
 Budd-Chiari syndrome
 Primary sclerosing cholangitis (adults)

De-novo autoimmune hepatitis
Nodular regenerative hyperplasia
Lymphoproliferative disease

Hepatitis
 Viral (e.g. Epstein–Barr virus, cytomegalovirus, hepatitis A–E, adenovirus, HSV, HHV6)
 Drug-induced
 Non-specific histological hepatitis

Immunological (e.g. rejection)

Graft-vs.-host disease

O'Grady et al., 1992; Gane et al., 1994; Rosenthal et al., 1997; *Vilca-Melendez* et al., 1997; Kerkar et al., 1998; Pinna et al., *1999; Hadzic* et al., 2000; Kauffman et al., 2000; Vajro et al., *2000; Gupta* et al., 2001; Hubscher, 2001; Rai et al., 2001

---

planted into children. Certain indications for pediatric liver transplantation are associated with a variable but definite risk of recurrent disease in the graft. These include hepatic malignancy (see Chapter 18), autoimmune hepatitis (which is associated with a recurrence rate of 20–30% and may respond to increased immuno-

suppression or progress to cirrhosis and graft failure) (Hubscher, 2001), primary sclerosing cholangitis (Rai *et al.*, 2001), hepatitis B and C (although recurrence of hepatitis B infection in children transplanted for fulminant HBV infection is unusual) (O'Grady *et al.*, 1992), Langerhans cell histiocytosis (Hadzic *et al.*, 2000) and giant-cell hepatitis with autoimmune hemolytic anemia (Vilca Melendez *et al.*, 1997).

Irrespective of the initial indication for transplantation, an autoimmune hepatitis may develop *de novo* despite maintenance immunosuppression (Kerkar *et al.*, 1998; Gupta *et al.*, 2001). The condition presents months to years after OLT with a transaminitis, elevated IgG levels and positive autoantibodies. It shows a variable response to treatment with prednisolone and azathioprine, and may progress to end-stage liver disease. Nodular regenerative hyperplasia, which has been linked with azathioprine, may develop in the graft in young adults and cause portal hypertension (Gane *et al.*, 1994).

In adults, approximately 20–40% of protocol biopsies that are performed as part of routine annual review have histological features of chronic hepatitis for which no definite cause can be identified. Rosenthal *et al.* (1997) examined protocol biopsies of transplanted livers in immunosuppressed but otherwise healthy children with normal biochemical liver function. Histological changes consisting of scattered, mild to moderate, portal and/or parenchymal mononuclear cell infiltrates were common. Mild fibrosis and focal pericholangitis were observed in less than 10% of specimens.

Graft-vs.-host disease (GvHD) is a rare complication which may occur when a large number of donor lymphocytes are transplanted with the liver. After solid organ transplantation, GvHD has two principal presentations – humoral and cellular. Antibody production by passenger B-lymphocytes in the donor liver from a nonidentical ABO living donor may cause hemolysis

(Kunimasa *et al.*, 1998). In the cellular type of GvHD, mature donor T-cells are activated by alloantigens expressed by the host. The symptoms after liver transplantation are identical to those that occur after bone-marrow transplantation, except that the liver is spared because it lacks host antigens (Pinna *et al.*, 1999). Diarrhea, fever, skin rashes and pancytopenia are the main features, and there may be evidence of coexisting CMV infection. The diagnosis may be suspected on the basis of bone-marrow examination, and confirmed by the demonstration of donor and recipient HLA chimerism after typing peripheral blood lymphocytes. GvHD has a poor prognosis despite treatment with immunosuppressive agents, including antithymocyte globulin (Bhaduri *et al.*, 1990). Fatal septic complications are common.

The risk of GvHD is higher in living-related liver transplantation where the donor and recipient are homozygous at all HLA loci, because engrafted passenger lymphocytes can react to recipient HLA antigens inherited from the other parent (Whitington *et al.*, 1996).

Complications of immunosuppressive therapy

INFECTION

Infectious complications are common during the first 3 months post transplant. Risk factors for early infection include poor graft function, prolonged intensive-care/ventilator dependence, gut perforation, acute liver failure, retransplantation and age under 1 year (Saint-Vil *et al.*, 1991; Garcia *et al.*, 1998; Bouchut *et al.*, 2001). Infections within 1 month are mostly bacterial, and the commonest sites are respiratory, bloodstream (especially catheter related) and abdominal (Garcia *et al.*, 1998; Bouchut *et al.*, 2001). Viral infections, particularly with CMV and Epstein–Barr virus (EBV), are a common cause of late infection.

Bacterial infection

The majority of children will have at least one bacterial infection during their postoperative recovery, particularly if they experience surgical complications. Gram-positive infections of indwelling venous catheters may be reduced by meticulous catheter care and replacement of the line after 5 days. Gram-negative sepsis has become less common with the use of prophylactic antibiotics during and after transplant. The presence of Gram-negative organisms and *Candida* species in peritoneal fluid postoperatively should suggest the possibility of bowel perforation, biliary leakage or graft ischemia. Increasing problems are being encountered with antibiotic-resistant organisms such as vancomycin-resistant *Enterococcus*. Cholangitis, intra-abdominal collections and subphrenic abscess tend to present after the first postoperative week, and may be delayed if clinical signs are masked by immunosuppressive drugs (Muiesan and Heaton, 1998). After removal of abdominal drains, most fluid collections adjacent to the cut surface of a reduced or split liver will be reabsorbed spontaneously, but ultrasound-guided aspiration is useful if there are concerns about infection or a bile leak.

Fungal infection

Liver transplant recipients are at risk of fungal sepsis because of immunosuppression, invasive monitoring devices and the need for multiple or prolonged courses of broad-spectrum antibiotics (Tollemar, 1998). Fungal sepsis is more likely to occur in association with hepatic artery thrombosis, intestinal perforation or acute liver failure, or after retransplantation. The majority of cases are due to infection with *Candida* species, but *Aspergillus*, *Cryptococcus*, *Coccidioides* and *Histoplasma*, although less common, may also occur and are associated with a high mortality rate. Prophylaxis against *Candida* sepsis with fluconazole or nystatin is routine in most units. Fungal sepsis should be suspected in any transplant patient with a fever and a high white blood count who is receiving appropriate antibiotics. Diagnosis is often difficult and delayed. Early treatment of suspected infection is advisable, particularly since systemic or invasive fungal sepsis is associated with a high mortality. Amphotericin B is the mainstay of treatment in most cases.

Viral infection

Central to the mechanism of action of the calcineurin inhibitors, cyclosporine and tacrolimus, is the inhibition of cytotoxic T-cell responses. Consequently, these agents inhibit the host's immune response to viral infections such as herpes simplex, varicella zoster, CMV, EBV, human herpes virus 6 and adenovirus. Adenovirus pneumonitis and hepatitis and disseminated CMV disease are among the most severe and life-threatening complications after OLT.

The incidence of CMV disease has decreased with improved management of immunosuppression and the use of prophylactic regimens for high-risk recipients (e.g. a CMV-seronegative recipient receiving a CMV-positive graft). Children are at increased risk because the majority are CMV-seronegative prior to transplantation, and primary CMV infection from latent virus in the donor allograft subsequently affects more than 70% of cases and has a small but significant mortality (Mellon *et al.*, 1993). In CMV-seropositive pediatric recipients, evidence of reactivation of CMV occurs in up to 60% of cases. CMV infection may be symptomatic (CMV disease) or asymptomatic. Disease usually manifests as malaise, fever, leucopenia and arthralgia, but it may cause hepatitis, enteritis, pneumonitis or chorioretinitis.

Intensely immunosuppressed patients, such as those receiving monoclonal antibodies (e.g. OKT3) or high-dose mycophenolate mofetil, and those undergoing retransplantation, are at greater risk of CMV disease. The introduction of ganciclovir, in tandem with reduced immunosuppression, has transformed the course and prognosis of CMV infection. Without prophylaxis, the peak incidence of disease is around 1 month post transplant (Abu-Nader and Patel, 2000). Prophylaxis can delay or prevent the development of CMV infection. More recently, the use of quantitative assays for CMV DNA using polymerase chain reaction technology has enabled the detection of high-level antigenemia, and pre-emptive therapy with ganciclovir in such cases can prevent progression to CMV disease.

EBV infection is common in childhood, and is characterized by latency, liver involvement and a potential for reactivation. The clinical features in a normal host, which include lymphadenopathy, pharyngitis, tonsillitis, hepatitis and splenomegaly, may be more severe in the immunocompromised patient, with an increased risk of atypical lymphocyte transformation and proliferation. The virus infects and stimulates B-lymphocytes, and in the presence of T-cell inhibition in immunosuppressed hosts there is a proliferation of EBV-infected lymphocytes which can lead to malignant transformation. After OLT, EBV may manifest as a primary infection from a positive donor or reactivation of a previous infection. In children, EBV reactivation occurs in up to 50% of cases and primary infection in 70–80% of cases (Breinig et al., 1987; Smets et al., 2000). EBV infection or reactivation typically occurs within 3–4 months of the transplant, but can cause late graft dysfunction more than 1 year after transplantation. It presents with a spectrum of clinical features ranging from the asymptomatic, through a mononucleosis-like illness to malignant lymphoma. As with CMV infection, there is a correlation between high-level antigenemia (detected by polymerase chain reaction technology) and the development of EBV disease in children within the first year after OLT (McDiarmid et al., 1998). Those who develop symptomatic EBV infection (i.e. EBV disease) (Smets et al., 2000) appear to be particularly at risk of developing EBV-related post-transplant lymphoproliferative disease (PTLD). Young, previously EBV-naive children are most at risk.

Hepatitis B and hepatitis C infections are uncommon indications for transplantation in childhood, but recurrence may be a cause of late graft dysfunction. Adenovirus infection may cause fulminant hepatitis or necrotizing pneumonitis in the early post-transplantation period. Serotypes 1, 2 and 5 are most commonly implicated, and type 5 is often responsible for the development of hepatitis, which is associated with a mortality rate of up to 45% (Michaels et al., 1992). Influenza A and B viruses are common viral pathogens associated with respiratory tract infections. They typically occur in winter, and in any given year one strain of either virus predominates. Immunosuppressed patients should receive the inactivated influenza vaccine annually. Respiratory syncytial virus is the commonest cause of bronchiolitis

in young children, but it seldom causes life-threatening complications in the transplant patient. Ribavirin has been used in severe cases.

Although not a complication of immunosuppression, virally-induced acute liver failure may be associated with another important complication after OLT. Bone-marrow failure, resulting in aplastic anemia, may complicate the progress of up to 10% of children presenting with acute liver failure (Tung et al., 2000). In those with presumed non A, non-C viral hepatitis or parvovirus-induced acute liver failure, the proportion is even higher. In some cases the aplastic anemia may not become apparent until after an urgent OLT has been performed. Treatment is largely supportive, but administration of antithymocyte globulin and granulocyte colony-stimulating factor may hasten marrow recovery. Bone-marrow transplantation is occasionally required.

Late infections

These may be classified as persistent infections, community-acquired infections and opportunistic infections associated with immunosuppression (Muiesan and Heaton, 1998). Late opportunistic bacterial infections include Legionnaires' disease and tuberculosis. Children from ethnic minorities are at increased risk of developing tuberculosis. The risk of mycobacterial infection in the King's College Hospital series was estimated to be 1–2%, with onset between 1 month and 5 years after transplantation (Verma et al., 2000). Both Mycobacterium tuberculosis and atypical mycobacteria can cause skin, lymph node, pulmonary or miliary disease. The possibility of tuberculosis should be considered in any immunosuppressed child with an unusual or persistent chest infection.

Atypical pneumonia due to Pneumocystis carinii presents with fever, a dry cough and hypoxia, and should be treated with high-dose cotrimoxazole. Children with poor graft function, high levels of immunosuppression and chronic rejection appear to be at greater risk of this opportunistic infection. However, late infection is occasionally seen in the absence of these risk factors. Central nervous system infection with toxoplasmosis is rare, but should be considered in any child with evidence of seroconversion and neurological symptoms and signs. A reduction in immunosuppression and treatment with pyrimethamine/sulfadiazine or high-dose penicillin usually leads to resolution.

Intestinal infection by Cryptosporidium is a rare cause of cholangiopathy in pediatric liver transplant recipients. In a series from Belgium, three out of 461 pediatric liver transplant recipients developed diffuse cholangitis associated with intestinal carriage of Cryptosporidium (Campos et al., 2000). They were treated with paramomycin in conjunction with reduced immunosuppression. Biliary reconstruction was needed in all three cases, and biliary cirrhosis requiring retransplantation developed in one patient.

DRUG TOXICITY AND SIDE-EFFECTS

Liver transplantation for the patient and their family involves exchanging the inevitably fatal outcome of chronic liver disease for the potentially life-threatening complications of immunosuppression. For most patients, immunosuppression is lifelong, but after the first year it can usually be maintained at relatively low levels. Surveillance of patients for complications of their immunosuppressive therapy is important for ensuring long-term survival and quality of life. Major side-effects associated with cyclosporine and tacrolimus are described in Chapter 29. Both drugs exhibit a similar profile of side-effects, but the use of cyclosporine is associated with hirsutism, gingival hyperplasia and a higher incidence of hypertension, whereas the use of tacrolimus may be associated with a slightly higher incidence of diabetes mellitus and neurotoxicity. The two drugs share a large number of important drug interactions.

Nephrotoxicity

Renal insufficiency is a very significant long-term complication. Long-term nephrotoxicity is largely secondary to the immunosuppressive agents cyclosporine and tacrolimus. Cyclosporine toxicity is mediated by vasoconstriction of the renal vasculature. Later, chronic arteriolar changes may be associated with the development of irreversible interstitial fibrosis. Glomerular filtration appears to stabilize in the majority of patients, despite progressive pathological changes evidenced by compensatory hypertrophy of undamaged glomeruli. Cyclosporine dose reduction in acute renal insufficiency results in improvement in renal function. Chronic cyclosporine nephrotoxicity is less reversible, but alteration of immunosuppressive regimens is still worthwhile several years after OLT in those with calcineurin-inhibitor-related nephrotoxicity (Aw et al., 2001).

Children appear to suffer a progressive decrease in glomerular filtration rate after OLT (McDiarmid et al., 1990; McDiarmid, 1996). This decrease may be as much as 20–50% in half of the cases at 2–4 years after transplantation. Tacrolimus and cyclosporine have similar nephrotoxic properties, and both are associated with hypertension, hyperkalemia, hypomagnesemia and metabolic acidosis. Initially, tacrolimus was thought to cause a higher incidence of renal dysfunction, but subsequent follow-up using lower drug concentrations has shown that the incidence of nephrotoxicity following liver transplantation is similar for both drugs (Berg et al., 2001).

Hypertension

The proportion of pediatric patients with chronic hypertension after OLT is lower than that in adults, but hypertension still represents a significant long-term management problem that may contribute to the development of renal impairment (Muiesan and Heaton, 1998). The onset of hypertension is early, often within a few weeks of starting cyclosporine or tacrolimus and steroids.

The incidence of hypertension appears to decline during the first year post transplant, and by 1–2 years after OLT only 6% of children remain on antihypertensive treatment (McDiarmid et al., 1990). However, this proportion increases to 16% after 3 years as a consequence of ongoing cyclosporine nephrotoxicity. Cyclosporine-induced hypertension results in a loss of the nocturnal fall in blood pressure. It does not necessarily progress, but it may still cause organ damage, particularly in children who were normotensive prior to the transplant. Cyclosporine appears to have a direct effect on the endothelium, and a variety of mediators have been implicated in association with impaired sodium excretion and the resultant increase in intravascular volume. Tacrolimus also induces hypertension, but the incidence appears to be lower than with cyclosporine. This may be partly related to a lower steroid exposure in patients who receive primary tacrolimus immunosuppression (Jain et al., 2000).

Optimal therapy for post-transplant hypertension in the pediatric patient has yet to be defined. First-line measures include dietary sodium restriction, a reduction in steroid dose, and treatment with calcium-channel blockers such as nifedipine. Other antihypertensive agents, particularly beta-blockers, are effective but can potentiate hyperlipidemia. Angiotensin-converting-enzyme inhibitors are less effective and should be used with caution in the presence of renal impairment.

Cardiomyopathy

Tacrolimus-induced hypertrophic cardiomyopathy has been reported to be a rare but serious complication that is seen almost exclusively among pediatric patients (Nakata et al., 2000). The development of cardiomyopathy is correlated with high tacrolimus trough levels. Other factors which may contribute to this disorder include fluid overload, hypertension, steroid therapy and renal dysfunction. The myocardial hypertrophy can be reversed by lowering the trough level of tacrolimus or converting to cyclosporine or sirolimus (Pappas et al., 2000).

Hyperlipidemia

After liver transplantation, hyperlipidemias have been described in 40–50% of patients, but they tend to be less severe than those observed after heart or kidney transplantation. This may be because most hyperlipidemias are caused by abnormalities in the metabolism of lipoproteins (the plasma transporters of triglycerides and cholesterol), and these proteins are synthesized by the transplanted liver. Cyclosporine, tacrolimus and steroid therapy have all been implicated. Lipid profiles have been systematically studied in only a small number of children after liver transplantation (Hyams et al., 1989; Granot, 1998; Siirtola et al., 2001). Mild to moderate hypertriglyceridemia and variable effects on high-density lipoproteins have been recorded. Lipid-lowering drugs have rarely been required, but control of additional cardiovascular risk factors, such as systemic hypertension, is important.

Oral complications

Gingival hyperplasia occurs in a significant number of children who receive cyclosporine, and is exacerbated by the concurrent administration of nifedipine. Gingival changes occur most rapidly during the first 6 months after starting cyclosporine, and they appear to be due to a connective tissue response by fibroblasts. Meticulous oral hygiene should be encouraged prior to liver transplantation. If gingival hyperplasia becomes established, dental hygiene is important in order to avoid recurrent bacteremia and septicemia. All dental procedures after OLT must be protected with prophylactic antibiotics. Gingival hyperplasia regresses after conversion to tacrolimus.

Hair growth

A common side-effect of cyclosporine is hypertrichosis, which is not seen with tacrolimus therapy. Some patients, particularly girls, find the excessive hair growth distressing, and conversion to tacrolimus may prevent difficulties with compliance.

Diabetes mellitus

The incidence of hyperglycemia during the early postoperative period is higher in patients who are receiving tacrolimus than in those treated with cyclosporine. Follow-up studies in adults have revealed a similar incidence of diabetes mellitus in both groups (Pichlmayr *et al.*, 1997).

Benign skin lesions

Viral warts are relatively common in pediatric recipients of solid organ transplants. Ingelfinger *et al.* (1991) reported the successful eradication of warts in only 30% of pediatric renal transplant recipients. It is likely that drug-induced suppression of cell-mediated and (to a lesser extent) humoral immunity predisposes to the problem. The type of human papillomavirus responsible tends to be the same as that in the general population.

POST-TRANSPLANT LYMPHOPROLIFERATIVE DISEASE

Several major risk factors for the development of PTLD are frequently present in pediatric OLT recipients, namely young age, primary EBV infection, EBV-positive donors transplanted into EBV-naive recipients and, in some cases, the requirement for intensive immunosuppression (e.g. with monoclonal antibodies) (McDiarmid *et al.*, 1998). Most instances of PTLD are driven by EBV-infected lymphocytes, and this complication is now one of the leading causes of morbidity and mortality after the early post-transplant period. The incidence of PTLD in children after OLT is 3–4% with cyclosporine therapy, 6–13% with tacrolimus therapy (although this figure may be lower with current levels of immunosuppression), and even higher after treatment with OKT3 for steroid-resistant rejection. Furthermore, PTLD occurs earlier after primary tacrolimus immunosuppression (mean 13 months) than after cyclosporine (mean 50 months) (Younes *et al.*, 2000). Primary EBV infection is a greater risk factor for the development of PTLD than reactivation.

The clinical picture of PTLD ranges from a well-localized polyclonal B-cell proliferation with a good prognosis to a disseminated monoclonal malignant non-Hodgkin's lymphoma with a high mortality. Almost any organ system can be involved, but gastrointestinal involvement is relatively common in children. The condition is defined by signs and symptoms of EBV disease (e.g. lymphadenopathy, fever, hepatitis, tonsillitis, diarrhea, gastrointestinal bleeding, weight loss), the presence of EBV DNA in peripheral blood detected by polymerase chain reaction, and a tissue biopsy (e.g. lymph nodes, liver, tonsils) with histological features of PTLD. Patients with central nervous system involvement tend to have isolated disease. Microscopic or macroscopic involvement of the

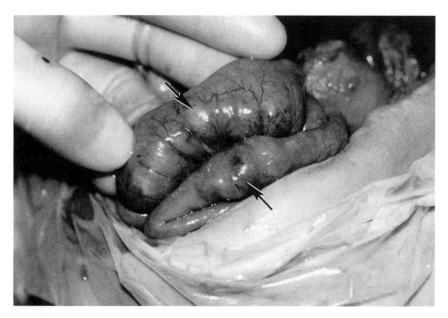

Figure 30.9 *Post-transplant lymphoproliferative disease affecting the gut of a 1-year-old boy after retransplantation for chronic rejection. Ulcerating lymphoid plaques were visible in the small bowel at laparotomy.*

allograft occurs in up to 20% of cases. Macroscopically, PTLD may appear as solid tumor, diffuse infiltration, or enlargement of native lymphoid tissue. In the gastrointestinal tract, ulcerating mucosal lesions on the mesenteric border may penetrate the muscularis propria, leading to perforation and peritonitis (Figure 30.9). The microscopic appearance of PTLD is that of a diffuse proliferation of lymphoid cells that can be characterized on the basis of the degree of lymphocyte heterogeneity.

The mainstay of treatment involves stopping or drastically reducing immunosuppression in an attempt to restore the host's cytotoxic T-cell response to EBV (Starzl et al., 1984; McDiarmid et al., 1998). Antiviral agents such as ganciclovir are often used in addition to inhibit viral replication, but their effectiveness is uncertain. Most patients respond to this approach. Some of those with tumors will show disease regression after reduction of immunosuppression, but other therapies, such as chemotherapy, interferon and high-titer EBV immunoglobulin, are required in those with progressive disease (Cacciarelli et al., 1998; Younes et al., 2000). The overall mortality rate for PTLD is at least 20%, and survivors are at increased risk of both acute and chronic rejection (Newell et al., 1996; Cacciarelli et al., 1998). Serial monitoring of EBV-PCR after OLT and pre-emptive reduction of immunosuppression in those with a high viral load before the onset of clinical disease may be a useful preventive strategy (McDiarmid et al., 1998; Kogan-Liberman et al., 2001). EBV serology is not helpful when following the course of EBV infection or disease after OLT in children, and apart from pretransplant testing of donors and recipients it has been abandoned altogether in some centers (McDiarmid et al., 1998).

OTHER MALIGNANCIES

An increased risk of malignancy is well described in patients taking immunosuppressive agents after solid organ transplantation. In adults, the risk of developing neoplasia in the first 10 years after renal transplantation is estimated to be 14%. By 20 years this is 40%, compared with a 6% cumulative risk of neoplasia in an age-matched control population (London et al., 1995). More than half of the lesions are skin malignancies. Liver transplant recipients seem to have a different pattern of risk, which may reflect differences in the level or type of immunosuppression and the length of follow-up. The incidence of lymphoma after liver transplantation is higher than that after renal transplantation (Penn, 1990; Nalesnik et al., 1993).

Several mechanisms have been proposed for the development of post-transplant malignancies, including the reduced ability of a depressed immune system to destroy malignant cells, direct DNA damage caused by drugs such as azathioprine and cyclosporine, and the oncogenic potential of viral infections such as EBV, herpes and papillomaviruses. Long-term surveillance and prevention of post-transplant malignancies are essential. The level of immunosuppression should be reduced to the lowest level that is compatible with good allograft function. Viral infections may require pre-emptive therapy. Excessive exposure to ultraviolet radiation from sunlight should be avoided, and the use of effective sunscreens should be encouraged.

NON-COMPLIANCE

During long-term follow-up after OLT, most centers attempt to reduce the overall level of immunosuppression. Steroids can be rapidly tapered to low doses which do not cause growth retardation, and the dosage of other drugs can be reduced in order to minimize side-effects and optimize compliance. Monotherapy with tacrolimus or cyclosporine is possible, although late acute rejection is a hazard (Dunn et al., 1994). Lifelong treatment was initially thought to be necessary in all patients, but the observation that 15% of 10-year survivors of liver transplantation had stopped taking their immunosuppression for more than 5 years without developing rejection led to a re-evaluation of this concept (Starzl et al., 1993). The liver appears to be inherently more tolerant than other solid organs, and the fact that there is a two-way migration of cells following transplantation is well documented. This cell migration has been proposed as a possible mechanism of inducing graft acceptance and tolerance. However, for the majority of patients immunosuppression must be maintained, and inadvertent withdrawal of therapy may precipitate intractable rejection with the risk of retransplantation and death. Non-compliance is a particular problem in teenagers, especially those who are completely well and who were transplanted in early childhood. It is a cause of late mortality in this age group (Sudan et al., 1998).

Nutritional complications

Protein-energy malnutrition is commonly encountered in children with end-stage liver disease, and it adversely affects post-transplant morbidity and mortality (see Chapter 5). Linear growth in most children is stunted at the time of transplantation. Reduced growth and short stature have a negative influence on the psychosocial development of a child. Even when sufficient calories are delivered, lean body mass may not increase because of alterations in energy metabolism and resistance to growth hormone.

Liver transplantation itself may be followed by various nutritional sequelae. A dramatic improvement in growth is often seen after transplantation, particularly in infants, which enables them to catch up, although height catch-up may take many years (Viner et al., 1999; van Mourik et al., 2000). Nevertheless, poor linear growth after pediatric OLT is well recognized and is more likely to occur in children who are older at the time of transplant (Peeters et al., 1996). Suggested causes include chronic corticosteroid therapy, poor graft function and multiple operations. Sarna *et al.* (1997) noted that growth accceleration was not observed in patients with chronic rejection or impaired graft function.

Various strategies have been developed for improving linear growth in children after solid organ transplantation. The best results have been seen after discontinuing corticosteroids and instigating recombinant human growth hormone (rhGH) therapy. No major side-effects have been reported with rhGH treatment, but the response is variable (Ramaccioni *et al.*, 2000). The rhGH-induced increase in height is greater in children who are treated at an early stage rather than at a late pubertal stage. Certain children, such as those with Alagille's syndrome, cannot achieve normal growth after transplantation, regardless of the level of steroid use or nutritional replacement (Bucuvalas *et al.*, 1994).

Like adults, children are also at risk of metabolic bone disease after OLT. Regardless of preoperative bone density, which may be reduced as a result of chronic cholestasis or malnutrition, liver transplant recipients initially lose bone mass after OLT (Ramaccioni *et al.*, 2000). However, with good graft function, bone mineral density gradually normalizes between 6 months and 2 years later (Argao *et al.*, 1994). The use of calcium and vitamin D supplements, advice about physical activity, and limitation of corticosteroid therapy may all contribute to a reduced risk of fractures in the preoperative and early post-transplant period (Hill *et al.*, 1995).

Neurological complications

Neurological complications are common in the early post-transplant period, and include the following:

- seizures (secondary to drug toxicity, hepatic encephalopathy, hypomagnesemia, hypocalcemia, infections);
- encephalopathy;
- strokes (thrombotic or hemorrhagic) (Mawk *et al.*, 1988);
- central pontine myelinolysis.

The sequelae of these complications are often a cause of significant long-term morbidity. Central pontine myelinolysis occurs in critically ill patients with severe preoperative hyponatremia (< 120 mmol/L), and may be precipitated by too rapid correction of the plasma sodium concentration (Estol *et al.*, 1989; Wszolek *et al.*, 1989). In this setting, the diagnosis should be considered in any patient who develops a marked change in mental status or a focal neurological deficit several days after OLT.

Many children experience minor neurotoxicity due to cyclosporine or tacrolimus, usually soon after transplantation. Varying degrees of tremor are common and usually resolve after dose reduction. Headache, paresthesiae and insomnia can be particularly troublesome.

Headache is associated with high trough levels, and will respond to dose reduction. Seizures may be precipitated by toxicity secondary to drug interactions, and they may be exacerbated by hypomagnesemia.

Central nervous system involvement by PTLD or opportunistic infection may occur as a later complication.

Psychosocial problems

The psychological, social and general health problems associated with successful transplantation are only gradually beginning to be recognized (see Chapter 6). Quality of life after transplantation is dependent on good graft function and an absence of recurring complications which require repeated hospital admission. With modern immunosuppressive regimens, children now take fewer medications and spend less time in hospital after OLT. Resolution of the symptoms and signs of chronic liver disease and associated metabolic bone disease improves development and social interaction (Zitelli *et al.*, 1988). More than 75% of the children are in age-appropriate school classes or only slightly behind. Studies by Stewart *et al.* (1991, 1992) showed that developmental outcome at 1 year after OLT was more likely to be delayed in children whose liver disease began in infancy but who were older at the time of transplantation. Earlier transplantation in such children may be advantageous, for neurodevelopmental outcome (van Mourik *et al.*, 2000).

Many families experience great difficulty in adjusting to the new situation after transplantation. There remain long-term anxieties about the child's prognosis and well-being. Family life may remain focused on the 'ill' child, and attempts to correct this imbalance can cause problems. Parents express persistent fears, even in the long term, of immunological rejection, unwanted side-effects of treatment, becoming overprotective, and continuing medical and social costs.

DONOR COMPLICATIONS AFTER LIVING-RELATED LIVER TRANSPLANTATION

The exact role of living-related liver transplantation (LRLT) in centers that offer cadaveric liver transplantation has yet to be established (Malago *et al.*, 1997). It can provide a valuable option for the family of a seriously ill child who has little time to wait for a suitable cadaveric graft, and it can have a positive impact on the overall mortality of children who are awaiting liver transplantation. Advantages over cadaveric reduced or split-liver transplantation include optimal timing of OLT, a short period of graft preservation, good early function, and excellent patient survival rates (Otte *et al.*, 1998; Broering *et al.*, 2001). *In-situ* liver splitting in the cadaveric donor offsets some of these advantages.

Furthermore, recent results indicate that the short- and long-term outcomes of LRLT do not differ significantly from those of cadaveric split-liver transplantation (Broering *et al.*, 2001). Moreover, LRLT exposes the donor to complications which must be carefully considered in the overall equation. Reported donor hazards include a morbidity of 5–10% from bleeding, bile leakage, incisional hernia, peptic ulceration and pulmonary embolism. Although only one donor death has been documented in the literature after more than 1000 left lateral segment living-related donations, the actual mortality rate is almost certainly higher (Strong, 1999).

SURVIVAL AND LONG-TERM COMPLICATIONS AFTER LIVER TRANSPLANTATION

Post-transplant complications have a profound impact on survival. Short- and long-term outcomes are discussed in detail in Chapter 31, but in so far as these relate to complications, they will be discussed briefly in this section. When analyzing survival statistics it is important to interpret the data cautiously, recognizing the multitude of frequently interrelated variables that affect outcome. These include the type and match of the graft, age and status of the patient, underlying diagnosis, donor factors, duration of cold ischemia, and type and intensity of immunosuppression, to name just a few. Added to this are less tangible variables such as an institution's learning curve.

An important predictor of early outcome is the *medical urgency* of the transplant, i.e. the patient's United Network for Organ Sharing (UNOS) status. The UNOS grades patients awaiting OLT such that status 1 indicates a patient in intensive care with liver failure and an anticipated survival of less than 7 days, status 2B denotes a hospitalized patient with complications from liver disease (e.g. variceal bleeding, hepatorenal syndrome, refractory ascites, etc.) and status 3 reflects the need for continuous medical care but not necessarily hospitalization. In experienced transplant centers, young *age* is not predictive of outcome (Colombani *et al.*, 1996; Bonatti *et al.*, 1997; van der Werf *et al.*, 1998). Data from the European Liver Transplant Registry (1988–99), which draws on more than 3500 pediatric transplants, shows a marginal increase in survival in children older than 2 years compared with younger ones, but no difference in graft survival rates between these two groups (Figure 30.10). Actuarial survival rates at 1, 5 and 10 years were 80%, 75% and 71%, respectively. The figures for patient and graft survival from the UCLA pediatric program (1984–97), which pertain to 569 transplants, are similar with patient survival rates of 82%, 78% and 76%, respectively (Goss *et al.*, 1998).

Transplantation for *acute liver failure* is associated with a consistently poorer outcome than OLT for chronic liver disease. For patients under 2 years of age in the European Registry, 1- and 10-year survival rates are approximately 80% and 74%, respectively, for chronic liver disease but only 64% and 44%, respectively, for acute liver failure. For elective liver transplantation there is no significant difference in patient and graft survival between full-size and reduced or split cadaveric liver grafts (Sieders *et al.*, 1999). Graft and patient survival rates after pediatric OLT are lower in *gender-mismatch* groups, particularly for male recipients of female organs (Francavilla *et al.*, 1998). Most of the differences are apparent within 3 months of the transplant, suggesting that gender mismatch may influence early complication rates. The results of LRLT are similar or only slightly better than those for cadaveric transplants (Emond *et al.*, 1993a; Drews *et al.*, 1997; Otte *et al.*, 1999; Revillon *et al.*, 1999; Broering *et al.*, 2001). Surprisingly, the incidence of acute rejection and immunosuppression requirements are not less, but the quality of the graft, the short cold ischemic time and the planned nature of the procedure are advantageous.

The influence of *donor age* on survival after pediatric OLT is controversial. McDiarmid *et al.* (2000), using data from the UNOS Scientific Registry, found that 3-year graft survival rates were significantly lower in children receiving adult rather than pediatric donor grafts. However, most of the difference in outcome was evident at 3 months post transplant, after which the survival curves were parallel up to 3 years. Others have suggested that grafts from older donors can perform comparatively well (Otte, 2001).

There are few reports of long-term outcome and late mortality after liver transplantation in children (Goss *et al.*, 1998; Muiesan and Heaton, 1998; Sudan *et al.*, 1998; Ryckman *et al.*, 1999). Sudan *et al.* (1998) studied a cohort of 263 children who were transplanted between 1985 and 1995 and followed up for a mean period of more than 5 years. There were 23 late deaths, of which nine were due to graft failure (four with chronic rejection, three with late biliary complications and two with recurrent disease), and eight were due to infection (five in previously healthy children who experienced a sudden onset of sepsis at home, two after percutaneous cholangiography, and one after appendicectomy). Two of the eight children who died of septic complications had previously undergone splenectomy. This highlights the importance of antibiotic prophylaxis for invasive procedures and after splenectomy, and prompt antibiotic treatment of fever in immunosuppressed patients. The third most important cause of late death was non-compliance, which occurred in four cases but accounted for the majority of deaths at between 10 and 17 years of age. There was only one late death from PTLD, the majority of these deaths occurring in the first year after transplantation.

Ryckman *et al.* (1999) reported the outcome of 150 children after OLT. There were 33 deaths, but more than half of these occurred within 3 months of transplantation. During a mean follow-up period of 69 months, a

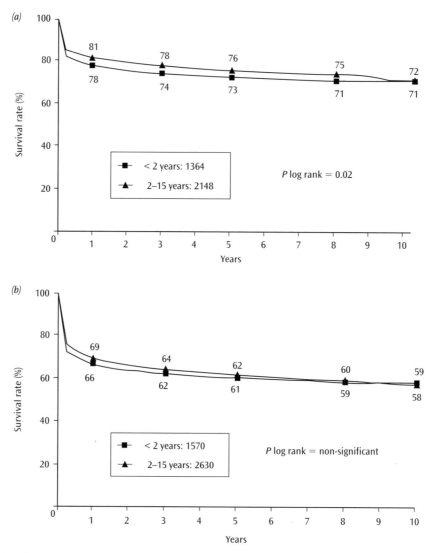

Figure 30.10 *(a) Patient and (b) graft survival data for pediatric liver transplantation according to recipient age (European Liver Transplant Registry data: January 1988 to December 1999).*

further 15 children (10%) died, largely due to complications of immunosuppression and sepsis. There were two septic deaths related to retransplantation, and two deaths due to pneumocystis pneumonia. PTLD was responsible for late mortality in three patients, but contributed to one further death. In contrast to the findings of Sudan *et al.* (1998), chronic rejection leading to allograft failure only contributed to two of the deaths.

Retransplantation

Historically, retransplantation has been necessary in 15–25% of children (Bilik *et al.*, 1992; Langnas *et al.*, 1993; Hamada *et al.*, 1995; Newell *et al.*, 1998; Achilleos *et al.*, 1999; Sieders *et al.*, 1999). The principal reasons have been hepatic artery thrombosis, primary non-function, and acute and chronic rejection, all of which have declined in recent years. Retransplantation rates are simi-

lar for reduced and split livers (Rela *et al.*, 1998), but are lower after LRLT (Emond *et al.*, 1993a; Hattori *et al.*, 1998). Retransplantation is strongly correlated with lower survival rates (Goss *et al.*, 1998; Newell *et al.*, 1998; Achilleos *et al.*, 1999; Sieders *et al.*, 2000b), particularly when undertaken urgently. An individual patient's likelihood of survival declines by 10–20% with the first retransplant, and the gap widens with each successive attempt (Goss *et al.*, 1998; European Liver Transplant Registry, 1999). Postoperative sepsis is a common hazard. However, repeated transplantation may be worthwhile despite the increased hazards associated with recipient hepatectomy, infection and the potential need for creative organ revascularization techniques (Schindel *et al.*, 2000). In the presence of multi-organ failure, retransplantation is associated with a dismal outcome (Esquivel *et al.*, 1987). Late elective retransplantation at 5 or more years is associated with a better prognosis, with the results approaching those expected from primary transplantation.

Key references

European Liver Transplant Registry, December 1999; http://www.eltr.org

A useful website containing a wide range of information on liver transplantation in children and adults, with up-to-date outcome statistics.

Goss JA, Shackleton CR, McDiarmid SV et al. Long-term results of pediatric liver transplantation: an analysis of 569 transplants. *Annals of Surgery*, 1998; **228**: 411–20.

An analysis of late complications and outcomes from a highly experienced pediatric liver transplant center.

McDiarmid SV, Jordan S, Lee GS et al. Prevention and pre-emptive therapy of post-transplant lymphoproliferative disease in pediatric liver recipients. *Transplantation* 1998; **66**: 1604–11.

Post-transplant lymphoproliferative disease remains a major concern in pediatric liver transplantation. The UCLA group outlines their successful strategy for reducing the risks of PTLD under primary tacrolimus immunosuppression by reacting to quantitative EBV PCR titers.

SPLIT Research Group. Studies of pediatric liver transplantation (split): year 2000 outcomes. *Transplantation* 2001; **72**: 463–76.

An analysis of survival, outcome and major complications after pediatic liver transplantation in centers in the USA and Canada since December 1995.

REFERENCES

Abu-Nader R, Patel R. Current management strategies for the treatment and prevention of cytomegalovirus infection in solid organ transplant recipients. *BioDrugs* 2000; **13**: 159–75.

Achilleos OA, Mirza DF, Talbot D et al. Outcome of liver retransplantation in children. *Liver Transplant Surgery* 1999; **5**: 401–6.

Angstadt J, Jarrell B, Maddrey W et al. Hemolysis in ABO-incompatible liver transplantation. *Transplantation Proceedings* 1987; **19**: 4595–7.

Argao EA, Balistreri WF, Hollis BW et al. Effect of orthotopic liver transplantation on bone mineral content and serum vitamin D metabolites in infants and children with chronic cholestasis. *Hepatology* 1994; **20**: 598–603.

Aw MM, Samaroo B, Baker AJ et al. Calcineurin-inhibitor related nephrotoxicity – reversibility in paediatric liver transplant recipients. *Transplantation* 2001; **72**: 746–9.

Bartosh SM, Alonso EM, Whitington PF. Renal outcomes in pediatric liver transplantation. *Clinical Transplantation* 1997; **11**: 354–60.

Berg UB, Ericzon B, Nemeth A. Renal function before and long after liver transplantation in children. *Transplantation* 2001; **72**: 631–7.

Bhaduri B, Tan K, Humphreys S. et al. Graft-versus-host disease after orthotopic liver transplantation in a child. *Transplantation Proceedings* 1990; **22**: 2378–80.

Bhatnagar V, Dhawan A, Chaer H et al. The incidence and management of biliary complications following liver transplantation in children. *Transplantation International* 1995; **8**: 388–91.

Bilik R, Yellen M, Superina RA. Surgical complications in children after liver transplantation. *Journal of Pediatric Surgery* 1992; **27**: 1371–5.

Bonatti H, Muiesan P, Connelly S et al. Hepatic transplantation in children under 3 months of age: a single centre's experience. *Journal of Pediatric Surgery* 1997; **32**: 486–8.

Bonham CA, Kapur S, Geller D et al. Excision and immediate revascularization for hepatic artery pseudoaneurysm following liver transplantation. *Transplantation Proceedings* 1999; **31**: 443.

Bouchut JC, Stamm D, Boillot O, Lepape A, Floret D. Postoperative infectious complications in paediatric liver transplantation: a study of 48 transplants. *Paediatric Anaesthesia* 2001; **11**: 93–8.

Breinig MK, Zitelli B, Starzl TE. Epstein–Barr virus, cytomegalovirus and other viral infections in children after liver transplantation. *Journal of Infectious Diseases* 1987; **156**: 273.

Broering DC, Mueller L, Ganschow R et al. Is there still a need for living-related liver transplantation in children? *Annals of Surgery* 2001; **234**: 713–22.

Bucuvalas JC, Horn JA, Carisson L et al. Growth hormone insensitivity associated with elevated circulating growth hormone binding protein in children with Alagille syndrome and short stature. *Journal of Clinical Endocrinology and Metabolism* 1994; **76**: 1477–82.

Cacciarelli TV, Esquivel CO, Moore DH et al. Factors affecting survival after orthotopic liver transplantation in infants. *Transplantation* 1997; **64**: 242–8.

Cacciarelli TV, Green M, Jaffe R et al. Management of post-transplant lymphoproliferative disease in pediatric liver transplant recipients receiving primary tacrolimus (FK506) therapy. *Transplantation* 1998; **66**: 1047–52.

Campos M, Jouzdani E, Sempoux C et al. Sclerosing cholangitis associated with cryptosporidiosis in liver-transplanted children. *European Journal of Pediatrics* 2000; **159**: 113–15.

Chaib E, Friend P, Jamieson NV, Calne RY. Biliary tract reconstruction: comparison of different techniques after 187 paediatric liver transplants. *Transplant International* 1994; **7**: 39–42.

Chardot C, Herrera JM, Debray D et al. Portal vein complications after liver transplantation for biliary atresia. *Liver Transplant Surgery* 1997; **3**: 351–8.

Chardot C, Nicoluzzi JE, Janssen M et al. Use of mycophenolate mophetil as rescue therapy after pediatric liver transplantation. *Transplantation* 2001; **71**: 224–9.

Cho JH, Bhatnagar V, Andreani P *et al.* Chronic rejection in pediatric liver transplantation. *Transplantation Proceedings* 1997; **29**: 452–3.

Colombani PM, Cigarroa FG, Schwarz K *et al.* Liver transplantation in infants younger than 1 year of age. *Annals of Surgery* 1996; **223**: 658–62.

de Ville de Goyet J, Alberti D, Clapuyt P *et al.* Direct bypassing of extrahepatic portal venous obstruction in children: a new technique for combined hepatic portal revascularization and treatment of extrahepatic portal hypertension. *Journal of Pediatric Surgery* 1998a; **33**: 597–601.

de Ville de Goyet J, Struye de Swielande Y, Reding R, Sokal EM, Otte JB. Delayed primary closure of the abdominal wall after cadaveric and living related donor liver graft transplantation in children: a safe and useful technique. *Transplant International* 1998b; **11**: 117–22.

Drews D, Sturm E, Latta A *et al.* Complications following living-related and cadaveric liver transplantation in 100 children. *Transplantation Proceedings* 1997; **29**: 421–3.

Dunn SP, Falkenstein K, Lawrence JP *et al.* Monotherapy with cyclosporin for chronic immunosuppression in pediatric liver transplant recipients. *Transplantation* 1994; **57**: 544–7.

Egawa H, Inomata Y, Uemoto S *et al.* Hepatic vein reconstruction in 152 living-related donor liver transplantation patients. *Surgery* 1997a; **121**: 250–7.

Egawa H, Tanaka K, Uemoto S *et al.* Relief of hepatic vein stenosis by balloon angioplasty after living-related donor liver transplantation. *Clinical Transplantation* 1997b; **11**: 56–9.

Egawa H, Uemoto S, Inomata Y *et al.* Biliary complications in pediatric living-related liver transplantation. *Surgery* 1998; **124**: 901–10.

Emond JC, Heffron TG, Kortz EO *et al.* Improved results of living-related liver transplantation with routine application in a pediatric program. *Transplantation* 1993a; **55**: 835–40.

Emond JC, Heffron TG, Whitington PF, Broelsch CE. Reconstruction of the hepatic vein in reduced-size hepatic transplantation. *Surgery, Gynecology and Obstetrics* 1993b; **76**: 11–17.

Esquivel CO, Koneru B, Todo S *et al.* Is multiple organ failure a contraindication for liver transplantation in children? *Transplantation Proceedings* 1987; **19 (Supplement 3)**: 47–8.

Estol CJ, Faris AA, Martinez AJ, Ahdab-Barmada M. Central pontine myelinolysis after liver transplantation. *Neurology* 1989; **39**: 493–8.

European Liver Transplant Registry, December; http://www.eltr.org

Francavilla R, Hadzic N, Heaton ND *et al.* Gender matching and outcome after pediatric liver transplantation. *Transplantation* 1998; **66**: 602–5.

Funaki B, Rosenblum JD, Leef JA, Hackworth CA, Szymski GX, Alonso EM. Angioplasty treatment of portal vein stenosis in children with segmental liver transplants: mid-term results. *American Journal of Roentgenology* 1997; **169**: 551–4.

Gaetano AM, Cotroneo AR, Maresca G *et al.* Color Doppler sonography in the diagnosis and monitoring of arterial complications after liver transplantation. *Journal of Clinical Ultrasound* 2000; **28**: 373–80.

Gane E, Portmann B, Saxena R, Wong P, Ramage J, Williams R. Nodular regenerative hyperplasia of the liver graft after liver transplantation. *Hepatology* 1994; **20**: 88–94.

Garcia S, Roque J, Ruza F *et al.* Infection and associated risk factors in the immediate postoperative period of pediatric liver transplantation: a study of 176 transplants. *Clinical Transplantation* 1998; **12**: 190–7.

Garcia-Gallont R, Bar-Nathan N, Shaharabani E *et al.* Hepatic artery thrombosis in pediatric liver transplantation: graft salvage after thrombectomy. *Pediatric Transplantation* 1999; **3**: 74–8.

Goss JA, Shackleton CR, McDiarmid SV *et al.* Long-term results of pediatric liver transplantation: an analysis of 569 transplants. *Annals of Surgery* 1998; **228**: 411–20.

Granot E. Lipoprotein changes in children after liver transplantation: mild hypertriglyceridemia and a decrease in HDL3/HDL2 ratio. *Hepatology* 1998; **27**: 175–80.

Gupta P, Hart J, Millis JM, Cronin D, Brady L. *De novo* hepatitis with autoimmune antibodies and atypical histology. *Transplantation* 2001; **71**: 664–8.

Hadzic N, Pritchard J, Webb D *et al.* Recurrence of Langerhans cell histiocytosis in the graft after pediatric liver transplantation. *Transplantation* 2000; **70**: 815–19.

Hall TR, McDiarmid SV, Grant EG *et al.* False-negative Duplex Doppler studies in children with hepatic artery thrombosis after liver transplantation. *American Journal of Roentgenology* 1990; **154**: 573–5.

Hamada H, Valayer J, Gauthier F, Yandza T, Takahashi H. Liver retransplantation in children. *Journal of Pediatric Surgery* 1995; **30**: 705–8.

Hattori H, Higuchi Y, Tsuji M *et al.* Living-related liver transplantation and neurological outcome in children with fulminant hepatic failure. *Transplantation* 1998; **65**: 686–92.

Heffron TG, Emond JC, Whitington PF *et al.* Biliary complications in pediatric liver transplantation. *Transplantation* 1992; **53**: 391–5.

Hill SA, Kelly DA, John PR. Bone fractures in children undergoing orthotopic liver transplantation. *Pediatric Radiology* 1995; **25 (Supplement 1)**: S112–17.

Hubscher SG. Recurrent autoimmune hepatitis after liver transplantation: diagnostic criteria, risk factors and outcome. *Liver Transplantation* 2001; **7**: 285–91.

Hyams JS, Treem WR, Andrews WS, Herbert PN. Lipid abnormalities in pediatric hepatic allograft recipients. *Journal of Pediatric Gastroenterology and Nutrition* 1989; **9**: 441–4.

Ingelfinger JR, Grupe WE, Topor M *et al.* Warts in a pediatric renal transplant population. *International Journal of Dermatology* 1991; **30**: 785–9.

Inomoto T, Nishizawa F, Sasaki H *et al.* Experiences of 120 microsurgical reconstructions of hepatic artery in living related liver transplantation. *Surgery* 1996; **119**: 20–6.

Jain A, Mazariegos G, Kashyap R *et al.* Comparative long-term evaluation of tacrolimus and cyclosporine in pediatric liver transplantation. *Transplantation* 2000; **70**: 617–25.

Kauffman HM, McBride MA, Delmonico FL. First report of the United Network for Organ Sharing Transplant Tumor Registry: donors with a history of cancer. *Transplantation* 2000; **70**: 1747–51.

Kawasaki S, Makuuchi M, Ishizone S *et al.* Liver regeneration in recipients and donors after transplantation. *Lancet* 1992; **339**: 580–1.

Kerkar N, Hadzic N, Davies ET *et al. De-novo* autoimmune hepatitis after liver transplantation. *Lancet* 1998; **351**: 409–13.

Kitabayashi K, Gores GJ, Krom RA. Arterial ketone body ratio in clinical liver transplantation. *Transplantation Proceedings* 1998; **30**: 4356–9.

Kiuchi T, Kasahara M, Uryuhara K *et al.* Impact of graft size mismatching on graft prognosis in liver transplantation from living donors. *Transplantation* 1999; **67**: 321–7.

Kogan-Liberman D, Burroughs M, Emre S, Moscona A, Shneider B. The role of quantitative Epstein–Barr virus polymerase chain reaction and preemptive immunosuppression reduction in pediatric liver transplantation: a preliminary experience. *Journal of Pediatric Gastroenterology and Nutrition* 2001; **33**: 445–9.

Kunimasa J, Yurugi K, Ito K *et al.* Hemolytic reaction due to graft-versus-host (GVH) antibody production after liver transplantation from living donors: report of two cases. *Surgery Today* 1998; **28**: 857–61.

Lallier M, St Vil D, Luks FI *et al.* Biliary tract complications in pediatric orthotopic liver transplantation. *Journal of Pediatric Surgery* 1993; **28**: 1102–5.

Langnas AN, Marujo W, Stratta RJ *et al.* Hepatic allograft rescue following arterial thrombosis. *Transplantation* 1991; **51**: 86–90.

Langnas AN, Inagaki M, Bynon JS *et al.* Hepatic retransplantation in children. *Transplantation Proceedings* 1993; **25**: 1921–2.

Lee J, Ben-Ami T, Yousefzadeh D. Extrahepatic portal vein stenosis in recipients of living-donor allografts: Doppler sonography. *American Journal of Roentgenology* 1996; **167**: 85–90.

Lo CM, Shaked A, Busuttil RW. Risk factors for liver transplantation across the ABO barrier. *Transplantation* 1994; **58**: 543–7.

London NJ, Farmery SM, Will EJ, Davison AM, Lodge JP. Risk of neoplasia in renal transplant patients. *Lancet* 1995; **346**: 403–6.

Lopez Santamaria M, Vazquez J, Gamez M *et al.* Donor vascular grafts for arterial reconstruction in pediatric liver transplantation. *Journal of Pediatric Surgery* 1996; **31**: 600–3.

Lyass S, Eid A, Jurim O. Coronary vein 'steal' and portal vein thrombosis after orthotopic liver transplantation. *Transplantation Proceedings* 2000; **32**: 702–3.

McDiarmid SV. Renal function in pediatric liver transplant patients. *Kidney International* 1996; **53 (Supplement)**: S77–84.

McDiarmid SV, Ettenger RB, Hawkins RA *et al.* The impairment of true glomerular filtration rate in long-term cyclosporine-treated pediatric allograft recipients. *Transplantation* 1990; **49**: 81–5.

McDiarmid SV, Klintmalm GBG, Busuttil RW. FK506 conversion for intractable rejection of the liver allograft. *Transplant International* 1993; **6**: 305–12.

McDiarmid SV, Jordan S, Lee GS *et al.* Prevention and pre-emptive therapy of post-transplant lymphoproliferative disease in pediatric liver recipients. *Transplantation* 1998; **66**: 1604–11.

McDiarmid SV, Davies DB, Edwards EB. Improved graft survival of pediatric liver recipients transplanted with pediatric-aged liver donors. *Transplantation* 2000; **70**: 1283–91.

Malago M, Rogiers X, Broelsch CE. Liver splitting and living donor technique. *British Medical Bulletin* 1997; **53**: 860–7.

Marcucci L, Shaked A, Maller ES *et al.* Supraceliac aortic pseudoaneurysms after liver transplantation in infants. *Transplantation* 1999; **68**: 1617–19.

Mawk JR, Shaw BW, Wood RP, Williams L. Neurosurgical complications of pediatric liver transplantation. *Childs Nervous System* 1988; **4**: 26–9.

Mazariegos GV, O'Toole K, Mieles LA *et al.* Hyperbaric oxygen therapy for hepatic artery thrombosis after liver transplantation in children. *Liver Transplant Surgery* 1999; **5**: 429–36.

Mazariegos GV, Garrido V, Jaskowski-Phillips S *et al.* Management of hepatic venous obstruction after split-liver transplantation. *Pediatric Transplantation* 2000; **4**: 322–7.

Mellon A, Shepherd RW, Faoagali JL *et al.* Cytomegalovirus infection after liver transplantation in children. *Journal of Gastroenterology and Hepatology* 1993; **8**: 540–4.

Michaels MG, Green M, Wald ER *et al.* Adenovirus infection in pediatric liver transplant recipients. *Journal of Infectious Diseases* 1992; **165**: 170–4.

Migliazza L, Lopez Santamaria M, Murcia J *et al.* Long-term survival expectancy after liver transplantation in children. *Journal of Pediatric Surgery* 2000; **35**: 5–8.

Millis JM, Seaman DS, Piper JB *et al.* Portal vein thrombosis and stenosis in pediatric liver transplantation. *Transplantation* 1996; **62**: 748–54.

Mondragon RS, Karani JB, Heaton ND *et al.* The use of percutaneous transluminal angioplasty in hepatic artery stenosis after transplantation. *Transplantation* 1994; **57**: 228–31.

Muiesan P, Heaton ND. Liver transplantation. In: Stringer MD, Oldham KT, Mouriquand PDE, Howard ER (eds) *Pediatric surgery and urology: long-term outcomes.* Philadelphia, PA: WB Saunders Co., 1998; 745–64.

Nakata Y, Yoshibayashi M, Yonemura T *et al.* Tacrolimus and myocardial hypertrophy. *Transplantation* 2000; **69**: 1960–2.

Nalesnik MA, Randhawa P, Demetris AJ *et al.* Lymphoma resembling Hodgkin disease after post-transplant lymphoproliferative disorder in a liver transplant recipient. *Cancer* 1993; **72**: 2568–73.

Newell KA, Alonso EM, Whitington PF *et al.* Post-transplant lymphoproliferative disease in pediatric liver transplantation. Interplay between primary Epstein–Barr virus infection and immunosuppression. *Transplantation* 1996; **62**: 370–5.

Newell KA, Millis JM, Bruce DS *et al.* An analysis of hepatic retransplantation in children. *Transplantation* 1998; **65**: 1172–8.

O'Grady JG, Smith HM, Davies SE *et al.* Hepatitis B virus reinfection after orthotopic liver transplantation. *Journal of Hepatology* 1992; **14**: 104–11.

Oh CK, Pelletier SJ, Sawyer RG *et al.* Uni- and multivariate analysis of risk factors for early and late hepatic artery thrombosis after liver transplantation. *Transplantation* 2001; **71**: 767–72.

Otte JB. The availability of all technical modalities for pediatric liver transplant programs. *Pediatric Transplantation* 2001; **5**: 1–4.

Otte JB, de Ville de Goyet J, Reding R *et al.* Pediatric liver transplantation: from the full-size liver graft to reduced split and living related liver transplantation. *Pediatric Surgery International* 1998; **13**: 308–18.

Otte JB, Reding R, de Ville de Goyet J *et al.* Experience with living related liver transplantation in 63 children. *Acta Gastroenterologica Belgica* 1999; **62**: 355–62.

Pappas PA, Weppler D, Pinna AD *et al.* Sirolimus in pediatric gastrointestinal transplantation: the use of sirolimus for pediatric transplant patients with tacrolimus-related cardiomyopathy. *Pediatric Transplantation* 2000; **4**: 45–9.

Pastacaldi S, Teixeira R, Montalto P, Rolles K, Burroughs AK. Hepatic artery thrombosis after orthotopic liver transplantation: a review of nonsurgical causes. *Liver Transplantation* 2001; **7**: 75–81.

Payen DM, Fratacci MD, Dupuy P *et al.* Portal and hepatic arterial blood flow measurements of human transplanted liver by implanted Doppler probes: interest for early complications and nutrition. *Surgery* 1990; **107**: 417–27.

Peclet MH, Rykman FC, Pedersoen SH *et al.* The spectrum of bile duct complications in pediatric liver transplantation. *Journal of Pediatric Surgery* 1994; **29**: 214–19.

Peeters PM, Sieders E, ten Vergert EM *et al.* Analysis of growth in children after orthotopic liver transplantation. *Transplant International* 1996; **9**: 581–8.

Penn I. Cancers complicating organ transplantation. *New England Journal of Medicine* 1990; **323**: 1767–9.

Pichlmayr R, Winkler M, Neyhaus P *et al.* Three-year follow-up of the European Multicenter Tacrolimus (FK506) Liver Study. *Transplantation Proceedings* 1997; **29**: 2499–502.

Pinna AD, Weppler D, Berho M *et al.* Unusual presentation of graft-versus-host disease in pediatric liver transplant recipients: evidence of late and recurrent disease. *Pediatric Transplantation* 1999; **3**: 236–42.

Ploeg RJ, D'Alessandro AM, Knechtle SJ *et al.* Risk factors for primary dysfunction after liver transplantation – a multivariate analysis. *Transplantation* 1993; **55**: 807–13.

Rai RM, Boitnott J, Klein AS, Thuluvath PJ. Features of recurrent primary sclerosing cholangitis in two consecutive liver allografts after liver transplantation. *Journal of Clinical Gastroenterology* 2001; **32**: 151–4.

Ramaccioni V, Soriano HE, Arumugam R, Klish WJ. Nutritional aspects of chronic liver disease and liver transplantation in children. *Journal of Pediatric Gastroeuterology and Nutrition* 2000; **30**: 361–7.

Reichert PR, Renz JF, Rosenthal P *et al.* Biliary complications of reduced-organ liver transplantation. *Liver Transplant Surgery* 1998; **4**: 343–9.

Rela M, Muiesan P, Bhatnagar V *et al.* Hepatic artery thrombosis after liver transplantation in children under 5 years of age. *Transplantation* 1996; **9**: 1355–7.

Rela M, Vougas V, Muiesan P *et al.* Split liver transplantation: King's College Hospital experience. *Annals of Surgery* 1998; **227**: 282–8.

Revillon Y, Michel JL, Lacaille F *et al.* Living-related liver transplantation in children: the 'Parisian' strategy to safely increase organ availability. *Journal of Pediatric Surgery* 1999; **34**: 851–3.

Reyes J, Jain A, Mazariegos G *et al.* Long-term results after conversion from cyclosporine to tacrolimus in pediatric liver transplantation for acute and chronic rejection. *Transplantation* 2000; **69**: 2573–80.

Rosenthal P, Emond JC, Heyman MB *et al.* Pathological changes in yearly protocol liver biopsy specimens from healthy pediatric liver recipients. *Liver Transplant Surgery* 1997; **3**: 559–62.

Ryckman FC, Alonso MH, Bucuvalas JC, Balistreri WF. Long-term survival after liver transplantation. *Journal of Pediatric Surgery* 1999; **34**: 845–50.

Saint-Vil D, Luks FI, Lebel P *et al.* Infectious complications of pediatric liver transplantation. *Journal of Pediatric Surgery* 1991; **26**: 908–13.

Salt A, Noble-Jamieson G, Barnes ND *et al.* Liver transplantation in 100 children: Cambridge and King's College Hospital series. *British Medical Journal* 1992; **304**: 416–21.

Sarna S, Ronnholm K, Laine J *et al.* Mechanisms and treatment of growth retardation in children with liver transplants. *Transplantation Proceedings* 1997; **29**: 447–8.

Schindel DT, Dunn SP, Casas AT *et al.* Pediatric recipients of three or more hepatic allografts: results and technical challenges. *Journal of Pediatric Surgery* 2000; **35**: 297–300.

Shackleton CR, Goss JA, Swenson K *et al.* The impact of microsurgical hepatic arterial reconstruction on the outcome of liver transplantation for congenital biliary atresia. *American Journal of Surgery* 1997; **173**: 431–5.

Shaked A, Vargas J, Csete ME *et al.* Diagnosis and treatment of bowel perforation following pediatric orthotopic liver transplantation. *Archives of Surgery* 1993; **128**: 994–9.

Shaw BW, Iwatsuko S, Bron K, Starzl TE. Portal vein grafts in hepatic transplantation. *Surgery, Gynecology and Obstetrics* 1985; **161**: 67–8.

Sieders E, Peeters PM, Ten Vergert EM *et al.* Analysis of survival and morbidity after pediatric liver transplantation with full-size and technical-variant grafts. *Transplantation* 1999; **68**: 540–5.

Sieders E, Peeters PM, Ten Vergert EM *et al.* Early vascular complications after pediatric liver transplantation. *Liver Transplantation* 2000a; **6**: 326–32.

Sieders E, Peeters PM, Ten Vergert EM *et al.* Prognostic factors for long-term actual patient survival after orthotopic liver transplantation in children. *Transplantation* 2000b; **70**: 1448–53.

Siirtola A, Solakivi T, Jokela H *et al.* Hypertriglyceridemia and low serum HDL cholesterol are common in children after liver transplantation. *Transplantation Proceedings* 2001; **33**: 2449.

Smets F, Bodeus M, Goubau P *et al.* Characteristics of Epstein–Barr virus primary infection in pediatric liver transplant recipients. *Journal of Hepatology* 2000; **32**: 100–4.

Smyrniotis V, Andreani P, Muiesan P *et al.* Diaphragmatic nerve palsy in young children following liver transplantation. *Transplant International* 1998; **11**: 281–3.

Soliman T, Langer F, Puhalla H *et al.* Parenchymal liver injury in orthotopic liver transplantation. *Transplantation* 2000; **69**: 2079–84.

Soubrane O, El Meteini M, Devictor D, Bernard O, Houssin D. Risk and prognostic factors of gut perforation after orthotopic liver transplantation for biliary atresia. *Liver Transplant Surgery* 1995; **1**: 2–9.

Srinivasan P, Vilca-Melendez H, Muiesan P, Prachalias A, Heaton ND, Rela M. Liver transplantation with monosegments. *Surgery* 1999; **126**: 10–12.

Starzl TE, Nalesnik M, Porter KA *et al.* Reversibility of lymphomas and lymphoproliferative lesions developing under cyclosporin-steroid therapy. *Lancet* 1984; **i**: 583–7.

Starzl TE, Demetris AJ, Trucco M *et al.* Cell migration and chimerism after whole organ transplantation: the basis of graft acceptance. *Hepatology* 1993; **17**: 1127–52.

Stevens LH, Emond JC, Piper JB *et al.* Hepatic artery thrombosis in infants. *Transplantation* 1992; **53**: 396–9.

Stewart SM, Hiltebreitel C, Nici J *et al.* Neuropsychological outcome of pediatric liver transplantation. *Pediatrics* 1991; **87**: 367–76.

Stewart SM, Campbell RA, McCallon D, Waller DA, Andrews WS. Cognitive patterns in school-age children with end-stage liver disease. *Journal of Developmental and Behavioral Pediatrics* 1992; **13**: 331–8.

Stringer MD, Marshall MM, Muiesan P *et al.* Survival and outcome after hepatic artery thrombosis complicating pediatric liver transplantation. *Journal of Pediatric Surgery* 2001; **36**: 888–91.

Strong RW. Whither living donor liver transplantation? *Liver Transplant Surgery* 1999; **5**: 536–8.

Sudan DL, Shaw BL, Langnas AN. Causes of late mortality in pediatric liver transplant recipients. *Annals of Surgery* 1998; **227**: 289–95.

Tan KC, Yandza T, de Hemptinne B *et al.* Hepatic artery thrombosis in pediatric liver transplantation. *Journal of Pediatric Surgery* 1988; **23**: 927–30.

Tisone G, Gunson BK, Buckels JA, McMaster P. Raised hematocrit: a contributing factor to hepatic artery thrombosis following liver transplantation. *Transplantation* 1988; **46**: 162–3.

Tissieres P, Pariente D, Chardot C *et al.* Postshunt encephalopathy in liver-transplanted children with portal vein thrombosis. *Transplantation* 2000; **70**: 1536–9.

Tollemar J. Fungal infections in solid organ transplant recipients. In: Lippincott-Raven Publishers, Bowden B, Ljungman S, Paya J (eds) *Transplant infections in transplantation.* Philadelphia, PA: 1998: 339–50.

Tung J, Hadzic N, Layton M *et al.* Bone marrow failure in children with acute liver failure. *Journal of Pediatric Gastroenterology and Nutrition* 2000; **31**: 557–61.

Vajro P, DeVincenzo A, Lucariello S *et al.* Unusual early presentation of Gilbert syndrome in pediatric recipients of liver transplantation. *Journal of Pediatric Gastroenterology and Nutrition* 2000; **31**: 238–43.

van der Werf WJ, D'Alessandro AM, Knechtle SJ *et al.* Infant pediatric liver transplantation results equal those for older pediatric patients. *Journal of Pediatric Surgery* 1998; **33**: 20–3.

van Mourik ID, Beath SV, Brook GA *et al.* Long-term nutritional and neurodevelopmental outcome of liver transplantation in infants aged less than 12 months. *Journal of Pediatric Gastroenterology and Nutrition* 2000; **30**: 269–75.

Verma A, Dhawan A, Wade JJ *et al.* Mycobacterium tuberculosis infection in pediatric liver transplant recipients. *Pediatric Infectious Disease Journal* 2000; **19**: 625–30.

Verzaro R, Nishida S, Angelis M, Khan F, Tzakis A. Thoraco-abdominal bypass graft with liver retransplantation for the treatment of a pseudoaneurysm of the supraceliac aorta after liver transplantation. *Pediatric Transplantation* 2001; **5**: 64–8.

Vickers CR, O'Connor HJ, Quintero GA *et al.* Delayed perforation of the esophagus after variceal sclerotherapy and hepatic transplantation. *Gastrointestinal Endoscopy* 1989; **35**: 459–61.

Vilca-Melendez H, Rela ZM, Baker AJ *et al.* Liver transplant for giant-cell hepatitis with autoimmune haemolytic anaemia. *Archives of Disease in Childhood* 1997; **77**: 249–51.

Vilca-Melendez H, Vougas V, Muiesan P *et al.* Bowel perforation after paediatric orthotopic liver transplantation. *Transplant International* 1998; **11**: 301–4.

Viner RM, Forton JT, Cole TJ, Clark IH, Noble-Jamieson G, Barnes ND. Growth of long-term survivors of liver transplantation. *Archives of Disease in Childhood* 1999; **80**: 235–40.

Whitington PF, Rubin CM, Alonso EM *et al.* Complete lymphoid chimerism and chronic graft-versus-host-disease in an infant recipient of a hepatic allograft from an HLA-homozygous parental living donor. *Transplantation* 1996; **62**: 1516–19.

Wolf DC, Freni MA, Boccagni P *et al.* Low-dose aspirin therapy is associated with few side-effects but does not prevent hepatic artery thrombosis in liver transplant recipients. *Liver Transplant Surgery* 1997; **3**: 598–603.

Wszolek ZK, McComb RD, Pfeiffer RF *et al.* Pontine and extrapontine myelinolysis following liver transplantation. Relationship to serum sodium. *Transplantation* 1989; **48**: 1006–12.

Yanaga K, Makowka L, Starzl TE. Is hepatic artery thrombosis after liver transplantation really a surgical complication? *Transplantation Proceedings* 1989; **21**: 3511–13.

Yandza T, Anteur F, Gauthier O *et al.* Reoperative procedures following pediatric liver transplantation. *Transplantation Proceedings* 1992; **24**: 1963–4.

Yandza T, Gauthier F, Valayer J. Lessons from the first 100 liver transplantations in children at Bicetre Hospital. *Journal of Pediatric Surgery* 1994; **29**: 905–11.

Yokoyama I, Tzakis AG, Imventarza O *et al.* Pediatric liver transplantation from neonatal donors. *Transplant International* 1992; **5**: 205–8.

Younes BS, McDiarmid SV, Martin MG *et al.* The effect of immunosuppression on post-transplant lymphoproliferative disease in pediatric liver transplant patients. *Transplantation* 2000; **70**: 94–9.

Zamboni F, Franchello A, David E *et al.* Effect of macrovesicular steatosis and other donor and recipient characteristics on the outcome of liver transplantation. *Clinical Transplantation* 2001; **15**: 53–7.

Zitelli BJ, Miller JW, Gartner JC *et al.* Changes in lifestyle after liver transplantation. *Pediatrics* 1988; **82**: 173–80.

31

Short- and long-term outcomes

STEPHEN P DUNN AND ADELA T CASAS-MELLEY

OVERVIEW

The parents of children who require liver transplantation are primarily concerned about the answer to the question 'What chance does my child have of surviving a liver transplant and having a normal life?' Answering that question is not easy. Short-term outcomes for children are now readily available through the Internet for liver transplant centers within the USA at www.unos.org (Department of Health and Human Services, 1999). However, an individual child's possible risk or benefit cannot be easily determined from these data. Long-term outcomes are even more difficult to predict for an individual child. In recent years a few reports have been published with follow-up results for approximately 10 years or less (Abbasoglu et al., 1997; Seaberg et al., 1997; Goss et al., 1998a; Burdelski et al., 1999; Cacciarelli et al., 1999; Ryckman et al., 1999; Migliazza et al., 2000). In general, their purpose is to report average results, with some attempt to demonstrate the improvements in outcome over time. Helpful as the generalities of short- and long-term outcomes for liver transplantation are to the public, there is little that will answer the question of outcomes for the individual child.

The level of complexity involved in answering the question about outcome for an individual child involves many areas. Liver transplant is still a relatively new therapy and has only been widely available for the past two decades. During that time there have been dramatic changes in surgical techniques, immunosuppression, organ availability and organ distribution. In general, liver transplant results have improved (Burdelski et al.,

1999; Migliazza et al., 2000). Higher-risk patients are now being transplanted with results equal to the outcomes for low-risk patients who were transplanted in the past. The highest risk of mortality occurs in the first 3 months post transplant. Children who are still alive 1 year after transplant have a greater than 90% chance of being alive and well 10 years later (Migliazza et al., 2000). Improving short-term outcomes should result in improved long-term outcomes. Each new cohort of children with an improved short-term outcome becomes the most relevant group to follow for long-term outcomes. Unfortunately, for the most recent liver transplant recipients there has not been sufficient time since transplantation for adequate long-term evaluation. Even for children with the longest follow-up there has not been enough time since transplant for them to be followed through a normal lifespan. At best, the currently available long-term patient and graft survival data are depressed by the short-term outcomes of the past. A search for possible outcomes for the individual child must be sensitive both to current outcomes and to the factors which affect those outcomes.

New surgical techniques have dramatically increased the availability of donor livers for children (Reding et al., 1999). Due to the young age of the average child who requires a liver transplant and the relative paucity of size-appropriate liver donors, techniques for creating transplantable livers from larger allografts have been developed, significantly decreasing mortality while patients are waiting to be transplanted. The initial results obtained from reduced-size or split donor organs were not as good as those currently being reported. At present, outcomes from all of the techniques which increase the number of organs available to children are yielding similar results (Sieders *et al.*, 1999).

Immunosuppression has improved significantly since cyclosporine A treatment began in the late 1970s. Recent immunosuppressive management has led to acute rejection rates which are less than 50% of those seen in the past (Alvarez *et al.*, 2000). Graft survival rates of 90% at 1 year have now been achieved (Reding *et al.*, 1999). Outcomes after liver transplantation in children are dependent on immunosuppressive management, and should improve with better understanding of the immune response, immunosuppressive medications and immune modulation.

Organ donation and allocation have improved dramatically since liver transplantation first became clinically relevant (Department of Health and Human Services, 1999). Public awareness of organ donation has increased significantly, as have the numbers of donated organs. An efficient and fair national distribution program in the USA has replaced an archaic system of organ allocation. Children have benefited from this system by gaining equal status with adult recipients. Current short-term outcomes benefit from the effective functioning of the national organ and distribution network.

Distinct liver disease categories that lead to liver transplantation have a profound effect on the outcome of liver transplantation. Hepatocellular carcinoma requiring liver transplantation has perhaps the worst 5-year prognosis, being roughly one-third of the survival rate for patients with alpha-1-antitrypsin deficiency (Seaberg *et al.*, 1997; Department of Health and Human Services, 1999). Fulminant hepatic failure has the worst short-term prognosis (Seaberg *et al.*, 1997; Department of Health and Human Services, 1999). Furthermore, the outcome of liver transplantation for any liver disease etiology is dependent on the extent or progression of an individual child's illness. Children with any liver disease that requires life-supporting treatment have roughly two-thirds the survival rate of similar children whose disease does not require life-supportive measures at the time of the transplant (Seaberg *et al.*, 1997; Department of Health and Human Services, 1999).

Age at the time of transplant can have a significant effect on short-term outcomes. Historically, survival for children under 1 year of age at the time of transplant was less than that for older children (Kelly, 1998; Department of Health and Human Services, 1999). With improvements in liver transplantation, only children under 3 months of age remain at higher risk than older individuals (Colombani *et al.*, 1996; Bonatti *et al.*, 1997; VanderWerf *et al.*, 1998; Woodle *et al.*, 1998; Cox *et al.*, 1999; Saing *et al.*, 1999).

Long-term outcomes for children are available up to 10 years, but cannot be simply measured by patient and graft survival. Quality of life, intellectual function, psychosocial adjustment, complications, growth and development and general health are important measures that must be considered as well. Recurrence of primary liver disease, chronic rejection and late complications are also important aspects of long-term outcomes. All of these factors need to be addressed when evaluating long-term outcomes.

The short- and long-term outcomes of liver transplantation are available to us in general terms. Short-term results have shown a striking improvement, and long-term results are encouraging and should improve further. Accurate risk assessment of an individual child is hampered by the absence of a reliable mechanism with which to assess that child's risks. Risk assessment for the individual child should factor in the liver disease and its severity, the condition of the child at transplantation and their age, the type or combination of immunosuppressive agents and their side-effects, and the long-term complications of transplant recipients.

SHORT-TERM OUTCOMES OF LIVER TRANSPLANTATION IN CHILDREN

Death on the waiting-list

An accurate review of short-term outcomes would be incomplete if it did not address the sometimes hidden mortality of those children who die of the complications of their liver disease while waiting for a transplant. These children have many of the characteristics that increase mortality after transplantation. Age less than 1 year is a significant risk factor for waiting-list mortality (Department of Health and Human Services, 1999). This is due to the acuity of their illness and the lack of size-appropriate donors. Acute hepatic failure is a significant risk factor for death while on the waiting-list (Goss *et al.*, 1998b). Death rates on the waiting-list may be as high as 20% (Department of Health and Human Services, 1999; Emre *et al.*, 1999). Children with decompensated liver disease are at very high risk of death. In their pivotal study of risk factors for death while on the waiting-list, Malatack and his colleagues demonstrated conclusively the relationship between hepatic decompensation and decreased survival (Malatack *et al.*, 1987). In that report, children with serum cholesterol below 100 mg/dl and indirect bilirubin greater than 6 mg/dl, both of which represent findings of hepatocellular failure, had a greater than 75% likelihood of death within 6 months. This study laid the foundation for an objective system which would prioritize children for transplantation, favoring those who had the greatest risk of death while on the waiting-list. Recently, Reding and colleagues demonstrated that the Malatack score accurately predicted those with decreased survival post transplant. Further development of Malatack's research and the work of others should finally allow us to predict risk both preoperatively and postoperatively for an individual child (Reding *et al.*, 1999).

UNOS data

The United Network for Organ Sharing (UNOS) became the recipient of the initial contract awarded by the Health Resources Administration of the USA. As mandated by their contract, UNOS maintains a scientific registry with accurate information with regard to solid organ transplantation in the USA from 1987 until the present. These data can be obtained by contacting the United Network for Organ Sharing through its website at www.unos.org.

Data are available for pediatric liver transplant recipients from 1987 to 1999 (Department of Health and Human Services, 1999). Liver transplant outcomes are reported both overall and by individual centers. Data are reported by time periods and reflect the general trend towards improving results. At present, only 5-year follow-up data are available. Outcomes are reported by age groups, although subclassification is limited. For example, all children under 1 year of age at transplantation are reported as a group. Outcomes are reported by disease categories, recipient age, race and blood type, clinical status at transplant and type of transplant (primary transplant vs. retransplant). Some generalizations can be made for the relatively short-term outcomes (5-year follow-up) reported. Children under 1 year of age when transplanted, those on life support or of UNOS status 1, those with acute hepatic failure and those receiving a retransplant have a poorer prognosis than their peers. In general, graft survival rates are approximately 10% lower than patient survival rates at 1 year (Table 31.1).

For example, one would evaluate the short-term outcomes for a child with biliary atresia. This is the commonest diagnosis leading to liver transplantation in childhood. One-year patient and graft survival rates for children with biliary atresia are 91% and 81%, respectively. UNOS data do not currently allow the combination of risk factors that an individual child might possess. If the child had biliary atresia, was less than 6 months of age and on life support at the time of transplantation, the outcome would not be as good as that for all children with biliary atresia. Young age and critical condition lower the likelihood of this child's recovery below the reported outcomes at 1 year for all children. Similarly, but in the opposite direction, the lowest-risk children with biliary atresia will have a better survival than the results for all children with biliary atresia. Helpful as the generalizations of the UNOS data are, at present it is not possible to evaluate the risk for individual children.

Variables that affect short-term outcomes

Many variables affect the short-term outcomes of liver transplantation in children. These include age at transplant, the child's overall clinical condition, the liver disease and its severity, immunosuppression and postoperative complications.

Liver disease in childhood is most commonly caused by biliary atresia (Cox et al., 1999). This disease affects the very young and, due to its prevalence, it decreases the average age at liver transplant for all children to approximately 5 years. Over 40% of children are under 2 years of age when transplanted. Many of these children come to transplant at less than 1 year of age. Historically, children weighing less than 10 kg or under 1 year of age have had poor outcomes from liver transplantation. The results for these children continue to lag behind those of older children, but many centers now report outcomes with patient and graft survival rates of 80–90% and 70–80%, respectively, at 1 year (Colombani et al., 1996; Kelly, 1998; VanderWerf et al., 1998; Department of Health and Human Services, 1999). These results are almost identical to those for adult patients. Children over the age of 1 year have a prognosis that is generally better than that of adults (Department of Health and Human Services, 1999). However, among those under 1 year old there is a subgroup of children less than 3 months of age who have an excess mortality. Few

Table 31.1 *UNOS data: percentage patient/graft survival, 1996–99*

	3 months	1 year	3 years	5 years
Condition at transplant				
Life support	79/71	74/65	65/54	62/50
Hospitalized	90/85	86/78	77/67	72/61
Diagnosis				
Biliary atresia	91/85	86/75	85/69	84/67
Acute hepatic failure	84/78	81/74	73/60	70/57
Malignant neoplasm	96/88	87/77	52/47	41/36
Recipient age				
< 1 year	91/78	87/74	83/60	82/58
1–5 years	91/80	87/73	83/70	82/69
6–10 years	92/83	87/75	85/72	83/69

reports exist regarding this group (Bonatti et al., 1997; Woodle et al., 1998). Berquist and Cox reported a 30% patient survival rate at 1 year in children under 3 months of age at transplant (Cox et al., 1999). The authors' own experience would confirm this decreased value, with 50% patient survival in six cases. The excess mortality in this group is associated with their small size, the resulting technical complexity, and the severity of their illness at the time of transplant. The waiting-list mortality rate in these children is also excessive. In contrast to older children, the commonest diagnosis in this age group is neonatal hepatitis (Cox et al., 1999). This disease and metabolic diseases that occur in the newborn result in rapid onset of hepatocellular dysfunction (Bonatti et al., 1997; Woodle et al., 1998; Cox et al., 1999). These extremely ill babies require aggressive management and early liver transplantation in order to achieve success. The lack of size-appropriate donors for these children is a critical variable. The living-donor liver transplant experience of the Japanese centers has resulted in identification of the optimal hepatic allograft size as a percentage of recipient body weight. This range is 0.8–6% of the total body weight of the recipient (Tanaka et al., 1996). The adult left lateral liver segment may be too large for the small recipient (Kawasaki et al., 1993). For children under 4 kg in weight, the scarcity of donors is even more acute. Between 60% and 100% require a segmental graft (Bonatti et al., 1997; Woodle et al., 1998). Increased graft loss and patient mortality are seen in these cases, although the etiology of graft loss is unclear.

The condition of the child at the time of transplant has an impact on short-term outcomes (Seaberg et al., 1997; Department of Health and Human Services, 1999). UNOS data show the decrease in survival of liver transplant recipients who are on life support when transplanted, compared with those who are simply hospitalized (Department of Health and Human Services, 1999). These data, although not specific to children, are confirmed by the outcomes of children in the European Split Liver Database (de Ville de Goyet, 1995). Children who were critically ill at the time of transplant had patient and graft survival rates that were 17% and 22%, respectively, below those of children who were stable. In a recent review of the single-center experience at Pittsburgh Children's Hospital, graft survival rates decreased from 81% for stable patients to 67.5% for critically ill children, and the risk of graft loss increased by 2.2-fold (Cacciarelli et al., 1999). Graft loss was secondary to recipient death in half of the cases, with sepsis being the most frequent cause of death. Data from the Pitt-UNOS database for over 3000 pediatric liver transplant recipients document a decreased patient survival rate at 6 months (64% vs. 81%) and 1 year (62% vs. 80%) for recipients on life support compared with children in the intensive-care unit when transplanted (Seaberg et al., 1997). Critical illness at the time of liver transplant significantly increases the risk of death postoperatively.

The liver disease which causes the need for liver transplantation has an important impact on short-term outcomes. Children with fulminant hepatic failure have an increased death rate and graft loss rate compared with other children (Alper et al., 1998; Goss et al., 1998b; Hattori et al., 1998; Emre et al., 1999). Fulminant hepatic failure is a rather uncommon disease in children, representing only a few per cent of all children who require transplantation. It is a lethal disease that results in death in approximately 80% of children if they are not transplanted (Saing et al., 1999). The disease is fulminant, often resulting in complete hepatic failure, hepatic coma and brain death within a few days or weeks. Most children require intensive-care support prior to transplant. The decreased survival rate may be associated with the overall deterioration in these children prior to transplant, which frequently results in sepsis, renal failure and brain injury (Alper et al., 1998). Most centers have experienced the unsatisfactory results of transplanting a child in fulminant hepatic failure, only to have the new liver work well and the recipient experience permanent neurological injury (Bonatti et al., 1997; Goss et al., 1998). Monitoring of intracranial pressure prior to transplant can aid the identification of children who will not benefit from liver transplantation (Alper et al., 1998). Alper reported poor outcomes in children with cerebral edema secondary to acute hepatic failure (Alper et al., 1998). Improving waiting-list and postoperative morbidity and mortality depends on early referral to a liver transplant center, aggressive supportive care and transplantation prior to irreversible brain injury (Alper et al., 1998; Goss et al., 1998b; Hattori et al., 1998; Emre et al., 1999).

Children with primary hepatic malignancy who must be treated with liver transplantation show decreased survival rates at 5 years, primarily due to disease recurrence (Superina and Bilik, 1996; Seaberg et al., 1997; Al-Qabandi et al., 1999; Department of Health and Human Services, 1999). These results are based on a relatively small number of reports and a small number of patients in each report (see Chapter 18). Patient survival rates at 1 year are nearly the same as for all pediatric liver transplant indications but decrease by approximately 15–20% at 5 years due to death resulting from tumor recurrence (Seaberg et al., 1997). Long-term tumor-free survival is common in those patients who are free of tumor after 3 years (Superina and Bilik, 1996; Al-Qabandi et al., 1999; Laine et al., 1999). Transplantation for hepatoblastoma, the commonest primary hepatic malignancy in childhood, is uncommon. Hepatic resection prior to transplantation may be a risk factor for recurrence post transplant (Superina and Bilik, 1996). Improvements in chemotherapy and patient selection may lead to improved long-term outcomes.

Children with Alagille's syndrome have multi-organ involvement associated with paucity of intrahepatic bile ducts (Emerick *et al.*, 1999). In total, 80% of children have peripheral pulmonary/artery stenosis (Quiros-Tejeira *et al.*, 1999). When the latter is associated with intracardiac defects, survival after liver transplantation may be compromised (Emerick *et al.*, 1999). Serious heart disease is a risk factor in children with Aligille's syndrome who do not require liver transplantation.

Postoperative complications can adversely effect short-term outcomes after liver transplantation (see Chapter 30). Primary non-function occurs when the transplanted hepatic allograft does not function adequately to sustain normal metabolic demands (Ploeg *et al.*, 1993; Deschenes *et al.*, 1998). This results in rapid onset of multisystem injury with acute renal failure, hepatic coma, coagulopathy and metabolic derangements (including severe acidosis, hypoglycemia and hyperammonemia). Immediate retransplantation is the treatment of choice, but may not be possible due to lack of an available donor. The overall incidence of primary non-function is 0.6–22% (Busuttil and Klintmalm, 1996). Survival of children who experience primary non-function is not well documented. Newell and colleagues reported patient and graft survival rates of 62% and 58%, respectively, for children who were retransplanted due to primary non-function (Newell *et al.*, 1998). Hepatic artery thrombosis is another postoperative complication that adversely affects short-term outcome. Approximately 75% of children with hepatic artery thrombosis require retransplantation, and the retransplant mortality rate is 50% (Rela *et al.*, 1996). Grafts that undergo hepatic artery thrombosis may be salvaged if hepatic artery embolectomy and graft re-arterialization can be achieved in a timely manner. The rate of graft loss due to hepatic artery thrombosis is approximately 5–10% (Reding *et al.*, 1999; Sieders *et al.*, 1999). Although many other medical and surgical complications can and do occur after liver transplantation in children, most of them do not directly affect short-term outcomes.

The child who receives a liver transplant must take lifelong immunosuppressive medication to prevent allograft rejection. The US multicenter trial of cyclosporine vs. tacrolimus as primary immunosuppression after liver transplantation was one of the first studies to include children (McDiarmid *et al.*, 1995). This study showed no difference in patient or graft survival rates at 1 year in children on cyclosporine or tacrolimus. The incidence of acute rejection and steroid-resistant rejection was higher in the cyclosporine group. A subsequent study of the micro-emulsion formulation of cyclosporine reported a decreased rate of graft rejection (Alvarez *et al.*, 2000). Recently, McAllister and colleagues reported greatly improved patient and graft survival rates in adults receiving tacrolimus and sirolimus with rapid steroid weaning (McAllister *et al.*, 2000). However, a large multicenter randomized study showing improved short-term patient or graft survival rates for children with any of the current immunosuppressive regimens has not yet

been published. It does appear that the rates of chronic rejection are lower on tacrolimus-based therapy for children compared with those for children who are receiving cyclosporine-based therapy (McDiarmid *et al.*, 1998a; Cacciarelli *et al.*, 1999; Cox *et al.*, 1999; Reding *et al.*, 1999). The decreased incidence of late graft loss due to chronic rejection has improved long-term graft survival rates in children on tacrolimus. The incidence of Epstein–Barr virus-associated lymphoproliferative disease is higher in children who are receiving tacrolimus-based therapy (McDiarmid *et al.*, 1998a). This may be a source of long-term morbidity or mortality for this group. Although long-term effects of immunosuppression may decrease the rate of graft loss, the short-term outcomes resulting from commonly used immunosuppressive regimens that utilize tacrolimus or cyclosporine are very similar.

LONG-TERM OUTCOMES OF LIVER TRANSPLANTATION IN CHILDREN

Overview

Data on the long-term outcomes of liver transplantation are difficult to obtain. Many articles are starting to appear in the literature that report 10-year follow-up of children after successful liver transplantation (Abbasoglu *et al.*, 1997; Seaberg *et al.*, 1997; Goss *et al.*, 1998a; Burdelski *et al.*, 1999; Cacciarelli *et al.*, 1999; Ryckman *et al.*, 1999; Migliazza *et al.*, 2000). These data are useful for several reasons. They demonstrate the stable survival curves for patients and grafts which occur approximately 1 year post liver transplant, and the general improvement in outcomes for all patients who have been transplanted in more recent times. However, a 10-year follow-up is much shorter than the full lifespan of a child, and the current data are inadequate for evaluation of the benefits of liver transplantation and its risks.

A review of the available literature leads us to some broad and preliminary conclusions. After liver transplant, most children enjoy a good quality of life with excellent liver function (Burdelski *et al.*, 1999). Pretransplant central nervous system deficits may not resolve post transplant. However, most children have normal intellectual function (Wayman *et al.*, 1997; Kennard *et al.*, 1999). Those who have been exposed to prolonged or high total-dose corticosteroids may show irreversible growth impairment (McDiarmid *et al.*, 1999). Protocols which wean steroids more rapidly have been associated with normal growth and few increased problems with rejection (Reding, 2000). Allografts that are lost late are usually lost to infectious complications, immunosuppression-related problems or surgical complications, and not to recurrent liver disease (Sudan *et al.*, 1998; Ryckman *et al.*, 1999). Those children who require late retransplant have decreased survival rates compared with children who receive a primary transplant (Newell et al., 1998).

As children live longer and normal life expectancy is possible, attention has turned to the long-term effects of immunosuppression. The major calcineurin inhibitors currently in use, namely cyclosporine and tacrolimus, have a similar nephrotoxicity, which is significant in over 50% of children who are transplanted (McDiarmid, 1996). Lymphoproliferative disease is currently the commonest post-transplant malignancy after liver transplantation (Penn, 1994). Tacrolimus, although it lowers the rate of acute and chronic rejection, has been associated with increased rates of lymphoproliferative disease (Goss et al., 1998a; McDiarmid et al., 1998a). Strategies for diagnosing and treating Epstein–Barr virus infection seem to decrease the overall incidence of lymphoproliferative disease (McDiarmid et al., 1998a). New immunosuppressive regimens must be evaluated in terms of the incidence of lymphoproliferative disease as well as their immunosuppressive effects. The effect of current immunosuppressive agents on pregnant women and their fetuses is also an important issue. A growing body of data shows that many women have already carried pregnancies to completion successfully without grave danger to themselves or their babies (Wu et al., 1998)

Causes of late patient and graft loss

Several articles have reviewed the long-term outcomes of children after liver transplantation. Magliazzi and colleagues demonstrated that children who are alive 1 year after liver transplant have survival rates at 3, 5 and 10 years of 95%, 93% and 93%, respectively (Migliazza et al., 2000). Sudan and colleagues reported a 10-year actuarial patient survival rate of 84% for those alive at 1 year post transplant (Sudan et al., 1998). In contrast to adults, where late death or graft loss is commonly due to recurrent liver disease or patient death from stroke or heart disease, late death in children is usually due to graft failure or sepsis (Sudan et al., 1998; Ryckman et al., 1999). In Sudan's report, 39% of late deaths were directly related to graft failure and a further 35% were due to infection. Graft failure was secondary to chronic rejection in 44% of cases, biliary complications in 33% and recurrent disease in 22% of cases. Alarmingly, the commonest cause of graft loss leading to death in adolescents was non-compliance with medication. Ryckman and colleagues found that 73% of late deaths were caused by sepsis (Ryckman et al., 1999). Complications of immunosuppression contributed to over 50% of these cases. Sudden and unanticipated sepsis occurred in one-third of deaths, with pneumonia being the commonest infection. Late deaths in these reports contrast sharply with causes of mortality for all children

(Sudan et al., 1998). Unlike the general pediatric population, where trauma or accidents account for 40% of deaths between the ages of 1 and 14 years, there were no late deaths due to trauma or accidents. Sepsis as a cause of death in the general pediatric population is less common than cancer, congenital anomalies, homicide, heart disease or suicide. Vigilant care of the ill liver transplant child is the most important step in addressing the risk of sepsis.

The rate of late graft loss due to chronic rejection has decreased from approximately 15% to approximately 4% (Burdelski et al., 1999). This is largely due to the use of tacrolimus as primary or rescue therapy. Recent changes in cyclosporine formulation (micro-emulsion formulation) have also led to decreased rates of acute rejection and steroid-resistant rejections which are strongly associated with chronic rejection (Alvarez et al., 2000). Additional agents, such as sirolimus, may be used in combination with tacrolimus or cyclosporine to lower the rates of acute and chronic rejection (McAllister et al., 2000). Decreasing rates of chronic rejection should improve graft survival unless larger amounts of immunosuppression decrease patient survival due to complications of over-suppression.

Children who lose their transplanted livers are at higher risk of death following retransplantation. Newell and colleagues reported survival rates of less than 50% for children who were retransplanted for chronic rejection (Newell et al., 1998). Nicolette and colleagues reported a much higher survival rate of 83%. However, several patients required more than one retransplant (Nicolette et al., 1998). The retransplant procedure is frequently challenging. Schindel and colleagues reported the results of several patients who required three or more liver transplants. Increased recipient hepatectomy times and increased donor organ cold storage time require careful planning in these cases. The short-term outcome was 71% for patient and graft survival (Schindel et al., 2000).

Recurrent primary liver disease can occur in children. The diseases which may recur are hepatitis B and C and autoimmune hepatitis. In Caccamo's report, seven out of eight children who were alive at 1 year post transplant and who had hepatitis C prior to transplant had recurrent hepatitis C (Caccamo et al., 1998). Two of them died of the recurrent hepatitis C complication, one was retransplanted and four showed ongoing signs of chronic active hepatitis. McDiarmid and colleagues reported on 13 children who developed hepatitis C after liver transplantation (McDiarmid et al., 1998b). Eleven of them developed chronic active hepatitis and one developed cirrhosis. Treatment with interferon was beneficial for only two patients, while four cases required retransplantation. Three of these developed rapid recurrence of disease and subsequently died. Although 76% of these children were alive at the time of the report, most of them had chronic active hepatitis. Acquisition of hepatitis C at the time of transplant may occur from blood products or the donor liver. Acquisition rates are directly related to the volume of blood transfused (Nowicki et al., 1994).

Autoimmune hepatitis is a rare disease in childhood, representing approximately 2% of the indication for liver transplantation (Goss et al., 1998a). Unfortunately, the rate of recurrence of autoimmune hepatitis post transplant is high. Birnbaum and colleagues reported recurrence in five out of six children, three of whom required retransplantation during the first year (Birnbaum et al., 1997). These three children had recurrent autoimmune hepatitis in their second allografts. This experience is worse than that seen in adults, where the recurrence rate is approximately 25% (Ratziu et al., 1999). Birnbaum noted that the use of tacrolimus did not prevent recurrent disease.

Hepatic failure secondary to hepatitis B is rare in the USA, especially now that hepatitis B vaccination is widely practised. The author has had only two children transplanted for hepatitis B. Both of them have remained healthy with normal liver function on chronic treatment with hepatitis B hyperimmune globulin. The experience with hepatitis B in adults suggests a low rate of recurrence for patients who receive hepatitis B hyperimmune globulin on a long-term basis (Samuel et al., 1991).

Growth, development and quality of life

Children with hepatic failure suffer from severe growth disturbance. Viner and McDiarmid reported mean height standard deviation scores of −1.22 and −1.72, respectively, in their pediatric liver failure patients prior to transplant (McDiarmid et al., 1999; Viner et al., 1999). Growth disturbance is a result of malnutrition, inanition, metabolic bone disease, vitamin deficiency and liver disease (Kelly, 1997). Children with liver disease have low levels of insulin-like growth factor (Infante et al., 1998). Growth hormone does not correct this deficiency when administered to the child with liver disease (Bucuvalas et al., 1997). Successful transplantation with good graft function is the best treatment for growth failure due to liver disease. Growth after transplant is directly affected by the total steroid dose and maintenance steroid use (Birnbaum et al., 1997). McDiarmid and colleagues reported poor improvement in height standard deviation scores for children in whom steroids were maintained chronically (McDiarmid et al., 1999). Viner and colleagues reported mean height standard deviation scores at 5 and 7 years post transplant and at final height to be −1.5, −0.84 and −0.55, respectively, for children who were weaned from steroids (Viner et al., 1999). The mean height of those who had no more growth potential was at the 27th percentile for adult height. Growth acceleration begins when alternate-day steroids are started, and it continues to accelerate after steroids have been discontinued (Reding, 2000). Low rates of allograft rejection are seen with steroid withdrawal after 7 months (Reding, 2000). Those who were withdrawn at 3 months and 7 months showed acute rejection rates of 27% and 13%, respectively, compared with 7% when withdrawn at 18 months (Reading, 2000). Viner and others have noted that children with the greatest potential for catch-up growth and ability to reach normal height were transplanted when they were very young (Kelly, 1997; Viner et al., 1999). Some children with Alagille's syndrome have shown continued slow growth post transplant even with good hepatic function (Kelly, 1997). Growth hormone secretion and insulin-like growth factor levels return to normal after liver transplantation (Infante et al., 1998). Sarna and colleagues reported that growth hormone administered to severely growth-delayed children who were on steroids after liver transplantation was successful in improving height standard deviation scores (Sarna et al., 1996).

Severe liver disease is associated with developmental delays in young children. Wayman and colleagues found that prior to liver transplant, infants with biliary atresia had low average mental and psychomotor development (Wayman et al., 1997). Their test results decreased 3 months post transplant but had returned to pretransplant levels by 1 year post transplant. At that time, 35% of the post-transplant group were developmentally delayed. This is consistent with the report of Kennard and colleagues, who found that 18% of children after transplant had an IQ of < 70, 26% had learning problems and 56% were functioning within their cognitive ability, which was within the normal range (Kennard et al., 1999). Kennard notes that 38% of the children who were functioning below their cognitive ability had never received special services. This may be in part due to the young age of many of these children and the effort required to elicit these developmental delays. Recognition of the risk these children have for developmental delay should lead to more widespread testing and early intervention. Deutsch and colleagues detected a significant percentage of children with severe sensorineural hearing loss post liver transplant (Deutsch et al., 1998). In total, 12% of the children studied had sensorineural hearing loss. At risk were those children with short bowel syndrome and hyperalimentation-associated liver disease and those under 2 years of age who were exposed to high total doses of amikacin. Recognition and appropriate care of these children will enable them to deal with this deficit and achieve acceptable integration into adult life.

Quality of life can be difficult to assess. Apajasalo and colleagues compared childhood transplant recipients with normal controls using a well-described health-related quality-of-life assessment tool (Apajasalo et al., 1997). Health-related quality of life was similar to that of controls for adolescents, but lower than that of controls for those in the 8–11 years age group. This may have been due to an earlier age at transplant for this group, or to more complicated illness and growth disturbance seen in this age group. Emotional evaluation showed that adolescent transplant patients have a significantly better status than controls. The reasons for the improved emotional scores in these patients cannot readily be ascertained. Decreased health-related quality of life may be secondary to limitations, which may be addressed when they are discovered.

Pregnancy poses special risks for the transplant recipient. Changes due to pregnancy may alter the immunological balance that characterizes stable transplant recipients. Immunosuppressive agents may be toxic to the developing fetus. Wu and colleagues reported on 22 successful pregnancies in 16 women who had received liver transplants (Wu et al., 1998). In total, 23 healthy babies were born (one set of twins) with an average gestation of 38 weeks and fetal weight of 2876 ± 589 g. No congenital abnormalities or unusual infections were identified. Three deliveries were premature, including the twin birth. All of the children appeared to be growing and developing normally. One steroid-sensitive rejection occurred, but otherwise there were no transplant-related complications.

Late complications

Long-term effects of immunosuppression increase the incidence of lymphoproliferative disease (LPD) in children. After liver transplantation, lymphoproliferative disease occurs in 4–11% of recipients and may be as high as 22% in those children who are treated with sequential therapy for rejection, including cyclosporine, pulse steroids, OKT3 and tacrolimus (McDiarmid, 1998). Children who are young, Epstein–Barr virus (EBV)-seronegative and receive a seropositive donor organ are at highest risk for LPD (Sokal et al., 1997). Early detection of EBV viremia by polymerase chain reaction allows for a decrease in immunosuppression and treatment with acyclovir or ganciclovir to limit progression to monoclonal malignancy (Green et al., 1998). Most transplantation centers decrease immunosuppression gradually over time in order to decrease the possibility of over-suppression and development of EBV-associated LPD (McDiarmid et al., 1998a). Screening by EBV polymerase chain reaction has become standard at most centers. Early detection and tapering of immunosuppression have lowered the risk of progression of LPD to frank lymphoma (Green et al., 1998; McDiarmid et al., 1998a). Although EBV infection occurs early in the post-transplant course of most seronegative children, not all children with LPD present in the first year post transplant (Burdelski et al., 1999). Late presentation, especially with extranodal involvement, has been reported (Renard et al., 1991). Even with an aggressive approach leading to early discovery of EBV infection in the first year post transplant, late-presenting cases of LPD may be missed. Early diagnosis and decrease or withdrawal of immunosuppressive therapy may lead to successful outcomes (McDiarmid et al., 1998a). Patients with tumor presentation will usually require chemotherapy in addition to decreasing immunosuppression (Giez-Chamorro et al., 2000).

The calcineurin inhibitors in common use for long-term immunosuppression are nephrotoxic in a dose-dependent manner (McDiarmid, 1996). Children on tacrolimus after liver transplant were found to have glomerular filtration rates of 43 mL/minute/1.73 m^2 compared with those on cyclosporine, who had rates of 49 mL/minute 1.73 m^2 (McDiarmid, 1996). Earlier estimates of decreases in glomerular filtration rate by cyclosporine were approximately 50%. Andrews and colleagues reported a decrease in creatinine clearance, measured by inulin clearance, over 4 years of cyclosporine treatment in children (Andrews et al., 1991). A similar result was found by McDiarmid (1996). In that study, 50% of children with a glomerular filtration rate of < 50 mL/minute/1.73 m^2 required antihypertensive therapy. Bartosh and colleagues found abnormal creatinine clearance in one-third of children (Bartosh et al., 1997). At 1 year, 28% of them required antihypertensive medication. Both tacrolimus and cyclosporine resulted in a tubulopathy which caused magnesium wasting and metabolic acidosis (McDiarmid, 1996). Approximately 20% of the authors' patients require long-term bicarbonate administration. The immunosuppressive agents mycophenolate mofetil and rapamycin have no nephrotoxicity. Rapamycin in combination with tacrolimus has given low rejection rates, allowing for a reduction in the amount of nephrotoxic drug used (McAllister et al., 2000). It is hoped that renal function will be preserved by this approach, but long-term outcome data are not available.

SUMMARY

Children who receive liver transplants today face a brighter and more well-characterized future than ever before. For the individual child and his or her parents, much cannot be answered. We still do not have an accepted risk assessment model for the individual child, and we do not know the long-term risks of transplantation for the life of a child. However, our general knowledge allows us to give useful general answers, and some day we shall have better ones.

Key references

Burdelski M, Nolkemper D, Ganschow R et al. Liver transplantation in children: long-term outcome and quality of life. *European Journal of Pediatrics* 1999; **158**: S34–42.

An excellent current review of the late outcomes of liver transplantation in children.

Cox KL, Berquist WE, Castillo RO. Current issues in liver transplantation. Paediatric liver transplantation: indications, timing and medical complications. *Journal of Gastroenterology and Hepatology* 1999; **14**: S61–6.

Very complete but brief review of the important issues in pediatric liver transplantation.

Newell KA, Millis JM, Bruce DS et al. An analysis of hepatic retransplantation in children. *Transplantation* 1998; **65**: 1172–8.

An important current review of the negative effects of retransplantation on outcomes.

Reding R, de Ville de Goyet J, Delbeke I et al. Pediatric liver transplantation with cadaveric or living related donors: comparative results in 90 elective recipients of primary grafts. *Journal of Pediatrics* 1999; **134**: 280–6.

An excellent current review of the impact of living donor transplantation on children with liver disease.

Department of Health and Human Services. *United Network for Organ Sharing. 1999 annual report.* Richmond, VA: United Network for Organ Sharing, 1999.

Data on transplantation outcomes in the USA.

REFERENCES

Abbasoglu O, Levy MF, Brkic BB et al. Ten years of liver transplantation. *Transplantation* 1997; **64**: 1801–7.

Al-Qabandi W, Jenkinson HC, Buckels JA et al. Orthotopic liver transplantation for unresectable hepatoblastoma: a single center's experience. *Journal of Pediatric Surgery* 1999; **34**: 1261–4.

Alper G, Jarjour IT, Reyes JD et al. Outcome of children with cerebral edema caused by fulminant hepatic failure. *Pediatric Neurology* 1998; **18**: 299–304.

Alvarez F, Atkinson PR, Grant DR et al. NOF-11: a one-year pediatric randomized double-blind comparison of neoral versus sandimmune in orthotopic liver transplantation. *Transplantation* 2000; **69**: 87–92.

Andrews W, Agrant B, Fyock B et al. The effect of cyclosporine A on long-term renal function in pediatric liver transplant recipients. *Transplantation Proceedings* 1991; **23**: 1252–3.

Apajasalo M, Rautonen J, Sintonen H et al. Health-related quality of life after organ transplantation in childhood. *Pediatric Transplantation* 1997; **1**: 130–7.

Bartosh SM, Alonso EM, Whitington PF et al. Renal outcomes in pediatric liver transplantation. *Clinical Transplantation* 1997; **11**: 354–60.

Birnbaum AH, Benkov KJ, Pittman NS et al. Recurrence of autoimmune hepatitis in children after liver transplantation. *Journal of Pediatric Gastroenterology and Nutrition* 1997; **25**: 20–5.

Bonatti H, Muiesan P, Connelly S et al. Hepatic transplantation in children under 3 months of age: a single centre's experience. *Journal of Pediatric Surgery* 1997; **32**: 486–8.

Bucuvalas JC, Horn JA, Chernausek SD. Resistance to growth hormone in children with chronic liver disease. *Pediatric Transplantation* 1997; **1**: 73–9.

Burdelski M, Nolkemper D, Ganschow R et al. Liver transplantation in children: long-term outcome and quality of life. *European Journal of Pediatrics* 1999; **158**: S34–42.

Busuttil RW, Klintmalm GB. *Transplantation of the liver*, 1st edn. Philadelphia, PA: WB Saunders Co., 1996.

Caccamo L, Colledan M, Rossi G. Post-hepatitis primary disease does not influence 6-year survival after liver transplantation beyond 1 year. *Transplantation International* 1998; **11**: S212–20.

Cacciarelli TV, Dvorchik I, Mazariegos GV et al. An analysis of pretransplantation variables associated with long-term allograft outcome in pediatric liver transplant recipients receiving primary tacrolimus (FK506) therapy. *Transplantation* 1999; **68**: 650–5.

Colombani PM, Cigarroa FG, Schwarz K et al. Liver transplantation in infants younger than 1 year of age. *Annals of Surgery* 1996; **223**: 658–64.

Cox KL, Berquist WE, Castillo RO. Current issues in liver transplantation. Paediatric liver transplantation: indications, timing and medical complications. *Journal of Gastroenterology and Hepatology* 1999; **14**: S61–6.

Department of Health and Human Services. *United Network for Organ Sharing. 1999 annual report*, Richmond, VA: United Network for Organ Sharing, 1999.

Deschenes M, Belle SH, Krom RAF et al. Early allograft dysfunction after liver transplantation. *Transplantation* 1998; **66**: 302–10.

Deutsch ES, Bartling V, Lawenda B et al. Sensorineural hearing loss in children after liver transplantation. *Archives of Otolaryngology Head and Neck Surgery* 1998; **124**: 529–33.

de Ville de Goyet J. Split liver transplantation in Europe – 1988 to 1993. *Transplantation* 1995; **59**: 1371–6.

Emerick KM, Rand EB, Goldmuntz E et al. Features of Alagille syndrome in 92 patients: frequency and relation to prognosis. *Hepatology* 1999; **29**: 822–9.

Emre S, Schwartz ME, Shneider B et al. Living-related liver transplantation for acute liver failure in children. *Liver Transplantation and Surgery* 1999; **5**: 161–5.

Giez-Chamorro A, Jimenez C, Moreno-Giez E *et al.* Management and outcome of liver recipients with post-transplant lymphoproliferative disease. *Hepato-Gastroenterology* 2000; **47**: 211–19.

Goss JA, Shackleton CR, McDiarmid SV *et al.* Long-term results of pediatric liver transplantation. An analysis of 569 transplants. *Annals of Surgery* 1998a; **228**: 411–20.

Goss JA, Shackleton CR, Maggard M *et al.* Liver transplantation for fulminant hepatic failure in the pediatric patient. *Archives of Surgery* 1998b; **133**: 839–46.

Green M, Cacciarelli TV, Mazariegos GV *et al.* Serial measurement of Epstein–Barr viral load in peripheral blood in pediatric liver transplant recipients during treatment for post-transplant lymphoproliferative disease. *Transplantation* 1998; **66**: 1641–4.

Hattori H, Higuchi Y, Tsuji M *et al.* Living-related liver transplantation and neurological outcome in children with fulminant hepatic failure. *Transplantation* 1998; **65**: 686–92.

Infante D, Tormo R, Castro de Kolster C *et al.* Changes in growth, growth hormone, and insulin-like growth factor-1 (IGF-I) after orthotopic liver transplantation. *Pediatric Surgery International* 1998; **13**: 323–6.

Kawasaki S, Makuuchi M, Matsunami H *et al.* Preoperative measurement of segmental liver volume of donors for living related liver transplantation. *Hepatology* 1993; **18**: 1115–20.

Kelly DA. Post-transplant growth failure in children. *Liver Transplantation and Surgery* 1997; **3**: S32–9.

Kelly DA. Nutritional factors affecting growth before and after liver transplantation. *Pediatric Transplantation* 1997; **1**: 80–4.

Kelly DA. Current results and evolving indications for liver transplantation in children. *Journal of Pediatric Gastroenterology and Nutrition* 1998; **27**: 214–21.

Kennard B, Stewart S, Phelan-McAulitte D *et al.* Academic outcome in long-term survivors of pediatric liver transplantation. *Developmental and Behavioral Pediatrics* 1999; **20**: 17–23.

Laine J, Jalanko H, Saarinen-Pihkala UM *et al.* Successful liver transplantation after induction chemotherapy in children with inoperable, multifocal primary hepatic malignancy. *Transplantation* 1999; **67**: 1369–72.

McAllister V, Gzo Z, Peltescian K *et al.* Sirolimus-tacrolimus combination immunosuppression. *Lancet* 2000; **355**: 375–7.

McDiarmid SV. Renal function in pediatric liver transplant patients. *Kidney International* 1996; **49**: S77–84.

McDiarmid SV. The use of tacrolimus in pediatric liver transplantation. *Journal of Pediatric Gastroenterology and Nutrition* 1998; **26**: 90–102.

McDiarmid S, Busuttil R, Ascher N *et al.* KF 506 (tacrolimus) compared with cyclosporine for primary immunosuppression after pediatric liver transplantation. *Transplantation* 1995; **59**: 530–40.

McDiarmid SV, Jordan S, Lee GS *et al.* Prevention and pre-emptive therapy of post-transplant lymphoproliferative disease in pediatric liver recipients. *Transplantation* 1998a; **66**: 1604–11.

McDiarmid SV, Conrad A, Ament ME *et al.* De novo hepatitis C in children after liver transplantation. *Transplantation* 1998b; **66**: 311–18.

McDiarmid S, Gornbein JA, DeSilva PJ *et al.* Factors affecting growth after pediatric liver transplantation. *Transplantation* 1999; **67**: 404–11.

Malatack J, Schaid D, Urbach A *et al.* Choosing a pediatric recipient for orthotopic liver transplantation. *Journal of Pediatrics* 1987; **111**: 479–89.

Migliazza L, Santamarie ML, Murcia J *et al.* Long-term survival expectancy after liver transplantation in children. *Journal of Pediatric Surgery* 2000; **35**: 5–8.

Newell KA, Millis JM, Bruce DS *et al.* An analysis of hepatic retransplantation in children. *Transplantation* 1998; **65**: 1172–8.

Nicolette LA, Reichard KW, Falkenstein K *et al.* Results of transplantation for acute and chronic hepatic allograft rejection. *Journal of Pediatric Surgery* 1998; **33**: 909–12.

Nowicki MJ, Ahmad N, Heubi JE *et al.* The prevalence of hepatitis C virus (HCV) in infants and children after liver transplantation. *Digestive Diseases and Sciences* 1994; **39**: 2250–4.

Penn I. Post-transplant malignancies in pediatric organ transplant recipients. *Transplantation Proceedings* 1994; **26**: 2763–5.

Ploeg RJ, D'Alessandro AM, Knechtle SJ *et al.* Risk factors for primary dysfunction after liver transplantation – a multivariate analysis. *Transplantation* 1993; **55**: 807–13.

Quiros-Tejeira RE, Ament ME, Heyman MD *et al.* Variable morbidity in Alagille syndrome: a review of 43 cases. *Journal of Pediatric Gastroenterology and Nutrition* 1999; **29**: 431–7.

Ratziu V, Samuel D, Sebagh M *et al.* Long-term follow-up after liver transplantation for autoimmune hepatitis: evidence of recurrence of primary disease. *Journal of Hepatology* 1999; **30**: 131–41.

Reding R. Steroid withdrawal in liver transplantation. Benefits, risks and unanswered questions. *Transplantation* 2000; **70**: 405–10.

Reding R, de Ville de Goyet J, Delbeke I *et al.* Pediatric liver transplantation with cadaveric or living related donors: comparative results in 90 elective recipients of primary grafts. *Journal of Pediatrics* 1999; **134**: 280–6.

Rela M, Muiesan P, Bhatnagar V *et al.* Hepatic artery thrombosis after liver transplantation in children under 5 years of age. *Transplantation* 1996; **61**: 1355–7.

Renard T, Andrew SW, Foster M. Relationship between OKT$_3$ administration, EBV seroconversion and the lymphoproliferative syndrome in pediatric liver transplant recipients. *Transplantation Proceedings* 1991; **23**: 1473–6.

Ryckman FC, Alonso MH, Bucuvalas JC *et al.* Long-term survival after liver transplantation. *Journal of Pediatric Surgery* 1999; **34**: 845–50.

Saing H, Fan ST, Chan KL *et al.* Liver transplantation in infants. *Journal of Pediatric Surgery* 1999; **34**: 1721–4.

Samuel D, Bismuth A, Mathieu D *et al.* Passive immunoprophylaxis after liver transplantation in HBs Ag-positive patients. *Lancet* 1991; **337**: 813–19.

Sarna S, Sipila I, Ronnholm K *et al.* Recombinant human growth hormone improves growth in children receiving glucocorticoid treatment after liver transplantation. *Journal of Clinical Endocrinology and Metabolism* 1996; **81**: 1476–82.

Schindel DT, Dunn SP, Casas AT *et al.* Pediatric recipients of three or more hepatic allografts: results and technical challenges. *Journal of Pediatric Surgery* 2000; **35**: 297–302.

Seaberg EC, Belle SH, Beringer KC *et al.* Long-term patient and retransplantation-free survival by selected recipient and donor characteristics: an update from the Pitt-UNOS liver transplant registry. *Clinical Transplant* 1997; **34**: 15–28.

Sieders E, Peeters PMJG, TenVergert EM *et al.* Analysis of survival and morbidity after pediatric liver transplantation with full-size and technical-variant grafts. *Transplantation* 1999; **68**: 540–5.

Sokal E, Autunes H, Bequin C *et al.* Early signs and risk factors for the increased incidence of Epstein–Barr virus-related post-transplant lymphoproliferative disease in pediatric liver transplant recipients treated with tacrolimus. *Transplantation* 1997; **64**: 1438–42.

Sudan DL, Shaw BW, Langnas AN. Causes of late mortality in pediatric liver transplant recipients. *Annals of Surgery* 1998; **227**: 289–95.

Superina R, Bilik R. Results of liver transplantation in children with unresectable liver tumors. *Journal of Pediatric Surgery* 1996; **31**: 835–9.

Tanaka A, Tanaka K, Tokuka A. Graft size-matching in living related partial liver transplantation in relation to tissue oxygenation and metabolic capacity. *Transplantation International* 1996; **9**: 15–22.

VanderWerf WJ, D'Alessandro AM, Knechtle SJ *et al.* Infant pediatric liver transplantation results equal those for older pediatric patients. *Journal of Pediatric Surgery* 1998; **33**: 20–3.

Viner RM, Forton JTM, Cole TJ *et al.* Growth of long-term survivors of liver transplantation. *Archives of Disease in Childhood* 1999; **80**: 235–40.

Wayman KI, Cox KL, Esquivel CO. Neurodevelopmental outcome of young children with extrahepatic biliary atresia 1 year after liver transplantation. *Journal of Pediatrics* 1997; **131**: 894–8.

Woodle ES, Millis JM, So SKS *et al.* Liver transplantation in the first three months of life. *Transplantation* 1998; **66**: 606–9.

Wu A, Nashan B, Messner U *et al.* Outcome of 22 successful pregnancies after liver transplantation. *Clinical Transplantation* 1998; **12**: 454–64.

Pancreas

32

Embryology of the pancreas

PATRICIA COLLINS

TIMING OF DEVELOPMENT

Our understanding of the timing of human development is based largely on the work of Streeter (1942) and, more recently, of O'Rahilly and Müller (1987). Both research groups studied the Carnegie Collection of Embryos in the USA and contributed to the staging system of human embryos which is commonly used. The majority of modern studies on human embryos and fetuses establish the age of specimens using data originally generated from the Carnegie Collection. It should be pointed out that extrapolating age from crown–rump or foot length is an inexact method, and thus that the times of development of body systems vary at the very least by ± 2 days. Gestational dates in this section, given as post-ovulatory days or weeks, are based on development from fertilization, which is considered to be as close as possible to ovulation. It should be borne in mind that this time-scale is 2 weeks less throughout than the obstetric time-scale, which dates pregnancy from the last menstrual period.

MORPHOGENESIS OF THE PANCREAS

The main morphological features of the development of the pancreas are presented in Table 32.1 and Figure 32.1. The pancreas forms as a result of the fusion of two pan-

creatic buds (dorsal and ventral) which arise from the distal foregut. Due to the craniocaudal progression of development, the dorsal pancreas develops ahead of the ventral pancreas, which arises as an evagination from the early bile duct. When the stomach and duodenum undergo rotation, there is repositioning of the origin of the common bile duct within the duodenal wall. The common bile duct and ventral pancreas rotate clockwise about a longitudinal axis, moving dorsally until the ventral pancreatic bud comes into contact with the dorsal bud (Figure 32.2). The ventral pancreatic bud thus moves from a position within the ventral mesoduodenum to a position in the dorsal mesoduodenum.

Three-dimensional anatomical reconstruction of the ventral and dorsal pancreata have confirmed the portion of the mature pancreas that is derived from each primordium (Uchida et al., 1999). The dorsal pancreas forms the anterior part of the head of the pancreas and the body and tail of the pancreas. The ventral pancreas forms the posterior part of the head of the pancreas and the posterior part of the uncinate process. Uchida et al. (1999) noted that the uncinate process consisted of the ventral pancreas alone in three out of eight human pancreata, and of both the dorsal and ventral pancreas in the remaining five specimens (Figure 32.3). This finding differs from the traditional view that the ventral pancreas forms all of the uncinate process and extends across the front of the superior mesenteric vein and to the left. Uchida et al. (1999) observed that the ventral pancreas stopped short of covering the anterior aspect of the

Table 32.1 *Time-scale of the morphological development of the human pancreas*

Stage	Days/weeks post-ovulation	Somite pairs	Crown–rump length (mm)	Description of development
6	13 days			Primitive streak appears
10	22 days	4–12	1.5–3	Head and tail folding, foregut formed
11	24 days	13–20	2.5–4.5	Notochord moves out of the endoderm layer, but remains in contact with dorsal layer of endoderm
12	26 days	21–29	3–5	Notochord separated from the endoderm by dorsal aortae. First appearance of dorsal pancreatic bud, dorsal and slightly higher than the liver, as a region of increased proliferative activity
		25–28		The foregut lengthens, increasing the distance between the lung buds and hepatic diverticulum
13	28 days	30+	4–6	The ventral pancreatic region may just be distinguished in some embryos as a region of increased proliferative activity
14	32 days		5–7	First appearance of ventral pancreatic bud as an evagination of the bile duct at this stage and stage 15
15	33 days		7–9	First appearance of ventral pancreatic bud as an evagination of the bile duct at this stage and stage 14. Dorsal pancreas elongates
16	37 days		8–11	Bile duct and ventral pancreas migrate to posterior side of duodenum
17	41 days		11–14	Ventral and dorsal pancreata fuse, each retaining their original ducts. Ventral pancreatic duct still connected to bile duct
20	50 days			*Data above from O'Rahilly and Müller (1987)*

Stages stop at stage 23, 56–57 days or 8 weeks

	9–10 weeks			Scattered polyhormonal endocrine cells within walls of pancreatic ducts
	11–15 weeks			Endocrine cells have clustered into immature polyhormonal islets
	16–29 weeks			Insulin can be detected in monohormonal cells in the core of the islets
	24 weeks			Islets still in direct contact with pancreatic ducts
	30 weeks onwards			Three monohormonal cell types present – insulin, glucagon and somatostatin. Polymorphic islets continue to develop
				Data from Bocian-Sobtowska et al. (1999)

superior mesenteric vein and was only related to its right lateral surface.

The ventral pancreas maintains characteristic macroscopic, histological and immunohistochemical features that are distinct from the dorsal pancreas. It has smaller and more closely packed lobuli which facilitate macroscopic differentiation. It has a lower fat content than the dorsal pancreas, and this facilitates its identification on ultrasonography and computed tomography in some cases. Pancreatic polypeptide-secreting cells (γ-cells) are more prevalent in the ventral than the dorsal pancreas. However, there are no marked differences in the numbers of α, β and δ cells between the two pancreata (Uchida *et al.*, 1999).

The dorsal and ventral pancreatic duct systems fuse so that most of the dorsal duct drains into the proximal part of the ventral duct to form the main pancreatic duct (of Wirsung) of the mature pancreas. The proximal remnant of the dorsal duct usually persists as an accessory duct (of Santorini), draining either into the duodenum or into the main duct. The fusion of the ducts occurs mainly in the postnatal period. Around 85% of infants have patent accessory ducts, compared with 40% of adults. Non-fusion of the ducts, known as pancreas divisum, is present in about 10% of all individuals (Githens, 1989).

Initially the body of the pancreas extends posteriorly into the dorsal mesoduodenum and then cranially into the dorsal mesogastrium. With rotation of the stomach, this part of the dorsal mesogastrium becomes

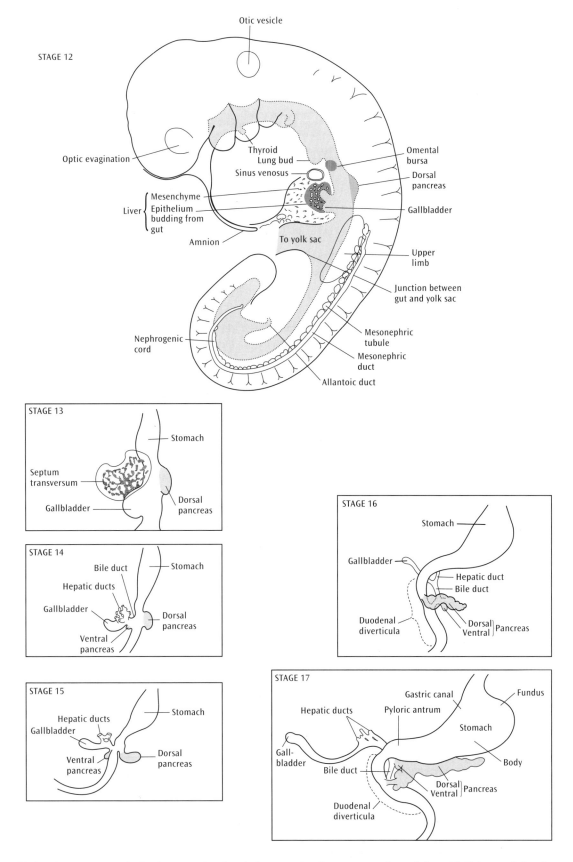

Figure 32.1 *Human pancreatic development. A series of diagrams showing reconstructions of the epithelial core of the alimentary canal, based on embryos in the Carnegie Collection in Washington. Note that the dorsal pancreas is present at stage 12 (not shown. The ventral pancreas can be seen initially at stages 14 and 15. Posterior migration of the ventral pancreatic bud occurs from stage 16. From O'Rahilly and Müller (1987).*

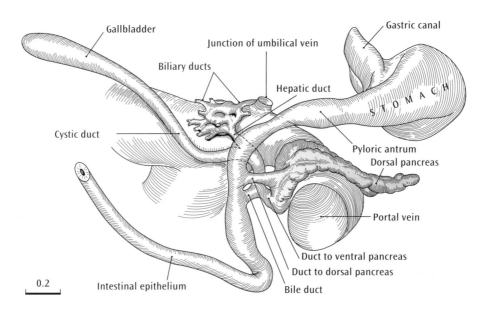

Figure 32.2 *Reconstruction of the epithelial core of the two pancreatic ducts, typical of stage 17. The dorsal pancreas still has its original duct, and the ventral pancreas still gains access to the duodenum via the bile duct. From O'Rahilly and Müller (1987).*

directed to the left, forming the posterior wall of the lesser sac. The posterior layer of this part of the dorsal mesogastrium fuses with the parietal layer of the peritoneum, and the pancreas becomes mainly retroperitoneal. This fusion of the dorsal mesogastrium does not include the portion containing the tail of the pancreas, which passes into the lienorenal ligament. The anterior border of the pancreas subsequently provides the main line of attachment for the posterior leaves of the greater omentum.

ORIGIN OF PANCREATIC ENDODERM

Endoderm, from which the pancreas develops, arises from invagination of cells through the most rostral end of the primitive streak – the primitive or Hensen's node. Epiblast cells which form the surface of the early embryonic disc undergo proliferation and, in the caudal portion of the disc, migrate in the midline through the

primitive streak to form a layer deep to the epiblast. The time and position at which epiblast cells pass through the streak affects their future developmental fate. Cells that ingress through the primitive node give rise to the axial cell lines, notochord and medial half of the somites, as well as all of the endodermal population (Selleck and Stern, 1991). Initially, the endoderm cells are mainly in the midline interspersed with presumptive notochordal cells. The endodermal cells displace the visceral hypoblast which initially forms the roof of the primitive yolk sac by changing their morphology from a cuboidal epithelium immediately after ingression to a squamous arrangement (Tam and Beddington, 1999). In this way the hypoblast cells are pushed into the secondary yolk sac wall.

The earliest endodermal population which ingresses via the primitive streak contributes to the prechordal (prochordal) plate. This region, which lies rostral to the invaginated notochordal cells, gives rise to the buccopharyngeal membrane and, towards the edge of the embryonic disc, an area of endoderm which will become

Figure 32.3 *(a) Schematic representation of the pancreas based on sections cut from A to I. Cut surfaces are shown below. The contribution made by the ventral pancreas to the total gland is denoted by shading. The ventral pancreatic bud gives rise to the posterior part of the head of the pancreas. CBD, common bile duct; PD, main pancreatic duct; WD, duct of Wirsung, derived from the ventral pancreatic bud; SD, duct of Santorini, derived from the dorsal pancreatic bud. (b) Anterior view and (c) posterior view in schematic reconstruction of the ventral pancreas alone. The ventral pancreas is located in the posterior part of the pancreas and in the uncinate process. It relates to the right lateral surface of the superior mesenteric vein and extends behind the superior mesenteric vein to the left. It does not extend across the anterior surface of the superior mesenteric vein to the left. D, duodenum; PV, portal vein–superior mesenteric vein; CBD, common bile duct; GB, gallbladder. Reproduced from Uchida T, Takeda T, Ammori BJ, Suda K, Takahashi T. Three-dimensional reconstruction of the ventral and dorsal pancreas: a new insight into anatomy and embryonic development. Journal of Hepatobiliary and Pancreatic Surgery 1999; 6: 176–80.*

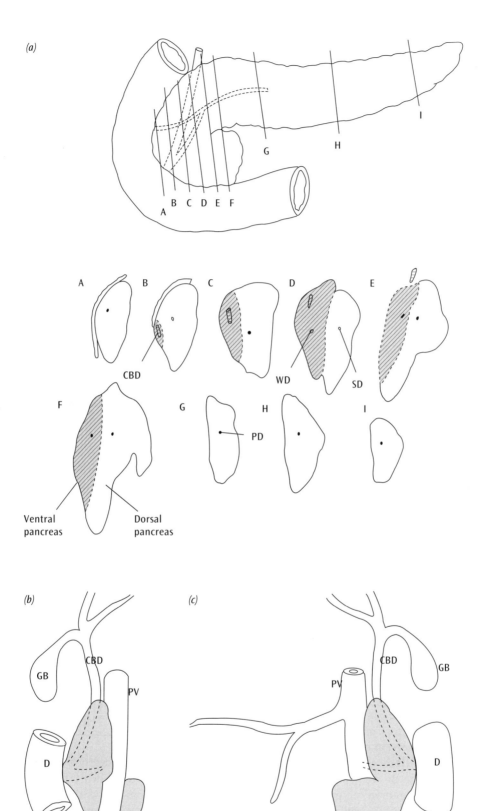

(a)

A B C D E F   G   H   I

CBD

WD   SD

F   Ventral pancreas   Dorsal pancreas   G   H   PD   I

(b)   (c)

GB   CBD   PV   CBD   GB

D   PV   D

Anterior view   Posterior view

the ventral wall of the foregut. The way in which the earliest invaginating endodermal cells give rise to the cell line from which the foregut develops is not yet clear. The foregut will produce glands associated with the head and neck via pharyngeal pouch development, and it also produces the respiratory tract and the esophagus, stomach and duodenum, as well as the liver, bile duct and pancreas. Early contact with the notochord is important for the early induction of this process.

The notochordal plate roofs the secondary yolk sac and the early gut in the midline until stage 10. The notochordal plate becomes increasingly U-shaped and the edges of the 'U' fuse to form the notochord proper. At the same time, the endoderm becomes continuous across the midline of the secondary yolk sac. The close relationship between the foregut endoderm and the notochord continues until the laterally placed, paired dorsal aortae fuse into a single midline aorta. Local mesenchymal proliferations then further separate the endoderm and notochord.

Experimental removal of the notochord prevents the expression of genes that are required for pancreatic development and function in the early chick embryo (Kim *et al.*, 1997). The proximity of the notochord to the dorsal endoderm is essential. However, the interactions which are necessary for dorsal pancreatic induction do not seem to be required for the first steps of ventral pancreas development. The endoderm that is responsive to the influence of the notochord is very discrete, as endoderm caudal to the pancreatic region does not respond to the notochordal signals.

The regions of the gut can be defined after head and tail folding. Head folding begins at stage 9, when neurulation causes the enlarging brain vesicles to rise above the surface ectoderm. The portion of the embryonic disc rostral to the buccopharyngeal membrane, containing the pericardial region of intra-embryonic celom, moves to lie ventral to the developing brain. The previously flat endoderm is now modified into a deep tube, the primitive foregut.

By definition, the mid-gut is that portion of the gut that is in broad connection to the yolk sac. However, this definition is vague. It can be appreciated that the delineation of cells into fore- or mid-gut involves broad morphological descriptors made at a very early but unspecified stage of development. There are no studies which suggest whether the foregut–mid-gut boundary separates persistent cell populations or whether it encompasses a common cell population. As the pancreas develops from both ventral and dorsal portions of the distal foregut, the specificity of the foregut–mid-gut junction is important, since whereas the distinction between fore- and mid-gut is esoteric for dorsal derivatives, there is a sharp junction between somatic and extra-embryonic cells at the end of the ventral wall of the foregut in the early embryo (O'Rahilly and Müller, 1987).

ORIGIN OF PANCREATIC MESENCHYME

Just before the formation of the head fold, spaces appear between the mesenchyme cells rostral to the buccopharyngeal membrane and within the cranial lateral plate mesenchyme. The mesenchymal cells at the edges of the spaces form an epithelium. The spaces coalesce to form a horseshoe-shaped cavity within the mesenchymal layer. This is the intra-embryonic celom. The most rostral portion of the intra-embryonic celom will form the pericardial cavity. This migrates ventrally with head folding, retaining contact with the ventral surface of the foregut. The two arms of the horseshoe-shaped celom form tubular conduits between the pericardial cavity and the peritoneal cavity around the developing mid-gut. These tubes are termed pericardial-peritoneal canals, and they lie laterally on each side of the foregut. The celomic epithelium is generally a site of cell proliferation, producing mesenchymal populations which become associated with the body wall and midline viscera. The medial wall of each pericardial-peritoneal canal adjacent to the foregut, the splanchnopleuric layer, produces mesenchymal populations which invest the developing lungs, the developing esophagus (thoracic and abdominal), and the diaphragm, stomach, duodenum and dorsal pancreas. The different developmental characteristics of each of these organs will be determined by permissive and instructive interactions with the local mesenchyme.

The mesenchyme that is situated ventral to the foregut is mainly derived from the septum transversum. This cell population was initially found at the most rostral end of the embryonic disc. With head folding it moves ventrally to lie caudal to the pericardial cavity. The septum transversum is mainly involved in the development of the sinusoids of the liver. However, it also gives rise to the fibrous pericardium and the diaphragm. Evagination of the ventral pancreatic bud will be into the lower portions of septum transversum-derived mesenchyme and into ventral splanchnopleuric mesenchyme from the pericardial-peritoneal canals.

EPITHELIAL–MESENCHYMAL INTERACTIONS WHICH GIVE RISE TO THE PANCREAS

Although there are some descriptions of the morphological development of the pancreas based on human studies, most of the studies on cellular interactions are based on animal experiments, especially involving rat and mouse tissue (Kritzik *et al.*, 2000) Therefore it is valuable to have comparative data on the relative developmental time-scales of the pancreas in these species, as shown in Table 32.2.

Pancreatic endoderm requires the presence of pancreatic mesenchyme for normal morphogenesis and differentiation. Experiments separating the two have indicated

Table 32.2 *Comparison table of human, rat and mouse development during the somite period*

Somites	Human (stage)	Human (days)	Mouse (days)	Rat (days)
8–14	10	22	8.5–9	9–10
13–20	11	24	9–9.5	10.5
21–29	12	26	9.5–10.25	11–11.5
30–39	13	28	10.25–10.75	11.5–12
40–45	14	32	11–11.5	12
	15	33		12.25
	16	37		12.5–13
	17	41		13
	18	44		13.5
	19	48		14
	20	51		15
	21	52		15.25
	22	54		15.5
	23	57		16

that a permissive interaction occurs between the two tissue types (Wessells, 1977). The pancreatic endoderm gives rise to the ductal cells throughout the gland, to the enzyme-secreting exocrine cells arranged in acini, and to the endocrine cells arranged in the islets of Langerhans (Miralles *et al.*, 1998a). The pancreatic mesenchyme produces the connective tissue cell lines and smooth muscle within the pancreas (Figure 32.4). Angiogenic mesenchymal cells invade all splanchnic mesenchymal populations to produce blood and lymphatic vessels (Colen *et al.*, 1999). Neural populations are derived from neural crest cells.

Recent experimental studies (summarized in Figure 32.5) have aimed to identify which factors in the mesenchyme are necessary for the appropriate epithelial branching morphogenesis, for acinar and exocrine cell differentiation, and for islet and endocrine cell maturation (Gittes *et al.*, 1996). This work and other studies (Miralles *et al.*, 1998b) indicate that the presence of pancreatic mesenchyme or follistatin, a soluble protein that is present in pancreatic mesenchyme, will support the differentiation of pancreatic epithelium into acinar structures but seems to repress the development of islets. Culture of pancreatic epithelium under adult mouse renal capsule or in supplemented three-dimensional gels specifically encourages the development of islet tissue and suggests that whereas islet formation may be a default pathway for pancreatic epithelium, this is repressed by the presence of pancreatic mesenchyme.

The ductal branching pattern and acinar structure of the pancreas which produces the species-specific morphology is thus determined by the pancreatic mesenchyme (Figure 32.6). The early endocrine cell population is found in the walls of the ducts. These cells proliferate and move out of the duct walls into the surrounding mesenchyme to form primitive islets (Figures 32.7 and 32.8). The process of islet differentiation con-

sists of two phases (Bocian-Sobkowska *et al.*, 1999). Phase I, which occurs from weeks 9–15 in human fetuses, is characterized by the proliferation of polyhormonal cells. Phase II (from week 16 onwards) is characterized by the differentiation of monohormonal cells. The first cells to differentiate are β-cells producing insulin and amylin, followed by α-cells producing glucagon, and δ-cells producing somatostatin after 30 weeks. During phase II, islet growth occurs centripetally, forming zonular islets.

The demonstration of cells containing all four hormones in fetal life has led to the hypothesis that the four islet cell types differentiate sequentially from a common pluripotent progenitor stem cell (Yamaoka and Itakura, 1999). This sequence begins with cells which coexpress peptide tyrosine tyrosine (PYY) and glucagon from E9.5 in the mouse. Figure 32.9 shows the putative cell lineage of the pancreatic islets.

FACTORS THAT REGULATE PANCREATIC DEVELOPMENT

There has been an explosion of studies on genes and transcription factors that control pancreatic development (Sanches *et al.*, 1998; Moutgomery *et al.*, 1999), particularly in the last five years, mainly because understanding of the control of development of the islets of Langerhans may provide a route for initiating regeneration of the pancreas in diabetes (Larsson, 1998; Yamaoka and Itakura, 1999). Much of the research is aimed at identifying the sequences of genes that control early induction of the pancreatic primordium and then later differentiation of the cells into exocrine and endocrine lineages (Ahlgren *et al.*, 1996; Crisera *et al.*, 1999). The speed of advances in this area of research is demonstrated by the myriad

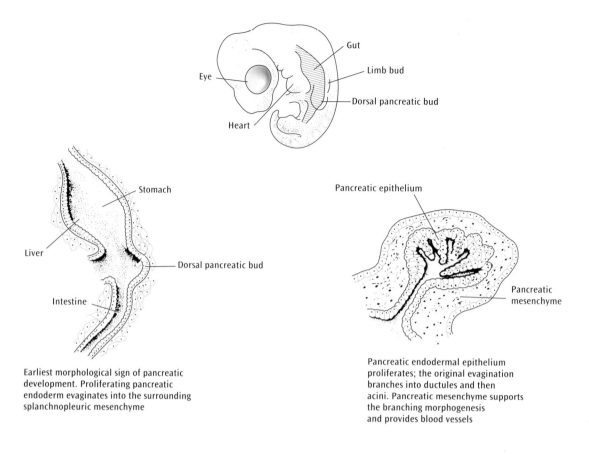

Earliest morphological sign of pancreatic development. Proliferating pancreatic endoderm evaginates into the surrounding splanchnopleuric mesenchyme

Pancreatic endodermal epithelium proliferates; the original evagination branches into ductules and then acini. Pancreatic mesenchyme supports the branching morphogenesis and provides blood vessels

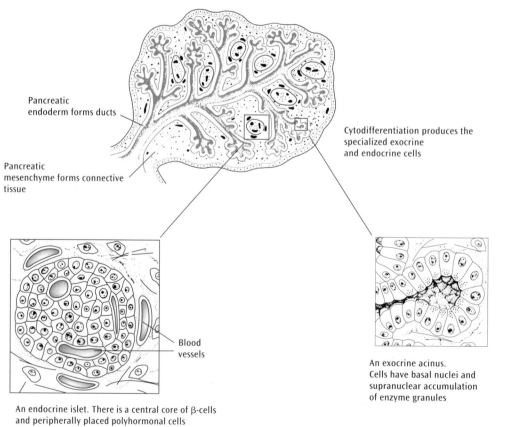

Cytodifferentiation produces the specialized exocrine and endocrine cells

An endocrine islet. There is a central core of β-cells and peripherally placed polyhormonal cells

An exocrine acinus. Cells have basal nuclei and supranuclear accumulation of enzyme granules

Figure 32.4 *Pancreatic tissue development. Reproduced from Wessels (1977).*

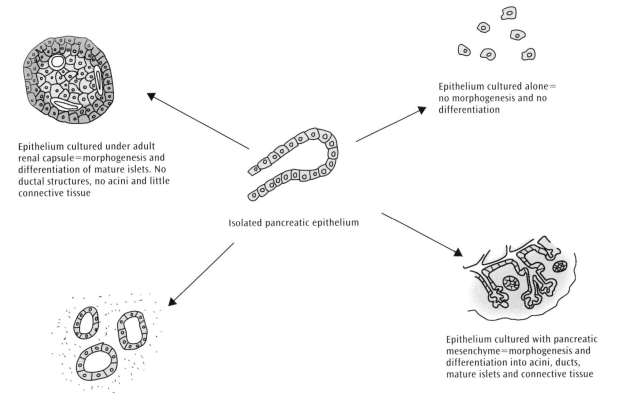

Epithelium cultured alone=
no morphogenesis and no
differentiation

Epithelium cultured under adult
renal capsule=morphogenesis and
differentiation of mature islets. No
ductal structures, no acini and little
connective tissue

Isolated pancreatic epithelium

Epithelium cultured with pancreatic
mesenchyme=morphogenesis and
differentiation into acini, ducts,
mature islets and connective tissue

Epithelium cultured in a basement-
membrane-rich gel (Matrigel)=morphogenesis
of epithelial cysts and differentiation of polarized,
secretory cells. Endocrine cells loosely associated
with cysts. No acini

Figure 32.5 *Culture experiments indicating the necessity for pancreatic mesenchyme or mesenchymal factors for morphogenesis and differentiation of pancreatic epithelia. Based on Gittes* et al. *(1996).*

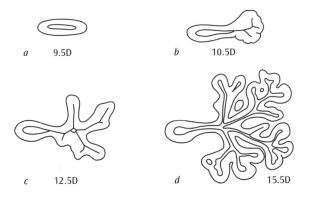

a   9.5D   *b*   10.5D

c   12.5D   *d*   15.5D

Figure 32.6 *Ductal branching pattern of the pancreatic bud in the mouse. After Slack (1995). D, days of gestation.*

Figure 32.7 *Transition of islet distribution in pancreatic lobules in the human. (a) Fetal pancreas. (b) Neonatal pancreas. (c) Adult pancreas. Each shows one lobule. Islets remain in contact with the ducts during the fetal period and gradually become separated from the ducts, dispersing in the lobule as the pancreas grows. I, periductal islets next to the duct; I' (shaded), islets separated from the duct and surrounded by the acinar tissue; D, pancreatic duct. Reproduced from Watanabe* et al. *(1999).*

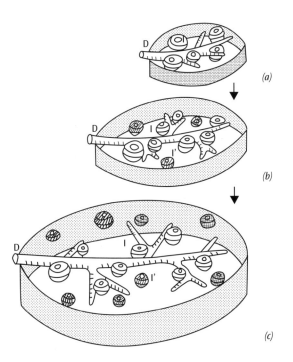

(a)

(b)

(c)

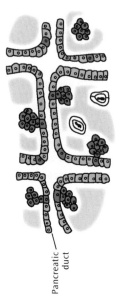

Pancreatic duct

9–10 weeks

1 Scattered cell stage.
Single polyhormonal cells in walls of pancreatic ducts.

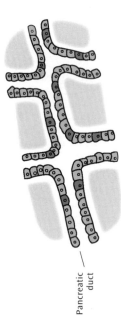

Pancreatic duct

11–15 weeks

2 Immature polyhormonal islet stage.
Groups of polyhormonal cells in and outside walls of pancreatic ducts.

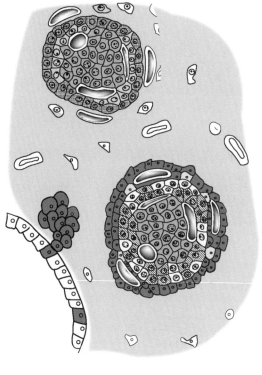

16–29 weeks

3 Insulin monohormonal core islet stage.
Cells containing only insulin form the central core, surrounded by glucagon, somatostatin and pancreatic polypeptide-positive polyhormonal cells. Stage characterized by extensive vascularization of fetal islets.

30 weeks onwards

4 Polymorphic islet stage.
Three monohormonal cell types producing insulin, glucagon and somatostatin. The most external polyhormonal cells react for glucagon, somatostatin and pancreatic polypeptide. All arrangements observed in earlier stages are present.

Key

Hormonal status of the cells at each stage:

polyhormonal
insulin–monohormonal
glucagon and weak somatostatin
glucagon–monohormonal
somatostatin–monohormonal
pancreatic polypeptide–monohormonal
glucagon, somatostatin and pancreatic polypeptide

Figure 32.8 *Development of the pancreatic endocrine cells in the human fetus. Based on Bocian-Sobkowska et al. (1999).*

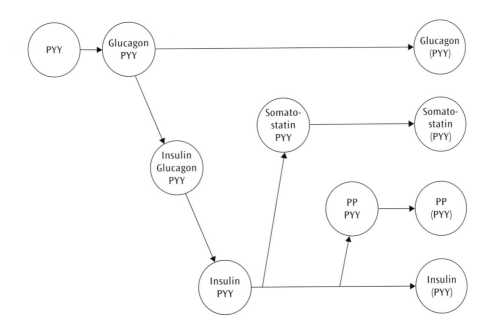

Figure 32.9 *Putative cell lineage of pancreatic islets. PYY, peptide YY; PP, pancreatic polypeptide. After Yamaoka and Itakura (1999).*

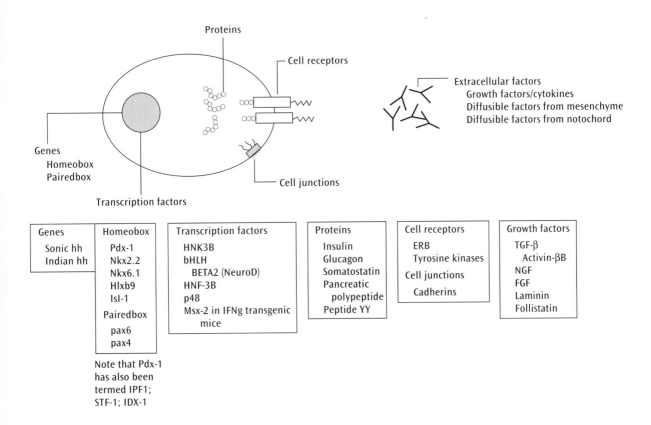

Genes	Homeobox	Transcription factors	Proteins	Cell receptors	Growth factors
Sonic hh	Pdx-1	HNK3B	Insulin	ERB	TGF-β
Indian hh	Nkx2.2	bHLH	Glucagon	Tyrosine kinases	Activin-βB
	Nkx6.1	BETA2 (NeuroD)	Somatostatin	Cell junctions	NGF
	Hlxb9	HNF-3B	Pancreatic	Cadherins	FGF
	Isl-1	p48	polypeptide		Laminin
		Msx-2 in IFNg transgenic	Peptide YY		Follistatin
	Pairedbox	mice			
	pax6				
	pax4				

Note that Pdx-1
has also been
termed IPF1;
STF-1; IDX-1

Figure 32.10 *Factors that influence pancreatic development and their location at the cellular level.*

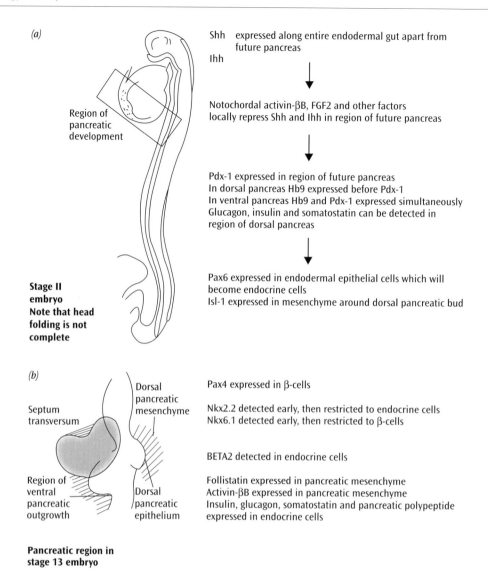

(a)

Region of pancreatic development

Stage II embryo
Note that head folding is not complete

Shh expressed along entire endodermal gut apart from future pancreas
Ihh

Notochordal activin-βB, FGF2 and other factors locally repress Shh and Ihh in region of future pancreas

Pdx-1 expressed in region of future pancreas
In dorsal pancreas Hb9 expressed before Pdx-1
In ventral pancreas Hb9 and Pdx-1 expressed simultaneously
Glucagon, insulin and somatostatin can be detected in region of dorsal pancreas

Pax6 expressed in endodermal epithelial cells which will become endocrine cells
Isl-1 expressed in mesenchyme around dorsal pancreatic bud

(b)

Septum transversum

Dorsal pancreatic mesenchyme

Region of ventral pancreatic outgrowth

Dorsal pancreatic epithelium

Pancreatic region in stage 13 embryo

Pax4 expressed in β-cells

Nkx2.2 detected early, then restricted to endocrine cells
Nkx6.1 detected early, then restricted to β-cells

BETA2 detected in endocrine cells

Follistatin expressed in pancreatic mesenchyme
Activin-βB expressed in pancreatic mesenchyme
Insulin, glucagon, somatostatin and pancreatic polypeptide expressed in endocrine cells

Figure 32.11 *Factors that influence pancreatic development and their location in the embryo. (a) Early pancreatic development. (b) Later pancreatic development.*

names and codes for the genes and transcription factors. As fast as one research team finds a specific gene, it may also have been identified contemporaneously by another group but given a different name. There is then a slowing of progress as teams identify that their protein is the same as that found by the other groups. Many of the genes which are identified in pancreatic development are ubiquitous throughout the embryo and illustrate basic developmental processes that are seen in all embryonic body systems. Thus the deletion of these genes in null transgenic animals affects many body systems, and the resulting phenotype demon-

strates the extent to which the embryo can catch up or cope with this perturbation. The main genes and transcription factors involved in pancreatic development (Kritzik *et al.*, 1999; Li *et al.*, 1999; Dohrmann *et al.*, 2000) are summarized in Figures 32.10 and 32.11, and the consequences of their deletion are summarized in Table 32.3. The recent proliferation of review articles on pancreatic development indicates the necessity for reflection on progress so far and its evaluation in terms of specific gains for pancreatic development alone (Slack, 1995; Edlund, 1999; St-Onge *et al.*, 1999; Yamaoka and Itakura, 1999; Bramblett *et al.*, 2000).

Table 32.3 *Consequences of gene deletions in transgenic animal experiments*

Transcription factor	First detected in embryo	Detected in adult	Null mutant mouse characteristics
Shh			Ectopic expression of Shh in the pancreatic bud converts the pancreatic mesenchyme into intestinal mesenchyme and inhibits spleen development
Pdx-1	8.5	β-cells	Absence of pancreas. Pancreatic differentiation arrested at early stage
Isl-1	9.0	β, α, δ, PP-cells	Absence of endocrine cells; dorsal pancreatic mesenchyme deleted. Amylase-producing exocrine cells present
Pax6	9.0–9.5	β, α, δ, PP-cells	Absence of α-cells producing glucagon. β-, γ- and δ-cells present, but remain disorganized throughout exocrine tissue
Pax4	9.5	β, δ, PP-cells	Absence of β-cells producing insulin, and δ-cells producing somatostatin. Increase in α-cells producing glucagon
Nkx6.1	9.0–9.5	β-cells	
Nkx2.2	9.5	β, α, PP-cells	Islet mass reduced
BETA2/NeuroD	9.5	β, α, δ, PP-cells	Numbers of β-, α- and δ-cells decrease by nearly 75%, 40% and 20%, respectively. Endocrine cells aggregate as small clusters and fail to form mature islets
p48	10	Exocrine cells	Absence of exocrine cells. Endocrine cells found in the spleen

Key references

Edlund H. Pancreas: how to get there from the gut? *Current Opinions in Cell Biology* 1999; **11**: 663–8.

This paper discusses models for patterning and induction of pancreatic cell lines.

Slack JMW. Developmental biology of the pancreas. *Development* 1995; **121**: 1569–80.

An overview of pancreatic development, which includes concepts of growth control of the embryonic and post-natal pancreas.

St-Onge L, Wehr R, Gruss P. Pancreas development and diabetes. *Current Opinions in Genetics and Development* 1999; **9**: 295–300.

A comprehensive account of the transcription factors that are essential for pancreatic development.

Uchida T, Takada T, Ammori BJ, Suda K, Takahashi T. Three-dimensional reconstruction of the ventral and dorsal pancreas: a new insight into anatomy and embryonic development. *Journal of Hepatobiliary and Pancreatic Surgery* 1999; **6**: 176–80.

This paper shows a three-dimensional reconstruction of ventral and dorsal pancreatic development and illustrates the differences between these parts.

REFERENCES

Ahlgren U, Jonsson J, Edlund H. The morphogenesis of the pancreatic mesenchyme is uncoupled from that of the pancreatic epithelium in IPF1/PDX1-deficient mice. *Development* 1996; **122**: 1409–16.

Bocian-Sobkowska J, Zabel M, Wozniak W, Surdyk-Zasada J. Polyhormonal aspect of the endocrine cells of the human fetal pancreas. *Histochemistry and Cell Biology* 1999; **112**: 147–53.

Bramblett DE, Huang HP, Tsai MJ. Pancreatic islet development. *Advances in Pharmacology* 2000; **47**: 255–315.

Colen KL, Crisera CA, Rose MI, Connelly PR, Longaker MT, Gittes GK. Vascular development of the mouse embryonic pancreas and lung. *Journal of Pediatric Surgery* 1999; **34**: 781–5.

Crisera CA, Longaker MT, Gittes GK. Molecular approaches to understanding organogenesis. *Seminars in Pediatric Surgery* 1999; **8**: 109–18.

Dohrmann C, Gruss P, Lemaire L. Pax genes and the differentiation of hormone-producing endocrine cells in the pancreas. *Mechanisms of Development* 2000; **92**: 47–54.

Edlund H. Pancreas: how to get there from the gut? *Current Opinions in Cell Biology* 1999; **11**: 663–8.

Githens S. Development of duct cells. In: Lebenthal E (ed.)

Human gastrointestinal development New York; Raven Press, 1989: 669–83.

Gittes GK, Galante PE, Hanahan D, Rutter WJ, Debas HT. Lineage-specific morphogenesis in the developing pancreas: role of mesenchymal factors. *Development* 1996; **122**: 439–47.

Kim SK, Hebrok M, Melton DA. Notochord-to-endoderm signaling is required for pancreas development. *Development* 1997; **124**: 4243–52.

Kritzik MR, Jones E, Chen Z *et al.* PDX-1 and Msx-2 expression in the regenerating and developing pancreas. *Journal of Endocrinology* 1999; **163**: 523–30.

Kritzik MR, Krahl T, Good A *et al.* Expression of ErbB receptors during pancreatic islet development and regrowth. *Journal of Endocrinology* 2000; **165**: 67–77.

Larsson L. On the development of the islets of Langerhans. *Microscopy Research and Technique* 1998; **43**: 284–91.

Li H, Arber S, Jessell TM, Edlund H. Selective agenesis of the dorsal pancreas in mice lacking homeobox gene Hlxb9. *Nature Genetics* 1999; **23**: 67–70.

Miralles F, Battelino T, Czernichow P, Scharfman R. TGF-β plays a key role in morphogenesis of the pancreatic islets of Langerhans by controlling the activity of the matrix metalloproteinase MMP-2. *Journal of Cell Biology* 1998a; **143**: 827–36.

Miralles F, Czernichow P, Scharfman R. Follistatin regulates the relative proportions of endocrine versus exocrine tissue during pancreatic development. *Development* 1998b; **25**: 1017–24.

Montgomery RK, Mulberg AE, Grand RJ. Development of the human gastrointestinal tract: twenty years of progress. *Gastroenterology* 1999; **116**: 702–31.

O'Rahilly R, Müller F. *Developmental stages in human embryos*. Washington, DC: Carnegie Institution of Washington, 1987.

Sanches D, Moriscot C, Marchand S, Fredouille C, Figarella C, Guy-Crotte O. Developmental gene expression and immunohistochemical study of the human endocrine pancreas during fetal life. *Hormone Research* 1998; **50**: 258–63.

Selleck MAJ, Stern CD. Fate mapping and cell lineage analysis of Hensen's node in the chick embryo. *Development* 1991; **112**: 615–26.

Slack JMW. Developmental biology of the pancreas. *Development* 1995; **121**: 1569–80.

St-Onge L, Wehr R, Gruss P. Pancreas development and diabetes. *Current Opinions in Genetics and Development* 1999; **9**: 295–300.

Streeter GL. Developmental horizons in human embryos. Descriptions of age group XI, 13 to 20 somites, and age group XII, 21 to 29 somites. *Contributions to Embryology* 1942; **30**: 211–45.

Tam PPL, Beddington RSP. Establishment and organization of germ layers in the gastrulating mouse embryo. In: McLaren A (ed.) *Ciba Foundation Symposium 165*. Chichester: John Wiley & Sons, 1992: 27–49.

Uchida T, Takada T, Ammori BJ, Suda K, Takahashi T. Three-dimensional reconstruction of the ventral and dorsal pancreas: a new insight into anatomy and embryonic development. *Journal of Hepatobiliary and Pancreatic Surgery* 1999; **6**: 176–80.

Watanabe T, Yaegashi H, Koizumi M, Toyota T, Takahashi T. Changing distribution of islets in the developing human pancreas: a computer-assisted three-dimensional reconstruction study. *Pancreas* 1999; **18**: 349–54.

Wessells NK. *Tissue interactions and development*. Menlo Park, CA: Benjamin/Cummings, 1977.

Yamaoka T, Itakura M. Development of pancreatic islets (review). *International Journal of Molecular Medicine* 1999; **3**: 247–61.

33

Congenital abnormalities

EDWARD R HOWARD

DEVELOPMENT OF THE PANCREAS

Despite the complex embryology of the pancreas (see Chapter 32), serious congenital abnormalities are remarkably rare. Briefly, the pancreas develops from two buds which arise from dorsal and ventral aspects of the distal foregut (duodenum). The ventral pancreas rotates clockwise around the duodenal axis to coalesce with the developing dorsal pancreas on the left side of the duodenum. The ducts of the dorsal and ventral portions of the pancreas fuse so that the distal portion of the main pancreatic duct (Wirsung) is formed from the embryological dorsal duct, whereas the proximal portion of the main duct represents the original ventral duct. The residual proximal portion of the dorsal duct remains as the accessory duct (Santorini), which drains separately into the duodenum.

Many of the congenital abnormalities of the pancreas can be understood as malrotations of the ventral pancreas (annular pancreas) or as abnormal fusion of the dorsal and ventral duct systems (pancreas divisum). The most commonly reported congenital abnormalities are listed in Box 33.1. (Abnormalities of pancreatic and bile duct union are also discussed in Chapter 10, and congenital islet cell hyperplasia is described in Chapter 35.)

Box 33.1 *Congenital abnormalities of the pancreas*

Agenesis
Hypoplasia
Common pancreaticobiliary channels
Abnormal bile duct insertion into fourth part of
    duodenum
Pancreatic duct strictures
Annular pancreas
Ectopic pancreas (abdominal and extra-abdominal)
Unilocular and multiple simple cysts
Dermoid and teratomatous cysts
Enteric duplication cysts

AGENESIS AND HYPOPLASIA

Complete absence of the whole pancreas is a lethal condition which has been reported very rarely (Mehes *et al.*, 1976; Lemons *et al.*, 1979; Voldsgaard *et al.*, 1994). It is associated with intrauterine growth retardation, hyperglycemia, diabetic coma and meconium ileus.

Congenital absence of the islets of Langerhans is also accompanied by intrauterine growth retardation due to insulin deprivation, and death during the neonatal period. Dodge and Laurence (1977) described a small-for-dates male infant who died at 40 hours of age. A brother of this individual died a similar death at 48 hours of age, and the authors suggested a possible X-linked form of inheritance.

Agenesis of acinar tissue occurs in association with the Schwachman syndrome, an autosomal-recessive disorder that is characterized by exocrine pancreas insufficiency, growth retardation, metaphyseal dysostosis and bone-marrow dysfunction (Marseglia et al., 1998). Although there are nutritional problems secondary to the pancreatic abnormality, mortality is related to recurrent infections and susceptibility to leukemia. Treatment with bone-marrow transplantation is now advocated for high-risk patients. Agenesis of the dorsal pancreas has been described in association with diabetes mellitus by Lechner and Read (1966), Wang et al. (1990) and Wildling et al. (1993). The latter reported dorsal agenesis in a mother and her two sons, suggesting possible genetic mechanisms for the abnormality. This abnormality has now been described on ultrasound scans and CT, (Wildling et al., 1993), as well as on MR pancreatography (Macari et al., 1998).

Leese et al. (1989) reviewed 20 cases of dorsal pancreatic agenesis and pointed out that the commonest presentation is of recurrent acute pancreatitis of the ventral pancreas with the subsequent development of exocrine pancreatic insufficiency.

PATTERNS OF DUCTAL ANATOMY

Many variations of the 'normal' anatomical pattern of the dorsal and ventral ducts occur (Skandalakis et al., 1993). For example, the accessory duct of Santorini, which opens into the duodenum via the minor papilla, may be absent, hypoplastic or the dominant route for pancreatic secretions. There is no connection between the accessory duct and the main duct in approximately 10% of pancreatic duct studies, and the minor papilla is absent in 30% of cases. However, variations in ductal anatomy are rarely of clinical significance.

The pattern of the junction of the bile duct and the terminal portion of the pancreatic duct is also very variable, and it is clinically significant (see Chapter 10). The extrahepatic bile duct is developed from the duct of the ventral pancreas, and initially the junction of the two ducts lies outside the wall of the developing duodenum. As fetal development proceeds, the junction moves towards the duodenal lumen (Wong and Lister, 1981). Arrest of this process results in an abnormally long 'common' pancreaticobiliary channel which remains outside the sphincter mechanism of the ampulla of Vater. Free reflux of pancreatic juice into the biliary tract is therefore possible, particularly as the excretion pressure in the pancreatic duct exceeds that of the common bile duct by at least two- or threefold. Long 'common' channels of

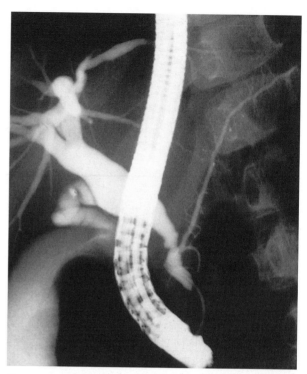

Figure 33.1 *Fusiform dilatation of the common bile duct with long common pancreaticobiliary channel in an 8-year-old girl. The pancreatic duct is of normal size (ERCP).*

this type are associated with recurrent episodes of pancreatitis, and are observed in 70–75% of choledochal cysts, although they may also occur as single abnormalities (Figure 33.1).

Komi et al. (1992) studied the radiological appearance of 51 cases of choledochal cyst and classified the abnormal pancreaticobiliary junctions into three main types. They reported that an abnormal dilatation of the pancreatic duct in association with a 'common' channel could be associated with recurrent pancreatitis even after disconnection of the bile duct from the pancreatic duct by hepaticojejunostomy (Figure 33.2).

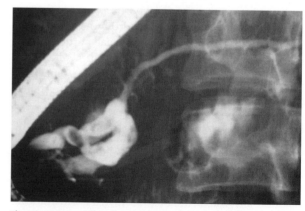

Figure 33.2 *Dilated pancreatic ducts, containing calculi, within the head of the pancreas of a 15-year-old girl. A choledochal cyst had been previously excised.*

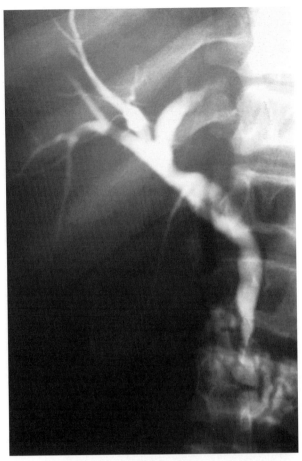

Figure 33.3 *Operative cholangiogram in a 15-year-old boy with recurrent abdominal pain and a dilated common bile duct opening via a stenosed ampulla into the fourth part of the duodenum.*

ANOMALOUS INSERTION OF THE COMMON BILE DUCT

Insertion of the common bile duct into the third or fourth portions of the duodenum has been reported in 1.3% of adults (Auld and Thomson, 1985) (Figure 33.3). Although the abnormality rarely causes symptoms, Doty *et al.* (1985) described an association with pancreatitis in two girls aged 2.5 and 3 years. In addition to the abnormal drainage of the bile duct, both patients had long common pancreaticobiliary channels measuring 10 and 27 mm. Complete diversion of bile via hepaticojejunostomy operations resulted in relief from symptoms in both cases.

PANCREAS DIVISUM

A failure of the embryological coalescence of the dorsal and ventral ducts may result in a ductal pattern known as pancreas divisum, the history of which has been reviewed exhaustively by Stern (1986). The ducts remain separate, with persistence of the entire dorsal duct, which empties into the duodenum via the accessory papilla (Figures 33.4a and b). Variants of the divisum abnormality have been classified by Warshaw *et al.* (1990). The classification includes a filamentous connection between the dorsal and ventral ducts and a complete absence of the ventral duct. The prevalence of this anatomical pattern ranges from 0.3 to 5.8% in patients undergoing endoscopic retrograde cholangiography (ERCP) to 5–14% in postmortem studies (Millbourn, 1950, 1959/60; Berman *et al.*, 1960).

The importance of the abnormality lies in its possible relationship with recurrent pancreatitis (see Chapter 34). The concept of a 'dominant dorsal duct syndrome' has been suggested to represent a functional obstruction to pancreatic secretion through a relatively small accessory duct sphincter (Warshaw *et al.*, 1990), and beneficial results from surgical enlargement of the accessory sphincter in children have now been reported (Adzick *et al.*, 1989; Sanada *et al.*, 1995; O'Rourke and Harrison, 1998).

CONGENITAL DUCT STRICTURES

Postmortem studies have demonstrated congenital strictures of the main pancreatic ducts in 3% of subjects (Birnstingl, 1959). These strictures have been most commonly reported at the junction of the ventral and dorsal ducts, with dilatation of the distal ducts (Figure 33.5). Secondary pancreatitis may be the presenting feature, and distal duct drainage using the operation of pancreaticojejunostomy is the treatment of choice (Turner, 1983; Leese *et al.*, 1989; Tagge *et al.*, 1991).

ANNULAR PANCREAS

The term annular pancreas is applied to the complete encirclement of the second part of the duodenum by a band of pancreatic tissue which may be associated with either partial or complete obstruction of the duodenum (Figure 33.6). The abnormality occurs with a frequency of 1 in 20 000 births (Lehman and O'Connor, 1985), and was observed in 8–21% of cases of neonatal duodenal obstruction which proved to be secondary to either stenosis or atresia of the duodenal lumen (Young and Wilkinson, 1968; Fonkalsrud *et al.*, 1969; Bailey *et al.*, 1993).

The annulus varies in morphology from case to case, and ranges from a structure which is completely separate from the duodenal surface to a mass of pancreatic tissue that is intimately associated with the muscle coat of the duodenal wall. Occasional familial cases have been described, and an autosomal-dominant or X-linked type

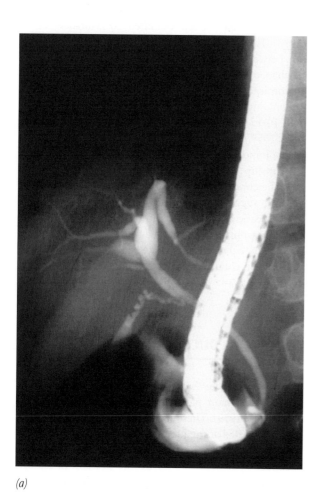

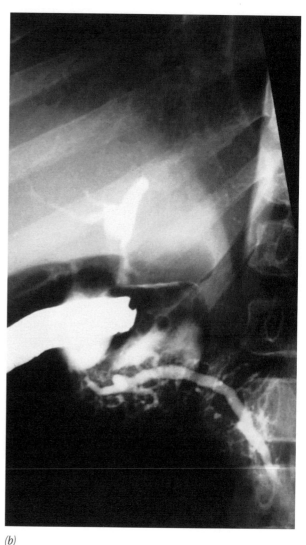

(a)   (b)

Figure 33.4 *Pancreas divisum, presenting as pancreatitis in a 9-year-old boy. (a) ERCP via the ampulla of Vater. The common bile duct is outlined together with a very small remnant of the ventral pancreatic duct. (b) Pancreatogram via the minor papilla. The pancreatic duct is dilated up to the papilla.*

of inheritance has been suggested (Hendricks and Sybert, 1991; Rogers *et al.*, 1993; Claviez *et al.*, 1995). The sexes are affected equally in infancy, and 20% of cases are associated with Down syndrome.

Lecco (1910) proposed that an annular pancreas is the result of a disturbance in the rotation of the ventral bud, which rotates around the duodenum to fuse with the dorsal bud (see Figure 33.6 and Chapter 32). Fixation of the tip of the ventral bud to the duodenal wall, before the onset of rotation during week 5 of development, is believed to be the most likely explanation (Gray and Skandalakis, 1972), and the ventral origin of the annulus has been confirmed immunohistochemically (Dowsett *et al.*, 1989). Approximately one-third of the cases of annular pancreas are symptomatic from duodenal obstruction during the neonatal period, and this figure rises to 50% before the end of the first year of life.

Older patients with annular pancreas may present with pancreatitis rather than duodenal obstruction. This association was first reported by Drey (1957) in 14 out of 62 adults (23%) whose ages ranged from 23 to 37 years. There was a male predominance of 78% in this adult series, which is in contrast to the equal sex incidence observed during infancy. Pancreatolithiasis has also been documented in at least five adults with the malformation (Yogi *et al.*, 1999). Occasional cases of pancreatitis have been recorded in children who had an annular pancreas associated with either a common pancreaticobiliary channel (Komura *et al.*, 1993) or a pancreas divisum (Tagge *et al.*, 1991). The latter authors noted that up to 36% of the previous reports of patients with annular pancreas described an associated pancreas divisum.

Peptic ulcers have also been observed in patients with annular pancreas (Kiernan *et al.*, 1980) and, like pancre-

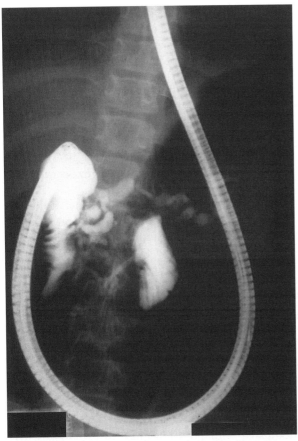

Figure 33.5 *Congenital pancreatic duct stricture in the head of the pancreas of an 11-year-old girl who presented with pancreatitis.*

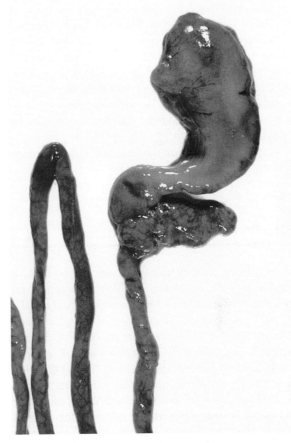

Figure 33.6 *Annular pancreas. Postmortem specimen from a 1-week-old infant who had died of aspiration pneumonia.*

atitis, may be the cause of recurrent abdominal pain and vomiting.

Ductal anatomy within an annular pancreas is variable, but in many cases a large duct runs clockwise around the duodenum to enter the duct of Wirsung within the head of the pancreas. Surgical division of the annulus might therefore result in a pancreatic fistula, and is contraindicated in the surgical treatment of any associated duodenal obstruction (see Figure 35.2).

The diagnosis of annular pancreas associated with duodenal obstruction may be suggested antenatally by a maternal presentation with polyhydramnios. This presentation has been reported in 17–75% of cases (Girvan and Stephens, 1974; Spigland and Yazbeck, 1990). The diagnosis may be confirmed by antenatal ultrasonography (Pachi *et al.*, 1989; Akhtar and Guiney, 1992).

In the newborn period the typical 'double-bubble' sign of gastric and duodenal obstruction is visible on a plain upright X-ray of the abdomen, and contrast studies are rarely necessary for diagnosis. However, barium studies are useful in older patients, and ring-like constrictions of the duodenum were observed in seven out of nine adults who had presented with symptoms of partial duodenal obstruction, or of pancreatitis secondary

to annular pancreas (Kiernan *et al.*, 1980). ERCP may aid diagnosis in older children and adults by imaging periduodenal pancreatic ducts within the annulus (Glazer and Margulis, 1979).

Jadvar and Mindelzun (1999) evaluated the usefulness of various imaging modalities in seven adult patients. Upper gastrointestinal contrast studies confirmed narrowing of the duodenum, whilst contrast-enhanced CT allowed direct visualization of the annular pancreatic tissue. The report also confirmed the value of ERCP in demonstrating pancreatic ducts within the annulus.

More recent investigations include magnetic resonance cholangiopancreatography (MRCP), which is now widely used as a non-invasive diagnostic test for abnormalities of the pancreaticobiliary system. Hidaka *et al.* (1998) used the technique successfully to visualize the pancreatic duct within an annular portion of pancreas in an adult. Diagnosis has also been achieved using endoscopic ultrasound (Gress *et al.*, 1996).

The surgical management of annular pancreas in childhood is mostly concerned with relief of any associated duodenal obstruction. A duodenoduodenostomy is the operation of choice, and long-term survival rates are described as excellent. For example, Bailey *et al.* (1993)

reported survival in 93% of 138 infants. However, Spigland and Yazbeck (1990) described morbidity in 70% of 33 infants, which included persistent megaduodenum and blind-loop syndrome, bile and gastro-esophageal reflux, and cholestatic jaundice. Many of these problems were related to chronic dilatation and muscular hypertrophy of the proximal duodenum, and a reduction duodenoplasty is now recommended in infants with severe duodenal dilatation to reduce the complication rate.

As stated previously, division of the annulus is not recommended because of the risk of pancreatic fistula from severed pancreatic ducts (Ravitch and Woods, 1950).

ECTOPIC PANCREATIC TISSUE

Islands of pancreatic heterotopic tissue may be found at many sites, both within and outside the abdomen, and have been reported in 1–2% of autopsies (Caberwal et al., 1977). Analysis of 212 examples of the abnormality (Dolan et al., 1974) showed that 80–90% of the sites were in the stomach, duodenum or jejunum. Rarer locations included the ileum (Figure 33.7), Meckel diverticulum, colon, gallbladder, extrahepatic bile ducts (Schu et al., 1988), splenic hilus and ampulla of Vater (Laughlin et al., 1983). Ectopic pancreas was mistaken for a granuloma of the umbilicus in a 13-month-old male infant (Caberwal et al., 1977). Affected sites outside the abdomen have included the distal esophagus, and Biceno et al. (1981) suggested that this might have resulted from transplantation of pancreatic cells during the embryological rotation and fusion of the dorsal and ventral pancreatic buds. An alternative explanation may be provided by the differentiation of totipotent endodermal cells lining the gut or vitello-intestinal duct in the early embryo.

Although in most cases islands of ectopic pancreatic tissue remain asymptomatic, they may occasionally cause complications. The simple presence of a mass of ectopic tissue may cause obstruction – for example, at the ampulla of Vater (Laughlin et al., 1983) and in the pyloric canal (Hayes-Jordan et al., 1998). The latter was reported in a 2-day-old infant, and was initially mistaken for hypertrophic pyloric stenosis.

Pancreatitis may also occur within ectopic tissue, and has been reported in the jejunum (Rubesin et al., 1997), duodenum (Chung et al., 1994), jejunal mesentery (Fam et al., 1982) and gallbladder (Quizilbash, 1976). Ectopic pancreatitis may be accompanied by concomitant inflammation within the main pancreas.

Other recorded complications have included upper gastrointestinal hemorrhage (Schurmans and De Baere, 1980) and malignant transformation in ectopic pancreas within the mesocolon of a 13-year-old girl (Ishikawa et al., 1990). Histology of the latter lesion showed a well-encapsulated lesion of both solid and papillary neoplasm.

The treatment of symptomatic ectopic pancreatic tissue is surgical, and examples include Meckel diverticulectomy and segmental resection of stomach or bowel.

CONGENITAL PANCREATIC CYSTS

Compared with post-inflammatory pseudocysts, true congenital cysts of the pancreas are extremely rare, and their incidence has been calculated to be around 0.007% (Rosato and Mackie, 1963). Auringer (1993) collected 21 pediatric reports with a female predominance of 11 out of 13 cases in which the sex was stated. True cysts, which may be unilocular or multiple, are lined by cuboidal or flattened epithelium and are believed to arise from anomalous development of the pancreatic ductal system. They may be associated with other abnormalities, such as polydactyly, anorectal malformations, polycystic kidneys and thoracic dystrophy. Dermoids and cystic teratomata may also occur within the pancreas.

Unilocular cysts (FIGURES 33.8A AND B)

A collected series of 20 cases included six cases in adults aged 35–56 years and 14 cases in children aged 6 weeks to 10 years (Mao et al., 1992). The presentation in these cases included asymptomatic abdominal mass, pyloric obstruction, pancreatitis, ascites and splenic vein thrombosis. Antenatal cases have also been reported either as incidental findings during routine antenatal ultrasonography, or presenting with an associated polyhydramnios (Baker et al., 1990).

Symptomatic cysts are treated by either excisional surgery or internal drainage procedures. Surgery is also recommended for asymptomatic cysts of significant size to confirm or exclude a diagnosis of cystadenoma, which has premalignant potential (Howard, 1998).

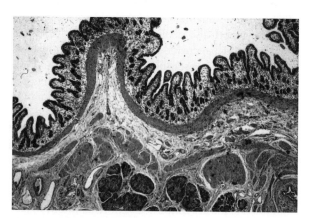

Figure 33.7 *Darkly staining ectopic pancreas within the muscle coats of ileum resected from a newborn infant with ileal atresia.*

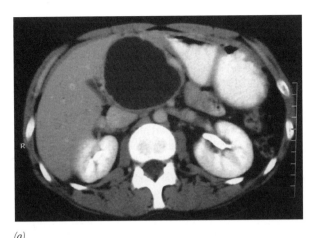
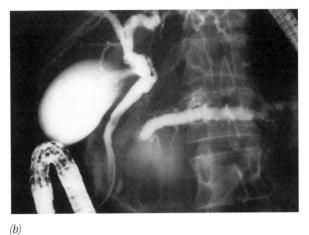

(a)   (b)

Figure 33.8 *Congenital 'simple' cyst in the head of the pancreas. (a) CT scan showing smooth-walled cyst confined to the head of the pancreas. (b) ERCP showing distortion of the common bile duct and compression of the pancreatic duct by the cyst. The cyst is faintly opacified with contrast.*

Polycystic disease

Multiple cysts may occur as an isolated pancreatic abnormality. Mares and Hirsch (1977) reported the case of a 20-month-old girl who presented with increasing abdominal distension and a palpable mass in the epigastrium. Angiography showed an avascular mass, and at surgery multiple cysts lined by cuboidal epithelium were found in the head of the pancreas. The largest cyst was treated successfully by cystoduodenostomy. A similar case concerned a 4-month-old girl with a palpable, asymptomatic mass in the left hypochondrium, which was caused by an area of polycystic disease in the tail of the pancreas (Auringer *et al.*, 1993).

Multiple cysts of the pancreas may also be identified as part of the autosomal-dominant condition known as Hippel–Lindau's syndrome (polycystic disease affecting the kidney, pancreas, liver and cerebellum in association with retinal angiomas). A review of 426 patients of all ages with this syndrome revealed multiple pancreatic cysts in 55 cases (Howard, 1998).

Dermoid and teratomatous cysts

Typical dermoid cysts containing structures derived from ectoderm, such as sebaceous material, hair, teeth and hair follicles, have been described in the pancreas on at least four occasions. These cases have been summarized by Howard (1998) and differentiated from cystic teratomas, which contain structures derived from all three embryonic germinal layers, and which have also been reported in the pancreas (Mester *et al.*, 1990). Complete surgical excision is the treatment of choice for these lesions.

ENTERIC DUPLICATION CYSTS

Although these lesions are not true congenital lesions of the pancreas itself, their close relationship with the gland and their common presentation with pancreatitis justify their inclusion in this chapter.

Histologically, the structure of the wall of enteric duplications shows tissues such as epithelium, submucosa and smooth muscle typical of normal bowel. Enteric cysts related to the pancreas may also contain high levels of amylase, and may be either confined within the pancreas or related more closely to adjacent stomach or duodenum.

Siddiqui *et al.* (1998) described four patients, aged 13 months to 4 years, who were shown to have enteric duplications entirely within the pancreatic head. They had presented with pancreatitis ($n = 2$), gastritis secondary to hypergastrinemia ($n = 1$) and pleural effusion ($n = 1$). The authors recommended that possible investigations should include abdominal ultrasonography (which may reveal peristalsis in the cyst wall), ERCP, angiography, CT or MRCP. They also recommended intraoperative ultrasonography as a useful technique for accurate localization of the cyst during surgery. All four of their cases were treated by complete cyst excision after incision of the overlying pancreas. Histology showed the cysts to be lined by gastric, duodenal or respiratory mucosa. The authors recommended excisional surgery, as malignant change has been reported in a duodenal duplication cyst (Falk *et al.*, 1991). The report includes reference to a literature search, which identified 14 further cases of enteric duplication confined within the pancreatic head.

Other foregut duplications may involve the pancreas. Johnstone *et al.* (1991) described a case of gastric duplication communicating with pancreatic ducts and associated with recurrent pancreatitis. Similarly, Akers *et al.*

(1972) described a gastric duplication lying on the head of the pancreas which had presented as pancreatitis associated with a posterior peptic perforation of the cyst on to the pancreas gland.

Moss *et al.* (1996) described a gastric duplication of the antrum in a 9 year-old-girl which communicated with an inflamed aberrant pancreatic lobe. The authors usefully added nine other cases of gastric duplication communicating with the pancreas, and they emphasized the difficulty involved in diagnosing these lesions. Recorded complications of gastric duplications include pancreatitis (caused by mucus and debris from the duplication blocking the pancreatic ductal system) and hemorrhage (from peptic ulceration).

Key references

Bailey PV, Tracy TF, Connors RH, Mooney DP, Lewis JE, Weber TR. Congenital duodenal obstruction: a 32-year review. *Journal of Paediatric Surgery* 1993; **28**: 92–5.

This is a major review of 138 newborn infants with duodenal obstruction and associated defects. Although only a minority of the infants had an annular pancreas, the paper is a very useful reference for the problems which can follow surgical correction of the obstructed duodenum.

Howard JM. Congenital cysts of the pancreas. In: Beger HG, Warshaw AL, Buchler MW *et al.* (eds) *The pancreas*. Oxford: Blackwell Science, 1998: 1427–31.

This is a major review of a rare problem, which includes several illustrative case histories.

Skandalakis LJ, Rowe JS, Gray SW, Skandalakis JE. Surgical embryology and the anatomy of the pancreas. *Surgical Clinics of North America* 1993; **73**: 661–97.

A succinct and clear review of the basic embryology and anatomy of the pancreas, with a useful reference list.

Stern C. A historical perspective on the discovery of the accessory duct of the pancreas, the ampulla of Vater and pancreas divisum. *Gut* 1986; **27**: 203–12.

This review places the original observations on pancreas divisum in the seventeenth century, and reviews the contributions of Santorini and Vater to our understanding of the fundamental anatomy of the pancreas and other congenital variations in anatomy. A very interesting and useful historical review.

Tagge EP, Smith SD, Raschbaum GR, Newman B, Wiener ES. Pancreatic ductal abnormalities in children. *Surgery* 1991; **110**: 709–16.

A review of the presentation and management of 12 children with a wide range of congenital pancreatic abnormalities.

REFERENCES

Adzick NS, Shamberger RC, Winter HS, Hendren WH. Surgical treatment of pancreas divisum causing pancreatitis in children. *Journal of Pediatric Surgery* 1989; **24**: 54–8.

Akers DR, Favara BE, Franciosi RA, Nelson JM. Duplications of the alimentary tract: report of three unusual cases associated with bile and pancreatic ducts. *Surgery* 1972; **71**: 817–23.

Akhtar J, Guiney EJ. Congenital duodenal obstruction. *British Journal of Surgery* 1992; **79**: 133–5.

Auld CD, Thomson JWW. The common bile duct and its anomalies. *Journal of the Royal College of Surgeons of Edinburgh* 1985; **30**: 248–50.

Auringer ST, Ulmer JL, Sumner TE, Turner CS. Congenital cyst of the pancreas. *Journal of Pediatric Surgery* 1993; **28**: 1570–1.

Bailey PV, Tracy TF, Connors RH, Mooney DP, Lewis JE, Weber TR. Congenital duodenal obstruction: a 32-year review. *Journal of Pediatric Surgery* 1993; **28**: 92–5.

Baker LL, Hartman GE, Northway WH. Sonographic detection of congenital pancreatic cysts in the newborn: report of a case and review of the literature. *Pediatric Radiology* 1990; **20**: 488–90.

Berman LG, Prior JT, Abramow SM, Ziegler DD. A study of the pancreatic duct system in man by the use of vinyl acetate casts of postmortem preparations. *Surgery, Gynecology and Obstetrics* 1960; **110**: 391–403.

Biceno LI, Grases PJ, Gallego S. Tracheobronchial and pancreatic remnants causing esophageal stenosis. *Journal of Pediatric Surgery* 1981; **16**: 731–2.

Birnstingl M. A study of pancreatography. *British Journal of Surgery* 1959; **47**: 128–39.

Caberwal D, Kogan SJ, Levitt SB. Ectopic pancreas presenting as an umbilical mass. *Journal of Pediatric Surgery* 1977; **12**: 593–5.

Chung JP, Lee SI, Kim KW *et al.* Duodenal ectopic pancreas complicated by chronic pancreatitis and pseudocyst formation – a case report. *Journal of Korean Medical Science* 1994; **9**: 351–6.

Claviez A, Heger S, Bohring A. Annular pancreas in two sisters. *American Journal of Medical Genetics* 1995; **58**: 384.

Dodge JA, Laurence KM. Congenital absence of islets of Langerhans. *Archives of Disease in Childhood* 1977; **52**: 411–13.

Dolan RV, ReMine WH, Dockerty MB. The fate of heterotopic pancreatic tissue. A study of 212 cases. *Archives of Surgery* 1974; **109**: 762–5.

Doty J, Hassal E, Fonkalsrud EW. Anomalous drainage of the common bile duct into the fourth portion of the duodenum. *Archives of Surgery* 1985; **120**: 1077–9.

Dowsett JF, Rode J, Russell RC. Annular pancreas: a clinical, endoscopic and immunohistochemical study. *Gut* 1989; **30**: 130–5.

Drey NW. Symptomatic annular pancreas in the adult. *Annals of Internal Medicine* 1957; **46**: 750–72.

Falk GL, Young CJ, Parker J. Adenocarcinoma arising in a duodenal duplication cyst: a case report. *Australian and New Zealand Journal of Surgery* 1991; **61**: 551–3.

Fam S, O'Briain DS, Borger JA. Ectopic pancreas with acute inflammation. *Journal of Pediatric Surgery* 1982; **17**: 86–7.

Fonkalsrud EW, de Lorimier AA, Hays DM. Congenital atresia and stenosis of the duodenum. *Pediatrics* 1969; **43**: 79–83.

Girvan DP, Stephens CA. Congenital intrinsic duodenal obstruction: a twenty-year review of its surgical management and consequences. *Journal of Pediatric Surgery* 1974; **9**: 833–9.

Glazer GM, Margulis AR. Annular pancreas: etiology and diagnosis using endoscopic retrograde cholangiopancreatography. *Radiology* 1979; **133**: 303–6.

Gray SW, Skandalakis JE. *Embryology for surgeons.* Philadelphia, PA: WB Saunders, 1972.

Gress F, Yiengpruksawan A, Sherman S *et al*. Diagnosis of annular pancreas by endoscopic ultrasound. *Gastrointestinal Endoscopy* 1996; **44**: 485–9.

Hayes-Jordan A, Idowu O, Cohen R. Ectopic pancreas as the cause of gastric outlet obstruction in a newborn. *Pediatric Radiology* 1998; **28**: 868–70.

Hendricks SK, Sybert VP. Association of annular pancreas and duodenal obstruction – evidence for Mendelian inheritance? *Clinical Genetics* 1991; **39**: 383–5.

Hidaka T, Hirohashi S, Uchida H *et al*. Annular pancreas diagnosed by single-shot MR cholangiopancreatography. *Magnetic Resonance Imaging* 1998; **16**: 441–4.

Howard JM. Congenital cysts of the pancreas. In: Beger HG, Warshaw AI, Buchler MW *et al*. (eds) *The pancreas.* Oxford: Blackwell Science, 1998: 1427–31.

Ishikawa O, Ishiguro S, Ohhigashi H *et al*. *American Journal of Gastroenterology* 1990; **85**: 597–601.

Jadvar H, Mindelzun RE. Annular pancreas in adults: imaging features in seven patients. *Abdominal Imaging* 1999; **24**: 174–7.

Johnstone DW, Forde KA, Markowitz D, Green PHR, Farman J, Markowitz M. Gastric duplication cyst communicating with the pancreatic duct: a rare cause of recurrent abdominal pain. *Surgery* 1991; **109**: 97–100.

Kiernan PD, ReMine SG, Kiernan PC, ReMine WH. Annular pancreas. *Archives of Surgery* 1980; **115**: 46–50.

Komi N, Takehara H, Kunimoto K, Miyoshi Y, Yagi T. Does the type of anomalous arrangement of pancreatobiliary ducts influence the surgery and prognosis of choledochal cyst? *Journal of Pediatric Surgery* 1992; **27**: 728–31.

Komura J, Yano H, Tanaka T, Tsura T. Annular pancreas associated with pancreatobiliary maljunction in an infant. *European Journal of Pediatric Surgery* 1993; **3**: 244–7.

Laughlin EH, Keown ME, Jackson JE. Heterotopic pancreas obstructing the ampulla of Vater. *Archives of Surgery* 1983; **118**: 979–80.

Lecco TM. Zur morphologie des pankreas annulare.

Sitzunsberichte der kaiserlichen Akademie der Wissenschaffen. Wien 1910; **119**: 391–406.

Lechner GW, Read RC. Agenesis of the dorsal pancreas in an adult diabetic presenting with duodenal ileus. *Annals of Surgery* 1966; **163**: 311–14.

Leese T, Chiche L, Bismuth H. Pancreatitis caused by congenital anomalies of the pancreatic ducts. *Surgery* 1989; **105**: 125–30.

Lehman GA, O'Connor KW. Coexistence of annular pancreas and pancreas divisum: ERCP diagnosis. *Gastrointestinal Endoscopy* 1985; **31**: 25–8.

Lemons JA, Ridenour R, Orsini EN. Congenital absence of the pancreas and intrauterine growth retardation. *Pediatrics* 1979; **64**: 255–7.

Macari M, Giovanniello G, Blair L, Krinsky G. Diagnosis of agenesis of the dorsal pancreas with MR pancreatography. *American Journal of Roentgenology* 1998; **170**: 144–6.

Mao CY, Greenwood S, Wagner S, Howard JM. Solitary true cysts of the pancreas in an adult. *International Journal of Pancreatology* 1992; **12**: 181–6.

Mares AJ, Hirsch M. Congenital cysts of the head of the pancreas. *Journal of Pediatric Surgery* 1977; **12**: 547–52.

Marseglia GL, Bozzola M, Marchi A, Ricci A, Touraine JL. Response to long-term hGH therapy in two children with Schwachman–Diamond syndrome associated with GH deficiency. *Hormone Research* 1998; **50**: 42–5.

Mehes K, Vamos K, Goda M. Agenesis of pancreas and gallbladder in an infant of incest. *Acta Paediatrica Academiae Scientiarum Hungaricae* 1976; **17**: 175–6.

Mester M, Trajber HJ, Compton CC, de Carmargo HAS Jr, de Almeida PCC, Hoover HC Jr. Cystic teratomas of the pancreas. *Archives of Surgery* 1990; **125**: 1215–18.

Millbourn E. On the excretory ducts of the pancreas in man with special reference to their relations with each other, to the common duct and to the duodenum. *Acta Anatomica* 1950; **9**: 1–34.

Millbourn E. Calibre and appearance of the pancreatic ducts and relevant clinical problems. *Acta Chirurgica Scandinavica* 1959/60; **118**: 286–303.

Moss RL, Ryan JA, Kozarek RA, Hatch EI. Pancreatitis caused by a gastric duplication communicating with an aberrant pancreatic lobe. *Journal of Pediatric Surgery* 1996; **31**: 733–6.

O'Rourke RW, Harrison MR. Pancreas divisum and stenosis of the major and minor papillae in an 8-year-old girl: treatment by dual sphincteroplasty. *Journal of Pediatric Surgery* 1998; **33**: 789–91.

Pachi A, Maggi E, Giancotti A, Torcia F, De Prosperi V. Ultrasound diagnosis of fetal annular pancreas. *Journal of Perinatal Medicine* 1989; **17**: 361–4.

Quizilbash AH. Acute pancreatitis occurring in heterotopic pancreatic tissue within the gallbladder. *Canadian Journal of Surgery* 1976; **19**: 413–14.

Ravitch MM, Woods AC. Annular pancreas. *Annals of Surgery* 1950; **132**: 1116–27.

Rogers JC, Harris DJ, Holder T. Annular pancreas in a mother and daughter. *American Journal of Medical Genetics* 1993; **45**: 116.

Rosato FE, Mackie JA. Pancreatic cysts and pseudocysts. *Archives of Surgery* 1963; **86**: 551–6.

Rubesin SE, Furth EE, Birnbaum BA, Rowling SE, Herlinger H. Ectopic pancreas complicated by pancreatitis and pseudocyst formation mimicking jejunal diverticulitis. *British Journal of Radiology* 1997; **70**: 311–13.

Sanada Y, Yoshizawa Y, Chiba M, Nemoto H, Midorikawa T, Kumada K. Ventral pancreatitis in a patient with pancreas divisum. *Journal of Pediatric Surgery* 1995; **30**: 665–7.

Schu W, Copeland R, Fromm D, Elbadawi A. Obstruction of the common hepatic duct by ectopic pancreas. *New York State Journal of Medicine* 1988; **88**: 197–8.

Schurmans J, De Baere H. Upper gastrointestinal hemorrhage caused by ectopic pancreas. *Acta Clinica Belgica* 1980; **35**: 233–7.

Siddiqui AM, Shamberger RC, Filler RM, Perez-Atayde AR, Lillehei CW. Enteric duplications of the pancreatic head: definitive management by local resection. *Journal of Pediatric Surgery* 1998; **33**: 1117–21.

Skandalakis LJ, Rowe JS, Gray SW, Skandalakis JE. Surgical embryology and the anatomy of the pancreas. *Surgical Clinics of North America* 1993; **73**: 661–97.

Spigland N, Yazbeck S. Complications associated with surgical treatment of congenital intrinsic duodenal obstruction. *Journal of Pediatric Surgery* 1990; **25**: 1127–30.

Stern C. A historical perspective on the discovery of the accessory duct of the pancreas, the ampulla of Vater and pancreas divisum. *Gut* 1986; **27**: 203–12.

Tagge EP, Smith SD, Raschbaum GR, Newman B, Wiener ES. Pancreatic ductal abnormalities in children. *Surgery* 1991; **110**: 709–16.

Turner LJ. Chronic pancreatitis and congenital strictures of the pancreatic duct. *American Journal of Surgery* 1983; **145**: 582–4.

Voldsgaard P, Kryger-Baggesen N, Lisse I. Agenesis of pancreas. *Acta Paediatrica; 1994; 83*: 791–3.

Wang JT, Lin JT, Chuang CN *et al*. Complete agenesis of the dorsal pancreas – a case report and review of the literature. *Pancreas* 1990; **5**: 493–7.

Warshaw AL, Simeone JF, Schapiro RH, Flavin-Warshaw B. Evaluation and treatment of the dominant dorsal duct syndrome (pancreas divisum redefined). *American Journal of Surgery* 1990; **159**: 59–66.

Wildling R, Schnedl WJ, Reisinger EC *et al*. Agenesis of the dorsal pancreas in a woman with diabetes mellitus and in both of her sons. *Gastroenterology* 1993; **104**: 1182–6.

Wong KC, Lister J. Human fetal development of the hepato-pancreatic duct junction – a possible explanation of congenital dilatation of the biliary tract. *Journal of Pediatric Surgery* 1981; **16**: 139–45.

Yogi Y, Kosai S, Higashi S, Iwamura T, Setoguchi T. Annular pancreas associated with pancreatolithiasis: a case report. *Hepatogastroenterology* 1999; **46**: 527–31.

Young DG, Wilkinson AW. Abnormalities associated with neonatal duodenal obstruction. *Surgery* 1968; **63**: 832–6.

34

Pancreatic anatomy

MOHAMED RELA

INTRODUCTION

The pancreas lies in the upper part of the abdomen immediately behind the peritoneum of the posterior abdominal wall. It is a fixed organ lying transversely between the second part of the duodenum and the hilum of the spleen. When normal, the gland is soft in consistency with a finely lobulated surface. It is related to the lesser sac above and anteriorly and to the greater sac below. The root of the transverse mesocolon runs anterior to the pancreas, separating the lesser sac above from the greater sac below. The pancreas can therefore be accessed through both the lesser sac and the greater sac by entering the retroperitoneum above or below the transverse mesocolon, but it is usually approached from above in order to prevent damage to the middle colic vessels. Posteriorly the pancreatic bed in the retroperitoneal space consists of an area between the hilum of the right kidney and the hilum of the spleen. From right to left the structures related to the pancreas posteriorly are the hilum of the right kidney, the inferior vena cava, the portal and superior mesenteric veins, the aorta, the left kidney, the left adrenal and the hilum of the spleen.

For descriptive purposes, the pancreas is arbitrarily divided into five parts, namely the head, neck, body, tail and uncinate process (Figure 34.1). The head and tail lie in the paravertebral gutters, while the neck and body are

curved boldly forward over the inferior vena cava and aorta at the level of the first lumbar vertebra.

HEAD AND UNCINATE PROCESS

The head of the pancreas is that part of the gland that lies to the right of the superior mesenteric artery and vein, within the C-shaped concavity of the duodenum with which it shares its blood supply. On the anterior surface of the head, the transverse mesocolon is very short, and therefore the hepatic flexure of the colon itself appears to be closely related to the gland. Exposure of the anterior surface of the head is achieved by mobilizing the hepatic flexure downwards by dividing the peritoneal attachments of the colon laterally and superiorly. The head is loosely attached posteriorly, and this plane is avascular and easily entered during the Kocher maneuver used to mobilize the duodenum and the head of the pancreas. The posterior surface of the head is deeply indented and sometimes tunneled by the terminal part of the bile duct.

The uncinate process extends downwards and backwards from the inferior margin of the head, and passes behind the portal vein and superior mesenteric vessels and in front of the aorta and inferior vena cava. In the sagittal section (Figure 34.2) the uncinate process is located between the superior mesenteric artery and the

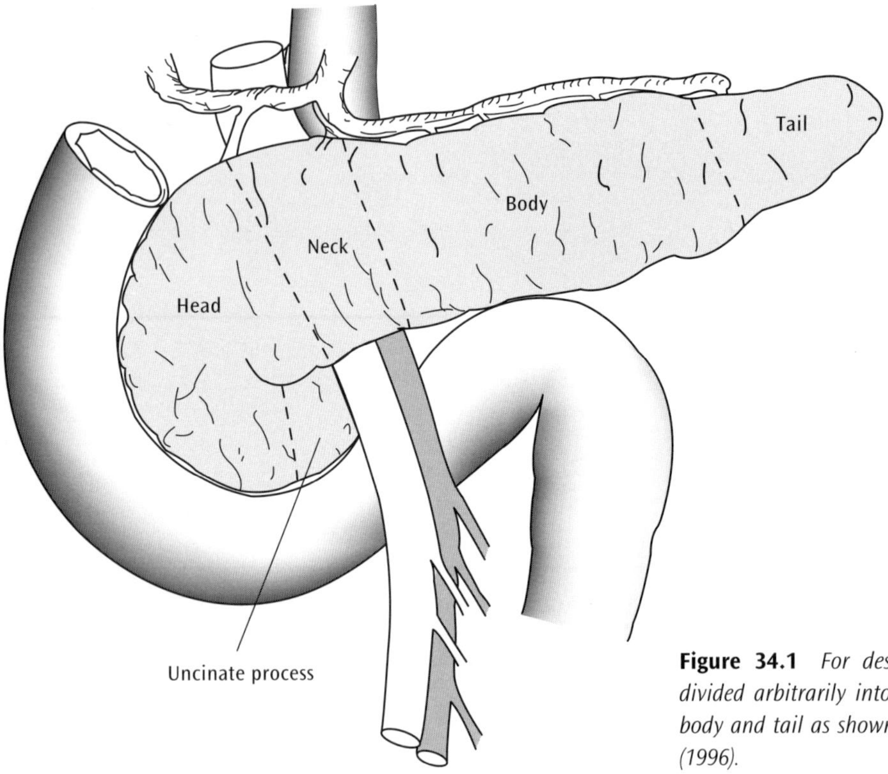

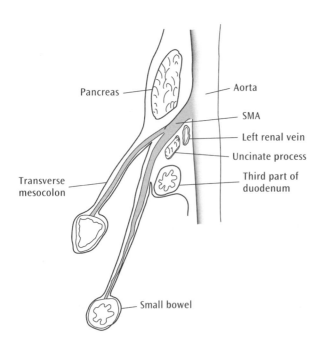

Uncinate process

Figure 34.1 *For descriptive purposes the pancreas is divided arbitrarily into the head, uncinate process, neck, body and tail as shown. Modified from Carter and Russell (1996).*

Pancreas —
Aorta

SMA

Left renal vein

Uncinate process

Transverse mesocolon

Third part of duodenum

Small bowel

Figure 34.2 *Saggital section of pancreas. The uncinate process is shown at the level of the superior mesenteric artery. More laterally the transverse mesocolon splits into two leaves to cover the anterior and inferior borders. SMA, superior mesenteric artery. Modified from Skandalakis et al. (1987).*

aorta, with the left renal vein above and the third part of the duodenum below. The uncinate process may be very short or sometimes well developed, encircling the superior mesenteric vessels completely. Short vessels from the superior mesenteric vessels supply the uncinate process, and these need to be ligated carefully in order to avoid injury to the superior mesenteric vessels during resection of the head of the pancreas. Retraction of these vessels during ligation may lead to torrential bleeding directly from the superior mesenteric artery, which is difficult to identify.

THE NECK

The neck is that portion of the pancreas which lies over the superior mesenteric vessels. Posterior to the neck the portal vein is formed by the confluence of the superior mesenteric and splenic veins. There are no direct veins draining from the back of the neck into the anterior part of the portal vein or superior mesenteric vein. Therefore the plane between the neck and the portal vein can be safely entered during resection of the head. The superior mesenteric artery emerges from the inferior border of the neck and passes over the uncinate process. The celiac axis divides into its main branches over the superior border of the neck. The splenic artery passes almost vertically downwards from its origin for approximately 1 cm, before passing to the left to run along the superior border of the body. It gives off the dorsal pancreatic artery close to its origin. At the time of retrieval of the pancreas for transplantation, the splenic artery should be divided at its origin, to prevent injury to the dorsal pancreatic artery.

THE BODY AND TAIL

The body of the pancreas lies to the left of the superior mesenteric vessels. It is triangular in cross-section with a broad anterior and posterior surface and a narrow inferior surface (Figure 34.2). Anteriorly, the body is covered by the peritoneal layer of the posterior wall of the lesser sac, which separates the stomach from the pancreas. It is common to find a number of avascular bands between the front of the pancreas and the back of the stomach. The body of the gland terminates in a short tail, which passes forwards and ends in the splenic hilum. The body and tail of the pancreas are approached by entering the lesser sac, either by widely dividing the gastrocolic omentum with contained vessels, or by reflecting the greater omentum from the transverse colon through the congenital avascular plane. The avascular bands between the stomach and the pancreas are then divided to expose the pancreas.

Anteriorly the body is also related to the transverse mesocolon, which separates into its two layers, one leaf covering the anterior surface and the other covering the inferior surface. The transverse mesocolon is short on the right and relatively long over the left side of the gland, with the middle colic vessels running between the two leaves. As one passes to the left of the gland, the transverse mesocolon is attached to the inferior border of the body, and this part of the pancreas can also be approached from below by opening an avascular window in the mesocolon, taking care not to damage the middle colic vessels. Posteriorly, the body is related to the left crus of the diaphragm, the left adrenal gland, the left renal vessels and the left kidney. The plane between these posterior structures and the pancreas is avascular, and the body with the splenic vein can be lifted forwards without undue difficulty. When performing this maneuver care must be taken not to injure the friable left adrenal gland. The splenic vein is embedded in the body of the pancreas posteriorly, and numerous small and short veins drain from the pancreas into the vein. During resection of the body of the pancreas, these must be ligated carefully in order to avoid injury to the splenic vein if the spleen is to be preserved. The splenic artery runs a tortuous course along the upper border of the gland.

The tail of the pancreas reaches the hilum of the spleen and, together with the splenic artery and the beginning of the splenic vein, the two layers of spleno-renal ligament envelop it. This peritoneal reflection is continuous with the gastrosplenic ligament, and care must therefore be taken when mobilizing the tail of the pancreas to prevent damage to the short gastric vessels.

PANCREATIC DUCTS

The main pancreatic duct (Wirsung) is a continuous tube leading from the tail to the head, gradually increasing in diameter as it receives tributaries along its length. It drains the tail, body, neck and upper part of the head of the pancreas, and joins the bile duct at the ampulla of Vater. The accessory pancreatic duct (Santorini) drains the uncinate process and the lower part of the head, and crosses the main pancreatic duct to open into the duodenum at the minor duodenal papilla. Within the gland, both ducts lie anterior to the major pancreatic vessels and can be palpated when distended. They can be opened from the anterior surface of the gland (Puestow's procedure). Because of the developmental origin of the two ducts, several variations are encountered within the head of the pancreas, the commonest of which are as follows. In 60% of glands both ducts open into the duodenum, the accessory duct draining approximately 2 cm above the main duct. In 30% of glands the main pancreatic duct carries the entire secretion and the accessory duct ends blindly. The accessory duct carries the entire secretion in 10% of cases, the main duct being small or absent in the head of the gland.

BLOOD SUPPLY

The pancreas is supplied with blood from both the celiac trunk and the superior mesenteric artery (Figure 34.3). In general, the blood supply is greatest to the head, less to the body and tail, and least to the neck. The head is supplied from above by the gastroduodenal artery, which divides into anterior and posterior superior pancreaticoduodenal arteries. These vessels pass downwards with the curve of the duodenum and anastomose with the anterior and posterior branches of the inferior pancreaticoduodenal branch of the superior mesenteric artery. This vessel can be quite short and, during the final stages of resection of the head of the pancreas, traction on the specimen can pull the superior mesenteric artery, resulting in damage to it. The pancreaticoduodenal arcades that are formed on the anterior and posterior part of the head of the pancreas supply the second and third part of the duodenum. Despite this the duodenum can be preserved after division of the pancreaticoduodenal arteries in the operation of duodenum-preserving total pancreatectomy.

The splenic artery supplies the body and the tail of the pancreas as it courses along the upper border. The dorsal

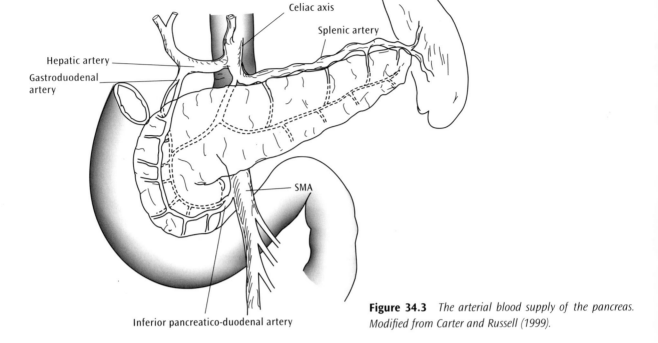

Celiac axis

Splenic artery

Hepatic artery

Gastroduodenal
artery

SMA

Inferior pancreatico-duodenal artery

Figure 34.3 *The arterial blood supply of the pancreas. Modified from Carter and Russell (1999).*

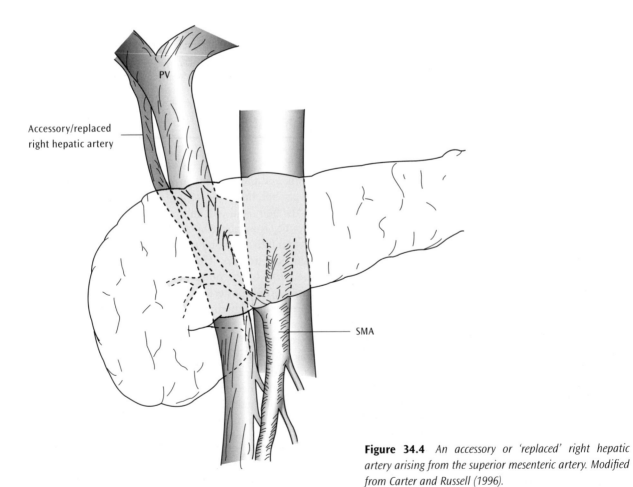

PV

Accessory/replaced
right hepatic artery

SMA

Figure 34.4 *An accessory or 'replaced' right hepatic artery arising from the superior mesenteric artery. Modified from Carter and Russell (1996).*

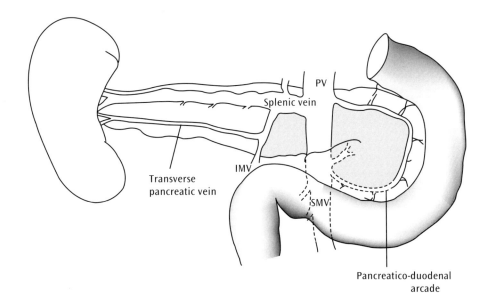

Figure 34.5 *The veins of the pancreas parallel the arteries and lie superficial to them. They drain into the portal vein (PV), superior mesenteric vein (SMV) and splenic vein. Modified from Skandalakis et al. (1987).*

pancreatic artery is a significant branch of the splenic artery, and it divides into a right and left branch. The right branch supplies the back of the head and the uncinate process, and the left branch (transverse pancreatic artery) supplies the body and tail of the pancreas. There is a rich anastomosis between the transverse pancreatic artery and branches of the splenic artery along the length of the pancreas.

Anomalies in the arterial supply to the liver may pose problems during pancreatic surgery. The commonest anomaly is the presence of an accessory or replaced right hepatic artery arising from the superior mesenteric artery in up to 30% of individuals. This branch is given off as a right branch of the superior mesenteric artery, and courses behind the head of the pancreas, emerging on its upper border to the right of the portal vein behind the common bile duct (Figure 34.4). This may be identified by palpating for pulsation just behind the common bile duct. When present, this artery can easily be separated from the head of the pancreas during resection. Occasionally the inferior pancreaticoduodenal artery can arise from the aberrant right hepatic artery. This has implications during multi-organ retrievals for organ transplantation, when both the pancreas and the liver are being used for transplantation. In such cases, the replaced or accessory right hepatic artery should be divided at the upper border of the duodenum, preserving the blood supply to the head, which in whole-pancreas transplantation is entirely dependent on the inferior pancreaticoduodenal arcade.

In general, the veins of the pancreas parallel the arteries and lie superficial to them. They drain into the portal vein, superior mesenteric vein and splenic vein (Figure 34.5).

LYMPHATIC DRAINAGE

The lymphatic vessels from the pancreas follow the course of the arteries. Eleven groups of lymph nodes draining the pancreas have been designated superior head, superior body, inferior head, inferior body, anterior pancreaticoduodenal, posterior pancreaticoduodenal, splenic, portal, celiac, mesenteric and para-aortic. Knowledge of these lymph-node groups is essential in order to standardize lymph-node dissection during radical resection of the pancreas for malignancy (Deki and Sato, 1988).

REFERENCES

Carter DC, Russell RCG. Surgical anatomy of the pancreas. In: Carter D, Russell RCG, Pitt HA, Bismuth H (eds) *Hepatobiliary and pancreatic surgery*. London: Chapman and Hall, 1996: 447–53.

Deki H, Sato T. An anatomic study of the peripancreatic lymphatics. *Surgical and Radiologic Anatomy* 1988; **10**: 121–35.

Skandalakis JE, Gray SW, Skandalakis LJ. Surgical anatomy of the pancreas. In: Howard JM, Jordan GL Jr, Reber HA (eds) *Surgical diseases of the pancreas*. Philadelphia, PA: Lea and Febiger, 1987: 11–36.

Endoscopic retrograde cholangiopancreatography (ERCP)

STEVEN L WERLIN AND ANDREW TAYLOR

INTRODUCTION

Endoscopic retrograde cholangiopancreatography (ERCP) is a specialized procedure that combines the skills of gastrointestinal endoscopy and interpretive fluoroscopy for diagnostic and therapeutic management of pancreatic and biliary tract disorders. This procedure, which has been applied in adult patients for more than 30 years, is now an accepted modality for use in children.

McCune and colleagues (McCune et al., 1968) reported the first successful cannulation of the ampulla of Vater in 1968 using a forward-viewing endoscope. Side-viewing duodenoscopes became available in the 1970s. The first successful ERCP in a child, involving the use of the adult-size duodenoscope in a 3.5-month-old, 6.0 kg infant with cholestasis, was reported by Waye in 1976. Smaller-diameter duodenoscopes (7.5–9.0 mm) have subsequently been developed. Although improvement in the design of these duodenoscopes has allowed the use of ERCP in children at major pediatric referral centers throughout the world, published experience remains relatively limited.

The feasibility of ERCP in young children and infants has been repeatedly demonstrated in case reports and small series, and has been reviewed by Werlin (1994). The safety and clinical outcomes of both diagnostic and therapeutic interventions have not been critically examined in large numbers of pediatric patients. Even the two largest series combined (Brown et al., 1993; Guelrud et al., 1997) include only 356 patients. Table 35.1 summarizes the data, including age range, indications and rates of complications, from some of the larger published pediatric series.

Guidelines for the use of ERCP in children have recently been developed by the North American Society for Pediatric Gastroenterology and Nutrition (Fox et al., 2000). These guidelines review the technical aspects of the procedure and the fluoroscopic, procedure-room and equipment requirements. The details of patient preparation and sedation are also summarized. The importance of appropriate training of the endoscopist is reviewed. Antibiotic prophylaxis is recommended for patients with high-risk cardiovascular conditions, including prosthetic valves, a history of endocarditis, systemic-pulmonary shunt, and synthetic vascular grafts less than 1 year old, and for any patient with an obstructed bile duct or pancreatic pseudocyst.

RISKS AND COMPLICATIONS

The subject of ERCP-related complications in adults has been extensively reviewed (Aliperti, 1996). The major risks and complications of ERCP in children are the same as for adults, and include pancreatitis, hemorrhage, infection and perforation, although due to the small numbers of patients in pediatric series, the relative risk of these complications in children is not well established (for a summary, see Box 35.1). Only one pediatric death following ERCP has been reported (Reiman and Koch, 1978).

Table 35.1 *Pediatric ERCP series*

Author	Patients (n)	Procedures (n)	Age range	Indications (% of total) Biliary	Pancreatitis	Pain	Therapeutic (%)	Complications (%) Pancreatitis	Hemorrhage	Infection
Cotton and Lange (1982)	20	25	7–16 years	20	50	30	5	0	0	0
Buckley and Connon (1990)	42	42	1–19 years	36	43	21	12	5	2	0
Guelrud et al. (1991)	32	32	16–150 days	100	0	0	0	0	0	0
Putnam et al. (1991)	38	42	14 months–19 years	36	64	0	0	8	0	0
Brown (1993)	92	121	4 months–19 years	20	77	3	NR	3	0	2.5
Brown and Goldschmiedt (1994)	25	42	22 months–19 years	64	36	0	68	8	0	0
Guelrud et al. (1994)	51	NR	1–18 years	0	100	0	35	8	0	0
Mitchell and Wilkinson (1994)	40	40	6–80 weeks	100	0	0	0	0	0	0
Ohnuma et al. (1997)	73	75	8–300 days	100	0	0	0	0	0	0
Guelrud et al. (1999a)	264	264	< 1 year–15 years	75	25	0	NR	1	0	0
Hsu et al. (2000)	22	34	1.5–17 years	0	100	0	0	2	0	0
Linuma et al. (2000)	50	50	25–274 days	100	0	0	100	0	0	0
Teng et al. (2000)	42	50	57 days–15 years	64	36	0	12	0	0	1
Ohnuma et al. (1997)	73	75	8–300 days	100	0	0	0	0	0	0

NR, not reported.

Box 35.1 *Complications of ERCP*

Cholangitis
Cholecystitis
Complications of anesthesia/sedation
Fever
Hemorrhage
Ileus
Infection
Intramural dye injection
Pain
Pancreatitis
Perforation

Pancreatitis, the commonest complication of ERCP, occurred in up to 8% of patients in the larger pediatric series. This compares with rates of 3–7% reported in adults (Aliperti, 1996). In our series (Brown *et al.*, 1993) (121 procedures), the overall complication rate was 11.6%. Pancreatitis occurred in four cases (3.3%). Adults and children undergoing *therapeutic* ERCP are at increased risk for post-ERCP pancreatitis, which occurred in 17% of patients in one pediatric series (Guelrud *et al.*, 1994). Although the pathogenesis of this complication is not well understood, it may be related to repeated duct cannulation and injection, prolonged manometry catheter infusion into the pancreatic duct and mechanical irritation of the papilla or pancreatic duct orifice. The use of octreotide to prevent post-ERCP pancreatitis is controversial, and is not practised in our units (Andriulli *et al.*, 2000).

In adults, hemorrhage and perforation occur in 0.7–2.0% and 0.3–0.6% of procedures, respectively. ERCP-related bacteremia may occur following 15% of diagnostic procedures and 27% of therapeutic procedures in adults (Aliperti, 1996). These complications have rarely been reported in children.

A multicenter prospective study of complications in adults undergoing endoscopic sphincterotomy found an overall complication rate of 9.8% (Freeman *et al.*, 1996). The most frequent complications included pancreatitis (5.4%), hemorrhage (2.0%), cholangitis (1.0%), cholecystitis (0.5%) and perforation (0.3%). Failed or inadequate biliary drainage is a major risk factor for cholangitis. There have been no such studies in children.

Stent occlusion occurs in 20–30% of patients within 3 months of insertion, and the rate of stent migration for both biliary duct and pancreatic duct stents is approximately 5.0% (Aliperti, 1996). The long-term complications of sphincterotomy or use of stents in pediatric patients are not known. The incidence of complications associated with therapeutic interventions, such as sphincterotomy or stent placement, is not known for children.

Contraindications to ERCP include unstable cardiovascular, pulmonary or neurological conditions, or suspected bowel perforation. Esophageal stricture is a relative contraindication depending on the severity of the stricture. Coagulopathy is a relative contraindication, which should be corrected prior to ERCP if possible. Medications that might affect platelet function, such as aspirin or non-steroidal anti-inflammatory drugs, should be discontinued several days prior to the procedure.

DIAGNOSTIC AND THERAPEUTIC INDICATIONS

Although the indications for ERCP are similar for children and adults, the relative frequency of each indication differs. For example, children are much more likely to have indications related to congenital abnormalities or trauma than to malignancy. Indications related to biliary lithiasis or to prior surgery are less common in children. Magnetic resonance imaging cholangiopancreatography (MRCP) can provide high-quality non-invasive imaging of biliary and pancreatic ducts in adults, and has eliminated the need for diagnostic ERCP in some settings (Fulcher and Turner, 1999). Initial reports of the results of MRCP in children (Hirohashi *et al.*, 1997; Yamataka *et al.*, 1997; Ernst *et al.*, 1998; Miyazaki *et al.*, 1998) are very promising, but further study is needed to compare accuracy and utility with ERCP for specific disorders. ERCP provides high-resolution imaging of duct anatomy and permits sampling of tissue and fluid as well as therapeutic intervention.

Pancreatic indications

Pancreatic indications for diagnostic and therapeutic ERCP are listed in Box 35.2. ERCP may be used to identify intrinsic (e.g. anomalous pancreaticobiliary junction) and extrinsic (e.g. gallstones) causes of persistent or recurrent acute pancreatitis, to evaluate complications of chronic pancreatitis, and to treat mechanical obstruction or fluid collections. Abnormal findings are present in the majority of children who are investigated for presumed idiopathic recurrent pancreatitis.

Developmental anomalies identifiable by pancreatography have been associated with recurrent pancreatitis. The commonest of these is pancreas divisum (Warshaw *et al.*, 1990), which is found in 5–10% of the general population (Figure 35.1) (see Figure 33.4). Endoscopic sphincterotomy of the minor papilla has led to improvement in approximately 75% of adult patients with recurrent acute attacks of pancreatitis associated with pancreas divisum (Lehman and Sherman, 1995), which is comparable with the outcome following surgical sphincteroplasty. Improved outcome has been reported after endoscopic therapy in children, but the data are limited to a small number of case reports (Brown *et al.*,

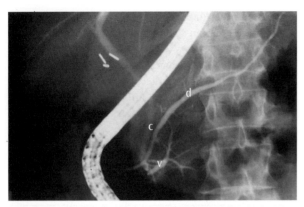

Figure 35.1 *Pancreas divisum. Contrast has been injected into the ventral duct (v) and dorsal duct (d) with no communication. The distal common bile duct (c) is also partly filled.*

Box 35.2 *Pancreatic indications for ERCP in children*

Diagnostic indications
Evaluation of known or suspected developmental pancreatic anomalies
Pancreatic mass
Pancreatic trauma
Preoperative evaluation
Unexplained persistent acute, recurrent acute or chronic pancreatitis

Therapeutic indications
Pancreatic duct obstruction (stenosis, stricture, stone, disruption)
Pseudocyst drainage

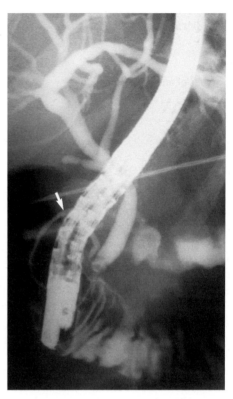

Figure 35.2 *Annular pancreas. During biliary tract injection, a segment of the common bile duct (arrow) encircles the partially contrast-filled duodenum.*

1993; Kozarek *et al.*, 1993; Brown and Goldschmiedt, 1994; Guelrud *et al.*, 1994; Lemmel *et al.*, 1994; Fox *et al.*, 1995; Graham *et al.*, 1998).

Other anomalies, such as anomalous union of the pancreaticobiliary ductal system (Mori *et al.*, 1993), annular pancreas (Figure 35.2) (Guelrud *et al.*, 1994), dorsal pancreatic agenesis (Guelrud *et al.*, 1994) and duodenal duplications (Lang *et al.*, 1994), have also been associated with recurrent attacks of pancreatitis in children, and may be demonstrated by ERCP.

Early ERCP is used to assess the integrity of the pancreas following abdominal trauma when ductal transection is considered or when fluid collections fail to resolve after conservative therapy (Rescorla *et al.*, 1995). If the ductal system is intact, the patient can be managed conservatively. Transection of the duct is treated surgically or endoscopically by placement of a transpapillary stent (Kozarek *et al.*, 1993).

If a pseudocyst fails to resolve following an attack of pancreatitis, ERCP should be obtained for drainage or to provide diagnostic information for planning surgical or percutaneous radiological drainage (Figure 35.3).

Endoscopic options include a nasocystic drainage catheter, transpapillary endoprosthesis (stent), transmural cyst duodenostomy or cyst gastrostomy, and combination therapy with transmural and transpapillary drainage. Definitive therapy has been achieved in up to 76% of adult patients, with a complication rate of about 15% (Cremer *et al.*, 1989; Barthet *et al.*, 1995; Binmoeller *et al.*, 1995; Catalano *et al.*, 1995; Lehman, 1995; Smits *et al.*, 1995). Successful endoscopic drainage has been reported in children (Brown *et al.*, 1993; Kozarek *et al.*, 1993; Guelrud *et al.*, 1994; Lemmel *et al.*, 1994; Graham *et al.*, 1998), but experience is insufficient to allow conclusions to be drawn on either the efficacy or the safety of this procedure in children. In our institution we typically drain pseudocysts percutaneously.

ERCP is helpful in the evaluation and treatment of chronic pancreatitis as it provides detailed information about anatomical changes in both the main pancreatic duct and its side branches that may be used to confirm the diagnosis (Figures 35.4 and 35.5). The major indication for therapeutic ERCP in patients with chronic pancreatitis is the presence of stones within a dilated pancreatic duct. Recent adult studies (Dumonceau *et al.*, 1996; Smits *et al.*, 1996) suggest that 80–100% of patients with either partial or complete clearance of intraductal stones enjoy immediate relief of pain (Figure 35.6). As with other therapeutic interventions, pediatric

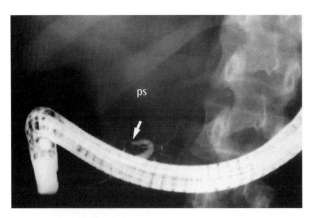

Figure 35.3 *Endoscopic retrograde pancreatogram as a road-map to surgery. A 17-year-old had continued pain and pseudocyst formation following pancreatitis. Filling of the main pancreatic duct demonstrates complete duct occlusion at the pancreatic neck (arrow). There is subtle extravasation into a large pseudocyst (ps).*

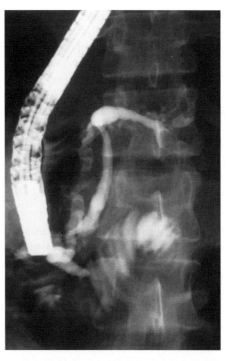

Figure 35.5 *Hereditary pancreatitis. A 17-year-old boy had recurrent bouts of pancreatitis. Endoscopic retrograde pancreatography shows the typical changes of hereditary pancreatitis, with an irregular, ectatic duct system as well as large faceted intraductal concretions.*

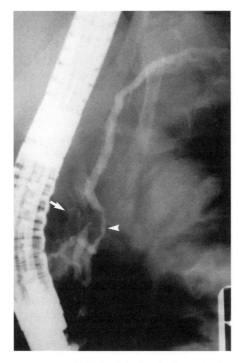

Figure 35.4 *ERCP prior to surgery. A 12-year-old girl presented with pancreatitis and elevated liver function tests. At ERCP there was severe focal common bile duct stricture (arrow) and a moderately narrowed irregular main pancreatic duct (arrowhead). This patient had no risk factors for pancreatitis, and eventually underwent surgery for non-alcoholic duct-destructive pancreatitis.*

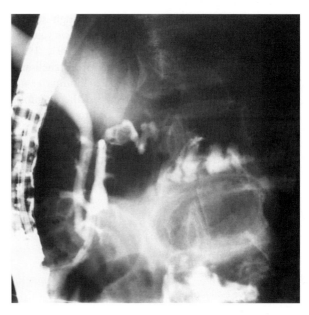

Figure 35.6 *Pancreatic duct stone. This 8-year-old girl has concretions behind a focal pancreatic neck stricture. This stricture is most probably related to a prior traumatic event.*

experience is limited (Kozareck et al., 1993; Guelrud et al., 1994; Graham et al., 1998; Hsu et al., 2000).

In the absence of intraductal stones, endoscopic sphincterotomy may be considered as an alternative to surgical sphincteroplasty in the presence of obstructive findings, including intermittent or persistent ductal dilatation or abnormally prolonged dilatation following provocative testing (e.g. secretin stimulation) (Tulassay et al., 1991). The outcomes of this procedure in pediatric patients have not been established.

Biliary indications

The biliary indications for ERCP in children are summarized in Box 35.3. Diagnostic tests such as abdominal ultrasound or CT, liver biopsy, biliary scintigraphy and biochemical testing do not always distinguish between intrahepatic cholestasis due to neonatal hepatitis and biliary atresia. Rapid diagnosis and treatment of structural causes of neonatal cholestasis, such as biliary atresia, choledochal cyst, choledocholithiasis, paucity or hypoplasia of intrahepatic bile ducts, neonatal sclerosing cholangitis and congenital bile duct strictures are important in order to minimize ongoing liver injury. Ultimately, a cholangiogram or surgical exploration is often required. ERCP offers a relatively non-invasive alternative to percutaneous transhepatic or transcholecystic cholangiography, or open surgical cholangiography. If normal biliary anatomy is demonstrated, a surgical procedure may be avoided. Although several authors have reported a high positive predictive value of ERCP in this setting (Guelrud et al., 1991, 1997; Wilkinson et al., 1991; Derkx et al., 1994; Mitchell and Wilkinson, 1994; Ohnuma et al., 1997; Linuma et al., 2000), endoscopic findings which suggest the diagnosis of biliary atresia include absence of contrast in the bile

duct despite filling of the pancreatic duct, and partial filling of the common bile duct with abnormal termination. Endoscopic investigation of neonatal cholestasis remains controversial. ERCP may have value in selected circumstances for clarifying the cause of neonatal cholestasis, but since the cause of cholestasis in most infants can be determined without ERCP, at this time the latter cannot be recommended as part of the routine evaluation of such infants.

ERCP can be used to confirm the diagnosis of a choledochal cyst (Chaudhary et al., 1996) and to assist surgical planning (Yamashiro et al., 1993). The cholangiographic finding of a long common channel or anomalous pancreaticobiliary junction has been frequently associated with and may contribute to the etiology of choledochal cyst (Guelrud et al., 1999a). Choledocholithiasis with bile duct obstruction may mimic the findings of choledochal cyst in young infants (Fox et al., 1997), and should be excluded by cholangiography.

ERCP may be indicated for children with suspected sclerosing cholangitis or cholangiopathy in association with inflammatory bowel disease (Figure 35.7), histiocytosis X, HIV infection (Figure 35.8) (Yabut et al., 1996) or other immunodeficiency states and cystic fibrosis (Figure 35.9). ERCP is also indicated to evaluate strictures arising from operative injury, abdominal trauma, and extrinsic compression due to chronic fibrosing pancreatitis or tumors (either benign or malignant).

ERCP is used to perform sphincter of Oddi manometry in adults and children with suspected biliary dyskinesia or sphincter of Oddi dysmotility (Guelrud et al., 1999b). However, given the lack of normal control data in children, minimal published experience and inherent technical difficulties with the test, the clinical application and reliability of this test in children are not known.

Based on studies in adult patients (Neoptolemos et al., 1988; Fan et al., 1993; Fölsch et al., 1997), ERCP within 24–48 hours of presentation is indicated in acute biliary pancreatitis when a stone is identified in the common bile duct, or when biliary obstruction or cholangitis is evident. Early endoscopic intervention and biliary drainage reduce the morbidity of suppurative cholangitis without significantly affecting the course of pancreatitis in adult patients (Baillie, 1997; Fölsch et al., 1997). Although similar outcome studies in children have not been reported, our unpublished experience confirms the published studies in adults.

Endoscopic sphincterotomy and stone extraction for choledocholithiasis is the most commonly employed biliary intervention in children. This has been performed successfully in infants as young as 2 months of age (Guelrud et al., 1992; Wilkinson and Clayton, 1996; Tarnasky et al., 1998). Endoscopic papillary balloon dilatation is an alternative technique to sphincterotomy for removal of common bile duct stones (Komatsu et al., 1998). This sphincter-preserving technique is appealing for younger patients, for whom the long-term risks of

---

Box 35.3 *Biliary indications for ERCP in children*

Diagnostic indications
Biliary stricture
Choledocholithiasis
Choledochal cyst
Dilated intrahepatic or extrahepatic bile duct
Persistent bile leak
Preoperative evaluation
Primary sclerosing cholangitis
Sphincterotomy
Unexplained cholestasis of infancy

Therapeutic indications
Biliary pancreatitis associated with obstructive jaundice
Stent placement
Stone extraction
Stricture dilatation

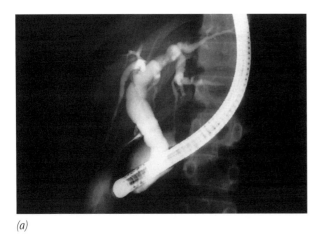

(a)

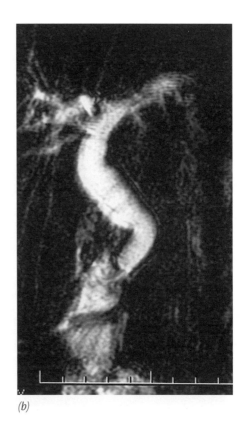

Figure 35.7 *Primary sclerosing cholangitis (PSC) in a 14-year-old boy with ulcerative colitis. (a) This endoscopic retrograde cholangiogram illustrates the typical features of PSC, with the scattered smooth strictures without prestenotic dilatation. These changes are best demonstrated in the intrahepatic duct system with mild mucosal irregularity in the dilated extrahepatic duct. (b) MRCP in the same patient does not give the same detail for small branch disease, but it does reveal the tight distal common duct stricture that was obscured by the ERCP endoscope.*

(b)

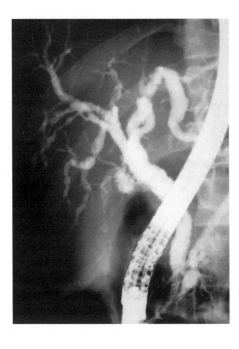

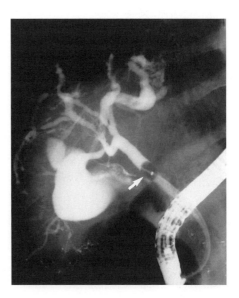

Figure 35.8 *AIDS cholangiopathy. This cholangiogram illustrates two main features of AIDS cholangitis. The first is the diffuse strictures present in the intrahepatic biliary tree, which superficially simulates primary sclerosing cholangitis. The second is the distal common duct stricture, which may raise the possibility of sphincter of Oddi dysfunction. However, the AIDS stricture is longer than the sphincter of Oddi dysfunction stricture.*

Figure 35.9 *Cystic fibrosis. This endoscopic retrograde cholangiogram was obtained with a balloon-tip catheter (arrow) to ensure adequate filling of the intrahepatic biliary tract. The intrahepatic biliary tree has areas of strictures related to a combination of secondary sclerosing cholangitis from bouts of obstruction as well as cirrhosis. Inspissated bile results in concretions that are seen as intraductal filling defects. The distal common bile duct is smoothly narrowed by extrinsic pressure related to the enlarged, fatty-replaced pancreas.*

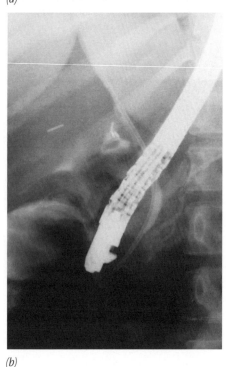

(a)

(b)

Figure 35.10 *Diagnosis and treatment of bile leakage at endoscopic retrograde cholangiogram. This 18-year-old woman has recently undergone laparoscopic cholecystectomy with increasing abdominal pain and ascites. (a) At endoscopic retrograde cholangiogram extravasation is found at the cystic duct stump (arrow). (b) In the same setting, a 7 FG biliary stent was placed without the need for a sphincterotomy. Two weeks later the stent was removed and the stump leak healed.*

sphincterotomy are still unknown. However, published experience with this technique in children is limited (Tarnasky *et al.*, 1998), and the risk of pancreatitis may be higher than following sphincterotomy (Bergman and Huibregtse, 1998). Strictures associated with congenital and acquired lesions in the biliary system have been successfully treated in children by transendoscopic balloon dilatation and placement of endoprostheses or stents (Bickerstaff *et al.*, 1989; Guelrud *et al.*, 1989; Brown and Goldschmiedt, 1994; Gold *et al.*, 1995; Sebesta *et al.*, 1995). Biliary endoprostheses may also be used to treat acute or chronic bile leaks or fistula following abdominal trauma or surgical injury, such as following a cholecystectomy (Figure 35.10) (Prasad *et al.*, 2000).

CONCLUSION

ERCP is a valuable diagnostic and therapeutic modality in children with known or suspected pancreatic or hepatobiliary disease. Indications for ERCP in children are similar to those in adults. An experienced endoscopist should perform the procedure in a medical environment that is optimal for the care of children. If a pediatric gastroenterologist with such training and experience is not available, the procedure should be performed applying the combined knowledge and expertise of a pediatric gastroenterologist and an experienced endoscopist (usually an adult gastroenterologist and a radiologist). Based on the limited data available, the safety and efficacy of therapeutic interventions appear to be comparable in children and adults.

Key references

Aliperti G. Complications related to diagnostic and therapeutic endoscopic retrograde cholangiopancreatography. *Gastrointestinal Endoscopy Clinics of North America* 1996; **6**: 379–407.

A thorough review of the complications of ERCP.

Brown CW, Werlin SL, Geenen JE, Schmalz M. The diagnostic and therapeutic role of endoscopic retrograde cholangiopancreatography in children. *Journal of Pediatric Gastroenterology and Nutrition* 1993; **17**: 19–23.

Guelrud M, Carr-Locke DL, Fox VL. *ERCP in pediatric practice: diagnosis and treatment.* Oxford: Isis Medical Media Ltd, 1997.

The largest pediatric series of ERCP in children.

Graham KS, Ingram JD, Steinberg SE, Narkewicz MR. ERCP in the management of pediatric pancreatitis. *Gastrointestinal Endoscopy* 1998; **47**: 492–5.

This small study demonstrates that ERCP changed the management of 50% of a group of children with pancreatitis.

REFERENCES

Aliperti G. Complications related to diagnostic and therapeutic endoscopic retrograde cholangio-pancreatography. *Gastrointestinal Endoscopy Clinics of North America* 1996; **6**: 379–407.

Andriulli A, Leandro G, Niro G *et al.* Pharmacologic treatment can prevent pancreatic injury after ERCP: a meta-analysis. *Gastrointestinal Endoscopy* 2000; **51**: 1–7.

Baillie J. Treatment of acute biliary pancreatitis. *New England Journal of Medicine* 1997; **336**: 286–7.

Barthet M, Sahel J, Bodiou-Bertei C, Bernard J-P. Endoscopic transpapillary drainage of pancreatic pseudocysts. *Gastrointestinal Endoscopy* 1995; **42**: 208–13.

Bergman JJGHM, Huibregtse K. What is the current status of endoscopic balloon dilation for stone removal? *Endoscopy* 1998; **30**: 43–5.

Bickerstaff KI, Britton BJ, Gough MH. Endoscopic palliation of malignant biliary obstruction in a child. *British Journal of Surgery* 1989; **76**: 1092–3.

Binmoeller KF, Seifert H, Walter A, Soehendra N. Transpapillary and transmural drainage of pancreatic pseudocysts. *Gastrointestinal Endoscopy* 1995; **42**: 219–24.

Brown CW, Werlin SL, Geenen JE, Schmalz M. The diagnostic and therapeutic role of endoscopic retrograde cholangiopancreatography in children. *Journal of Pediatric Gastroenterology and Nutrition* 1993; **17**: 19–23.

Brown KO, Goldschmiedt M. Endoscopic therapy of biliary and pancreatic disorders in children. *Endoscopy* 1994; **26**: 719–23.

Buckley A, Connon J. The role of ERCP in children and adolescents. *Gastrointestinal Endoscopy* 1990; **36**: 369–72.

Catalano MF, Geenen JE, Schmalz MJ, Johnson GK, Dean RS, Hogan WJ. Treatment of pancreatic pseudocysts with ductal communication by transpapillary pancreatic duct endoprosthesis. *Gastrointestinal Endoscopy* 1995; **42**: 214–18.

Chaudhary A, Dhar P, Sachdev A *et al.* Choledochal cysts – differences in children and adults. *British Journal of Surgery* 1996; **83**: 186–8.

Cotton P, Lange N. Endoscopic retrograde cholangio-pancreatography in children. *Archives of Disease in Childhood* 1982; **57**: 131–6.

Cremer M, Deviere J, Engelholm L. Endoscopic management of cysts and pseudocysts in chronic pancreatitis: long-term follow-up after 7 years of experience. *Gastrointestinal Endoscopy* 1989; **35**: 1–9.

Derkx HHF, Huibregtse K, Taminiau JJA. The role of endoscopic retrograde cholangiopancreatography in cholestatic infants. *Endoscopy* 1994; **26**: 724–8.

Dumonceau JM, Deviere J, Le Moine O *et al.* Endoscopic pancreatic drainage in chronic pancreatitis associated with ductal stones: long-term results. *Gastrointestinal Endoscopy* 1996; **43**: 547–55.

Ernst O, Gottrand F, Calvo M *et al.* Congenital hepatic fibrosis: findings at MR cholangiopancreatography. *American Journal of Roentgenology* 1998; **170**: 409–12.

Fan S-T, Lai ECS, Mok FPT, Lok C-M, Zheng S-S, Wong J. Early treatment of acute biliary pancreatitis by endoscopic papillotomy. *New England Journal of Medicine* 1993; **328**: 228–32.

Fölsch UR, Nitsche R, Lüdtke R, Hilgers RA, Creutzfeldt W. German Study Group on Acute Biliary Pancreatitis. Early ERCP and papillotomy compared with conservative treatment for acute biliary pancreatitis. *New England Journal of Medicine* 1997; **336**: 237–42.

Fox VL, Lichtenstein DR, Carr-Locke DL. Incomplete pancreas divisum in children with recurrent pancreatitis. *Gastrointestinal Endoscopy* 1995; **41**: 337.

Fox VL, Carr-Locke DL, Hardy S, Israel E, Share J. Transient bile duct obstruction mimicking choledochal cyst in infants. *Gastrointestinal Endoscopy* 1997; **45**: AB60.

Fox VL, Werlin SI, Heyman MB. Endoscopic retrograde cholangiopancreatography in children. Subcommittee on Endoscopy and Procedure of the Patient Care Committee of the North American Society for Pediatric Gastroenterology and Nutrition. *Journal of Pediatric Gastroenterology and Nutrition* 2000; **30**: 335–42.

Freeman ML, Nelson DB, Sherman S *et al.* Complications of endoscopic biliary sphincterotomy. *New England Journal of Medicine* 1996; **335**: 909–18.

Fulcher AS, Turner MA. MR pancreatography: a useful tool for evaluating pancreatic disorders. *Radiographics* 1999; **19**: 5–24.

Gold DM, Stark B, Pettei MJ, Levine JJ. Successful use of an internal biliary stent in Caroli's disease. *Gastrointestinal Endoscopy* 1995; **42**: 589–92.

Graham KS, Ingram JD, Steinberg SE, Narkewicz MR. ERCP in the management of pediatric pancreatitis. *Gastrointestinal Endoscopy* 1998; **47**: 492–5.

Guelrud M, Nendoza S, Zager A, Noguera C. Biliary stenting in an infant with malignant obstructive jaundice. *Gastrointestinal Endoscopy* 1989; **35**: 259–61.

Guelrud M, Jaen D, Mendoza S, Plaz J, Torres P. ERCP in the diagnosis of extrahepatic biliary atresia. *Gastrointestinal Endoscopy* 1991; **37**: 522–6.

Guelrud M, Mendoza S, Jaen D, Plaz J, Machuca J, Torres P. ERCP and endoscopic sphincterotomy in infants and children with jaundice due to common bile duct stones. *Gastrointestinal Endoscopy* 1992; **38**: 450–3.

Guelrud M, Mujica C, Jaen D, Plaz J, Arias J. The role of ERCP in the diagnosis and treatment of idiopathic recurrent pancreatitis in children and adolescents. *Gastrointestinal Endoscopy* 1994; **40**: 428–36.

Guelrud M, Carr-Locke DL, Fox VL. *ERCP in pediatric practice: diagnosis and treatment.* Oxford: Isis Medical Media Ltd, 1997.

Guelrud M, Morera C, Rodriquez M, Prados JG, Jaén D. Normal and anomalous pancreaticobiliary union in children and adolescents. *Gastrointestinal Endoscopy* 1999a; **50**: 189–93.

Guelrud M, Morera C, Rodriquez M, Jaen D, Pierre R. Sphincter of Oddi dysfunction in children with recurrent pancreatitis and anomalous pancreaticobiliary union: an etiologic concept. *Gastrointestinal Endoscopy* 1999b; **50**: 194–9.

Hirohashi S, Hirohashi R, Uchida H *et al*. Pancreatitis: evaluation with MR cholangiopancreatography in children. *Radiology* 1997; **203**: 411–15.

Hsu RK, Draganov P, Leung JW *et al*. Therapeutic ERCP in the management of pancreatitis in children. *Gastrointestinal Endoscopy* 2000; **51**: 396–400.

Komatsu Y, Kawabe T, Toda N *et al*. Endoscopic papillary balloon dilation for the management of common bile duct stones: experience of 226 cases. *Endoscopy* 1998; **30**: 12–17.

Kozarek R, Christie D, Barklay G. Endoscopic therapy of pancreatitis in the pediatric population. *Gastrointestinal Endoscopy* 1993; **39**: 665–9.

Lang T, Berquist W, Rich E *et al*. Treatment of recurrent pancreatitis by endoscopic drainage of a duodenal duplication. *Journal of Pediatric Gastroenterology and Nutrition* 1994; **18**: 494–6.

Lehman GA. Endoscopic management of pancreatic pseudocysts continues to evolve. *Gastrointestinal Endoscopy* 1995; **42**: 273–5.

Lehman GA, Sherman S. Pancreas divisum. Diagnosis, clinical significance and management alternatives. *Gastrointestinal Endoscopy Clinics of North America* 1995; **5**: 145–70.

Lemmel T, Hawes R, Sherman S *et al*. Endoscopic evaluation and therapy of recurrent pancreatitis and pancreato-biliary pain in the pediatric population. *Gastrointestinal Endoscopy* 1994; **40**: 54.

Linuma Y, Narisawa R, Iwafuchi M *et al*. The role of endoscopic retrograde cholangiopancreatography in infants with cholestasis. *Journal of Pediatric Surgery* 2000; **35**: 545–9.

McCune W, Shorb P, Moscovitz H. Endoscopic cannulation of the ampulla of Vater: a preliminary report. *Annals of Surgery* 1968; **167**: 752–6.

Mitchell SA, Wilkinson ML. The role of ERCP in the diagnosis of neonatal conjugated hyperbilirubinemia. *Gastrointestinal Endoscopy* 1994; **40**: A55.

Miyazaki T, Yamashita Y, Tang Y, Tsuchigame T, Takahashi M, Sera Y. Single-shot MR cholangiopancreatography of neonates, infants and young children. *American Journal of Roentgenology* 1998; **170**: 33–7.

Mori K, Nagakawa T, Ohta T *et al*. Pancreatitis and anomalous union of the pancreaticobiliary ductal system in childhood. *Journal of Pediatric Surgery* 1993; **28**: 67–71.

Neoptolemos JP, Carr-Locke DL, London NJ, Bailey IA, James D, Fossard DP. Controlled trial of urgent endoscopic retrograde cholangiopancreatography and endoscopic sphincterotomy versus conservative treatment for acute pancreatitis due to gallstones. *Lancet* 1988; **2**: 979–83.

Ohnuma N, Takahashi H, Tanabe M, Yoshida H, Iwai J. The role of ERCP in biliary atresia. *Gastrointestinal Endoscopy* 1997; **45**: 365–70.

Prasad H, Poddar U, Thapa B, Bhasin D, Rao KLN, Singh K. Endoscopic management of post-laparoscopic cholecystectomy bile leak in a child. *Gastrointestinal Endoscopy* 2000; **51**: 506–7.

Putnam PE, Kocoshis SA, Orenstein SR, Schade RR. Pediatric endoscopic retrograde cholangiopancreatography. *American Journal of Gastroenterology* 1991; **86**: 824–30.

Reiman JF, Koch H. Endoscopy of the biliary tract and the pancreas in children. *Endoscopy* 1978; **10**: 166.

Rescorla FJ, Plumley DA, Sherman S, Scherer LR III, West KW, Grosfeld JL. The efficacy of early ERCP in pediatric pancreatic trauma. *Journal of Pediatric Surgery* 1995; **30**: 336–40.

Sebesta C, Schmid A, Kier P *et al*. ERCP and balloon dilation is a valuable alternative to surgical biliodigestive anastomosis in the long common channel syndrome in childhood. *Endoscopy* 1995; **27**: 709–10.

Smits ME, Rauws EAJ, Tytgat GNJ, Huibregtse K. The efficacy of endoscopic treatment of pancreatic pseudocysts. *Gastrointestinal Endoscopy* 1995; **42**: 202–7.

Smits M, Rauws EAJ, Tytgat GHJ, Huibregtse K. Endoscopic treatment of pancreatic stones in patients with chronic pancreatitis. *Gastrointestinal Endoscopy* 1996; **43**: 556–60.

Tarnasky PR, Tagge EP, Hebra A *et al*. Minimally invasive therapy for choledocholithiasis in children. *Gastrointestinal Endoscopy* 1998; **47**: 189–92.

Teng R, Yokohata K, Utsunomiya N, Takahata S, Nabae T, Tanaka M. Endoscopic retrograde cholangio-pancreatography in infants and children. *Journal of Gastroenterology* 2000; **35**: 39–42.

Tulassay Z, Jakab Z, Vadász A *et al*. Secretin provocation ultrasonography in the diagnosis of papillary obstruction in pancreas divisum. *Gastroenterologisches Journal* 1991; **51**: 47–50.

Warshaw A, Simeone J, Schapiro R. Evaluation and treatment of the dominant dorsal duct syndrome (pancreas divisum redefined). *American Journal of Surgery* 1990; **159**: 59–66.

Waye JD. Endoscopic retrograde cholangiopancreatography in the infant. *American Journal of Gastroenterology* 1976; **65**: 461–3.

Werlin SL. Endoscopic retrograde cholangiopancreatography in children. *Gastrointestinal Endoscopy Clinics of North America* 1994; **4**: 161–78.

Wilkinson ML, Clayton PT. Sphincterotomy for jaundice in a neonate. *Journal of Pediatric Gastroenterology and Nutrition* 1996; **23**: 507–9.

Wilkinson ML, Mieli-Vergani G, Ball C, Portmann B, Mowat AP. Endoscopic retrograde cholangiopancreatography in infantile cholestasis. *Archives of Disease in Childhood* 1991; **66**: 121–3.

Yabut B, Werlin SL, Havens P, Bohorfoush S, Brown CW, Harb J. Endoscopic retrograde cholangiography in children with

HIV infection. *Journal of Pediatric Gastroenterology and Nutrition* 1996; **23**: 624–7.

Yamashiro Y, Sato M, Shimizu T, Oguchi S, Miyano T. How great is the incidence of truly congenital common bile duct dilatation? *Journal of Pediatric Surgery* 1993; **28**: 622–5.

Yamataka A, Kuwatsuru R, Shima H *et al*. Initial experience with non-breath-hold magnetic resonance cholangiopancreatography: a new non-invasive technique for the diagnosis of choledochal cyst in children. *Journal of Pediatric Surgery* 1997; **32**: 1560–2.

36

Acute and chronic pancreatitis and pancreatic trauma

WALTER PEGOLI Jr

Pancreatitis in childhood is an uncommon clinical entity. However, it must be considered in every child who manifests acute or chronic abdominal pain of uncertain etiology. The overall prognosis in children is good, but in cases complicated by multi-organ system failure there may be significant morbidity and mortality.

CLASSIFICATION

The term pancreatitis describes a wide variety of inflammatory conditions of the pancreas. The commonest system of classification distinguishes between acute and chronic forms of pancreatitis. In the acute form, the inflammatory process is for a defined duration and pancreatic function and morphology are restored after the attack. However, in chronic pancreatitis, the inflammatory process results in non-reversible changes in pancreatic morphology, and can lead to long-term dysfunction.

ACUTE PANCREATITIS

Acute pancreatitis is best described as an inflammatory condition of the pancreas caused by the activation, extracellular release and enzymatic digestion of the gland. The exact mechanism that triggers the acute inflammatory process is unclear. It has been proposed that initiating events activate pancreatic proteases, which in turn lead to a cascade effect. It is thought that activated zymogens, mainly trypsin, are able to activate other enzymes that result in autodigestion of the pancreas and surrounding soft tissues (Lampel and Kern, 1977). There is digestion of cell membranes, edema, coagulation, necrosis and injury to the peripancreatic vasculature. There may be interstitial glandular necrosis and saponification of the soft tissues surrounding the gland if the process continues unabated.

The primary event that leads to intrapancreatic proteolytic enzyme activation and release is unclear. An early popular hypothesis implicated pancreatic ductal hypertension as the initiating event. According to this hypothesis, continued secretion into an obstructed duct leads to rupture of small ducts, extravasation of pancreatic juices into the substance of the gland, and subsequent intraparenchymal activation of enzymes (Buntam et al., 1978). Recent studies have shown that oxygen free radicals may play an important role in the development of acute inflammation. Nonaka and colleagues have found increased amounts of lipid peroxidation products in the bile and pancreatic tissues of patients suffering from acute pancreatitis (Nonaka et al., 1990). In addition, treatment with acetylcysteine, a well-known radical scavenger, resulted in improvement when administered to patients with multisystem organ failure secondary to acute pancreatitis. Therefore it seems reasonable to assume that oxygen free radicals are generated in patients with acute pancreatitis, and that they may play a role in the inflammatory process.

Etiology

The known etiologies of acute pancreatitis in the pediatric age group are extensive. In adults, the commonest causes of acute pancreatitis are biliary tract disease and alcoholism. In contrast, the causes of acute pancreatitis in childhood are quite diverse. The commonest etiologies are trauma, multisystem organ failure, and drugs (Jordan and Ament, 1977; Weizman and Durie, 1988) (Box 36.1). Viral infections, congenital anomalies of the pancreas and biliary tract disease are also causes of acute pancreatitis in children. The commonest congenital anatomic pancreatic etiology is considered to be pancreas divisum (Eichelberger *et al.*, 1982). Pancreas divisum exists when the dorsal and ventral pancreatic ducts fail to fuse during embryogenesis, which results in aberrant pancreatic parenchymal drainage. Most of the pancreatic parenchyma is normally drained by the ventral duct. However, in pancreas divisum the dorsal duct drains most of the pancreatic mass, which is structurally unable to cope with the increased flow volume.

Cholelithiasis and choledocholithiasis in children are frequently associated with obesity or hemolytic disorders (e.g. hereditary spherocytosis, beta-thalassemia and sickle-cell disease) (Rescorla and Grosfeld, 1991) (see Chapter 13). The initiating event is thought to be transient obstruction of the pancreatic duct by a gallstone in the common bile duct at the ampulla of Vater. The attack is usually transient, and resolution commences at the time of stone dislodgement and passage into the gastrointestinal tract.

Drugs may be implicated in up to 25% of cases of acute pancreatitis. Drugs that cause pancreatitis in clinical practice include L-asparaginase, azathioprine, mercaptopurine and valproic acid (Mallory and Kern, 1980).

Among the metabolic disorders, hypertriglyceridemia and inborn errors of hepatic metabolism are the most frequently described causative factors in childhood pancreatitis (Steinberg and Tenner, 1994).

Clinical manifestations

The diagnosis of acute pancreatitis is based on the clinical history, physical examination, laboratory test results and diagnostic imaging. There is a spectrum of disease severity ranging from mild pancreatitis with almost no systemic upset through to fatal necrotizing pancreatitis. Severe acute pancreatitis is characterized by organ failure (pulmonary, renal or circulatory) and/or pancreatic collections (pancreatic necrosis, abscess or pseudocyst). Various clinical scoring systems have been used in adults to predict severe disease with a worse prognosis. These include the Glasgow criteria, APACHE II scores and

---

Box 36.1 *Causes of acute pancreatitis in childhood*

Trauma
  Blunt abdominal trauma (accidental/non-accidental)
  Iatrogenic (i.e. post splenectomy or ERCP)

Systemic disease
  Reye's syndrome
  Hemolytic–uremic syndrome
  Crohn's disease
  Kawasaki's disease

Drugs
  Azathioprine
  L-asparaginase
  Sulphonamides
  Sulfasalazine
  Thiazides
  Frusemide
  Estrogens
  Tetracycline
  Valproic acid
  Steroids
  Acetaminophen
  Alcohol

Infections
  Viral
    Measles
    Mumps
    Epstein–Barr virus
    Coxsackie B
    Influenza A

Metabolic disorders
  Hypercalcemia
  Hyperlipidemia
  Uremia
  Alpha-1-antitrypsin deficiency
  Organic acidemias

Vasculitis
  Systemic lupus erythematosus
  Henoch–Schönlein purpura

Pancreatic disorders
  Cystic fibrosis (and CFTR gene mutations)
  Pancreas divisum
  Duplication cyst

Biliary disorders
  Gallstones
  Choledochal cyst
  Pancreaticobiliary duct malunion

Duodenal disorders
  Duplication cyst
  Duodenal web

Shock states
  Severe hypotension
    Cardiopulmonary bypass
    Hypothermia

Miscellaneous
  Hereditary
  Idiopathic

C-reactive protein measurements (Mayer et al., 1984; Wilson et al., 1990; Bradley, 1993). These systems have not been evaluated on a similar scale in children because acute pancreatitis is much less frequent and the etiology is more variable. However, hypovolemic shock in children is a predictor of severe disease (Berney et al., 1996), and the Glasgow criteria may be of some relevance (Ziegler et al., 1988).

The cardinal symptom of pancreatitis is abdominal pain, which is often epigastric in location and radiates through to the back. The pain is usually of sudden onset, is aggravated by eating, and is often associated with nausea and vomiting, which may occasionally be bilious. Fever, when present, is low grade (less than 38.5°C). On physical examination, the child may manifest signs of hypovolemia secondary to third-space fluid losses. Tachycardia, tachypnea and hypotension may be present in more severe cases.

The abdomen is often distended and diffusely tender. Guarding and focal rebound tenderness may be present in the epigastrium. Bowel sounds are often absent. An epigastric mass may be palpable secondary to pancreatic phlegmon development or the presence of a pseudocyst. A bluish color is evident around the umbilicus (Cullen's sign) or in the flanks (Grey Turner's sign) in patients with severe pancreatitis. This represents a combination of ascites, and blood that has been diverted to those areas from the retroperitoneum in patients with necrotizing hemorrhagic pancreatitis. The pulmonary manifestations in some patients may include a left-sided pleural effusion, or in more severe cases a respiratory distress-like syndrome.

Diagnostic studies

An elevated white blood cell count is a frequent finding in patients with acute pancreatitis. However, in the absence of complications, white blood cell counts over 12 000/mm³ are unusual. The hematocrit may be elevated secondary to dehydration, or low as a result of pancreatic or retroperitoneal blood loss in necrotizing pancreatitis. Hypocalcemia occurs in approximately 15% of patients. Liver function tests are usually normal, but mild elevation of serum bilirubin levels (less than 2 mg/dL) may be seen. An elevated transaminase concentration is typically associated with gallstone pancreatitis.

Measurement of serum amylase is the commonest test for diagnosing acute pancreatitis, but hyperamylasemia is not specific (Gwozdz et al., 1990). Serum amylase activity may be elevated in other abdominal conditions, such as appendicitis, intestinal perforation, salpingitis and acute cholecystitis. The serum amylase concentration usually rises to more than three times normal values within 6 hours of the acute episode. It usually peaks within 48 hours, and may remain elevated for several days (Schmidt and Schmidt, 1990). The level of serum amylase does not correlate with the severity of the episode of pancreatitis. Determination of amylase iso-enzymes has also been used to increase diagnostic accuracy by identifying the tissue from which the amylase originates (Lorentz, 1987).

Other pancreatic enzymes have been measured in an attempt to improve the diagnostic accuracy of serum amylase determinations. Serum lipase may be more reliable than amylase for diagnosing acute pancreatitis. The pancreas is the main source of lipase in the blood, and therefore lipase determination offers higher sensitivity and specificity in the diagnosis of acute pancreatitis (Gumaste et al., 1992).

Radiological studies

Plain radiographs of the chest and abdomen may reveal dilatation of an isolated loop of intestine (duodenum, jejunum or transverse colon) adjacent to the pancreas (sentinel loop). A left-sided pleural effusion may be seen on chest X-ray (Ranson, 1985).

Ultrasonography may be used to identify hepatobiliary and pancreatic abnormalities (Cox et al., 1980). Gallstones are easily identified by ultrasound examination, as well as an edematous, swollen pancreas, peripancreatic fluid collections or pseudocysts. Serial ultrasound examinations may be useful when following the clinical course of patients with protracted or complicated pancreatitis or pseudocysts. However, in approximately 20% of patients ultrasound examination is precluded by the presence of overlying bowel gas. Computed tomography (CT) is considered to be the imaging procedure of choice in acute pancreatitis (Hill and Huntington, 1990). CT of the pancreas may identify edema, phlegmon, acute pseudocyst or abscess (Figure 36.1). The adequacy of pancreatic perfusion can be estimated if the CT scan is performed without and then with intravenous contrast material at least 2–3 days after the onset of disease. A viable pancreas 'enhances' as contrast material flows through it, whereas lack of enhancement suggests pancreatic necrosis (Figure 36.2). These findings represent a major advance in the diagnosis and management of patients with complicated acute pancreatitis. Patients with significant pancreatic necrosis are more likely to develop pancreatic infection and require surgical intervention. If bacterial infection is suspected, as evidenced by necrosis with peripancreatic air, a percutaneous needle may be introduced into the collection and material aspirated. Fungal or bacterial growth is proof of a surgical infection, and is an indication for laparotomy and drainage (Rattner et al., 1992).

Endoscopic retrograde cholangiopancreatography (ERCP) is rarely indicated in acute pancreatitis. However, it is recommended as an early diagnostic test in patients with blunt abdominal trauma associated with

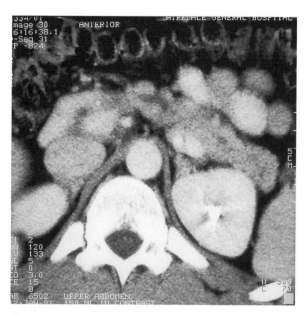

Figure 36.1 *CT scan with intravenous contrast demonstrating diffuse pancreatic swelling secondary to acute pancreatitis (associated with influenza A infection in this 16-year-old boy).*

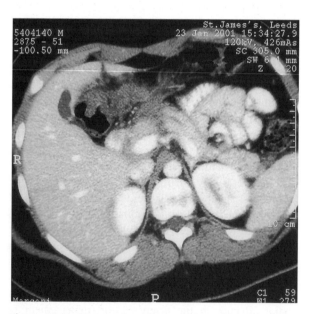

Figure 36.2 *CT scan of a 15-year-old boy with acute pancreatitis. After contrast enhancement, an area of pancreatic necrosis is clearly visible in the neck of the gland.*

progressive hyperamylasemia. Delineation of biliary and pancreatic ductal anatomy by ERCP is necessary during the planning of subsequent surgical intervention (Cotton, 1980). In particular, children with recurrent acute pancreatitis should be investigated by ERCP. If pancreas divisum is demonstrated, endoscopic sphincterotomy may be curative (Neblett and O'Neill, 2000).

Treatment

The treatment of acute, uncomplicated pancreatitis is medical and is directed towards alleviation of shock by restoration of fluid and electrolyte balance, the avoidance of secretory stimulation of the pancreas, and the treatment of pain. Intravenous crystalloids are administered in order to maintain normal intravascular volume. In addition, complete bowel rest is initiated, and nasogastric suction should be instituted to prevent emesis (Fuller *et al.*, 1981). Total parenteral nutrition is traditionally used to support patients with severe acute pancreatitis, but nasojejunal feeding may be advantageous in some cases (Wyncoll, 1999).

Although antibiotic therapy has been used in patients with acute pancreatitis, prophylactic antibiotics such as high-dose cefuroxime or imipenem are probably only beneficial in cases of acute necrotizing pancreatitis (Wyncoll, 1999). Anticholinergics, gastric acid secretory agents, glucagon, somatostatin and inhibitors of proteolytic enzymes have shown no beneficial effects in patients with acute pancreatitis (Steinberg and Schlesselman, 1987; Wyncoll, 1999). More recent studies in adults with Lexipafant, a platelet-activating-factor antagonist, have shown no effect on the incidence of organ failure in severe acute pancreatitis, but a reduction in local pancreatic complications (Johnson *et al.*, 2001).

Parenteral analgesia is an important part of the treatment of pain in acute pancreatitis – adequate pain relief is essential. Narcotics and non-steroidal anti-inflammatory drugs may alleviate the pain, but opiate analgesia may worsen the pain of acute pancreatitis by inciting spasm of the sphincter of Oddi. Traditionally, meperidine rather than morphine has been used because the latter is thought to induce ampullary spasm.

Peritoneal lavage has been used in adults with severe pancreatitis, and intraperitoneal fluid to remove toxins and various metabolites from the peritoneal cavity and minimize their systemic absorption. However, similar trials have not been conducted in children, and several centers have not found lavage to be helpful in the management of patients with acute pancreatitis (Synn *et al.*, 1987). The potential benefits of other specific therapeutic interventions, such as selective decontamination of the gut, are still being evaluated (Wyncoll, 1999).

Surgical treatment

Surgical treatment is contraindicated in cases of uncomplicated acute pancreatitis. However, patients with septic complications of the pancreas may require surgical intervention. Infected pancreatic necrosis is difficult to recognize clinically. Patients with sterile necrosis may manifest fever, leukocytosis, abdominal tenderness and pure sepsis. However, sterile necrosis may be managed expectantly. Infection is assumed to be present if gas bubbles are present on CT scan. CT-guided aspiration is then indicated. The commonest organisms include a mixed flora of *Escherichia coli*, *Bacteroides*, *Staphylococcus* and *Candida albicans*. Therefore broad-spectrum antibiotics should be used initially in these cases. Definitive management is surgical. Infected necrotic material should be widely debrided at operation, and the involved areas should be drained with a large sump drain. Reoperation is commonly required. In the most severe cases, an open abdominal technique may be necessary (Raffensperger, 1990).

CHRONIC PANCREATITIS

The principal symptom in patients with chronic pancreatitis is recurrent abdominal pain. The pain is located in the epigastric region, and radiates to the back. The pain is similar to that of acute pancreatitis in an acute exacerbation. The painful episodes may initially last from a few days to several weeks, with pain-free intervals lasting from weeks to months. Typically, the pain-free intervals become shorter. This chronic relapsing course is associated with varying degrees of exocrine and endocrine pancreatic dysfunction.

Weight loss is a factor in most of these patients, because food usually worsens the pain, and consequently intake is voluntarily restricted. Malabsorption secondary to pancreatic insufficiency may be present. Patients may also complain of bulky, malodorous stools (Reker, 1987). Pancreatic ductal rupture may rarely cause ascites and/or a pleural effusion.

Etiology

The causes and pathophysiology of chronic pancreatitis in children are not understood. The commonest causes are trauma, biliary tract disease and intrinsic anomalies of the pancreaticobiliary system. The commonest of these anomalies include pancreas divisum and pancreaticobiliary malunion (see Chapters 10 and 33). The rare variant of fibrosing pancreatitis is discussed in Chapter 37. Hereditary pancreatitis is also a cause of recurrent acute and chronic pancreatitis. Inherited as an autosomal-dominant condition, the underlying defect is now known to be related to mutations in the trypsinogen gene (located on chromosome 7) which render trypsinogen relatively resistant to autolysis (Whitcomb, 1999).

Diagnostic studies

In contrast to acute pancreatitis, laboratory studies in chronic pancreatitis are not particularly helpful. Pancreatic endocrine and exocrine function in chronic pancreatitis is impaired. However, the degree of impairment may be assessed by blood tests (amylase and lipase), stool tests (fecal fat and chymotrypsin/elastase) and pancreatic function tests (secretin stimulation) (Layer and Holtmann, 1994).

Diagnostic imaging

The classic finding on plain abdominal radiographs in patients with chronic pancreatitis is calcification. The diagnosis of chronic pancreatitis is made when calcifications are present.

In children, ultrasonography is valuable in the diagnosis of patients with chronic pancreatitis. Biliary and pancreatic ductal dilatation can be easily identified. Complications such as pseudocysts, calculi and ascites may be seen.

A CT scan may be helpful in the identification of pseudocysts and cystic communications within the pancreatic substance. It can provide precise information about the size and configuration of the pancreas (Figure 36.3), which may be useful as a guide during surgical intervention (Balthazar and Chako, 1990).

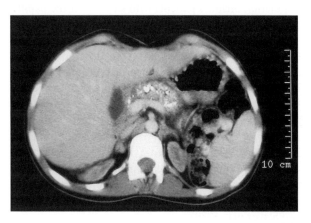

Figure 36.3 *CT scan demonstrating extensive calcification of the pancreas in a 12-year-old girl with chronic pancreatitis.*

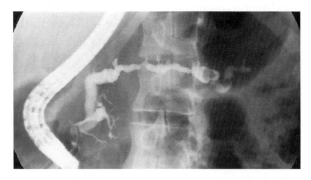

Figure 36.4 *An ERCP demonstrating severe pancreatic duct irregularities, dilatation and luminal filling defects in a 14-year-old girl with chronic pancreatitis.*

ERCP has become an important tool in the diagnosis and management of patients with chronic pancreatitis (see Chapter 34). Information about abnormalities in ampullary and ductal anatomy can be obtained. The ampulla may be stenotic, while the main pancreatic duct may be dilated, stenosed or obstructed (Kozarek and Traverso, 1996) (Figure 36.4). Variations in ductal anatomy diagnosed by ERCP are important when planning subsequent surgical drainage procedures.

Surgical treatment

The commonest indication for surgery in patients with chronic pancreatitis is to alleviate pain, although other complications may require operative intervention (Box 36.2). The operations for patients with chronic pancreatitis fall into two categories. The first of these consists of drainage procedures that attempt to bypass segments of ductal obstruction. The second category is that of pancreatic resections to remove diseased pancreatic tissue.

The general indication for the use of pancreatic drainage procedures is pancreatic ductal strictures, which are either isolated or multiple. A subset of this population includes patients with stenoses of the papilla of Vater. Sphincteroplasty can be useful in a carefully selected subgroup of the population where there is no evidence of intrapancreatic ductal obstruction (Jones et al., 1969). In those instances where multiple intrapancreatic strictures exist, the longitudinal pancreaticojejunostomy (Puestow procedure) may be used to decompress the pancreatic duct. The duct is opened throughout the length of the pancreas and anastomosed side to side with a Roux-en-Y limb of jejunum. This technique results in the relief of pain in 80–97% of children in the short term. However, pain returns unpredictably in 25–50% of patients after 3–5 years (White and Slavotinek, 1979).

Pancreatic resection should be considered for pain relief if the pancreatic duct is unsuitable for drainage procedures, or if previous drainage procedures have failed. Pancreatic resection (subtotal or total) or the Whipple pancreaticoduodenectomy are rarely indicated in children (Guillemin et al., 1971). The Whipple operation may be performed if the disease is isolated in the head of the pancreas. Subtotal and total pancreatectomy

can result in significant alterations in digestive and absorptive functions. These operations are associated with significant morbidity and mortality, and should be reserved for cases of intractable pain when there is diffuse parenchymal damage.

PSEUDOCYSTS

Pancreatic pseudocysts are localized collections of fluid that do not have an endothelial lining but contain high concentrations of pancreatic enzymes. Pseudocysts commonly occur as a complication of pancreatitis after pancreatic injury or duct obstruction (Hough et al., 1994). The cysts may be located within the pancreatic substance or in the juxtapancreatic regions surrounding the gland. Most of the time they are located in the lesser sac, anterior to the gland and posterior to the stomach (Brooks, 1983) (Figure 36.5). Rarely, pancreatic pseudocysts are found in the mediastinum (Crombleholme et al., 1990). Pseudocysts lack a true epithelial lining, in contrast to true pancreatic cysts, which are lined by epithelium. In patients with acute pancreatitis, pseudocysts should be suspected if the patient fails to improve after 5–7 days of conservative management. Chronic pseudocyst formation may be associated with vomiting (non-bilious or bilious) secondary to obstruction of the stomach or duodenum.

Classic conservative management involves supportive therapy for a 6-week period (Sanfey et al., 1994). Most pseudocysts resolve spontaneously. However, a small proportion of them require drainage. They may be drained internally or externally by a minimally invasive method that uses radiographic guidance. Internal surgical drainage is based on the location of the pseudocyst relative to the intestinal tract. Those cysts that are located in the lesser sac behind the stomach may be drained via cyst gastrostomy. Other pseudocysts, most commonly located in the distal two-thirds of the pancreas, may require Roux-en-Y decompression (Wade, 1985). There is rarely an indication for resection in the pediatric age group, but distal

---

Box 36.2 *Indications for surgery in chronic pancreatitis*

Pain
Obstruction of common bile duct
Intestinal obstruction
Pseudocyst
Splenic or portal vein obstruction with portal
  hypertension

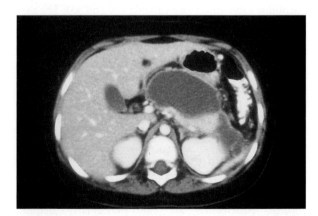

Figure 36.5 *A CT scan showing a pancreatic pseudocyst complicating acute pancreatitis in a 10-year-old girl.*

pancreatic resection may be indicated if the body or tail contains multiple small cysts (Yellin *et al.*, 1972).

Complications such as infection or bleeding in untreated pseudocysts may be indications for early intervention. The preferred method of decompression is internal drainage in the stable patient. In unstable patients, external percutaneous drainage may be undertaken. However, external drainage is associated with a higher rate of recurrence and fistula formation than is internal drainage (Cooney and Grosfeld, 1976).

PANCREATIC TRAUMA

Pancreatic injury is a relatively uncommon result of trauma, but may be the source of major morbidity. Recognition of injury is often delayed because of the retroperitoneal location of the gland. Once the possibility of injury has been considered, diagnosis is often difficult and the spectrum of pathology is diverse.

Etiology

The commonest mechanism of injury to the pancreas is blunt abdominal trauma (Raminofsky, 1987). The gland is injured by direct-force compression of the gland against the vertebral body. Bicycle-handlebar injury, pedestrian injury, motor-vehicle accidents and child abuse are the commonest causes of pancreatic injury (Smith *et al.*, 1988).

Diagnosis

Most often the diagnosis of pancreatic injury is made during the evaluation of a child who has sustained blunt abdominal trauma. In patients with isolated pancreatic injury, because of the retroperitoneal location of the organ, the physical finding of abdominal tenderness may be absent. However, over time, pain becomes manifest in the epigastrium. Enzymes are released from the retroperitoneum into the peritoneal cavity if there is significant glandular injury. The abdominal pain becomes diffuse under these circumstances, and is often accompanied by nausea and vomiting.

Serum amylase is the most useful biochemical marker of pancreatic injury. However, amylase is also produced by other organs and may be elevated in cases of internal injury or salivary gland injury as a result of facial trauma. Analysis of amylase isoenzymes by electrophoresis or chromatography may increase the specificity of any case determination in the multiply injured child (Bouwman *et al.*, 1984). Perhaps more important than an isolated elevation of serum amylase activity is the trend of serial determinations. A trend towards progressive elevation is suggestive of significant injury, while elevation followed by declining levels is suggestive of contusion (Greenlee *et al.*, 1984). Lipase originates primarily in the pancreas, and its levels can be elevated in glandular injury. However, Lifton *et al.* (1974) reported that elevated levels of serum lipase are not better indicators of pancreatic trauma than elevated levels of serum amylase.

The initial evaluation of the injured child begins with a primary survey. A CT scan is the diagnostic modality of choice in the hemodynamically stable child with suspected abdominal injury. The abdominal CT scan, with oral and intravenous contrast, can detect intestinal and solid-organ injuries with an acceptable specificity and sensitivity (Karp *et al.*, 1981). However, the sensitivity of CT examinations in cases of pancreatic injury is not as high.

ERCP can serve as a useful adjunct to CT examination in cases of suspected pancreatic injury (Rescorla *et al.*, 1995) (see Chapter 34). In selected cases, ERCP may be used to evaluate and identify ductal injury (Barkin *et al.*, 1988) (Figure 36.6). ERCP may provide useful

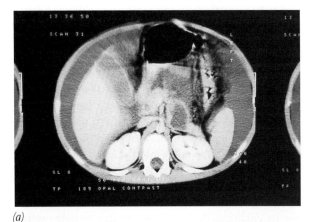

(a)

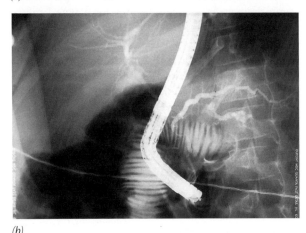

(b)

Figure 36.6 *(a) A CT scan demonstrating pancreatic ascites and an intrapancreatic cyst in a 9-year-old boy following blunt abdominal trauma. (b) A subsequent ERCP on the same patient demonstrating a pancreatic duct injury in the region of the pancreatic neck. Note the extravasation of contrast material from the ruptured duct.*

information to guide the surgeon if ductal disruption is identified, and it may allow continued non-operative management if none is detected. Due to the retroperitoneal position of the gland, ultrasound examination and diagnostic peritoneal lavage have a limited role in the determination of injury to the pancreas.

Management

Initial management of the injured child requires evaluation of airway, breathing and circulation. After resuscitation, resuscitated stabilized patients with a suspected abdominal injury should be evaluated with an abdominal and pelvic CT scan. Patients who are found to have pancreatic injury may be classified into subtypes dependent on the presence of injury to the parenchyma, major ducts or duodenum (Feliciano and Lowe, 1990) (Table 36.1).

In children with abdominal pain, an elevated serum amylase level and a normal abdominal/pelvic CT scan, non-operative management is recommended. Treatment consists of bed rest, nothing by mouth and intravenous fluids. Nasogastric-tube decompression to prevent gastric distension and H_2-blockers to inhibit pancreatic secretion have not shown any clinical benefit (Fuller *et al.*, 1981).

In patients with abdominal trauma who require laparotomy, the pancreas should be evaluated after life-threatening injury has been controlled. The commonest conditions that necessitate emergency laparotomy are hemodynamically significant injuries to the spleen and liver and bowel perforation. Adequate exploration of the entire gland requires entry into the lesser sac to evaluate the body and tail, and a Kocher maneuver to expose the head of the pancreas.

The operative strategy is based on the extent of injury to the parenchyma, ducts and duodenum. Simple external sump drainage is adequate therapy for a type I injury. Distal pancreatectomy is the procedure of choice for cases of distal transection of the gland, or parenchymal injury with ductal injury type II (Figure 36.7). In patients with type III injuries with major ductal disruption, a distal pancreatectomy may be performed if 20–40% of the pancreatic tissue remains *in situ*. However, if the injury requires extensive parenchymal resection, the proximal pancreas can be closed and the distal gland drained with a Roux-en-Y pancreaticojejunostomy. Pancreaticoduodenal type IV

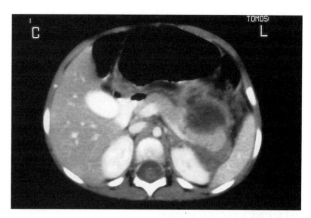

Figure 36.7 *A CT scan showing a pancreatic pseudocyst overlying the tail of the pancreas where a traumatic fracture of the gland is clearly visible (type II pancreatic ductal injury).*

injuries may require pancreaticoduodenectomy. Several authors have described procedures that divert enteric and biliary content away from the area of injury, and externally drain pancreatic secretions as a temporizing measure, only to return at a later date when formal reconstruction may be performed safely (Berne *et al.*, 1974; Flynn *et al.*, 1990).

Complications associated with pancreatic injury in children are rare. Pseudocysts that are noted after non-operative management generally resolve spontaneously. Some pseudocysts may require drainage (see the above section on chronic pancreatitis). Pancreatic fistulas can complicate an operative procedure, but most fistulas will close with time if the pancreatic ductal anatomy is normal. Bowel rest, total parenteral nutrition and octreotide may help to encourage resolution. Persistent high-output fistulas are associated with ductal obstruction/injury and warrant further investigation via pancreatography. Persistent debilitating fistulas will require internal drainage.

Key references

Raminofsky ML. Pancreatic abdominal trauma. *Pediatric Annals* 1987; **16**: 318–26.

A seminal article on pancreatic trauma in children, written by a renowned pediatric trauma surgeon.

Rescorla F, Grosfeld JL. Pancreatitis. In: Schiller M (ed.) *Pediatric surgery of the liver, pancreas and spleen*. Philadelphia, PA: WB Saunders, 1991.

An excellent review of surgical pathology that may accompany or result from pancreatic inflammation.

Wyncoll DL. The management of severe acute necrotising pancreatitis: an evidence-based review of the literature. *Intensive Care Medicine* 1999; **25**: 146–56.

An evidence-based review of severity scoring systems and the management of acute severe pancreatitis in adults.

Table 36.1 *Classification of pancreatic injury*

Type	Pancreatic injury
I	Contusion/laceration without ductal injury
II	Distal transection or parenchymal injury with ductal injury
III	Proximal transection or parenchymal injury with probable ductal injury
IV	Combined pancreatic and duodenal injury

REFERENCES

Balthazar EJ, Chako AC. Computed tomography of pancreatic masses. *American Journal of Gastroenterology* 1990; **85**: 343–9.

Barkin JS, Ferstenberg RM, Panullo W *et al*. Endoscopic retrograde cholangiopancreatography in pancreatic trauma. *Gastrointestinal Endoscopy* 1988; **34**: 102–5.

Berne CJ, Donovan AJ, White GJ. Duodenal 'diverticularization' for duodenal and pancreatic injury. *American Journal of Surgery* 1974; **127**: 503–7.

Berney T, Belli D, Bugmann P *et al*. Influence of severe underlying pathology and hypovolemic shock on the development of acute pancreatitis in children. *Journal of Pediatric Surgery* 1996; **31**: 1256–61.

Bouwman DL, Weaver DL, Walt AJ. Serum amylase and its isoenzymes: clarifications of their implications in trauma. *Journal of Trauma* 1984; **24**: 573–8.

Bradley EL. A clinically based classification of acute pancreatitis. *Archives of Surgery* 1993; **128**: 586–90.

Brooks JR. Pseudocysts of the pancreas. In: Brooks JR (ed.) *Surgery of the pancreas*. Philadelphia, PA: WB Saunders, 1983.

Buntam WL, Wood JB, Woolley MM. Pancreatitis in childhood. *Journal of Pediatric Surgery* 1978; **13**: 143–7.

Cooney DR, Grosfeld JL. Operative management of pancreatic pseudocysts in infants and children: a review of 75 cases. *Annals of Surgery* 1976; **182**: 590–6.

Cotton PB. Congenital anomaly of pancreas division as cause of obstructive pain and pancreatitis. *Gut* 1980; **21**: 105–14.

Cox KL, Ament ME, Sample WF *et al*. The ultrasonic and biochemical diagnosis of pancreatitis in children. *Journal of Pediatrics* 1980; **96**: 407–11.

Crombleholme TM, deLorimier AA, Adzick NS *et al*. Mediastinal pancreatic pseudocysts in children. *Journal of Pediatric Surgery* 1990; **25**: 843–8.

Eichelberger MR, Hoelzer DJ, Koop CE. Acute pancreatitis: the difficulties of diagnosis and therapy. *Journal of Pediatric Surgery* 1982; **17**: 244–54.

Feliciano P, Lowe DK. Pancreatic trauma. In: Maull KI (ed.) *Advances in trauma*. Chicago, IL: Mosby Year Book, 1990: 101–2.

Flynn WJ Jr, Cryer HG, Richardson JD. Reappraisal of pancreatic and duodenal injury management based on injury severity, *Archives of Surgery* 1990; **125**: 1539–41.

Fuller RK, Loveland JP, Frankel MH. An evaluation of the efficacy of nasogastric suction treatment in alcoholic pancreatitis. *American Journal of Gastroenterology* 1981; **75**: 349–53.

Greenlee T, Murphy K, Ram MD. Amylase isoenzymes in the evaluation of trauma patients, *Annals of Surgery* 1984; **50**: 637–40.

Guillemin G, Cuilleret J, Michel A *et al*. Chronic relapsing pancreatitis. Surgical management including 63 cases of pancreaticoduodenectomy. *American Journal of Surgery* 1971; **122**: 802–7.

Gumaste V, Dave P, Sereny G. Serum lipase: a better test to diagnose acute alcoholic pancreatitis. *American Journal of Medicine* 1992; **92**: 239–42.

Gwozdz GP, Steinberg WM, Werner M *et al*. Comparative evaluation of the diagnosis of acute pancreatitis based on serum and urine enzyme assays. *Clinica Chimica Acta* 1990; **197**: 243–54.

Hill MC, Huntington DK. Computed tomography and acute pancreatitis. *Gastroenterology Clinics of North America* 1990; **19**: 811–42.

Hough DM, Stephens DH, Johnson CD, Binkovitz LA. Pancreatic lesions in von Hippel–Lindow disease: prevalence, clinical significance and CT findings. *American Journal of Roentgenology* 1994; **162**: 1091–4.

Johnson CD, Kingsnorth AN, Imrie CW *et al*. Double-blind, randomised, placebo-controlled study of a platelet-activating-factor antagonist, lexipafant, in the treatment and prevention of organ failure in predicted severe acute pancreatitis. *Gut* 2001; **48**: 62–9.

Jones SA, Steedman RA, Keller TB, Smith LL. Transduodenal sphincteroplasty (not sphincterotomy) for biliary and pancreatic disease. *American Journal of Surgery* 1969; **118**: 292–306.

Jordan SC, Ament ME. Pancreatitis in children and adolescents. *Journal of Pediatrics* 1977; **91**: 211–16.

Karp MP, Cooney DR, Berger PE *et al*. The role of computed tomography in the evaluation of blunt abdominal trauma in children. *Journal of Pediatric Surgery* 1981; **16**: 316–23.

Kozarek RA, Traverso LW. Endotherapy for chronic pancreatitis. *International Journal of Pancreatology* 1996; **19**: 93–102.

Lampel M, Kern LT. Acute interstitial pancreatitis in the rat induced by excessive doses of a pancreatic secretogogue. *Virchows Archiv Pathological Anatomy and Histopathology* 1977; **373**: 97–117.

Layer P, Holtmann G. Pancreatic enzymes in chronic pancreatitis. *International Journal of Pancreatology* 1994; **15**: 1–11.

Lifton LJ, Slickers KA, Pragay DA *et al*. Pancreatitis and lipase: a re-evaluation with five-minute turbidimetric lipase determination. *Journal of the American Medical Association* 1974; **229**: 47–50.

Lorentz K. Iso-amylase measurement with monoclonal antibody test strips. *Journal of Clinical Chemistry and Clinical Biochemistry* 1987; **25**: 309–11.

Mallory A, Kern F Jr. Drug-induced pancreatitis: a critical review. *Gastroenterology* 1980; **78**: 813–20.

Mayer AD, McMahon MJ, Bowen M, Cooper EH. CRP: an aid to assessment and monitoring in acute pancreatitis. *Journal of Clinical Pathology* 1984; **37**: 207–11.

Neblett WW, O'Neill JA. Surgical management of recurrent pancreatitis in children with pancreas divisum. *Annals of Surgery* 2000; **231**: 899–908.

Nonaka A, Manabe T, Kyogku T *et al*. Changes in lipid peroxide and oxygen radical scavengers in caerulein-induced acute pancreatitis: imbalance between the offense and defense systems. *Digestion* 1990; **47**: 130–37.

Raffensperger JG. Pancreatitis. In: *Swenson's pediatric surgery*, 5th edn. Norwalk, CT: Appleton and Lange, 1990.

Raminofsky ML. Pancreatic abdominal trauma. *Pediatric Annals* 1987; **16**: 318–26.

Ranson JHC. Acute pancreatitis. In: Schwartz SI, Ellis H (eds) *Maingot's abdominal operations*, 8th edn. Norwalk, CT: Appleton-Century-Crofts, 1985.

Rattner DW, Legermate DA, Lee MJ *et al*. Early surgical debridement of symptomatic pancreatic necrosis is beneficial irrespective of infection. *American Journal of Surgery* 1992; **163**: 105–9.

Reker H. Chronic pancreatitis: etiology, diagnosis and pathology. In: Howard JM, Jordan GL, Pelser HA (eds) *Surgical diseases of the pancreas*. Philadelphia, PA: Lea and Febiger, 1987: 496–521.

Rescorla F, Grosfeld JL. Pancreatitis. In: Schiller M (ed.) *Pediatric surgery of the liver, pancreas and spleen*. Philadelphia, PA: WB Saunders, 1991.

Rescorla F, Plumley DA, Sherman S *et al*. The efficacy of early ERCP in pediatric pancreatic trauma. *Journal of Pediatric Surgery* 1995; **30**: 336–40.

Sanfey H, Aguilar M, Jones RS. Pseudocysts of the pancreas: a review of 97 cases. *American Surgeon* 1994; **60**: 661–8.

Schmidt E, Schmidt FW. Advances in the enzyme diagnosis of pancreatic diseases. *Clinical Biochemistry* 1990; **23**: 383–94.

Smith SD, Nakayama DK, Ganitt N *et al*. Pancreatic injury in childhood due to blunt trauma. *Journal of Pediatric Surgery* 1988; **23**: 610–14.

Steinberg WM, Schlesselman SE. Treatment of acute pancreatitis: comparison of animal and human studies. *Gastroenterology* 1987; **93**: 1420–27.

Steinberg W, Tenner S. Acute pancreatitis. *New England Journal of Medicine* 1994; **330**: 1198–210.

Synn AY, Mulvihill SJ, Fonkalsrud EW. Surgical management of pancreatitis in childhood. *Journal of Pediatrics* 1987; **22**: 628–32.

Wade JW. Twenty-five-year experience with pancreatic pseudocysts. Are we making progress? *American Journal of Surgery* 1985; **149**: 705–8.

Weizman Z, Durie PR. Acute pancreatitis in childhood. *Journal of Pediatrics* 1988; **113**: 24–9.

Whitcomb DC. Hereditary pancreatitis: new insights into acute and chronic pancreatitis. *Gut* 1999; **45**: 317–22.

White TT, Slavotinek AH. Results of surgical treatment of chronic pancreatitis. Report of 142 cases. *Annals of Surgery* 1979; **189**: 217–24.

Wilson C, Heath DI, Imrie CW. Prediction of outcome in acute pancreatitis: a comparative study of APACHE II. Clinical assessment and multiple factor scoring systems. *British Journal of Surgery* 1990; **77**: 1260–4.

Wyncoll DL. The management of severe acute necrotising pancreatitis: an evidence-based review of the literature. *Intensive Care Medicine* 1999; **25**: 146–56.

Yellin AE, Vecchione TR, Donovan AJ. Distal pancreatectomy for pancreatic trauma. *American Journal of Surgery* 1972; **124**: 135–42.

Ziegler DW, Long JA, Philippart AI, Klein MD. Pancreatitis in childhood. *Annals of Surgery* 1988; **207**: 257–61.

37

Pancreatic tumors and related disorders

MARK D STRINGER

INTRODUCTION

Pancreatic tumors in children are both rare and diverse. They may be broadly classified into neoplasms of epithelial (exocrine or endocrine) or non-epithelial origin and non-neoplastic tumors (Table 37.1). The rarity of these lesions is highlighted by reports of larger series from around the world (Table 37.2). Grosfeld et al. (1990) and Jaksic et al. (1992) were able to identify a total of only 19 pediatric pancreatic neoplasms over a 20-year period in two major centers in North America. These tumors are similarly infrequent in Europe and Asia (Jung et al., 1999; van Dooren et al., 2000). Japanese autopsy data indicate that pancreatic malignancy accounts for less than 0.2% of deaths from malignant disease in children (Tsukimoto et al., 1973).

Pancreatic neoplasms may be benign or malignant, and solid or cystic, with exocrine or endocrine components. Tumor imaging is best achieved with a combination of ultrasound (US), computed tomography (CT) and magnetic resonance imaging (MRI). Endoscopic ultrasound scanning, endoscopic retrograde cholangiopancreatography (ERCP), angiography and sophisticated endocrine investigations are occasionally needed.

Complete tumor excision is the goal of surgery and, depending on the type of tumor and its location, this is usually achieved by local excision, distal pancreatectomy or pancreaticoduodenectomy. Postoperative drainage of the pancreatic bed is advisable. In all cases, the pancreas can be fully exposed via a transverse upper abdominal incision, and full evaluation of the gland itself, the duodenal wall and surrounding structures, regional lymph nodes and the liver must be undertaken prior to tumor resection. Intraoperative ultrasonography, cholangiography and/or frozen-section histology may be helpful. Linear stapling devices are useful for transection of the bowel (and the pancreas in distal pancreatectomy).

Pancreaticoduodenectomy is necessary for complete excision of most malignant lesions in the head of the pancreas, and this may be undertaken as a conventional Whipple procedure or as a pylorus-preserving pancreaticoduodenectomy (Figure 37.1). Both operations are associated with a low mortality but a significant morbidity. Early complications such as anastomotic leakage (especially pancreatic) may be fatal, and delayed gastric emptying commonly prolongs recovery. Late complications include stomal ulceration, cholangitis and diabetes mellitus (Yamaguchi et al., 1999).

Despite the tendency of malignant exocrine pancreatic tumors to present late because of their anatomical location, they generally have a more favorable outcome than their adult counterpart. Papillary solid and cystic tumors in particular are associated with a good overall prognosis.

PANCREATIC EXOCRINE NEOPLASMS

Cystadenomas

Only a few examples of this pancreatic tumor have been recorded in children (Gundersen and Janis, 1969;

Table 37.1 *Classification of pancreatic tumors in children*

	Benign	Malignant
Exocrine	Adenoma Cystadenoma (serous/mucinous)	Adenocarcinoma Pancreatoblastoma Acinar-cell carcinoma
	Papillary solid and cystic tumor	
Endocrine	Insulinoma (β-cell) Gastrinoma (G-cell) Vipoma Glucagonoma (α-cell) Somatostatinoma (δ-cell) Non-functioning islet-cell tumors Carcinoid	
Non-epithelial	Lymphangioma Teratoma (dermoid) Fibrous histiocytoma	Rhabdomyosarcoma Lymphoma
	Hemangioendothelioma	
Metastases		
Non-neoplastic	Cysts • congenital (single or multiple), alimentary duplication cyst • acquired (cystic fibrosis, hydatid, hamartoma, tropical fibrocalcareous disease) Pseudocysts Inflammatory pseudotumor Pancreatic abscess	

Table 37.2 *Larger published series of pancreatic neoplasms in children*

Author	Geographical origin	Study period	*n*	Tumor types
Grosfeld *et al.* (1990)	Ohio and Indianapolis	1969–89	13	Benign: insulinoma (*n* = 5), cystadenoma (*n* = 2) Malignant: ductal adenocarcinoma, acinar-cell carcinoma, pancreatoblastoma, papillary solid and cystic tumor, rhabdomyosarcoma (*n* = 2)
Jaksic *et al.* (1992)	Toronto	1971–91	6	Benign: insulinoma Malignant: papillary solid and cystic tumor (*n* = 3), pancreatoblastoma, insulinoma
Jung *et al.* (1999)	Seoul	1984–97	11	Malignant: papillary solid and cystic tumor (*n* = 6) pancreatoblastoma (*n* = 5)

Grosfeld *et al.*, 1970; Jenkins and Othersen, 1992). There were no pediatric cases in a French multicenter series of 398 cystadenomas/cystadenocarcinomas collected during a 13-year period (Le Borgne *et al.*, 1999). Serous cystadenomas have no malignant potential in children, but present a diagnostic challenge; some of them are composed of a few large cysts, whilst most consist of microcysts. An association with cytomegalovirus infection has been reported (Chang *et al.*, 1980). Mucinous cystadenomas are often large and multilocular, contain gelatinous, mucinous fluid, and have the potential to progress to mucinous cystadenocarcinomas. In contrast to intraductal papillary-mucinous tumors (which have not been reported in children), they do not communicate with the pancreatic duct. Biopsy is necessary to confirm the nature of the cyst, and mucinous lesions must be completely excised. Both symptomatic recurrence and sarcomatous degeneration in the wall of a mucinous cystadenoma have been described after incomplete excision (Gundersen and Janis, 1969; Grosfeld *et al.*, 1990).

(a)   (b)

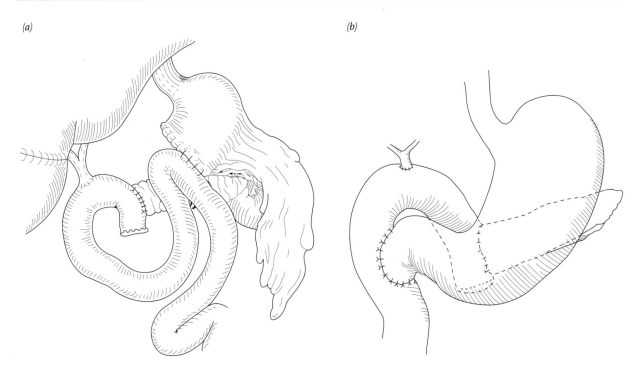

Figure 37.1 *(a) Conventional surgical reconstruction after Whipple pancreaticoduodenectomy. (b) Surgical reconstruction after pylorus-preserving pancreaticoduodenectomy. The pancreatic remnant may be implanted into the end of the jejunal loop or directly into the stomach as an alternative to the end-to-side anastomosis shown.*

Pancreatoblastoma

Until Horie *et al.* (1977) suggested the term 'pancreato-blastoma', this malignant embryonal pancreatic tumor was known as 'infantile carcinoma of the pancreas'. The tumor has subsequently been found to possess both pancreatic exocrine and endocrine differentiation. Lesions are large (up to 20 cm in diameter), solid and encapsulated, with a lobulated appearance due to the presence of fibrous septa. Central areas of hemorrhage and necrosis may be present. They are more often located in the head of the pancreas (embryologically derived from ventral pancreatic anlage).

Histologically, there is acinar differentiation and characteristic foci of squamous epithelium. Immuno-histochemical staining may be positive for alpha-1-antitrypsin, alpha-fetoprotein (AFP) and carcino-embryonic antigen. The tumor is well encapsulated early on, but subsequently metastasizes to lymph nodes, liver and lung. In advanced cases, the tumor invades the surrounding viscera and the portal vein and encases the celiac or superior mesenteric vessels (Vossen *et al.*, 1998; Gupta *et al.*, 2000). Horie *et al.* (1977) suggested that pancreatoblastomas arising from the embryonic dorsal anlage of the pancreas were less likely to be encapsulated and were more prone to behave aggressively and have a worse prognosis.

Pancreatoblastoma most often occurs in young children (typically under 10 years of age). Presentation is with an abdominal mass, epigastric pain and occasionally vomiting or jaundice. This tumor is occasionally found in association with Beckwith–Wiedemann syndrome, when it tends to be cystic (Drut and Jones, 1988). There is one report of inappropriate ACTH secretion resulting in Cushing syndrome (Passmore *et al.*, 1988). The serum concentration of AFP (and to a lesser extent lactate dehydrogenase) is raised in some patients, and can be useful in diagnosis and monitoring (Iseki *et al.*, 1986). However, serum AFP levels may also be elevated in association with pancreatic acinar cell carcinoma and ductal adenocarcinoma.

Imaging studies (ultrasound, CT and MRI) show a heterogenous, lobulated tumor with well-defined margins, but its precise anatomical origin can be difficult to determine (Montemarano *et al.*, 2000). The tumor often shows enhancement on CT images, and there may be evidence of tumor hemorrhage, necrosis, calcification and/or cystic change (Chun *et al.*, 1997; Gupta *et al.*, 2000; Kohda *et al.*, 2000). Fine-needle aspiration cytology has been used in diagnosis (Silverman *et al.*, 1990).

Complete surgical excision usually requires partial pancreatectomy or pancreaticoduodenectomy depending on the tumor location (Rich *et al.*, 1986). Complete excision of tumors affecting the head of the pancreas may occasionally be possible without formal pancreaticoduodenectomy, but less radical resections should not be undertaken at the expense of local recurrence (Vossen *et al.*, 1998).

The prognosis for patients with completely resected tumors is good (Willnow *et al.*, 1996). For non-resectable or metastatic tumors, preliminary biopsy and combination chemotherapy should precede any attempt at excisional surgery (Inomata *et al.*, 1992). A wide variety of chemotherapeutic agents has been used (Vossen *et al.*, 1998; Defachelles *et al.*, 2001), and cis-platin and doxorubicin may be superior (Defachelles *et al.*, 2001), but the prognosis in such cases is generally very poor (Chun *et al.*, 1997). Radiotherapy may be use-ful for locally recurrent or incompletely resected tumors (Griffin *et al.*, 1987), and resection of a solitary hepatic metastasis can be worthwhile (Grosfeld *et al.*, 1990).

Pancreatic carcinoma

In children, the term pancreatic carcinoma has often been used to describe a variety of malignant pancreatic tumors, including pancreatoblastoma, ductal adenocar-cinoma, acinar-cell carcinoma, and papillary solid and cystic tumors (Kissane, 1982). Although these are all malignant pancreatic neoplasms, pancreatoblastoma and papillary tumors have distinct clinical and histolog-ical features and will therefore be considered separately. This section deals with pancreatic ductal adenocarci-noma (the tumor type observed in most adults with pan-creatic cancer) and pancreatic acinar-cell carcinoma, which is proportionally more common in children than in adults (Lack *et al.*, 1983).

Both of these tumors tend to present late with abdom-inal pain and/or a mass, vomiting, anorexia and weight loss. Obstructive jaundice is occasionally seen (more often with ductal adenocarcinoma). Both tumors are rare in childhood, but acinar-cell cancers have been described in small children and ductal adenocarcinoma has been reported in adolescents. Tumor spread is to lymph nodes and the liver. Serum AFP, carcino-embry-onic antigen or human chorionic gonadotrophin may be elevated in some patients, and there may be evidence of anemia and mildly elevated plasma amylase levels.

On cross-sectional imaging, acinar-cell tumors are often encapsulated, whilst ductal cancers are poorly demarcated. Histology varies from poorly differentiated to well-differentiated tumors with ducts and acini. Ductal adenocarcinomas are usually positive for carcino-embryonic antigen on immunohistochemistry. Acinar-cell carcinomas typically have periodic acid–Schiff positive cytoplasmic granules on light microscopy and evidence of zymogen granules on ultrastructural studies.

Treatment is by radical surgical excision, which usu-ally involves distal pancreatectomy or pancreaticoduo-denectomy, depending on tumor location. Although there are occasional reports of long-term survivors after radical surgery (Vane *et al.*, 1989), the overall prognosis of ductal adenocarcinoma in children, as in adults, is poor (Lack *et al.*, 1983). Some reports of pancreatic can-cers in children have suggested a reasonably good prog-nosis (Camprodon and Quintanilla, 1984), but closer scrutiny suggests that these cases were actually more favorable tumors, such as papillary solid and cystic tumor of the pancreas (Wetzel, 1984). Nevertheless, aci-nar-cell cancers in children do appear to have a better prognosis than ductal adenocarcinomas (Kissane, 1982; Lack *et al.*, 1983; Klimstra *et al.*, 1992).

Papillary solid and cystic tumor

Numerous terms have been used to describe this low-grade malignant pancreatic neoplasm, including papil-lary cystic tumor, pseudopapillary and solid tumor, papillary and solid tumor, and Frantz's tumor. Histochemical and morphological studies indicate that the tumor has acinar, ductal and endocrine components, suggesting that it may originate from a pluripotential embryonic stem cell.

The tumor is found predominantly in young women. Less than 25% of patients are under 20 years of age (Wang *et al.*, 1998). The tumor may have a higher inci-dence in Africa and Asia (Jung *et al.*, 1999). Fewer than 10% of all cases are boys, although this pronounced male bias may be less obvious in children (Jung *et al.*, 1999). The youngest reported patient was 2 years old. Papillary solid and cystic tumors are typically large, with a mean diameter of 10 cm (Wang *et al.*, 1998). They usually pre-sent with either abdominal pain and/or a mass. Presentation after minor abdominal trauma is relatively common (Jaksic *et al.*, 1992; Ky *et al.*, 1998; Wang *et al.*, 1998; Jung *et al.*, 1999), and occasionally this may precipitate tumor rupture (Figure 37.2) (Todani *et al.*, 1988). Jaundice and acute pancreatitis have been described, but are exceptionally uncommon (Branchereau *et al.*, 2000).

Imaging studies (ultrasound, CT and MRI) show a well-circumscribed, encapsulated mass in the pancreas with variable degrees of central hemorrhage, calcifica-tion and cystic degeneration. Histological diagnosis may be obtained by ultrasound-guided percutaneous needle biopsy (Jaksic *et al.*, 1992) or by open tumor biopsy (which can be performed at the time of planned surgical excision). Fine-needle aspiration cytology may be a use-ful alternative (Bondeson *et al.*, 1984), but is not consis-tently diagnostic (Ky *et al.*, 1998). Lymphoma should be specifically excluded prior to resectional surgery.

Macroscopically, papillary solid and cystic tumors of the pancreas are round and surrounded by a prominent fibrous capsule; two-thirds of them are located in the body or tail of the gland. On cut section there are often areas of hemorrhage, cystic degeneration and calcifica-tion. Invasive or metastatic disease is uncommon, but the tumor can infiltrate the portal vein, duodenum and spleen and be associated with liver and lymph-node metastases, particularly in adult patients (Horisawa *et al.*, 1995).

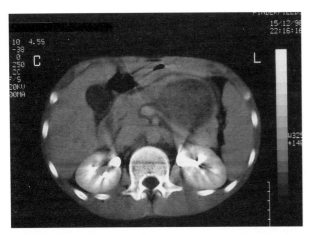

Figure 37.2 *Papillary pancreatic tumor in a 12-year-old boy who presented with abdominal pain and a mass following minor blunt abdominal trauma. At operation the tumor had ruptured posteriorly. He remains well and disease-free 4 years after a distal pancreatectomy.*

Microscopically, rather uniform oval cells are present in solid areas, and adjacent cells are arranged in sheets around discrete fibrovascular cords containing thin-walled blood vessels (Plate 16). Capsular invasion may be noted. Venous invasion and nuclear abnormalities are histological markers of the tumor's malignant potential (Nishihara *et al.*, 1993).

Immunohistochemical stains may be positive for cytokeratin, vimentin, neuron-specific enolase and alpha-1-antitrypsin (Plate 17) (Wunsch *et al.*, 1997; Wang *et al.*, 1998). Hormone receptors have been identified in some tumors (progesterone more often than estrogen receptors), but their presence was not correlated with prognosis (Lee *et al.*, 1997; Wunsch *et al.*, 1997).

Papillary solid and cystic tumors of the pancreas should be treated by complete surgical excision. This usually requires a distal pancreatectomy for body and tail tumors, or pancreaticoduodenectomy if the tumor is in the head of the pancreas. Tumor clearance is essential, but wide margins are not necessary. Metastatic tumor deposits should be removed where feasible (Jaksic *et al.*, 1992). An ultrasonic dissector may be useful for separating the portal vein (Snajdauf *et al.*, 1999). The spleen can usually be preserved unless there is direct tumor involvement. After distal pancreatectomy, a persistent cystic area adjacent to the pancreatic remnant may represent a pseudocyst rather than tumor recurrence (Wang *et al.*, 1998; Snajdauf *et al.*, 1999).

The prognosis for completely resected tumors is generally excellent, but long-term follow-up is essential. In the literature review undertaken by Wang *et al.* (1998), three out of 20 patients under 20 years of age who were treated by local tumor excision experienced tumor recurrence between 8 and 10 years later, whereas only one out of 44 patients of the same age undergoing more extensive resections developed a recurrence during a similar time period. Although rare, recurrent disease or distant metastases in the lung, liver or skin may develop years after tumor resection, when further surgery may still be successful (Horisawa *et al.*, 1995).

PANCREATIC ENDOCRINE NEOPLASMS

These rare tumors arise from cells within the islets of Langerhans which represent only 2% of the pancreatic mass. Benign and malignant, functioning and non-functioning, and isolated and multiple tumors exist. Functioning tumors produce identifiable syndromes, whereas non-functioning lesions usually present with abdominal pain and/or a mass. Many endocrine tumors are small (< 1 cm in diameter), making localization difficult despite modern methods of imaging. Consequently, a variety of additional investigative techniques need to be employed when managing these neoplasms. Endoscopic (Anderson *et al.*, 2000) and intraoperative ultrasonography (Telander *et al.*, 1986) are helpful for detecting small tumors which would be impalpable at surgery. Selective angiography is used less often than previously, but venous sampling using a transhepatic venous catheter may be useful for localizing the tumor to the body or tail rather than to the head of the pancreas.

Complete tumor excision is the goal of therapy in most cases, but is not always possible. In cases of malignant pancreatic neuroendocrine tumors with metastatic disease confined to the liver, liver transplantation should be considered if complete excision of the primary tumor is possible (Lobe *et al.*, 1992).

Insulinoma

The most frequent islet cell is the β-cell, which secretes insulin, and insulinoma is the commonest pancreatic endocrine tumor in children. Most occur after the age of 4 years. Approximately 90% of these tumors are benign, and most of them are solitary (Grosfeld *et al.*, 1990). Insulinomas are well-circumscribed tumors and may be found throughout the pancreas. They typically present with symptoms of hypoglycemia, which may include behavioral problems and seizures. Investigations demonstrate fasting hypoglycemia with inappropriately high insulin levels. Measurement of the circulating C-peptide fragment helps to exclude an exogenous source of insulin. Preoperative tumor localization may be achieved by CT (generally for tumors measuring 1 cm or more in diameter), MRI and/or transhepatic portal venous sampling. The tumor may occasionally be ectopic to the pancreas. Accurate localization should avoid the need for blind pancreatic resection.

At operation, insulinomas appear pink, firm and well encapsulated. The pancreas should be carefully palpated and examined by intraoperative ultrasound to exclude multifocal tumors. Benign insulinomas can be treated by enucleation (Vane *et al.*, 1989). After successful surgery, rebound hyperglycemia may occur in the early postoperative period. Malignant lesions should be treated by resection of the primary tumor and metastases where possible combined with chemotherapy.

Gastrinoma

Neoplasia of the gastrin-producing islet G-cells causes Zollinger–Ellison syndrome, which is characterized by hypergastrinemia and severe peptic ulceration. Most gastrinomas arise in the pancreas, but they occasionally develop at extrapancreatic sites such as the duodenum, stomach or liver (Thompson *et al.*, 1989). These tumors tend to grow slowly in children, but two-thirds of them are malignant, with the potential for liver metastases (Grosfeld *et al.*, 1990). Multifocal tumors are found in as many as 30% of patients, and particularly those with type 1 multiple endocrine neoplasia (MEN).

Gastrinomas cause peptic ulcer disease which is severe, located at unusually distal sites in the duodenum and jejunum, poorly responsive to treatment, and recurrent. Ulceration may be accompanied by diarrhea and steatorrhea due to lipase and bile-salt inactivation by excess gastric acid. The disease is more common in boys, and the youngest reported patient to date was 5 years of age (Grosfeld *et al.*, 1990; Wilson, 1991).

The diagnosis of gastrinoma is confirmed by a markedly elevated fasting serum gastrin level. For those tumors which cannot be localized by CT, MRI or endoscopic ultrasound, interventional radiological techniques can be used. Injection of secretin into the gastroduodenal artery provokes gastrin secretion, which can be measured in efferent veins (Imamura *et al.*, 1987). At operation, a careful search is made for tumor in the pancreas, duodenal wall and lymph nodes. Excision alone may be curative if the tumor is solitary and there is no evidence of metastases. For malignant lesions, resection of involved lymph nodes and liver metastases is potentially useful because the tumor is often slow growing. For those with residual disease, the alternatives are medical control of peptic ulceration with high-dose H_2-blockers or proton-pump inhibitors, subcutaneous octreotide or total gastrectomy. Long-term survival (>25 years) is possible after total gastrectomy even if there is persistent hypergastrinemia (Thompson *et al.*, 1989; Wilson, 1991).

Vipoma

Excessive secretion of vasoactive intestinal polypeptide (VIP) stimulates the intestinal mucosa to secrete fluid and electrolytes into the intestinal lumen, and increases intestinal motility. Vipomas therefore cause a syndrome of profuse watery diarrhea, hypokalemia and achlorhydria (WDHA syndrome), which may be accompanied by abdominal pain and vomiting.

Plasma VIP levels are markedly elevated and hypokalemia is often profound (Brenner *et al.*, 1986). In children, VIP-secreting tumors such as ganglioneuromas and neuroblastomas occur much more frequently than pancreatic vipomas (Grosfeld *et al.*, 1990). After correction of fluid and electrolyte imbalance, the diarrhea can be controlled by steroids, prostaglandin inhibitors or somatostatin. Tumor resection is then necessary, but pancreatic vipomas are often malignant.

Other pancreatic endocrine neoplasms

Glucagonomas, which cause diabetes mellitus, a migratory erythematous rash and weight loss in adults, and *somatostatinomas*, which cause diabetes mellitus, steatorrhea and cholelithiasis in adults, have not been reported in children. *Carcinoid tumors* which can arise in the pancreas in children are extremely rare but may be malignant (van Dooren *et al.*, 2000).

Islet-cell adenomas can occur as part of type 1 MEN syndrome in which the pituitary, parathyroid and pancreatic glands are affected. This condition may be inherited in an autosomal-dominant fashion, or it may occur sporadically. Pancreatic involvement is multifocal with functioning or non-functioning tumors (Figure 37.3). For example, there may be more than 10 insulinomas, which are sometimes as small as 2 mm in diameter. A 95% pancreatectomy may be warranted in such cases, together with sonographic identification and enucleation of any adenomas that remain in the pancreatic remnant (Telander *et al.*,

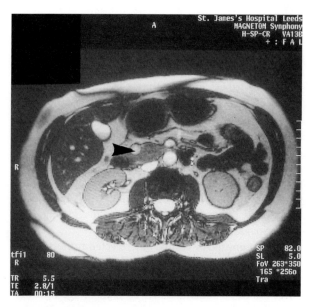

Figure 37.3 *A patient with MEN 1 and a non-functioning pancreatic tumor (arrowed) prior to pancreatectomy. (Reproduced courtesy of Dr Ashley Guthrie.)*

1986). Von Hippel–Lindau disease (a genetic condition that is characterized by retinal hemangiomas, cerebellar cysts or tumors and pheochromocytoma) may also be complicated by islet-cell adenomas.

Malignant islet-cell tumors may be functioning (e.g. insulin or gastrin) or non-functioning, and have been reported in children in association with MEN type 1 and tuberous sclerosis (Verhoef *et al.*, 1999). Non-functioning islet-cell carcinomas, which may appear cystic, are more common in children than in adults, and are often large at presentation, with distant metastases (Grosfeld *et al.*, 1970).

NON-EPITHELIAL PANCREATIC NEOPLASMS

A variety of non-epithelial pancreatic neoplasms have been reported in children, but they are all exceptionally rare. They include benign hemangioendothelioma (Horie *et al.*, 1985), lymphangioma (a multilocular, serous or chylous fluid-filled cystic tumor which is amenable to complete excision and is associated with a good prognosis) (Paal *et al.*, 1998) and dermoid cyst (a mature benign teratoma which is usually large and lined by squamous epithelium) (Assawamatiyanont and King, 1977; Mester *et al.*, 1990). Non-Hodgkin's lymphoma in the pancreas is an unusual cause of obstructive jaundice in childhood. Biopsy followed by chemotherapy usually provides effective treatment (Pietsch *et al.*, 2001).

NON-NEOPLASTIC PANCREATIC TUMORS

Many of these are cystic lesions. Non-neoplastic epithelial-lined pancreatic cysts are most often developmental in origin. They are usually small and asymptomatic, do not communicate with the duct system (and therefore do not contain fluid rich in pancreatic enzymes), and are more often confined to the body or tail of the pancreas. Very occasionally they are large and complex (Mares and Hirsch, 1977) or cause symptoms such as abdominal distension or acute pancreatitis (Shieh *et al.*, 1994). Multiple congenital cysts may be found in association with polycystic kidney disease or von Hippel–Lindau disease (Seitz *et al.*, 1987; Flaherty and Benjamin, 1992). In cystic fibrosis, pancreatic cysts develop as a result of mucinous obstruction of pancreatic ducts (Ade-Ajayi *et al.*, 1997). Cysts may also be acquired in chronic pancreatitis. Other cystic lesions in the pancreas in children include pancreatic hamartoma (Flaherty and Benjamin, 1992) and alimentary tract duplication cysts (either in the stomach or duodenum and communicating with the pancreatic duct, or buried within the pancreas itself). Complete local resection of enteric duplication cysts in the pancreatic head is possible, thereby avoiding the complications of more radical procedures (Siddiqui *et al.*, 1998).

These lesions must be distinguished from benign and malignant cystic tumors, post-inflammatory pseudocysts and parasitic cysts. If there is no suspicion of neoplasia, small asymptomatic cysts do not require treatment. Large or symptomatic lesions usually require excision, although marsupialization is an option for simple congenital cysts.

There are two pancreatic solid lesions that occur in children which may easily be confused with pancreatic neoplasia.

- *Pancreatic inflammatory pseudotumor:* These are unusual lesions composed of myofibroblasts (Stringer *et al.*, 1992). Symptoms are dependent on the tumor's location, and may be accompanied by a microcytic anemia, hypergammaglobulinemia and elevated inflammatory markers. Imaging studies do not allow a precise diagnosis, which depends on histology. Although there are reports of spontaneous regression and response to steroids, most symptomatic lesions require complete excision (Morris-Stiff *et al.*, 1998).

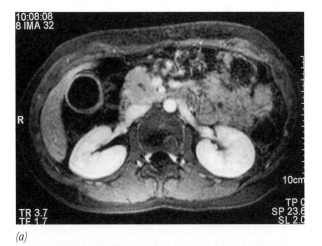

(a)

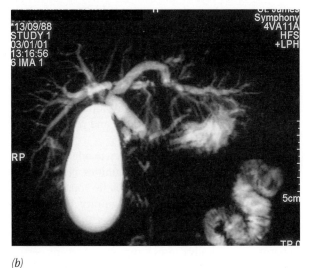

(b)

Figure 37.4 *a and b.* *Magnetic resonance imaging of fibrosing pancreatitis associated with obstructive jaundice in a 12-year-old boy. Note the expansion of the pancreatic head and dilated biliary tree.*

- *Fibrosing pancreatitis:* Typically, this condition presents with obstructive jaundice due to extrinsic compression of the common bile duct within the head of the pancreas. Affected patients show no evidence of previous acute or chronic pancreatitis, cystic fibrosis or sclerosing cholangitis. Plasma amylase levels are normal or only slightly elevated. Abdominal ultrasound and CT show diffuse pancreatic enlargement, predominantly in the head of the pancreas (Figure 37.4). Ultrasound-guided percutaneous pancreatic biopsy shows fibrosis and acinar-cell atrophy. The cause of fibrosing pancreatitis is not known, but a viral etiology was implicated in one report (Sylvester *et al.*, 1998). The condition can be successfully treated by temporary endoscopic placement of a common bile duct stent which can be removed a few months later, since the biliary obstruction is self-limiting. Pancreatic fibrosis progresses to pancreatic atrophy, which may cause exocrine and less commonly endocrine insufficiency. Biliary–enteric bypass has been undertaken in some cases (Amerson and Ricketts, 1996).

HYPERINSULINEMIC HYPOGLYCEMIA OF INFANCY

Insulin is synthesized, stored and secreted by pancreatic β-cells located within the islets of Langerhans. Hyperinsulinism is the commonest cause of severe or recurrent hypoglycemia in infancy. This condition was previously known as nesidioblastosis because it was considered to be caused by persistent fetal islet-cell budding in the infant pancreas, but since this histological feature can be seen in normoglycemic infants, alternative terms have been suggested. These include persistent hyperinsulinemic hypoglycemia of infancy, congenital hyperinsulinism, pancreatic microadenomatosis, islet-cell dysregulation syndrome and islet-cell dysmaturation syndrome. The term *hyperinsulinemic hypoglycemia of infancy* (HHI) is used here to describe this entity, which includes several conditions with a highly variable age of onset, severity and responsiveness to medical treatment.

HHI is a rare condition with an incidence of 1 in 50 000 live births in outbred communities. However, the condition is as frequent as 1 in 2500 live births in societies with a high rate of consanguinity (e.g. in the Arabian peninsula) (Aynsley-Green *et al.*, 2000). The unregulated secretion of insulin in pancreatic β-cell hyperplasia classically causes symptoms of severe, persistent hypoglycemia within hours or days after birth. Neurological features such as jitteriness, irritability, poor feeding or convulsions are common. Early diagnosis and appropriate treatment are critical in order to prevent hypoglycemic damage to the neonatal brain. Imaging studies are rarely helpful, and diagnosis is based on the following criteria:

- inappropriately raised plasma insulin levels in the presence of hypoglycemia (laboratory blood glucose < 2.6 mmol/L);
- a high glucose requirement to maintain normoglycemia (> 10 mg/kg/minute);
- lack of ketone-body production during hypoglycemia (no ketonuria).

It should be noted that a normal plasma insulin concentration in the presence of hypoglycemia is inappropriate. Plasma ammonia levels should also be measured, as these can be markedly elevated in a small proportion of infants (Stanley *et al.*, 1998).

Hyperinsulinism must be distinguished from well-defined clinical conditions associated with hypoglycemia, such as Beckwith–Wiedemann syndrome (Munns and Batch, 2001), maternal diabetes mellitus, sulphonylurea poisoning and perinatal asphyxia.

Etiology, pathogenesis and genetics

HHI is clinically and genetically heterogeneous, but in recent years major advances have been made in understanding the molecular and genetic basis of the condition. Insulin secretion is regulated and influenced by many interacting biochemical pathways. At a cellular level the critical mechanisms are summarized in Figure 37.5 (Glaser *et al.*, 2000). The resting membrane potential of the β-cell is maintained by ATP-sensitive potassium channels (K_{ATP}). When plasma glucose levels increase, it enters the β-cell via a specific membrane-bound glucose transporter (GLUT-2), and is phosphorylated by the enzyme glucokinase. Ultimately this leads to the production of ATP, which causes the K_{ATP} channels to close. Depolarization of the cell membrane occurs and an influx of calcium ions activates insulin secretion. Different genetic mutations are responsible for defective steps in this pathway, but all of them result in uncontrolled insulin secretion and hypoglycemia.

In 1994, the genetic mutation for HHI was localized to chromosome 11 (Thomas *et al.*, 1995a), and later that year mutations in the sulphonylurea receptor gene (SUR1) were implicated (Aguilar-Bryan *et al.*, 1995; Thomas *et al.*, 1995b). The SUR1 is a subunit of the β-cell membrane's ATP-dependent potassium channel. Soon after this discovery, the gene encoding the inward rectifying potassium channel (Kir6.2) was cloned, and it was found that the product of this gene together with SUR1 formed the β-cell K_{ATP} channel. Mutations in the genes encoding the two subunits of the K_{ATP} channel (particularly SUR1) and in others affecting the β-cell enzymes glucokinase and glutamate dehydrogenase (GDH) account for as many as half of the cases of HHI (Glaser *et al.*, 2000). However, no genetic etiology has yet

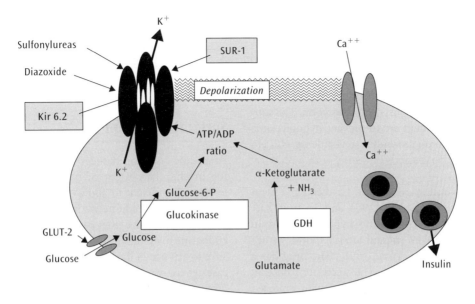

Figure 37.5 *The major pathways responsible for glucose regulation of insulin secretion (from Glaser* et al.*, 2000). Hyperinsulinism can be caused by mutations in the genes encoding the four proteins highlighted within boxes. The K_{ATP} channel is composed of two subunits (the inward-rectifying potassium channel and the sulphonylurea receptor) encoded by their respective genes. Glucokinase is the rate-limiting step in the metabolism of glucose, and thus regulates changes in the intracellular ATP/ADP ratio in response to extracellular glucose concentrations. See text for details. Reproduced by kind permission of the author and* Archives of Disease in Childhood.

been determined for many other cases. Familial cases of HHI are well described in the literature, and autosomal-recessive inheritance has been postulated in most of them (Thornton *et al.*, 1991; Woolf *et al.*, 1991).

The histopathology of the pancreas in HHI is variable, with no single pathognomonic feature (Rahier *et al.*, 2000). Two variants of HHI must be distinguished, namely diffuse involvement of the pancreas and focal adenomatous hyperplasia (DeLonlay-Debeney *et al.*, 1999; Rahier *et al.*, 2000). The picture is confused by the fact that, in some patients, both diffuse and focal pathologies apparently coexist (Schonau *et al.*, 1991; Spitz *et al.*, 1992). The diffuse form is associated with β-cells that have abnormal, large nuclei and abundant cytoplasm not seen in the focal form, and with experience, this feature can be detected on intraoperative frozen-section histology (Rahier *et al.*, 2000). In neonates and infants, macroscopic identification of focal lesions is often impossible (in contrast to the pancreatic adenomas seen in older children and adults). The focal lesions are also histologically distinct from the insulinomas in that they are composed of apparently normally organized islets.

The distribution of these two variants may have a genetic and geographical basis, since in some European centres up to one-third or more of cases of HHI are related to focal disease (Fekete *et al.*, 1997). A genetic distinction between focal and diffuse forms seems likely. DeLonlay-Debeny *et al.* (1997, 1999) have demonstrated a specific loss of the maternal allele at the 11p15 chro-

mosomal region in focal adenomatous hyperplasia, which is associated with loss of a tumor suppressor gene. In affected cases this genetic abnormality has been combined with an SUR1 mutation on the paternal allele. In diffuse forms of HHI, the precise cause of hyperinsulinism is uncertain, but it is not related to an increased β-cell mass (Rahier *et al.*, 2000).

The β-cell defect in HHI is not corrected with the passage of time, despite the disappearance of spontaneous hypoglycaemia. Leibowitz *et al.* (1995) demonstrated that some children with HHI show impaired insulin responses to glucose and a lack of suppressibility of endogenous insulin secretion years after clinical remission. The β-cell may therefore be on course for premature failure in HHI, and this may be accelerated by pancreatic resection. Medical follow-up of these patients must therefore extend into adulthood, since childhood 'cure' of the condition may simply represent a phase of remission prior to subsequent endocrine failure. Although timely surgical intervention can be important in preventing hypoglycemic brain injury, it may also hasten subsequent pancreatic insufficiency.

Medical treatment

The initial aim in the medical management of HHI is the maintenance of normoglycemia. This may be achieved by using frequent high-calorie enteral feeds, but more often demands the administration of intravenous glucose which may need to be given at a rate of 15–20 mg/kg/minute or more. This usually requires the insertion of a central venous catheter. Once the blood glucose concentration has been stabilized, drug therapies can be instituted in an attempt to reduce insulin secretion and limit the need for excess carbohydrate intake. Patients should be referred to specialist centers early on. The subsequent aims of treatment are to prevent hypoglycemia and, with the minimum morbidity, to enable the child to safely tolerate normal periods of fasting with a practical feeding regimen.

Diazoxide, an insulin antagonist, has been the main therapeutic agent for HHI since 1964, and has been particularly successful in controlling hyperinsulinism in infants and children who present after 1 month of age (Grant et al., 1986; Horev et al., 1991). The drug has a direct action on K_{ATP} channels. The maximum dose of diazoxide is 20 mg/kg/day. Grant et al. (1986) reported spontaneous remission of hyperinsulinism in seven children after 2 to 14 years of diazoxide treatment, but a very variable success rate has been reported by other researchers (Touati et al., 1998; DeLonlay-Debeney et al., 1999). Diazoxide has numerous side-effects, including fluid retention, cardiomyopathy and congestive heart failure, hirsutism and (rarely) blood dyscrasia. Chlorthiazide is a useful addition to diazoxide treatment, since it has both a synergistic action in relation to hyperinsulinism and diuretic effects.

Other agents that have been used alone or in combination to treat HHI include growth hormone (Hocking et al., 1986), glucagon (Bougnères et al., 1985), nifedipine (Aynsley-Green et al., 2000), octreotide, phenytoin, streptozotocin, cyproheptadine and hydrocortisone. Glucagon injection leads to a glycemic response through hepatic mobilization of glycogen, and can be useful in an emergency, but may result in rebound hypoglycemia. Octreotide, a long-acting somatostatin analog, can only be administered by subcutaneous injection or intravenous infusion. Potential side-effects include vomiting, diarrhea, steatorrhea, abdominal distension, gallstones and cramps, growth impairment and (rarely) adrenal suppression. Tolerance may develop over time. Nevertheless, successful long-term medical management of HHI has been reported with octreotide (Glaser et al., 1993).

Current medical therapy alone is effective in controlling hyperinsulinism in a variable proportion of affected infants and children, ranging from 22% (Haddad and Mathew, 1996) to 75% (Grant et al., 1986). This disparity is partly explained by the different age groups of patients in the various studies, and by variations in clinical phenotype. For example, some inherited forms of HHI in Arabic and Finnish children are particularly resistant to medical treatment and require early surgery. Infants with severe hypoglycemia who present within days after birth often have more severe disease, whilst infants who present after the first few months of life tend to be more responsive to pharmacological therapy. Surgical intervention is necessary if medical management is unsuccessful. This should be considered at an early stage in order to minimize the risk of hypoglycemic injury to the developing brain.

Surgical treatment

Pancreatic resection reduces the mass of β-cells producing insulin. The extent of pancreatic resection should ideally be sufficient to allow control of hyperinsulinism (with or without adjunctive medical therapy), but not so radical as to leave the patient with exocrine and/or endocrine insufficiency. In practice, this is a difficult balance to achieve in the long term. Infants with diffuse disease generally require a 95% pancreatectomy, but in focal disease good glycemic control is possible with less radical surgery.

Preoperative percutaneous transhepatic pancreatic venous sampling can identify focal areas of insulin hypersecretion within the pancreas (DeLonlay-Debeney et al., 1999). This requires expert interventional angiography under general anesthesia, and multiple blood sampling in splenic, mesenteric, portal and pancreatic veins with measurement of insulin, glucose and C peptide. During the procedure, the blood glucose level needs to be maintained at 2.5–3.0 mmol/L by glucose infusion to promote maximal insulin release. In the Paris series of 52 neonates with hyperinsulinism who were seen during a 14-year period, there were 30 cases with diffuse disease and 22 cases with focal adenomatous islet-cell hyperplasia (pancreatic head, $n = 9$; neck, $n = 3$; body, $n = 8$; tail, $n = 2$). Clinical manifestations were similar in both groups. Using selective venous catheterizaton and localized sampling, focal disease was correctly identified preoperatively in 17 out of 22 cases and diffuse disease in 17 out of 30 cases. Seven cases were incorrectly characterized as focal. Armed with this preoperative information and aided by intraoperative frozen-section histology, the extent of pancreatic resection could be tailored to the type of disease. In focal hyperplasia, excellent control of hyperinsulinism was possible with partial pancreatectomy, whereas 13 out of 30 infants with diffuse disease had persistent hypoglycemia despite near total pancreatectomy (and eight had diabetes mellitus).

The extent of pancreatic resection is best described in relation to anatomical landmarks as shown in Figure 37.6 (Spitz, 1994). Consistency between surgical reports is important, since the degree of resection may otherwise differ markedly between surgeons, explaining the widely different success rates for apparently similar operative procedures. Reyes et al. (1993) have demonstrated that these planes of excision actually underestimate the extent of pancreatic resection as determined by pediatric autopsy specimens. In recent years, a so-called 95% resection has become the standard procedure for diffuse

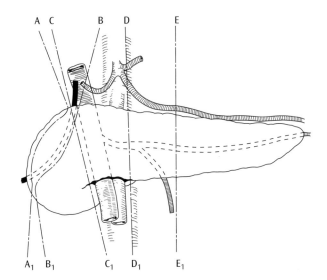

Figure 37.6 *Extent of pancreatic resection for HHI. An 80% resection extends just to the right of the superior mesenteric/portal vein (C–C₁), and a 95% resection only leaves pancreatic tissue between the common bile duct and the duodenum and a sliver of pancreatic tissue on the concavity of the duodenal wall (B–B₁). Reproduced from Spitz (1994) with kind permission of Chapman and Hall.*

islet-cell hyperplasia in most units (Plate 18), although this remains a controversial subject. During surgery, care must be taken to avoid injury to the common bile duct, which usually lies on the posterior aspect of the head of the gland, but may lie within the substance of the pancreas. Bile duct injury has been reported by several authors (Spitz *et al.*, 1992; Haddad and Mathew, 1996; Nihoul-Fekete *et al.*, 2001). In the author's experience, drainage of the pancreatic bed after 95% pancreatectomy is not required.

After successful surgery, the infant's glucose requirement usually falls dramatically and insulin may need to be given temporarily or permanently. Limited regrowth of the pancreatic remnant has been demonstrated (Aynsley-Green *et al.*, 1981; Schonau *et al.*, 1991), but the extent of pancreatic regeneration is unpredictable (Schonau *et al.*, 1991; Cade *et al.*, 1998b).

In the future it may be possible to harvest β-cells from pancreatectomy specimens from patients with HHI and genetically engineer them for subsequent autotransplantation (Shepherd *et al.*, 2000).

Outcome after pancreatic resection

The literature suggests that less than a 95% pancreatectomy for HHI with diffuse islet-cell hyperplasia is associated with a significant failure rate (Gough, 1984). In some cases, recurrent hypoglycemia can be successfully managed with medical treatment, but further pancreatic resection is often required if the initial resection was less

than 95%. The long-term outcome after pancreatic resection (and in HHI generally) is influenced by neurological handicap, endocrine and exocrine insufficiency, recurrent hypoglycemia, feeding difficulties and psychosocial aspects of the condition (Cade and Stringer, 1998).

Thomas and colleagues published two extensive reviews of the literature spanning the years 1934–76 and 1977–87, respectively (Thomas *et al.*, 1977, 1988). In their first review of 72 neonates and infants undergoing < 90% pancreatectomy, one-third of the patients required supplementary treatment postoperatively to maintain normoglycemia. A total of 13 patients (18%) needed further pancreatic resections, six of whom were rendered insulin-dependent diabetics. The overall mortality rate was 10%, and in survivors the incidence of mental retardation was 54%. Although it was not statistically significant, there was a positive temporal correlation between the duration of hypoglycemia prior to surgery and the incidence of mental retardation. In their second review of 165 neonates and infants from 1977 to 1987, 76% of cases underwent < 90% pancreatectomy as the primary surgical procedure, and 28% of these went on to require a further pancreatic resection for persistent hyperinsulinism. The remaining 40 patients (24%) had a ≥ 95% pancreatectomy as the primary procedure, and only two (5%) needed a further pancreatic resection. Three (7.5%) were rendered diabetic. The mortality rate was 2.5% (one death) and the incidence of mental retardation was 12.5%.

Since 1988 there have been several further studies of long-term pancreatic function after surgical treatment of HHI (Dunger *et al.*, 1988; Schonau *et al.*, 1991; Spitz *et al.*, 1992; Rother *et al.*, 1994; Leibowitz *et al.*, 1995; Parashar *et al.*, 1995; Haddad and Mathew, 1996; Soliman *et al.* 1996; Cade *et al.*, 1998b; Cresto *et al.*, 1998). These results are summarized in Table 37.3 and Table 37.4. There was no operative mortality. Considerably more patients developed recurrent hypoglycemia than those undergoing further pancreatic resection, since most of these cases responded to medical treatment. Table 37.4 needs to be interpreted cautiously, since the different groups of patients have been followed up for different periods (and the incidence of pancreatic endocrine and exocrine insufficiency increases with time), and the age mix of the patients (and thus the pathology) varies in different centers.

From these data it is evident that mental retardation continues to be a significant complication of HHI. To what extent this figure can be reduced by more aggressive blood sugar control and early surgery is uncertain. Surgical resection of the pancreas is a major undertaking, but can be achieved with no mortality and minimal morbidity in this age group, and should not be considered a last resort in the management of HHI. Clinicians must be aware of the potential for subclinical hypoglycemia during follow-up that might contribute to

Table 37.3 Outcome after pancreatic resection for HHI in infants and children (1988–98)

Author	Number of children	Pancreatectomy (%)	Further resection	Clinical status	Median/mean follow-up (years)	Endocrine function	Exocrine function
Dunger et al. (1988)	7	95	No	NA	1–2	1 diabetic GTT	1 pancreatic supplements
	3	75	No	NA	9–11	3 normal GTT	3 normal
Schonau et al. (1991)	4	88–95	No	Normal	0.3–2.6	4 normal GTT and HbA$_{1c}$	4 normal fecal chymotrypsin / No steatorrhea
Spitz et al. (1992)	21	95	1 → 95%	3 neurological deficit	1–10	1 IDDM	2 pancreatic supplements
Rother et al. (1994)	8	90–95	No	2 mild MR	12.7	8 normal HbA$_{1c}$	8 normal fecal fat
Leibowitz et al. (1995)	8	80–95	No	NA	10.2	5 IDDM / 1 NIDDM	NA
Parashar et al. (1995)	7	80	2 → 95%	3 developmental delay	0.2–22	Normal	1 pancreatic supplements
	4	95	No	2 developmental delay	1.8–9.5	3 IDDM	2 pancreatic supplements
Haddad and Mathew (1996)	12	95	1 → 100%	1 developmental delay	0.75–9	1 IDDM	NA
	1	85	No	Normal	9	Normal	NA
	1	99	No	Normal	7	1 IDDM	NA
Soliman et al. (1996)	7	95–98	No	1 mild MR	4.6	3 IDDM and 2 impaired GTT	7 normal fecal fat
Cade et al. (1998)	6	85–95	No	2 developmental delay	4.3	1 IDDM	1 pancreatic supplements
Cresto et al. (1998)	10	70–95	2 → 100%	5 impaired	2–22	1 IDDM	2 steatorrhea

NA, data not available.
GTT, glucose tolerance test; MR, mental retardation; IDDM, insulin-dependent diabetes mellitus; NIDDM, non-insulin-dependent diabetes mellitus; SD, = standard deviation.

Table 37.4 Summary of outcomes after pancreatic resection for HHI (1988–98)

Pancreatectomy (%)	Number of patients	Further resection (%)	IDDM (%)	Exocrine failure (%)	Mental retardation (%)
≤75	4	1	1	1	NA
75–90	18	2	6	1	3
91–95	69	3	5	7	14
>95	8	0	4 (50)	0	1 (25)
Total	99	6 (6)	16 (16)	11 (11)	18 (18)

NA, data not available.

overall decreased intellectual performance (Cresto *et al.*, 1998).

The incidence of pancreatic exocrine failure partly depends on whether this is biochemically or clinically determined and on the length of follow-up. The incidence of insulin-dependent diabetes mellitus also increases with time (Leibowitz *et al.*, 1995). Feeding difficulties have been relatively neglected in these patients. HHI itself may be complicated by foregut dysmotility (Cade *et al.*, 1998a), and further feeding problems may arise from the use of supplementary feeding techniques.

Key references

DeLonlay-Debeney P, Poggi-Travert F, Fournet JC *et al.* Clinical features of 52 neonates with hyperinsulinism. *New England Journal of Medicine* 1999; **340**: 1169–75.

A unique experience of 52 infants with HHI due to focal or diffuse β-cell hyperplasia seen in Paris during a 14-year period. Particularly valuable are the details of preoperative selective venous sampling techniques and surgical modifications of the extent of pancreatic resection based on these findings in combination with detailed intraoperative histology.

Glaser B, Thornton P, Otonkoski T, Junien C. Genetics of neonatal hyperinsulinism. *Archives of Disease in Childhood* 2000; **82**: F79–86.

A fascinating account of the recent genetic and molecular discoveries which are beginning to elucidate the different conditions underlying the clinical picture of HHI.

Spitz L, Bhargava RK, Grant DB, Leonard JV. Surgical treatment of hyperinsulinaemic hypoglycaemia in infancy and childhood. *Archives of Disease in Childhood* 1992; **67**: 201–5.

An account of the technique and results of 95% pancreatectomy for HHI from Great Ormond Street Hospital, London.

REFERENCES

Ade-Ajayi N, Law C, Burge DM, Johnson C, Moore I. Surgery for pancreatic cystosis with pancreatitis in cystic fibrosis. *British Journal of Surgery* 1997; **84**: 312.

Aguilar-Bryan L, Nichols CG, Wechsler SW *et al.* Cloning of the β-cell high-affinity sulfonylurea receptor: a regulator of insulin secretion. *Science* 1995; **268**: 422–5.

Amerson JL, Ricketts RR. Idiopathic fibrosing pancreatitis: a rare cause of obstructive jaundice in children. *American Surgeon* 1996; **62**: 295–9.

Anderson MA, Carpenter S, Thompson NW *et al.* Endoscopic ultrasound is highly accurate and directs management in patients with neuroendocrine tumors of the pancreas. *American Journal of Gastroenterology* 2000; **95**: 2271–7.

Assawamatiyanont S, King AD Jr. Dermoid cysts of the pancreas. *American Surgeon* 1977; **43**: 503–4.

Aynsley-Green A, Polak JM, Bloom SR *et al.* Nesidioblastosis of the pancreas: definition of the syndrome and the management of the severe neonatal hyperinsulinaemic hypoglycaemia. *Archives of Disease in Childhood* 1981; **56**: 496–508.

Aynsley-Green A, Hussain K, Hall J *et al.* Practical management of hyperinsulinism in infancy. *Archives of Disease in Childhood* 2000; **82**: F98–107.

Bondeson L, Bondeson AG, Genell S, Lindholm K, Thorstenson S. Aspiration cytology of a rare solid and papillary epithelial neoplasm of the pancreas. Light and electron microscopic study of a case. *Acta Cytologica* 1984; **28**: 605–9.

Bougnères P-F, Landier F, Garnier P, Job J-C, Chaussain J-L. Treatment of insulin excess by continuous subcutaneous infusion of somatostatin and glucagon in an infant. *Journal of Pediatrics* 1985; **106**: 792–4.

Branchereau S, Fabre M, Ait Ali Slimane M *et al.* Solid pseudopapillary tumor of pancreas. *Medical and Pediatric Oncology* 2000; **35**: 378.

Brenner RW, Sank LI, Kerner MB *et al.* Resection of a vipoma of the pancreas in a 15-year-old girl. *Journal of Pediatric Surgery* 1986; **21**: 983–5.

Cade A, Stringer MD. Nesidioblastosis. In: Stringer MD, Oldham KT, Mouriquand PDE, Howard ER (eds) *Pediatric surgery and urology: long-term outcomes.* Philadelphia, PA: WB Saunders Co., 1998: 447–53.

Cade A, Abel G, Stringer MD, Milla P, Puntis JWLP. Foregut dysmotility complicating persistent hyperinsulinaemic hypoglycaemia of infancy. *Journal of Pediatric Gastroenterology and Nutrition* 1998a; **27**: 355–8.

Cade A, Walters M, Puntis JWL, Arthur RJ, Stringer MD. Pancreatic exocrine and endocrine function following pancreatectomy for persistent hyperinsulinaemic hypoglycaemia of infancy. *Archives of Disease in Childhood* 1998b; **79**: 435–9.

Camprodon R, Quintanilla E. Successful long-term results with resection of pancreatic carcinoma in children: favorable prognosis for an uncommon neoplasm. *Surgery* 1984; **95**: 420–6.

Chang CH, Perrin EV, Hertzler J, Brough AJ. Cystadenoma of the pancreas with cytomegalovirus infection in a female infant. *Archives of Pathology and Laboratory Medicine* 1980; **104**: 7–8.

Chun Y, Kim W, Park K, Lee S, Jung S. Pancreatoblastoma. *Journal of Pediatric Surgery* 1997; **32**: 1612–15.

Cresto JC, Abdenur JP, Bergada I, Martino R. Long-term follow-up of persistent hyperinsulinaemic hypoglycaemia of infancy. *Archives of Disease in Childhood* 1998; **79**: 440–4.

Defachelles AS, Martin de Lasalle E, Boutard P *et al.* Pancreatoblastoma in childhood: clinical course and therapeutic management of seven patients. *Medical and Pediatric Oncology* 2001; **37**: 47–52.

DeLonlay-Debeney P, Fournet JC, Rahier J et al. A somatic deletion of the imprinted 11p15.1 region in sporadic persistent hyperinsulinemic hypoglycemia of infancy is specific for focal adenomatous hyperplasia and endorses partial pancreatectomy. Journal of Clinical Investigation 1997; 4: 802–7.

DeLonlay-Debeney P, Poggi-Travert F, Fournet JC et al. Clinical features of 52 neonates with hyperinsulinism. New England Journal of Medicine 1999; 340: 1169–75.

Drut R, Jones MC. Congenital pancreatoblastoma in Beckwith–Wiedemann syndrome: an emerging association. Pediatric Pathology and Laboratory Medicine 1988; 8: 331–9.

Dunger DB, Burns C, Ghale GK, Muller DPR, Spitz L, Grant DB. Pancreatic exocrine and endocrine function after subtotal pancreatectomy for nesidioblastosis. Journal of Pediatric Surgery 1988; 23: 112–15.

Fekete CN, Brunelle F, Rahier J, di Benedetto V, Brusset MC, Saudubray JM. Surgical treatment in permanent hyperinsulinaemic hypoglycaemia (HIH) in neonates and infants: what is the place of elective partial pancreatectomy? Abstracts from the Second European Congress of Paediatric Surgery, Madrid, May 1997.

Flaherty MJ, Benjamin DR. Multicystic pancreatic hamartoma: a distinctive lesion with immunohistochemical and ultrastructural study. Human Pathology 1992; 23: 1309–12.

Glaser B, Hirsch HJ, Landau H. Persistent hyperinsulinemic hypoglycaemia of infancy: long-term octreotide treatment without pancreatectomy. Journal of Pediatrics 1993; 123: 644–50.

Glaser B, Thornton P, Otonkoski T, Junien C. Genetics of neonatal hyperinsulinism. Archives of Disease in Childhood 2000; 82: F79–86.

Gough MH. The surgical treatment of hyperinsulinism in infancy and childhood. British Journal of Surgery 1984; 71: 75–8.

Grant DB, Dunger DB, Burns EC. Long-term treatment with diazoxide in childhood hyperinsulinism. Acta Endocrinologica (Supplement) 1986; 279: 340–5.

Griffin BR, Wisbeck WM, Schaller RT, Benjamin DR. Radiotherapy for locally recurrent infantile pancreatic carcinoma (pancreatoblastoma). Cancer 1987; 60: 1734–6.

Grosfeld JL, Clatworthy HW, Hamoudi AB. Pancreatic malignancy in children. Archives of Surgery 1970; 101: 370–5.

Grosfeld JL, Vane DW, Rescorla FJ, McGuire W, West KW. Pancreatic tumors in childhood: analysis of 13 cases. Journal of Pediatric Surgery 1990; 25: 1057–62.

Gundersen AE, Janis JF. Pancreatic cystadenoma in childhood: report of a case. Journal of Pediatric Surgery 1969; 4: 478–81.

Gupta AK, Mitra DK, Berry M et al. Sonography and CT of pancreatoblastoma in children. American Journal of Roentgenology 2000; 174: 1639–41.

Haddad MJ, Mathew PM. Role of initial near total (95%) pancreatectomy in persistent neonatal hyperinsulinism (PNH). European Journal of Pediatric Surgery 1996; 6: 82–5.

Hocking MD, Newell SJ, Rayner PHW. Use of human growth hormone in treatment of nesidioblastosis in a neonate. Archives of Disease in Childhood 1986; 61: 706–7.

Horev Z, Ipp M, Levey P, Daneman D. Familial hyperinsulinism: successful conservative management. Journal of Pediatrics 1991; 119: 717–20.

Horie A, Yano Y, Kotoo Y et al. Morphogenesis of pancreatoblastoma, infantile carcinoma of the pancreas: report of two cases. Cancer 1977; 39: 247–54.

Horie H, Iwasaki I, Iida H et al. Benign hemangioendothelioma of the pancreas with obstructive jaundice. Acta Pathologica Japonica 1985; 35: 975–9.

Horisawa M, Niinomi N, Sato T et al. Frantz's tumor (solid and cystic tumor of the pancreas) with liver metastasis: successful treatment and long-term follow-up. Journal of Pediatric Surgery 1995; 30: 724–6.

Imamura M, Takahashi K, Adachi H et al. Usefulness of selective arterial secretion injection test for localization of gastrinoma in the Zollinger–Ellison syndrome. Annals of Surgery 1987; 205: 230–9.

Inomata Y, Nishizawa T, Takasan H, Hayakawa T, Tanaka K. Pancreatoblastoma resected by delayed primary operation after effective chemotherapy. Journal of Pediatric Surgery 1992; 27: 1570–2.

Iseki M, Suzuki T, Koizumi Y et al. Alpha-fetoprotein-producing pancreatoblastoma. A case report. Cancer 1986; 57: 1833–5.

Jaksic T, Yaman M, Thorner P, Wesson DK, Filler RM, Shandling B. A 20-year review of pediatric pancreatic tumors. Journal of Pediatric Surgery 1992; 27: 1315–17.

Jenkins JM, Othersen HB. Cystadenoma of the pancreas in a newborn. Journal of Pediatric Surgery 1992; 27: 1569.

Jung S-E, Kim D-Y, Park K-W et al. Solid and papillary epithelial neoplasm of the pancreas in children. World Journal of Surgery 1999; 23: 233–6.

Kissane JM. Tumors of the exocrine pancreas in childhood. In: Humphrey GB, Grindey GB, Dehner LP, Acton RT, Pysher TJ (eds) Pancreatic tumors in children. The Hague: Martinus Nijhoff Publishers, 1982: 100–29.

Klimstra DS, Heffess CS, Oertel JE, Rosai J. Acinar-cell carcinoma of the pancreas. A clinicopathologic study of 28 cases. American Journal of Surgical Pathology 1992; 16: 815–37.

Kohda E, Iseki M, Ikawa H et al. Pancreatoblastoma. Three original cases and review of the literature. Acta Radiologica 2000; 41: 334–7.

Ky A, Shilyansky J, Gerstle J et al. Experience with papillary and solid epithelial neoplasms of the pancreas in children. Journal of Pediatric Surgery 1998; 33: 42–4.

Lack EE, Cassady JR, Levey R, Vawter GF. Tumors of the exocrine pancreas in children and adolescents. A clinical and pathological study of eight cases. American Journal of Surgical Pathology 1983; 7: 319–27.

Le Borgne J, de Calan L, Partensky C et al. Cystadenomas and cystadenocarcinomas of the pancreas: a multi-institutional retrospective study of 398 cases. *Annals of Surgery* 1999; **230**: 152–68.

Lee WY, Tzeng CC, Che RM *et al*. Papillary cystic tumors of the pancreas: assessment of malignant potential by analysis of progesterone receptor, flow cytometry, and ras oncogene mutation. *Anticancer Research* 1997; **17**: 2587–91.

Leibowitz G, Glaser B, Higazi AA, Salameh M, Cerasi E, Landau H. Hyperinsulinemic hypoglycemia of infancy (nesidioblastosis) in clinical remission: high incidence of diabetes mellitus and persistent β-cell dysfunction at long-term follow-up. *Journal of Clinical Endocrinology and Metabolism* 1995; **80**: 386–92.

Lobe TE, Vera SR, Bowman LC *et al*. Hepatico-pancreaticogastroduodenectomy with transplantation for metastatic islet cell carcinoma in childhood. *Journal of Pediatric Surgery* 1992; **27**: 227–9.

Mares AJ, Hirsch M. Congenital cysts of the head of the pancreas. *Journal of Pediatric Surgery* 1977; **12**: 547–52.

Mester M, Trajber HJ, Compton CC *et al*. Cystic teratomas of the pancreas. *Archives of Surgery* 1990; **125**: 1215–18.

Montemarano H, Lonergan GJ, Bulas DI, Selby DM. Pancreatoblastoma: imaging findings in 10 patients and review of the literature. *Radiology* 2000; **214**: 476–82.

Morris-Stiff G, Vujanic GM, Al-Wafi A, Lari J. Pancreatic inflammatory pseudotumour: an uncommon childhood lesion mimicking a malignant tumor. *Pediatric Surgery International* 1998; **13**: 52–4.

Munns CFJ, Batch JA. Hyperinsulinism and Beckwith–Wiedemann syndrome. *Archives of Disease in Childhood* 2001; **84**: F67–9.

Nihoul-Fekete CL, Cretolle C, Brunelle F *et al*. *Partial elective pancreatectomy is curative in focal form of permanent hyperinsulinemic hypoglycemia of infancy (PHHI): a report of 45 cases*. Paper presented at British Association of Paediatric Surgeons XLVIII Annual International Congress, London, July 2001.

Nishihara K, Nagoshi M, Tsuneyoshi M *et al*. Papillary cystic tumors of the pancreas. Assessment of their malignant potential. *Cancer* 1993; 71: 82–92.

Paal E, Thompson LD, Heffess CS. A clinicopathologic and immunohistochemical study of ten pancreatic lymphangiomas and a review of the literature. *Cancer* 1998; **82**: 2150–8.

Parashar K, Upadhyay V, Corkery JJ. Partial or near total pancreatectomy for nesidioblastosis? *European Journal of Pediatric Surgery* 1995; **5**: 146–8.

Passmore SJ, Berry PJ, Oakhill A. Recurrent pancreato-blastoma with inappropriate adrenocorticotrophic hormone secretion. *Archives of Disease in Childhood* 1988; **63**: 1494–6.

Pietsch JB, Shankar S, Ford C, Johnson JE. Obstructive jaundice secondary to lymphoma in childhood. *Journal of Pediatric Surgery* 2001; **36**: 1792–5.

Rahier J, Guiot Y, Sempoux C. Persistent hyperinsulinaemic hypoglycaemia of infancy: a heterogenous syndrome

unrelated to nesidioblastosis. *Archives of Disease in Childhood* 2000; **82**: F108–12.

Reyes GA, Fowler CL, Pokorny WJ. Pancreatic anatomy in children: emphasis on its importance to pancreatectomy. *Journal of Pediatric Surgery* 1993; **28**: 712–15.

Rich RH, Weber JL, Shandling B. Adenocarcinoma of the pancreas in a neonate managed by pancreato-duodenectomy. *Journal of Pediatric Surgery* 1986; **21**: 806–8.

Rother KI, Matsumoto MS, Rasmussen NH, Schwenk WF. Long-term follow-up of children who underwent subtotal pancreatectomy as infants for hyperinsulinemic hypoglycemia. *Pediatric Research* 1994; **35**: 106A.

Schonau E, Deeg KH, Huemmer HP, Akcetin YZ, Bohles HJ. Pancreatic growth and function following surgical treatment of nesidioblastosis in infancy. *European Journal of Pediatrics* 1991; **50**: 550–3.

Seitz ML, Shenker IR, Leonidas JC, Nussbaum MP, Wind ES. Von-Hippel Lindau in an adolescent. *Pediatrics* 1987; **79**: 632–7.

Shepherd RM, Cosgrove KE, O'Brien RE *et al*. Hyperinsulinism of infancy: towards an understanding of unregulated insulin release. *Archives of Disease in Childhood* 2000; **82**: F87–97.

Shieh CS, Eng HL, Huang SC *et al*. Congenital pancreatic cyst presenting as acute pancreatitis in an adolescent. *Journal of Pediatric Gastroenterology and Nutrition* 1994; **18**: 490–3.

Siddiqui AM, Shamberger RC, Filler RM, Perez-Atayde AR, Lillehei CW. Enteric duplications of the pancreatic head: definitive management by local resection. *Journal of Pediatric Surgery* 1998; **33**: 1117–20.

Silverman JF, Holbrook CT, Pories WJ *et al*. Fine-needle aspiration cytology of pancreatoblastoma with immunocytochemical and ultrastructural studies. *Acta Cytologica* 1990; **34**: 632–40.

Snajdauf J, Pycha K, Rygl M *et al*. Papillary cystic and solid tumor of the pancreas – surgical therapy with the use of CUSA, and a review of the pediatric literature. *European Journal of Pediatric Surgery* 1999; **9**: 416–19.

Soliman AT, Alsalmi I, Darwish A, Asfour MG. Growth and endocrine function after near total pancreatectomy for hyperinsulinaemic hypoglycaemia. *Archives of Disease in Childhood* 1996; **74**: 379–85.

Spitz L. Surgery for hyperinsulinaemic hypoglycaemia. In: Spitz L, Coran AG (eds) *Pediatric surgery*, 5th edn. London: Chapman & Hall, 1994: 618–22.

Spitz L, Bhargava RK, Grant DB, Leonard JV. Surgical treatment of hyperinsulinaemic hypoglycaemia in infancy and childhood. *Archives of Disease in Childhood* 1992; **67**: 201–5.

Stanley CA, Lieu TK, Hsu BY *et al*. Hyperinsulinism and hyperammonemia in infants with regulatory mutations of the glutamate dehydrogenase gene. *New England Journal of Medicine* 1998; **338**: 1352–7.

Stringer MD, Ramani P, Yeung CK *et al*. Abdominal inflammatory myofibroblastic tumors (inflammatory pseudotumours) in children. *British Journal of Surgery* 1992; **79**: 1357–60.

Sylvester FA, Shuckett B, Cutz E, Durie PR, Marcon MA. Management of fibrosing pancreatitis in children presenting with obstructive jaundice. *Gut* 1998; **43**: 715–20.

Telander RL, Charboneau JW, Haymond MW. Intraoperative ultrasonography of the pancreas in children. *Journal of Pediatric Surgery* 1986; **21**: 262–6.

Thomas CG, Underwood LE, Carney CN, Dolcourt JL, Whitt JJ. Neonatal and infantile hypoglycemia due to insulin excess: new aspects of diagnosis and surgical management. *Annals of Surgery* 1977; **185**: 505–17.

Thomas CG, Cuenca RE, Azizkhan RG, Underwood LE, Carney CN. Changing concepts of islet-cell dysplasia in neonatal and infantile hyperinsulinism. *World Journal of Surgery* 1988; **12**: 598–609.

Thomas PM, Cote GJ, Hallman DM, Mathew PM. Homozygosity mapping, to chromosome 11p, of the gene for familial persistent hyperinsulinemic hypoglycemia of infancy. *American Journal of Human Genetics* 1995a; **56**: 416–21.

Thomas PM, Cote GJ, Wohllk N *et al.* Mutations in the sulphonylurea receptor gene in familial persistent hyperinsulinemic hypoglycemia of infancy. *Science* 1995b; **268**: 426–9.

Thompson NW, Vinik AI, Eckhauser FE. Microgastrinomas of the duodenum. A cause of failed operations for the Zollinger–Ellison syndrome. *Annals of Surgery* 1989; **209**: 396–404.

Thornton PS, Sumner AE, Ruchelli ED, Spielman RS, Baker L, Stanley CA. Familial and sporadic hyperinsulinism: histopathologic findings and segregation analysis support a single autosomal recessive disorder. *Journal of Pediatrics* 1991; **119**: 721–4.

Todani T, Shimada K, Watanabe Y *et al.* Frantz's tumor: a papillary and cystic tumor of the pancreas in girls. *Journal of Pediatric Surgery* 1988; **23**: 116–21.

Touati G, Poggi-Travaer F, Ogier de Baulney H *et al.* Long-term treatment of persistent hyperinsulinemic hypoglycemia of infancy with diazoxide: a retrospective review of 77 cases and analysis of efficacy-predicting criteria. *European Journal of Pediatrics* 1998; **157**: 628–33.

Tsukimoto I, Watanabe K, Lin J *et al.* Pancreatic carcinoma in children in Japan. *Cancer* 1973; **31**: 1203–7.

van Dooren MF, Hakvoort-Cammel FG, Madern GC. Malignant pancreatic tumors in children: three case reports. *Medical and Pediatric Oncology* 2000; **35**: 379 (S-23).

Vane DW, Grosfeld JL, West KW, Rescorla FJ. Pancreatic disorders in infancy and childhood: experience with 92 cases. *Journal of Pediatric Surgery* 1989; **24**: 771–6.

Verhoef S, van Diemen-Steenvoorde R, Akkersdijk WL *et al.* Malignant pancreatic tumor within the spectrum of tuberous sclerosis complex in childhood. *European Journal of Pediatrics* 1999; **158**: 284–7.

Vossen S, Goretzki PE, Goebel U, Willnow V. Therapeutic management of rare malignant pancreatic tumors in children. *World Journal of Surgery* 1998; **22**: 879–82.

Wang KS, Albanese C, Dada F, Skarsgard ED. Papillary cystic neoplasm of the pancreas: a report of three pediatric cases and literature review. *Journal of Pediatric Surgery* 1998; **33**: 842–5.

Wetzel WJ. Successful long-term results with resection of pancreatic carcinoma in children (letter). *Surgery* 1984; **96**: 946–7.

Willnow U, Willberg B, Schwamborn D, Korholz D, Gobel U. Pancreatoblastoma in children. Case report and review of the literature. *European Journal of Pediatric Surgery* 1996; **6**: 369–72.

Wilson SD. Zollinger–Ellison syndrome in children: a 25-year follow-up. *Surgery* 1991; **110**: 696–703.

Woolf DA, Leonard JV, Trembath RC, Pembrey ME, Grant DB. Nesidioblastosis: evidence for autosomal-recessive inheritance. *Archives of Disease in Childhood* 1991; **66**: 529–30.

Wunsch LP, Flemming P, Werner U, Gluer S, Burger D. Diagnosis and treatment of papillary cystic tumor of the pancreas in children. *European Journal of Pediatric Surgery* 1997; **7**: 45–7.

Yamaguchi K, Tanaka M, Chijiiwa K *et al.* Early and late complications of pylorus-preserving pancreato-duodenectomy in Japan 1998. *Journal of Hepatobiliary and Pancreatic Surgery* 1999; **6**: 303–11.

Index

Page numbers in **bold** type refer to figures; those in *italic* refer to tables or boxed material